Comprehensive Review of Geriatric Psychiatry—II

Second Edition

Comprehensive Review of Geriatric Psychiatry—II

Second Edition

Edited by

Joel Sadavoy, M.D., F.R.C.P.C.
Lawrence W. Lazarus, M.D.
Lissy F. Jarvik, M.D., Ph.D.
George T. Grossberg, M.D.

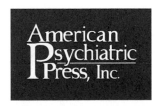

Washington, DC
London, England

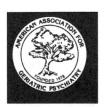

Sponsored by the
American Association
for Geriatric Psychiatry

Note: The authors have worked to ensure that all information in this book concerning drug dosages, schedules, and routes of administration is accurate as of the time of publication and consistent with standards set by the U.S. Food and Drug Administration and the general medical community. As medical research and practice advance, however, therapeutic standards may change. For this reason and because human and mechanical errors sometimes occur, we recommend that readers follow the advice of a physician who is directly involved in their care or the care of a member of their family.

Books published by the American Psychiatric Press, Inc., represent the views and opinions of the individual authors and do not necessarily represent the policies and opinions of the Press or the American Psychiatric Association.

Copyright © 1996 American Association for Geriatric Psychiatry
ALL RIGHTS RESERVED
Manufactured in the United States of America on acid-free paper
99 98 97 96   4 3 2 1

American Psychiatric Press, Inc.
1400 K Street, N.W., Washington, DC 20005

Library of Congress Cataloging-in-Publication Data
Comprehensive review of geriatric psychiatry—II / edited by Joel
    Sadavoy . . . [et al.]. — 2nd ed.
    Includes bibliographical references and index.
    ISBN 0-88048-723-2
    1. Geriatric psychiatry.   I. Sadavoy, Joel, 1945-
    [DNLM: 1. Mental Disorders—in old age.   WT 150 C737 1996]
RC451.4.A5C634   1996
618.97'689—dc20
DNLM/DLC
for Library of Congress   95-43308
                                                                                CIP

British Library Cataloguing in Publication Data
A CIP record is available from the British Library.

Contents

Section I
The Aging Process
Jeffrey Foster, M.D., Section Editor

Section III
Psychiatric Disorders of the Elderly
Gabe Maletta, M.D., Section Editor

Section IV
Treatment
Barnett S. Meyers, M.D., Section Editor

Section V
Medical-Legal, Ethical, and Financial Issues
Gary L. Gottlieb, M.D., M.B.A., Section Editor

Section VI
Self-Assessment: Questions & Answers
Jonathan Lieff, M.D., Section Editor

Contributors

Marilyn S. Albert, Ph.D.   Associate Professor, Harvard University; Director, Gerontology Research Unit, Massachusetts General Hospital, Harvard Medical School, Boston, Massachusetts

Cathy A. Alessi, M.D.   Assistant Professor of Medicine, UCLA Multicampus Program in Geriatrics and Gerontology; Director, Geriatric Evaluation and Management Services, Geriatric Research, Education, and Clinical Center, Sepulveda Veterans Affairs Medical Center, Sepulveda, California

George S. Alexopoulos, M.D.   Professor of Psychiatry, Cornell University Medical College; Director, Cornell Institute of Geriatric Psychiatry, The New York Hospital–Cornell Medical Center, Westchester Division, White Plains, New York

Roland M. Atkinson, M.D.   Professor of Psychiatry, Oregon Health Sciences University; Chief, Psychiatry Service, Portland VA Medical Center, Portland, Oregon

Christine K. Cassel, M.D.   Professor and Chairman, Department of Geriatrics and Adult Development, Mount Sinai Hospital, New York, New York

Carl I. Cohen, M.D.   Professor of Psychiatry and Director, Geriatric Psychiatry, State University of New York Health Science Center at Brooklyn, Brooklyn, New York

Bertram J. Cohler, Ph.D.   William Rainey Harper Professor of Social Sciences in The College and the Departments of Psychology (The Committee on Human Development), Psychiatry, and Education, University of Chicago, Chicago, Illinois

David K. Conn, M.B., F.R.C.P.C.   Assistant Professor of Psychiatry, University of Toronto; Psychiatrist-in-Chief, Baycrest Centre for Geriatric Care, North York, Ontario, Canada

Carl Eisdorfer, Ph.D., M.D.   Professor and Chairman of Psychiatry, University of Miami School of Medicine, Miami, Florida

Barry S. Fogel, M.D.   Professor of Psychiatry and Human Behavior, Brown University; Associate Director, Center for Gerontology and Health Care Research, Brown University, Providence, Rhode Island; Medical Director of Psychiatric Services, Eleanor Slater Hospital, Cranston, Rhode Island

Jeffrey Foster, M.D.   Clinical Associate Professor of Psychiatry, New York University Medical Center; Director, Geriatric Psychiatry Fellowship Program, New York University Medical Center, New York, New York

Linda Ganzini, M.D.   Associate Professor of Psychiatry, Oregon Health Sciences University; Director, Geriatric Psychiatry, Portland Veterans Affairs Medical Center, Portland, Oregon

Sylvia Gerson, Ph.D.   Department of Psychiatry and Behavioral Sciences, UCLA, Los Angeles, California

Marion Zucker Goldstein, M.D.   Clinical Associate Professor of Psychiatry and Internal Medicine, SUNY Buffalo, School of Medicine and Biomedical Sciences; Erie County Medical Center, Department of Psychiatry, Buffalo, New York

Gary L. Gottlieb, M.D., M.B.A.   Clinical Professor of Psychiatry, University of Pennsylvania School of Medicine; Director and Chief Executive Officer, Friends Hospital, Philadelphia, Pennsylvania

George T. Grossberg, M.D.   Professor and Chairman of Psychiatry and Human Behavior, Saint Louis University School of Medicine, St. Louis, Missouri

Barry Gurland, M.D.   Director and John E. Borne Professor of Clinical Psychiatry, Columbia University Center for Geriatrics and Gerontology in the Faculty of Medicine; New York State Psychiatric Institute, New York, New York

M. Jackuelyn Harris, M.D.   Assistant Professor of Psychiatry, University of California San Diego; San Diego Veterans Affairs Medical Center, Psychiatry Service, San Diego, California

Donald P. Hay, M.D.   Associate Professor of Psychiatry and Director of Inpatient Program and Late Life Mood Disorders Program, Division of Geriatric Psychiatry, Department of Psychiatry and Human Behavior, St. Louis University Medical School, St. Louis, Missouri

Linda K. Hay, Ph.D.   Assistant Professor of Psychiatry and Director of Psychological Services, Division of Geriatric Psychiatry, Department of Psychiatry and Human Behavior, St. Louis University Medical School, St. Louis, Missouri

Nathan Herrmann, M.D.   Assistant Professor and Head of Division of Geriatric Psychiatry, University of Toronto; Staff Psychiatrist, Sunnybrook Health Science Center, Toronto, Ontario, Canada

Daniel Holschneider, M.D.   Clinical Instructor, University of California, Los Angeles, UCLA Neuropsychiatric Institute and Hospital, Center for Health Sciences, Los Angeles, California

Lissy F. Jarvik, M.D., Ph.D.   Research Professor of Psychiatry, UCLA/NPI and H; Distinguished Physician (Emer.) Director, GET SMART and UPBEAT Programs, West Los Angeles Veterans Affairs Medical Center, Los Angeles, California

Dilip V. Jeste, M.D.   Professor of Psychiatry and Neurosciences, University of California San Diego; San Diego Veterans Affairs Medical Center, Psychiatry Service, San Diego, California

Ira R. Katz, M.D., Ph.D.   Professor of Psychiatry, University of Pennsylvania; Director, Section on Geriatric Psychiatry, Department of Psychiatry, University of Pennsylvania, Philadelphia; Philadelphia Veterans Affairs Medical Center, Philadelphia, Pennsylvania

Eleanor Lavretsky, M.D., Ph.D.   Department of Psychiatry and Behavioral Sciences, UCLA, Los Angeles, California

Lawrence W. Lazarus, M.D.   Assistant Professor of Psychiatry, Rush Medical College; Director, Geriatric Psychiatry Fellowship Program, Rush-Presbyterian St. Lukes Medical Center, Chicago, Illinois

Molyn Leszcz, M.D., F.R.C.P.C.   Associate Professor of Psychiatry, University of Toronto; Head, Psychotherapy Program, Department of Psychiatry, University of Toronto, Toronto, Ontario, Canada

Andrew Leuchter, M.D.   Associate Professor, University of California, Los Angeles; UCLA Neuropsychiatric Institute and Hospital, Center for the Health Sciences, Los Angeles, California

Elaine A. Leventhal, M.D., Ph.D.   Department of Medicine, University of Medicine and Dentistry of New Jersey, Robert Wood Johnson Medical School, New Brunswick, New Jersey

Jonathan Lieff, M.D.   Associate Clinical Professor of Psychiatry, Boston University Medical School, Boston, Massachusetts; Past President, American Association of Geriatric Psychiatry; Chief of Psychiatry, American Geriatric Service, St. Elizabeth Hospital, Geriatric Specialty Unit, Boston, Massachusetts

Benjamin Liptzin, M.D.   Professor and Deputy Chair of Psychiatry, Tufts University School of Medicine, Boston; Chair, Department of Psychiatry, Baystate Medical Center, Springfield, Massachusetts

David A. Loewenstein, Ph.D.   Associate Professor of Psychiatry, Wein Center for Alzheimer's Disease and Related Disorders of Aging, University of Miami School of Medicine; Mount Sinai Medical Center, Miami Beach, Florida

Charles F. Longino, Jr., Ph.D.   Professor of Sociology and Director of the Reynolds Gerontology Program, Wake Forest University; Professor of Public Health Sciences, Bowman Gray School of Medicine, Winston-Salem, North Carolina

Gabe Maletta, M.D.   Associate Professor of Psychiatry, University of Minnesota; Associate Chief of Staff, Geriatric and Extended Care, Veterans Affairs Medical Center, Minneapolis, Minnesota

Richard Margolin, M.D.   Assistant Professor of Psychiatry, Radiology and Psychology, Vanderbilt University Medical Center; Director, Division of Geriatric Psychiatry, Vanderbilt University, Nashville, Tennessee

Steven S. Matsuyama, Ph.D.   Department of Psychiatry and Behavioral Sciences, UCLA; West Los Angeles Veterans Affairs Medical Center, Brentwood Division, Los Angeles, California

Barnett S. Meyers, M.D. Associate Professor of Clinical Psychiatry, Cornell University Medical College; The New York Hospital–Cornell Medical Center, Westchester Division, White Plains, New York

Steven H. Miles, M.D. Associate Professor of Medicine and Ethics, University of Minnesota; Division of Geriatric Medicine, Department of Medicine, Medical School, University of Minnesota; Hennepin County Medical Center, Minneapolis, Minnesota

Maurice B. Mittelmark, Ph.D. Professor of Health Promotion, Centre of Health Promotion Research, University of Bergen, Bergen, Norway

Peter Moran, M.B., L.R.C.P., S.I. Lecturer of Psychiatry, Faculty of Medicine, University of Toronto; Staff Psychiatrist, Department of Psychiatry, Mount Sinai Hospital, Toronto, Ontario, Canada

Jeanne E. Nakamura, M.A. The Committee on Human Development, University of Chicago, Chicago, Illinois

Jane S. Paulsen, Ph.D. Assistant Professor of Psychiatry, University of California San Diego; San Diego Veterans Affairs Medical Center, Psychiatry Service, San Diego, California

Walter M. Potoczny, M.D., F.R.C.P.C. Assistant Professor of Psychiatry, University of Ottawa; Director, Geriatric Psychiatry Day Hospital, Royal Ottawa Hospital, Ottawa, Ontario, Canada

Stephen Read, M.D. Assistant Clinical Professor of Psychiatry and Biobehavioral Sciences, UCLA School of Medicine; Associate Director, UPBEAT Program, Veterans Affairs Medical Center, West Los Angeles, Los Angeles, California

Barry Reisberg, M.D. Professor of Psychiatry, New York University School of Medicine; Clinical Director, Aging and Dementia Research Center, New York University Medical Center, New York, New York

Domeena C. Renshaw, M.D. Professor of Psychiatry, Loyola University Chicago; Associate Chairman and Director, Sexual Dysfunction Program and CME Program, Loyola University Medical Center, Stritch School of Medicine, Maywood, Illinois

Charles F. Reynolds III, M.D.   Professor of Psychiatry and Neurology, University of Pittsburgh School of Medicine; Director, Sleep and Chronobiology Center, Western Psychiatric Institute and Clinic, Pittsburgh, Pennsylvania

Barry W. Rovner, M.D.   Associate Professor of Psychiatry, Thomas Jefferson University; Director, Division of Geriatric Psychiatry, Jefferson Medical College, Jefferson University, Philadelphia, Pennsylvania

Mark P. Rubert, Ph.D.   Research Assistant Professor of Psychiatry, Center on Adult Development and Aging, University of Miami School of Medicine, Miami, Florida

Joel Sadavoy, M.D., F.R.C.P.C.   Associate Professor of Psychiatry, University of Toronto; Psychiatrist-in-Chief, Joint Department of Psychiatry, Mount Sinai Hospital/Princess Margaret Hospital, Toronto, Ontario, Canada

Kenneth Sakauye, M.D.   Professor of Clinical Psychiatry, Louisiana State University; Louisiana State University Medical Center, Department of Psychiatry, New Orleans, Louisiana

Javaid I. Sheikh, M.D.   Associate Professor of Psychiatry and Director, Geriatric Psychiatry Program, Department of Psychiatry and Behavioral Sciences, Stanford University School of Medicine, Stanford; Chief of Psychiatry, Palo Alto Veterans Affairs Health Care System, Menlo Park Division, Menlo Park, California

Stephen R. Shuchter, M.D.   Professor of Clinical Psychiatry, University of California San Diego, San Diego; Director, UCSD Outpatient Psychiatric Services, San Diego, California

Ivan L. Silver, M.D.   Associate Professor of Psychiatry, University of Toronto; Staff Psychiatrist, Department of Psychiatry, Sunnybrook Health Science Centre, Toronto, Ontario, Canada

Gary W. Small, M.D.   Professor of Psychiatry and Biobehavioral Sciences, University of California, Los Angeles, School of Medicine; Neuropsychiatric Institute and Hospital; Chief, Geriatric Psychiatry Program of the West Los Angeles Veterans Affairs Medical Center, Los Angeles, California

Joel E. Streim, M.D.   Assistant Professor of Psychiatry, Section on Geriatric Psychiatry, Department of Psychiatry, University of Pennsylvania, Philadelphia, Pennsylvania

Marie-France Tourigny-Rivard, M.D., F.R.C.P.C., D.A.B.N.P.   Assistant Professor of Psychiatry, University of Ottawa; Clinical Director, Geriatric Psychiatry Program, Royal Ottawa Hospital, Ottawa, Ontario, Canada

Jürgen Unützer, M.D., M.A.   NRSA Fellow in Primary Care Psychiatry, University of Washington, Seattle, Washington

Jeff Victoroff, M.D.   Assistant Professor of Neurology, University of Southern California School of Medicine; Co-Director, Geriatric Neurology Clinic, Rancho Los Amigos Medical Center, Downey, California

Robert C. Young, M.D.   Associate Professor of Psychiatry, Cornell University Medical College, New York; The New York Hospital–Cornell Medical Center, Westchester Division, White Plains, New York

George H. Zimny, Ph.D.   Professor of Psychiatry and Human Behavior, Saint Louis University School of Medicine, St. Louis, Missouri

Sidney Zisook, M.D.   Professor of Psychiatry, School of Medicine; Director, Residency Training Program, University of California San Diego, San Diego, California

Preface

The preparation of a second edition of the *Comprehensive Review of Geriatric Psychiatry* was stimulated by the continuing growth of knowledge in geriatric psychiatry. In its first edition, the book became one of the standards for the field. For the second edition, approximately one-third of the book was completely rewritten, and all the remaining chapters were revised and updated. The topics of genetics, normal aging, ethnocultural and sociodemographic aspects of aging, self and experience across the second half of life, Alzheimer's disease, grief and bereavement, mood disorders, anxiety disorders, personality and somatoform disorders, geriatric consultation-liaison psychiatry, and medicolegal and ethical issues are included in the newly written material. In addition, most of the questions in the self-assessment section are new.

As in the first edition, we have striven for clarity, completeness, and conciseness. This approach is in keeping with the intent that the book be particularly useful for mental health professionals involved in the care of elderly people who require a focused but comprehensive review of the field. Consequently, this text will be of value to psychiatrists, psychiatric residents, geriatricians, geriatric residents, psychologists, social workers, nurses, and other mental health workers.

The production of this book relied heavily on the unstinting effort of the contributors and section editors to whom we express our sincere thanks. The book could not have been completed without the skillful organization and manuscript preparation of Tammy LePage, who was responsible for coordinating the project with the help of Janissa Williams. It is also timely to redress an omission from the first edition and to offer the deep thanks of the editors for the work of Malarie Feldman, who was responsible for coordinating and preparing the manuscript for the first edition.

Introduction

New Clinical Perspectives on Aging

Geriatrics and geriatric psychiatry are at a historic turning point. The increase of clinical interest and research activity in the area of aging has been a catalyst for academic developments in geriatric psychiatry and in geriatrics as a whole (Rowe et al. 1987) during the last quarter of the 20th century. Before 1978 there had been only a single specialty training program in geriatric psychiatry; but in the following decade, the number of geriatric psychiatry specialty training programs grew to more than 30, including nearly one-fourth of the medical schools in the United States (Cohen 1989). Similarly, every medical school in Canada provides mandatory training in geriatric psychiatry to all psychiatric residents. Since the mid-1970s, three areas of significant conceptual growth have become particularly apparent: 1) differentiating changes of normal aging from symptoms of illness in later life, 2) the modifiability of illness in later life, and 3) the modifiability of normal aging for better functioning.

Differentiating Changes of Normal Aging From Symptoms of Illness in Later Life

If one fails to distinguish illness from normal aging, then clinical symptoms are overlooked and dismissed as inevitable concomitants of the aging process; as a result, treatment options then fail to be considered. As the influence of gerontology became increasingly evident in the mid-1970s, challenging questions were raised about illness versus normal aging. Nowhere is this occurrence better illustrated than in the case of Alzheimer's disease. Many people saw senility as their fate in growing old, an unavoidable concomitant of aging. However, two types of evidence began to throw into question that point of view. First, longitudinal psychometric data began to accumulate, documenting that many older persons maintained high levels of cognitive functioning. When speed was not a factor, some of them—especially those who were healthy—showed improvement in performance during their 80s. The second line of evidence came from neurochemistry and led to new hypotheses about a deficiency of the neurotransmitter acetylcholine in the brains of "senile" older adults (Cohen 1989), thus pointing to the presence of disease as opposed to a scheduled developmental event in one's later years. Concepts of depression similarly evolved and were no longer viewed as going with the normal territory of aging; similar changes occurred in the perspectives on other disorders in older adults.

The Modifiability of Illness in Later Life

Once clinicians and researchers began to recognize the role of illness in producing some of the mental changes of later life, the next step was to appreciate its modifiability, especially the modifiability of mental illness in late life. Growing clinical experience and new research methodologies showed that depression in elderly patients did respond to psychopharmacology and psychotherapy. Moreover, new views on treatment emerged even for Alzheimer's disease with the awareness of the modifiability of excess disability states, including alterable, comorbid conditions (e.g., depression and delusions) that compound dysfunction (Group for the Advancement of Psychiatry Committee on Aging 1988).

Modifiability of Normal Aging for Better Functioning

The growth of understanding about how much functional decline in later life is attributable to disorder rather than to development has made it increasingly difficult to determine exactly what changes do indeed represent normal aging. However, in practical terms the distinction may no longer be important, because it is becoming apparent that even normal changes may be modified to enhance effective functioning in later life. For example, even though there is agreement among researchers that reaction time increases with aging, new data indicate that the rate of reaction in later life can be improved with practice. Thus, an investigation of the effects of videogame play on responses of elderly adults reported improvement in both the speed and the accuracy of responses following a 7-week training program (Clark et al. 1987). Such research should put to rest the negative stereotype about "old dogs and new tricks," and it is at the same time highly relevant to the development of interventions to promote mental health.

The Capacity to Change and the Significance of Time in Later Life

Particularly in the domain of psychiatric treatment, perspectives on time have a major influence on practitioner behavior. To the extent that the service provider feels that the patient has only a limited amount of time left, treatment planning may be compromised. Neither doubt about time left nor skepticism about the capacity to change in later life stands up to clinical experience. The significance of time and the capacity to change in old age are captured by Somerset Maugham (1938) in an observation on the behavior of the elder Cato approximately 20 centuries ago: "When I was young, I was amazed at Plutarch's statement that the elder Cato began, at the age of eighty, to learn Greek. I am amazed no longer. Old age is ready to undertake tasks that youth shirked because they would take too long" (p. 297). With people over 85 representing the fastest growing age group, most older adults have much time left for both life and treatment in their later years. This optimism is reflected in the potential for change that is evident in geriatric patients who undertake psychodynamically oriented psychotherapy late in life (Sadavoy and Leszcz 1987).

The Special Knowledge of Geriatric Psychiatry

The special knowledge of geriatric psychiatry needs to be examined along two planes: 1) as it relates to elderly patients and 2) as it relates to aging per se (Cohen 1988; Lazarus 1988). From the perspective of elderly patients, the focus of geriatric psychiatry ranges from attention to special, later-life problems (e.g., late-onset schizophrenia and Alzheimer's disease) to interventions (e.g., retirement counseling and geriatric psychopharmacology) and service settings (e.g., geriatric assessment units and nursing homes). The general perspective on aging of geriatric psychiatry, however, is less well appreciated. It is through this perspective that geriatric psychiatry makes contributions not only to older patients but to all age groups.

In any field, whenever a problem can be examined in a new light, the opportunity for new insights presents itself. The longitudinal view developed through research on elderly subjects has helped to shed new light on mental disorders affecting the young as well as the old. For example, why is it that the group of late-onset schizophrenic persons pass through so much of the life cycle before first developing psychosis? Moreover, by studying this group of individuals, new information may be gained about schizophrenia independent of age. What might be learned about schizophrenia, in general, by studying it in people who grow old with the disorder but experience an attenuation (burnout) of its symptoms with aging?

Another example comes from research in geriatric depression. An early theory of depression, the catecholamine hypothesis, stated that the mood disorder resulted from a central deficit in the neurotransmitter norepinephrine. Meanwhile, studies on the aging brain revealed that monoamine oxidase (MAO) levels *increased* with advancing years. Because MAO reduces norepinephrine levels, all older adults should be depressed, and increasingly so over time. However, epidemiological studies show that this is not the case.

These findings from research on aging, together with other evidence incompatible with the catecholamine hypothesis, have helped generate newer theories of depression, such as the "dysregulation hypothesis," that postulates disruption in mechanisms that regulate the activity of neurotransmitters rather than their levels (Siever and Davis 1985).

The 70-Year Follow-Up

Much can be learned by following a given disorder over time to study its natural history. The problem for the researcher is that doing so takes time. The geriatric patient offers a modified shortcut in this process. If an older patient is being followed for major depression or chronic schizophrenia, one has the opportunity to look back, via the patient's history, to examine the course of the illness over a period of decades—at times, over a period of 70 or more years. This is a unique opportunity offered only by geriatric patients, who provide us the opportunity to expand our understanding of mental disorders across the life cycle.

Interaction of Mental and Physical Health Phenomena

A clinical dimension that distinguishes older patients, in general, from younger ones is the greater likelihood of experiencing more than one concurrent illness in later life, including coexistent mental health and physical impairments. Accordingly, geriatric patients provide one of the best windows on mechanisms underlying the influence of mental illness on physical condition and, conversely, on the influence of somatic disorder on mental condition. It is through the geriatric patient that one most commonly comes into clinical contact with that elusive "whole person" in a biopsychosocial context (Jarvik 1983).

Certificate of Added Qualifications in Geriatric Psychiatry

The American Board of Psychiatry and Neurology administered the first examination for a certificate of added qualifications in geriatric psychiatry in April of 1991. The fifth annual exam is planned in November of 1996. As of this writing, more than 1,200 psychiatrists have obtained added qualifications in geriatric psychiatry. Several factors have led to the historic movement toward developing the first new area of special competence in American psychiatry (since child psychiatry) in nearly three decades.

The dramatic growth in numbers of people ages 65 and older, who now comprise >12% of the population or more than 30 million people, has resulted in a historically new challenge for society. Moreover, the group of people 85 and older is expected to increase six- to sevenfold by the middle of the 21st century, at which time it will number more than 15 million. Everyone who will be 85 in 2050 is alive today.

As the aging population has grown, so have the numbers of psychiatrists interested and specializing in care of elderly people. By the late 1980s, the total number of American psychiatrists was approximately 35,000. A decade earlier, relatively few psychiatrists expressed interest in working with older adults. However, formal surveys taken during the 1980s found more than 5,000 psychiatrists providing active treatment to elderly patients, with an indication of that number being on the rise (Cohen 1989). Moreover, the need for training in this area prompted a dramatic growth in the number of postresidency training programs in geriatric psychiatry. With the dramatic growth between 1978 and 1988 in the number of postresidency specialty training programs in geriatric psychiatry, American psychiatry reached a critical mass of training programs consistent with subspecialization.

The number of research projects on mental health and aging has soared since the mid-1970s, significantly stirred in the United States by the establishment of the Center on Aging at the National Institute of Mental Health and the National Institute on Aging—the latter with a budget of one-fourth of a billion dollars in 1990. By then, support in the United States for Alzheimer's disease research alone had reached more than $130 million annually. Early in 1980, the growth of knowledge was marked by the publication of major texts on mental health and aging and on geriatric psychiatry; since then, separate texts have been written for almost every one of the chapters in the original comprehensive works (i.e., separate geriatric texts now exist on depression, schizophrenia, Alzheimer's disease, psychotherapy, and psychopharmacology).

Medicare can be described as national health insurance for America's older adults. However, for more than a generation since its inception—from the early 1960s to the late 1980s—Medicare provided very little coverage for outpatient services for community-dwelling, older adults, which group includes 95% of people ages 65 and older. Consequently patients were discouraged from using mental health services and practitioners were discouraged from providing them. Psychiatry's previous low visibility vis-à-vis elderly patients did not help in attempts to secure improved patient benefits. Psychiatry's new statement about interest, knowledge, and skills in the area of geriatric psychiatry, made by its movement toward developing added qualifications, in all likelihood influenced the granting of new psychiatric benefits under Medicare as the 1980s came to a close.

The American public has been growing increasingly sophisticated in its knowledge and expectations of geriatric health care. By so doing, it has been influencing the profession to pay greater attention to specialization, thereby, to a degree, responding to consumer demand. Public pressure is enhanced further when families themselves form organizations to better highlight need and focus attention in various areas. For example, the Alzheimer's Association in the United States, formed in 1980, now has more than 200 local chapters across the country.

The goal of the added qualifications process is to allow the general practitioner of psychiatry to add qualifications, not to establish a new guild within a guild. The added qualifications process in geriatric psychiatry is an attempt to strengthen both academic leadership and the capacity of the general psychiatrist to address mental illness in geriatric patients. It should strengthen both fellowship training in geriatric psychiatry and the development of geriatric psychiatry rotations in general residency training. A similar situation exists in both internal medicine and family practice. Ideally, this process will lead to significant growth of expert faculty in geriatric psychiatry; significant growth of research focused on mental health and mental illness in older adults; improved psychogeriatric skills of psychiatrists in general; improved psychogeriatric skills for practitioners in all fields who work with older patients; enhanced public awareness of the nature of mental illness in later life and its modifiability through the application of psychogeriatric interventions; and heightened awareness in policymakers of the state-of-the-art in psychogeriatrics, leading to the development of increasingly effective policies addressing mental health needs of older persons (Cohen 1989). A direct result of the added qualifications process has been the development of Accreditation Council for Graduate Medical Education (ACGME)-approved, postgraduate residencies in geriatric psychiatry. As of this writing, approximately 40 programs have met ACGME criteria for training geriatric psychiatry in the United States.

The Beginning

The Bible described King David as having a depression (Psalms 31:9–12):

> Be gracious unto me, O Lord, for I am in distress;
> Mine eye wasted away with vexation, yea, my soul and my body.
> For my life is spent in sorrow, and my years in sighing;
> My strength faileth because of mine iniquity, and my bones are wasted away.
> Because of all mine adversaries I am become a reproach, yea....
> I am forgotten as a dead man out of mind;
> I am like a useless vessel.

Thus, we know that the history of geriatric psychiatry is rooted in biblical times.

The Maximes of PtahHaty described dementia (depressive pseudo-dementia) in the seventh century B.C. (Loza and Milad, unpublished data, 1989):

> Sovereign my master the old age is here, senility has descended in me, the weakness of my childhood is renewed, so I sleep all the time. The arms are weak, the legs have given up following the heart that has become tired. The mouth is mute, it can no longer speak, the eyes are weak, the ears are deaf, the nose is blocked, it can no longer breathe. The taste is completely gone. The spirit is forgetful. It can no longer remember yesterday. The bones ache in the old age, getting up and sitting down are both difficult. What was nice has become bad. What causes senility in men is bad in every way.

Yet examples of good mental health in the elders of ancient Egypt also exist (Loza and Milad 1989). The statue of Nebenterou, son of the high priest of the Twelfth Dynasty (950–730 B.C.) bore the following engraving: "I have spent my life in happiness, without the worry of illness…. I have outlived my contemporaries. May this happen to you too."
Evidence of attempts to treat dementia have been found in the Edwin Smith papyrus, as well as the Magical Papyri.

During the Coptic Era (Loza and Milad 1989) (A.D. second to seventh centuries), Father Jean Cassien described a paranoid psychosis in a French monk in his book *Les Conferences des Peres du Desert*. The monk ultimately kills himself in a delusional state.

Plato observed that older people did not have an increasing anxiety about death. He believed that reductions in the power of impulses led to the sense of tranquillity and greater freedom to pursue philosophy and intellectual endeavors. In 44 B.C., at the age of 62, Cicero wrote an essay on senescence (*De Senecute*) in which he described the problems and goals for older people. He acknowledged ageism in Roman society while stressing the value of older people in administrative and intellectual pursuits. Cicero echoed Plato's ideas about diminishing sexual pleasure and greater acceptance of death in old age. He also described the severe regression that can occur with dementia, a condition he viewed with abhorrence.

Modern Clinical Geriatric Psychiatry

In the Middle Ages, Esquirol differentiated dementia (loss of mental faculties) from amentia (mental retardation). However, he did not believe that dementia was an irreversible process. Berios differentiated depression and dementia in the 19th century based on his book, *Montpelier.*

In the early years of psychoanalysis, Freud was pessimistic about the application of psychoanalytic techniques to the treatment of "older people" (people over 40). When Freud was 42 he wrote "Sexuality in the Aetiology of the Neuroses" (Freud 1898/1953), in which he stated "With persons who are too far advanced in years, it [psychoanalytic method] fails because, owing to the accumulation of material, so much time would be required so that the end of the cure would be reached at a period of life in which much importance is no longer attached to nervous health" (p. 245). Subsequently, he recognized that his statements were based on his limited number of cases, predominantly of hysteria and obsessional neurosis.

Twenty years later, however, Abraham (1927) described his years of employing psychoanalytic techniques in the treatment of older people: He said that it would seem incorrect today to deny the possibility of exercising a curative influence upon the neurosis in the period of involution and rather it is the task of psychoanalysis to inquire under what conditions the method of treatment can attain results in the later years.

Abraham described a successful treatment of a melancholic man age 50 who had been institutionalized several times. This man was the first of several patients Abraham treated who were in their middle years. He concluded that the age at which the neurosis breaks out is of greater importance than the age at which treatment has begun (Abraham 1927).

At around the same time, Sandor Ferenczi (1955) described psychodynamic changes in later life, which include a decreased ability to sublimate, increasing narcissism, and often a more negative and hostile approach to life. Ferenczi theorized that in old age there is a reversion to the discharge of pregenital impulses including voyeurism, exhibitionism, and a tendency to masturbate—which he termed "underdistinguished" anal and urethral eroticism.

In 1906, two revolutionary monographs were written. One was the classic description of dementia by Alzheimer (1906). The other was written by Gaupp (Barraclough 1989), who differentiated dementias from nondementias (mainly depression). Although some nondementias ended in dementia, Gaupp observed that most did not.

Hitler's ascension in Germany prompted the relocation to the United Kingdom of two very important individuals in the field of geriatric psychiatry. In the decades after World War II, Felix Post and Sir Martin Roth made major contributions to the field of geriatric psychiatry. Under the guidance and direction of Dr. Aubrey Lewis, Felix Post assumed the first geriatric psychiatric position in England in 1947 at the Bethlem Hospital. By 1950–1951,

Post had developed an entire ward of people over age 60. Among his trainees were David Kay, who made major contributions to the understanding of the epidemiology of mental disorders in late life, and Raymond Levy and Tom Arie, who have continued in Post's tradition. Levy was the first professor of the Department of Psychiatry of Old Age at Maudsley, and Arie chaired the Division of Health Care of the Aged in Nottingham.

Post, Roth, Kay, and Hopkins intensively studied older patients who were hospitalized in the 1950s and determined that there was no evidence that depressed patients without brain symptoms subsequently developed them (Barraclough 1989; Post 1965). Roth's research, in distinguishing between affective and organic disorders, turned up a small group with paranoid symptoms (hallucinations and delusions) in otherwise well-maintained personality in late life (paraphrenia).

Around the same time, T. K. Henderson of Edinburgh and Duncan McMillan of Nottingham were working intensively with older people with mental disorders. McMillan focused on integration of services with a strong social-psychiatric approach. He played a major role in the development of respite care to meet the need of families who had people with depression or dementia living with them. McMillan emphasized the importance of ready access to appropriate levels and intensity of service based on the patient's and family's needs. In the United States, the first relevant treatise on geriatric psychiatry was written by Benjamin Rush in 1805, titled "An Account of the State of the Body and the Mind in Old Age; With Observation on Its Diseases and Remedies" (Busse 1989).

Hall published *Senescence: The Last Half of Life* in 1922. One of his findings included the observation, based on questionnaires, that older people did not become more fearful of death. In 1914, Nascher published a textbook titled *Geriatrics: The Diseases of Old Age and Their Treatment*, thereby establishing a new name for the field. Nascher, who is considered the father of geriatrics in America, continued his interest in the field. His final paper, "The Aging Mind," published in 1944, described the characteristics of chronic brain syndrome. Nascher hypothesized that there was a genetic etiology of chronic brain syndrome.

Organized Geriatric Psychiatry

In the late 1930s, voices all over the world spoke of the need to establish a gerontological society. Before that time, a great deal of emphasis had been placed on how to extend the human life span, with little attention to careful and thoughtful study of the aging process. Shock (1988) and Busse (1989) wrote detailed reviews of the history of the International Association of Gerontology (IAG), established in Liège, Belgium, in 1950. The IAG has supported regular, well-attended conferences all over the world addressing many gerontological issues, including mental health and mental illness.

In the 1940s and 1950s, several other major national and international geriatric organizations were founded. The American Geriatric Society was founded in 1942 and began to publish *The Journal of the American Geriatric Society* in 1953. The Gerontological Society of America was founded in 1945 and began to publish the *Journal of Gerontology* in 1946. At that time, however, the number of investigators involved in research on aging was extremely small.

Three other developments in geriatric psychiatry in the United States began in the 1950s and picked up momentum in the following decades. The Group for the Advancement of Psychiatry (GAP) was founded in 1946 with the following goals: "to collect and appraise significant data in the field of psychiatry, mental health and human relations; to re-evaluate old concepts and to develop and test new ones; and to apply the knowledge thus obtained for the promotion of mental health in group human relations" (GAP 1950, p. 6). *The Problem of the Aged Patient in the Public Psychiatric Hospital* was GAP's first geropsychiatric monograph, published in 1950 by the Committee on Hospitals (GAP 1950).

The GAP Committee on Aging was established in the early 1960s by Jack Weinberg, future president of the American Psychiatric Association (APA). A second treatise, *Psychiatry and the Aged: An Introductory Approach*, was published in 1965 (GAP 1965). Other monographs addressed issues related to community mental health (GAP 1971), curriculum development (GAP 1983), and psychotherapy of Alzheimer's disease (GAP 1988).

In 1954, longitudinal studies on aging began at Duke University. These studies led to a series of books based on research findings, many taken from the longitudinal data (Busse and Pfeiffer 1969; Palmore 1970, 1974). Busse established the first geriatric psychiatry training program at Duke University Medical Center in 1965. In the late 1960s, Carl Eisdorfer, Eric Pfeiffer, Adrian Verwoerdt, and others began to make major contributions to the field of geriatric psychiatry, under the leadership of Ewald (Bud) Busse.

The Boston Society for Gerontologic Psychiatry (BSGP) was founded by a group of psychoanalytically oriented psychiatrists—Martin Berezin,

Stanley Cath, David Blau, and Ralph Kahana, among others—with a special interest in developmental issues related to aging. The BSGP's semi-annual, half-day workshops became the primary source of intellectual stimulation for budding geriatric psychiatrists across the country. Papers from BSGP's symposia were published in three books in the 1960s (Berezin and Cath 1965; Levin and Kahana 1967; Zinberg and Kaufman 1963). Subsequently, BSGP created *The Journal of Geriatric Psychiatry* in 1967 and has continued this publication uninterrupted since that time. In the 1970s the inspiration provided by BSGP stimulated similar groups in Chicago, Houston, New York, and greater Washington, DC.

During the late 1950s and 1960s psychotropic medication was introduced; this medication provided unprecedented pharmacological relief from depression, anxiety, and psychosis. Chlorpromazine (Thorazine), lithium carbonate, imipramine hydrochloride (Tofranil), chlordiazepoxide hydrochloride (Librium), and diazepam (Valium) were introduced or developed.

In the mid-1960s, APA created a small component on aging, with particular interest in community geriatric psychiatry, under the leadership of Alexander Simon. It was not until 1979, however, that APA played a major role in the development of the field.

The 1960s also marked the inception of several Great Society programs, including Medicare and Medicaid, which allowed more older people to receive inpatient psychiatric services. Unfortunately, outpatient services were severely limited by a $250 annual cap, which remained until 1988.

The 1970s

The 1970s marked a significant worldwide increase in psychogeriatric services and training. In France, Jean-Marie Leger, professor and chairman of the Department of Psychiatry at the University of Limoges, started a psychogeriatric service that included community psychiatry, inpatient and outpatient psychiatric services, and an outreach program. All medical students rotated through the psychogeriatric service. Soon, newly trained French psychiatrists developed satellites with similar services in other parts of France. French geropsychiatrists have frequently divided into psychoanalytic versus organic camps. Doctor Henri Ey of Bonneval began to bridge this gap with an integrated approach.

In Switzerland, two psychogeriatric centers were established in French-speaking areas. After Junat established a substantial program in Geneva, Dr. Christian Mueller similarly established a service and academic component in Lausanne. The effects of aging on schizophrenia and other psychiatric disorders were studied by Luc Ciompi (1972), who found an unusually high percentage of dementia in elderly schizophrenic people.

In the late 1960s, Kiloh emigrated from Newcastle in the United Kingdom to Sydney, Australia. Kiloh was a general psychiatrist with a special interest in electroencephalography. Dr. D. K. Henderson, a research psychiatrist, established a division of psychogeriatric research, and Edmund Chiu of Melbourne conducted research on dementias that are uncommonly seen. These three spawned a new generation of Australian psychogeriatricians.

The decade from 1965 to 1975 marked the establishment in the United States of three major federal agencies devoted to gerontology. In 1965, the new Administration on Aging was established with the specific purpose of developing and coordinating services and research initiatives for elderly people. In 1971, the second White House Conference on Aging took place, leading to specific recommendations that catalyzed the formation of the National Institute of Mental Health (NIMH) Center for Studies of the Mental Health of the Aging, as well as the National Institute on Aging (NIA) (White House Conference on Aging 1981). NIA was assigned responsibility for promoting, coordinating, and supporting research regarding normal aging, as well as pathology and problems of elderly persons. NIA's mandate from Congress included conducting research in behavioral and social sciences, as well as biological and biomedical sciences. Robert Butler, a geriatric psychiatrist with extensive clinical, research, and teaching experience, was NIA's first director. In its first decade, more than 100 new researchers were trained (Butler 1977).

NIMH had sponsored research on the mental health of the aging on a limited basis between 1960 and 1976 (U.S. Department of Health, Education, and Welfare 1977). Under the energetic and creative leadership of its first chief, Dr. Gene Cohen, the NIMH Center for Studies of the Mental Health of the Aging grew rapidly as it carried out its mandate to support and coordinate research, clinical training projects, and research training. Geropsychiatric training, fellowship programs, continuing education, demonstration curricula and training projects, and inservice training all flourished. In 1976, the Secretary of Health, Education, and Welfare appointed Eric Pfeiffer to establish an agenda on the needs of the mental health of older Americans. President Carter in 1977 established a task panel regarding mental health and mental illness in late life. Both reports were published in 1978 (U.S. Department of Health, Education, and Welfare 1979).

By 1978 there was a clear need for an American organization with a specific focus on geriatric psychiatry. Although the field had been developing significantly since the late 1940s, the increasing number of older people, the concomitant number of older persons with psychiatric disorders—particularly depressions and dementias—and the larger base of knowledge mandated the establishment of a forum in which to exchange ideas. The interest level of professionals regarding older people had significantly increased, with growing efforts to provide services to older people (Finkel 1979).

In late 1978, Sanford Finkel assembled a group of 15 nationally recognized leaders in the field of geriatric psychiatry to discuss the establishment of a national organization, the American Association for Geriatric Psychiatry (AAGP). This organizational meeting occurred at the 1978 annual meeting of APA, the theme of which centered on aging. The initial goals of the organization were as follows:

- To provide a focus for dissemination of information to the psychiatrists who care for the elderly. (A primary mechanism would be the publication of a newsletter that would provide information regarding mental health issues and elderly people.)
- To increase the attention of APA on the field of aging with particular reference to services, training, research, and policy development. (AAGP also wished to advocate the establishment of a significant component on aging in APA.)
- To encourage throughout the country the development of local societies concerned with mental health aspects of aging. The first AAGP newsletter included "A Rationale for the Creation of an American Psychiatric Association Council on Aging" (Finkel 1978).

In its first year, AAGP accomplished its first and third goals, and AAGP representatives successfully solicited the assistance of Alan Stone, president-elect of APA, to support the establishment of an APA Council on Aging. On February 23, 1979, the APA created a Council on Aging, effective September 1979. Also in 1979, Congress held the first national legislative conference on the mental health of older Americans.

The 1980s

In 1980, two major textbooks were published in the field of geriatric psychiatry: *The Handbook of Mental Health and Aging* and *A Handbook of*

Geriatric Psychiatry (Birren and Sloane 1980; Busse and Blazer 1980). They appropriately reflected and started a veritable explosion in information and knowledge in the field of geriatric psychiatry.

The APA Council on Aging, working in close collaboration with AAGP, focused on several important issues of the time: psychiatric services, reimbursement options, Alzheimer's disease, the interface of medicine and psychiatry in geriatrics, the White House Conferences on Aging of 1981 and 1991, postgraduate education, nursing homes, geriatric psychiatry in the public sector, minorities, forensic psychiatric issues, and psychotropic medication for older people (Baker et al. 1985; Finkel et al. 1981; Moak et al. 1989). Chairpersons of the council were Jack Weinberg, Charles Gaitz, Charles Wells, Sanford Finkel, Charles Shamoian, Gene Cohen, and Jerome Yesavage.

At the same time, AAGP was becoming a major force on the national scene. As the decade progressed, membership approached 1,000 psychiatrists. AAGP began publishing a newsletter six times per year, and a variety of new programs were instituted. Some of the major accomplishments of AAGP included an active advocacy role with the American Board of Psychiatry and Neurology to achieve "added qualifications" in geriatric psychiatry at the same time. This event followed the decision, 3 years earlier, of the American Board of Internal Medicine and the American Board of Family Practice to offer certificates of added qualifications in geriatrics in 1988. In anticipation of this major landmark event, AAGP edited and published a syllabus of geriatric psychiatry (Lazarus 1988). AAGP presidents in the 1980s included Sanford Finkel, Eric Pfeiffer, Alvin Levenson, Lissy Jarvik, Elliott Stein, Charles Shamoian, Lawrence Lazarus, and George Grossberg.

The 1980s also marked the substantial growth of lay organizations concerned with elderly people. In addition to the continued growth of the American Association for Retired Persons and the National Council on Aging, the Alzheimer's Disease and Related Disorders Association (ADRDA) was organized to meet an increasing human need and pursue the following goals:

- To better serve Alzheimer's patients and other patients with dementia and their families (ADRDA's goals included supporting research into diagnosis, therapies, causes, and cures for Alzheimer's disease).
- To aid and organize family support groups in their own localities so as to give assistance, encouragement, and education to afflicted families.
- To sponsor educational forums.

- To dispense information to both lay and professional people with Alzheimer's disease.
- To advise government agencies (federal and state) of the needs of afflicted families as well as the need for extensive research on a nationwide scale.
- Most important, to offer assistance, when needed in any manner whatsoever, to those afflicted and their loved ones.

The cause of patients with dementia and their families has been furthered substantially by the publication of *The 36-Hour Day*, written by Nancy Mace and geriatric psychiatrist Peter Rabins (Mace and Rabins 1981).

In 1980, child psychiatrist Arthur Kornhaber established the Foundation for Grandparenting. This group emphasizes the relationship between grandparent and grandchild as a meaningful, healthy, and positive relationship. Among its accomplishments, the foundation has brought to the attention of legislators the need to establish the legal right for grandparents and grandchildren to maintain contact after the middle generation has divorced (Kornhaber and Woodward 1981).

The 1981 White House Conference on Aging established a number of sound recommendations based on the multidisciplinary mini-conference on the Mental Health of Older Americans (White House Conference on Aging 1981). The action group to implement the recommendations did some careful research on community mental health centers and the general problems of underserving the elderly (Fleming et al. 1984). Furthermore, the White House Conference recommendation to expand mental health benefits was finally implemented in 1988. At the end of the decade, outpatient psychiatric benefits increased from $250 a year to $1,100 a year (50% of $500 versus 50% of $2,200). Psychologists became eligible for reimbursement under certain conditions. In addition, under the leadership of Margaret Heckler, Secretary of Health and Human Services, Alzheimer's disease centers in various sections of the country were created and psychiatrists treating patients with dementia were reimbursed without an annual maximum when providing medical therapy and medication to elderly patients with dementia.

Congress passed Public Law 99-660 in 1986, authorizing a Council on Alzheimer's Disease, as well as a panel on Alzheimer's disease with a primary goal of creating a major services research program in the area of Alzheimer's disease and related dementias. Meanwhile, research budgets for aging and mental health increased annually in both NIA and the NIMH Center for Studies of the Mental Health of the Aging.

International activities also grew rapidly. The World Psychiatric Association section on geriatric psychiatry increased its visibility with meetings in Europe and North America. In Sweden, much progress was made in diagnostic tests for Alzheimer's disease and other dementias (Steen and Bucht 1988), and in Japan, dementia research expanded with special emphasis on diagnosis, pathology, and caretaker support (Homma and Hasegawa 1989).

In 1988, the Royal College of Physicians in London created its first examination for a diploma in geriatric medicine. The examination was not for "geriatric specialists," but rather for physicians who were general practitioners and who wished to have special expertise in geriatric medicine. An extensive psychogeriatric program was established in Nottingham, United Kingdom, under the leadership of Tom Arie, a geriatric psychiatrist who has developed a comprehensive system of training for medical students, physicians, nurses, and other geriatric health care professionals (Arie et al. 1985).

The Canadian Psychiatric Association developed a division on aging in the 1970s. The Canadian Geriatric Association also was active in the 1970s, and both groups continued their activities into the 1980s. The first Canadian division of geriatric psychiatry for the training of geriatric psychiatrists was established at the University of Toronto in 1978 under the leadership of Dr. Abraham Miller. In 1981, the Royal College of Physicians and Surgeons of Canada gave its first examination for certification in geriatric medicine, and in 1983 the college mandated that all psychiatric training programs include psychogeriatric experience (Reichenfeld 1987).

The World Health Organization (WHO) has had a long-standing interest in psychogeriatrics, having published an early monograph (1972b) which elaborated the extent of the potential problems of psychopathology in later life, organizational services, research, epidemiology, and training (Henderson and MacFadyen 1985). WHO has made efforts to stimulate the production of self-help guides and has developed monographs on drugs and senile dementia as well as mental health care (WHO 1972a, 1983, 1984, 1985). Other areas of exploration in psychogeriatrics include assessing mental health care needs in the community and attention to diagnostic classification. Currently, there is a great deal of interest in these dementias with focus on improving clinical drug evaluation and other therapeutic interventions. The World Assembly on Aging met in Vienna in 1982 to determine an international policy on many issues related to aging, including psychogeriatrics (United Nations 1983).

The major thrust for international collaboration in psychogeriatrics in the 1980s came from the International Psychogeriatric Association (IPA). The fledgling organization began as the "Nottingham 1980 Club," following an annual 2-week psychogeriatric conference for geriatric psychiatrists, internists, and general practitioners engaged in psychogeriatric clinical work. The course was devised and supervised by Tom Arie. Shortly after the 1980 meeting, two Canadians, Imre Fejer and Hans Reichenfeld, sought to establish an international organization. After collaboration with Dr. A. Ashour of Ain Shams Medical School in Egypt, Cairo became the site of the first meeting of the IPA: the International Conference for the Mental Health of the Elderly. As a result of the meeting, the Egyptian medical schools in Cairo incorporated geriatrics into their training, and the Egyptian Medical Association developed a special committee on geriatrics. The conference was marred by Mideast politics, and subsequently the small international group was temporarily divided by factions. However, unified support was established by the late 1980s. Under the strong leadership of Presidents Manfred Bergener, Gustav Bucht, and Kazuo Hasegawa, and with publication of a newsletter and later a journal (*International Psychogeriatrics*) and two annual conferences, the organization has grown significantly and has played a role in the founding of national psychogeriatric societies in Japan, Italy, and Sweden.

During the 1980s, there was also rapid growth in the number of journals in geriatric psychiatry, including the establishment of *The International Journal of Geriatric Psychiatry* (Elaine Murphy, editor), *International Psychogeriatrics* (Gene Cohen, editor), *Comprehensive Gerontology* (Alvar Svanborg, editor), *The Journal of Alzheimer's Disease and Related Disorders* (Lissy Jarvik, editor), and *The Journal of Cross-Cultural Anthropology* (Jay Sokolovsky, editor), to name but a few. Pharmaceutical companies have become increasingly interested and involved as the world's population ages. The Sandoz Research Awards in Gerontology were established in 1984, and the Bayer Psychogeriatric Research Awards were established in 1989. Sandoz, Bristol-Myers, Bayer, Hoffmann-LaRoche, Upjohn, Mead-Johnson, Charter Medical, and many others have sponsored educational and research activities.

Other ideas that developed in the 1980s included the concept of the teaching nursing home (Schneider et al. 1985); age-associated memory impairment as a condition of "normal aging"; and new assessment scales, including the Global Deterioration Scale (Reisberg et al. 1982), the Geriatric Depression Scale (Sheikh et al. 1986), and a variety of brief mental status measurements (of which the Mini-Mental State Exam [Folstein et al. 1975] remains the most popular). The use of sophisticated equipment for diagnostic purposes (e.g., nuclear magnetic resonance, magnetic resonance imaging, positron-emission tomography, and single photon emission computed tomography) has risen rapidly in our technologically oriented world (Margolin and Daniel 1990). Furthermore, the use of electronics and electronic gadgets has played an increasing role in supporting the mental health of elderly people (Lieff 1990; Stein 1990).

The 1990s

As we approach the year 2000, geriatric psychiatry continues to thrive. The first half of the decade was marked by a variety of important events and emerging trends including the inauguration of the *American Journal of Geriatric Psychiatry,* the official journal of the AAGP (Gene Cohen, editor).

Four additional major textbooks appeared in the late 1980s and early 1990s: *Geriatric Psychiatry* (Busse and Blazer 1989), *Textbook of Geriatric Neuropsychiatry* (Coffey and Cummings 1994), *Principles and Practice of Geriatric Psychiatry* (Copeland et al. 1994), and the first edition of *Comprehensive Review of Geriatric Psychiatry* (Sadavoy et al. 1991). A variety of specialty texts began to appear as well, including *Geriatric Psychiatry and Psychopharmacology* (Jenike 1989), *Anxiety in the Elderly* (Salzman and Lebowitz 1991), and *Problem Behaviors in Long-Term Care* (Szwabo and Grossberg 1993). A major event was the publication of the fourth edition of the *Diagnostic and Statistical Manual of Mental Disorders* by the APA in May of 1994 with its greater emphasis and direction of dementias, whether of the Alzheimer's type or vascular dementia.

The AAGP continued its growth with over 1,300 members by 1995. The organization was also streamlined for efficiency and for the first time opened its own office with a full-time executive director in 1994. Presidents in the early part of the decade included Barnett Meyers, Jonathan Lieff, Alan Siegal, Gary Gottlieb, and Ira Katz.

The NIMH Center on Aging continued its leadership role under the direction of Barry Lebowitz. A major event was the first NIMH Consensus Conference on Late-Life Depression in 1991. During the early 1990s, Gene Cohen was appointed as acting director of NIA, with Dan Blazer serving as president of the American Geriatric Society.

The APA Council on Aging became an increasingly important voice under the leadership of Burt Reifler, who also chaired the national Alzheimer's Daycare Initiative funded by the Robert Wood Johnson Foundation. For the first time, a permanent seat on the Council on Aging was created for the past president of AAGP, further enhancing collaboration. Important issues of the early 1990s included parity in reimbursement for mental disorders, the special problems of psychiatric disturbances in the nursing home, the impact of managed care on geropsychiatric services, and the United States' debate concerning national health care reform.

After multiple delays, the White House Conference on Aging was finally held in May 1995. A Mini White House Conference on Aging and Mental Health held in Washington, DC, in February of 1995 under the auspices of the AARP developed consensus recommendations relative to increasing funds for research and research training in mental health and aging, promoting parity of coverage, and increasing public and professional awareness relative to aging and mental health.

Further indications of the arrival of geriatric psychiatry in the 1990s included a growth in endowed chairs in geriatric psychiatry and the trend for nationally recognized geriatric psychiatrists to assume chairs of major departments of psychiatry.

On the international front, IPA continued its growth with over 1,300 members representing more than 60 countries. Under the presidency of Sanford Finkel, IPA joined the World Health Organization in 1992 and its journal *International Psychogeriatrics* increased its frequency of publication to quarterly with regular special monographs on issues such as delirium and geriatric suicide.

In 1991, the Canadian Academy of Geriatric Psychiatry was formed. Under the leadership of its founding executive Drs. Joel Sadavoy (founding president) and J. Kenneth LeClair and Marie-France Tourigny-Rivard, the organization set out to establish, promote, and develop excellence in geriatric psychiatry in Canada. In contrast to the AAGP, this group began as a subspecialty organization with formal training and/or defined practice in geriatric psychiatry required for full members. Since its inception, the academy has established a national fellowship program to develop leadership in geriatric psychiatry and national guidelines for training in geriatric psychiatry that have been adopted by all the medical schools in Canada and has advanced continuing medical education through its annual scientific meeting and a national visiting professorship program.

The pharmaceutical industry continued its strong support of psychogeriatrics through its work with AAGP and IPA. A special initiative begun in 1990 with funding from the Mead Johnson division of Bristol-Myers Squibb was the AAGP Fellowship in Geriatric Psychiatry, funding five PGYIII and PGYIV psychiatry residents each year to attend the AAGP Annual Symposium and facilitating their involvement in AAGP. This competitive award has served its purpose of identifying future leaders in the field. A similar award was established in Canada by Solvay-Kingswood and the CAGP.

Other initiatives to encourage the growth of research in geriatric psychiatry included the NIMH-funded AAGP Summer Research Colloquium for young investigators and the establishment by AAGP of annual junior and senior investigator awards through the active AAGP Research Committee.

Major developments during the early 1990s relative to geriatric psychiatry included

- The growing recognition of Alzheimer's disease as a psychiatric disorder and the increasing role of psychiatry in the nursing home, in particular, the decreased use of physical restraints in long-term care.
- The notion of rational use of psychotherapeutic agents in elderly people with more geriatric studies occurring before Food and Drug Administration approval of new psychotherapeutic medications.
- The introduction of many new drugs, including the first drug to treat Alzheimer's disease, the selective serotonin reuptake inhibitors (SSRIs), and antipsychotic and anxiolytic/sedative-hypnotic agents with improved safety and side effect profiles.

Other emerging trends that had an impact on psychogeriatrics in the early 1990s included

- The growing role of managed care, which often eliminated mental health benefits.
- The need to control health care spending and the trend toward shorter hospital stays with increased use of day treatment, day hospital, and outpatient settings.
- The growing role of physician extenders such as nurse clinicians and physician assistants in geriatric psychiatry and the trend on the part of managed care providers to see psychotherapy as primarily the domain of psychologists and social workers.

In the chapters that follow, the reader will be provided with state-of-the-art knowledge in the growing field of psychogeriatrics as well as insights into trends that will have an impact on the field in the years ahead.

References

Abraham K: The applicability of psychoanalytic treatment to patients at an advanced age, in Selected Papers on Psychoanalysis. Edited by Abraham K. London, Hogarth Press, 1927, pp 312–317

Alzheimer A: A characteristic disease of the cerebral cortex, in The Early Story of Alzheimer's Disease. New York, Raven Press, 1906

American Psychiatric Association: Diagnostic and Statistic Manual of Mental Disorders, 4th Edition. Washington, DC, American Psychiatric Association, 1994

Arie T, Jones R, Smith C: The educational potential of old age psychiatric services, in Recent Advances in Psychogeriatrics. Edited by Arie T. Edinburgh, Churchill Livingstone, 1985

Baker FN, Pen IN, Yesavage JY: An Overview of Legal Issues in Geriatric Psychiatry. Washington, DC, American Psychiatric Press, 1985

Barraclough B: Conversations with Felix Post: part II. Psychiatric Bulletin 13:114–119, 1989

Berezin MA, Cath SH (eds): Geriatric Psychiatry: Grief, Loss, and Emotional Disorders in the Aging Process. New York, International Universities Press, 1965

Birren J, Sloane B: Handbook of Mental Health and Aging. Englewood Cliffs, NJ, Prentice-Hall, 1980

Busse EW: The myth, history, and science of aging, in Geriatric Psychiatry. Edited by Busse EW, Blazer DG. Washington, DC, American Psychiatric Press, 1989, pp 3–34

Busse EW, Blazer DG (eds): Handbook of Geriatric Psychiatry. New York, Van Nostrand Reinhold, 1980

Busse EW, Blazer DG (eds): Geriatric Psychiatry. Washington, DC, American Psychiatric Press, 1989

Busse EW, Pfeiffer E (eds): Behavior and Adaptation in Late Life. Boston, MA, Little, Brown, 1969

Butler RN: Mission of the National Institution on Aging. J Am Geriatr Soc 25:97–103, 1977

Ciompi L: The outcome of late life psychiatric disorders. J Geriatr Psychiatry 39:789–794, 1972

Clark JE, Lanphear AK, Riddick CC: The effects of videogame playing on the response selection processing of elderly adults. J Gerontol 4:82–85, 1987

Coffey CE, Cummings JL (eds): Textbook of Geriatric Neuropsychiatry. Washington, DC, American Psychiatric Press, 1994

Cohen GD: The Brain in Human Aging. New York, Springer, 1988

Cohen GD: The movement toward subspecialty status for geriatric psychiatry in the United States. International Psychogeriatr 1:201–205, 1989

Copeland JRM, Abou-Saleh MT, Blazer DG (eds): Principles and Practice of Geriatric Psychiatry. London, Wiley, 1994

Ferenczi S: A contribution to the understanding of the psychoneuroses of the age of involution, in Selected Papers: Problems and Methods of Psychoanalysis,

Vol III: Final Contributions to the Problems and Methods of Psychoanalysis. Edited by Ferenczi S. New York, Basic Books, 1955

Finkel SI: The rationale for the creation of an American psychiatric council on aging. AAGP Newsletter 1:5, 1978

Finkel SI: Experience of a private practice psychiatrist working with the elderly in the community. Int J Mental Health 8:147–172, 1979

Finkel SI, Borson S, Shamoian C, et al: The American Psychiatric Association Task Force Report on the 1981 White House Conference on Aging. Washington, DC, American Psychiatric Association, 1981

Fleming AS, Buchanan JG, Santos JF: Report on the Survey of Community Health Centers by the Action Committee to Implement the Mental Health Recommendations of the 1981 White House Conference on Aging. Chicago, IL, The Retirement Research Foundation, 1984

Folstein, M, Folstein S, McHugh PR: Mini-Mental State: a practical method of grading the cognitive state of patients for the clinician. J Psychiatr Res 12:189–198, 1975

Freud S: My views on the past plagued by sexuality in the aetiology of the neuroses (1898), in The Complete Psychological Works of Sigmund Freud, Vol VI. Edited by Ernest Jones. London, Hogarth Press, 1953

Group for the Advancement of Psychiatry: The Problem of the Aged Patient in the Public Psychiatric Hospital (GAP Report No 14). New York, Group for Advancement of Psychiatry, 1950

Group for the Advancement of Psychiatry: Psychiatry and the Aged: An Introductory Approach (GAP Report No 59). New York, Group for Advancement of Psychiatry, 1965

Group for the Advancement of Psychiatry: Mental Health and Aging: Approaches to Curriculum Development (GAP Report No 114). New York, Mental Health Materials Center, 1983

Group for the Advancement of Psychiatry: The Psychiatric Treatment of Alzheimer's Disease (GAP Report No 125). New York, Brunner/Mazel, 1988

Group for the Advancement of Psychiatry, Committee on Aging: The Aged and Community Mental Health: A Guide to Program Development (GAP Report No 81). New York, Group for Advancement of Psychiatry, 1971

Group for the Advancement of Psychiatry, Committee on Aging: The Psychiatric Treatment of Alzheimer's Disease. New York, Brunner/Mazel, 1988

Hall GS: Senescence: The Last Half of Life. New York, Appleton, 1922

Henderson JH, MacFadyen DM: Psychogeriatrics and the programmes of the World Health Organization, in Recent Advances in Psychogeriatrics. Edited by Arie T. Edinburgh, Churchill Livingstone, 1985

Homma A, Hasegawa K: Recent developments in gerontopsychiatric research on age-associated dementia in Japan. Int Psychogeriatr 1:31–50, 1989

Jarvik L: The impact of immediate life situations on depression, illness, and loss, in Depression and Aging. Edited by Bresla D, Haig MR. New York, Springer, 1983, pp 114–120

Jenike MA: Geriatric Psychiatry and Psychopharmacology. St. Louis, MO, Mosby–Year Book, 1989

Kornhaber A, Woodward KL: Grandparents/Grandchildren: The Vital Connection. Garden City, NY, Anchor Press/Doubleday, 1981

Lazarus LW (ed): Essentials of Geriatric Psychiatry. New York, Springer, 1988

Levin S, Kahana RJ: Psychodynamic Studies on Aging, Creativity, Reminiscing, and Dying. New York, International Universities Press, 1967

Lieff J: High technology and geriatric psychiatry, in Clinical and Scientific Psychogeriatrics. Edited by Bergener M, Finkel S. New York, Springer, 1990, pp 112–135

Mace NL, Rabins PV: The 36-Hour Day. Baltimore, MD, Johns Hopkins University Press, 1981

Margolin R, Daniel D: Neuroimaging in geropsychiatry, in Clinical and Scientific Psychogeriatrics. Edited by Bergener M, Finkel S. New York, Springer, 1990, pp 162–186

Maugham S: The Summing Up. London, William Heinemann, 1938

Moak GS, Stein EM, Rubin JEV: The Over-50 Guide to Psychiatric Medications. Washington, DC, American Psychiatric Press, 1989

Nascher IL: Geriatrics: The Diseases of Old Age and Their Treatment. Philadelphia, PA, P Blokiston's Son, 1914

Nascher IL: The aging mind. Medical Record 157:669, 1944

Palmore E (ed): Normal Aging: Reports From the Duke Longitudinal Study, 1955–1969. Durham, NC, Duke University Press, 1970

Palmore E (ed): Normal Aging: II. Durham, NC, Duke University Press, 1974

Post F: The Clinical Psychiatry of Late Life. Oxford, UK, Pergamon, 1965

Reichenfeld HF: Geriatric psychiatry north of the border. AAGP Newsletter 9:11–12, 1987

Reisberg B, Ferris SH, DeLeon MJ, et al: The Global Deterioration Scale for assessment of primary degenerative dementia. Am J Psychiatry 139:1136–1139, 1982

Rowe JW, Grossman E, Bond E: The Institute of Medicine Committee on Leadership for Academic Geriatric Medicine: academic geriatrics for the year 2000. N Engl J Med 316:1425–1428, 1987

Sadavoy J, Lazarus LW, Jarvik L (eds): Comprehensive Review of Geriatric Psychiatry. Washington, DC, American Psychiatric Press, 1991

Sadavoy J, Leszcz M: Treating the Elderly With Psychotherapy: The Scope for Change in Later Life. New York, International Universities Press, 1987

Salzman C, Lebowitz BD (eds): Anxiety in the Elderly. New York, Springer, 1991

Schneider EL, Wendland CJ, Zimmer AW, et al: The Teaching Nursing Home—A New Approach to Geriatric Research, Education, and Clinical Care. New York, Raven, 1985

Sheikh JI, Yesavage JA, Brink PL: Geriatric Depression Scale (GDS): recent evidence and development of a short version, in Clinical Gerontology: A Guide to Assessment and Intervention. Edited by Brink TL. New York, Haworth Press, 1986

Shock NW: The International Association of Gerontology: A Chronicle—1950 to 1986. New York, Springer, 1988

Siever LJ, Davis KL: Overview: toward a dysregulation hypothesis of depression. Am J Psychiatry 142:1017–1031, 1985

Steen B, Bucht G: Psychogeriatrics in Sweden. IPA Newsletter 5:23–25, 1988

Stein E: Gadgets and other high-tech devices for use with the elderly, in Clinical and Scientific Psychogeriatrics. Edited by Bergener M, Finkel S. New York, Springer, 1990

Szwabo PA, Grossberg GT (eds): Problem Behaviors in Long-Term Care. New York, Springer, 1993

SECTION I

The Aging Process

Barry Gurland, M.D.

Epidemiology of Psychiatric Disorders

E pidemiology can contribute to learning about psychiatric problems in relation to aging by the study of the variation in frequency and course of psychiatric problems between subgroups of aging persons. Frequency is usually expressed as prevalence (over a period of time or at a single point in time) or incidence (new cases or episodes during a period of time, usually a year). More complex strategies of epidemiology are required for the discovery of the profiles of current (e.g., age) or antecedent (e.g., education) characteristics that are unique to persons with a given psychiatric problem and the range of outcomes that occur under prevailing conditions of service delivery.

Subgroups of persons can be delineated in any manner that offers promise of revealing variation in frequencies of psychiatric problems or of their associated characteristics. Analysis of the characteristics of those subgroups and their circumstances can identify clinical and public health challenges and can lead to an understanding of the forces that govern the origin and course of psychiatric problems.

Peter Cross, M.Phil., assisted in the collation of literature for review.

Characteristics that are commonly used to define subgroups of persons or the associations of psychiatric problems, include the residential and service context (e.g., community or institution or type of health services), demography (e.g., age, gender, or race), and exposure to other probable risk factors (e.g., life events, social supports, or medical illness). Each of these characteristics can be measured crudely or can be refined (e.g., by detailing types of medical illness or the social network) to allow the examination of a promising hypothesis. Other informative characteristics may be derived from service use and outcomes in various service settings. Psychiatric problems in epidemiological reports are often taken to mean diagnostic groups, usually restricted to those meeting criteria in a nomenclature, such as DSM-IV (American Psychiatric Association 1994), but may be expanded to refer to symptom levels that are of clinical interest or are linked to the functional consequences of psychiatric disorder.

Epidemiological Issues That Span Psychiatric Problems

Epidemiology makes little sense if it is restricted to mustering subgroups and counting problems; it is the analysis of the circumstances surrounding variation that carries etiologic, clinical, and organizational implications for geriatric psychiatry. The need for treatment of psychiatric problems in a defined population should be estimated with a level of accuracy that would guide, not mislead, policy and organization of services. It is also important to interpret epidemiological evidence in the light of information on the benefits of treatment, likelihood of contacts of cases with health care resources during the course of the problem, the proportion of cases receiving inappropriate treatment, and availability of informal sources of care. In addition, it is desirable to know the rates of recovery and relapse with and without treatment, the frequency and severity of the consequences of failing to adequately treat the problem, and the extent to which disposition and treatment are determined by overlap between psychiatric problems and the frequency of types of comorbidity. Moreover, barriers and resistances to access, compliance with treatment recommendations, quality and cost of care, and human resources considerations also have a bearing on estimations of fulfilled and unfulfilled needs for treatment.

Given the protean applications of epidemiology and its ubiquitous relevance to psychiatric problems in aging, there is a likelihood of redundancy between this chapter on epidemiology and corresponding sections of the chapters on particular psychiatric problems. To minimize redundancy, in this chapter I focus on epidemiological issues that are best addressed by scanning across specific psychiatric problems; exploration in-depth of the epidemiology of specific conditions is left to other chapters. Therefore, in this chapter, I have grouped psychiatric problems under residential, service, and other risk factor contexts. This approach should illustrate the contribution of epidemiology in drawing attention to the extent and location of the need for treatment of psychiatric problems and opportunities for early and preventive intervention. Other chapters will give a more pointed and substantive account of the nature of specific psychiatric disorders and their effective treatment.

Community, Residential, and Service Settings

Community Residents

It is evident from the prevalent data that psychiatric problems are frequent during the period conventionally designated as containing the older age groups (starting at age 65). In elderly people living within a community (i.e., samples representative of all noninstitutionalized persons age 65 years or older in a geographic area), depressions conforming to DSM-IV criteria (major depression, dysthymia, cyclothymic disorder, and atypical depression) are between 2% and 4% (Myers et al. 1984; Weissman et al. 1991) of the population, with major depression accounting for less than 1% (Blazer et al. 1980); however, if all persons with depressive symptomatology of clinical interest are included, the rates rise to between 10% and 15% (Blazer and Williams 1980; Gurland et al. 1983) or even higher. In the combined Epidemiologic Catchment Area (ECA) samples, persons ages 65 years and older comprised 6.3% of major depressions and dysthymias and 12.9% of subclinical depressions (versus 14.7% and 19.9% for those 18–24 years) (Johnson et al. 1992). The prevalence of mild to more severe depressed mood, based on the Beck Depression Inventory, for elderly people ages 65 years or older within a community, was 5.2% (Palinkas et al. 1990). In an urban community study of elderly people, a significant level of depressive symptoms was found (Kennedy et al. 1990) in 17% of elderly people by Center for Epidemiologcal Studies depression scale (CES-D) criteria (about one-third meeting criteria for major depression). Among United Kingdom community residents, ages 60 years and older, approximately 15.9% were found to be clinically depressed in an inner city area (G. Livingston et al. 1990) and another study found 9% of cognitively intact elderly patients were diagnosable as having major depression (O'Connor and Roth 1990). Of elderly patients not depressed at baseline in a longitudinal study, 11.2% were newly depressed 2 years later (Kennedy et al. 1990).

Anxiety disorders, including panic, phobic, obsessional, and somatization disorders, range in elderly people within a community from 4% upward (Blazer et al. 1991; Eaton et al. 1991; Karno and Golding 1991; Swartz et al. 1991), with the most common form being agoraphobia, especially in older women (Turnbull and Turnbull 1985).

Anxiety disorders affect more than 7% of adults in the United States according to the results of the ECA surveys (Regier et al. 1990); dropping from 7.7% for 18- to 24-year-old persons to 5.5% for those 65 years or older. The subgroup of phobias is the most common and again shows diminished frequency for those 65 years or older, although still 4.8% for 1-month prevalence. Panic disorders are low in prevalence compared with the other anxiety disorders. Prevalence of phobic disorders in a community survey of United Kingdom urban elderly people was 10% (Lindesay 1991a). Phobic cases from the latter community survey had multiple fears and an increased prevalence of other neurotic symptoms. Agoraphobia was commonly of late onset, with onset tied to comorbid physical illness or other traumatic incident and to moderate to severe social impairments. Specific fears were more often of early onset and less disabling.

Active symptoms among individuals with schizophrenia who have grown old, together with late-onset persistent paranoid states, are noted in less than 0.5% of the population (Keith et al. 1991), although obtrusive behaviors may suggest a more frequent presence (Kay 1975). It has been claimed that, with highly sensitive measures, paranoid features can be found in as many as 11% of elderly patients (Lowenthal 1964; Savage et al. 1977).

About 7.5% of all older adults have progressive dementias; about two-thirds of these patients reside in the community (Gurland and Cross 1982), although this proportion can drop to one-half or less where the capacity of long-term care facilities is large (Bland et al. 1988). In a United States metropolitan community, among those ages 65 years and older, the estimated prevalence of Alzheimer's disease was 2.0%; multi-infarct dementia, 2.0%; and mixed dementia, 0.5% (Folstein et al. 1991). In a United

Kingdom community study, approximately 4% of those ages 60 years or older were classified as having dementia (G. Livingston et al. 1990). Complaints of memory problems are common in elderly people residing in a community, but most of those who complain have neither dementia nor depression (G. Livingston et al. 1990). In elderly people residing in a community, age 70 years and older, concurrent major depressive disorder occurred in 5% of dementias, especially among those with the multi-infarct and Parkinson's disease subtypes of dementia; except for extreme apathy, symptoms were similar to cognitively intact elderly patients with major depression (O'Connor and Roth 1990).

Dementias are characterized by impaired ability to perform the activities of daily living (ADLs). Even in early or mild dementia, errors in verbal recall, visuospatial recall, object function recognition, and object identification are good predictors of decline in performance of ADLs (Flicker et al. 1991); apraxias are also indicative of a decline in performance of ADLs (Edwards et al. 1991). A significant correlation has been found between Mini-Mental State Exam (Folstein et al. 1975) scores and the ADL measures of functional abilities. Conversely, information on ADLs may increase the specificity and sensitivity of the diagnosis of dementia (Warren et al. 1989). However, when medical illness is ruled out in patients with progressive dementias, cognitive scores explain only about one-third of the variance in instrumental ADLs and physical ADLs and much less in the patients with milder dementia. Therefore, cognitive and ADL function must be assessed separately (Reed et al. 1989).

In surveys of a representative sample of the general older population, Alzheimer's disease alone usually accounts for a majority of cases of dementia (Copeland et al. 1992; Letenneur et al. 1993; Launer and Hofman 1992). Another substantial subtype is caused by multi-infarcts or other cerebrovascular disorders (Folstein et al. 1991). Both subtypes may be present, and it may be often difficult to establish whether the pathology of Alzheimer's disease or multi-infarcts predominates. The residual group amounts to about 15% and includes dementias or states of cognitive impairment associated with well-recognized neurological diseases (e.g., Huntington's chorea or parkinsonism) and a variety of causes that may be treatable (e.g., increased intracranial pressure; systemic effects from metabolic, toxic, or anoxic conditions; and altered mood). These proportions of subtypes of dementia may vary depending on the ethnic, racial, and cultural characteristics of the population. Blacks and socially disadvantaged groups have been reported to have higher proportions of the multi-infarct subtype than do non-Latino whites (Heyman et al. 1991).

Alcohol abuse and dependence is detected by community surveys in about 1% to 2% of elderly people; the rate is higher than this in men and lower in women (Bland et al. 1988; Holzer et al. 1984; Kramer et al. 1985; Weissman et al. 1985).

Methodological problems and solutions surrounding underestimation of alcohol (and illicit drug consumption) in surveys of older adults are discussed by Mishara and McKim (1993). G. Livingston and King (1993) offer the explanation that very low rates found in some surveys are caused by the poor economic status of the particular elderly population under study and the limit that restricted income imposes on ability to obtain quantities of alcohol. Atkinson (1994) agrees that higher economic status increases the likelihood of a late onset to alcoholism. The age bracket for defining an older population will also greatly affect the prevalence rate. In a study of community-residing persons ages 45 years and older by Nakamura et al. 1990, 15% were found to be severe drinkers.

Psychiatric inpatients.   Among short-stay psychiatric inpatients, depressions that meet DSM-IV criteria are common. In many such settings, one-half of all admissions meet the criteria for major depression.

Early studies reported that a minority (about 10%) of patients who were first admitted to inpatient units after the age of 60 had late-onset symptoms closely related to schizophrenia (Kay and Roth 1961). More recent reports indicate that in long-stay psychiatric centers, such as state psychiatric hospitals, there are a disproportionate number of elderly patients—as much as half the resident population (Goodman and Siegel 1986). A substantial proportion (35%–60%) of these elderly patients are first admitted during early adulthood with a diagnosis of schizophrenia. Late-onset schizophrenia, as a proportion of all schizophrenic admissions, varies from about 10% (less for men and more for women) to as high as one-third of first admissions ages 45 to 64 years (Goodman and Siegel 1986). In three developed countries, cohorts first discharged from psychiatric hospitals in the late 1960s to early 1970s had a prevalence of the onset of schizophrenia after age 40 years of around 25%–44% and after 60 years of age of around 6%–12% (Eaton et al. 1992). Between 1970 and 1986, the proportion of patients with schizophrenia admitted to state hospitals who were self-payers or covered by private insurance decreased, whereas the proportion of patients who were black increased. However, age was not a special factor in these changing admission patterns (Thompson et al. 1993). Patients with schizophrenia ages 65 years or older who have aged in long-stay public hospitals are characterized by deficit states with negative symptoms and thought disorder and more negative but fewer positive symptoms than younger patients (Soni and Mallik 1993). These features are in large part determined by selective retention, although poor self-care and decreased social interaction might be aggravated by a long-term institutional effect (Simpson et al. 1989; Wing 1989).

Nursing homes. The great majority of nursing home residents have a psychiatric problem in the form of a disorder, mainly depression or dementia, or a behavioral disturbance (Burns et al. 1988; Rovner et al. 1986); the need for suitably trained staff in these locations is pressing. Residents in nursing homes and congregate apartment residences were found to have a 15.7% prevalence of major depression and a 16.5% prevalence for minor depressive symptoms (Parmelee et al. 1992). The incidence of major depression at the end of 1 year was 6.6% and was higher in persons with pre-existing minor depression than in those with no depression. These incidence rates are many times higher than comparable results of community surveys. Half or more of the long-stay residents in nursing homes have Alzheimer's disease or related dementia (Burns et al. 1988). Individuals with schizophrenia may be placed in nursing homes, especially if chronic medical problems have supervened. A diagnosis of schizophrenia, based on information obtained from staff and records, has been reported in about 6% of nursing home residents with an average age of 79 years (Burns et al. 1988).

The Omnibus Budget Reconciliation Act of 1987 (OBRA 87) attempted sweeping changes in admission and retention criteria for residents in Medicare- or Medicaid-certified nursing homes (Eichmann et al. 1992). Eichmann et al. noted, by extrapolation from a 1985 national survey, that 21% of residents were diagnosed as having a nonorganic mental illness (depression, anxiety, and personality disorders); a further 32% had only an organic disorder; and 33% had no mental disorder. Only a very small proportion of elderly people with a mental disorder were actually receiving mental health treatment at the time of the 1985 National Nursing Home Survey (Burns et al. 1993). Smith and Jensen (1990) pointed out that OBRA 87 seeks to divert patients with mental illness to other sites with better access to appropriate treatment. Under OBRA 87 regulations, 18% of residents might have to be discharged; 31% of these patients are estimated to have disabling symptoms of depression, anxiety, or worry, and 40% require some mental health treatment. Nevertheless, Eichmann et al. (1992) noted that those who would remain in nursing homes after OBRA 87 might still include about one-third who could have a diagnosis mandated to receive mental health care. Nonorganic disorders might become less common among residents, but given the high rates of depression and anxiety among those eligible for residency by virtue of dependencies (three or more ADL impairments), the frequency of behaviors such as aggression and screaming, and the requirements to increase active mental health treatment where needed, nursing homes might have to deliver more intensive mental health care than at present.

OBRA 87 was implemented in 1990 and has led to several responsive initiatives. For example, Ray et al. (1993) addressed the requirement for reduction of unnecessary use of antipsychotic drugs, previously reported to be administered to about one-fifth of nursing home residents, mostly for control of the disturbing behaviors of dementia. Through education of staff in the use of behavioral techniques, the number of days on which antipsychotic medications were given to the residents was reduced by 72%, whereas days of application of physical restraints were also decreased; behavioral problems did not increase in frequency as antipsychotic medication was withdrawn.

Medical services.   Some psychiatric problems of elderly patients are encountered more frequently in medical than in psychiatric settings. In ambulatory medical settings, anxiety and depressive disorders are common, especially atypical rather than major depressions (Sireling et al. 1985) and depressions accompanying acute and chronic medical disorders (Kukull et al. 1986; O'Riordan et al. 1989). Depression as a nosological entity, and as a symptom syndrome not meeting diagnostic criteria, is the most frequently encountered psychiatric condition in primary medical care (Blacker and Clare 1988; Coulehan et al. 1990a; Katon et al. 1990). Katon and Schulberg (1992) concluded in their review of studies that major depression occurs in about 5%–10% of primary care patients. Reported rates will vary depending on the level of severity that is required for a symptom syndrome to fulfill the criteria for diagnosis (Blacker and Clare 1987), with subcase-level syndromes being more common (Katon and Schulberg 1992). An admixture of anxiety symptoms of varying degree of prominence is common (Goldberg et al. 1987).

Depression of all types, including clinically significant depression, is increased in the presence of a wide variety of functional impairments (Katon et al. 1993; Turner and McLean 1989; Turner and Noh 1988) and physical illnesses (Turner and Wood 1985; Wells et al. 1993) and tends to improve as physical status improves (von Korff et al. 1990). The causal direction is uncertain and has been argued both ways (Wells et al. 1992).

Haley et al. (1985) noted gender differences in response to disability and physical illness, with depression being a reaction to pain in women and to functional impairment in men. Depression rates decline with age despite the association with physical illness and disability (Turner and Wood 1985). Depression is also associated with the accumulation of life events and constant strain and is moderated by higher levels of mastery and social support (Turner and Noh 1988).

Patients in primary medical care, judged by research evaluation to be suitable for a trial of antidepressants, nonetheless often go untreated (Katon et al. 1992). Depression as a syndrome or diagnosable disorder is often chronic, although potentially responsive to antidepressants, in medical settings (Katon and Schulberg 1992; Katon and Sullivan 1990). Detection rates may improve as a result of the National Institute of Mental Health's efforts, intensified in 1988, to raise awareness of practitioners and patients about the opportunities to effectively treat depressive disorders (Regier et al. 1988). Because of the frequency of depression in medical settings and the close association of suicide, suicide risk can and should be assessed in medical settings (Goldberg 1987).

Depression may amplify (i.e., increase the severity, awareness, and reporting of) the symptoms of physical illness (Barsky et al. 1988). Somatic symptoms could potentially confound the diagnosis of major depression, especially if the patient emphasizes the somatic rather than the mood symptoms of depression or complains principally about the symptoms of an accompanying physical illness (Katon 1987). In these circumstances, information from screening instruments has been shown to increase recognition and treatment of depression by the primary care physician (Magruder-Habib et al. 1990). However, Coulehan et al. (1988) did not find this diagnosis in a primary medical care setting to be accompanied by an excess loading of somatic symptoms. Somatization disorder occurs in approximately 5% to 10% of primary care patients (Katon and Russo 1989) and is frequently accompanied by a depressive disorder. Multiplicity of pains raises the likelihood that a depressive disorder is present (Dworkin et al. 1990). Finch et al. (1992) found that 10% of patients admitted to an acute geriatric care unit had a depressive illness and a further 30% had some milder but clinically significant symptoms.

As reviewed by Liberto et al. (1992), rates of excess alcohol consumption and associated problems in various hospital and outpatient medical settings for samples of patients ages 60 years or over range from 5% (in a primary medical care setting) to 44% (in some more psychiatrically oriented units). In as many as one-third of elderly patients ill enough to be admitted to an acute psychiatric ward, alcohol abuse had gone previously undetected by medical staff (Mears and Spice 1993).

Delirium (confusional state), which is often caused by factors surrounding medical illness, is common in acute medical settings, occurring in more than 25% of general medical inpatients (Knight and Folstein 1977; McCartney and Palmateer 1985) and rehabilitation inpatients (Garcia et al. 1984) It occurs even more commonly in neurology service populations (DePaulo and Folstein 1978). Symptoms of delirium may be mistaken for dementia but are distinguishable, and the underlying condition is usually treatable.

Demographic Groups

Age. Rates of dementia rise steeply with age (Folstein et al. 1991) and reach more than 20% in those patients over age 80. The prevalence of Alzheimer's disease and other dementias increases even through the most advanced ages (Fratiglioni et al. 1991). Incidence varies from less than 1% annually at age 70 to about 4% annually at age 85. Although the prevalence rate of dementia reaches beyond 20% over age 80, the extent to which this scourge threatens the average person is better conveyed by the lifetime risk: about one in three for men who survive to age 85 years (Sluss et al. 1981) and probably in the same range for women. As an exception to the rule, among persons ages 65 years or older in a rural community of Korea, the prevalence of mild impairment did not increase prominently with aging (Park and Ha 1988).

Apart from cognitive impairment, the prevalence of most psychiatric disorders remains flat or decreases as people age (Bland et al. 1988; Kramer et al. 1985; Weissman et al. 1985). Depression (at least major depression such as dysthymia) appears to plateau after age 65 years or, arguably, decreases with further aging (Comstock and Helsing 1976; Dewey et al. 1993; Eaton and Kessler 1981; Frerichs et al. 1981; Gurland 1976; Myers et al. 1984; Robins et al. 1984). However, Palinkas et al. (1990) report that rates of depression may rise with age. Manic states occur less commonly with advancing age and are often found—even in first episodes—to be associated with central nervous system lesions in this age group. The incidence of phobic disorders does not drop off much with age, at least in men; obsessive-compulsive disorder may increase in older women (Eaton et al. 1991).

Depression in older age groups has possibly been undercounted in surveys because of the confounds of physical comorbidity and age-specific presentation of symptoms. There have been calls for revision of criteria for the diagnosis of depression in the older person, especially with supervening physical illness (Rosen et al. 1987). There may be poor agreement between different definitions of endogenous depression applied to elderly patients (Gallagher-Thompson et al. 1992). These doubts about survey diagnosis reflect on the usefulness of survey information, such as the ECA data on age and rates of depression. The reported rates of affective disorders in older age groups do not tally with previous prevalence studies, and the confounds of physical illness may have been inadequately discounted (Snowdon 1990).

The claims that rates of major and other types of depression do not rise with advancing age, if accepted, might imply that older persons are able to cope well with physical illness and other age-related insults. Some studies have suggested that elderly people are less prone to blame themselves regarding their disability (Felton and Revenson 1987) and more likely to receive calmly the reality or possibility of life-threatening illness such as cancer (F. Cohen 1980; Mages and Mendelsohn 1979). Older adults may be viewed as a band of survivors who have learned to cope with adverse circumstances, perhaps because certain negative events are sufficiently common at this age to acquire a normative value (they are "on time") (Neugarten and Datan 1973). Events such as physical illness tend to be more chronic than acute and perhaps are less stressful for that reason (Kennedy et al. 1990) as age increases. On the other hand, individuals with earlier onset depression may be vulnerable to premature death or institutionalization and hence might not enter the cohort of elderly people residing within the community, or—a more optimistic view—they might receive treatment that prevents new episodes from occurring in later life. Perhaps, neurobiological changes with age make the older person less vulnerable to depression with or without a stressor such as a disability. It has been suggested, with reservations about the evidence, that successive cohorts of elderly people have shown progressively higher rates of depression and an earlier age of onset (Klerman et al. 1985).

Suicide rates increase with age in white men, rising to 0.06% in the very old (age 75 years and older) (National Center for Health Statistics 1987). This high rate of suicide stands in apparent contradiction to the notion of a flat age variation curve of depression (Cross and Gurland 1984), perhaps as a result of other characteristics of the cohort. Another cohort effect is possibly emerging as the oldest age groups grow in size, probably a reflection of the general tendency for the largest age groups in a population to be most at risk for suicide (see Lindesay 1991b). Suicides in the United States among elderly men increased between 1974 and 1987, and in general, suicide rates for elderly people, those age 75 years or older, were among the worst in the Western world (Pritchard 1992). Whether these historic changes are affected by socioeconomic forces is the subject of controversy (Lester 1993). Rates are higher among elderly white men than among women or black men. Risk of suicide peaks in women at about the time of menopause (Woodbury et al. 1988). Studies in both the United Kingdom (Hawton and Fagg 1990) and the United States (Pierce 1987) have shown that adults ages 65 years or older constitute approximately 4% to 6% of people who have attempted suicide and have been referred for treatment. With advancing age, prevalence of attempted suicide appears to decrease, but completed suicides increase (Hawton and Fagg 1990).

Distinctions between predictors of suicide attempts and completions are not marked in elderly people. Older adults attempting suicide are at high risk for a later completed suicide (Merrill and Owens 1990). The vast majority of people who have completed suicides had a preceding psychiatric condition, usually major depression with a late onset, often the first episode (Conwell et al. 1991; Draper 1994; Pierce 1987). In addition to the effects of depressive disorders, risk of suicide attempts and completions is accentuated in older adults who are divorced, alcoholic (Draper 1994; Hawton and Fagg 1990), recently bereaved, have a sense of loneliness and isolation (Vogel and Wolfersdorf 1989), or are seriously physically ill (Conwell et al. 1990; Nowers 1993), particularly if the illness is painful (Pierce 1987). Lifelong traits, such as incapacity for intimacy, feelings of helplessness, or intolerance for change, may heighten vulnerability (Lindesay 1991b). Access to means of suicide is important; in the United Kingdom between 1976 and 1987, there was a decline in the use of barbiturates and a substitution by non-opiate analgesics (Hawton and Fagg 1990).

It is widely accepted that schizophrenia and conditions related to schizophrenia, such as paranoid disorder or paraphrenia, may occur for the first time in late adulthood (45–64 years of age) or old age (Jeste 1993; Rabins et al. 1984; Volavka and Cancro 1986). As many as 20% of patients with schizophrenia have a late onset of symptoms, after mid-life (44 years) and even in older age groups. Early- and late-onset types of schizophrenia are similar in clinical presentation and outcome (Harris and Jeste 1988). Late-onset types have been reported to have a higher frequency of distinctive brain abnormalities on neuroimaging (e.g., high mean ventricle-to-brain ratio relative to healthy controls), neuropsychological deficits, and a higher female-to-male ratio than in younger schizophrenic patient groups (Rabins et al. 1987). However, using findings on the prevalence of awareness of the involuntary movements of tardive dyskinesia and addiction to tobacco as indicators of the integrity of specific brain structures, Sandyk and Awerbuch (1993) proposed that patients with late-onset schizophrenia have less damage to the dopaminergic and serotonergic neurons than patients with early-onset schizophrenia. These investigators infer from their findings that later onset would be less likely to induce a defect state and the consequent unfavorable prognosis. When symptoms result from a late-onset type of schizophrenia, a paranoid picture may predominate (Larson and Nyman 1970). The symptoms found in aging patients with schizophrenia, whose conditions began in earlier life, tend to become less vivid and disturbing to the patient and others as age advances (e.g., fewer positive symptoms). Eaton et al. (1992) support the view that schizophrenia follows a course of progressive amelioration over time, resulting in increasing intervals before rehospitalization. Possible explanations (see Soni and Mallik 1993) for the more favorable course of the late-onset types of schizophrenia range from changes in administrative practice to improved patient compliance with medications, early recognition of impending relapse, better family relationships, biological changes with age, improved adaptation and coping, fewer dopamine receptors (Andreasen et al. 1988), and diminished metabolic degradation of psychotropic drugs.

Grief and Eastwood (1993) found that psychiatric diagnoses on elderly patients in various hospital settings rarely invoked a category featuring paranoid labels, although the hospital records indicated that a high proportion of patients had paranoid symptoms. The investigators criticized current nosology as taking a haphazard approach to paranoid diagnoses. The term *paranoia* has had a long history of use in representing the clinical picture of well-organized delusional states with an onset late in life and without evident hallucinations or deterioration of thought processes, affect, or personality; *late paraphrenia* refers to a similar syndrome but with hallucinations (see Flint et al. 1991). For the past four decades, paraphrenia has been taken to refer to late-onset schizophrenia (Roth 1955). Current practice is to class these conditions under late-onset schizophrenia (DSM-IV) or, in the *International Classification of Diseases,* 10th revision (WHO 1991), under paranoid schizophrenia or persistent delusional disorder. This trend has been questioned by Almeida et al. (1992), who point to the frequency of organic factors and distinctive neuroimaging patterns in late-onset types of schizophrenia. Flint et al. (1991) also advocate the distinction between paranoia and paraphrenia on the grounds that the former was found in their series of elderly patients to have strikingly more clinically silent neurological disorders, especially cerebral infarction in the subcortical or frontal lobes, and to be less responsive to treatment. Lifelong isolation was characteristic of patients from either group who did not have evidence of infarction.

The majority of individuals with schizophrenia will achieve old age even though they have a higher death rate than the general population (Allebeck and Wistedt 1986). Most will be left with impaired functioning, including about one-third of the cohort who will have chronic or relapsing symptoms. However, about one-third of the survivors to old age will have recovered virtually completely (Ciompi 1985).

Overall frequency of excess alcohol consumption and associated problems diminishes with age (Atkinson 1994; Eaton et al. 1991; Holzer et al. 1984); almost one-half of persons over age 55 years have been found to be abstainers, around twice the rate of younger adults (Caracci and Miller 1991). Incidence also decreases with age (Eaton et al. 1989). Nevertheless, new cases do continue to occur; up to one-half of elderly patients with problem drinking have an onset in middle or late life (Atkinson 1994; Liberto et al. 1992). Alcohol abuse may increase again in very old men (Eaton et al. 1991). Cohort effects are probably the main determinants of age variation in alcohol consumption and associated problems (Glynn et al. 1985). Evidence contradicts the notion that late-onset alcoholism stems from an underlying associated psychiatric disorder more often than is the case for early-onset alcoholism (Atkinson et al. 1990; Schonfeld and Dupree 1991), although bereavement may tend to precede admission for elderly patients with problem drinking (Mears and Spice 1993). The course and outcome of alcoholism are somewhat better for late- than for early-onset alcoholism, with milder symptoms and more frequent spontaneous recovery (Atkinson 1994; Moos et al. 1991; Penn et al. 1989). Schonfeld and Dupree (1991) found that patients with late-onset cases of alcoholism, matched for age with patients with early-onset cases, were less frequently intoxicated, less likely to have delirium tremens or severe inner shakes, and more often complied with treatment. Fitzgerald and Mulford (1992) similarly noted that among drivers arrested for drinking, elderly people were more likely to complete treatment successfully. Yet, investigators caution, alcoholic problems may be responsible in elderly patients for falls, amnesia, incontinence, and injuries from accidents in the home (Mears and Spice 1993). Well-publicized reports of the protective action by light or moderate drinking against coronary artery disease might encourage more older adults to begin drinking; a critical and highly reserved review of the body of evidence supporting the alleged protective action was provided by Shaper (1990).

Age and comorbidity. Comorbidity would be a feature of psychiatric disorders in old age even if there were no causal relationship involved. The increase of concurrent physical and mental problems, beyond chance, with respect to depression and acute or chronic physical disorder is mentioned later. This increase occurs for other psychiatric disorders, such as manic states, as well.

The effect of age itself must be separated from that of accompanying difficulties such as changes in health and social support (Cappeliez 1988). Psychiatric problems in elderly patients occur in the context of physical, mental, and social aging. Among the population ages 65 years and older, a majority have at least one chronic physical disorder, but a minority are impaired in mobility or capacity to carry out the daily tasks of independent living (e.g., self-care and household chores) (Verbrugge 1990). Only about 5% of all older adults need to live in highly sheltered residences such as nursing homes, although this percentage increases sharply over the age of 80. There are changes in the speed and style of intellectual activities and slowing of the rate of new learning, but the great majority of older adults remain mentally active and competent. Those are the normal standards against which the causes, presentation, and consequences of psychiatric disorders at older ages are evaluated. Aging adds distinctive characteristics not only to the nature, presentation, and treatment of psychiatric problems, but also to the social milieu, a vital aspect of treatment. One-third of older adults live alone, but most have someone, usually a daughter or daughter-in-law, who assists in the support and management of treatment (Albert and Cattell 1994).

An important type of concurrence in older age is that of depression and intellectual impairment. In general, depressive disorders in the elderly patient, such as major depressions, are quite distinct in nature and natural history from the dementias such as Alzheimer's disease. Yet, depression and dementia syndromes are found to occur together even when diagnoses are carefully established. Setting aside those DSM-IV exclusionary criteria that bear on the presence of an organic etiology, major depression is found in cases of Alzheimer's disease and related dementias at high rates: up to 30% in some series (Larson et al. 1985). In these mixed conditions, the cognitive impairment component usually follows a progressively deteriorating course despite improvement in depression in response to treatment (McAllister and Price 1982; Rabins 1985). Pioneering studies (Kay 1962; Post 1972) found no increased risk of dementia in patients with late-onset depression; however, in about 10% of major depressions, a syndrome resembling dementia was noted to arise and be resolved when the depression remitted (Madden et al. 1952; Post 1975). This syndrome was termed *depressive pseudodementia* by some investigators, but it now falls under the wider rubric of treatable or reversible dementias. In the short term, depressions that are apparently primary in terms of their responsiveness to pharmacological interventions account for about 5% of cases referred for investigation of dementia and 20% of treatable dementia syndromes (Larson et al. 1985; Rabins 1985). It is now recognized that a proportion of cases of mixed depression and cognitive impairment do take a course of cognitive deterioration. The proportion ranges from a minority of about 20% (Rabins et al. 1984) to about one-half (Reding et al. 1985), or even a large majority if follow-up is long enough (Kral 1983). Reding et al. (1985) demonstrated that 57% (16 of 28) of older patients who had been referred to a dementia service, but who were found to have depression rather than dementia, nevertheless went on to develop frank dementia. Some investigators (e.g., Jacoby et al. 1980; 1983) have found brain changes (enlarged ventricles and reduced radiodensity) in patients with late-onset depression that do not occur in age-matched patients with early-onset depression. However, the changes do not include the pathology typical of Alzheimer's disease or multi-infarct dementias (Tomlinson et al. 1968). A conservative position to take is that the prognosis of depression is more guarded if cognitive impairment is concurrent.

Gender.   High rates of depression in older women have been widely reported (Palinkas et al. 1990). Computerized diagnosis (AGECAT) on elderly people residing in communities in New York and London showed rates for depression higher in women at all levels of diagnostic confidence except one (Copeland et al. 1987). Elderly people residing in communities in Liverpool and Zaragoza, Spain, had prevalence rates of depressive symptoms around 14% for women and 6% to 7% for men (Dewey et al. 1993).

Excessive use of alcohol in older age is greater in men than in women (Liberto et al. 1992). With education controlled, gender has been found to be significantly associated with prevalence of cognitive disorders (Yu et al. 1989). Folstein et al. (1991) found higher rates of Alzheimer's disease in women and of multi-infarct dementia in men. In community residents of Beijing, prevalence rates of moderate and severe dementia were higher in women (Li et al. 1989). Among elderly people in a rural community of Korea, prevalence rates of cognitive impairment (based on the Mini-Mental State Exam) were significantly higher in women (64%) than in men (33%)

(Park and Ha 1988). Women are not only purportedly more prone to develop dementia, but also to survive to extreme old age where the risk of developing dementia is highest.

Sociocultural factors.   Epidemiological data suggest higher rates of depression and dementia in certain socioeconomically disadvantaged older groups (Blazer et al. 1987; George et al. 1991). However, at present this finding must be taken to refer to depressive symptoms and poor performance on measures of cognitive performance; the implications for diagnosis and the need for treatment are not clear.

Ethnoracial differences in rates of psychiatric disorders of older age have also been noted, although the extent to which these are confounded by other social and economic factors is not clear. Caregivers of people with dementia were found to be more likely to have symptoms of depression if they were non-Hispanic whites than if they were black (Mintzer and Macera 1992). Rates of dementia, particularly of the Alzheimer's disease type, are reported as being relatively low in certain Asian groups. Among first-degree relatives of older adults without dementia, Jewish and Italian groups had a greater risk of progressive primary dementia than Chinese or Puerto Rican groups (Silverman et al. 1992). In community residents of Beijing, prevalence rates of moderate and severe dementia were 1.28% for ages 60–64 years and 1.82% for ages 65 years and over. Kua (1991) compared a survey in Singapore with a previous survey in Beijing and found that prevalence of dementia at ages 80–84 years in Singapore was 4.8%; in Beijing, 8.8%. In those persons over age 89 years, the Singapore rate was 12%; the Beijing rate, 16.7%. These rates for Asian groups are relatively low compared with survey results from the United States and the United Kingdom. The prevalence of multi-infarct dementia was higher than primary degenerative dementia in elderly Beijing residents (Li et al. 1989), and the 3-year incidence of multi-infarct dementia was higher than for primary degenerative dementia (Li et al. 1991), a reversal of the corresponding ratios for the United States and the United Kingdom. However, in probability samples of Chinese and Finnish adults, ages 65–74 years, mean scores on translated versions of the Mini-Mental State Exam were similar (Salmon et al. 1989). Elderly people, ages 65 and older, residing in a community in Japan had prevalence and incidence rates of dementia of 4.1% and 1.0%, respectively (Fukunishi et al. 1991).

The prevalence of dementia and the proportion of vascular dementias among community residents ages 65 years and older, as determined through diagnosis by a neurologist, was found to be higher in blacks than in whites (Heyman et al. 1991). In addition, a history of heart attacks, high blood pressure, diabetes, and stroke was reported more often by blacks than by whites in both patients with dementias and patients without dementias. Rates of dementia were also reported as higher in non-whites by Folstein et al. (1991). However, autopsy studies of hospitalized patients with histological Alzheimer's disease found rates 2.6 times higher among whites than blacks (de la Monte et al. 1989). In the latter study, dementia caused by Parkinson's disease was more frequent among whites, and dementia caused by multi-infarct and chronic alcohol abuse was higher among blacks. In neurologically normal controls, ages 60 and older, histological lesions of Alzheimer's disease were observed more frequently in whites than blacks.

Education.   Less education and a history of consistent unemployment appear to be associated with higher risk for developing dementia (Li et al. 1991). Rates of Alzheimer's disease have been found to be relatively greater in higher educated groups, and rates of multi-infarct dementia have been found to be greater in lower educated groups (Folstein et al. 1991). In contrast, prevalence of Alzheimer's disease and vascular dementia have been reported as not associated with gender or lower education, although lower educated groups did have increased rates of alcoholic dementia and unspecified types of dementia (Fratiglioni et al. 1991). A question about the interpretation of these results is raised by the possible effect of education on tests of cognitive status. In probability samples of Chinese and Finnish adults, ages 65–74 years, mean scores on translated versions of the Mini-Mental State Exam were noted to be confounded by education: approximately one-fourth of the Chinese subjects had no formal education. Moreover, cultural differences occurred on some individual test items even after controlling for education (Salmon et al. 1989). In studies of elderly people in Beijing (Li et al. 1989) and Shanghai communities (Murden et al. 1991), education was inversely related to Mini-Mental State Exam scores. Results were affected by education but not by race, although only certain test items were educationally related. Education-specific norms for cut scores have been proposed for middle school, high school, and college graduates (Uhlmann et al. 1991). Nevertheless, in the United Kingdom, among those with border zone or severely impaired cognitive scores, neither education nor social class influenced probability of diagnosis of dementia (O'Connor et al. 1991b).

Other Risk Factors

Depression. Life events have been observed to influence the outcome of depression in elderly patients (Murphy 1983). Elderly people, ages 65 and older, studied in the New Haven ECA survey (Oxman et al. 1992) were reinterviewed 3 years later to identify predictors of depression; baseline depression, loss of a spouse, and functional disability and its change were predictive. Also predictive were adequacy of emotional support and, at a lesser level, tangible support (help with tasks), confidants, visits from children, and changes in these factors. Green et al. (1992) based a 3-year follow-up on general practitioner lists and the incidence of depression as calculated from an AGECAT classification (i.e., depressive psychosis and neurosis together; more or less equivalent to DSM-III major depression and dysthymia). Depression was predicted principally by ratings of lack of satisfaction with life, loneliness, smoking, female gender, and bereavement within the previous 6 months; increasing age was not predictive.

The outcome of depression is also altered by the size, functioning, and perceived helpfulness and warmth of the patient's social network; the quality of social exchanges is more salient than the mere quantity of social interactions (George et al. 1989). Infrequency and other deficits in the extent and closeness of the person's social contacts, the expectation of help from that network, and the paucity of club or religious membership correlate with a higher risk of depression (Norris and Murrell 1990; Russell and Cutrona 1991; Stallones et al. 1990). It may be that stress precipitates depression, and ill health in general, in the presence of weak social supports. This weakness results in the older person placing greater demands on health services (Counte and Glandon 1991). The effect of social patterns on depression may work through the sense of control persons have over their lives, on the perception of being supported, and the nature of problem-solving communication at times of crisis (Ross and Mirowsky 1989) or through preventive actions (Russell and Cutrona 1991).

Alternatively, ineffective help from others, and failures in giving encouragement and assistance where and when needed, may expose the older person not only to the more immediate effects of stress but also to the depressing influence of sustained daily hassles over a long period of time (Russell and Cutrona 1991). Persons without a significant other with whom they can share their thoughts and feelings and from whom they can gather encouragement and comfort appear to be particularly vulnerable.

Bereavement. There is a strong clinical impression and research evidence (Blazer et al. 1987; Murphy 1982) that negative life events such as bereavement often (some say usually) precipitate episodes of depression. Depressive episodes and dysphoria are both increased by bereavement (B. M. Livingston et al. 1990).

In inner-city United Kingdom community residents, ages 60 years and older (G. Livingston et al. 1990), depression was associated with being widowed or single. For older persons, death of a spouse is more depressing than death of a parent or child (Norris and Murrell 1990). Elevated levels of depression have been found in widows preceding, and for up to 2 years following, bereavement (Harlow et al. 1991a, 1991b); only 10% of married women were high scorers on depression rating scales. A majority of widows (58%) had high scores on depression rating scales soon after bereavement, but most of the high scorers returned to prebereavement levels at 12 months. Symptoms of self-limiting grief are hard to distinguish from diagnostic symptoms of depression in the first 3 months after a loss (Zisook and Schuchter 1991; 1992). According to B. M. Livingston et al. (1990), about one in three bereaved persons with depression could meet criteria for major depression, although feelings of guilt and worthlessness are much less prominent than in nonbereaved persons with depression. Small social networks (e.g., fewer children in contact, living alone, and not being an active member of clubs or religious circles) and small size of the friendship network increased vulnerability to depression. However, friends had a long-term influence on depression (adjustment to single living), whereas families seemed to be a bigger help soon after bereavement (by providing emotional support). Yet, overall, health was a more powerful influence than social factors. Depression several months before bereavement predicted postbereavement depression and identified caregivers who might benefit from early intervention (Harlow et al. 1991a, 1991b).

Physical illness. Affective and anxiety disorders are associated with both acute and chronic limitations of physical functioning (Wells et al. 1988). The correlation of depression in older persons with physical illness or disability is especially striking (Kemp et al. 1987; Revenson and Felton 1985; Turner and Noh 1988). Increasing disability and deterioration in health are stronger predictors of depression than number of medical conditions, social support, and stress (Kennedy et al. 1990). This association holds true not only for the symptoms and syndromes of depression, but also for depression diagnoses such as major depression (Hall et al. 1980; Kinzie et al. 1986); risk for depression in the physically ill older patient is increased up to threefold. With some exceptions, the links between physical illness and depression are general and multiple rather than specific (Borson et al. 1986; Kukull et al. 1986). Nevertheless, there are convincing correlations between depression and particular medical conditions; the latter differ between the genders in some respects (Palinkas et al. 1990). Notable examples of depressogenic medical conditions are stroke, particularly left hemisphere lesions (Robinson et al. 1984), Parkinson's disease, cancer, and endocrine disorders (Finch et al. 1992). The potential for reciprocal influences between depression and physical illness could operate through the personal meanings of lost health and functioning, noncompliance with treatment, stress imposed by symptoms, increased vulnerability to physical illness through suppression of immune processes, cognitive impairment, concurrent aging effects on physical illness and neurotransmitter levels controlling mood, consequences of constricted lives and erosion of independence, increased sensitivity in reporting physical symptoms, degree of acuity and chronicity of the course of the physical condition, and side effects of medications. More than one-third of major depressions found in one community study were associated with medication use (Kinzie et al. 1986). Lists of particularly depressogenic drugs and diseases have been known for some time (Ouslander 1982) and point to the need to avoid nonessential medications.

Other life events. In a community study that included older adults with disabilities, it was found that cumulative life events and chronic strain had independent effects on depression (Turner and Noh 1988). Caregivers of persons with dementia, especially those who seek help, are prone to develop clinically diagnosable depression (Gallagher et al. 1989). Nevertheless, older subjects may have a more constricted set of salient life events than younger persons (Turner and Wood 1985).

Anxiety disorders. Agoraphobia in elderly people is commonly of late onset, is often precipitated by comorbid physical illness or other traumatic incident, and is characterized by moderate to severe social impairments; specific fears are more often of early onset and are less disabling (Lindesay 1991a). Relationships between phobic disorder and physical illness might arise from anxiety occasioned by the stress of physical illness; by virtue of the depressive effects of physical illness; through specific pathways associated with, for example, cardiovascular disorder, respiratory illness, or inner ear dysfunction; and through common roots in social class deprivations (Lindesay 1991a). It has also been suggested, although not replicated, that benzodiazepines might prolong phobic symptoms (S. I. Cohen 1992).

Paranoid states.   Most studies show that an abnormal personality (cold and querulous) and an unfavorable social milieu are a long prelude to the emergence of frank paranoid symptoms in old age (Christenson and Blazer 1989; Kay et al. 1976; Post 1966). Prior social isolation is common; the sufferers are often unmarried or have few children, although they usually manage an independent existence fairly well (Eisdorfer 1980).

Deafness also appears to be a predisposing influence for late-onset paranoid states (Cooper et al. 1976). The data are consistent across long-stay and recently admitted psychiatric patients and elderly people residing in a community. Deafness is more frequent, about threefold, in older persons with a late-onset paranoid disorder than in age-matched controls or patients with affective disorder. Hearing impairment is of a level that affects receptive communication in social situations and is quite severe on audiometric testing. Most intriguing is that the deafness is the conductive type associated with the sequelae of middle ear disease, not the type induced by aging processes. By its nature and by report, the deafness seems to begin many years before the onset of paranoid symptoms, although not prior to the stage of language acquisition. Deafness appears to predispose patients to paranoid disorder, even those without the typical vulnerable personality. The majority of studies are in line with these conclusions (Eastwood et al. 1985).

Cautions About Classification

Epidemiological data may reflect diverse methods of collection and case ascertainment (i.e., variations in wording of questionnaires, training of interviewers, use of an informant history, and the use of diagnostic hierarchies). There is often a lack of agreement among screens and diagnostic instruments for assessing depression, dementia, and other psychiatric disorders in elderly patients. Gender, education, and social class influence scores on tests of cognition (Burvill 1990). In an Australian survey of persons ages 70 years and older, diagnoses made by a psychiatrist, DSM-III criteria, and algorithms for clinically significant syndromes of depression and dementia were compared, with the conclusion that more precision and uniformity were needed (Kay et al. 1985). Computerized diagnoses (e.g., AGECAT) can be set to obtain consistent borderline and subcase designation of depression and dementia (Copeland et al. 1990). However, when a comparison of five operational methods for diagnosis of mild dementia among elderly patients, ages 75 years and older, was conducted in terms of agreements, prediction of cognitive deterioration over 3 years, and rejection of the influence of "nondementia" factors, the results were disappointing. Furthermore, the predictive value of a cutpoint on a brief cognitive scale was just as good as the more elaborate algorithms for diagnosis (Rosenman 1989). In a follow-up study of community residents with minimal dementia (cognitive impairment insufficient for a diagnosis of dementia proper), only 6 of 29 survivors after 1 year showed progressive intellectual deterioration, and 13 were reclassified as normal (O'Connor et al. 1990); after 2 years the initial test results had not predicted who declined (O'Connor et al. 1991a). Furthermore, only two of seven memory test items in the CAMDEX discriminated between adults with depression and older adults without depression (O'Connor et al. 1990). In a study of a representative sample of elderly people, ages 70 years and older, residing in a community, 25% of persons had mild dementia by one or more criteria; prevalence rates for mild dementia varied widely according to the criteria used (Mowry and Burvill 1988). As reviewed by Liberto et al. (1992), the validity of self-reported data on alcohol abuse and dependency also must be viewed with caution.

Because of the uncertainty occasioned by inconsistencies in the techniques of epidemiology, and by the limits on generalizing from one population and era to another, discretion must govern the interpretation of the findings reviewed here. With that discretion, these findings carry relevant messages for clinical practice, public health responses, and research directions.

Conclusion: Service Actions Suggested by Epidemiology

Epidemiological perspectives highlight the need for specially skilled professionals to care for elderly patients with psychiatric problems. Treatable problems are frequently encountered in the older population in the community and in the spectrum of clinical and residential settings. Age-relevant epidemiological understanding is required for diagnosis, evaluation of causes, administration of treatment, and longer term management. The epidemiological perspective can guide the acts of scouting for opportunities to reduce the risk of onset, persistence, and relapse of psychiatric problems. The discovery of precursors of a condition can suggest opportunities for preventive interventions.

The complex set of relations connecting depression and physical illness opens up several evident opportunities for intervention in gaining compliance, minimizing medication effects, enhancing motivation, strengthening physiological and physical functioning, and improving quality of life. Coexistent depression slows recovery from physical illness. Epidemiological data show that depression impedes recovery of function in medical conditions such as ischemic heart disease (Morgan 1983), stroke (Feibel and Springer 1982), and disability from a variety of causes (Gurland et al. 1988). Whether treating the physical illness may be a means of secondarily preventing the prolongation of the depression remains speculative.

Older persons with psychiatric problems do seek help but not necessarily appropriately or from psychiatrists. Lifetime prevalence of major depression and dysthymia, and subclinical depressive symptoms (not meeting diagnostic criteria, but having two or more of the eight symptoms of major depression), in the ECA-combined five communities, was associated with increased use of psychoactive medications (tranquilizers, hypnotics, or antidepressants) and treatment for emotional problems in medical and emergency department settings (Johnson et al. 1992). Depressive symptoms accounted for a greater proportion of this service use than did the diagnostic categories. Psychotropic medications, such as sedatives and hypnotics, are actively dispensed to the older patient by primary care physicians who are often the sole providers of professional care for patients with mental health problems (Ware 1986). Depending on the type of service, the likelihood of contact may be higher or lower for individuals with depressive symptoms than for those with diagnosable depression, but the size of the former group overshadows the latter and accounts for the disproportion in aggregate use of services (A. Mann, personal communication, 1993).

In a review by Finch et al. 1992, depression was mentioned as the first- or second-most frequent diagnosis among older patients referred to a psychiatrist. However, in general, the detection rate is low and implementation of treatment is still lower, possibly because of beliefs about the medical contraindications to antidepressants. There are reports that medical residents often lack adequate knowledge of the recognition and treatment of comorbid depression in physical illness (Rapp and Davis 1989). Elderly patients are less likely than younger patients to be evaluated and treated by a mental health specialist, even when there is contact with a health care center where specialist referrals are available and where the prevalence of psychiatric problems warranting conventional diagnosis is not decreased by age (Goldstrom et al. 1987).

If personal characteristics are prodromal signs of an eventual psychotic disorder, they may offer a means of intervention for high-risk groups. Long-range possibilities for prevention of some late-onset paranoid states are raised by epidemiological findings. The role of deafness, as a predisposing influence on late-onset paranoid states, is an epidemiological finding (Cooper et al. 1976) that has tantalized investigators seeking to turn it to a useful clinical purpose. That depression several months prior to bereavement can predict postbereavement status could be applied to selecting vulnerable caregivers for early intervention.

Although the dementias are, for the most part, not yet proven to be amenable to preventive strategies, consideration of the relative rates of the dementia subtypes and of conditions that can mimic dementia keep the issue of prevention open. In the future, new treatments may make early detection of dementia a therapeutic necessity. The figures presented on reversible dementias argue for vigilance in considering the possibility of a treatable cause in all new cases of dementia.

The compelling importance of the field of geriatric psychiatry stems not only from the growing number and proportion of elderly patients (especially the very old—over age 80 years), but equally from gains in longevity and active life expectancy. This change in the life span means that old age occupies a larger proportion (currently about 25%) of the average life. Consequently, the quality of life in old age and the influence of psychiatric problems on that quality are growing in relevance to the whole of a person's life. Prevention and treatment of psychiatric disorders can help older adults to fully enjoy their added years.

References

Albert SM, Cattell MG: Old Age in Global Perspective. New York, G. K. Hall, 1994, p 87

Allebeck P, Wistedt B: Mortality in schizophrenia. Arch Gen Psychiatry 43:650–653, 1986

Almeida OP, Howard R, Forstl H, et al: Late paraphrenia: a review. International Journal of Geriatric Psychiatry 7:543–548, 1992

American Psychiatric Association: Diagnostic and Statistical Manual of Mental Disorders, Fourth Edition. Washington, DC, American Psychiatric Association, 1994

Andreasen NC, Carson R, Diksic M, et al: Workshop on schizophrenia, PET and dopamine D_2 receptors in the human neostriatum. Schizophr

    Bull 14:471–481, 1988

Atkinson RM: Late onset problem drinking in older adults. International
    Journal of Geriatric Psychiatry 9:321–326, 1994

Atkinson RM, Tolson RL, Turner JA: Late versus early onset problem drink-
    ing in older men. Alcohol Clin Exp Res 14:574–579, 1990

Barsky AJ, Goodson JD, Lane RS, et al: The amplification of somatic symp-
    toms. Psychosom Med 50:510–519, 1988

Blacker CV, Clare AW: Depressive disorder in primary care. Br J Psychia-
    try 150:737–751, 1987

Blacker CV, Clare AW: The prevalence and treatment of depression in gen-
    eral practice. Psychopharmacology 95:S14–S17, 1988

Bland RC, Newman SC, Om H: Prevalence of psychiatric disorders in the
    elderly in Edmonton. Acta Psychiatr Scand 77:57–63, 1988

Blazer DG, Williams CD: Epidemiology of dysphoria and depression in
    an elderly population. Am J Psychiatry 137:439–444, 1980

Blazer DG, Hughes DC, George LK: The epidemiology of depression in
    an elderly community population. Am J Psychiatry 137:439–444, 1980

Blazer DG, Hughes DC, George LK: The epidemiology of depression in
    an elderly community population. Gerontologist 27:281–287, 1987

Blazer DG, Hughes D, George LK: Generalized anxiety disorder, in Psy-
    chiatric Disorders in America: The Epidemiologic Catchment Area
    Study. Edited by Robins LN, Regier DA. New York, Free Press, 1991,
    pp 180–203

Borson S, Barnes RA, Kukull WA, et al: Symptomatic depression in elderly
    medical outpatients, I: prevalence, demography, and health service
    utilization. J Am Geriatr Soc 34:341–347, 1986

Burns BJ, Larson DB, Goldstrom ID, et al: Mental disorder among nurs-
    ing home patients: preliminary findings from the National Nursing
    Home Survey pretest. International Journal of Geriatric Psychiatry
    3:27–35, 1988

Burns BJ, Wagner HR, Taube JE, et al: Mental health service use by the
    elderly in nursing homes. Am J Public Health 83:331–337, 1993

Burvill PW: The impact of criteria selection on prevalence rates. Fifth Con-
    gress of the International Federation of Psychiatric Epidemiology
    (1990, Montreal, Canada). Psychiat J Univ Ott 15:194–199, 1990

Cappeliez P: Some thoughts on the prevalence and etiology of depressive
    conditions in the elderly. Can J Aging 7:431–440, 1988

Caracci G, Miller NS: Epidemiology and diagnosis of alcoholism in the
    elderly (a review). International Journal of Geriatric Psychiatry 6:511–
    515, 1991

Christenson R, Blazer D: Epidemiology of persecutory ideation in an elderly population in the community. Am J Psychiatry 141:1088–1091, 1989

Ciompi L: Aging and schizophrenic psychosis. Acta Psychiatr Scand 71:93–105, 1985

Cohen F: Coping with surgery: information, psychological preparation, and recovery, in Aging in the 1980s: Psychological Issues. Edited by Poon LW. Washington, DC, American Psychological Association, 1980, pp 375–382

Cohen SI: Phobic disorders and benzodiazepines in the elderly (letter). Br J Psychiatry 160:135, 1992

Comstock GW, Helsing KJ: Symptoms of depression in two communities. Psychol Med 6:551–563, 1976

Conwell Y, Rotenberg M, Caine ED: Completed suicide at age 50 and over. J Am Geriatr Soc 38:640–644, 1990

Conwell Y, Olsen K, Caine ED, et al: Suicide in later life: psychological autopsy findings. Int Psychogeriatr 3:59–66, 1991

Cooper AF, Garside RF, Kay DWK: A comparison of deaf and non-deaf patients with paranoid and affective psychoses. Br J Psychiatry 129:532–538, 1976

Copeland JR, Gurland BJ, Dewey ME, et al: The distribution of dementia, depression and neurosis in elderly men and women in an urban community: assessed using the GMS-AGECAT package. International Journal of Geriatric Psychiatry 2:177–184, 1987

Copeland JR, Dewey ME, Griffiths-Jones HM: Dementia and depression in elderly persons: AGECAT compared with DSM-III and pervasive illness. International Journal of Geriatric Psychiatry 5:47–51, 1990

Copeland JRM, Dewey ME, Davidson IA, et al: Geriatric Mental State–AGECAT: prevalence, incidence and long-term outcome of dementia and organic disorders in the Liverpool Study of Continuing Health in the Community. Neuroepidemiology 11:84–87, 1992

Coulehan JL, Schulberg HC, Block MR, et al: Symptom patterns of depression in ambulatory medical and psychiatric patients. J Nerv Ment Dis 176:284–288, 1988

Coulehan JL, Schulberg HC, Block MR, et al: Depressive symptomatology and medical co-morbidity in a primary care clinic. Int J Psychiatry Med 20:335–347, 1990a

Coulehan JL, Schulberg HC, Block MR, et al: Medical comorbidity of major depressive disorder in a primary medical practice. Arch Intern Med 150:2362–2367, 1990b

Counte MA, Glandon GL: A panel study of life stress, social support, and the health services utilization of older persons. Med Care 29:348–361, 1991

Cross PS, Gurland BJ: Age, period, and cohort views of suicide rates of the elderly, in Suicide and the Life Cycle. Proceedings of the American Association of Suicidology 15th Annual Meeting, New York, April 1982. Edited by Pfeffer C, Richman J, New York, American Association of Suicidology, 1984, pp 70–71

de la Monte SM, Hutchins GM, Moore GW: Racial differences in the etiology of dementia and frequency of Alzheimer lesions in the brain. J Natl Med Assoc 81:644–652, 1989

DePaulo J, Folstein M: Psychiatric disturbances in neurological patients: detection, recognition, and course. Ann Neurol 4:225–228, 1978

Dewey ME, de la Camara C, Copeland JRM, et al: Cross-cultural comparison of depression and depressive symptoms in older people. Acta Psychiatr Scand 87:369–373, 1993

Draper BM: The elderly admitted to a general hospital psychiatry ward. Aust N Z J Psychiatry 28:288–297, 1994

Dworkin SF, von-Korff M, LeResche L: Multiple pains and psychiatric disturbance: an epidemiologic investigation. Arch Gen Psychiatry 47:239–244, 1990

Eastwood MR, Corbin S, Reed M, et al: Acquired hearing loss and psychiatric illness: an estimate of prevalence and co-morbidity in a geriatric setting. Br J Psychiatry 147:552–556, 1985

Eaton W, Kessler LG: Rates of symptoms of depression in a national sample. Am J Epidemiol 114:528–538, 1981

Eaton WW, Kramer M, Anthony JC, et al: The incidence of specific DIS/DSM-III mental disorders: data from the NIMH Epidemiologic Catchment Area Programs. Acta Psychiatr Scand 79:163–178, 1989

Eaton WW, Dryman A, Weissman MM: Panic and phobia, in Psychiatric Disorders in America: The Epidemiologic Catchment Area Study. Edited by Robins LN, Regier DA. New York, Free Press, 1991, pp 155–179

Eaton WW, Bilker W, Haro JM, et al: Long-term course of hospitalization for schizophrenia, II: change with passage of time. Schizophr Bull 18:229–241, 1992

Edwards DF, Baum CM, Deuel RK: Constructional apraxia in Alzheimer's disease: contributions to functional loss (Special Issue: The Mentally Impaired Elderly: Strategies and Interventions to Maintain Function). Physical and Occupational Therapy in Geriatrics 9:53–68, 1991

Eichmann MA, Griffin BP, Lyons JS, et al: An estimation of the impact of OBRA-87 on nursing home care in the United States. Hosp Community Psychiatry 43:781–789, 1992

Eisdorfer C: Paranoia and schizophrenic disorders in later life, in Handbook of Geriatric Psychiatry. Edited by Busse EW, Blazer DG. New York, Van Nostrand Reinhold, 1980, pp 329–337

Feibel JH, Springer CJ: Depression and failure to resume social activities after stroke. Arch Phys Med Rehabil 63:276–278, 1982

Felton BJ, Revenson TA: Age differences in coping with chronic illness. Psychologizing and Aging. Aging 2:164–170, 1987

Finch EJL, Ramsay R, Katona CLE: Depression and physical illness in the elderly. Clin Geriatr Med 8:275–287, 1992

Fitzgerald JL, Mulford HA: Elderly vs. younger problem drinker "treatment" and recovery experiences. Br J Addict 87:1281–1291, 1992

Flicker C, Ferris SH, Reisberg B: Mild cognitive impairment in the elderly: predictors of dementia. Neurology 41:1006–1009, 1991

Flint AJ, Rifat SL, Eastwood MR: Latent-onset paranoia: distinct from paraphrenia? International Journal of Geriatric Psychiatry 6:103–109, 1991

Folstein MF, Folstein SE, McHugh PR: Mini-Mental State: a practical method for grading the cognitive state of patients for the clinician. J Psychiatr Res 12:189–198, 1975

Folstein MF, Bassett SS, Anthony JC, et al: Dementia: a case ascertainment in a community survey. J Gerontol 46:M132–M138, 1991

Fratiglioni L, Grut M, Forsell Y, et al: Prevalence of Alzheimer's disease and other dementias in an elderly urban population: relationship with age, sex, and education. Neurology 41:1886–1892, 1991

Frerichs RR, Aneshensel C, Clark VA: Prevalence of depression in Los Angeles County. Am J Epidemiol 113:1669–1699, 1981

Fukunishi I, Hayabara T, Hosokawa K: Epidemiological surveys of senile dementia in Japan. Int J Soc Psychiatry 37:51–56, 1991

Gallagher D, Rose J, Rivera P, et al: Prevalence of depression in family caregivers. Gerontologist 29:449–456, 1989

Gallagher-Thompson D, Futterman A, Hanley-Peterson P, et al: Endogenous depression in the elderly: prevalence and agreement among measures. J Consult Clin Psychol 60:300–303, 1992

Garcia C, Tweedy J, Blass J: Underdiagnosis of cognitive impairment in a rehabilitation setting. J Am Geriatr Soc 32:339–342, 1984

George LK, Blazer DG, Hughes DC, et al: Social support and the outcome of major depression. Br J Psychiatry 154:478–485, 1989

George LK, Landerman R, Blazer DG, et al: Cognitive impairment, in Psychiatric Disorders in America: The Epidemiologic Catchment Area Study. Edited by Robins LN, Regier DA. New York, Free Press, 1991, pp 291–327

Glynn RJ, Bouchard GR, LoCastro JS, et al: Aging and generational effects on drinking behaviors in men: results from the Normative Aging Study. Am J Public Health 75:1413–1419, 1985

Goldberg DP, Bridges K, Duncan-Jones P, et al: Dimensions of neuroses seen in primary-care settings. Psychol Med 17:93–112, 1987

Goldberg RJ: The assessment of risk of suicide in the general hospital. Gen Hosp Psychiatry 9:446–452, 1987

Goldstrom IG, Burns BJ, Kessler LG, et al: Mental health services use by elderly adults in a primary care setting. J Gerontol 42:147–153, 1987

Goodman A, Siegel C: Elderly schizophrenic inpatients in the wake of deinstitutionalization. Am J Psychiatry 143:204–207, 1986

Green BH, Copeland JRM, Dewey ME, et al: Risk factors for depression in elderly people: a prospective study. Acta Psychiatr Scand 86:213–217, 1992

Grief C, Eastwood RM: Paranoid disorders in the elderly. International Journal of Geriatric Psychiatry 8:681–684, 1993

Gurland B: The comparative frequency of depression in various adult age groups. J Gerontol 31:283–292, 1976

Gurland B, Cross P: The epidemiology of psychopathology in old age: some clinical implications. Psychiatr Clin North Am 5:11–26, 1982

Gurland B, Copeland J, Kuriansky J, et al: The Mind and Mood of Aging. New York, Haworth, 1983

Gurland BJ, Wilder DE, Golden R, et al: The relationship between depression and disability in the elderly—data from the comprehensive assessment and referral evaluation (CARE), in Psychological Assessment of the Elderly. Edited by Wattis JP, Hindmarch I. London, Churchill Livingstone, 1988, pp 114–137

Haley WE, Turner JA, Romano JM: Depression in chronic pain patients: relation to pain, activity, and sex differences. Pain 23:337–343, 1985

Hall RCW, Gardner ER, Stickney SK, et al: Physical illness manifesting as psychiatric disease, II: analysis of a state hospital inpatient population. Arch Gen Psychiatry 37:989–995, 1980

Harlow SD, Goldberg EL, Comstock GW: A longitudinal study of risk factors for depressive symptomatology in elderly widowed and married women. Am J Epidemiol 134:526–538, 1991a

Harlow SD, Goldberg EL, Comstock GW: A longitudinal study of the prevalence of depressive symptomatology in elderly widowed and married women. Arch Gen Psychiatry 48:1065–1068, 1991b

Harris MJ, Jeste DV: Late-onset schizophrenia: an overview. Schizophr Bull 14:39–55, 1988

Hawton K, Fagg J: Deliberate self-poisoning and self-injury in older people. International Journal of Geriatric Psychiatry 5:367–373, 1990

Heyman A, Fillenbaum G, Prosnitz B, et al: Estimated prevalence of dementia among elderly black and white community residents. Arch Neurol 48:594–598, 1991

Holzer III CE, Robins LN, Myers JK, et al: Antecedents and correlates of alcohol abuse and dependence in the elderly, in Nature and Extent of Alcohol Problems Among the Elderly (Res Monogr 14, DHHS Publ No ADM-84-1321). Edited by Maddox G, Robins LN, Rosenberg N. Washington, DC, U.S. Government Printing Office, 1984, pp 217–244

Jacoby RJ, Levy R, Dawson JM: Computed tomography in the elderly, III: affective disorders. Br J Psychiatry 137:70–75, 1980

Jacoby RJ, Dolan R, Levy R, et al: Quantitative computed tomography in elderly depressed patients. Br J Psychiatry 143:124–127, 1983

Jeste DV: Late-onset schizophrenia. International Journal of Geriatric Psychiatry 8:283–285, 1993

Johnson J, Weissman MM, Klerman GL: Service utilization and social morbidity associated with depressive symptoms in the community. J Am Med Assoc 267:1478–1483, 1992

Karno M, Golding JM: Obsessive compulsive disorder, in Psychiatric Disorders in America: The Epidemiologic Catchment Area Study. Edited by Robins LN, Regier DA. New York, Free Press, 1991, pp 204–219

Katon W: The epidemiology of depression in medical care. Int J Psychiatry Med 17:93–112, 1987

Katon W, Russo J: Somatic symptoms and depression. J Fam Pract 29:65–69, 1989

Katon W, Schulberg HC: Epidemiology of depression in primary care. Special section: developing guidelines for treating depressive disorders in the primary care setting. Gen Hosp Psychiatry 14:237–247, 1992

Katon W, Sullivan M: Depression and chronic medical illness. J Clin Psychiatry 51:3–11, 1990

Katon W, von Korff M, Lin E, et al: Distressed high utilizers of medical care: DSM-III-R diagnoses and treatment needs. Gen Hosp Psychiatry 12:355–362, 1990

Katon W, von Korff M, Lin E, et al: Adequacy and duration of antidepressant treatment in primary care. Med Care 30:67–76, 1992

Katon W, Sullivan M, Russo J, et al: Depressive symptoms and measures of disability: a prospective study. J Affect Disord 27:245–254, 1993

Kay DWK: Outcome and course of death in mental disorders of old age. Acta Psychiatr Scand 38:249–276, 1962

Kay DWK: Schizophrenia and schizophrenia-like states in the elderly. Br J Psychiatry 9:18–24, 1975

Kay DWK, Roth M: Environmental and hereditary factors in the schizophrenias of old age ("late paraphrenia") and their bearing on the general problem of causation in schizophrenia. Journal of Mental Science 107:649–686, 1961

Kay DWK, Cooper AF, Garside RF, et al: The differentiation of paranoid from affective psychoses by patient's premorbid characteristics. Br J Psychiatry 129:207–215, 1976

Kay DWK, Henderson AS, Scott R, et al: Dementia and depression amongst the elderly living in the Hobart community: the effect of the diagnostic criteria on the prevalence rates. Psychol Med 15:771–788, 1985

Keith SJ, Regier DA, Rae DS: Schizophrenic disorders, in Psychiatric Disorders in America: The Epidemiologic Catchment Area Study. Edited by Robins LN, Regier DA. New York, Free Press, 1991, pp 33–52

Kemp BJ, Staples F, Lopez-Aqueres W: Epidemiology of depression and dysphoria in an elderly Hispanic population: prevalence and correlates. J Am Geriatr Soc 35:920–926, 1987

Kennedy GJ, Kelman HR, Thomas C: The emergence of depressive symptoms in late life: the importance of declining health and increasing disability. J Community Health 15:93–104, 1990

Kinzie JD, Lewinsohn P, Maricle R, et al: The relationship of depression to medical illness in an older community population. Compr Psychiatry 27:241–246, 1986

Klerman G, Lavori PW, Rice J, et al: Birth-cohort trends in rates of major depressive disorder among relatives of patients with affective disorder. Arch Gen Psychiatry 42:689–693, 1985

Knight EB, Folstein MF: Unsuspected emotional and cognitive disturbance in medical patients. Ann Intern Med 87:723–734, 1977

Kral V: The relationship between senile dementia (Alzheimer type) and depression. Can J Psychiatry 28:304–306, 1983

Kramer M, German PS, Anthony JC, et al: Patterns of mental disorders among the elderly residents of eastern Baltimore. J Am Geriatr Soc 33:236–245, 1985

Kua EH: The prevalence of dementia in elderly Chinese. Acta Psychiatr Scand 83:350–352, 1991

Kukull WA, Koepsell TD, Inui TS, et al: Depression and physical illness among general medical clinical patients. J Affect Disord 10:153–162, 1986

Larson C, Nyman G: Age of onset in schizophrenia. Hum Hered 20:241–247, 1970

Larson E, Reifler B, Sumi S, et al: Diagnostic evaluation of 200 elderly outpatients with suspected dementia. Gerontologist 40:536–543, 1985

Launer LJ, Hofman A: Studies on the incidence of dementia: the European Perspective. Neuroepidemiology 11:127–134, 1992

Lester D: Attempts to explain changing elderly suicide rate: a comment on Pritchard (letter to the editor). Int J Geriatr Psychiatry 8:435–440, 1993

Letenneur L, Fabrigoule D, Dartigues JF: Incidence and premonitory symptoms of dementia. Ann Med Psychol 151:670–672, 1993

Li G, Shen YC, Chen CH, et al: An epidemiological survey of age-related dementia in an urban area of Beijing. Acta Psychiatr Scand 79:557–563, 1989

Li G, Shen YC, Chen CH, et al: A three-year follow-up study of age-related dementia in an urban area of Beijing. Acta Psychiatr Scand 83:99–104, 1991

Liberto JG, Oslin DW, Ruskin PE: Alcoholism in older persons: a review of the literature. Hosp Community Psychiatry 43:975–984, 1992

Lindesay J: Phobic disorders in the elderly. Br J Psychiatry 159:531–541, 1991a

Lindesay J: Suicide in the elderly. Int J Geriatr Psychiatry 6:355–361, 1991b

Livingston BM, Kim K, Leaf PJ, et al: Depressive disorders and dysphoria resulting from conjugal bereavement in a prospective community sample. Am J Psychiatry 147:608–611, 1990

Livingston G, Hawkins A, Graham N, et al: The Gospel Oak Study: prevalence rates of dementia, depression and activity limitation among elderly residents in Inner London. Psychol Med 20:137–146, 1990

Livingston G, King M: Alcohol abuse in an inner city elderly population: the Gospel Oak Survey. International Journal of Geriatric Psychiatry 8:511–514, 1993

Lowenthal MF: Lives in Distress: The Paths of the Elderly to the Psychiatric Ward. New York, Basic Books, 1964

Madden JJ, Luhan JA, Kaplan LA, et al: Nondementing psychoses in older persons. JAMA 150:1567–1570, 1952

Mages NL, Mendelsohn GA: Effects of cancer on patients' lives: a personological approach, in Health Psychology. Edited by Stone GC, Cohen F, Adler NE. San Francisco, Jossey-Bass, 1979, pp 255–284

Magruder-Habib K, Zung WWK, Feussner JR: Improving physicians' recognition and treatment of depression in general medical care. Med Care 28:239–250, 1990

McAllister TW, Price TR: Severe depressive pseudodementia with and without dementia. Am J Psychiatry 139:626–629, 1982

McCartney JR, Palmateer L: Assessment of cognitive deficit in geriatric patients. J Am Geriatr Soc 33:467–471, 1985

Mears HJ, Spice C: Screening for problem drinking in the elderly: a study in the elderly mentally ill. Int J Geriatr Psychiatry 8:319–326, 1993

Merrill J, Owens J: Age and attempted suicide. Acta Psychiatr Scand 82:385–388, 1990

Mintzer JE, Macera CA: Prevalence of depressive symptoms among white and African-American caregivers of demented patients. Am J Psychiatry 149:575–576, 1992

Mishara BL, McKim W: Methodological issues in surveying older persons concerning drug use. Int J Addict 28:305–326, 1993

Moos RH, Brennan PL, Moos BS: Short-term processes of remission and nonremission among late-life problem drinkers. Alcohol Clin Exp Res 15:948–955, 1991

Morgan HG: General medical disorders, in Handbook of Psychiatry, Mental Disorders, and Somatic Illness. Edited by Lader MH. New York, Cambridge University Press, 1983, pp 14–36

Mowry BJ, Burvill PW: A study of mild dementia in the community using a wide range of diagnostic criteria. Br J Psychiatry 153:328–334, 1988

Murden RA, McRae TD, Kaner S, et al: Mini-Mental State Exam scores vary with education in blacks and whites. J Am Geriatr Soc 39:149–155, 1991

Murphy E: Social origins of depression in old age. Br J Psychiatry 141:135–142, 1982

Murphy E: The prognosis of depression in old age. Br J Psychiatry 142:111–119, 1983

Myers JK, Weissman MM, Tischler GL, et al: Six-month prevalence of psychiatric disorders in three communities, 1980 to 1982. Arch Gen Psychiatry 41:959–967, 1984

Nakamura CM, Molgaard CA, Stanford EP, et al: A discriminant analysis of severe alcohol consumption among older persons. Alcohol Alcohol 25:75–80, 1990

National Center for Health Statistics: Health Statistics of Older Persons,

United States, 1986. Vital and Health Statistics 25 (Series 3) (PHS Publ No 87-1409). Washington, DC, U.S. Department of Health and Human Services, Public Health Service, 1987

Neugarten BL, Datan N: Sociological perspectives on the life cycle, in Life-Span Developmental Psychology: Personality and Socialization. Edited by Baltes PB, Schaie KW. New York, Academic Press, 1973, pp 53–69

Norris FH, Murrell SA: Social support, life events, and stress as modifiers of adjustment to bereavement by older adults. Psychol Aging 5:429–436, 1990

Nowers M: Deliberate self-harm in the elderly: a survey of one London borough. International Journal of Geriatric Psychiatry 8:609–614, 1993

O'Connor DW, Roth M: Coexisting depression and dementia in a community survey of the elderly. Int Psychogeriatr 2:45–53, 1990

O'Connor DW, Pollitt PA, Roth M, et al: Memory complaints and impairment in normal, depressed, and demented elderly persons identified in a community survey. Arch Gen Psychiatry 47:224–227, 1990

O'Connor DW, Pollitt PA, Hyde JB, et al: The progression of mild idiopathic dementia in a community population. J Am Geriatr Soc 39:246–251, 1991a

O'Connor DW, Pollitt PA, Treasure FP: The influence of education and social class on the diagnosis of dementia in a community population. Psychol Med 21:219–224, 1991b

Omnibus Budget Reconciliation Act of 1987. P.L. 100–203, 101 Stat. 1330.

O'Riordan TG, Hayes JP, Shelley R, et al: The prevalence of depression in an acute geriatric medical assessment unit. International Journal of Geriatric Psychiatry 4:17–21, 1989

Ouslander JG: Physical illness and depression in the elderly. J Am Geriatr Soc 30:593–599, 1982

Oxman TE, Berkman LF, Kasl S, et al: Social support and depressive symptoms in the elderly. Am J Epidemiol 135:356–368, 1992

Palinkas LA, Wingard DL, Barrett-Connor E: Chronic illness and depressive symptoms in the elderly: a population-based study. J Clin Epidemiol 43:1131–1141, 1990

Park J, Ha JC: Cognitive impairment among the elderly in a Korean rural community. Acta Psychiatr Scand 77:52–57, 1988

Parmelee PA, Katz IR, Lawton MP: Incidence of depression in long-term care settings. J Gerontol Med Sci 47:M189–M196, 1992

Penn ND, Corrado OJ, Pitchfork LJ, et al: Blood alcohol levels in acute elderly admissions to hospital. Postgrad Med J 65:20–21, 1989

Pierce D: Deliberate self-harm in the elderly. International Journal of Geriatric Psychiatry 2:105–110, 1987

Post F: Persistent Persecutory States of the Elderly. London, Pergamon, 1966

Post F: The management and nature of depressive illness in late life: a follow-through study. Br J Psychiatry 212:393–404, 1972

Post F: Dementia, depression, and pseudo-dementia, in Psychiatric Aspects of Neurological Disease. Edited by Benson DF, Blumer D. New York, Grune & Stratton, 1975, pp 99–120

Pritchard C: Changes in elderly suicides in the USA and the developed world 1974–87: comparison with current homicide. International Journal of Geriatric Psychiatry 7:125–134, 1992

Rabins P: The reversible dementias, in Recent Advances in Psychogeriatrics. Edited by Arie T. London, Churchill Livingstone, 1985

Rabins P, Pauker S, Thomas J: Can schizophrenia begin after age 44? Compr Psychiatry 25:290–293, 1984

Rabins P, Pearlson G, Jayaram G, et al: Increased ventricle to brain ratio in late onset schizophrenia. Am J Psychiatry 144:1216–1218, 1987

Rapp SR, Davis KM: Geriatric depression: physician's knowledge, perceptions, and diagnostic practices. Gerontologist 29:252–257, 1989

Ray WA, Taylor JA, Meador KG, et al: Reducing antipsychotic drug use in nursing homes: a controlled trial of provider education. Arch Intern Med 153:713–721, 1993

Reding M, Haycox J, Blass J: Depression in patients referred to a dementia clinic: a three year prospective study. Arch Neurol 42:894–896, 1985

Reed BR, Jagust WJ, Seab JP: Mental status as a predictor of daily function in progressive dementia. Gerontologist 29:804–807, 1989

Regier DA, Hirschfeld RM, Goodwin FK, et al: The NIMH Depression Awareness, Recognition, and Treatment program: structure, aims, and scientific basis. Am J Psychiatry 145:1351–1357, 1988

Regier DA, Narrow WE, Rae DS: The epidemiology of anxiety disorders: the Epidemiologic Catchment Area (ECA) experience. J Psychiatr Res 24:3–14, 1990

Revenson TA, Felton BJ: Patients' perceptions of the stressor of chronic illness. Paper presented at the meeting of the Gerontology Society of America, New Orleans, November, 1985

Robins L, Holzer J, Weissman M, et al: Lifetime prevalence of specific psychiatric disorders in three sites. Arch Gen Psychiatry 41:949–958, 1984

Robinson RG, Kubos KL, Starr LB, et al: Mood disorders in stroke patients: importance of location of lesion. Brain 107:81–93, 1984

Rosen DH, Gregory RJ, Pollock D, et al: Depression in patients referred for psychiatric consultation: a need for a new diagnosis. Gen Hosp Psychiatry 9:391–397, 1987

Rosenman S: The validity of the diagnosis of mild dementia. Psychol Med 21:923–934, 1989

Ross CE, Mirowsky J: Explaining the social patterns of depression: control and problem solving or support and talking? J Health Soc Behav 30:206–219, 1989

Roth M: The natural history of mental disorder in old age. Journal of Mental Science 101:281–301, 1955

Rovner BW, Kafonek S, Fillip L, et al: Prevalence of mental illness in a community nursing home. Am J Psychiatry 143:1446–1449, 1986

Russell DW, Cutrona CE: Social support, stress, and depressive symptoms among the elderly: test of a process model. Psychol Aging 6:190–201, 1991

Salmon DP, Riekkinen PJ, Katzman R, et al: Cross-cultural studies of dementia: a comparison of Mini-Mental State Examination performance in Finland and China. Arch Neurol 46:769–772, 1989

Sandyk R, Awerbuch GI: Late-onset schizophrenia: relationship to awareness of abnormal involuntary movements and tobacco addiction. Int J Neurosci 71:9–19, 1993

Savage RD, Gaber LB, Britton PG, et al: Personality and Adjustment in the Aged. New York, Academic Press, 1977

Schonfeld L, Dupree LW: Antecedents of drinking for early- and late-onset elderly alcohol abusers. J Stud Alcohol 52:587–592, 1991

Shaper AG: Alcohol and mortality: a review of prospective studies. Br J Addict 85:837–847, 1990

Silverman JM, Li G, Schear S, et al: A cross-cultural family history study of primary progressive dementia in relatives of nondemented elderly Chinese, Italians, Jews and Puerto Ricans. Acta Psychiatr Scand 85:211–217, 1992

Simpson CJ, Hyde CE, Faragher EP: The chronically mentally ill in the community: a study of quality of care. Br J Psychiatry 154:77–82, 1989

Sireling LI, Paykel ES, Freeling P, et al: Depression in general practice: case thresholds and diagnosis. Br J Psychiatry 147:113–119, 1985

Sluss TK, Gruenberg EM, Kramer M: The use of longitudinal studies in the investigation of risk factors for senile dementia-Alzheimer type, in Epidemiology of Dementia. Edited by Mortimer JA, Schuman LM. New York, Oxford University Press, 1981, pp 132–154

Smith DA, Jensen S: OBRA—its effect on the mentally ill in South Dakota nursing homes. S D J Med 43:13–14, 1990

Snowdon J: The prevalence of depression in old age. International Journal of Geriatric Psychiatry 5:141–144, 1990

Soni SD, Mallik A: The elderly chronic schizophrenic inpatient: a study of psychiatric morbidity in "elderly graduates." International Journal of Geriatric Psychiatry 8:665–673, 1993

Stallones L, Marx MB, Garrity TF: Prevalence and correlates of depressive symptoms among older U.S. adults. Am J Prev Med 6:295–303, 1990

Swartz M, Landerman R, George LK, et al: Somatization disorder, in Psychiatric Disorders in America: The Epidemiologic Catchment Area Study. Edited by Robins LN, Regier DA. New York, Free Press, 1991, pp 220–257

Thompson JW, Belcher JR, DeForge BR, et al: Changing characteristics of schizophrenic patients admitted to state hospitals. Hosp Community Psychiatry 44:231–235, 1993

Tomlinson B, Blessed G, Roth M: Observations on the brains of non-demented old people. J Neurol Sci 7:331–356, 1968

Turnbull JM, Turnbull SK: Management of specific anxiety disorders in the elderly. Geriatrics 40:75–82, 1985

Turner RJ, McLean PD: Physical disability and psychological distress. Rehabilitation Psychology 34:225–242, 1989

Turner RJ, Noh S: Physical disability and depression. J Health Soc Behav 29:23–37, 1988

Turner RJ, Wood DW: Depression and disability: the stress process in a chronically strained population, in Research in Community and Mental Health, Vol 5. Greenwich, CT, JAI Press, 1985, pp 77–109

Uhlmann E, Richard F, Larson EB: Effect of education on the Mini-Mental State Examination as a screening test for dementia. J Am Geriatr Soc 39:876–880, 1991

Verbrugge LM: Longer life but worsening health? in The Nation's Health, 3rd Edition. Edited by Lee PR, Estes CL. Boston, MA, Jones & Bartlett, 1990, pp 14–34

Vogel R, Wolfersdorf M: Suicide and mental illness in the elderly. Psychopathology 22:202–207, 1989

Volavka J, Cancro R: The late onset schizophrenic disorders, in Aspects of Aging. Edited by Busse E. Philadelphia, PA, Smith Kline & French, 1986

von Korff M, Dworkin S, Le Resche L: Graded chronic pain status: an epidemiological evaluation. Pain 40:279–291, 1990

Ware JP: Use of outpatient mental health services by a general population with health insurance coverage. Hosp Community Psychiatry 37:1119–1125, 1986

Warren EJ, Grek A, Conn D, et al: A correlation between cognitive performance and daily functioning in elderly people. J Geriatr Psychiat Neurol 2:96–100, 1989

Weissman MM, Myers JK, Tischler GL, et al: Psychiatric disorders (DSM-III) and cognitive impairment among the elderly in the U.S. urban community. Acta Psychiatr Scand 71:366–379, 1985

Weissman MM, Bruse ML, Leaf PJ, et al: Affective disorders, in Psychiatric Disorders in America: The Epidemiologic Catchment Area Study. Edited by Robins LN, Regier DA. New York, Free Press, 1991, pp 53–80

Wells KB, Golding JM, Burnam MA: Psychiatric disorder and limitations in physical functioning in a sample of the Los Angeles general population. Am J Psychiatry 145:712–717, 1988

Wells KB, Burnam MA, Rogers W, et al: The course of depression in adult outpatients: results from the Medical Outcomes Study. Arch Gen Psychiatry 49:788–794, 1992

Wells KB, Rogers W, Burnam MA, et al: Course of depression in patients with hypertension, myocardial infarction, or insulin-dependent diabetes. Am J Psychiatry 150:632–638, 1993

Wing J: The concept of negative symptoms (Negative Symptoms in Schizophrenia Symposium). Br J Psychiatry 155:10–14, 1989

Woodbury MA, Manton KG, Blazer D: Trends in U.S. suicide mortality rates 1968 to 1982: race and sex differences in age, period and cohort components. Int J Epidemiol 17:356–362, 1988

World Health Organization: International Classification of Diseases, 10th Revision. Geneva, World Health Organization, 1991

Yu ES, Liu WT, Levy P, et al: Cognitive impairment among elderly adults in Shanghai, China. J Gerontol 44:S97–S106, 1989

Zisook S, Schuchter SR: Depression through the first year after the death of a spouse. Am J Psychiatry 148:1346–1352, 1991

Zisook S, Schuchter SR: Depression through the first year after the death of a spouse: reply (letter). Am J Psychiatry 149:580, 1992

Eleanor Lavretsky, M.D., Ph.D.
Steven S. Matsuyama, Ph.D.
Sylvia Gerson, Ph.D.
Lissy F. Jarvik, M.D., Ph.D.

Genetics of Geriatric Psychopathology

S everal of the neuropsychiatric disorders seen in the elderly tend to occur in multiple generations, suggesting a role for genetic factors in the etiology of these disorders. This observation is in accord with the increasing evidence that genes are major determinants of human behavior, either directly responsible for or underlying the susceptibility of an individual to certain forms of mental illness. Current investigations of the genetics of such disorders draw on a broad knowledge base rooted in fields as diverse as clinical psychiatry, protein chemistry, and genetics, ranging from population to molecular genetics. Application of molecular genetic techniques has led to the identification of the gene responsible for Huntington's disease, and this research has raised the hope that other disorders, such as Alzheimer's disease, schizophrenia, and bipolar disorder, will soon yield their genetic secrets. The increasing application of molecular genetic techniques promises further substantial progress in our understanding of the genetics of geriatric psychopathology.

The rapid rate at which molecular genetics has been developing is illustrated by the fact that one of its cornerstones, polymerase chain reaction, was unknown a mere 10 years ago. The continuing advances in recombinant DNA technology will allow rapid generation of information on individual genomes. By 1993, at least 2,600 genes had been mapped to specific chromosomes, and that number continues to increase. As ever-more disease-associated genes are identified, and as genetic testing becomes increasingly common, presymptomatic diagnosis will begin to affect the lives of countless individuals and their families. To be of help to their patients, therefore, psychiatrists will need to have in-depth knowledge of basic genetics. In Huntington's disease, for example, there is already a clear role for the genetically sophisticated psychiatrist in helping at-risk relatives confront the dilemma of *access* to the knowledge that they may harbor a gene that almost invariably dooms its carrier to a relentlessly progressing disease at a time when neither prevention nor effective therapeutic measures exist. Because it is controversial whether cognitive impairment and neurodegenerative disorders, such as Alzheimer's disease, are specific diseases or part of normal aging per se, today's geriatric psychiatrist needs to be familiar with the genetics of normal aging as well as the genetics of specific psychiatric disorders seen in old age.

In this chapter we attempt to provide a succinct guide to the baseline information necessary to enable geriatric psychiatrists to understand and apply advances in genetics as they are being made. To keep up-to-date in this rapidly evolving area, each reader will have to augment the contents of this chapter by perusal of the current literature.

Methodology in Psychiatric Genetics: Traditional Methods

The genetic information contained in cells that allows them to replicate and to carry out their biological functions is contained within their chromosomes, which are located in the cell nuclei. All human somatic cells (i.e., all cells other than gametes) contain duplicate sets of 22 different chromosomes, called *autosomes*. Because one member of each pair of autosomes is derived from the mother and the other from the father, the two members of the pair are not identical and are referred to as being *homologous*. An additional pair of chromosomes, the nonhomologous *X and Y sex chromosomes,* bring the total to 23 pairs.

Genes, the units of heredity, are arranged in a specific linear order, with each gene located at an identifiable position (*locus*) on a particular chromosome. The existence of genes was predicted in the 1860s by the Austrian monk Gregor Mendel on the basis of his breeding experiments with garden peas. Mendel's experiments led to the formulation of two laws that form the basis of genetics. The first law states that *alleles* (i.e., different genetic alternatives at the same locus on homologous chromosomes) segregate; the second states that different pairs of alleles *assort independently*. It is now known that this second law does not always hold (see later discussion).

Diversity in the human gene pool is achieved by sexual reproduction. Through the process of *meiosis,* each gamete (sperm or ovum) contains only half the chromosomes, and therefore only one copy of each allele. Thus, only one allele at a given locus is transmitted to each gamete from a parent. If both alleles are identical, the individual is homozygous, and if the alleles are different, the individual is heterozygous. When gametes join during fertilization, new combinations of genes are generated. Because there are 23 pairs of chromosomes, and because members of each pair assort independently, humans can generate 2^{23} different types of gametes. Additional diversity is achieved through the mechanism of *crossing over,* which occurs during gamete formation. In this process, parts of homologous chromosomes are exchanged.

Pedigrees and Family Studies

One of the oldest methods of genetic investigation begins with the *index case,* or *proband* (i.e., person with an illness through whom families are located). Family histories are then compiled and pedigrees are constructed. The assumption is that in a disorder with a genetic basis, there will be a correlation between the frequency of the disorder in relatives and their degree of genetic relatedness. Thus, the frequency of the disorder is expected to be higher in *first-degree* relatives (i.e., parents, siblings, and children), who share, on the average, 50% of their genes with the proband, than among *second-degree* relatives (i.e., grandparents, aunts, uncles, nieces, nephews), who share only about 25% of the genes.

The pedigree patterns seen with single gene defects reflect the chromosomal location of the gene locus (i.e., autosomal or X-linked) and the mode of transmission (dominant or recessive). The mode of transmission is readily determined if there is complete *penetrance* (i.e., all affected individuals manifest the illness) and complete *expressivity* (i.e., all affected individuals exhibit the same characteristic symptomatology). For single gene defects, there are four basic modes of transmission:

1. In *autosomal dominant* transmission, every affected person in the pedigree has an affected parent, who also has an affected parent, and so on, as far back as the disorder can be traced. The disorder will be present in about 50% of siblings and children, both male and female, of the affected individual. An example is Huntington's disease.

2. In *autosomal recessive* transmission, the most common scenario is that neither of the proband's parents has the disease, although both must have one copy of the mutant allele (i.e., both are "carriers"). Approximately 25% of the offspring, irrespective of their gender, will have the disease; 50% will be carriers; and 25% will not have inherited the responsible gene. Diseases with this mode of transmission include Wilson's disease, cystic fibrosis, and many inborn errors of metabolism, such as phenylketonuria. There are, at present, no examples from geriatric psychopathology of disorders with this mode of transmission.

3. In *X-linked dominant* transmission, a single mutant allele on one of the X chromosomes will determine the abnormal phenotype even in the presence of the normal allele on the other X chromosome. The offspring of an affected mother, regardless of whether it is a son or daughter, has a 50% chance of inheriting the mutant allele. By contrast, all daughters of affected fathers will be affected and none of their sons, because sons inherit only the father's Y chromosome. Few genetic disorders are classified as X-linked dominant; examples are vitamin D–resistant rickets and ornithine transcarbamylase (a liver enzyme) deficiency. These conditions are always much more severe in males.

4. In *X-linked recessive* transmission, the presence of identical mutant alleles on each of the two X chromosomes in women or of the mutant allele on the single X chromosome in men determines the abnormal phenotype. Thus, homozygosity is restricted to women. Heterozygous mothers do not manifest the disease but transmit the mutant allele to half their daughters and half their sons. The daughters with the mutant allele are carriers (asymptomatic), whereas the sons manifest the disease. A daughter may be affected if her mother is a carrier and her father has the disorder. Examples of disorders with this mode of transmission include hemophilia A, Duchenne's dystrophy, and Lesch-Nyhan syndrome. There are, at present, no examples from geriatric psychopathology of disorders with this mode of transmission.

Determination of the mode of inheritance is often complicated by reduced penetrance (i.e., some of those with the particular genotype fail to express it completely in their phenotype). Further, the clinical expression of a phenotype may differ in people who have the same genotype, and in this case the phenotype is said to have *variable expressivity*. Many single gene disorders are characterized by multiple phenotypic effects, and patients may differ in the extent to which they manifest the spectrum of the disorder as well as in the degree of severity of specific abnormalities. Complicating matters even more is the fact that *familial* does not necessarily mean *genetic*; some familial cases may be due to common environmental factors rather than an underlying genetic defect.

In addition to simple Mendelian patterns of transmission, *polygenic*, or *multifactorial*, inheritance has often been suggested in psychiatric disorders. In such inheritance, the phenotype is determined by the combined effects of many genes at different loci.

The mode of inheritance can be determined by a statistical method, *segregation analysis*, in which the pattern of observed frequency of illness in a family is compared with the pattern expected from the hypothesized mode of inheritance. The power of segregation analysis rests on accurate diagnosis, and this often presents major difficulties. Geriatric psychopathology is usually characterized by a wide range of symptoms, varying levels of severity, and a high frequency of comorbidity. As a consequence, there is lack of clarity at diagnostic boundaries. The effectiveness of this method is further compromised by etiologic heterogeneity. It may thus not be the best approach for investigating the genetics of psychopathology.

The family study method itself also has several limitations, including 1) *difficulties in obtaining accurate information*, especially for older individuals whose memory may be impaired and whose parents, siblings, and friends have died (i.e., no one may be left to provide information about the family); 2) *small family size*, making it difficult to determine the mode of inheritance; and 3) *selection bias* (on average, probands have been brought to the attention of investigators because of dramatic illnesses, often unusually severe, or because of multiple affected family members, and therefore, are not representative of the group afflicted with a given illness).

Twin Studies

Twin study methodology is a valuable research tool for understanding the genetic and environmental components in aging, survival, and disease. Twin studies are based on the natural occurrence of two genetically different types of twins: *monozygotic* (MZ), or one-egg, twins are genetically identical; *dizygotic* (DZ), or two-egg, twins share, on average, 50% of their genes, as do siblings. Twin studies assess the frequency with which members of a twin pair manifest a given trait or disease. If both twins manifest it, the pair is *concordant*; if only one member of the twin pair does, the pair is *discordant*. Concordance is expressed as a percentage derived from the following formula:

$$\text{Concordance} = \frac{\text{Number of co-twins with the disease}}{\text{Number of co-twins at risk}} \times 100$$

If genetic factors play a role in the etiology of a disorder, MZ twins will have a much higher concordance than DZ twins. On the other hand, if genetic factors are of minor importance (e.g., in a measles epidemic), the concordance for MZ and DZ twin pairs will be similar. The absence of 100% concordance in MZ twins suggests that environmental factors also play a role in the etiology of a disease.

Adoption Studies

Adoption studies are another approach to help clarify the relative importance of genetic and environmental influences. Such studies compare biological relatives raised apart or unrelated individuals raised together. Similarities between biological relatives raised apart are explained by shared genetic backgrounds, and similarities between unrelated individuals raised together are explained by shared environmental influences.

Although family, twin, and adoption studies may provide evidence for genetic factors, these methods do not provide information on the location of the genetic effect. Other approaches are needed for that purpose. As discussed below, molecular genetic technology has provided exciting new approaches. To begin to understand the principles of this technology, it is important to review some further fundamentals of genetics.

Further Fundamentals of Genetics: Basic Review

Molecular Genetics

The genetic material is DNA, a long polymerized structure composed of four kinds of nucleotides. Each nucleotide contains the five-carbon sugar deoxyribose, phosphoric acid, and one of four nitrogenous bases (adenine [A], thymine [T], guanine [G], and cytosine [C]). The DNA molecule consists of two polynucleotide chains in a double-helix configuration. Base pairing is precise and always complementary: A with T, and G with C. The DNA contains sequences that code for proteins as well as sequences that serve as regulatory domains (i.e., they regulate the amounts of specific proteins produced at any given moment throughout life). The sequence of the bases provides the code for the genetic information: the code is "read" in non-overlapping groups of three nucleotides (i.e., *codons*) from a fixed starting point.

Each codon specifies an amino acid, the building block of proteins. However, the code is *degenerate* (i.e., more than one codon codes for the same amino acid). Substitution of a single base alters only the codon in which the base is located and affects only that amino acid in the protein. Deletion or insertion of a single nucleotide changes the reading frame subsequent to that change, thus altering the amino acid sequence beyond the site of the mutation, which is likely to result in loss of protein function. The final products of gene expression are specific proteins. Differences in protein structure, together with differences in regulation, account for the range of biological diversity, including the diversity of disease processes.

The human genome contains approximately 3 billion nucleotides coding for an estimated 50,000–100,000 genes. Currently, more than 4,000 genes have been identified, and it is predicted that all genes will have been identified by the end of the next decade. One puzzle to be solved is that only about 3% of the total DNA in the human genome codes for proteins. Aside from regulatory sequences that affect gene expression, most of the remaining 97% currently has no known function and is labeled "junk DNA," a complex mix of different types of DNA. Recent investigations suggest that junk DNA contains regulatory gene sequences (outside the protein coding sequences) and is vital to the life of the cell (Nowak 1994). Further, some junk DNA appears to have a crucial function in maintaining the structure of chromosomes. Another type of junk DNA comprises *introns.* DNA segments coding for the proteins (i.e., *exons*) are interrupted by intervening segments (i.e., introns). In protein synthesis, the first step is transcription of DNA to a messenger ribonucleic acid (mRNA), which then represents a copy of the entire sequence of the gene. The mRNA is then processed (i.e., the introns are removed, which brings together the exons), and the processed mRNA (i.e., without introns) is then translated in protein.

In addition to the nucleus containing DNA, mitochondria in the cytoplasm contains DNA (mtDNA) that codes for mitochondrial genes. There has been recent interest in mitochondrial genetics because of increasing evidence for an association of mtDNA mutations with aging as well as neurodegenerative disorders such as Alzheimer's disease and Parkinson's disease (Wallace 1992).

The current molecular genetic approach involves localization, identification, and sequencing of the relevant gene and determination of the gene product and its normal function. These objectives are as yet unrealized. Recently, large collaborative groups of researchers, both in the United States and in Europe, joined forces to map the chromosomal locations of disease genes as a first step toward isolating them.

Mendel's second law does not hold up universally. It holds only for genes that reside on separate chromosomes or that are sufficiently distant from each other on the same chromosome to behave independently. Thus, genes do not always segregate independently; some of them remain associated in inheritance (i.e., they *cosegregate*).

Linkage Analysis

The propensity of some genes to remain associated in inheritance is called *linkage*, and this feature is the basis of the strategy used to localize a disease gene to a region of a specific chromosome. Once the position of the gene is known, it can be cloned and characterized. Thus, no prior knowledge of the nature of the disease gene is required. The pattern of transmission of a disease gene can be followed through families if *markers* (i.e., variants that mark nearby positions on the chromosome) close to the disease gene are available.

The transmission of a trait along with a known specific marker within families suggests that the two genes are located on the same chromosome in close proximity to each other. The closer the two loci are, the more frequently they are transmitted together; the farther apart they are, the more likely they are to form new combinations (i.e., *recombinations*). The recombination frequency provides a measure of distance between loci. Evidence for linkage is derived from statistical analysis of the observed association between two loci. That is, the probability of observing the segregation of the two loci (or combination of traits) over a range of recombination fractions when linkage (it is assumed) exists is compared with the probability of observing the two traits together in the absence of linkage (i.e., the loci are segregating independently). The logarithm of this ratio of likelihoods is the *lod score*. Lod scores are additive across families, and evidence for linkage is generally accepted if the lod score exceeds 3.0

(which indicates that linkage is at least 1,000 times more likely than no linkage).

Human genetic linkage analysis was revolutionized in 1978 with the application of molecular genetic techniques and the discovery of new types of markers based on large amounts of DNA base sequence variations (i.e., *polymorphisms*) that occur at random in the human genome. Most of the polymorphisms known at present are innocuous and have no known undesirable consequences.

The molecular genetic mapping technique utilizes *restriction enzymes* (endonucleases) that recognize specific short sequences of DNA (usually four to six base pairs) and cleave the DNA each time the recognition sequence occurs. This results in DNA fragments of distinct lengths. The fragments are then visualized by separating the DNA fragments on the basis of size by gel electrophoresis (smaller fragments move faster than larger ones). Further analysis of the DNA is carried out with the use of Southern blotting, a technique in which the DNA separated in the gel is denatured to single-stranded DNA, which is then transferred onto a membrane filter. The filter is incubated with a labeled DNA *probe* (i.e., a short section of DNA with a known chromosomal location); this probe combines (i.e., hybridizes with) only with its complementary sequence in a sea of noncomplementary DNA. This labeled complex can then be localized to a particular DNA fragment of a specific molecular weight. (In comparable techniques for RNA, known as Northern blotting, and for proteins, known as Western blotting, RNA and proteins, respectively, are separated on gels, transferred to membranes, and probed with the appropriately labeled RNA and specific protein antibodies, respectively.) A large variety of restriction enzymes with different sequence specificities are known. By using different restriction enzymes, one can construct a restriction map of the area that has been "recognized" by the probe of interest (Figure 2–1).

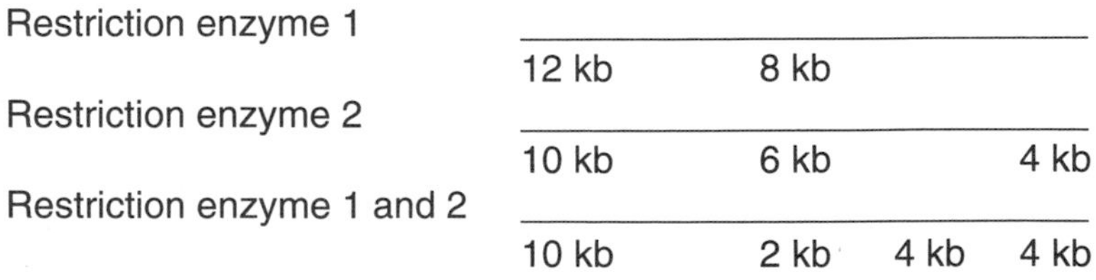

Restriction enzyme 1
_____
12 kb   8 kb

Restriction enzyme 2
_____
10 kb   6 kb   4 kb

Restriction enzyme 1 and 2
_____
10 kb   2 kb   4 kb   4 kb

Figure 2–1. Hypothetical restriction map of 20-kilobase DNA molecule. The map was constructed by use of two restriction enzymes, alone and in combination, resulting in different fragment lengths that indicate points of cleavage. See text for details.

For example, a 20-kilobase (kb) DNA molecule is cleaved into two fragments (12 and 8 kb) by one restriction enzyme (a single cleavage site). Cleavage of the same molecule with a second restriction enzyme (two cleavage sites) results in three fragments (10, 6, and 4 kb, respectively), indicating that DNA was cleaved at two sites. Simultaneous incubation of the molecule with both restriction enzymes results in two fragments of 10 and 2 kb, respectively, and two fragments of 4 kb. These patterns of cleavage suggest that the cleavage site for the first restriction enzyme occurs within the 6-kb fragment found with the second restriction enzyme and the linear arrangement of 10, 2, 4, and 4 kb, as shown in Figure 2–1.

Variations in the DNA base sequence (e.g., polymorphisms in the genome or mutation in the DNA recognition site) create or eliminate such recognition sites and lead to DNA fragments of varying lengths. Comparing such restriction maps for two different individuals gives restriction fragment length polymorphisms (RFLPs). These RFLPs behave as Mendelian traits and are, therefore, useful genetic markers. If the base change causing the polymorphism is in close proximity to the mutant gene, the polymorphism can be used to detect the disease gene. The advantage is that neither knowledge of the biochemical nature nor identification of the altered gene sequence responsible for the trait is necessary to locate the gene. Thus, mutations occurring in the regulatory domains of the gene can be mapped as well. The RFLP technique has led to the mapping of genes for cystic fibrosis and Huntington's disease.

Another important technological advance, the polymerase chain reaction (PCR), amplifies the DNA by chemical rather than biological proliferation and ensures an adequate amount of DNA for genetic analysis. Furthermore, PCR can amplify DNA obtained from frozen or fixed postmortem specimens as well as from tissue specimens mounted on slides, and thus may provide a source of DNA (otherwise unavailable) for linkage analysis from deceased relatives.

The PCR amplification of specific DNA segments from complex genomic DNA has simplified the study of sequence variation and transformed the way in which genetic analysis can be carried out. Recently, highly informative genetic markers have been developed that can detect multiple alleles. This contrasts with the RFLP technique in which genetic markers identifying RFLPs can detect only two alleles (the presence or absence of the recognition site). This latter method is called short tandem repeat (STR) polymorphism and is based on the variations in numbers of copies of a tandemly repeated DNA sequence of a few nucleotides. The most common STR polymorphism is the CA (cytosine, adenine) dinucleotide repeat. The CA repeats have numerous alleles and are randomly distributed in the genome making them ideal genetic markers for linkage studies. These repeats can be analysed by a method based on PCR.

Candidate Genes

The above linkage approach involves broad-based scanning of the entire genome, testing for linkage section by section. The goal is the eventual localization of disease genes. An alternative linkage strategy, and one that has been used with limited success in the study of neuropsychiatric disorders, is the study of a specific gene ("candidate" *gene*) that is suspected of involvement in a given disorder. Candidate genes from affected individuals can be cloned and sequenced to detect a genetic abnormality in the gene. Alternatively, and a much simpler approach, is to conduct linkage analysis of the candidate gene (based on normal variations in that region) to determine if the DNA around the gene is related to the presence or absence of disease. Examples of these genes include the dopamine receptor genes in schizophrenia and the beta-amyloid gene in Alzheimer's disease; the latter will be discussed later in this chapter.

Genetic Factors in Normal and Accelerated Aging

Cognitive Impairment With Advancing Age

The dementias represent the most frequent diagnoses in geriatric psychopathology. Rarely seen in those younger than 65 years, these disorders increase progressively with advancing age. One of the problems in the differential diagnosis of early dementia is the cognitive decline associated with normal aging. The forgetfulness of the elderly is proverbial, and decline in Wechsler Adult Intelligence Scale (WAIS; Wechsler 1981) scores is so pronounced that age-adjusted norms had to be developed. Impairment of memory that is more severe than that ordinarily seen in normal aging but that does not qualify for the diagnosis of dementia may belong in the diagnostic category of age-associated memory impairment (AAMI). Because not all older persons show either AAMI or other intellectual decline, the relationship between normal aging and mental decline requires further examination. If the pathophysiology of age-associated mental decline is similar to that of the dementias, our understanding of both is likely to be enhanced by insights gained from the study of the dementias. The geriatric psychiatrist needs to consider the mental changes associated with normal aging as well as AAMI in the differential diagnosis of dementia.

Community-dwelling elderly persons exhibit marked individual differences in memory and other cognitive functions—differences that are noticeable even among nonagenarians and centenarians. There is a paucity of data on genetic determinants of these individual differences and precise mechanisms have not as yet been defined. A longitudinal study of aging twins that antedated the modern era of molecular genetics indicated that in healthy MZ twins, similarities in cognitive functioning persist well into old age. To date, the relationship between age-related cognitive impairment and the dementias of old age remains obscure.

There is some evidence that even clinically asymptomatic cognitive decline is related to mortality. Although genes may play a significant role in determining human life span (e.g., the correlation between MZ twin partners for length of life is twice that seen in DZ pairs), their mechanisms of action and their relationship to cognitive decline have remained largely unexplored. By contrast, the role of genetic factors in premature aging is well established. Several of the progeria syndromes (accelerated aging) have been proposed as models of human aging. Among the classical progerias are Hutchinson-Gilford and Werner's syndromes, both of which are characterized by the premature aging of young individuals, making them look old and wizened. These progerias are genetic conditions with autosomal recessive inheritance. None of them results in an accelerated phenocopy of the entire aging process. An understanding of these disorders may facilitate our understanding of specific aspects of the aging process.

Hutchinson-Gilford syndrome is characterized by dwarfism and physical immaturity; affected individuals look like caricatures of the very old and wizened, with comparatively large heads. However, some features commonly associated with aging, such as tumors, cataracts, osteoporosis, and cognitive decline, are not increased. This syndrome has been described in all races and affects both sexes.

Werner's syndrome, first described in 1904, is associated with a characteristic and striking appearance: the face develops a tightly drawn and pinched expression with pseudoexophthalmos, a beak nose, protuberant teeth, and a recessive chin. Cataracts, hypogonadism, diabetes, and cancer often develop in these individuals. They look 20 to 30 years older than their chronological age, and their life span is shortened.

Although the premature aging seen in the progerias appears to spare mental functions, another genetic disorder, Down's syndrome, typically is closely associated with dementia. *Down's syndrome* is an autosomal disorder due primarily to an extra chromosome 21. The characteristic clinical findings include epicanthic folds, short neck, abnormal and low-set ears, brachycephaly, and hypotonia. Individuals with Down's syndrome appear older than their chronological age, with premature greying and hair loss, pigment deposition in skin, cataracts, and immune system changes. Infection, neurotransmitter abnormalities, endocrine dysfunction, and leukemia are increased in these patients. Down's syndrome has been of interest to those who are studying the genetics of aging as well as those studying dementia because persons with this syndrome who live beyond the age of 35 (and come to autopsy) have been found to exhibit the neuropathological lesions of senile plaques and neurofibrillary tangles that are characteristic of Alzheimer's disease, suggesting that the syndrome may be an appropriate model for the study of Alzheimer's disease. The clinical diagnosis of Alzheimer's disease in persons with Down's syndrome is complicated by the mental retardation, but a substantial proportion of these individuals (although not all of those with the neuropathological changes) do exhibit the clinical manifestations of Alzheimer's disease.

Both Werner's and Hutchinson-Gilford syndromes accelerate physical aging without clinical or neuropathological evidence of dementia or other typical histopathological changes of brain aging (e.g., changes in lipofuscin or amyloid). These conditions may entail greatly advanced aging of specific tissues such as vasculature or integument, other than the brain. Brain changes, by contrast, are appropriate for chronological age.

Cellular Aging Research

There is increasing evidence for genetically programmed cell death (i.e., cellular suicide). Developmental biologists have known that many cells must die in order for an embryo to mature normally—that, in fact, certain cells are programmed to die at certain points during development. Cells subject to programmed cell death exhibit a pattern of characteristic changes, referred to as *apoptosis*: the cells round up, the nuclear membrane breaks down, the chromatin condenses, the cellular membrane develops protuberances called "blebs," and the cells disintegrate.

The total number of genes that control programmed cell death is not known; however, researchers using the roundworm *Caenorhabditis elegans* are making progress toward elucidating the number of genes involved (Barinaga 1994). The advantages of studying *C. elegans* include a short life span (3-weeks, on average) and a total of a mere 1,090 cells (of which 131 die during development, leaving 959 cells in the adult)—characteristics that facilitate developmental biologists' attempts to trace cell lineages and to isolate mutants affecting life span. Two genes (ced-3 and ced-4) that cause cells to undergo programmed cell death have been identified; a programmed cell death protection gene (ced-9) has also been identified. When ced-9 is "on," it turns off ced-3 and ced-4 and cells survive. Conversely, in mutants in which the ced-9 gene has been inactivated, ced-3 and ced-4 are active, and cells undergo programmed cell death.

The applicability of findings in this simple model to the process in mammalian cells was recently clarified. When cloned and sequenced, the ced-9 gene was found to be 23% identical with the oncogene bcl-2, which has been shown to prevent apoptosis and extend B cell survival in living animals. Further, when bcl-2 was substituted for ced-9 in C. elegans, it was found that ced-9 mutants were prevented from committing suicide. Recently, it was found that ced-3 was similar to the protease interleukin-1 β–converting enzyme (ICE). When the ICE gene was transferred into rat cells, it induced cell death, but this cell death could be blocked by bcl-2 and by a cowpox virus gene (crmA), whose protein product inhibits the activity of ICE (Gagliardini et al. 1994). The results suggest that programmed cell death and other mechanisms that control it have been conserved in evolution from roundworms to humans. In a search for proteins that bind to the bcl-2 protein and help to protect cells from death, a protein called bax was identified (which is similar to bcl-2); bax contributes to cell death by altering the bcl-2:bax pair ratio, which determines whether a cell lives or dies. If bcl-2 is in excess, it binds bax as well as itself and the cell survives; if bax predominates, it binds all bcl-2 as well as itself and the cell dies. However, these two genes are not the only controllers of cell death. Knockout mice missing bcl-2 exhibit excessive cell death in some tissues (e.g., kidney and thymus), whereas in other tissues (e.g., nervous system), cells develop normally, suggesting that there are other cell death protection genes. Indeed, one candidate gene has been found that is related to bcl-2 and has been named bcl-x. This gene makes two proteins, a long form that protects cultured lymphocytes from death and a short form that seems to promote cell death. Continued research will uncover new pieces of the genetically programmed cell death puzzle. Programmed cell death may be involved in degenerative diseases of the brain, and inappropriate cell death may underlie the neuronal loss characteristic of dementias.

Genetics of Psychiatric Disorders of Old Age

The dramatic rise in life expectancy during this century has made it possible for a significant proportion of the population to reach an age at which degenerative diseases of the brain, particularly Alzheimer's disease, become common.

Alzheimer's Disease

Alzheimer's disease is the leading cause of dementia, affecting approximately 5% to 10% of those ages 65 and older. The prevalence of Alzheimer's disease increases significantly with age. Alzheimer's disease is a progressive and catastrophic neurodegenerative disorder of insidious onset, with impairment of memory, judgment, and other aspects of cognition and affect. Ultimately, there is physical deterioration with a gradual, relentless decline, usually leading to a severely debilitated state and death anywhere from 4 to 20 years after onset. The characteristic neuropathological lesions, first described in 1907 by Alois Alzheimer, are senile plaques and the neurofibrillary tangles. Senile plaques are complex structures consisting primarily of a core of abnormal aggregates of a small protein molecule known as beta-amyloid, surrounded by abnormal neurites, altered glial cells, and cellular debris. Neurofibrillary tangles are dense bundles of helically wound abnormal fibers composed of a modified form of a normally occurring neuronal protein, the microtubule-associated protein tau, and are found in the cytoplasm of neurons. Neither senile plaques nor neurofibrillary tangles alone are sufficient evidence on which to base a diagnosis of Alzheimer's disease, nor are they specific to this disease (they are known to occur in other chronic diseases of the brain, as well as in normal aging). Nonetheless, they have been considered pathognomonic when present with the appropriate clinical history.

Although the etiology of Alzheimer's disease is unclear, the current consensus is that advanced age, a positive family history of dementia, and the presence of apolipoprotein E allele 4 (*APOE-e4*) are risk factors for Alzheimer's disease, the second and third of which implicate a genetic component. In some families with a history of early-onset Alzheimer's disease (disease onset before age 60) and in multiple affected individuals, inheritance appears to be autosomal dominant with age-dependent penetrance. In other instances, several genes probably contribute to the etiology of Alzheimer's disease. Several factors have complicated the investigations of the genetics of Alzheimer's disease:

1. *The late age at onset of the disease.* Family members may die before or
   during the risk period, making it difficult to determine in any given
   individual whether the disease was genetically transmitted or a
   sporadic occurrence.
2. *The difficulty in getting an accurate clinical diagnosis.* Even when the
   most restrictive diagnostic criteria are used, 10% to 20% of patients
   who received a clinical diagnosis of Alzheimer's disease are judged to
   not have had the disease upon neuropathological examination at autopsy (Jarvik et al. 1995).
3. *The probability that the disease is genetically heterogeneous* (i.e., caused
   by different genes located on different chromosomes).

Family Studies

Evidence for the role of genetic factors in Alzheimer's disease has come from
a number of family studies. A survey of the world literature in 1985 located
a total of 13 studies (including cases of early and late onset) with information on familial risk for Alzheimer's disease (Matsuyama et al. 1985). The
risk for parents ranged from 1.5% to 34%, and that for siblings, from 2% to
20%. Data from eight studies also provided information on secondary cases:
113 out of 515 families (21.9%) reported at least one additional affected
family member. However, only 58 (11.3%) exhibited transmission through
two or more generations. Only one study, by a Swiss group, has provided
data for children; they were found to have a risk of approximately 4%.

The most likely genetic hypothesis is one of heterogeneity, with some
families exhibiting an autosomal dominant mode of inheritance and other
families exhibiting a pattern that supports a multifactorial model. Several
large family studies published since 1985 have reported a morbid risk
among first-degree relatives approaching 50% by the age of 90, which is
consistent with an autosomal dominant mode of inheritance. However,
the calculations of risk were based on a small number of individuals in the
oldest age groups, resulting in very large standard errors (the older the
age, the fewer individuals alive to be sampled). Segregation analysis of
Alzheimer's disease demonstrated familial patterns consistent with several possible modes of transmission, including an autosomal dominant
major gene, two or more major genes, and a polygenic background.

Twin Studies

Comparative studies of senescence in twins initiated by Kallmann and
colleagues in the 1940s provided the first data on Alzheimer's disease in

twins. To date, there have been reports on 50 MZ and 10 DZ twin pairs; overall concordance rates were 48% in MZ twin pairs and 30% in DZ twin pairs (Small et al. 1993). Although the small number of reported DZ twins precludes meaningful comparison of twin concordance rate between these two groups, the apparent discordance in half of the reported MZ twins argues in favor of significant nongenetic components in the etiology of Alzheimer's disease.

Early-Onset Alzheimer's Disease

Even though Alzheimer's disease is most prevalent among people over age 65 years, in a small percentage of patients the disease develops at an unusually young age, with some receiving the diagnosis in their 40s and 50s and some, even in their 30s. These cases are known as early-onset Alzheimer's disease, and various estimates place its frequency anywhere from 1% to 10% of Alzheimer's disease patients. As will be reviewed later in this section, molecular genetic evidence pointing to a genetic factor in the etiology of Alzheimer's disease has been obtained in families with a history of the early-onset form of this disease and with multiple affected individuals.

Amyloid gene studies. The central core of the senile plaques is amyloid, a 39– to 43–amino acid fragment known as the *beta-amyloid protein* (ßAP). It is derived by an abnormal protein-splitting process from a much larger, membrane-spanning glycoprotein, the *amyloid precursor protein* (APP). Thus, the APP gene was a candidate gene for Alzheimer's disease. Further, in light of the presence of Alzheimer's disease lesions in individuals with Down's syndrome, the search for the APP gene has focused on chromosome 21.

The APP gene has been identified as the site of mutations in some individuals with early-onset familial Alzheimer's disease (FAD). In 1991, a "missense" mutation resulting in a valine-to-isoleucine amino acid substitution at codon 717 was reported to cosegregate with the disease (in 2 of 17 early-onset FAD families), but this mutation was not found in unaffected family members (Goate et al. 1991). In subsequent studies by other investigators, several additional early-onset families were identified with the same amino acid substitution; two more families had other missense mutations at the same site (codon 717), one leading to a valine-to-glycine and the other to a valine-to-phenylalanine amino acid substitution. In addition, mutations at two adjacent codons (double mutation at codons 670 and 671) segregated with early-onset FAD in two related Swedish families

(Table 2–1; cf. review by Matsuyama [1995]). These mutations lie outside the ßAP domain of APP and may change the configuration of APP and facilitate abnormal cleavage of the amyloid protein, inducing increased formation and deposition of ßAP. Several hundred families, with both early- and late-onset Alzheimer's disease, have since been evaluated; it has been found that APP mutations are exceedingly rare and account for Alzheimer's disease in only a very small fraction of patients with early-onset FAD (Schellenberg et al. 1991).

Evidence that mutations within the APP gene may be the primary event initiating an illness has emerged from studies of other forms of amyloidosis that are not related to Alzheimer's disease (Table 2–1). For example, *hereditary cerebral hemorrhage with amyloidosis, Dutch type* (HCHWA-D) is a rare autosomal dominant condition that has been described in four families from two coastal villages in the Netherlands. HCHWA-D is characterized by recurrent intracerebral hemorrhages, caused by parenchymal deposits that resemble the immature plaques characteristically found in Alzheimer's disease and Down's syndrome, and results in severe disablement, mental impairment, and death between the ages of 45 and 65. The deposits have been shown to be composed of beta-amyloid protein. In 1990, a mutation in the APP gene was discovered, with the mutation leading to the substitution of glutamine for glutamate at codon 693 (Levy et al. 1990a). This mutation is in the ßAP domain. Recently, in another Dutch family, a mutation was reported in the adjacent codon, 692 (glycine substituted for alanine), that resulted in severe amyloid angiopathy and classical senile plaques (Hendriks et al. 1992). Interestingly, there is variable clinical expression in this family with family members presenting with either early-onset dementia or with recurrent cerebral hemorrhage. Exactly why these specific mutations lead to such severe cerebrovascular consequences is not clear. In addition, there are other syndromes with different forms of abnormal amyloid deposits. For example, *hereditary cerebral hemorrhage with amyloidosis, Icelandic type* (HCHWA-I) has been found in eight families in western Iceland. Like the Dutch variant, HCHWA-I is characterized by cerebral hemorrhages at a young age. However, in HCHWA-I, the amyloid deposit is not beta-amyloid; it is a variant of cystatin C, and the single amino acid substitution is leucine to glutamine (Ghiso et al. 1986). The gene for cystatin C is located on chromosome 20.

Another autosomal dominant form of systemic amyloidosis with central nervous system involvement, *familial amyloidosis of the Finnish type* (FAF), is characterized by extracelluar deposits of amyloid (especially in

Table 2–1. Point mutations in amyloidoses

Disease	Amyloid protein	Chromosome location	Abnormality
Alzheimer's disease	Beta-amyloid	21	Codon 717: Valine → isoleucine Valine → phenylalanine Valine → glycine Codons 670, 671[a]: Lysine → asparagine Methionine → leucine
Down's syndrome	Beta-amyloid	21	None detected
HCHWA-Dutch	Beta-amyloid	21	Codon 693: Glutamic acid → glutamine Codon 692: Alanine → glycine
HCHWA-Icelandic	Cystatin C	20	Leucine → glutamine
Familial amyloidosis of the Finnish type (FAF)	Gelsolin	9	Codon 187: Aspartic acid → asparagine
Transmissible dementias			
CJD	Prion	20	Codon 53: Octapeptide repeats: +2,4,5–9 Codon 178: Aspartic acid → asparagine Codon 200: Glutamic acid → lysine Codon 210: Valine → isoleucine
GSS	Prion	20	Codon 102: Proline → leucine Codon 117: Alanine → valine Codon 198: Phenylalanine → serine Codon 217: Glutamine → arginine

Note. HCHWA = hereditary cerebral hemorrhage with amyloidosis; CJD = Creutzfeldt-Jakob disease; GSS = Gerstmann-Sträussler-Scheinker disease.
[a]Double mutation.

the blood vessels and in the membranes of other tissues) and by clinical signs of polyneuropathy, the latter usually appearing after the third decade of life. The amyloid protein in FAF appears to be a variant of the protein gelsolin (the gene for which is on chromosome 9). A point mutation (G to A) at codon 187 results in an amino acid substitution of asparagine for aspartic acid (Haltia et al. 1990; Levy et al. 1990b).

Chromosome 21.   As mentioned above, chromosome 21 was an obvious candidate chromosome for study because of the well-known association between Down's syndrome and Alzheimer's disease, some evidence of which were reports of an increased frequency of Down's syndrome in families in which Alzheimer's disease occurs. In 1987, St. George-Hyslop and co-workers reported findings from a study of four families with early-onset Alzheimer's disease. Using molecular genetic techniques, the authors found preliminary evidence of positive linkage between a putative FAD gene and DNA markers on the proximal portion of chromosome 21. Both positive and negative results were obtained in subsequent linkage studies.

Chromosome 14.   In 1992, Schellenberg and co-workers reported evidence for another putative gene for early-onset FAD located on chromosome 14, three-quarters of the way down the long arm. Other groups have since confirmed linkage between early-onset FAD and chromosome 14. Families exhibiting linkage to chromosome 14 account for 70%–80% of early-onset familial cases. The early-onset FAD gene on choromosome 14 has been successfully cloned (Sherrington et al. 1995). DNA sequencing of this putative gene (S182) detected five different missense mutations in seven families. These mutations were present in Alzheimer's disease patients and some at-risk relatives but not in neurologically normal control subjects nor in asymptomatic family members (older by more than two standard deviations than the mean age at onset in their family). The gene appears to code for a transmembrane protein and may be involved in protein transport within cells or may be a receptor or channel protein.

There is another group of early-onset FAD patients, known as "Volga Germans." These families are descendants of Germans who settled along the Volga River in the 18th century and are thought to be genetically homogeneous with respect to FAD (Bird et al. 1988). The absence of linkage to either chromosome 21 or 14 in these patients suggests a third locus for early-onset AD.

Chromosome 1. In 1995, the gene for Alzheimer's disease in early-onset Volga Germans was localized to chromosome 1 (Levy-Lahad et al. 1995a), cloned, and sequenced. It is a homolog of the Alzheimer's disease gene on chromosome 14 (Levy-Lahad et al. 1995b) and, like S182, it has a seven-transmembrane domain; it is known as STM2 (second transmembrane gene associated with Alzheimer's disease). A missense mutation in codon 141 was found in affected individuals in five of seven families. Collectively, findings from the above studies have led to the conclusion that early-onset FAD is genetically heterogeneous.

Late-Onset Alzheimer's Disease

Chromosome 19. Although data on early-onset FAD have been rapidly accumulating, the majority of Alzheimer's disease patients (more than 75%) develop the disease after the age of 65. A group at Duke University led by Allen Roses reported evidence for linkage of late-onset FAD to chromosome 19 (Pericak-Vance et al. 1991) and, more recently, an association with the apolipoprotein E (APOE) locus (Corder et al. 1993). APOE has three major alleles: *APOE-e2, APOE-e3,* and *APOE-e4.* The *APOE-e3* allele is the most common, with more than 90% of the general population inheriting one copy, and around 60% inheriting two copies of the gene. By contrast, only about 30% in various control groups have at least one *APOE-e4* allele, compared with 80% of individuals with familial and 64% of individuals with sporadic late-onset Alzheimer's disease. Further, individuals with two copies of the *APOE-e4* allele are much more likely to manifest Alzheimer's disease, and they appear to develop it much earlier, than those who have no copies or one copy. The risk for Alzheimer's disease increased from 20% to 90% and mean age at onset decreased from 84 to 68 years with an increasing number of *APOE-e4* alleles. Homozygosity for *APOE-e4* was virtually sufficient to cause Alzheimer's disease by age 80. Since the initial report by Corder and co-workers, confirmation has been obtained by numerous other investigators in many different populations.

Recently, Small et al. (1995), in a positron emission tomography study of asymptomatic relatives at risk for familial Alzheimer's disease, reported significantly lower parietal metabolism and significantly higher left–right parietal asymmetry in those patients with compared with those patients without the *APOE-e4* allele. Patients with Alzheimer's disease had significantly lower parietal metabolism than at-risk relatives with *APOE-e4.* These results suggest an association of the *APOE-e4* allele with cerebral glucose metabolism in asymptomatic relatives at risk for Alzheimer's disease.

Other data support the direct involvement of *APOE-e4* in the pathogenesis of Alzheimer's disease (e.g., its product binds to beta-amyloid in the spinal fluid and, therefore, presumably in the brain). More recently, it was reported that *APOE-e4* has higher avidity in vitro for beta-amyloid than does the *APOE-e3* isoform, and that there is greater beta-amyloid staining evident in Alzheimer's disease patients with two *APOE-e4* alleles, as determined at autopsy, than in other Alzheimer's disease patients (Strittmatter et al. 1993). Thus, the *APOE-e4* gene variant appears to be the first genetic risk factor to have been identified for late-onset Alzheimer's disease; the only other general risk factors consistently associated with Alzheimer's disease have been age and a positive family history of dementia.

Roses and colleagues (Strittmatter et al. 1994) proposed that individuals with *APOE-e4* are at increased risk of Alzheimer's disease, not because of a deleterious effect of *APOE-e4*, but because of the absence of *APOE-e3*. The researchers suggest that *APOE-e3* stabilizes microtubules (protein filaments needed for normal neuronal functioning) by binding to tau, a microtubule-associated protein that is important in the polymerization and stabilization of microtubules and in maintaining cell integrity. Phosphorylation decreases the efficiency of tau, and hyperphosphorylated tau is the major constituent of the paired helical filaments that make up the neurofibrillary tangles. This hypothesis is provocative, partly because it reduces the role of ßAP, which many researchers believe causes the neurodegeneration in Alzheimer's disease. Roses' group believes that the beta-amyloid buildup in Alzheimer's disease is a side effect of the disorder, rather than a key to the disease. According to a recent report from the University of Washington (Jarvik et al. 1994), the risk of Alzheimer's disease for a given APOE genotype may be modified by non-APOE familial factors.

Multi-Infarct Dementia

Multi-infarct dementia, or vascular dementia (as referred to in DSM-IV [American Psychiatric Association 1994]), can be differentiated from Alzheimer's disease by its more sudden onset, focal neurological signs, patchy deterioration, and stepwise progressive decline in intellectual function. There is evidence to support a hereditary predisposition to this illness, and a few studies suggest an autosomal dominant mode of inheritance. However, it should be noted that the dementia is secondary to vascular disease, and vascular disease is related to environmental factors as well as to other conditions with genetic components (e.g., hypertension). Moreover, a substantial number of patients show the lesions of both vascular dementia and Alzheimer's disease further complicating the differential diagnosis.

Parkinson's Disease

Parkinson's disease is a movement disorder that usually begins in the fifth or sixth decade of life and is characterized by bradykinesia, muscular rigidity, tremor, and loss of postural reflexes. Patients with Parkinson's disease tend to have a significantly higher incidence of depression (often preceding any other symptoms) than do other physically disabled patients of similar age. Neuropathologically, there is neuronal loss, Lewy bodies in the substantia nigra, and a degeneration of dopaminergic tracts. Unfortunately, no satisfactory correlation has been found between the clinical symptoms and the neuropathological findings, and Parkinson's disease is not a well-defined nosologic entity. A substantial proportion of Parkinson's disease patients also have intellectual impairment. However, whether the dementia often associated with Parkinson's disease is due to Parkinson's disease or to the coexistence of Alzheimer's disease–type pathology continues to be the subject of research.

To confuse the issue even more, there is a separate clinical entity known as diffuse Lewy body disease (DLBD). Neuropathological findings in DLBD include subcortical and cortical Lewy bodies, cortical plaques, and, sometimes, occasional neurofibrillary tangles without either the marked neuronal loss or the severe brain atrophy characteristic of Alzheimer's disease. Clinically, DLBD is characterized by a combination of dementia with parkinsonian symptoms, mainly muscular rigidity. There are at least two forms of DLBD—common and pure—a classification made on the basis of neuropathological findings (Kosaka 1990). The pure form shows subcortical and cortical Lewy bodies without either senile plaques or neurofibrillary tangles. Clinically, patients with DLBD tend to show parkinsonian symptoms, sometimes tetraplegia; patients with this disease usually are young, and the male-to-female ratio is about 2:1. In the common form, numerous Lewy bodies are found in the cerebral cortex in combination with senile plaques and neurofibrillary tangles. Clinically, DLBD is characterized by memory deficit and psychotic symptoms at onset, average age at onset of 69, duration of approximately 6 years, and male predominance. Parkinsonian symptoms appear later in the course and are not found in all DLBD patients.

The role of genetic factors in the etiology of Parkinson's disease has been controversial, and, since 1983, the dominant hypothesis has been an environmental one, with the report that a simple pyridine derivative (*N*-methyl-4-phenyl-1,2,3,6-tetrahydropyridine, or MPTP) could simulate the syndrome. The environmental hypothesis was bolstered by the results of twin studies reporting 2.8% and 6.8% concordance rates for MZ and DZ twin pairs, respectively. Further, although family studies reported that approximately 15% of Parkinson's disease patients have an affected relative, the disease is common, with a lifetime incidence rate of 2.5%, and chance alone could account for this finding. In a critical review of family and twin studies, Golbe (1990) noted the shortcomings of the published studies, including possible diagnostic errors, no confirmation of secondary cases, and, as in most diseases of late onset, the lack of multigenerational data, all of which led him to suggest a reconsideration of the genetic hypothesis for Parkinson's disease. A subset of families in which Parkinson's disease occurs exhibit a transmission pattern consistent with an autosomal dominant pattern of inheritance with reduced penetrance and markedly age-related expression.

Patients with Parkinson's disease may exhibit a broad range of clinical manifestations that extend beyond those associated with the traditional concept of Parkinson's disease. A positron-emission tomography (PET) study of asymptomatic MZ and DZ co-twins reported increased concordance rates for nigral dysfunction in MZ compared with DZ twin pairs, providing new support for the existence of genetic factors in Parkinson's disease (Burn et al. 1990). Also, a number of pedigrees with autosomal dominant transmission of Lewy body parkinsonism have been described, all of which were confirmed histologically.

In most cases, Parkinson's disease is sporadic (non-familial), yet clinically and neuropathologically indistinguishable from the subset of familial Parkinson's disease cases described above. It is now hypothesized that the genetic factors in Parkinson's disease are susceptibility genes—that is, genes that increase an individual's susceptibility to environmental agents that lead to the clinical symptoms of Parkinson's disease. Molecular genetic approaches are being applied to locate Parkinson's disease susceptibility genes so that those individuals who are at high risk for Parkinson's disease can be identified. Further research may also expedite the identification of contributory environmental agents.

Huntington's Disease

Huntington's disease is a progressive neurodegenerative disorder of insidious onset (most often in the mid-30s) that is characterized by a gradual, progressive decline over 20 to 30 years until death. Age at onset varies, with reports of onset at ages under 20 as well as over 60, and early onset is often associated with more severe symptoms and a more rapid course. The disease is characterized clinically by choreiform movements (i.e., rapid, jerky, involuntary motions), dementia, and behavioral disturbances and neuropathologically by selective loss of neurons in the neostriatum. No effective treatment or means of prevention currently exists for this devastating disorder.

Huntington's disease exhibits an autosomal dominant pattern of inheritance with full penetrance. There is an equal probability of having inherited the Huntington's disease gene from the affected mother or father. A unique but currently unexplained feature of Huntington's disease is the influence of parental sex on age at onset. Children with juvenile onset almost always inherit the Huntington's disease gene from their father, and the later the onset of the disease, the more likely it is that maternal transmission occurred.

Reports of twins in the literature include 13 MZ twin pairs who were concordant for Huntington's disease, whereas only 1 of 5 DZ twin pairs was concordant. MZ twins had similar ages at onset, behavioral abnormalities, and clinical features, whereas DZ twins and siblings were dissimilar. No discordant MZ twin pairs have been reported.

In 1983, Huntington's disease became the first gene disorder to be linked to DNA markers on a chromosome using the molecular genetic technique of RFLPs with the result that the Huntington's disease gene was localized to the short arm of chromosome 4 (Gusella et al. 1983). Ten years later, an international research consortium formed to characterize the gene announced the successful cloning and sequencing of the gene (Huntington's Disease Collaborative Research Group 1993). At one end (5') of the gene were numerous repeats of a single trinucleotide sequence (CAG). The number of CAG repeats in the normal population varies between 6 and 37, whereas in Huntington's disease patients it ranges from 38 to 121. The number of repeats has been found to correlate with the age at onset and severity of the disease. Further, there is instability of the number of repeats during transmission, as successive generations reportedly show increasing numbers of repeats and the disease often appears earlier and with increased severity.

The nature of the Huntington's disease gene continues to remain elusive, but discovery of the gene increases the precision of presymptomatic testing of at-risk individuals. However, caution is warranted in light of a recent study of 1,022 affected individuals from 573 families in which 2.9%

($n = 30$) did not have the expanded trinucleotide repeat in the expected disease range (Andrew et al. 1994). In 10 (1.0%) the absence of this repeat was due to misdiagnosis; in 8 (0.8%), clerical error or sample mix-up; and in 12 (1.2%), to possible phenocopies for Huntington's disease (i.e., mutations in other genes presenting with a clinical phenotype similar to that of Huntington's disease). Thus, recent data suggest that genetic heterogeneity may underlie Huntington's disease despite the fact that it is a classic example of a human disease with clear autosomal dominant mode of transmission and complete penetrance.

Pick's Disease

Pick's disease is a rare presenile dementia. It is estimated that in the United States the ratio of Pick's disease to Alzheimer's disease diagnosis is 1:100. Pick's disease lasts for 2–10 years and is characterized by a progressive decline in memory and cognitive functioning. The clinical presentation has several similarities to that of Alzheimer's disease, including age at onset, slowly progressive course, and lack of focal neurological signs. Although early in its course Pick's disease can be differentiated from Alzheimer's disease by its characteristic pattern of personality changes and inappropriate social behavior, with relative absence of memory loss, later on it is difficult to distinguish from Alzheimer's disease. Final diagnosis rests on neuropathological examination and the presence of Pick bodies; senile plaques, neurofibrillary tangles, and granulovacuolar degeneration are usually not seen. Positron emission tomography studies indicate differences between Pick's disease and Alzheimer's disease, which may lead to more accurate in vivo diagnoses.

The largest systematic investigation on the heritable aspect of Pick's disease (Sjogren et al. 1952) reported an increased morbidity risk for parents (19%) and siblings (6.8%). The authors concluded that an autosomal dominant major gene with modifiers was the most likely mode of inheritance. In a longitudinal study of a single pedigree comprising six generations and including 25 patients with the clinical diagnosis of Pick's disease (14 autopsy confirmed) and 7 others in whom the diagnosis was considered likely, the findings were consistent with an autosomal dominant pattern of inheritance (Groen and Endtz 1982). Unfortunately, a thorough review of the literature by the above authors failed to find additional families, and the elucidation of the genetics of Pick's disease awaits systematic examinations of additional large families.

Transmissible Dementias

The transmissible dementias include kuru, Creutzfeldt-Jakob disease (CJD), and Gerstmann-Sträussler-Scheinker disease (GSS); these dementias exhibit clinical and neuropathological characteristics similar to those observed in scrapie, a transmissible neurodegenerative disease of goats and sheep. CJD and GSS are referred to collectively as *prion* (proteinaceous infectious agent) diseases and both have an infectious and a genetic component (Prusiner and Hsiao 1994). They are caused by a single common agent, a protease-resistant isoform of the prion protein (PrP). PrP is a normal brain constituent and is encoded by a gene (*PRNP*) located on the short arm of chromosome 20. Mutations found in the *PRNP* gene indicate that CJD and GSS are variants of one disease (see discussion below; also see Table 2–1). The prion diseases are of interest also in light of recent findings that some families with a clinical diagnosis of FAD actually have prion disease, with positive PrP and negative beta-amyloid staining of the amyloid plaques.

Creutzfeldt-Jakob disease. Creutzfeldt-Jakob disease is a rare disease (incidence of approximately 1 per 1,000,000) that usually manifests itself between the ages of 40 and 60. Two clinical types have been described: one characterized by rapidly progressing dementia, with death ensuing within 3 to 6 months, and the other characterized by a 1- or 2-year course (although there is one neuropathological confirmed report of an individual's having survived for 16 years). The first clinical symptoms may include dizziness, nervousness, vague physical complaints, apathy, irritability, confusion, and sometimes emotional lability, depression, or even psychotic symptoms. Eventually, most patients exhibit memory impairment and develop progressive dementia, cerebral ataxia, myoclonus, seizures, extrapyramidal signs, and involuntary movements. Pathological brain changes include spongiform encephalopathy with severe astrocytic gliosis. Neurofibrillary tangles and senile plaques characteristic of Alzheimer's disease are usually absent. However, in the 5% to 10% of CJD cases in which amyloid plaques are present, they appear stellate (similar to those seen in kuru) and they immunostain positive with the PrP antibody and negative with the beta-amyloid antibody.

Creutzfeldt-Jakob disease is usually sporadic, not familial, and there have been reports of unintentional iatrogenic disease transmission to humans via corneal transplants, administration of growth hormone, and neurosurgery. However, approximately 15% of CJD is familial, and pedigree studies suggest an autosomal mode of inheritance. In these cases, molecular genetic studies have focused on the *PRNP* gene and its protein product, PrP. Point mutations in the *PRNP* gene have been identified at codon 200 (lysine substituted for glutamine), at codon 210 (isoleucine instead of valine), at codon 53 (insertion of additional octapeptide repeats in the gene), and at codon 178 (asparagine instead of aspartic acid). Recently, the same mutation at codon 178 was also found in fatal familial insomnia (FFI), suggesting the possibility that a second genetic component modifies the expression of the codon 178 mutation. Indeed, DNA sequencing found that the coding region of *PRNP* has a polymorphism at codon 129 with two variant alleles, one coding for methionine and the other for valine, and that this determines the CJD (methionine) or FFI (valine) phenotype (Goldfarb et al. 1992). To date, no mutation in the *PRNP* gene has been demonstrated in sporadic cases.

Gerstmann-Sträussler-Scheinker disease.   Gerstmann-Sträussler-Scheinker disease is a very rare disease (incidence of 2–5 per 100 million) with mean age at onset of about 40 years (range = 19 to 66). Duration of illness prior to death ranges from 1 to 11 years and varies considerably within families. Two clinical forms of this disorder that have thus far been identified are *ataxic GSS*, in which cerebellar ataxia is the predominant feature and mild dementia develops later, and *dementing GSS*, in which patients present clinically with dementia, and pyramidal and parkinsonian symptoms and signs are predominant features. An atypical form of GSS, with dementia, ataxia, and parkinsonism, has also been described.

A distinctive neuropathological feature in GSS is the large number of unusual unicentric and multicentric amyloid plaques in the cerebrum and cerebellum (with few or no neurofibrillary tangles). The amyloid plaques are morphologically distinct from those observed in Alzheimer's disease, kuru, and CJD; they are immunoreactive with the PrP antibody, but not with the beta-amyloid antibody of Alzheimer's disease. However, neurofibrillary tangles, when present, are similar to those seen in Alzheimer's disease.

Gerstmann-Sträussler-Scheinker disease is usually familial, and transmission is consistent with an autosomal dominant mode of inheritance. As in CJD, molecular genetic studies have focused on the *PRNP* gene and its protein product. Point mutations in the *PRNP* gene in GSS are different from those found in CJD. They have been detected at codon 102 (ataxic GSS), codons 117 and 217 (dementing GSS), and codon 198 (atypical form), suggesting genetic heterogeneity in GSS. The demonstration of significant genetic linkage between the PrP codon 102 missense variant and the GSS phenotype strengthens the hypothesis of a causal relationship between PrP and the disease and suggests that the familial forms of prion disease are inherited.

Psychiatric Disorders in the Elderly (Nondementia)

Schizophrenia

Schizophrenia is a progressive mental disorder associated with disorganization of thought processes, delusions, hallucinations, and blunted affect and characterized by severe impairment of functioning. Evidence clearly indicates that genetic factors play a role in the development of schizophrenia; however, there also are important environmental contributions (Prescott and Gottesman 1993). In all likelihood, schizophrenia is not a single disease but, rather, comprises a group of disorders; genetic factors may play a more important role in some of these disorders than in others. Some researchers use the term "schizophrenia spectrum disorders" for conditions that do not meet all of the criteria for schizophrenia.

Systematic investigation of the genetic contribution to schizophrenia has been based on family, twin, and adoption studies. Family studies have shown an increased risk for schizophrenia in relatives of individuals with schizophrenia as compared with the general population: the risk for stepsiblings of a proband is the same as that for the general population, 0.35% to 2.85%; the risk for parents is 4% to 6%; for siblings, 10%; for children with one schizophrenic parent, 11% to 13%; and for children of two schizophrenic parents, 35% to 46%. Late-onset schizophrenia (i.e., onset after the age of 40 to 45) is characterized by a high female-to-male ratio, paranoid symptomatology, schizoid or paranoid traits in premorbid personality, and a tendency toward chronicity. A survey of family studies of late-onset schizophrenia (Harris and Jeste 1988) reported a combined mean prevalence of 7.2% in siblings and 2.9% in parents, prevalences that are slightly higher than those in the general population but lower than those for early-onset schizophrenia.

A clinical observation in one family linking schizophrenia and physical anomalies and subsequent cytogenetic analyses revealing a partial trisomy of chromosome 5 (i.e., an extra segment of chromosome 5 was inserted into chromosome 1) suggested this site on chromosome 5 as a candidate region for further linkage studies. Subsequent molecular genetic studies reported both positive and negative evidence for linkage to chromosome 5.

Recent data with additional markers and reanalysis of the earlier data do not provide evidence for the presence of a susceptibility gene for schizophrenia on chromosome 5.

Dopamine receptors and the limbic system are hypothesized to play an etiological role in schizophrenia. Genes for five dopamine receptors (D_1, D_2, D_3, D_4, and D_5) have been cloned and mapped to chromosome 11. These were obvious candidate genes to test for linkage to schizophrenia in families with multiple affected individuals. To date, no evidence for a susceptibility gene for schizophrenia on chromosome 11 has been obtained. Attempts to show linkage to other chromosomal regions have also been largely unsuccessful.

One cannot exclude the possibility that the absence of precise and reliable criteria for the diagnosis of schizophrenia has compromised the findings from these studies. At the moment, a major gene cannot explain the transmission of schizophrenia, but the possibility of such a gene's operating together with polygenic or familial environmental effects cannot be excluded, and the search for the schizophrenia gene(s) continues.

Mood Disorders

There are two major forms of mood disorders: unipolar and bipolar. Unipolar (or pure depressive) disorder may include single or recurrent episodes of depression, whereas bipolar (or manic depressive) disorder is associated with episodes of both depression and mania in the same patient. Two subtypes of bipolar disorder are bipolar I, depression with mania, and bipolar II, depression with hypomania.

Family studies have shown a higher incidence of unipolar and bipolar disorders in first-degree relatives of probands with unipolar and bipolar disorders compared with families of control subjects. Unipolar disorder is the most frequently diagnosed mood disorder in families of both bipolar and unipolar patients, suggesting a genetic overlap. However, the risk of bipolar disease is much higher in the relatives of bipolar patients. The overall morbidity risk for a mood disorder in relatives of probands with unipolar disorder is about 13% for parents, 15% for siblings, and 21% for children. The genetic component in bipolar disorder is even stronger: the morbidity risk for a mood disorder is about 22% for parents, 25% for siblings, 27% for children having one parent with bipolar disorder, and 50% to 75% for children whose parents both have a bipolar disorder.

The marked difference in concordance for mood disorders between MZ and DZ twins argues for heritability. In a study utilizing the Danish

Twin Registry, the concordance rate for bipolar disorder in MZ twins was 67% and in DZ twins, 20%, findings that are in agreement with other twin studies. The concordance rate was higher for bipolar (79%) than for unipolar (54%) MZ twin pairs, whereas the rates for these disorders were similar in DZ twin pairs (24% for bipolar and 19% for unipolar). Unipolar MZ twin pairs with three or more depressive episodes had 59% concordance, and unipolar MZ twin pairs with fewer than three depressive episodes had 33% concordance. Adoption studies also support the concept of a genetic basis for the aggregation of mood disorders in families. The prevalence of mood disorders in the biological relatives is higher than in the adoptive relatives of an affected individual. In one study of bipolar adoptees, mood disorders were found in 31% of biological parents of these probands, as compared with 2% in the biological parents of normal adoptees.

The exact mode of transmission of mood disorders remains unclear, although multifactorial and single-locus models have been widely tested. In one study (Gershon et al. 1982), investigators found a multifactorial model that fit the rates of illness in relatives of patients with mood disorders, but other authors have been unable to confirm this model. Most simple Mendelian single-locus models do not fit the existing data on familial prevalence of mood disorders. However, some studies have reported linkage of bipolar disease to color vision and blood group markers on the X chromosome. A recent study using DNA markers from the tip of the X chromosome (the Xq28 region) did not provide compelling evidence for linkage, but also did not rule out X linkage completely (Baron et al. 1993). Significant evidence for genetic linkage of bipolar disease with DNA markers at the tip of the short arm of chromosome 11 was reported in a large Old Order Amish kindred (Egeland et al. 1987). However, follow-up of family members and reanalysis failed to yield statistically significant evidence for a bipolar gene on chromosome 11. A recent report indicated that a gene predisposing to bipolar disorder in some families may be located on chromosome 18 (Berretini et al. 1994). The search for the gene(s) responsible for bipolar disease continues.

Schizoaffective Disorder

Patients with schizoaffective disorder exhibit symptoms of both schizophrenia and mood disorder. Several studies have shown that first-degree relatives of patients with schizoaffective illness tend to have a higher incidence of affective illness, particularly bipolar disorder, than schizophrenia. According to one report (Mendlewicz et al. 1980), the morbid risk for relatives of schizoaffective probands was 34.6% for mood disorder and 10.8% for schizophrenia. Gershon and colleagues' (1982) study of first-degree relatives of probands with schizoaffective disorder found that the morbid risk was 6.2% for schizoaffective disorder, 10.7% for bipolar I disorder, 6.1% for bipolar II disorder, and 14.5% for unipolar disorder, but only 3.6% for schizophrenia. Relatives of probands with schizoaffective disorder had the highest overall morbid risk for affective disorder in comparison with other proband groups (i.e., bipolar I, bipolar II, and unipolar depression). The probands with schizoaffective disorder also had more first-degree relatives with schizophrenia than did the other probands; however, the ratio of affective to schizophrenic disorders among these relatives was greater than 10:1. This suggests that schizoaffective disorder is related to both mood disorders and schizophrenia. Subsequent studies failed to find an increased prevalence of schizophrenia among the relatives of probands with schizoaffective disorder, bipolar type; however, the relative sof patients with schizoaffective disorder, depressive type, may be at higher risk for schizophrenia than for a mood disorder (Maj et al. 1991, Tsuang 1991). Further clarifiation is needed.

Anxiety Disorders

Anxiety disorders present serious problems in geriatric populations; however, accurate data on incidence and prevalence are lacking for the elderly. Data suggest a genetic contribution to the etiology of most anxiety disorders. Obsessive-compulsive disorder, agoraphobia, and specific and social phobias all demonstrate familial aggregation and appear to result from a combination of genetic and individual-specific environmental etiological factors. Panic disorder is much more prevalent among first-degree relatives of probands with this disorder (17%) than among control subjects without panic attacks (4%) (Kushner et al. 1992); however, panic disorder is relatively rare among the elderly. The heritability of the predisposition to phobias ranged from 30% to 40% in 2,163 female twins from a population-based registry (Kendler et al. 1992b). No epidemiological data on late-onset anxiety disorders or on genetic differences between early- and late-onset anxiety are available. There is as yet no candidate gene.

Alcohol and Substance Abuse

Alcohol and substance abuse, although less prevalent than among younger adults, do account for increased morbidity and mortality among the elderly.

In a recent study, Moos et al. (1994) reported mortality rates among late middle-aged and older (55+) substance abuse patients ($n = 21,139$) to be 2.64 times higher than expected. Family, twin, and adoption studies indicate a genetic component in alcoholism. Among adopted children born to parents of whom at least one was alcoholic, 20% were found to have manifested alcoholism before age 30 years, compared with 5% of adopted children born to nonalcoholic parents. A population-based twin study of alcoholism in women reported heritability of liability to alcoholism to be in the range of 50% to 60%, suggesting a major role for genetic factors (Kendler et al. 1992a). No data are available regarding the genetic contribution to late-onset substance abuse, including alcoholism, in comparison with that to early-onset disorder.

The reported association between the D_2 dopamine receptor (*DRD2*) allele *A1* and alcoholism remains controversial (Baron 1993). Interpretation of the existing data is difficult for numerous reasons, including the absence of agreed-upon criteria for alcoholic subtypes and measures of severity. Linkage studies have yielded negative results.

Summary

Family, twin, and adoption studies have provided evidence for genetic determinants in a variety of neuropsychiatric disorders that present in the elderly. The application of molecular genetic techniques has led to rapid and efficient screening of the genome for linkage. However, the linkage studies to date are based on small numbers of families and must be considered preliminary until follow-up data are obtained and additional families studied. Indeed, initial reports of linkage in some neuropsychiatric disorders (e.g., Alzheimer's disease, schizophrenia, and bipolar disorder) could not be confirmed. This inability to confirm these initial findings in subsequent studies can be attributed to new illness onset in previously unaffected family members as well as the application of more informative DNA markers. The dramatic successes of molecular genetics promise gene identification and the hornet's nest of ethical issues associated with reliable predictive presymptomatic testing (i.e., whether to offer testing and when, whom to test, and how to interpret the findings). Further, there is the expectation that dramatic breakthroughs in gene-based treatments of mental disorders are about to emerge. We tend to forget that there is a long road from enhanced understanding to effective treatment. Nonetheless, molecular genetic techniques are state-of-the-art and offer new hope to concerned relatives, basic scientists, and clinicians for increased understanding of geriatric psychiatry.

References

American Psychiatric Association: Diagnostic and Statistical Manual of Mental Disorders, 4th Edition. Washington, DC, American Psychiatric Association, 1994

Andrew SE, Goldberg YP, Kremer B, et al: Huntington disease without CAG expansion: phenocopies or errors in assignment? Am J Hum Genet 54:852–863, 1994

Barinaga M: Cell suicide: by ICE, not fire [Research News]. Science 263:754–756, 1994

Baron M: The D_2 dopamine receptor gene and alcoholism: a tempest in a wine cup (editorial)? Biol Psychiatry 34:821–823, 1993

Baron M, Freimer NF, Risch N, et al: Diminished support for linkage between manic depressive illness and X-chromosome markers in three Israeli pedigrees. Nat Genet 3:49–55, 1993

Berretini WH, Ferraro TN, Goldin LF, et al: Chromosome 18 DNA marker and manic-depressive illness: evidence for a susceptibility gene. Proc Natl Acad Sci U S A 91:5918–5921, 1994

Bird TD, Lampe TH, Nemens EJ, et al: Familial Alzheimer's disease in American descendants of the Volga Germans: probable genetic founder effect. Ann Neurol 23:24–31, 1988

Burn DJ, Mark MH, Playford ED, et al: Parkinson's disease in twins studied with ^{18}F-dopa and positron emission tomography. Neurology 42:1894–1900, 1990

Corder EH, Saunders AM, Strittmatter WJ, et al: Gene dose of apolipoprotein E type 4 allele and the risk of Alzheimer's disease in late onset families. Science 261:921–923, 1993

Egeland JE, Gerhard D, Pauls D, et al: Bipolar affective disorder linked to DNA markers on chromosome 11. Nature 235:783–787, 1987

Gagliardini V, Fernandez P-A, Lee RKK, et al: Prevention of vertebrate neuronal death by the crmA gene. Science 263:826–828, 1994

Gershon ES, Hamovit J, Guroff JJ, et al: A family study of schizoaffective, bipolar I, bipolar II, unipolar, and normal control probands. Arch Gen Psychiatry 39:1157–1167, 1982

Ghiso J, Jensson O, Frangione B: Amyloid fibrils in hereditary cerebral hemorrhage with amyloidosis of Icelandic type is a variant of γ-trace basic protein (cystatin C). Proc Natl Acad Sci U S A 83:2974–2978, 1986

Goate A, Chartier-Harlin MC, Mullan M, et al: Segregation of a missense mutation in the amyloid precursor protein gene with familial Alzheimer's disease. Nature 349:704–706, 1991

Golbe LI: The genetics of Parkinson's disease: a reconsideration. Neurology 40:7–14, 1990

Goldfarb LG, Petersen RB, Tabaton M, et al: Fatal familial insomnia and familial Creutzfeldt-Jakob disease: disease phenotype determined by a DNA polymorphism. Science 258:806–808, 1992

Groen JJ, Endtz LJ: Hereditary Pick's disease: second reexamination of a large family and discussion of other hereditary cases, with particular reference to electroencephalography and computerized tomography. Brain 105:443–459, 1982

Gusella JF, Wexler NS, Conneally PM, et al: A polymorphic marker genetically linked to Huntington's disease. Nature 306:234–238, 1983

Haltia M, Prelli F, Ghiso J, et al: Amyloid protein in familial amyloidosis (Finnish type) is homologous to gelsolin, an actin-binding protein. Biochem Biophys Res Commun 167:927–932, 1990

Harris MJ, Jeste DV: Late-onset schizophrenia: an overview. Schizophr Bull 14:39–55, 1988

Hendriks L, VanDuijn CM, Cras P, et al: Presenile dementia and cerebral hemorrhage linked to a mutation at codon 692 of the β-amyloid precursor protein gene. Nat Genet 1:218–221, 1992

Huntington's Disease Collaborative Research Group: A novel gene containing a trinucleotide repeat that is expanded and unstable on Huntington's disease chromosomes. Cell 72:971–983, 1993

Jarvik G, Goddard K, Kukull W, et al: ApoE and non-apoe genetic effects in Alzheimer disease (AD). Genet Epidemiol 11:298, 1994

Kendler KS, Heath AC, Neale MC, et al: A population-based twin study of alcoholism in women. JAMA 268:1877–1882, 1992a

Kendler KS, Neale MC, Kessler RS, et al: Generalized anxiety disorder in women. Arch Gen Psychiatry 49:267–272, 1992b

Kosaka K: Diffuse Lewy body disease in Japan. J Neurol 237:197-204, 1990

Kushner MG, Thomas AM, Bartels K, Beitman BD: Panic disorder history in the families of patients with angiographically normal coronary arteries. Am J Psychiatry 149:1563–1567, 1992

Levy E, Carman MD, Fernandez-Madrid IJ, et al: Mutation of the Alzheimer's disease amyloid gene in hereditary cerebral hemorrhage, Dutch type. Science 248:1124–1126, 1990a

Levy E, Haltia M, Fernandez-Madrid IJ, et al: Mutation in gelsolin gene in

Finnish hereditary amyloidosis. J Exp Med 172:1865–1867, 1990b

Levy-Lahad E, Wijsman E, Nemens E, et al: A familial Alzheimer's disease locus on chromosome 1. Science 269:970–973, 1995a

Levy-Lahad E, Wasco W, Poorkaj P, et al: Candidate gene for the chromosome 1 familial Alzheimer's disease locus. Science 269:973–977, 1995b

Maj M, Starace F, Pirossi R: A family study of DSM-III-R schizoaffective disorder, depressive type, compared with schizophrenia and psychotic and non-psychotic major depression. Am J Psychiatry 148:612–616, 1991

Matsuyama SS: Genetics of geriatric psychopathology, in Comprehensive Textbook of Psychiatry/VI, 6th Edition, Vol 2. Edited by Kaplan HI, Sadock BJ. Baltimore, MD, Williams & Wilkins, 1995, pp 2519–2527

Matsuyama SS, Jarvik LF, Kumar V: Dementia: genetics, in Recent Advances in Psychogeriatrics. Edited by Arie T. New York, Churchill Livingstone, 1985, pp 45–69

Mendlewicz J, Linkwosky P, Wilmotte J: Relationship between schizoaffective illness and affective disorders or schizophrenia: morbidity risk and genetic transmission. J Affec Disord 2:289–302, 1980

Moos RH, Brennan PL, Mertens JR: Mortality rates and predictors of mortality among late- middle-aged and older substance abuse patients. Alcohol Clin Exp Res 18:187–195, 1994

Nowak R: Mining treasures from "junk DNA" [Research News]. Science 263:608–610, 1994

Pericak-Vance MA, Bebout JL, Gaskell PC Jr, et al: Linkage studies in familial Alzheimer disease: evidence for chromosome 19 linkage. Am J Hum Genet 48:1034–1050, 1991

Prescott CA, Gottesman II: Genetically mediated vulnerability to schizophrenia. Psychiatr Clin North Am 16:245–267, 1993

Prusiner SB, Hsiao KK: Human prion diseases. Ann Neurol 35:285–295, 1994

Schellenberg GD, Anderson L, O'Dahl S, et al: APP_{717}, APP_{693}, and PRIP gene mutations are rare in Alzheimer disease. Am J Hum Genet 49:511–517, 1991

Schellenberg GD, Bird TD, Wijsman EM, et al: Genetic linkage evidence for a familial Alzheimer's disease locus on chromosome 14. Science 258:668–671, 1992

Sherrington R, Rogaev El, Liang Y, et al: Cloning of a gene bearing missense mutations in early-onset familial Alzheimer's disease. Nature 375:754–761, 1995

Sjogren T, Sjogren H, Lindgren AGH: Morbus Alzheimer and Morbus Pick: genetic, clinical and patho-anatomical study. Acta Psychiatria of Neurologica Scandinavica Supplementum 82:1–152, 1952

Small GW, Leuchter A, Mandelkern M, et al: Clinical, neuroimaging, and environmental risk differences in monozygotic female twins appearing discordant for dementia of the Alzheimer type. Arch Neurol 50:209–219, 1993

Small GW, Mazziotta JC, Collins MT, et al: Apolipoprotein E type 4 allele and cerebral glucose metablism in relatives at risk for familial Alzheimer disease. JAMA 273:942–947, 1995

St George-Hyslop PH, Tanzi RE, Polinsky R, et al: The genetic defect causing familial Alzheimer's disease maps on chromosome 21. Science 235:885–890, 1987

Strittmatter WJ, Saunders AM, Schmechel DE, et al: Apolipoprotein E: high-avidity binding to β-amyloid and increased frequency of type 4 allele in late-onset familial Alzheimer disease. Proc Natl Acad Sci U S A 90:1977–1981, 1993

Strittmatter WJ, Weisgraber KH, Goedert M, et al: Hypothesis: microtubule instability and paired helical filament formation in Alzheimer disease brain are related to apolipoprotein E genotype. Exp Neurol 125:163–171, 1994

Tsuang MT: Morbidity risks of schizophrenia and affective disorders among first-degree relatives of patients with schizoaffective disorders. Br J Psychiatry 158:165–170, 1991

Wallace DC: Mitochondrial genetics: a paradigm for aging and degenerative diseases? Science 256:628–632, 1992

Wechsler D: Wechsler Adult Intelligence Scale–Revised. San Antonio, TX, Psychological Corporation, 1987

C H A P T E R   3

Elaine A. Leventhal, M.D., Ph.D.

Biology of Aging

M any theories have been advanced to account for normal aging, and although none has gained wide acceptance, most investigators agree on some generalizations. Growth, development, and senescence are the essences of biology; they are not static stages in a natural history but represent the continuously changing processes of the life cycle. Normal aging or senescence is associated with declines in numbers of active metabolic cells, receptor numbers and affinities, and decrements in the regulation of cellular functions. Deterioration in overall reserve and declining ability to respond to stress and recover from illnesses represent losses in regenerative ability and degeneration in function that result eventually in death.

We can think of human aging in terms of multiple biological clocks that start to tick at conception and stop at death. Most cell proliferation peaks around birth, and virtually all growth ceases at puberty. A fraction of prenatal mitotic activity maintains homeostasis in the adult and allows response at times of heightened physiological demand caused by injury, infection, or other stress insults. For some tissues (e.g., the ovary), the aging clock starts in utero. Even though the fetal period is when the most dramatic growth and cell division occurs, it is also the time of greatest cell loss. Thus, the neonate ovary will contain one thousandth of the oocytes that initially populate the fetal gonad. When growth stops, normal aging begins. It is characterized by different, stem cell– and gender-specific rates of decline that translate into loss of replicative and repair ability. It is the innate biological plasticity and lifelong adaptive history that allows for personalized accommodation to changes in the regulation system of the body. Aging produces increasing heterogeneity among individuals.

The emotional and behavioral components of illness become as atypical in their presentation in the aging individual as the physical manifestations of illnesses. Therefore, it is important for the psychiatrist to understand the changes that lead to senescence and how these processes may determine how people behave as they age. The biological phenomena associated with caducity need to be understood to appreciate the degree of heterogeneity that is seen in clinical practice and to learn how to treat age-related behavioral changes that occur in both illness presentation and in the behaviors associated with illness and frailty. The examples here have been selected because of their relevance for clinical practice.

General Aging

How a person ages physically and psychologically reflects his or her unique biology—the genetic predispositions or relative invulnerability to certain chronic illnesses superimposed on individual biological clocks. It also is the effect of the external environment; exposure to trauma, infections, past diseases, and behaviors; and the health and illness practices that the individual has adopted during life.

As noted above, in biological senescence, there is a loss of cells and changes occur in many of the enzymatic activities within cells. Most enzymatic syntheses continue, although some rates of production and clearance may decline. In addition, a diminution may occur in receptor number or affinity for transmitters. The aging individual may be unable to respond to the demands for increased activity. Of the organ systems, the normal kidney, lung, and the skin age more rapidly than the heart and liver in both sexes, and the musculoskeletal system and the gonads become atrophic at different times during the life of men and women (Finch and Schneider 1985; Kenney 1989).

Age-related changes occur in body composition with up to an 80% decrease in muscle mass and an average 35% increase and a significant redistribution of body fat. Fat deposition accumulates around and within the viscera, whereas a loss of fat occurs on the surface. Thus, older people lose "insulation" and are more sensitive to extremes of ambient temperature than younger people (Kenney 1989).

Skin

The aging that occurs in the skin reflects genetically determined changes in physical structure, environmental exposures, and behaviors during life. Significant racial differences have been noted in the aging of the integument, with slower changes in the collagenous and elastic tissues seen in nonwhites. The skin atrophies with loss of the subcutaneous cushion of fat and the shrinkage of dermal appendages. There are fewer blood vessels in the skin, and the rate of healing slows. Elastin, the structural element responsible for the stretch in tissues, fragments with age. However, not all age-related changes represent cell or tissue loss or deterioration. Collagen accumulates, as evidenced by increased interstitial matrix formation. Wrinkles show the effects of age-related changes in elastin and collagen. Sun exposure accelerates fragmentation of skin elastin and contributes to increased collagen deposition. In whites, accompanying the lifetime accumulation of the effects of solar exposure, a loss of melanocytes occurs, leading to a decrease in pigmentation in the skin and increased vulnerability of the older person to further sun damage. People with prolonged tanning exposure have more wrinkles at earlier ages and a greater incidence of malignancies related to solar damage (Kligman et al. 1985).

Cardiovascular System

The age-related decline in the cardiovascular system has been thought to be the major determinant of decreased exercise tolerance and the resultant loss of conditioning and thus the major factor contributing to feelings of old age and decline in physical strength. However, more than heart and blood vessel deterioration is involved in the loss of energy reserve. There is a dependence as well on interactions between the musculoskeletal, pulmonary, and cardiovascular systems and on activity level and lifestyle. The biological complexities of these relationships become apparent when one examines the aging and gender differences in these particular organ systems.

In the heart, changes occur in the chambers, blood vessels, and valves. The ventricular myocardium and endocardial linings thicken, the ventricular cavities become smaller, and the amount of blood pumped per contraction decreases. An age-related rise in both systolic and diastolic blood pressure occurs that most likely reflects a reduction in aortic and arterial compliance (Cody et al. 1989). Heart rate slows. Studies of aging animals suggest that there are changes in extra-neuronal uptake mechanisms. In addition, presynaptic α_2-adrenoreceptor–mediated auto-regulation of norepinephrine decreases with age (Daly et al. 1989). The resulting physiological effects would be reflected in decreased adrenergic system control of cardiac function, decreased adaptation to stress, and increased epinephrine release into the plasma. Plasma epinephrine increases with age (Ziegler et al. 1976). Recent published findings indicate that this increase in epinephrine is most likely to reflect altered receptor sensitivity rather than an increase in transmitter release. Hypotheses to explain the decrease in heart rate suggest that downregulation or decreased responsiveness of adrenergic receptors on heart muscle occurs with age and that the catecholamine content of the heart declines because of decreases in receptor availability (Martinez et al. 1981; Mazzeo and Horvath 1987; Rappaport et al. 1981). Evidence also exists that baroreceptor modulation of heart rate diminishes.

To elucidate further the role of adrenergic function in humans, adrenergic receptivity has been studied in noncardiac tissues, namely lymphocyte membranes, where β-receptors are numerous and can be used as surrogates for β-receptor activity in other systems including cardiovascular structures. Receptor–binding site densities were increased in elderly individuals compared with younger subjects, but function, as reflected by both basal and stimulated adenosine 3', 5'-cyclic monophosphate (cAMP) generation, was lower in the older group. These studies support the hypothesis that receptor responsiveness is not the result of downregulation of receptor density but rather that the receptor numbers are increased with the deficit occurring in the regulatory mechanism that attempts to maintain cAMP levels (Gietzen et al. 1991). These anatomic, including neurohumoral, changes in the vascular system affect function by causing declines in cardiac output and a decrease in response to work demands (Lakatta 1987; Morley and Reese 1989; Rodeheffer et al. 1984; Simpson and Wicks 1988). Regular physical activity is associated with higher levels of plasma epinephrine and norepinephrine. This suggests that regular exercise acts to activate resting sympathetic nervous system tone. Note that the highest levels of norepinephrine are seen in fit elderly men. With alterations in lifestyle accompanying loss of fitness and weight gain, less norepinephrine may be available. This may be compatible with observations that aging organisms are less capable of making homeostatic adjustments in the absence of physiological stressors such as exercise (Poehlman et al. 1990).

Blood vessels narrow as endothelial linings thicken, and smooth muscle mass declines. Calcium may be deposited in vessel walls if intimal damage or medial necrosis is present. Thus, the blood vessels become more rigid, contributing to the slow elevation in blood pressure seen over time. In the absence of cardiovascular or renal disease, this may never reach the pathological range and an individual can be very old without hypertensive disease. When coronary artery disease is present along with normal cardiac aging, function is further compromised.

Women appear to have a slower rate of progression of arteriosclerotic disease before menopause while exposed to circulating estrogens. This advantage is reflected in the lower incidence of coronary artery disease in premenopausal women (National Center for Health Statistics 1982).

Respiratory System

The aging changes in the cardiovascular system are mirrored by the more rapid rate of functional decline in the respiratory system. All parts of the pulmonary system age, including lung tissue as well as the muscles, ribs, and vertebral column of the thoracic cage. There is less work capacity as skeletal muscles of the chest wall (along with smooth muscles in bronchi, diaphragm, and chest wall) weaken; collagen is deposited and elastin becomes fragmented. In women, the more rapid aging of the skeleton and the greater loss of muscle mass are important because of diminished exercise capacity and because of the greater vulnerability of women to fractures and possible immobilization.

The most common form of loss of bone mass, or osteopenia, is calcium demineralization, or osteoporosis. Osteoporosis can be especially prominent in the vertebral column of women, affecting posture and respiratory function. If the thoracic cage becomes smaller because of fractures of osteoporotic vertebrae, a decrease in chest capacity and thus in pulmonary function occurs. The bony changes will be discussed further in the section "Evaluation and Diagnosis." Within the lung, the alveolar septae are critical as the exchange sites for the gases oxygen and carbon dioxide. The lungs of older individuals have scattered areas of fibrosis or disruptions in the septae that interfere with gaseous exchange (Kenney 1989). These manifestations of "senile" emphysema may limit the amount of exercise and energy that can be expended even more than functional changes in the cardiovascular system described previously.

It is difficult to determine how much of the observed decline in respiratory function is age related and how much is environmentally induced, because most individuals are exposed to some degree of air pollution. No studies exist on nonsmokers living in nonpolluted environments, but the use of cigarettes or other inhaled substances probably exaggerates the above-described aging changes. Smoking-induced bronchitis and emphysema or chronic obstructive pulmonary disease (COPD) is characterized by an acceleration in fibrosis and septal damage leading to bullous formation. These disruptive changes in the alveolar walls result in decreased diffusion capacity, increased secretions, and an increased rate of chronic infection. COPD mimics and exaggerates the aging changes of senile emphysema and thus accelerates pulmonary aging in middle-aged smokers. These processes can be reversed or stabilized if smoking stops (Hermanson et al. 1988).

Aerobic exercise training has significantly positive cardiovascular, pulmonary, and behavioral effects (Blumenthal et al. 1989). After 4 months of training, healthy older men and women showed an 11.6% improvement in directly measured peak oxygen uptake (VO_2) and a 13% increase in anaerobic threshold, which is the amount of work tolerated before exercise-limiting ventilatory and metabolic change occurred. Anaerobic threshold is a reasonable reference for daily activity work capacity. In addition to aerobic fitness, they also found lower total and low-density lipoprotein (LDL) cholesterol levels and increases in high-density lipoprotein (HDL) levels. Changes in other physiological parameters included lowered systolic and diastolic blood pressures and the suggestion that bone mineral might be increased in these women at greater risk for fracture, though these latter data are not sufficiently convincing because of the insensitive methodology used (single-photon densitometry of the distal radius) and the short time covered by the study.

The other major problem in extrapolating from these subjects to most elderly individuals is that these study participants were healthy and had no concurrent diseases, a rare phenomenon in older individuals. However, this study is interesting because its findings are similar to other exercise studies in the literature and because it also looked at the psychological effects of exercise; subjects reported increased positive affect and felt better physically.

Musculoskeletal System

Skeletal aging involving the bones, muscles, ligaments, and tendons probably generates most of the common symptoms responsible for limitations of recreational activities, activities of daily living, and restrictions in job-related functions. Joint and muscle aches and stiffness characteristic of the arthritides are frequently ascribed to getting old (Prohaska et al. 1987). Both young and old patients, if attributing symptoms to getting old, delay seeking health care, although elderly people delay less long than younger patients with similar complaints (Cameron et al. 1993; Leventhal et al. 1993). These symptoms also lead to greater use of both prescription and nonprescription analgesics, many of which can have significant adverse side effects including gastrointestinal distress and bleeding and psychotropic side effects such as depression (Juby and Davis 1991).

Men maintain an advantage in greater musculoskeletal strength after pubescence, although with time, they lose significant muscle mass, as do women. Declines occur in skeleton mineralization at a rate of 0.8% to 1.0% each year during life for both men and women, but women show an increase in the rate of loss to between 8% and 10% per year around menopause and thus are at risk for osteoporosis-related fractures. This represents an approximate 10-year morbidity-free advantage for men, although men may become osteoporotic because of concurrent disease.

The gender-specific rate of demineralization has a complex metabolic etiology that includes the permissive effect of circulating estrogens and progesterone on the maintenance of vertebral trabecular bone. Thus postmenopausal women are more vulnerable to fractures of the vertebral spine than men of the same age. In contrast, calcium and vitamin D metabolism and weight-bearing activity may be more critical for the remodeling of the cortical bones of the extremities. Although both men and women are at risk for fractures of the long bones, women become more prone to fractures 10 years earlier than men. Because of the role of exercise and diet in maintaining bone integrity, regimens that include increased calcium intake and weight-bearing exercise along with estrogen replacement should show positive results in terms of bone density increases or slowing in the rate of demineralization. The evidence is controversial regarding the relationship between dietary intake of calcium and rates of bone loss or reversibility (Riggs et al. 1987), but much current research is directed toward finding tolerable and efficient treatments. One study indicates that weight-bearing exercise may have a positive effect on mineral content of the axial skeleton (Dalsky et al. 1988). However, the critical times to protect the skeleton and prevent the osteoporosis of old age probably are in childhood, adolescence, pregnancy, and lactation (Raiz 1988; Raiz and Kream 1983a, 1983b). Increased intake of calcium and foods containing vitamin D, weight-bearing exercise, and avoidance of excessive dieting and smoking are lifestyle behaviors to be encouraged.

Gastrointestinal Tract

In the oral cavity, aging changes are obvious. With time, the teeth show a reduction in dentine production, shrinkage and fibrosis of root pulp, and gingival retraction. Loss of bone density in the alveolar ridges is also seen and accelerates after tooth loss. An increase in caries occurs, especially of the root, that appears to be correlated with changes in bacterial content of the mouth and increased colonization with gram-positive facultative cocci replacing gram-negative anaerobic rods, although the population of fusospirochetal organisms remains unchanged. No aging-related changes have been observed in the salivary glands. Xerostomia, which is common in elderly people, is a disease caused by such problems as obstructing nasal disease leading to mouth breathing or mucous drying, drugs such as anticholinergics, and autoimmune diseases such as Sjögren's syndrome (Baum 1988). Primary aging in the esophagus is related to smooth muscle degeneration and results in a decrease in the amplitude of peristaltic movements, although overall esophageal function is largely preserved. The stomach shows evidence of impaired secretory capacity with maximal stimulated gastric acid production decreasing by 5 mEq/h per decade. Levels of serum gastrin increase, and levels of intrinsic factor decrease. Atrophic gastritis is common, often leading to vitamin B_{12} malabsorption, although reports of its incidence vary from 28% to 96% of elderly individuals. Most studies have small sample sizes, and many are descriptive studies of hospitalized patients; nevertheless, the incidence is probably sufficiently high that primary physicians need to be alert and look for vitamin B_{12} deficiency. Gastric emptying appears to be impaired only slightly (Geokas et al. 1985; Minaker et al. 1988).

Minimal changes in the small intestine and only a marginal reduction in mesenteric and splanchnic blood flow occur in the absence of vascular disease. The most significant decrease has been observed in the absorptive surface area, with loss of microvilli of the brush border and an associated decrease in enzymatic activities. The weight of the small intestine decreases as the mucosal surface area declines, yet there are minimal decreases in levels of function. Xylose, iron, and folate absorption remain normal, and although lipid and calcium absorption decline, the latter is probably related more to decreases in vitamin D availability and activity than changes in absorptive surface. With decreases in gastric acid, the sterility of the tract is jeopardized and larger numbers of coliforms are seen. Although absorption is largely preserved, when combined with poor intake and disease, malnutrition may result (Geokas et al. 1985).

Liver

The liver decreases modestly in weight and size from 4% to 2% of total body weight with aging. Hepatic blood flow shows a 1.5% fall per year so that there will be a 50% reduction during life. Most ingested drugs and metabolites absorbed from the small intestine and stomach pass through the liver. Some are unchanged, whereas others undergo metabolic detoxification by microsomal enzymes into water-soluble substances for renal excretion. With decreases in liver mass, decreases in the rate of biotransformation occur. This decrease in biotransformation is attributable to losses in cellular microsomal enzyme activity, primarily the CYP2D6 and CYP1A2 isoenzymes of cytochrome P450, and a decrease in blood flow. Thus, oxidation, or phase I of hepatic microsomal enzyme synthesis, is the principal metabolic pathway that diminishes with age, particularly in men. These functional changes result in a prolongation in the half-life of those metabolites and drugs that are inactivated by the liver and thereby an increase in the bioavailability of those that must undergo first-pass hepatic metabolism. For example, the benzodiazepines, tricyclics such as desipramine and imipramine, haloperidol, thioridazine, propafenone, perphenazine, and increasingly, the selective serotonin reuptake inhibitors, such as fluoxetine, paroxetine, and sertraline, appear to specifically inhibit CYP2D6. The significance of prescribing these drugs is obvious given the long half-life and potential for interactions with other commonly used drugs such as metaproterenol, calcium channel blockers, carbamazepine, cimetidine, and possibly warfarin, although the mechanism for warfarin is unknown. Conjugation, or phase II, remains largely unchanged (i.e., glucuronidation is not altered) (Geokas et al. 1985; Kenney 1989).

Large Bowel

Early studies indicated that the large bowel experiences alterations in flora in normal aging. Studies of transit time by ingestion of markers show that first markers will be passed in 3 days and 80% will appear by 5 days, with greater delays related to motility slowdown below the sigmoid (Geokas et al. 1985; Kenney 1989). Studies using more sensitive technologies have demonstrated that there are age-related changes in the intrinsic innervation of the gastrointestinal tract, with increased colonic transit time attributable to a decrease in intrinsic inhibitory nerve input to colonic circular smooth muscle. In addition, there are alterations in rectal function (Koch et al. 1991).

Endocrine System

Thyroid

Despite changes in thyroid physiology that occur over time, a euthyroid status is maintained with advancing age. Contrary to earlier studies, new evidence indicates that there are no age-related changes in circulating hormone levels, although daily production rates of T_4 and T_3 are reduced by about 25% and 33%, respectively. The changes are believed to be primarily attributable to a diminished availability of T_4 in peripheral tissues and decreased T_4 disposal rate. The decrease in T_3 is dependent on an overall age-related reduction in sequential demonoiodination of T_3 to diiodothyronine (Griffin 1991). Basal thyroid-stimulating hormone (TSH) secretion is reported to increase in persons over age 60 years, whereas the euthyroid state is maintained (Kabadi and Rosman 1986; Sawin et al. 1979), except in elderly men whose 24-hour mean TSH concentrations were approximately 50% lower than those of young men, whereas basal levels of T_4 remain normal and the circadian rhythm is preserved. Thyrotropin-releasing hormone (TRH)–induced TSH secretion also is lower, indicating a decrease in pituitary responsiveness to stimulation but a maintenance of chronobiological modulation (Van Coevorden et al. 1989). In a study of postmenopausal women, Rossmanith et al. (1992) demonstrated that T_4 serum concentrations were no different in younger or older postmenopausal women, although T_3 levels were decreased in older women. TSH and prolactin were secreted episodically, with considerable interindividual variabilities in both study groups. A tendency was noted for mean TSH to be higher in the older sample, suggesting that, given the depressed levels of T_3, the negative feedback on the hypothalamic-pituitary unit may be impaired. As with most metabolic studies, the number of study subjects was small and more exact clarifications of physiological mechanisms must await more extensive, carefully controlled studies; however, because the thyroid does not appear to respond to higher TSH levels by putting out more thyroid hormones, this study suggests that possible age-related changes important for homeostasis may occur in the thyroid-pituitary axis (i.e., decreased degradation of thyroid hormones with maintenance of normal serum thyroid hormone concentrations).

Recently, Sawin et al. (1991) reported on a small subset of ambulatory elderly individuals who were clinically euthyroid, not hyperthyroid, despite low levels of TSH demonstrated by a high-sensitivity assay. Overt hypothyroidism has been associated with various psychiatric conditions including dementia, organic and functional psychoses, and depression; however, controversy exists about the correlation of subclinical hypothyroidism with depression. Griffin (1991) reviewed most of the studies and reported that they are unconvincing and none adequately details a causal relationship. What is perhaps more interesting are findings that implicate the dopaminergic system in the suppression of the pulsatile secretion of TSH (Greenspan et al. 1991). A blunted nocturnal TSH pulsatile secretion is seen in elderly men when compared with the large (>160% increase) nocturnal peak exhibited by young subjects. These hormonal secretion patterns may be mediated by aging changes in day-night dopaminergic tone or regulation, because it appears that the circadian rhythm of TSH is tightly coupled with circadian pacemakers that regulate the sleep-wake cycles and body temperatures. Several studies have shown that these pacemakers and rhythms may be phase advanced in elderly individuals; the relationship to depression may lie in the dysregulation of the circadian rhythms (Greenspan et al. 1991).

Pancreas

Moderate anatomic changes occur in older individuals, with the pancreas fat deposition and shrinkage of islet cells. Although age-related impairment in glucose metabolism has been recognized for more than 60 years, only recently have the mechanisms begun to be investigated. Most studies show that modest impairments occur in glucose clearance in the response of healthy elderly individuals to oral or intravenous glucose challenges with circulatory insulin levels equivalent to or slightly higher than those from younger challenged individuals. Peripheral insulin resistance appears to play a significant role in carbohydrate intolerance. No evidence has been found to suggest changes in basal hepatic glucose production or changes in insulin receptor numbers or affinity. The controversy now focuses on how peripheral insulin becomes operational and the relative contributions of obesity, family history of diabetes, physical exercise, and the use of diabetogenic drugs in the development of senescent carbohydrate intolerance and the relationship to the neuroendocrine system. Thus the observed clearance abnormalities and insulin resistance in older people is probably related to many factors other than biological aging and may be influenced substantially by behaviors such as diet or exercise (Marchesini et al. 1987; Pacini et al. 1988).

Kidneys

The kidneys, as one of the two major excretory systems, function via passive glomerular filtration, active tubular secretion, and reabsorption and passive tubular diffusion. All of these functions decline significantly with age. The decrements in renal function, unrelated to concomitant disease in other organ systems, occur because of a progressive sclerosis of nephrons over time. Of particular importance are the age-related changes in renal blood flow that determine glomerular filtration rate (GFR) and tubular secretion, as well as the ability of the kidneys to compensate for abnormalities of acid, base, electrolyte, and free-water clearance. GFR declines by 40% to 50% during life. A modest reduction occurs in the capacity to conserve sodium, with increased osmoreceptor sensitivity that results in the release of more vasopressin from the posterior pituitary, leading to water retention. Elderly individuals are more prone to develop the syndrome of inappropriate antidiuretic hormone secretion (SIADH) (Rowe et al. 1976; Wesson 1969). When circulating levels of blood urea nitrogen (BUN) and creatinine rise before the 9th decade, it may be assumed that either the uremic individual is exhibiting accelerated renal aging or has some significant pathology superimposed on age-related changes in kidney function. If BUN is elevated while serum creatinine remains low, this may represent prerenal volume contraction indicative of other illness-related pathology without obligatory renal dysfunction (Finch and Schneider 1985; Kenney 1989). This decline in renal function has serious implications for the administration of drugs such as lithium and buspirone in elderly people.

Declines in renal function may effect erythropoiesis and contribute to a greater likelihood of anemia in elderly people. Measurements of erythropoietin in a large sample of healthy elderly individuals, compared with 1) elderly individuals with low hemoglobin and 2) younger control subjects, reveals that nonanemic elderly individuals have higher circulating erythropoietin than younger control men and reduced erythroid-forming cells in the marrow but enough function in available erythroid precursors to form sufficient red blood cells and avoid anemia. Increased circulating erythropoietin in nonanemic elderly people may be the mechanism that compensates for reduced hematopoiesis in the bone marrow of aging individuals. The lower levels of erythropoietin in elderly people with evidence of iron deficiency anemia may be partly attributable to less erythropoietin production by the kidney and decreased marrow responsiveness, even though the normal feedback mechanism may still be present (Kario et al. 1991).

Immune System

Many studies have been directed toward understanding the impact of aging on the normal immune system and its autoregulation. Therefore, it is useful to describe the system both anatomically and functionally to organize the frequently conflicting data in this area.

The immune system is arranged into a pool of fixed and circulating cells, including leukocytes, lymphocytes, monocytes, macrophages, and mast cells that move in and out of, or are fixed in, various lymphoid organs such as spleen, lymph nodes, Peyer's patches, and thymus. Leukocytes may have a more central role in immune function than previously assumed, but because age-relevant studies are few, these populations are not discussed here. The lymphocyte pool is made up of several subpopulations evolving from an ancestral stem cell in the bone marrow. These include the T cell line of antigen-responsive cells and effector cells that can kill antigen-specific target cells on direct contact; the B cell line of antigen-responsive cells and the immunoglobulin-producing plasma cells; and phagocytic mast cells fixed in tissues such as lymph nodes, lung, skin, and mucosa.

With increasing senescence, the total number of immune cells does not change, although increases in immature forms and decreases in germinal centers occur in the lymph nodes. Increases of plasma cells and lymphocytes in the bone marrow probably occur because of redistribution.

The total concentration of immunoglobulins is not altered, but there is a redistribution of immunoglobulin classes with increases in immunoglobulin A and immunoglobulin G and decreases in immunoglobulin M in serum (Hallgren et al. 1973). Although well-controlled studies on healthy humans are infrequent and much of the data on aging and immune function are conflicting and extrapolated from animal models, agreement exists that the actual numbers of some immune cells decline with age (Hausman and Weksler 1985; Makinodan and Hirokawa 1985). The major age-related cellular changes occur in the ratios of subpopulations of thymic-dependent T lymphocytes, with increases in immature cell forms

(T_3), and T-helper cells (T_4), and declines in suppressor or cytotoxic (T_8) cells and natural killer (NK) cells. There are less vigorous delayed-sensitivity reactions to common skin antigens, decreased immunity to virus infections, and graft-versus-host reactions (Leventhal and Burns 1987; Makinodan and Hirokawa 1985).

B cells show little change in total number, but responsiveness to stimulation by T cell–dependent antigens and to B cell mitogens declines. Those B cell functions that are not T cell dependent are relatively preserved, and there are essentially no changes in the functioning of adherent cells (macrophages) and monocytes between young and old subjects (Antonaci et al. 1984; Kim et al. 1985).

Of the glandular components, the thymus is critical for immune function. It provides the microenvironment for T cell differentiation, and as an endocrine organ, thymic stromal cells produce several hormones including the thymosins and thymopoietic factor. Aging in the thymus is dramatic and plays a critical role in immunosenescence. The anatomic patterns in the thymus remain unaltered until approximately age 9 years (prepuberty). By ages 11–13 years, the vasculature appears increasingly irregular, although parenchymal and perivascular nerves continue to be detectable in the capsule and proximal parts of the trabeculae until age 25. The nonlymphoid structures remain intact in the involuted thymus, but the lymphocytic portions, particularly in the cortex, become almost nonexistent. The hormonal activity responsible for lymphocytic maturation resides in epithelial cells that do not undergo involution, although these cells lose intimate contact with lymphocytes as the lymphoid elements atrophy. The decline in circulating levels of thymic hormone does not parallel the glandular lymphoid involution after puberty, and although hormonal levels peak before pubescence, they remain detectable until age 60 years before becoming essentially unmeasurable after ages 60–70 (Goldstein et al. 1979).

A humoral modulatory role has been observed for the sympathetic nervous system that appears to depend on sympathetic innervation of lymphoid organs augmented by plasma catecholamines of adrenal origin. Anatomic studies have demonstrated direct sympathetic innervation in fetal thymus and spleen. In both mice and humans, fibers in the adult thymus are abundant around blood vessels and in the parenchyma, encircling or relayed on Hassal's corpuscles (Ghali et al. 1980; Williams and Felton 1981; Williams et al. 1981).

The anatomic linkages between neural and immune systems briefly described above make clear that regulation and modulation of the immune system by the nervous system are complex. The linkages also indicate that many opportunities exist for disruption of intra- and intersystem regulatory mechanisms by various forms of internal and external stresses throughout life. Thus, the regulatory function of the intrinsic compartments within the immune system may be influenced by and dependent on a variety of nonimmune system factors, including psychological stress.

In one of the few longitudinal studies of the aging immune system, Goodwin et al. (1982) studied 279 subjects, all age 65 years and older, with a mean age of 72, taking no prescribed or over-the-counter drugs, and without serious medical diagnoses. They assayed delayed hypersensitivity, mitogen response, and autoantibody and circulating immune complexes and found that mitogen responses and delayed hypersensitive skin tests were depressed in healthy elderly people. Poor correlation was noted between the two assays (i.e., no relationship between measures of cellular immunity and autoimmunity), and no degree of correlation was observed between circulating immune complexes and other autoantibodies. These observations were noted despite the theory that loss of T-suppressor function leads to increasing autoimmunoglobulin levels. After exclusion of those subjects who developed serious illness, Goodwin et al. continued to find age-related decreases in cellular responses in repeat examinations after 2 years. These clinical observations are compatible with findings that, in older individuals, T cells have fewer surface receptors and B cells have fewer immunoglobulin markers. Thus, both cell types show declines in function with age, although there is no clear correlation with the development of specific diseases.

Gonads

Aging of the ovary begins in utero and continues throughout life. In females, potential germ cells reach maturation in the ovaries during gestation and undergo massive attrition during the latter half of fetal development, declining from a population of 10×10^6 cells at organogenesis of the ovary to 10^6 at birth. This steady decline in functional cell number continues until pubescence, when there remains a population of about 10,000 cells available for impregnation. The attrition of these cells continues, but at a slower rate, through the female reproductive period with its monthly cyclicity and interruptions for pregnancy (Nicosia 1983).

The maturation of germ cells and the production of hormones is controlled by a negative feedback loop between the brain and the gonads whereby the trophic hormones (luteinizing hormone [LH] and follicle-stimulating hormone [FSH]) secreted by the anterior pituitary regulate the follicular ripening of ova and the production of the gonadal hormones, estrogen (E_2) and progesterone. Follicles containing the mature ovum and capable of synthesizing E_2 and progesterone continue to decrease in number, so that at the climacteric, there are too few remaining to produce adequate circulating hormones to stimulate not only the gonad-dependent end organs such as the breasts and genitalia (and trabecular bone of the vertebrae) but also inadequate to participate in the negative feedback cycling with the pituitary. As estrogenic stimulation declines further, women begin to experience the symptoms of hormonal deficiency, including atrophy of the breasts and genitalia and vasomotor instability. The reduction in E_2 and progesterone results, finally, in the cessation of menstruation and an uninhibited production of the pituitary gonadotropic hormones. All women show elevations in circulating pituitary gonadotropic hormones (LH and FSH) after they enter the perimenopausal period between ages 40 and 55, the physiological significance of which is not clear (Barbo 1987; Mastroianni and Paulsen 1986). After menopause, with loss of the physiological protective effects of E_2 and progesterone, there is a greater vulnerability to stroke, coronary artery disease, and osteoporosis.

Men show minimal attrition of testicular structures or declines in hormonal synthesis and secretion. Potential sperm cells that were arrested in the testis at the spermatogonium stage remain at a primitive level into adulthood. The process of maturation to mature sperm continues throughout life, with declines occurring only in the 7th–8th decades. Hormonal function also remains relatively stable, and in many men, the negative feedback mechanisms with the anterior pituitary are unchanged until the 8th decade. Elevated gonadotropic hormones are rarely seen before age 70. In healthy men, a few individuals in their late 40s and 50s have elevated levels of FSH, but the majority do not have increased levels until their 70s (Stearns et al. 1974).

Nervous System

One of the effects of aging on the nervous system and its subsequent loss of function is the selective degeneration of neurons. Differences have been observed in the patterns of aging between the central and the peripheral nervous system, presumably because of random demyelination of long tracts. Although constant cell loss occurs, Terry et al.

(1987), using autopsy data from a large sample of elderly individuals without dementia, showed that both central and peripheral age-related neuronal loss is minimal. Using in vivo magnetic resonance images, Lim et al. (1992) found that elderly men without dementia had a significantly lower percentage of gray matter and a higher percentage of cerebral spinal fluid, with the percentage of white matter not significantly different for the control sample of young males. Clearly, despite neuronal loss, the brain has enormous reserve capacity for continued learning into old age (Baltheus 1989, 1991, 1992), although greater functional decline is noted in the peripheral nervous system. Cells disappear randomly throughout the cortex, but in other brain areas, there is clustered loss (i.e., there is a disproportionately greater loss of cells in the cerebellum, the locus ceruleus, the substantia nigra [Martin et al. 1989], and olfactory bulbs [Brody 1970, 1976]). Mild gait disturbances, sleep disruptions, and decreased smell and taste perception represent neuronal degeneration in these specific areas.

Neuroendocrine Function and Neurotransmitter Distribution

A great deal of attention has been paid to age-related changes in brain biochemistry, and many contemporary pharmacological interventions such as growth hormone (GH) and dopamine replacement using the metabolic precursor levodopa in individual's with Parkinson's disease are directed at extending function in systems beset with irreversible anatomic changes. The success of such interventions is dependent on understanding pituitary-endocrine axes and neurotransmitter metabolism and function. Although there are myriad identified neurotransmitters and much research on neuropeptides, behavior, and aging (Morley 1986), only a few of the age-relevant molecules are discussed below.

Pituitary

Growth Hormone

A flurry of lay interest has occurred in strategies to reverse aging using GH replacement in older men based on the assumption that, because aging is associated with decreases in GH, insulinlike growth factor-1 (IGF-1), and lean body mass and increased body fat, GH replacement could reverse these changes (Marcus et al. 1990; Rudman et al. 1990). It is premature to generalize about effective life extension on the basis of these studies (and variants using more physiological GH secretion stimulation by hypothalamic GH-releasing hormone [GHRH]) (Corpas et al. 1992).

Pituitary-Adrenocortical Axis

Numerous studies have investigated the preservation of function with age of the pituitary-adrenocortical axis in healthy young and old men. Basal mean 12-hour and 4-hour adrenocorticotropic hormone (ACTH) and cortisol values do not differ with age, and pulse analyses have revealed no differences for peak frequency, amplitude, or duration for either hormone thus examined (Waltman et al. 1991). Similar findings were obtained in a sample including women (Roberts et al. 1990), although some age and isolated gender differences to ACTH stimulation were observed. The individual variability highlights the problems mentioned earlier that come from extrapolation of data from a research methodology that is dependent on multiple measures in small samples (primarily of presumably healthy men). This dilemma is exemplified by the study by Greenspan et al. (1993). In three separate experiments, the authors examined the effects of age in the following subjects: 10 young men (ages 19–46 years) versus 8 older men (ages 69–83); 8 older men (ages 69–83) versus 7 older women (ages 62–86); and 12 healthy men (ages 21–86) versus 12 chronically ill men (ages 25–80). They found that both gender and age differences existed in basal and peak cortisol levels. Both levels were higher in young healthy men compared with older men. Basal, peak, and nadir levels of cortisol were 100% greater in women than in men, and the adrenal response was depressed with age in men. Another finding was that cortisol levels were 40% higher in men with a stable chronic disease than in men who were disease free. The clinical implication is that persistent elevation in circulating cortisol as a result of chronic stress may act as a negative modulator of symptoms and encourage disease development. If these data are reproducible, they are provocative and may offer the opportunity to explore the relationships between stress, the neuroendocrine system, the pituitary-adrenocortical axis, and chronic disease.

Acetylcholine

Acetylcholine (ACh) is widely distributed throughout the central and peripheral nervous system. It is synthesized from choline that is taken up at the presynaptic terminals and acetyl coenzyme A, which is synthesized in the mitochondria, in a reaction that is catalyzed by choline acetyltransferase (CAT). Choline uptake is the rate-limiting factor and shows significant decline with age, although whether the uptake decline reflects changes in number of septal or hippocampal neurons or specific biochemical defects in structure or activity of binding-site proteins is not clear. Of the numerous classes of neurotransmitters thus far identified, diminished ACh metabolism has been most closely associated with cognitive dysfunction. In healthy individuals, data on the metabolic activity of CAT are inconsistent; however, levels of the transmitter ACh consistently show no decline. This may reflect concurrent decreases in ACh release and CAT-mediated metabolism at the time that synthesis and precursor uptake are disappearing.

Another method of assessing age-related changes in ACh function is to examine ACh inactivation by acetylcholinesterase (AChE). Much inconsistency has been noted in reports of age-related changes in circulating levels of AChE, but reasonably good evidence exists that binding to cholinergic receptors declines with normal aging. This finding is independent of the cholinergic cell loss associated with dementia of the Alzheimer's type (Finch and Schneider 1985; E. G. McGeer and P. L. McGeer 1975). Sparks et al. (1992) found, looking at synaptic markers in the nucleus basalis of Meynert (chosen because of linkages to memory impairments in patients with dementia and its extensive radiation to cortical and subcortical targets), a significant decline of dopamine (DA), serotonin (5-HT) and metabolites, 5-hydroxyindoleacetic acid (5-HIAA), 5-HT binding, CAT and AChE activities, and DA turnover in individuals without dementia or chronic illness, with the largest declines noted early (<40 years). P. L. McGeer et al. (1984) reported a 65% reduction in CAT comparable to 68% loss of cholinergic neurons and a parallel decrease in AChE compatible with diminution of cholinergic function with age.

Dopamine

DA is widely distributed in the central nervous system, primarily associated with medium-length projections (tuberoinfundibular, incertohypothalamic, and medullary periventricular systems) and long projections of the ventral tegmental and substantia nigra DA cell groups to neostriatal and limbic targets. DA is synthesized from dietary tyrosine by hydroxylation to dihydroxyphenylalanine (dopa) catalyzed by tyrosine hydroxylase (TH) and then decarboxylated by dopa decarboxylase. The activity of TH is reported to remain stable, and many studies suggest that dopa decarboxylase declines throughout life after a sharp loss in childhood, impairing synthesis of DA. This report is consistent with findings that DA levels are decreased after midlife in autopsy studies of specific brain areas (e.g., striatum [Rogers and Bloom 1985; Sparks et al. 1992]) yet conflicts with in vivo studies (Sawle et al. 1990) of subjects using positron-emission tomography (PET) that find an absence of an aging effect in dopaminergic sites.

Plasma Catecholamines (Norepinephrine and Epinephrine)

Plasma norepinephrine represents a small proportion of norepinephrine released from postganglionic sympathetic neurons, because most is taken up or degraded locally, yet variations in circulating levels reflect biological responses to sympathetic nervous system (SNS) activity. For example, levels increase slightly with upright posture and volume depletion and greatly with severe exercise or stress such as surgery or hypoglycemia. The levels decrease with spinal anesthesia and drugs such as clonidine. Norepinephrine shares several enzymes of synthesis and catabolism with DA; thus the inconsistencies in the literature on DA hold as well for norepinephrine. Some human data exist, however, that permit us to make a few more definitive comments about norepinephrine, and these are discussed in the cardiovascular section.

Evidence exists that norepinephrine receptor concentrations decline (Schocken and Roth 1977). This has been documented in the locus ceruleus, where β-receptors show some area-specific declines (e.g., cerebellar purkinje cells and locus ceruleus [Brody 1970, 1976; E. G. McGeer and P. L. McGeer 1975]), yet norepinephrine from human cortex, striatum, hypothalamus, and thalamus does not appear altered (Rogers and Bloom 1985).

Supine baseline levels of plasma norepinephrine increase as a function of age, primarily in men during stresses such as those listed above, providing evidence that SNS activity increases with aging (Ziegler et al. 1976). Several explanations may exist for these findings. Either there is increased norepinephrine release from postganglionic sympathetic neurons or decreased clearance. However, because metabolic clearance rate and half-life are similar in young and old subjects, the variations noted may be attributable to changes in synthetic rate or reduced receptor sensitivity in elderly people (Vestal et al. 1979). Sympathetic nerve activity increases with age, compatible with elevated norepinephrine levels seen with advancing age, yet responsiveness of the system to hemodynamic stimulation including blockade are reduced in elderly individuals (Iwase et al. 1991).

No consistent findings of increased plasma levels of epinephrine with age are seen at rest or during SNS provocation. Although responses are similar across the age range, some data suggest that epinephrine clearance is amplified, resulting in increased adrenomedullary release of epinephrine (Lake et al. 1984). Thus, different effects of aging may occur on the central nervous system (CNS) regulation of postganglionic, sympathetic neurons, and adrenomedullary regulation.

Declines in β-receptors on nonnervous tissues (e.g., lymphocytes, myocardium, and adipocytes) have been demonstrated. The exact implications are not clear because several animal and human studies suggest that decreased responsiveness may represent declines in adenylate cyclase activity rather than receptor-binding abnormalities (Bertel et al. 1980; Rogers and Bloom 1985; Zahniser et al. 1988).

Serotonin

An accumulating body of evidence from animal studies exists implicating the serotonergic system in neurophysiological processes underlying learning and memory (Altman and Normile 1988). Sparks et al. (1992) found significant declines in nucleus basalis–based serotonin function including levels of 5-HT, 5-HIAA, and 5-HT binding with age. These data are consistent with similar findings from cortical region studies.

Peripheral Nervous System

In the periphery, random disruption of the myelin sheaths of the long nerves is seen. Physiological studies show modest change with age, including increases in surface baseline electromyogram at both the wrist and thumb. These may indicate a systemic change in motor unit composition modulated by changes in dermal thickness (Mortimer and Webster 1982). The slowing of motor function may reflect this loss, and nerve dysfunction may exaggerate myofibrillar losses. Thus, because of the interrelationship between nerves and muscles, muscle weakness may reflect not only myofibrillar loss but also disuse atrophy attributable to denervation (Kenney 1989).

Sense Organs

Vision

Minimal changes are noted in the retina of the eye, and thus minimal neurally determined changes in light perception, although some shrinkage in the size and sensitivity of visual fields appears to begin in the early 40s (Burg 1968). The major changes that do occur are in the transparent portions of the ocular system, and cataract development is inevitable if the individual lives long enough for the following changes to occur. Pigment is laid down in specific patterns in the lens over time and is coupled with increased rigidity of the lenticular proteins. It is this alteration in the normal molecular alignment that results in the formation of cataracts (Benedek 1971; Spector et al. 1974). The rate of opacification is individually determined and may be accelerated by diseases such as diabetes mellitus, hypoparathyroidism, myotonic dystrophy, and Wilson's disease or the use of drugs such as chlorpromazine or the corticosteroids. The world seen through a cataract is one of altered perception and sensory deprivation. Presbyopia, also important for visual acuity, is the standard marker of aging of the eye. It occurs as the muscles and ligaments supporting the lens become less taut and stretchable, compromising accommodation (Fisher 1973). Another common but pathological condition, macular degeneration or the appearance of age-related hyaline nodules in Bruch's membrane, leads to the development of subretinal neovascularization and the distortion of central visual fields with loss of visual acuity.

Hearing

Another sensory area in which significant change occurs is hearing. The ear loses its sensitivity with aging. Prolonged exposure to loud noise or heavy sound pollution may accelerate the rate of permanent damage to the hair cells of the cochlea. Because a genetic predisposition to hearing loss is known, the rates of decline in tone and speech discrimination may show significant individual variability. However, from ages 30 to 85, presbycusis, a decline in high-frequency perception, occurs in the oldest individuals compared with young persons with presumed perfect hearing. Decay in the hearing curves for women is less dramatic than that for men, although there still is significant falloff with age, supporting the assumption that the gender difference may be related to occupational exposure (Belal 1975; Gacek 1975). Note that most studies have been done with members of a cohort of older individuals who may have been exposed to significant noise during youth. Possibly, in the next few decades, frequency curves will show less of a dramatic decrement over time and the gender differences may disappear. It is interesting to speculate about what will happen to the hearing of the current cohort of adolescents who are constantly bombarded by sound from high-volume stereos or spend time in front of loud rock bands. They may have "old audiograms" in middle age.

Taste and Smell

Significant increases occur in taste threshold as a result of decreases in taste sensitivity during life. At birth, taste buds line the soft and hard palate, the buccal mucosa, and the tongue. A slow attrition of taste buds occurs during infancy, and at puberty palatal and buccal receptors are essentially lost. Taste perception becomes solely lingual and nasal; thus taste perception starts aging at adolescence. By ages 40 or 45 years, the tongue is an old organ. In addition, with the deterioration of the olfactory bulbs and the accompanying loss in the aromatic component of taste perception, a decline occurs in taste discrimination (Balogh and Lelkes 1961; El-Baradi and Bourne 1951; Schiffman et al. 1976). Hedonistic pleasure from the aromas of cooking and eating declines, bitter taste sensations predominate, and greater use of sugar and excessive salting of foods is needed to stimulate taste experiences. The impact of loss of taste discrimination on nutritional status and disease is just beginning to be elucidated.

Touch

Anatomic studies have demonstrated a continuous decrease in the cutaneous receptors during life. Meissner and Pacinian corpuscles, involved in touch and vibration, decrease in number and show morphological changes. Touch threshold increases as a function of age (Kenshalo 1977; Winkelmann 1965), and the number of touch spots per unit area of skin decreases by approximately 50% between the 2nd and 7th decade of life (Rong 1943). Stevens (1992), using two-point thresholds, confirmed that spatial acuity of the skin of the fingertip, which is critical in the perception of tactile patterns, deteriorates markedly with age and correlates with loss in density of distribution and morphology of Meissner's corpuscles, Merkel's discs, and Pacinian corpuscles (the former are the most likely candidates for mediation of spatial acuity). The latter also undergo morphological changes with age and may account for substantial loss of skin sensitivity to high-frequency vibration.

Proprioception

Aging results in degenerative changes and impaired postural reflexes, mild ataxias, and increased sway secondary to deficiencies in integrative function of the CNS with the cerebellum and the reticular formation along with disturbed perception of the vertical (Robinson and Conrad 1986). This perceptual sense is vitally important for ambulation and balance because older individuals, more than young persons, attempt to monitor their movements via afferent feedback. Proprioceptive information facilitates stretch reflexes that are necessary to convert limbs into fairly rigid pillars for support in walking and standing as well as ensuring awareness of limb orientation in space to guarantee proper foot placements (Isaacs 1983, 1985).

Studies of other non-CNS components vital for balance indicate that a significant age-related decline occurs in both active and passive motion-detection thresholds (Skinner et al. 1984) and joint kinesthetics (Skoglund 1973). If appears that such age-related changes are minimized if movements are patient initiated, although constrained movements are less accurately performed by elderly subjects (Stelmach and Worringham 1985).

Pain

Much research exists on pain that uses methodologies ranging from heat dolorimetry to dental pain elicited by the application of electrical stimuli to the tooth pulp (Clark and Mehl 1971; Corso 1971; Sherman and Robillard 1960). These studies show increasing thresholds with age. Although histological studies indicate that free nerve endings are reformed continuously (Montagna and Carlisle 1979), psychophysiological research has demonstrated that elderly people have diminished pain acuity. Careful dissection of the complex components of pain perception, including both perception of stimuli intensities and interpretation of meaning and implications of painful stimuli, indicates that central integration and interpretation of sensory effects rather than receptor changes are implicated in rising pain thresholds (Harkins and Chapman 1977).

Summary

Significant biological changes occur at different rates in different organ systems during life. Responsiveness to stress demands on the system become compromised, yet in the absence of significant chronic disease, functional independence can be maintained well into the ninth decade. Specific aspects of senescence are particularly relevant for the psychiatrist who must appreciate the limited reserve yet the remarkable resiliency of the elderly individual, the fragility of the immune response, and the increased vulnerability to medications of all types and, in particular, psychoactive drugs.

References

Altman HJ, Normile HJ: What is the nature of the role of the serotonergic nervous system in learning and memory: prospects for development of an effective treatment strategy for senile dementia. Neurobiol Aging 9:627–638, 1988

Antonaci S, Jirillo E, Ventura MT, et al: Non-specific immunity in aging: deficiency of monocyte and polymorphonuclear cell-mediated functions. Mech Ageing Dev 24:367–375, 1984

Balogh K, Lelkes K: The tongue in old age. Gerontolol Clin 3:38–54, 1961

Baltes PB: The many faces of human ageing: toward a psychological culture of old age. Psychol Med 21(4):837–854, 1991

Baltes PB, Reinhold K: Further testing of limits of cognitive plasticity: negative age differences in a mnemonic skill are robust. Developmental Psychology 28(1):121–125, 1992

Baltes PB, Sowarka D, Kliegel R: Cognitive training research on fluid intelligence in old age: what can older adults achieve by themselves? Psychol Aging 4(2):217–221, 1989

Barbo DM: The physiology of the menopause. Med Clin North Am 71:11–22, 1987

Baum BJ: Oral cavity, in Geriatric Medicine, 2nd Edition. Edited by Rowe JW, Besdine RW. Boston, MA, Little, Brown, 1988, pp 157–166

Belal A Jr: Presbycusis: physiological or pathological. J Laryngol Otol 89:1011–1025, 1975

Benedek GB: Theory of transparency of the eye. Appl Optics 10:459–473, 1971

Bertel O, Buhler FR, Kiowski W, et al: Decreased β-adrenoreceptor responsiveness as related to age, blood pressure and plasma catecholamines in patients with essential hypertension. Hypertension 2:130–136, 1980

Blumenthal JA, Emery GF, Madden DJ, et al: Cardiovascular and behavioral effects of aerobic exercise training in healthy older men and women. J Gerontol 44:147–157, 1989

Brody H: Structural changes in the aging nervous system. Interdisciplin Top Gerontol 1970, pp 7–9

Brody H: An examination of cerebral cortex and brainstem aging, in Neurobiology of Aging. Edited by Terry RD, Gershon S. New York, Raven, 1976, pp 177–181

Burg A: Lateral visual field as related to age and sex. J Appl Psychol 52:10–15, 1968

Cameron L, Leventhal EA, Leventhal H: Symptom representations and affect as determinants of care seeking in a community dwelling adult sample population. Health Psychology 12:171–179, 1993

Clark WC, Mehl L: Thermal pain: a sensory decision theory analysis of the effect of age and sex on d', various response criteria and 50% pain threshold. J Abnorm Psychol 78:202–212, 1971

Cody RJ, Torre S, Clark M, et al: Age-related hemodynamic, renal, and hormonal differences among patients with congestive heart failure. Arch Intern Med 149:1023–1028, 1989

Corpas E, Harman SM, Pineyro MA, et al: Growth hormone (GH)–releasing hormone (I-29) twice daily reverses the decreased GH and insulin-like growth factor-1 levels in old men. J Clin Endocrinol Metab 75:530–535, 1992

Corso JF: Sensory processes and age effects in normal adults. J Gerontol 26:90–105, 1971

Dalsky GP, Stocke KS, Ehsani AA, et al: Weight-bearing exercise training and lumbar bone mineral content in postmenopausal women. Ann Intern Med 108:824–828, 1988

Daly RN, Goldberg PB, Roberts J: The effect of age on presynaptic α_2 adrenoceptor autoregulation of norepinephrine release. J Gerontol 44:B59–B66, 1989

El-Baradi A, Bourne GH: Theory of taste and odors. Science 113:660–661, 1951

Finch CE, Schneider EL: Handbook of Biology of Aging, Vol 2. New York, Van Nostrand Reinhold, 1985

Fisher RF: Presbyopia and changes with age in the crystalline lens. J Physiol (Lond) 228:765–779, 1973

Gacek RR: Degenerative hearing loss in aging, in Neurological and Sensory Disorders in the Elderly. Edited by Fields WS. New York, Stratton, 1975, p 219–240

Geokas MC, Conteas CN, Majumdar APN: The aging gastrointestinal tract, liver and pancreas. Clin Geriatr Med 1:177–206, 1985

Ghali WM, Abdel-Rahman S, Hagib M, et al: Intrinsic innervation and vasculature of pre- and post-natal human thymus. Acta Anat 108:115–123, 1980

Gietzen DW, Goodman TA, Weiler PG, et al: Beta receptor density in human lymphocyte membranes: changes with aging? J Gerontol 46:B130–B134, 1991

Goldstein AL, Thurman GB, Low TLK, et al: Relationship of thymus development and function with life span and disease. Aging Series: Physiology and Cell Biology of Aging 8:51–80, 1979

Goodwin JS, Searles RP, Tung KSK: Immunological responses of a healthy elderly population. Clin Exp Immunol 48:403–410, 1982

Greenspan SL, Klibanski A, Rowe JW, et al: Age-related alterations in pulsatile secretion of TSH: role of dopaminergic regulation. Am J Physiol 260:E486–E491, 1991

Greenspan SL, Rowe JW, Maitland LA, et al: The pituitary-adrenal glucocorticoid response is altered by gender and disease. J Gerontol 48:M72–M77, 1993

Griffin JE: Review: hypothyroidism in the elderly. Am J Med Sci 299:334–345, 1991

Hallgren HM, Buckley CE, Gilbersten VA, et al: Lymphocyte phytohemagglutinin responsiveness, immunoglobulins and autoantibodies in aging humans. J Immunol 111:1101–1107, 1973

Harkins SW, Chapman RC: Age and sex differences in pain perception, in Pain in the Trigeminal Region. Edited by Anderson DJ, Matthews B. Amsterdam, Elsevier/North Holland Biomedical, 1977, pp 435–445

Hausman PB, Weksler ME: Changes in the immune response with age, in Handbook of the Biology of Aging, 2nd Edition. Edited by Finch CE, Schneider EL. New York, Van Nostrand Reinhold, 1985

Hermanson B, Omenn GS, Kronmal RA, et al: Beneficial six-year outcome of smoking cessation in older men and women with coronary artery disease. N Engl J Med 319:1365–1369, 1988

Isaacs B: Falls in old age, in Hearing and Balance in the Elderly. Edited by Hinchdiff R. New York, Churchill Livingstone, 1983, pp 373–388

Isaacs B: Clinical and laboratory studies of falls in old people: prospects for prevention. Clin Geriatr Med 1:513–524, 1985

Iwase S, Mano T, Watanabe T, et al: Age-related changes of sympathetic outflow to muscles in humans. J Gerontol 46:M1–M5, 1991

Juby A, Davis P: Psychological profiles of patients with upper gastrointestinal symptomatology induced by non-steroidal anti-inflammatory drugs. Ann Rheum Dis 50(4):211–213, 1991

Kabadi UM, Rosman PM: Thyroid hormone indices in adult healthy subjects: no influence of aging. J Am Geriatr Soc 36:312–316, 1986

Kario K, Matsuo T, Nakao K: Serum erythropoietin levels in the elderly. Gerontology 37:345–348, 1991

Kenney AR: Physiology of Aging: A Synopsis, 2nd Edition. Chicago, IL, Year Book Medical, 1989

Kenshalo DR: Age changes in touch, vibration, temperature, kinesthesis and pain sensitivity, in Handbook of the Psychology of Aging. Edited by Birren JE, Schaie KW. New York, Van Nostrand Reinhold, 1977, pp 562–579

Kim YT, Siskind GW, Weksler ME: Plaque-forming cell response of human blood lymphocytes, III: cellular basis of the reduced immune response in the elderly. Isr J Med Sci 21:317–322, 1985

Kligman AM, Grove GL, Balin AK: Aging of human skin, in Handbook of Biology of Aging, Vol 2. Edited by Finch CE, Schneider EL. New York, Van Nostrand Reinhold, 1985, pp 820–841

Koch TR, Carney JA, Go VLW, et al: Inhibitory neuropeptides and intrinsic innervation of descending human colon. Dig Dis Sci 36:712–718, 1991

Lakatta EG: Cardiovascular function and age. Geriatrics 42:84–94, 1987

Lake CR, Chernow B, Feuerstein G, et al: The sympathetic nervous system in man: its evolution and the measurement of plasma NE, in Norepinephrine. Edited by Ziegler MG, Lake CR. Baltimore, MD, Williams & Williams, 1984

Leventhal EA, Burns EA: Immune dysfunction in the elderly and the occurrence of cancer: aging and the insults of a lifetime of living, in Tumor Immunology and Immunoregulation by Thymic Hormones. Edited by Dammacco F. Milan, Masson, 1987, pp 41–56

Leventhal EA, Leventhal H, Schaefer P, et al: Conservation of energy, uncertainty reduction and swift utilization of medical care among the elderly. Journal of Gerontology: Psychological Sciences 48:P78–P86, 1993

Lim KO, Zipursky RB, Watts MC, et al: Decreased gray matter in normal aging: an in vivo magnetic resonance study. J Gerontol 47:B26–B30, 1992

Makinodan T, Hirokawa K: Normal aging of the immune system. Aging Series: Relations Between Normal Aging and Disease 28:117–132, 1985

Marchesini G, Cassarani S, Checchia GA, et al: Insulin resistance in aged man: relationship between impaired glucose tolerance and decreased insulin activity on branched-chain amino acids. Metabolism 36:1096–1100, 1987

Marcus R, Butterfield G, Holloway L, et al: Administration of recombinant growth hormone to elderly people. J Clin Endocrinol Metab 70:519–527, 1990

Martin WRW, Palmer MR, Patlak CS, et al: Nigrostriatal function in humans studied with positron emission tomography. Ann Neurol 26:535–542, 1989

Martinez JL, Vasquez BJ, Messing RB, et al: Age-related changes in the catecholamine content of peripheral organs in male and female F-344 rats. J Gerontol 36:280–284, 1981

Mastrioanni L, Paulsen CA: The Climacteric. New York, Plenum, 1986

Mazzeo RS, Horvath SM: A decline in myocardial and hepatic norepinephrine turnover with age in Fischer rats. Am J Physiol 252:E762–E764, 1987

McGeer EG, McGeer PL: Age changes in the human for some enzymes associated with metabolism of catecholamine, GABA and acetylcholine. Adv Behav Biol 16:287, 1975

McGeer PL, McGeer EG, Suzuki J, et al: Aging, Alzheimer's disease, and the cholinergic system of the basal forebrain. Neurology 34:741–745, 1984

Minaker KL, Bonis P, Rowe JW: Gastrointestinal system, in Geriatric Medicine, 2nd Edition. Edited by Rowe JW, Besdine RW. Boston, MA, Little, Brown, 1988, pp 495–512

Montagna W, Carlisle K: Structural changes in aging human skin. J Invest Dermatol 73:47–53, 1979

Morley JE: Neuropeptides, behavior and aging. J Am Geriatr Soc 34:52–62, 1986

Morley JE, Reese SS: Clinical implications of the aging heart. Am J Med 86:77–86, 1989

Mortimer JA, Webster DD: Comparison of extrapyramidal motor function in normal aging and Parkinson's disease, in The Aging Motor System (Advances in Neurogerontology, Vol 3). Edited by Mortimer JA, Pirozzolo FJ, Maletta GJ. New York, Praeger, 1982, pp 217–241

National Center for Health Statistics: Current estimates from the National Health Interview Survey, United States, 1982. Vital and Health Statistics, Series 10, No 150. Washington, DC, U.S. Government Printing Office, 1985

Nicosia SV: Morphological changes in the human ovary throughout life, in The Ovary. Edited by Serra GB. New York, Raven, 1983, pp 57–81

Pacini GM, Valerio A, Beccaro F, et al: Insulin sensitivity and β-cell responsivity are not decreased in elderly subjects with normal OGTT. J Am Geriatr Soc 36:317–323, 1988

Poehlman ET, MacAuliffe T, Danforth E: Effects of age and level of physical activity on plasma norepinephrine kinetics. Am J Physiol 258:E256–E262, 1990

Prohaska TR, Keller ML, Leventhal EA, et al: Impact of symptoms and aging attribution on emotions and coping. Health Psychology 6:495–514, 1987

Raiz LG: Local and systemic factors in the pathogenesis of osteoporosis. N Engl J Med 318:818–828, 1988

Raiz LG, Kream BE: Regulation of bone formation, part 1. N Engl J Med 309:29–33, 1983a

Raiz LG, Kream BE: Regulation of bone formation, part 2. N Engl J Med 309:83–89, 1983b

Rappaport EB, Young JB, Landsberg L: Impact of age on basal and diet-induced changes in sympathetic nervous system activity of Fischer rats. J Gerontol 36:152–157, 1981

Riggs BL, Wahner HW, Melton JL, et al: Dietary calcium intake and rates of bone loss in women. J Clin Invest 80:979–982, 1987

Roberts NA, Barton RN, Horan MA: Aging and the sensitivity of the adrenal gland to physiological doses of ACTH in man. J Endocrinol 126:507–513, 1990

Robinson BE, Conrad C: Falls and falling, in Geriatric Medicine Annual. Edited by Ham RJ. Oradell, NJ, Medical Economics, 1986, pp 198–212

Rodeheffer RJ, Gerstenblith G, Becker LC, et al: Exercise cardiac output is maintained with advancing age in healthy human subjects: cardiac dilatation and increased stroke volume compensate for a diminished heart rate. Circulation 69:203–213, 1984

Rogers J, Bloom FE: Neurotransmitter metabolism and function in the aging central nervous system, in Handbook of the Biology of Aging. Edited by Finch CE, Schneider EL. New York, Van Nostrand Reinhold, 1985, pp 645–691

Rong H: Altersveranderungen des beruhrungssinnes. Acta Physiol Scand 6:343–352, 1943

Rossmanith WG, Szilagyi A, Scherbaum WA: Episodic thyrotropin (TSH) and prolactin (PRL) secretion during aging in postmenopausal women. Horm Metab Res 24:185–190, 1992

Rowe JW, Andres R, Tobin JD, et al: The effect of age on creatinine clearance in man: a cross-sectional and longitudinal study. J Gerontol

31:155–163, 1976

Rudman D, Feller AG, Nagraj HS, et al: Effect of human growth hormone in men over 60 years old. N Engl J Med 323:1–6, 1990

Sawin CT, Chopra D, Azizi F, et al: The aging thyroid: increased prevalence of elevated serum thyrotropin levels in the elderly. J Am Med Assoc 242:247–250, 1979

Sawin CT, Geller A, Kaplan MM, et al: Low serum thyrotropin (thyroid-stimulating hormone) in older persons without hyperthyroidism. Arch Intern Med 151:165–168, 1991

Sawle GV, Colebatch JG, Shah A, et al: Striatal function in normal aging: implications for Parkinson's disease. Ann Neurol 28:799–804, 1990

Schiffman SS, Moss J, Erickson RP: Thresholds of food odors in the elderly. Exp Aging Res 2:389–398, 1976

Schocken DD, Roth GS: Reduced β-adrenergic receptor concentrations in aging man. Nature 26:856–858, 1977

Sherman ED, Robillard E: Sensitivity to pain in the aged. Can Med Assoc J 83:944–947, 1960

Simpson DM, Wicks R: Spectral analysis of heart rate indicates reduced baroreceptor-related heart rate variability in elderly persons. J Gerontol 43:M21–M24, 1988

Skinner HB, Barrack RI, Cook SD: Age-related decline in proprioception. Clin Orthop 184:208–211, 1984

Skoglund S: Joint receptors and kinaesthesis, in Handbook of Sensory Physiology, Vol 2. Edited by Iggo A. Berlin, Springer-Verlag, 1973, pp 111–136

Sparks DL, Hunsaker JC, Slevin JT, et al: Monoaminergic and cholinergic synaptic markers in the nucleus basalis of Meynert (nbM): normal age-related changes and the effect of heart disease and Alzheimer's disease. Ann Neurol 31:611–620, 1992

Spector A, Li S, Sigelman J: Age dependent changes in the molecular size of human lens proteins and their relationship to light scatter. Invest Ophthalmol 13:795–798, 1974

Stearns EL, MacDonnell JA, Kaufman BJ, et al: Declining testicular function with age. Am J Med 57:761–766, 1974

Stelmach CE, Worringham CJ: Sensorimotor deficits related to postural stability: implications for falling in the elderly. Clin Geriatr Med 3:679–694, 1985

Stevens JC: Aging and spatial acuity of touch. J Gerontol 47:35–40, 1992

Terry RD, De Teresa R, Hansen LAS: Neocortical cell counts in normal adult aging. Ann Neurol 21:530–539, 1987

Van Coevorden A, Laurent E, Decoster C, et al: Decreased basal and stimulated thyrotropin secretion in healthy elderly men. J Clin Endocrinol Metab 69:177–185, 1989

Vestal RE, Wood AJJ, Shand DG: Reduced β-adrenoreceptor sensitivity in the elderly. Clin Pharmacol Ther 26:1181–1186, 1979

Waltman C, Blackman MR, Chrousos GP, et al: Spontaneous and glucocorticoid-inhibited adrenocorticotropic hormone and cortisol secretion are similar in healthy young and old men. J Clin Endocr Metab 73:495–502, 1991

Wesson LG: Physiology of the Human Kidney. New York, Grune & Stratton, 1969

Williams JM, Felton DL: Sympathetic innervation of murine thymus and spleen: a comparative histofluorescence study. Anat Rec 199:531–542, 1981

Williams JM, Peterson RG, Shea PA, et al: Sympathetic innervation of murine thymus and spleen: evidence for a functional link between the nervous and immune systems. Brain Res Bull 6:83–94, 1981

Winkelmann RK: Nerve changes in aging skin. Adv Biol Skin 6:51–62, 1965

Zahniser NR, Parker DC, Bier-Laning CM, et al: Comparison between the effects of aging on antagonist and agonist interactions with β-adrenergic receptors on human mononuclear and polymorphonuclear leukocyte membranes. J Gerontol 43:M151–M157, 1988

Ziegler MG, Lake CR, Kopin IJ: Plasma noradrenaline increases with age. Nature 261:333–335, 1976

C H A P T E R 4

Mark P. Rubert, Ph.D.
Carl Eisdorfer, Ph.D., M.D.
David A. Loewenstein, Ph.D.

Normal Aging: Changes in Sensory/Perceptual and Cognitive Abilities

Psychological changes with aging are the product of alterations in anatomy and physiology as well as changes in social status (e.g., retirement) and interpersonal status (e.g., loss of friends or spouse). In addition, traumata show cumulative effects with age and may directly or indirectly affect performance (e.g., occupational noise exposure is associated with hearing loss). Certain environmental stressors, such as financial problems, crime, reduced standard of living, and other life-stage problems (e.g., moving to a new living situation), are also more likely to occur as one grows older. Factors such as exercise, diet, health care utilization, and other socioeconomic and cultural differences between older and younger people result in life-style differences and cohort effects that appear as age-related changes in late life. Generalizations about age-related changes can be made, but one must be careful as individual differences also increase with age (Eisdorfer and Mintzer 1988).

In part, the changes that occur with aging are the result of gradual declines in the function of various organ systems, with many organ systems losing function at the rate of about 1% per year after age 30. However, the effects of aging are not solely the result of biological changes. Increasing age is also associated with changes in cognitive function as a result of reduction of the number of neurons within the brain, increased stress on organ systems vital to blood circulation, and decreased sensory and perceptual abilities. These changes alter vision, taste, and cognitive capacity, but these changes occur to a much lesser extent than is commonly believed and may be mitigated to some extent by initial ability, practice, exercise, medication, or other life-style changes (La Rue 1992; Loewenstein and Eisdorfer 1992; Zarit and Zarit 1987).

Sensation and Perception

As people age, all five of their senses decline in acuity (Zarit and Zarit 1987). Vision and auditory loss are frequently the most problematic for older persons (Loewenstein and Eisdorfer 1992; Orr 1991). For example, a reduction in visual acuity can result in decreased independence by affecting an individual's ability to drive an automobile and navigate familiar and unfamiliar locations. As vision grows worse, an individual can also lose the ability to read and to pursue hobbies such as needlepoint. Similarly, decreased hearing can limit an individual's autonomy and can lead to increased isolation from others.

Normal elderly individuals typically experience a number of visual changes, including decreased accommodation, decreased acuity, decreased color sensitivity, and decreased depth perception, and the incidence of visual problems and blindness increases with age. Approximately 92% of older people wear glasses to help them cope with some of these changes (Hull 1989). Older people also require higher levels of illumination to discern an item than does someone in their 20s. In practical terms, this means that older people have to get much closer to highway signs before they can read them at night (Sivak et al. 1981). There is also a decline in the sensitivity of visual perception of motion. Trick and Silverman (1991) studied 95 subjects ages 25 to 80 and found that motion sensitivity declined at the rate of about 1% per decade, but the work of Gilmore et al. (1992) suggests that this decline can be found only in elderly women.

The most common cause of visual problems in older adults is cataracts (opacification of the lens). In fact, about 50% of adults over age 40 show signs of developing cataracts (Heath 1992). Other common visual disorders associated with aging are glaucoma, macular degeneration, and diabetic retinopathy.

Hearing also declines over a life span; about 50% of persons over age 75 (Plomp 1978) and about 70% of the residents of nursing homes (Ciurlia-Guy et al. 1993) have some degree of hearing loss. Presbycusis is associated with aging and results from sensorineural damage that occurs during life due to noise trauma, exposure to ototoxic subjects, and genetic factors (Nadol 1993). This type of hearing loss results in decreased perception of high frequencies, difficulty in localizing signals, and decreased pitch discrimination. This often leads to difficulty understanding the speech of others, especially when environmental conditions are unfavorable (e.g., noisy rooms with long reverberations). The interaction between age and living in a noisy, industrialized society may help to explain why there is an increase in hearing loss (deafness) from 2.8% of the population at age 55 to 15% by age 75 (Rockstein and Sussman 1979).

The impact of visual and auditory changes in elderly individuals has not received much attention from researchers. Blindness or severe visual impairments can curtail rewarding activities and force minimal social interaction if a person is unable to leave home without assistance. Therefore, it is important to improve an individual's vision and thus their quality of life, perhaps with simple aids such as a high-powered magnifying glasses or surgery to remove cataracts.

Although hearing loss is not significantly related to social isolation (Norris and Cunningham 1981; Powers and Powers 1978) or paranoia (Moore 1981; Thomas et al. 1983) as has been suggested in the past, hearing is important for safety (e.g., smoke alarms, running water) and pleasure (e.g., listening to grandchildren). Hearing might be enhanced with unilateral or bilateral hearing aids. Corso (1985) presented several additional methods to enhance a person's ability to perceive speech sounds, such as cochlear implants for individuals with profound hearing impairment.

Elderly individuals are also likely to have age-related declines in olfaction and taste (Ship and Weiffenbach 1993), but these sensory-perceptual changes also have received limited attention. Individual declines in olfaction (Doty et al. 1984) vary widely and the olfactory anatomy atrophies significantly (Bhatnagar et al. 1987). Olfaction not only plays an important role in the enjoyment of foods and beverages, but it also can provide important information about the environment, such as the detection of smoke or spoiled food. Russell et al. (1993) reported on data gathered from over 1 million respondents to the National Geographic smell survey. The survey suggested that perception of spicy and musky odors is relatively stable with age, but that perception of sweet and fruity odors declines with age.

Other age-related changes associated with aging that contribute to taste difficulties are substantial loss of lingual papillae, which results in reduced perception of sweet and salty tastes, decreases in salivation that limit the dispersal of the agents about the mouth that can reduce the perception of flavoring agents, and upper dentures that can cover the secondary taste areas (Nelson and Franzi 1992). In sum, it is likely that these changes in olfaction and taste are linked to the common complaint of many older individuals that food no longer tastes or smells right.

There is some evidence that adults in their 60s to 70s have less sensitivity in their palms (Kenshalo 1977) and feet (Skre 1972). In addition, studies suggest differences in the perception of pain and painful stimuli associated with aging (Sturgis et al. 1987). These somatosensory changes can lead to burns from hot water or appliances. In addition, falls can occur when an older individual moves from a slick floor surface (e.g., tile) to a surface that offers more resistance (e.g., carpet) or when using stairs.

Cognitive Abilities

The study of the intellectual changes resulting from normal psychological aging is challenging. For example, longitudinal studies with the elderly have inherent difficulties with cohort effects as a result of an enhanced probability of disease associated with older age and an increased likelihood of attrition through illness or death. In addition, educational attainment, widespread social practices such as specific child-rearing customs, and even exposure to certain illnesses make it difficult to study individuals in different age and ethnocultural groups, because cohort effects can confound or bias many of the dependent measures (Loewenstein and Eisdorfer 1992). These difficulties notwithstanding, the results of research indicate that most of the supposed intellectual declines associated with aging are a function of psychomotor slowing, declines in sensory/perceptual abilities, and the increased anxiety that older people often display in formal testing situations.

Intellectual Functions

Extensive literature on changes in intellectual performance with aging indicates that abilities peak in the 30s, plateau through the 50s or early 60s, and then begin a slow, but increasingly rapid decline in the late 70s (Botwinick 1977; Cunningham 1987; Schaie 1980). However, changes in intelligence as a function of age may be confounded by cohort effects, as many of these studies were cross-sectional in design (Loewenstein and Eisdorfer 1992; Rabbitt 1979). Studies using a longitudinal design may also overestimate or underestimate changes in intellectual performance caused by the effects of attrition and reactivity (Schaie 1988).

Despite the belief that older adults are unable to learn new information, or the "you can't teach an old dog new tricks" hypothesis, research shows that older adults are able to learn and can benefit from encoding strategies. They also can benefit from longer exposure to the to-be-remembered stimuli and may benefit from techniques designed to enhance their motivation. Spar and La Rue (1990) concluded that cognitive functions such as attention span; everyday communication skills; lexical, phonological, and syntactic knowledge; discourse comprehension; and simple visual perception remain preserved in older adults. On the other hand, selective attention, cognitive flexibility, and the ability to shift cognitive sets, naming objects, verbal fluency, more complex visuoconstructive skills, and logical analysis may decrease with age.

No consensus exists as to at what age these cognitive abilities decline, and a recent study of 25,140 American workers found that when the effects of experience, education, and occupational type were controlled for statistically, the age of the subject accounted for little of the variance in ability test scores, whereas race accounted for much of the variance (Avolio and Waldman 1994). This finding suggests that the intellectual decline associated with aging found in many studies may be the result of other influences (i.e., ethnoracial variables and their mediation of social and environmental variables) that interact with cognitive/intellectual functioning in middle and old age. Moreover, interindividual variability in performance on intelligence and memory tasks increases with advancing age (Christensen et al. 1994).

Cross-sectional data on the intellectual functioning of 1,628 community-dwelling individuals ages 29 to 88 were recently reported by Schaie and Willis (1993). Their sample population is well educated (mean years of education was 14.3 ± 3.06) with good jobs (most frequent occupations were skilled trades, clerical sales, managerial jobs, and semiprofessional jobs) and middle incomes (average family income was $23,200 ± $9,606). They reported age-related performance declines beginning around age 50 for inductive reasoning, spatial orientation, verbal memory, and perceptual speed. Differences in numeric and verbal abilities appeared in the later 60s. Performance of subjects in their 80s was the worst for all tasks, with the largest performance decline in the perceptual speed tasks and the least in the vocabulary tasks.

Hultsch et al. (1992) examined the rate of decline in a sample of 328 noninstitutionalized men and women ages 55 to 86. They controlled for differences in individual capacities by assessing the intraindividual effects of aging while also evaluating the changes that could be attributed to cohort effects. Age-related declines were found in working memory, verbal fluency, and world knowledge, even when cohort effects were controlled for statistically.

A two-factor model of intelligence has been proposed (Horn and Cattell 1967; Horn and Donaldson 1976). This model attempts to account for the differential decline in intelligence by distinguishing between *crystallized* and *fluid* abilities. Crystallized abilities are represented by knowledge acquired during the person's lifetime, and, as indicated above, several studies indicate that these abilities improve or remain consistent until late in life. In contrast, fluid abilities are represented by the ability to solve new tasks by the acquisition of new knowledge and new skills.

Such differences in types of abilities can also help to explain the lack of consistent findings on the relationship of age to work performance. Given the declines in inductive reasoning, spatial orientation, verbal memory, and perceptual speed, one could expect that the work performance of the older person would decline. However, both a review of the literature (Rhodes 1983) and a meta-analysis of 65 studies (McEvoy and Cascio 1989) failed to find a clear relationship between age and work performance, although those studies generally did not discriminate between the nature of the job and the years of experience the individual had performing that job. Years of job experience leads to the crystallization of abilities such that they do not decline much with age, and, in fact, elderly individuals may demonstrate improvement with age as a result of the years of practice.

Older workers performing jobs that require more fluid abilities should demonstrate more impairment. One example of how this change in fluid ability can impact an older individual can be found in a study by Czaja and Sharit (1993) that compared the abilities of 65 women ages 25 to 70 years to learn a "new" computer-based task. They found that increased age was associated with longer response times and a greater number of errors. Older subjects also felt the task was more difficult and more tiring. Another study found that skilled older typists did not show an age-related slowing in their motor performance but that unskilled older typists (fluid ability) were slower than younger unskilled typists (Bosman 1993).

In a series of studies, Eisdorfer and colleagues demonstrated that heightened autonomic nervous system (ANS) activity was associated with a slowing and/or reduction in response rate among older men compared with younger men in a learning task (Eisdorfer 1968; Eisdorfer et al. 1970). Prior experience with a similar task or the use of blocking agents reduced the differences between the two age groups. Women (Eisdorfer and Service 1967) and men with high verbal abilities did not show similar age-related deficits (Wilkie and Eisdorfer 1977). Health factors were also suggested as covariates by Eisdorfer and Wilkie (1973) and Wilkie and Eisdorfer (1973), who reported that heightened blood pressure or nearness to death and recent medical history were factors in predicting declining intellectual performance. Other data on hypertensive individuals, however, have suggested that the effect of blood pressure may be more equivocal (Perez-Stable et al. 1992).

The concept of *brain reserve capacity,* used to account for intra-individual differences in response to head injury and dementia, may also be relevant to the study of normal aging. Many researchers have noted that there are large individual differences in response to aging, in both the biological and cognitive systems. The concepts of reserve capacity and threshold in dementia are taken from the Newcastle studies, which first raised the possibility of individual differences to account for differences between postmortem findings and other measures of dementia (Blessed et al. 1968; Roth et al. 1967). Satz (1993) reviewed the research in brain reserve capacity and reported that studies have found that bright, well-educated patients—factors that are presumably reflective of higher levels of reserve capacity—retained more of their abilities in the face of organic impairments relative to less-educated patients. Future studies on normal aging may evaluate the construct of brain reserve capacity.

Memory Functions

When older adults complain about their cognitive functions, they most often cite difficulties with memory (Guterman et al. 1993; Williams et al. 1983). Indeed, mnemonic functions are among the most significant of all age-related losses cited by elderly persons. Although there are changes in memory associated with aging, the actual deterioration among healthy adults is not nearly as extensive as once thought (Zarit and Zarit 1987). Probably, the failure to appreciate that memory impairment was the result of Alzheimer's disease or other medical or neuropsychiatric conditions led to the erroneous belief that significant memory problems were a normal result of aging. There are three general types of memory that are differentially affected by normal aging: primary, secondary, and tertiary memory.

Primary memory is a time-limited temporary capacity store that can be maintained only through practice or rehearsal. If one were to ask the directory assistance operator for an unfamiliar phone number, one might hold the number in primary memory with a bit of rehearsal long enough to dial the party that one wished to call. However, if one were to ask that individual to remember the phone number 3 hours later, they would likely draw a blank. Primary memory appears to play an important role (through practice and rehearsal) in retaining things that are needed while permitting the relinquishing of trivial information that does not have any long-term purpose. Although Craik (1977) demonstrated that older people may be slower in accessing information from primary stores, tasks such as digit span appear to be performed equally well in older and younger adults (Botwinick 1977; Craik 1977).

Secondary memory is the ability to acquire new information and is probably the most susceptible to the effects of aging. For example, older adults are usually more sensitive to distractors on divided attention tasks (Craik 1977), quick pacing of material (Monge and Hultsch 1971), and the amount of material presented to them at one time (Light et al. 1982). It has been hypothesized that this reduction in the ability to learn new material may be related in part to degeneration of the hippocampus and a decrease in the efficacy or abundance of neurotransmitters, such as acetylcholine (La Rue 1992; Loewenstein et al. 1989).

Although older people generally show significant improvement in their performance when provided memory encoding strategies that appear to be typically employed by younger subjects, it appears that the initial benefits afforded by these strategies are not permanent because older adults tend to stop using the techniques that they have learned (Anschutz et al. 1987; Scogin and Bienas 1988). Perhaps reinforcement paradigms that emphasize rehearsal and use of these newly learned skills would prove beneficial. In any case, tools to enhance the efficacy of encoding may be beneficial in creating a greater sense of personal control, self-efficacy, and the reassurance that occasional memory lapses are normal (La Rue 1992). Boyarsky and Eisdorfer (1972) showed that learning in older individuals may be less efficient because they are more likely to learn peripheral and nonrelevant material, whereas younger subjects are more task oriented.

In addition to encoding, retrieval of new information is also more difficult for older people. It is difficult to determine whether older adults apply less effort at retrieval, have more difficulties accessing stored traces, or whether weakly encoded material by definition is more difficult to retrieve. Eisdorfer's (1972) finding that errors of omission occur more frequently than errors of commission in older men compared with younger men suggest that fear of failure may also play a role in the performance of older men. The older men showed heightened and more persistent autonomic nervous system activity during learning and postlearning than the younger men.

Tertiary, or remote, memory is those memories that have been stored and consolidated over long periods. Examples of such memory are one's birthdate, wedding anniversary, or a historical event (e.g., the assassination of a prominent national figure). Clinicians have been long aware that remote memories are clearer and more readily accessible to older adults than more recent memories, where there has been less exposure to the to-be-remembered material or fewer opportunities to rehearse or more strongly encode the information. Tertiary memories are probably more resistant to changes within the brain because they often represent personal, salient, or emotionally laden memory traces that have been recalled a number of times and are widely connected to a vast array of other neuronal networks and thus easier to access. Tertiary memory is perhaps one of the most difficult processes to measure because it is not possible to control for exposure or rehearsal of the to-be-remembered material. However, there is general consensus that tertiary memory is poorer among older subjects (Howes and Katz 1988; Warrington and Sanders 1971).

In summary, older adults exhibit the greatest memory problems in secondary memory with difficulties in encoding as well as retrieval processing. In contrast, primary and tertiary memory functions appear to be much better preserved in older adults.

Cognition and Health

The probability of having from one or more chronic medical conditions increases with age such that 80% of individuals over age 65 will have at least one chronic disease. In addition, changes in immune system functioning leave older adults more susceptible to infections (Spar and La Rue 1990). Few studies have attempted to evaluate the relationship between health and cognitive functioning, although there have been a number of studies that showed impairment in cognition and memory processes due to depression (for a review see Salzman and Gutfreund [1986]).

Studies have found substantial correlations between subjective health status and functional status in older adults (Ferraro 1980) and physical examinations or physician ratings (La Rue et al. 1979; Maddox and Douglass 1973), but it does *not* appear that there is a strong relationship between physical health and cognition. Lawton (1986) reviewed a number of studies that reported relationships between various measures of health and cognition. He found low correlations between self-rated health and reports of health problems with various gross measures of global cognitive functioning. In contrast, Perlmutter and Nyquist (1990) recently reported significant relationships between self-reported health status and intelligence as measured by the Wechsler Adult Intelligence Scale. They found that a significant portion of the variance in memory span and fluid intelligence was accounted for by self-reported health status. Hultsch et al. (1993) also found a significant relationship between self-reported health and measures of time processing, working memory, and text memory, but these relationships were of limited practical importance because they accounted for only 1% to 3% of the variance. Despite these modest effects, they argue that self-reported physical health is an important moderator of the effects of age on an individual's performance on a wide range of cognitive measures. However, at least one study reported that controlling for self-reported health had little effect on age-related differences in performance on four cognitive measures (Salthouse et al. 1990).

Cultural Differences

The findings reported in the preceding section on cognition are largely the result of research on populations that do not contain minority subjects. However, it is well known that the results of intelligence tests are influenced by the cultural background of the individual being tested (Pick 1980). Moreover, Holtzman, Diaz-Guerrero, and Swartz (1975) compared Anglo-American children to Mexican children (ages 6 to 18) and found a number of age-by-culture interactions in cognitive abilities, several of which indicated that the initial advantages of the Mexican children were reversed as they grew older.

Despite the importance of cultural variables, surprisingly few studies have addressed the patterns of cognitive decline among elders in various ethnic and cultural groups (Loewenstein and Rubert 1992; Valle 1989). Applying traditional normative data to these populations may be seriously misleading because measures of semantic memory and language measures may be biased against those individuals for whom English is a second language (Lopez and Taussig et al. 1991). For example, healthy Spanish-speaking elderly persons in the United States had a lower performance on verbal fluency tests, such as the Controlled Word Association Test (Benton and Hamsher 1977), even when the test was administered in the patient's native language (Loewenstein and Rubert 1992; Taussig et al. 1992), perhaps because the relative frequency of a word beginning with a certain letter of the alphabet is not equivalent in English and Spanish or because Spanish-speakers must also decide whether or not a phonologically correct word also begins with the correct letter.

A major challenge facing researchers is the establishment of normative data bases that take education, gender, age, sociological and cultural background, and the applicability of tests, testing situations, and test administrators into account (Loewenstein and Rubert 1992). However, even with normative data for a given measure that appears to be adequate, the measure may still not be valid. Some ethnoracial groups may be unwilling to participate in normative studies, and, even when they do, it is often extremely difficult to adequately account for the impact of the immigration experience and sociopolitical influences such as discriminatory laws and practices. Loewenstein et al. (1993) contend that a measure may be culturally biased because 1) a measure developed for an English-speaking population may not be salient or meaningful to other populations, and 2) the frequency of "correct" responses may vary based on the cultural background of the group studied. In addition, immigrant cultural groups may vary from similar groups in their native homeland. Geisinger (1992) has recommended the inclusion of formal measures of acculturation when individuals from other cultures are assessed with psychological tests.

Functional Changes

Although age-related changes in sensation and perception, intellectual abilities, and memory are significant in themselves, the ability to perform functions for personal care (activities of daily living [ADL]) and functions necessary for maintaining an independent residence (instrumental activities of daily living [IADL]) are *critical* indicators of an individual's ability to live independently (Loewenstein and Rubert 1992). Moreover, declines in functional status have been found to be significantly associated with death or nursing home placement (Ribbon et al. 1992).

Loewenstein et al. (1989) developed the Direct Assessment of Functional Status (DAFS), a measure that directly assesses an older person's ability to perform several instrumental activities of daily living (e.g., telling time, orientation to date, using the telephone, preparing a letter for mailing, writing a check, making change, or shopping for groceries) and activities of daily living (e.g., eating, dressing, and grooming). Older adults typically do not have difficulties performing the IADLs and ADLs that they have successfully performed in the past unless they have significant cognitive deterioration caused by conditions such as Alzheimer's disease, significantly impaired physical or mental health, and/or significant perceptual impairments (Loewenstein et al. 1992).

Crimmins and Saito (1993) examined the determinants of functional change for more than 2 years in 3,169 noninstitutionalized elderly people ages 70 or older. At the initial assessment, they found that less than 10% of their subjects reported difficulty in performing their IADLs (3.1% to 9.3%), and with the exception of reporting difficulty walking, less than 8% reported difficulty in performing their ADLs (1.0% to 7.6%). Two years later, the reported increase in difficulty performing IADLs ranged from 3.3% to 6.0%. For ADLs, the reported increase ranged from 2.1% to 6.9%, except for walking difficulties, which increased by 9.9%. Myers et al. (1993) assessed changes in the speed of functional performance of 46 persons over 1 year. They found declines in the time it took for a person to open bottles with safety tops (line up the arrows and push down/pull up before turning), remove a pill from a blister pack, boil water for soup, put away a bowl, and walk a distance of 12 feet.

Exercise and Aging

Physicians have been encouraged to tell their older patients to adopt a program of regular exercise (Hall 1992), because several studies have shown that a regular program of aerobic exercise can slow or reverse age-related declines in cardiovascular function and musculoskeletal fitness (Evans and Campbell 1993; Kannel et al. 1986; Warren et al. 1993). Aerobic exercise has also been associated with beneficial changes in performance of cognitive tasks, such as simple and choice reaction time tasks (Bashore 1989; Spirduso and Clifford 1978). However, these benefits may not extend to memory processes. Two studies that examined the effects of aerobic exercise on attention and memory retrieval found no differences in the performance of the aerobic exercise group compared with an anaerobic group and waiting-list control subjects (Blumenthal and Madden 1988; Madden et al. 1989).

One area of cognitive function where age-related differences in performance are typically found is in attentional capacity. Attentional capacity is typically assessed by divided attention tasks, where subjects are required to simultaneously perform two tasks. An interesting study performed by Hawkins et al. (1992) evaluated the effect of exercise on attentional processes. They first compared the performances of younger adults (ages 20–35) and older adults (ages 65–74) on a time-sharing task that required subjects to process two tasks simultaneously and an attentional flexibility task where subjects had to switch attention between two sequential tasks. The younger adults were more efficient on the time-sharing task and able to switch their attention more rapidly compared with the older adults. Next, the same tasks were given to 37 older subjects, 18 of whom were assigned to a 10-week aerobic exercise program. The older exercisers performed significantly better on the time-sharing and attentional tasks compared with the control subjects. The authors suggested that these changes may be the result of enhanced cardiovascular sufficiency.

Wisdom and Creativity

Although many age-related declines in cognition produce a rather negative picture of the cognitive effects of aging, there are areas in which researchers have begun to look for improvement, or at least lack of decline, with age. In particular, we usually hope to become wiser as we grow older, and many artists, writers, and composers remain productive throughout their lives.

Both wisdom and creativity are difficult concepts to define and quantify. One significant study on wisdom was performed by Baltes and colleagues (see Baltes 1993 for a review), who postulated that wisdom is related to crystallized intelligence, and they have attempted to objectively quantify wisdom based on one's level of performance on specific tasks. They asked people to solve life problems and scored their performance according to five wisdom criteria (factual knowledge, procedural knowledge, life-span contextualism, value relativism, and uncertainty). They also attempted to delineate three categories they felt facilitated the acquisition of wisdom: general personal conditions, specific expertise conditions, and facilitative life contexts. They propose that wisdom-related knowledge, particularly expertise-related knowledge, is established and refined during the life span by the tasks of life management, life planning, and life review. Smith and Baltes (1990) compared younger and older adults on wisdom-related tasks and found no significant differences in their performance.

Baltes (1993) also reported the findings of a study in which older people were nominated for participation in the study based on their wisdom. Subjects were asked to respond to two scenarios. The first scenario was that a 60-year-old businesswoman who had just opened her own business learns that her son has been left with two small children. The second was that someone gets a call from a good friend who states that he or she has decided to commit suicide. The subjects are then asked to state what they should do in each situation, and their responses were scored according to Baltes's wisdom criteria. No negative effects for age were found, but there was also little evidence of increased wisdom among those nominated for their wisdom compared with the control subjects. However, Baltes notes that the wisdom nominees did handle the more difficult suicide scenario better. In addition, age-related increases in wisdom were reported in another study that defined wisdom in terms of the ability to solve problems that one faces in everyday life (Cornelius and Caspi 1987).

As creativity is most often measured by performance on various standardized psychometric tests, it is not surprising to find that most investigations of age-related creativity show a decline with age (McCrae et al. 1987). However, most of these studies are cross-sectional and may suffer cohort effects, and the validity of many of the creativity measures ranges from modest to poor (Simonton 1990). Moreover, Simonton (1990) has suggested that creativity and wisdom may converge late in life, when individuals create products such as musical compositions that reflect wisdom in their design and content. In summary, the complex concepts of wisdom and creativity are difficult to quantify and study and more research is needed in these areas.

Conclusions

In this chapter, we have examined a number of the normal psychological changes that appear to be associated with aging. Sensory/perceptual changes result in diminished visual and auditory acuity and alterations in olfaction and taste. The ability to shift cognitive set rapidly, psychomotor speed, reaction time, verbal fluency, complex visuoconstructive skills, and logical analysis skills appear to decrease with age. Although older adults may have more difficulty with novel tasks, especially tasks that require quick psychomotor responding, the notion that increasing age is associated with significant decreases in intellectual and memory abilities is simply incorrect.

Normal elderly people do not experience significant cognitive deterioration. Primary and tertiary memory remain relatively intact with aging. Secondary memory, or the ability to encode, store, consolidate, and retrieve new material, appears to be more difficult for healthy older adults, but they do appear to benefit from learning and cuing strategies that are consistently used.

Moreover, much of the existing research on normal aging is cross-sectional in design, and potentially more ecologically valid longitudinal studies may be confounded by cohort effects. Many of the measures are not adequately validated for older adults and suffer from cultural bias. This situation is particularly problematic given the rapid growth of ethnoracial minority groups, particularly in the older adults, in the United States (U.S. Census 1990).

Physical health appears to have a significant impact on cognitive functioning, but few studies have addressed the impact of physical health on cognition. Studies have indicated that cardiovascular fitness can be significantly improved in older people with a simple program of regular aerobic exercise, and this improvement in cardiovascular function may also be associated with improvements in cognition.

To put these changes in a broader framework, it appears that the ability of an individual to perform at any time depends on 1) the person's ability at that point in time, 2) the level of performance needed from the system(s), and 3) the reserve capacity of the individual. For example, some elderly people may cope successfully with the demands of driving a car on a city street at 30 mph but, because of slower reaction time or visual problems associated with aging, be unable to cope with the demands of driving on the highway at 55 mph or faster. For other elderly people, the demands of highway driving will not overtax their abilities, and they will cope well with the demands of such tasks quite well. Finally, although the study of wisdom and creativity in older individuals has only just begun, it appears that wisdom and creativity may increase as one gets older and gains life experience.

References

Anschutz L, Camp CJ, Markley RP, et al: Remembering mnemonics: a three-year follow-up on the effects of mnemonics training in elderly adults. Exp Aging Res 13:141–143, 1987

Avolio BJ, Waldman DA: Variations in cognitive, perceptual, and psycho-motor abilities across the working life span: examining the effects of race, sex, experience, education, and occupational type. Psychol Aging 9:430–442, 1994

Baltes PB: The aging mind: potential and limits. Gerontologist 33:580–594, 1993

Bashore T: Age, physical fitness and mental processing speed, in Annual Review of Gerontology and Geriatrics. Edited by Lawton MP. New York, Springer, 1989, pp 120–144

Benton A, Hamsher K: Multilingual Aphasia Examination. Iowa City, University of Iowa, 1977

Bhatnagar NP, Kennedy RC, Baron G, et al: Number of mitral cells and the bulb volume in the aging human olfactory bulb: a quantitative morphological study. Anat Rec 218:73–87, 1987

Blessed G, Tomlinson BE, Roth M: Association between quantitative measures of dementing and senile change in the cerebral grey matter of elderly subjects. Br J Psychiatry 114:797–811, 1968

Blumenthal JA, Madden DJ: Effects of aerobic exercise training, age, and physical fitness on memory search performance. Psychol Aging 3:280–285, 1988

Bosman EA: Age-related differences in the motoric aspects of transcription typing skill. Psychol Aging 8:87–102, 1993

Botwinick J: Intellectual abilities, in Handbook of the Psychology of Aging. Edited by Birren JE, Schaie KW. New York, Van Nostrand Reinhold, 1977, pp 580–605

Boyarsky RE, Eisdorfer C: Forgetting in older persons. J Gerontol 27:254–258, 1972

Christensen H, Mackinnon A, Jorm AF, et al: Age differences and interindividual variation in cognition in community-dwelling elderly. Psychol Aging 9:381–390, 1994

Ciurlia-Guy E, Cashman M, Lewsen B: Identifying hearing loss and hearing handicap among chronic care elderly people. Gerontologist 33:644–649, 1993

Cornelius SW, Caspi A: Everyday problem-solving in adulthood and old age. Psychol Aging 2:144–153, 1987

Corso JF: Communication, presbycusis, and technological aids, in The Aging Brain: Communication in the Elderly. Edited by Ulatowska HK. Boston, MA, College Hill Press, 1985

Craik FIM: Age differences in human memory, in Handbook of the Psychology of Aging. Edited by Birren JE, Schaie KW. New York, Van Nostrand Reinhold, 1977, pp 384–420

Crimmins EM, Saito Y: Getting better and getting worse: transitions in functional status among older Americans. J Aging Health 5:3–36, 1993

Cunningham WR: Intellectual abilities and age, in Annual Review of Gerontology and Geriatrics. Edited by Schaie KW. New York, Springer, 1987, pp 117–134

Czaja SJ, Sharit J: Age differences in the performance of computer-based work. Psychol Aging 8:59–67, 1993

Doty RL, Shaman P, Applebaum SL, et al: Smell identification ability: changes with age. Science 226:1441–1443, 1984

Eisdorfer C: Arousal and performance: experiments in verbal learning and a tentative theory, in Human Behavior and Aging: Recent Changes in Research Theory. Edited by Talland G. New York, Academic Press, 1968, pp 189–216

Eisdorfer C: Autonomic changes in aging, in Aging and the Brain. Edited by Gaitz CM. New York, Plenum, 1972

Eisdorfer C, Mintzer J: Performance and aging: an integrative biopsychosocial paradigm, in Crossroads in Aging. London, Academic Press, 1988, pp 189–203

Eisdorfer C, Service C: Verbal role learning and superior intelligence in the aged. J Gerontol 22:158–161, 1967

Eisdorfer C, Wilkie F: Intellectual changes with advancing age, in Intellectual Functioning in Adults. Edited by Jarvik LF, Eisdorfer C, Blum J. New York, Springer, 1973, pp 21–29

Eisdorfer C, Nowlin J, Wilkie F: Improvement of learning in the aged by modification of autonomic nervous system activity. Science 170:1327–1329, 1970

Evans WJ, Campbell WW: Sarcopenia and age-related changes in body composition and functional capacity. J Nutr 123:465–468, 1993

Ferraro KF: Self-ratings of health among the old and old-old. J Health Soc Behav 21:377–383, 1980

Geisinger KF: Fairness and selected psychometric issues in psychological testing of Hispanics, in Psychological Testing of Hispanics. Edited by Geisinger KF. Washington, DC, American Psychological Association, 1992

Gilmore GC, Wenk HE, Naylor LA, et al: Motion perception and aging. Psychol Aging 4:643–653, 1992

Guterman A, Loewenstein D, Gamez E, et al: Stressful life experiences in the early detection of Alzheimer's disease: potential limitations associated with the estimation of illness duration. Behavior, Health and Aging 3:43–49, 1993

Hall NK: Health maintenance and promotion, in Primary Care Geriatrics:

A Case-Based Approach, 2nd Edition. Edited by Ham RJ, Sloane PD. St. Louis, MO, Mosby-Year Book, 1992

Hawkins HL, Kramer AF, Capaldi D: Aging, exercise and attention. Psychol Aging 4:643–653, 1992

Heath JM: Vision, in Primary Care Geriatrics: A Case-Based Approach, 2nd Edition. Edited by Ham RJ, Sloane PD. St. Louis, MO, Mosby-Year Book, 1992

Holtzman WH, Diaz-Guerrero R, Swartz JD: Personality Development in Two Cultures. Austin, University of Texas Press, 1975

Horn JL, Cattell RB: Age differences in fluid and crystallized intelligence. Acta Psycholog 26:107–129, 1967

Horn JL, Donaldson G: On the myth of intellectual decline in adulthood. Am Psychol 31:701–719, 1976

Howes JL, Katz AN: Assessing remote memory with an improved public events questionnaire. Psychol Aging 3:142–150, 1988

Hull R: Incidence of selected language, speech and hearing disorders among the elderly, in Communication Disorders in Aging. Edited by Hull R, Griffin KM. Newbury Park, CA, Sage, 1989

Hultsch DF, Hertzog C, Small BJ, et al: Short-term longitudinal change in cognitive performance in later life. Psychol Aging 7:571–584, 1992

Hultsch DF, Hammer M, Small BJ: Age differences in cognitive performance in later life: relationships to self-reported health and activity life style. Journal of Gerontology: Psychological Sciences 48:1–11, 1993

Kannel W, Belanger A, D'Agostino R, et al: Physical activity and physical demand on the job and risk of cardiovascular disease and death: the Framingham study. Am Heart J 112:820–825, 1986

Kenshalo DR: Age changes in touch, vibration, temperature, kinesthesis, and pain sensitivity, in Handbook of the Psychology of Aging. Edited by Birren JE, Schaie KW. New York, Van Nostrand Reinhold, 1977, pp 562–579

La Rue A: Aging and Neuropsychological Assessment. New York, Plenum, 1992

La Rue A, Bank L, Jarvik L, et al: Health in old age: how do physicians' ratings and self-ratings compare? J Gerontol 8:108–115, 1979

Lawton MP: Contextual perspectives: psychosocial influences, in Clinical Memory Assessment of Older Adults. Edited by Poon LW, Crook T, Davis KL, et al. Washington, DC, American Psychological Association, 1986

Light LL, Zelinski EM, Moore M: Adult age differences in reasoning from new information. J Exp Psychol Learn Mem Cogn 8:435–447, 1982

Loewenstein DA, Eisdorfer CE: Issues in geriatric research, in Research in Psychiatry: Issues, Strategies and Methods. Edited by George Hsu LK, Hersen M. New York, Plenum, 1992

Loewenstein DA, Rubert MP: The NINCDS-ADRDA neuropsychological criteria for the assessment of dementia: limitations of current diagnostic guidelines. Behav Health Aging 2:113–121, 1992

Loewenstein DA, Ardila A, Roselli M, et al: Comparative functional performance in Hispanic and non-Hispanic populations. Paper presented to the Annual Gerontological Society of America Meetings, Minneapolis, MN, 1989

Loewenstein DA, Rubert MP, Berkowitz-Zimmer N, et al: Neuropsychological test performance and prediction of functional capacities in dementia. Behavior Health Aging 2:149–158, 1992

Loewenstein DA, Argüelles T, Barker WW, et al: A comparative analysis of neuropsychological test performance of Spanish-speaking and English-speaking patients with Alzheimer's disease. J Gerontol 48:142–149, 1993

Lopez SR, Taussig FM: Cognitive-intellectual functioning of Spanish-speaking impaired and nonimpaired elderly: implications for culturally sensitive assessment—psychological assessment. J Consult Clin Psychol 3:448–454, 1991

Madden DJ, Blumenthal JA, Allen PA, et al: Improving aerobic capacity in healthy older adults does not necessarily lead to improved cognitive function. Psychol Aging 4:307–320, 1989

Maddox GL, Douglass EB: Self-assessment of health: a longitudinal study of elderly subjects. J Health Soc Behav 14:87–93, 1973

McCrae RR, Arenberg D, Costa PT: Declines in divergent thinking with age: cross-sectional, longitudinal, and cross-sequential analyses. Psychol Aging 2:130–137, 1987

McEvoy GM, Cascio WF: Cumulative evidence of the relationship between employee age and job performance. J Appl Psychol 74:11–17, 1989

Moore NC: Is paranoid illness associated with sensory deficits in the elderly? J Psychosom Res 25:69–74, 1981

Monge R, Hultsch D: Paired associate learning as a function of adult age and the length of anticipation and inspection intervals. J Gerontol 26:157–162, 1971

Myers AM, Holliday PJ, Harvey KA, et al: Functional performance measures: are they superior to self-assessments? Journals of Gerontology: Medical Sciences 48:196–206, 1993

Nadol JB: Hearing loss. N Engl J Med 329:1092–1102, 1993

Nelson RC, Franzi LR: Nutrition, in Primary Care Geriatrics: A Case-Based Approach, 2nd Edition. Edited by Ham RJ, Sloane PD. St. Louis, MO, Mosby-Year Book, 1992

Norris ML, Cunningham DR: Social impact of hearing loss in the aged. J Gerontol 36:727–729, 1981

Orr AL: The psychosocial aspects of aging and vision loss. Journal of Gerontological Social Work 17:1–14, 1991

Perez-Stable EJ, Coates TJ, Halliday R, et al: The effects of mild diastolic hypertension on the results of tests of cognitive function in adults 22 to 59 years of age. J Gen Intern Med 7:19–25, 1992

Perlmutter M, Nyquist L: Relationships between self-reported physical and mental health and intelligence performance across adulthood. Journals of Gerontology: Psychological Sciences 45:145–155, 1990

Pick AD: Cognition: psychological perspectives, in Handbook of Cross-Cultural Psychology: Basic Processes, Vol 3. Edited by Trandis HC, Lonner W. Boston, MA, Allyn & Bacon, 1980, pp 117–153

Plomp R: Auditory handicap of hearing impairment and the limited benefit of hearing aids. J Acoust Soc Am 63:533–549, 1978

Powers JK, Powers EA: Hearing problems of elderly persons: social consequences and prevalence. Journal of the American Speech and Hearing Association 20:79–83, 1978

Rabbitt PMA: Some experiments and a model for changes in attentional selectivity with old age, in Brain Function in Old Age. Edited by Hoffmeister F, Muller C. Berlin, Springer-Verlag, 1979

Rhodes SR: Age-related differences in work attitudes and behavior: a review and conceptual analysis. Psychol Bull 93:328–367, 1983

Rockstein MJ, Sussman M: Biology of aging. Belmont, CA, Wadsworth, 1979

Roth M, Tomlinson BE, Blessed G: The relationship between quantitative measures of dementia and of degenerative changes in the cerebral grey matter of elderly subjects. Proc Roy Soc Med 60:254–260, 1967

Ribbon DB, Si AL, Kimpau S: The predictive validity of self-report and performance-based measures of function and health. Journals of Gerontology: Medical Science 47:106–110, 1992

Russell MJ, Cummings BJ, Profitt BF, et al: Life span changes in the verbal categorization of odors. Journals of Gerontology: Psychological Sciences 48:49–53, 1993

Salthouse TA, Kausler DH, Saults JS: Age, self-assessed health status, and cognition. Journals of Gerontology: Psychological Sciences 45:156–160, 1990

Salzman C, Gutfreund MJ: Clinical techniques and research strategies for studying depression and memory, in Clinical Memory Assessment of Older Adults. Edited by Poon LW, Crook T, Davis KL, et al. Washington, DC, American Psychological Association, 1986

Satz P: Brain reserve capacity on symptom onset after brain injury: a formulation and review of the evidence for threshold theory. Neuropsychology 7:273–295, 1993

Schaie KW: Intelligence and problem solving, in Handbook of the Psychology of Aging. Edited by Birren JE, Schaie KW. New York, Van Nostrand Reinhold, 1980, pp 39–58

Schaie KW: Internal validity threats in studies of adult cognitive development, in Cognitive Development in Adulthood: Progress in Cognitive Development Research. Edited by Howe ML, Brainerd CJ. New York, Springer-Verlag, 1988, pp 241–272

Schaie KW, Willis SL: Age difference patterns of psychometric intelligence in adulthood: generalizability within and across ability domains. Psychol Aging 8:44–55, 1993

Scogin F, Bienas JL: A three-year follow-up of older adult participants in a memory skills training program. Psychol Aging 3:334–337, 1988

Ship JA, Weiffenbach JM: Age, gender, medical treatment and medication effects on smell identification. Journals of Gerontology: Medical Science 48:26–32, 1993

Simonton DK: Creativity and wisdom, in Handbook of the Psychology of Aging, 3rd Edition. Edited by Birren JE, Schaie KW. New York, Academic Press, 1990

Sivak M, Olson PL, Pastalan LA: Effect of driver's age on nighttime legibility of highway signs. Hum Factors 23:59–64, 1981

Skre H: Neurological signs in a normal population. Acta Neurol Scand 48:575–606, 1972

Smith J, Baltes PB: Wisdom-related knowledge: age/cohort differences in response to life-planning problems. Dev Psychol 26:494–505, 1990

Spar JE, La Rue A: Concise Guide to Geriatric Psychiatry. Washington, DC, American Psychiatric Press, 1990

Spirduso WW, Clifford P: Replication of age and physical activity effects on reaction time and movement time. J Gerontol 43:23–30, 1978

Sturgis ET, Dolce JJ, Dickerson PC: Pain management in the elderly, in Handbook of Clinical Gerontology. Edited by Carstensen LL, Edelstein BA. New York, Pergamon, 1987, pp 190–203

Taussig IM, Henderson VW, Mack W: Spanish translation and validation of a neuropsychological battery: performance of Spanish- and English-speaking Alzheimer's disease patients and normal comparison subjects, in Hispanic Aged Mental Health. Edited by Brink TL. New York, Haworth, 1992

Thomas PD, Hunt WC, Garry PJ, et al: Hearing acuity in a healthy elderly population: effects on emotional, cognitive and social status. J Gerontol 38:321–325, 1983

Trick GL, Silverman SE: Visual sensitivity to motion: age-related changes and deficits in senile dementia of the Alzheimer's type. Neurology 41:1437–1440, 1991

U.S. Bureau for the Census: Census of the Population and Housing. Summary Tape File 3A. Washington, DC, U.S. Government Printing Office, 1990

Valle R: Cultural and ethnic issues in Alzheimer's disease family research, in Alzheimer's Disease Treatment and Family Stress: Directions for Research (DHHS Publ No ADM-89-1569). Edited by Light E, Lebowitiz BD. Washington, DC, U.S. Government Printing Office, 1989, pp 122–154

Warren BJ, Nieman DC, Dotson RG, et al: Cardiorespiratory responses to exercise training in septuagenarian women. Int J Sports Med 14:60–65, 1993

Warrington EK, Sanders HI: The fate of old memories. Q J Exp Psychol 23:432–442, 1971

Wilkie F, Eisdorfer C: Systemic diseases and behavioral correlates in the aged, in Intellectual Functioning in Adults. Edited by Jarvik L, Eisdorfer C, Blum J. New York, Springer, 1973, pp 83–91

Wilkie F, Eisdorfer C: Sex, verbal ability and pacing differences in serial learning. J Gerontol 32:63–67, 1977

Williams A, Denney NW, Schadler M: Elderly adults' perception of their own cognitive development during the adult years. Int J Aging Hum Dev 16:147–158, 1983

Zarit JM, Zarit SH: Molar aging: the physiology and psychology of normal aging, in Handbook of Clinical Gerontology. Edited by Carstensen LL, Edelstein BA. New York, Pergamon, 1987, pp 18–32

CHAPTER 5

Charles F. Longino, Jr., Ph.D.
Maurice B. Mittelmark, Ph.D.

Sociodemographic Aspects

S ociodemographic aspects of mental health and mental illness are particularly important in geriatric psychiatry as a social context for individual cases. Concurrent with biologically based changes in health, old age also brings many important socially induced changes that have the potential for producing negative or positive effects on both the physical and mental well-being of older persons. These social changes include altered marriage and family patterns, living arrangements, work behaviors, economic status, and social support. Neither the psychiatric therapist nor the researcher can afford to ignore the sociodemographic aspects of old age when considering the older patient, client, or subject. To do so is to ignore the setting in which the condition is nurtured and the epidemiological connections to age, gender, race, ethnicity, work, economic status, and marital and residential relationships. These are the primary social factors that condition health and mental health. The physical and mental conditions that make illness more or less likely, and coping more or less successful, are rooted partly in sociodemographic factors.

Social and Demographic Characteristics

There are several sources of current statistics on the older population. Unless otherwise specified, however, this review and summary of social

and demographic characteristics is drawn from a 1991 report jointly produced by the U.S. Senate Special Committee on Aging, the American Association of Retired Persons, the Federal Council on the Aging, and the U.S.
Administration on Aging, entitled *Aging America: Trends and Projections.*

Age and Aging

America is growing older, and it is doing so at an accelerated rate. At the
beginning of the 20th century, fewer than 1 in 10 Americans were ages 55
or older and only 1 in 25 was age 65 or older. By 1990, 1 in 5 was at least 55
and 1 in 8 was at least 65. With each passing decade before 1990, there
were about 20% more persons ages 65 and older in the population, but in
the 1990s and in the first decade of the next century, this growth will slow
to about 10% because of the low fertility rates during the Great Depression in the 1930s. The surge of baby boomers (those born between 1946
and 1964) entering old age after the Depression cohort will cause the over-
65 population to more than double. By 2030, there will be as many persons over 65 as under 18 (about 20% of the total population each), and
the median age of all Americans is expected to be 43. The proportion of
the United States population over age 85 will grow from 1% in 1990 to 5%
in 2050. More people are surviving into their 10th and 11th decades as
well. The Census Bureau estimates that there were about 61,000 persons
ages 100 years or older in 1990, and there will be more than 100,000 by the
end of the decade. If members of the present geriatric psychiatry student
cohort have a 30-year career, the proportion and number of older persons
in the United States population will have doubled by the time they retire
from practice. Even if the proportion seeking psychiatric services remains
constant during this period, the number of patients or clients will more
than double. The major surge, however, will not occur until after 2010.

Although the overall number of the elderly in the United States is growing, not all sex, race, and ethnic groups are equally represented in the total
population of older persons. Women continue to live longer than men, so
the ratio of women to men varies dramatically with age. Men slightly outnumbered women in all age groups under 35 in 1990, but in the 65+ age
group, there were 18.3 million women and only 12.6 million men. Thus
elderly women outnumber elderly men by a ratio of 3:2. In 1990, 13% of
whites were ages 65 or older, compared with only 8% of blacks, 7% of
persons of other races, and 5% of Hispanics. However, when racial, nationality, and language categories are compared, it is important to remember that these categories have heterogeneous populations.

The overall aging of the United States population is, of course, related to increased life expectancy. A child born in 1900 had a life expectancy of 47.3 years; in 1960, this figure had grown to 69.6 years, and in 1987 it was 75.0 years. The increases in life expectancy during the first five decades of this century were due largely to the decreased infant mortality rate and reduced mortality from infectious diseases. By contrast, the increases in life expectancy since the 1960s are due largely to lower mortality rates among middle-aged and older individuals. Persons who were 65 years of age in 1987 could expect to live, on average, an additional 16.9 years. The gap in life expectancy for men and women appears to be decreasing slightly.

In 1990, the United States ranked behind several other countries in life expectancy at birth, with Canada, France, Germany, Italy, Japan, Sweden, and the United Kingdom all having longer life expectancies. Life expectancy at birth is sensitive to infant mortality rates, which are higher in the United States than in many of these countries.

Work and Retirement

As people live longer, they spend more time in several of life's major phases, most notably education, work, and retirement. Before World War II, retirement was the domain of a privileged few, but it has now become an institutionalized expectation, and there appears to be increasing acceptance of it as a desired social status (Atchley 1991).

On the whole, labor force and retirement patterns have been different for men and women. Since 1900, the average time spent by women in the labor force has increased from 6.3 to 29.4 years and from 13% of the life span to 38%. Retirement is currently an issue for a growing number of women, and the proportion of women entering retirement will increase dramatically with the aging of the "baby boom generation" into the next century.

Retirement is not a single concept. Age 65 has been considered the "normal retirement age" in the United States since the Social Security Act was passed in 1935. Since 1950, however, fewer than half of all men were still working at age 64. In addition, most private pensions provide benefits for eligible employees before age 65, a trend that accelerated in the 1960s and 1970s (U.S. Department of Labor, Bureau of Labor Statistics 1989). At the other extreme, many people continue to work full or part time after they begin receiving retired worker benefits. Are these individuals retired? One 1987 study found that nearly one-fourth of Americans continued to work during retirement (Iams 1987). The younger an individual is at retirement (except for those who retire because of a disability), the more likely it is that he or she will continue to work (Ullmann et al. 1991).

Studies indicate that people retire for a variety of reasons, including poor health, the availability of Social Security or private pension benefits, the retirement of a spouse, and the opportunity to participate in leisure and volunteer pursuits. Downturns in the economy and corporate mergers and bankruptcies can also induce unanticipated early retirement. However, most workers retire when they feel they can afford to do so (Quinn and Burkhauser 1990). Thus, persons without pensions or sizable personal savings, including those who do not own a home, are likely to remain in the labor force longer than persons who have such resources.

As a result of these factors, professionals and self-employed persons have greater variation in their age at retirement than workers employed by businesses and corporations. More individuals in the first two groups (especially self-employed persons) can afford early retirement. Among professionals, job satisfaction is often high, encouraging phased-in retirement or retirement at a later age. Workers employed by corporations who seek earlier retirement are more frequently motivated by health problems. Understanding retirement requires understanding the links between persons and their jobs (Atchley 1991; Ullmann et al. 1991).

Although retirement is becoming more normative in our society than it once was and the percentage of Americans retiring at earlier ages has increased, unemployment still remains a serious problem for many who want to remain in the labor force. Also, individuals ages 65 or older tend to be without work or underemployed for longer periods than do younger persons. They frequently must accept entry-level salaries and work for employers who offer few, if any, employee benefits. The U.S. Department of Labor reported that in 1986 there were 273,000 persons ages 60 and older who were unemployed and looking for work; approximately 91,000 of these were 65 or older. Because those who are not working and have ceased looking for employment are not counted as unemployed, the estimates of unemployment among older persons are low. If all discouraged workers were included, the number of unemployed individuals ages 60 and older in 1989 would have been 404,000. This represents 1 in 20 of all persons in this age cohort (U.S. Senate Special Committee on Aging 1991).

Economic Resources, Income, and Expenditures

Persons ages 65 and older in America tend to have lower incomes than those under 65. Moreover, the median income decreases with increasing age. In 1989 the median income of families with a head of household age 25 to 64 was $36,058. For those with a head of household age 65 or older, the median income was $22,806, or about one-third less. Furthermore, income differentials increase as age differences increase. For example, in 1989 persons in family units with a head of household ages 85 and older had median incomes of $17,600, which is about one-half the median income of family units with a head of household age 25 to 64 (U.S. Bureau of the Census 1990).

Surveys of income adequacy show that high proportions of older persons feel that their income is adequate, even when objectively it is low (Streib 1985). Liang and Fairchild (1979) found in an analysis of six national samples of elderly people that feelings of relative deprivation affected their financial satisfaction more than current income. Their sense of income adequacy was strengthened by comparing themselves with others their age who had less adequate incomes.

From the viewpoint of cash income alone, older age is usually accompanied by a reduction in economic resources. Despite this, older adults are only slightly more likely than younger adults to be below or just above the poverty level. In 1989, 11.4% of persons ages 65 and older were living in poverty, compared with 10.2% of persons ages 18 to 64. Elderly individuals were somewhat more likely than nonelderly individuals to have incomes just above the poverty threshold. Of families headed by someone age 65 years or older, 28% were living near the poverty level, compared with 22% of families headed by someone younger than 65. To keep these poverty rates in perspective, it should be remembered that the poverty rate in elderly individuals declined from 28.5% in 1966 to 14.6% in 1974 and 11.4% in the 1980s. The highest poverty rates are associated with minority women living alone. In 1990, three-fifths of elderly black women living alone had incomes below the poverty level.

Not surprisingly, the clear disparity in income among whites, blacks, and Hispanics carries over into old age. Among whites over 65, 9.4% are in families with incomes below the poverty threshold compared with 30.8% of African Americans and 20.6% of Hispanics. The personal and social challenges encountered by racial and ethnic minorities in American society are numerous, but perhaps none have more serious consequences for health and social well-being than those associated with low socioeconomic status (U.S. Senate Special Committee on Aging 1991).

Since the 1970s, a particularly steep decline in the role of earnings as a source of income has been offset by an increase in the role of assets and pensions. This shift was most pronounced for older couples between 1978 and 1984, when earnings dropped from 30% to 21% of income, while assets increased from 18% to 27% and pensions held nearly constant, increasing from 14% to 16% of total income. Social Security represents 79% of total income for poor couples and approximately 36% for nonpoor couples. In-kind health benefits are of particular significance to elderly persons, because 95% of noninstitutionalized elderly persons in 1989 were covered by Medicare.

Elderly individuals generally consume fewer goods and services than nonelderly individuals and spend slightly higher proportions of their budgets on essentials. In 1989, persons ages 65 and older spent 59% of their consumption dollars on housing, food, and medical care, compared with only 50% spent by younger persons on these items. The one service or commodity that elderly persons spend more on in actual dollars and as a percentage of total expenditures than nonelderly persons is health care. The major health expense for elderly households in 1989 was health insurance, including Medicare. Even though they had lower incomes and fewer household members, elderly individuals spent more than twice as much as their younger counterparts on health insurance, prescription drugs, and medical supplies.

Economic resources strongly influence the quality of life of persons in their later years, as they do for all individuals. The combination of economic resources and living arrangements, however, determines adequate or inadequate support in later life.

Marital Status and Living Arrangements

Marital status, family patterns, and living arrangements vary greatly between men and women ages 65 and older. Most older men (75%) live in family settings; the proportion for women living in such settings is much lower (40%). According to the 1990 census, nearly one-half of all women ages 65 and older were widows (U.S. Bureau of the Census 1990).

Approximately 8.3 million persons ages 65 and older were living alone in 1986; 80% of these (6.6 million) were women. Among all noninstitutionalized elderly individuals in 1989, only 16% of the men lived alone, compared with 41% of women (National Center for Health Statistics 1987; U.S. Senate Special Committee on Aging 1991). There is a trend away from intergenerational living arrangements that increases the proportion of individuals living alone even among the very old. The proportion of persons over 85 living with children in 1990 was 10.5%, down from 16.4% in 1980. During that decade, the percentage in this advanced age category living alone rose from 29.7% to 36.8% (Longino 1994).

Geographical Distribution and Mobility

The largest number of older people reside in the states with the largest populations; for the nation, more than half live in just nine states: California, New York, Florida, Pennsylvania, Texas, Illinois, Ohio, Michigan, and New Jersey, in that order. Elderly populations are heavily concentrated in areas within states, not in entire state populations. These areas have certain characteristics: some have been abandoned by young people in search of education and jobs, and others attract large numbers of retirees as migrants. The former consist largely but not entirely of small towns in the Midwest and New England, and the latter consist largely but not entirely of resort communities along the southern Atlantic Coast, in the Southwest, and along the Pacific Coast. The suburbs are also "aging"; in 1980, for the first time more elderly individuals lived in the suburbs than in the central cities.

Older individuals tend to remain where they have spent most of their adult lives. About 5% of all persons ages 60 and older will move in any 5-year period; by comparison, more than one-third of persons in their early 20s will move during that same period.

Interstate migration is focused. Of the nearly 1.7 million Americans ages 60 and older who moved out of state between 1975 and 1980, nearly half went to one of five states: Florida, California, Arizona, Texas, and New Jersey, in that order. Florida is in a class by itself, receiving one-fourth of all interstate migrants ages 60 and older. Most long-distance moves are life-style motivated and involve married couples who have recently retired. Much smaller migrations in the reverse direction have been detected, with retirees returning from the Sunbelt to the major "sending" states; migrants in these counterstreams tend to be, on average, a few years older, widowed, and more often living dependently or in institutions after their arrival than migrants in streams to the major destination states such as Florida. Older people move for different reasons at different times. Early moves tend to be amenity seeking; later ones are more often health or social support related (Longino 1990).

Health and Mental Health
Characteristics and Behavior

Economic and social resources strongly affect the ability to cope with health issues in old age, and demographic factors are associated with uneven distribution of these resources. Sociodemographic discussions of this topic are usually organized around the concepts of mortality and morbidity, disability, perceived health status, mental health, and psychosocial well-being. Throughout the following review, it is the distribution of characteristics in the older population or subpopulation, not the health or mental health of individuals, that is the focus. Because health professionals do not see a cross section of the population in their work, they may assume that elderly persons, as a category, have poorer health than they actually do.

Mortality and Morbidity

Heart disease, cerebrovascular disease, and atherosclerosis together account for almost half of all deaths among those 65 to 74 years old and for two-thirds of all deaths among those ages 85 and older (Brody et al. 1987). Malignant neoplasms account for 3 of every 10 deaths among those 65 to 74 years old, but for just 1 of every 10 deaths among those 85 and older (Brody et al. 1987).

Extensive information on the chronic conditions experienced by the population ages 65 and older is available from the 1991 National Health Interview Survey, from which the data presented here are abstracted (National Center for Health Statistics 1992). By far the most prevalent chronic condition is arthritis, with the highest prevalence (63%) found among women 75 years and older. As a point of comparison, the most prevalent circulatory disease in women, hypertension, affects about 40% of those ages 75 and older. Among Americans ages 65 and older, arthritis is much less prevalent among men (39%) than among women (56%) and slightly more common among whites (49%) than among blacks (47%).

After arthritis, the most common chronic conditions among those 65 and older are hypertension (31%–45%), poor hearing (22%–44%), heart disease (26%–30%), orthopedic impairments (16%–18%), cataracts (14%–17%, depending on gender and race), diabetes (9%–18%), and sinusitis (11%–16%).

These conditions are found in similar proportions of men and women and of whites and blacks, with several notable exceptions: men and whites are more likely to experience hearing problems than are women and blacks, blacks are twice as likely as whites to have diabetes, and women and blacks are more likely to have hypertension than are men and whites. These differences are also observed among those 75 and older.

Disability

Disability refers to limitations in one's capacity to perform normal activities of daily living (ADLs), such as managing personal hygiene. Evidence suggests that disability rates among elderly individuals appear to be decreasing, probably because of a combination of factors, including better medical care, more effective health education efforts, and improved health behaviors, among other reasons (Manton et al. 1993). If the disability rate continues to decrease, this will reduce, though by no means eliminate, the projected increase in number of disabled Americans. In 1985 it was estimated that 20% of older Americans were disabled, but because of the changing demographic profile of the United States, the proportion of disabled elderly persons is projected to increase to about 30% by the year 2060 (Manton 1989).

The presence of three or more limitations in ADLs, particularly personal care limitations such as dressing and bathing, is widely considered to be a marker for an increased risk of institutionalization. This situation is more prevalent among nonwhites (14%) than among whites (9%), among women (12%) than among men (6%), and among those 85 years and older (30%) than among those 75 to 84 years old (13%) (Van Nostrand et al. 1993).

The number of days spent in bed during a year is also a good indicator of poor health, functional loss, and disability. Data from the National Health Interview Survey showed wide variations among older Americans. Almost two-thirds of people ages 65 to 74 indicated they had not been confined to bed at any time in the year prior to being interviewed, and only 7.8% reported being bedfast for a month or more. By contrast, 13.4% of those ages 85 and older had been confined to bed for a month or more, and 3.4% said they were in bed constantly. However, only 1.4% of all noninstitutionalized persons ages 65 and older reported being in bed all the time (Dawson et al. 1987).

Perceived Health Status

Self-assessed health is a strong predictor of mortality among elderly individuals (Idler and Kasl 1991). Data from the National Health Interview

Survey indicated that most older adults perceive themselves to be in good health. When asked to make self-assessments of their physical well-being, 70% of those ages 65 and older reported that their health was excellent, very good, or good (National Center for Health Statistics 1987). Similarly, Warheit et al. (1986) observed that 71% of men and 67% of women ages 60 and older rated their physical health as excellent or good. Both of these studies found a linear relationship between positive self-assessment of physical health and higher income. In the study by Warheit et al. (1986), negative physical health self-assessments were highly correlated with psychiatric symptom scores.

Mental Health and Psychosocial Well-Being

The most definitive research on the prevalence of psychiatric disorders in the general population has been produced by the Epidemiologic Catchment Area (ECA) projects conducted under the aegis of the National Institute of Mental Health (Eaton and Kessler 1985). The ECA findings are based on a probability sample of 18,571 persons ages 18 and older, including 5,702 persons ages 65 and older, residing in five different sites in the United States. The ECA projects obtained DSM-III diagnoses (American Psychiatric Association 1980) by means of the Diagnostic Interview Schedule (DIS) (Robins et al. 1981).

In this population-based study, 15% of participants had at least one DIS/DSM-III–diagnosed disorder. People ages 65 and older had the lowest lifetime rates of any age group. They also had the lowest 1-month prevalence rates (any occurrence over a lifetime) for almost all individual disorders. The one exception was severe cognitive impairment, which was present in 5% of all respondents ages 65 and older, in 3% of those ages 65 to 74, and in 16% of those ages 85 and older. Women of all age groups had higher rates than men for most disorders; the major exceptions were alcohol and drug abuse.

Sociodemographic Aspects
of Self-Destructive Behavior

The health habits and risk profiles of the American population, including older women and men, have improved steadily since the 1960s (Manton 1991). Nevertheless, much disease among elderly individuals remains potentially preventable. The intentional and unintentional self-destructive behaviors that contribute directly and indirectly to the onset and progression of physical and psychiatric illness are of special relevance to geriatric psychiatry. Four such behaviors—suicide, setting fires, tobacco use, alcohol use—will be considered here.

Suicide

Age trends in the incidence of suicide are widely disparate for men and women, with rates for older men that are two to seven times those for older women (Wolf and Rivera 1992). There is little systematic evidence about risk factors for suicide among older persons, although social isolation, physical and mental illness, and the availability of means (e.g., gunshot is the most common means of suicide among older men) have been suggested as among the most important. The primary medical care setting may offer special opportunities for prevention, because the majority of older adult suicides are preceded by a visit to a physician (Wolf and Rivera 1992).

Fires

Poverty is one of the strongest risk factors for fatality in a residential fire, and cigarettes cause almost half of all fires and one-fourth to one-half of residential fire deaths (Wolf and Rivera 1992). The potential for prevention efforts is substantial: Many fire deaths are caused by smoke inhalation, and smoke detectors reduce the potential of death or severe injury in 8 of 10 fires.

Tobacco Use

Smoking rates among persons ages 65 and older vary widely across the United States; for example, older adults in Boston smoke at twice the rate of their Iowan counterparts: 25% versus 13% among men and 20% versus 9% among women (Cornoni-Huntley et al. 1987). The prevalence of tobacco use declines sharply with age; only 1% to 7% of those ages 85 and older report tobacco use (Cornoni-Huntley et al. 1987). Substantial epidemiological evidence suggests that quitting tobacco use even in old age may have important health benefits, including greater longevity and improved physical and physiological functioning (U.S. Department of Health and Human Services 1990). However, too many physicians fail to counsel older patients to stop tobacco use, perhaps because of a lack of appreciation of the potential for health improvement in the older adult (Forciea 1989).

Alcohol Use

There is substantial variability in alcohol use patterns among elderly Americans. Alcohol use rates (30-day prevalence) among persons ages 65 and older in Iowa were reported to be two-thirds to one-half those observed in Boston (46% versus 68% among men and 23% versus 47% among women, respectively) (Cornoni-Huntley et al. 1987). The prevalence of alcohol use declines with age, although not as markedly as the prevalence of tobacco use (Dufour et al. 1990).

Mechanisms Linking the Social Environment to Health Status

Social environment is a significant determinant of physical and psychiatric health status in the older adult population. It has long been observed that the condition of marriage imparts a protective effect on health, with married persons living substantially longer and healthier lives than unmarried persons. More recent research has extended this finding to the social network beyond the marriage dyad, exploring the direct and indirect mechanisms through which social support protects health and social isolation jeopardizes it.

Low levels of social contact and involvement have been associated prospectively with higher mortality from all causes (Berkman and Syme 1979; Blazer 1982; Cohen et al. 1987; Hanson et al. 1989; Hirdes and Forbes 1992; House et al. 1982; Kaplan et al. 1988; Orth-Gomer and Johnson 1987), cardiovascular disease (Berkman and Syme 1979; Kaplan et al. 1988; Orth-Gomer and Johnson 1987), ischemic heart disease (Berkman and Syme 1979; Kaplan 1988; Orth-Gomer et al. 1988), myocardial infarction (Ruberman et al. 1984), and cancer (Berkman and Syme 1979).

Although the epidemiological evidence of a positive, independent association between poor support and increased disease is impressive, little is known about the mechanisms that link social ties and disease. One difficulty has been the absence of a comprehensive etiological model to guide research. However, Ostergren (1991) has provided just such a model of the progression of chronic disease, integrating social environment, psychological functioning, and physiological responsiveness and incorporating five key constructs, as follows:

1. Stress as a physiological response to environmental threats (Selye 1936)

2. The psychological urge to act on or adapt to stressors (Ostergren 1991)
3. Coping with stressors by using resources in the physical and social environments (Lazarus 1966; Lazarus and Folkman 1984)
4. The accumulation either of mastery in dealing with stressors or strain owing to an inability to deal with stressors (Karasek and Theorell 1990)
5. Increased susceptibility to specific pathological agents as a consequence of inadequate coping resources and activation of specific aspects of stress physiology, such as increased blood pressure and heart rate (Cassel 1976)

Sociodemographic aspects of this process seem fairly evident: Potential stressors abound in disadvantaged environments. In such environments, a heightened state of vigilance is adaptive in the short term but probably maladaptive in the long run. The availability of resources in the immediate physical and social environment is determined to a degree by income, race, age, living arrangements, and educational attainment. Poor, minority, elderly, and isolated individuals have relatively few resources. Inadequate education in problem solving reduces coping effectiveness. It is sadly ironic that those who live in the most perilous environments are also those with the least adequate psychological, social, and physical resources to adapt to such environments.

As summarized by Adler and colleagues (1993), socioeconomic status, whether measured by income, occupation, or education, is a strong, consistent, and independent predictor of morbidity and mortality. Compared with persons with high socioeconomic status, individuals with low socioeconomic status are less exposed to health information, practice fewer health-enhancing behaviors, are exposed to more environmental pathogens, experience more physical danger and hardship and more stress-provoking events throughout life, and adjust less well to stress.

Caregiving

One of the most stressful situations many older adults will ever encounter is providing daily care to a disabled spouse or other individual. Being an elderly care provider exemplifies the dilemma of encountering chronic stressors with inadequate coping resources. For the caregiver, a lifetime's accumulation of strain, physical frailty, dwindling financial resources, and shrinking social networks reduce the capacity to deal with the daily care needs of another. The resulting psychiatric morbidity has been well documented. Providing care to a disabled individual results in physical, financial, and emotional strain. There is developing evidence that for some caregivers at least, such strain is associated both with psychiatric symptomatology (e.g., depression) and with clinically determined psychiatric illness (Cohen and Eisdorfer 1988; Schulz et al. 1988). The consequences may well extend beyond the caregiver. For the care receiver, the loss of a key social resource (the breakdown of a spouse caregiver, for example) may result in institutionalization.

Summary

The current elderly population is more socially advantaged than were their parents. Longevity has been dramatically extended, retirement years have increased, economic resources are more abundant and secure, and health care is available for most persons ages 65 and older. The data also indicate that, although racial and ethnic minorities still lag behind whites in most indicators of physical and social well-being, some changes that are occurring have the potential to reduce the current discrepancies in life expectancy and years in retirement. However, in other areas, especially those associated with economic resources, large disparities continue to exist and to perpetuate many of the differences in health and health-related behaviors among racial and ethnic groups in the United States.

Most older Americans perceive their physical health as good or excellent; these perceptions are confirmed by objective data on personal and social functioning and by information on numbers of days spent in bed. Furthermore, both physical and mental health self-assessments have been found to be good predictors of the mental health status of older persons and of their use of mental health services as well.

The self-perception of mental health and psychosocial well-being of the vast majority of older persons has been found to be positive. However, many elderly individuals living in community settings have mental health problems severe enough to require assistance from mental health professionals. Yet only a small percentage of those in need receive treatment and care. The recognition of mental health problems by primary physicians, accompanied by referrals to mental health specialists, would increase service rates and improve the psychiatric status of many older persons.

In this chapter we have attempted to show the connectedness between sociodemographic and health factors as they, in many combinations, affect psychosocial well-being in old age. It is important that the geriatric psychiatrist consider the sociodemographic dimension of physical and mental health for two reasons. First, such knowledge protects the clinician from inadvertently assuming that the patient's sociodemographic characteristics and health are normal because of a false understanding of population characteristics. Second, it sensitizes the mental health professional to sociodemographic factors in the patient's social environment, cues that can powerfully affect both diagnosis and treatment.

References

Adler NE, Boyce WT, Chesney MA, et al: Socioeconomic inequalities in health. JAMA 268:3140–3145, 1993

American Psychiatric Association: Diagnostic and Statistical Manual of Mental Disorders, 3rd Edition. Washington, DC, American Psychiatric Association, 1980

Atchley RC: Social Forces and Aging. Belmont, CA, Wadsworth, 1991

Berkman L, Syme SL: Social networks, host resistance, and mortality: a nine year follow-up study of Alameda County residents. Am J Epidemiol 109:186–204, 1979

Blazer D: Social support and mortality in an elderly community population. Am J Epidemiol 115:684–694, 1982

Brody JA, Brock DB, Williams TF: Trends in the health of the elderly population. Annu Rev Public Health 8:211–234, 1987

Cassel J: The contribution of the social environment to host resistance. Am J Epidemiol 104:107–123, 1976

Cohen D, Eisdorfer C: Depression in family members caring for a relative with Alzheimer's disease. J Am Geriatr Soc 36:885–889, 1988

Cohen CI, Teresi J, Holmes D: Social networks and mortality in an inner-city elderly population. Int J Aging Hum Dev 24:257–269, 1987

Cornoni-Huntley J, Brock DB, Ostfeld AM, et al: Established Populations for Epidemiologic Studies of the Elderly Resource Data Book (NIH Publ No PHS-86-2443). Washington, DC, U.S. Department of Health and Human Services, Public Health Service, National Institutes of Health, 1987

Dawson D, Hendershot G, Fulton J: Aging in the eighties: functional limitations of individuals 65 and older (Advance Data No 133). Rockville, MD, National Center for Health Statistics, June 1987

Dufour MC, Colliver J, Grigson MB, et al: Use of alcohol and tobacco, in Health Status and Well-Being of the Elderly. Edited by Cornoni-

Huntley JC, Huntley RR, Feldman JJ. Oxford, England, Oxford University Press, 1990, pp 172–183

Eaton W, Kessler L (eds): Epidemiologic Field Methods in Psychiatry: The NIMH Epidemiologic Catchment Area Program. New York, Academic Press, 1985

Forciea MA: Nutrition, alcohol, and tobacco in late life, in Practicing Prevention For The Elderly. Edited by Mourey RL, et al. Philadelphia, PA, Hanley & Belfus, 1989, pp 98–105

Hanson BS, Isacsson SO, Janzon L, et al: Social network and social support influence mortality in elderly men: the prospective population study of "men born in 1914" Malmo, Sweden. Am J Epidemiol 130:100–111, 1989

Hirdes JP, Forbes WF: The importance of social relationships, socioecomonic status and health practices with respect to mortality among healthy, Ontario males. J Clin Epidemiol 5:175–182, 1992

House J, Robbins C, Metzner H: The association of social relationships and activities with mortality: prospective evidence from the Tecumseh Community Health Study. Am J Epidemiol 116:123–140, 1982

Iams H: Jobs of persons working after receiving retired-worker benefits. Social Security Bulletin 50, 1987

Idler EL, Kasl S: Health perceptions and survival: do global evaluations of health status really predict mortality? J Gerontol 46:355–365, 1991

Kaplan GA: Social contacts and ischemic heart disease. Ann Clin Res 20:131–136, 1988

Kaplan GA, Salonen JT, Cohen RD, et al: Social connections and mortality from all causes and from cardiovascular disease: prospective evidence from eastern Finland. Am J Epidemiol 128:370–380, 1988

Karasek R, Theorell T: Healthy Work: Stress, Productivity, and the Reconstruction of Working Life. New York, Basic Books, 1990

Lazarus RS: Psychological Stress and the Coping Process. New York, McGraw-Hill, 1966

Lazarus RS, Folkman S: Stress, Appraisal, and Coping. New York, Springer Publishing, 1984

Liang J, Fairchild TJ: Relative deprivation and perception of financial adequacy among the aged. J Gerontol 34(5):746–759, 1979

Longino CF: Geographical distribution and migration, in Handbook on Aging and the Social Sciences. Edited by Binstock RH, George LK. Orlando, FL, Academic Press, 1990, pp 45–63

Longino CF: State profiles of the oldest Americans in 1990: decade cohort changes and the disabled. Final report submitted to the American

Association of Retired Persons Andrus Foundation. Winston-Salem, NC, Reynolds Gerontology Program, Wake Forest University, December 1994

Manton KG: Epidemiological, demographic, and social correlates of disability among the elderly. Milbank Quarterly 67 (suppl 1):13–58, 1989

Manton KG: The dynamics of population aging: demography and policy analysis. Milbank Quarterly 69:309–338, 1991

Manton KG, Corder LS, Stallard E: Estimates of change in chronic disability and institutional incidence and prevalence rates in the U.S. population from the 1982, 1984, and 1989 National Long-Term Care Survey. J Gerontol 48:S153, 1993

National Center for Health Statistics: Estimates From the National Health Interview Survey, U.S., 1986 (Vital Health Statistics Series 10, No 164; DHHS Publ No PHS-87-1592). Hyattsville, MD, U.S. Department of Health and Human Services, October 1987

National Center for Health Statistics: Current estimates from the National Health Interview Survey, 1991 (Vital Health Statistics Series 10, No 184, DHHS Publ No PHS-93-1512). Hyattsville, MD, U.S. Department of Health and Human Services, December 1992

Orth-Gomer K, Johnson JV: Social network interaction and mortality: a six year follow-up study of a random sample of the Swedish population. J Chron Dis 40:949–957, 1987

Orth-Gomer K, Unden AL, Edwards ME: Social isolation and mortality in ischemic heart disease. Acta Med Scand 224:205–215, 1988

Ostergren P: Psychosocial Resources and Health (PhD thesis). Malmo, Sweden, Lund University, Department of Community Health Sciences, 1991

Quinn, JF, Burkhauser, RV: Work and retirement, in Handbook on Aging and the Social Sciences. Edited by Binstock RH, George LK. Orlando, FL, Academic Press, 1990, pp 307–327.

Robins LN, Helzer SE, Croughan J, et al: National Institute of Mental Health diagnostic interview schedule: its history, characteristics, and validity. Arch Gen Psychiatry 38:381–389, 1981

Ruberman W, Weinblatt E, Goldberg JD, et al: Psychosocial influences after myocardial infarction. N Engl J Med 311:552–559, 1984

Schulz R, Tompkins CA, Rau MT: A longitudinal study of the psychosocial impact of stroke on primary support persons. Psychol Aging 3:131–141, 1988

Selye H: A syndrome produced by diverse noctuous agents. Nature 138:32, 1936

Streib GF: Social stratification and aging, in Handbook of Aging and the Social Sciences, 2nd Edition. Edited by Binstock RH, Shanas E. New York, Van Nostrand Reinhold, 1985, pp 339–368

Ullmann SG, Holtmann AG, Longino CF: Early retirement: a descriptive and analytical study. Final report submitted to the American Association of Retired Persons Andrus Foundation. Coral Gables, FL, Center on Adult Development, University of Miami, June 1991

U.S. Bureau of the Census: Current Population Reports (Series P-60). Washington, DC, U.S. Government Printing Office, 1990

U.S. Bureau of the Census: Marital Status and Living Arrangements: March 1989. Current Reports (Series P-20, No 445). Washington, DC, U.S. Government Printing Office, June 1990

U.S. Department of Health and Human Services: The Health Benefits of Smoking Cessation: A Report of the U.S. Surgeon General, 1990 (DHHS Publ No CDC-90-8416). Washington, DC, U.S. Department of Health and Human Services, Public Health Service, Centers for Disease Control, Center for Chronic Disease Prevention and Health Promotion, Office of Smoking and Health, 1990

U.S. Department of Labor, Bureau of Labor Statistics: Labor Market Problems of Older Workers. Washington, DC, U.S. Department of Labor, 1989

U.S. Senate Special Committee on Aging, the American Association of Retired Persons, the Federal Council on the Aging, and the U.S. Administration on Aging: Aging America: Trends and Projections. Washington, DC, U.S. Government Printing Office, 1991

Van Nostrand JF, Furner SE, Suzman R (eds): Health Data on Older Americans: United States, 1992. National Center for Health Statistics. Vital Health Statistics 3(27), 1993

Warheit G, Bell R, Schwab J: An epidemiologic assessment of mental health problems in the southeastern U.S., in Community Surveys of Psychiatric Disorders. Edited by Weissman M, Myers J, Ross C. Brunswick, NJ, Rutgers University Press, 1986

Wolf ME, Rivera FP: Nonfall injuries in older adults. Annu Rev Public Health 13:509, 1992

Bertram J. Cohler, Ph.D.
Jeanne E. Nakamura, M.A.

Self and Experience Across the Second Half of Life

S tudy of personality across the second half of life has been marked by two concerns: 1) the extent to which changes taking place in psychological functions across later life may lead to increased problems managing the tasks of everyday life, and 2) the extent to which the daily round continues to support the experience of morale and personal integrity or coherence. Missing in much of this discussion is a view of aging as a part of the expectable course of life. There is little comparable concern that the course of childhood, youth, or earlier adulthood be marked by "success" leading to optimized functioning. This emphasis on issues of successful aging, at least in part, reflects a more general concern in our culture with continued personal mobility and maintenance of interpersonal autonomy. The increasing need to have to depend on others to complete such activities of everyday living as grocery shopping is a major source of lowered morale in later life. Concern with successful aging may also be a consequence of the linear manner in which we understand the course of life.

In this chapter we consider aging in terms of the course of life as a whole, focusing on expectable changes in experience of self and others that serve as the background against which to understand both psychopathology and directed psychotherapeutic intervention. It is particularly important to view changes taking place across the second half of life in terms of expectable changes occurring both within lives over time and within the larger context of American culture. American culture has portrayed the course of life as linear, with a beginning, middle, and end. Within this linear life story, later life is often assumed to be a time of decline, perhaps marked by struggle, accompanied by the loss of such formerly sustaining activities as career. Just as in stories, in which the conclusion is expected to resolve the conflict posed within the plot, later life is assumed to resolve concerns enduring across a lifetime and to provide enhanced coherence or integrity, making possible a "good" death. However, study has suggested that this portrait of age and decline does not accurately represent the lives of older adults in contemporary society. In this chapter we review evidence that suggests that later life is marked by its own achievements and problems and that, at least until very late life, health and activity provide important sources of satisfaction and morale.

Aging, Social Timing, and the Course of Life

The term *aging* is often equated with a negative state of decline and senescence, implying loss, infirmity, and limitation. Viewing the second half of life from this perspective, some investigators have sought examples of older adults who are apparently more resilient, even when confronted with the presumed impact of aging represented as decline and deficit. Studies such as those of Baltes and Baltes (1990) or Rowe and Kahn (1987) focus on means used to resist the presumed experience of decline and deficit. However, expectable changes taking place across the second half of life are not different in kind from those taking place at other points in the course of life. There is little discussion of "successful" adolescence, although it is often claimed that this stage in the course of life is accompanied by a particular sense of personal crisis (Erikson 1950; Freud 1936). Studies of the expectable course of adolescence (Csikszentmihalyi and Larson 1984; Offer and Offer 1975; Offer and Sabshin 1984) show that a crisis view of adolescence conflicts with the reality of lives portrayed by adolescents. In a similar manner, a view of later life as a time of decline and infirmity conflicts with reports on the lives of older adults (Bengtson et al. 1985; Clausen 1993; Schaie 1981).

Aging is too often posed as a negative concept that implies loss and decline. Viewed from a life-course perspective, aging refers to the socially constructed and psychologically experienced passage of time. Birren and

Renner (1977) have defined aging as ". . . regular changes that occur in mature genetically representative organisms living under representative environmental conditions as they advance in chronological age" (p. 4).

The important aspect of this definition is that aging is a process beginning in early adulthood and continuing across the course of life. As Birren and Renner (1977) have noted, age may be understood in terms of 1) biological-functional changes in capacity relevant to the length of the life span; 2) psychological-functional age, or capacity to maintain continued adaptation to the environment; and 3) social age, or place in a shared definition of lives over time.

The Order of Life Changes

Since Durkheim's (1912/1963) discussion of the social origins of thought, it has been acknowledged that experiences of particular persons cannot be understood apart from the larger social order that structures and gives meaning to such experiences. It is precisely the social definition of the course of life that transforms the study of the life span or life cycle into the study of the life course. There is explicit recognition that changes with age are governed by shared definitions of expectable life events. Expected changes at particular ages are a function of the shared understandings of the length of finitude of lives and of the required progression or transitions through institutionally and informally defined social roles (Elder and Rockwell 1979; Neugarten and Hagestad 1976; Sorokin and Merton 1937). Role transitions may be "on time," according to shared understandings, or may happen "too early" or "too late" in terms of the shared timetable.

Normative and eruptive changes or events must both be understood in a larger sociohistorical context (Hultsch and Plemons 1979). To a large extent, particular adverse events that affect large numbers of persons, such as the Great Depression (Elder 1974, 1979; Elder and Rockwell 1979), natural disasters, or social cataclysms (e.g., wars or assassinations of national leaders), lead to feelings of shared participation in social experiences that create social bonds, distinguishing persons who have endured these events from those who have not. Furthermore, these sociohistorical events color responses to subsequent events (Elder 1974, 1979).

Sociohistorical events may affect the social timing of life events for many members of a cohort, leading to variations in the sense individuals have of being "on" or "off" time. As both men and women come to marry later in adulthood, the sense of the expectable age at which one becomes a parent shifts; the sense of being "on" or "off" time is always relative to that of other members of the same cohort, although there is a biological ceiling on the course of life engendered by the biosocial facts of the human life cycle. Retirement may be viewed increasingly as appropriate for persons during their late 60s or early 70s, rather than during their mid-60s, but earlier retirement, characteristic of Japanese society (Plath 1980), would be considered "off-time" across successive cohorts within this society.

As contrasted with "on-time" or expectable role transitions, off-time events may lead to decreased morale. By their nature, these events occur suddenly and provide little opportunity for advance preparation. Discovery of a life-threatening illness in a spouse or offspring may provide some opportunity for preparing for loss and change. However, the absence of others experiencing similar losses makes the anticipatory grief all the more difficult. Not only is there little realistic opportunity for preparing for the experience of grief, but in addition, even with the support of an informal self-help group, there are not "consociates" who have already negotiated this change. Both suddenness and timing make early, off-time life changes particularly difficult to negotiate.

Some events, such as marriage, may happen late, whereas other events, such as widowhood, may happen early. In general, it is those events that take place unexpectedly early, such as adolescent pregnancy or widowhood in early to middle life, that are likely to lead to decreased morale. Both women and, particularly, men widowed "off-time early" report prolonged struggles with an overwhelming sense of loss (Glick et al. 1974; Wortman and Silver 1990). Some off-time life changes may have a paradoxical impact. Lopata (1979, 1982) and Neugarten and Hagestad (1976) have noted that the impact of widowhood is different in women who become widows in their late 60s and 70s and women who become widows in their 30s and 40s.

Even when understood as changes taking place across the second half of life, including the long period of life after retirement, there is little evidence that older adulthood is more likely to be characterized by an experience of decline and decrement in personal and intellectual functioning than younger stages of life (George 1980; Perlmutter 1983; Salthouse 1989, 1990; Schaie 1990a, 1993). Butler and Lewis (1977) have documented the problems posed in understanding aging that stem from a view of the second half of life as a period of decline and infirmity. It is important both to understand the second half of life in terms of the expectable course of life and to focus on factors determining response to expectable and eruptive life changes that are most characteristic of this particular point in the course of life.

After adults have attained a characteristic adult role portfolio (Hagestad 1974), eruptive and normative events continue to interact with events resulting from the vicissitudes of adult roles, within particular cohorts, changing across the life course of life itself. For example, with the advent of late life, the number of possible role transitions diminishes, leading to a reduction in the number of expectable normative transitions. Although older persons are more at risk for some kinds of expectable events, such as the death of long-time friends and relatives and loss of morale as a result of unexpected adverse events happening among friends and kindred, in general there are fewer unexpected adverse life events serving as sources of distress among older adults (Goldberg and Comstock 1980; Lazarus and DeLongis 1983; Lowenthal et al. 1975; Uhlenhuth et al. 1974).

Although losses at older ages may be particularly poignant and remaining adverse life changes may be at least as painful as those already experienced, the expectable nature of the losses has different significance for adjustment (e.g., widowhood is more expectable for a women in her late 70s or 80s than for a woman her 30s) (Wortman and Silver 1987, 1990). In the same manner, older adults who lose an adult offspring find such losses particularly painful, because it is expected that their offspring will outlive them. However, this finding regarding the age-related prevalence of stressful life events must be understood within particular sociohistorical circumstances and recognizing the changing significance of a past loss across the course of life. Among older persons who have lost family members as a result of world wars, such losses may reduce stressful life events in old age because they have taken place much earlier in the course of life. With much adversity already having occurred, little remains to afflict these older adults. At the same time, however, earlier loss of an offspring takes on additional significance for those older adults who are otherwise socially isolated and have few formal resources available beyond the family.

Personal Adjustment and Life Changes

Across the adult years, transition into and out of expectable adult roles appears to have less impact on morale than is commonly assumed. Datan et al. (1981) and Neugarten and Datan (1974b) have shown that expectable or "on-time" menopause among women has little impact on personal adjustment. Bengtson and Robertson (1985) have shown that continuing intergenerational contact, even when in the context of caregiving, need not adversely affect morale. Numerous studies have shown that the transition from work to retirement does not necessarily adversely affect the morale or the physical health of most workers (Kasl 1984; Wan 1984), even though some of those employed anticipate that they will worry more about their health after they retire than while still working (Ekerdt and Bosse 1982). M. Lieberman and Peskin (1992) and Wortman and Silver (1990) have shown that on-time, expectable transition to widowhood has little long-term impact on the mental health of widows. However, gender must be considered in understanding this transition; although women widowed at an expectable age (mid- to late 70s) seem to recover from the immediate loss within about a year, older men do not show a similar capacity to recover from grief.

The manner in which persons cope with these events often changes their personal significance (Fisseni 1985; Maas 1985). Less is known about the factors that permit persons to remain resilient, even when confronted by adversity, than about those factors that may lead to distress and psychopathology (Cohler 1987; Cohler, Stott, Musik 1995; Vaillant 1993). Whitbourne (1985) has reviewed findings regarding the interplay of social timing and life changes, emphasizing the multiple factors from social circumstances and family values to the unique life history, all of which enter into both present understanding and response to adversity. Whitbourne's review stressed the significance of considering life changes across the course of life in terms of resources available for withstanding the impact of adverse life changes. This approach, closely identified with empirical studies by Lazarus and Folkman (1984), Lowenthal et al. (1975), and Vaillant (1993), focuses on the manner in which problems are approached and the extent to which persons are able to accurately evaluate and appropriately respond to challenges that are presented to them.

However, one possible problem with this approach, when understood from the perspective of the second half of life, is that it assumes an active, problem-centered mode of response that may be more appropriate to life changes taking place across middle age than to those associated with later life. Although Folkman and Lazarus (1980), Lazarus and DeLongis (1983), and McCrae and Costa (1990) maintain that coping processes are stable across the adult years and not affected by age, both the mode of measurement and the restricted age range (only up to age 65) in these studies qualify the assertion that age and coping approach are unrelated. Indeed, findings reported by Brim and Ryff (1979), Cohler and Lieberman (1980), Hultsch and Plemons (1979), and M. Lieberman and Falk (1971) suggest that older adults may respond to adversity in ways different from those of younger adults.

Middle-age adults tend to use reminiscence about the past in an effort to solve problems, whereas older adults rely on reminiscence in an effort to 1) become reconciled to problems and make peace with present reality and 2) cope with problems using emotion-focused rather than problem-focused solutions (Lazarus and Folkman 1984). Older adults tend to look inward somewhat more or to depend on a confidante rather than family members such as offspring in the effort to resolve problems in their present life. Indeed, Lazarus and DeLongis (1983) recognized that there are changes with age in the experience of life changes; older adults may become less distressed than younger counterparts when confronting health crises owing to the interplay of place in the course of life and a shifting perspective on the very concept of mortality or the finitude of life (Marshall 1975, 1986; Munnichs 1966). Older adults are apparently better able to confront these issues of mortality than their younger counterparts (Zweibel and Cassel 1989; Zweibel and Lydens 1990).

When there is little to be attained by active coping efforts, efforts to manage life circumstances may be less effective than renewed focus on the personal significance of this experience. Indeed, Kohut (1978) suggested that increased use of reminiscence and other modes of providing self-comfort and integrity might be the most effective responses to coping with surgery and other hospitalizations. This capacity to effectively use reminiscence and other so-called emotion-focused modes of coping with adversity and distress (Lazarus and Folkman 1984) appears to be somewhat less difficult to attain among older persons than among their younger counterparts. Since the time of Butler's (1963) initial formulation, much of the literature has shown that the capacity to use reminiscence as a mode of comforting is particularly characteristic of later life (Haight 1991), although a life-threatening illness such as cancer or acquired immunodeficiency syndrome (AIDS) appears to promote a similar self-comforting use of reminiscence at younger ages (Borden 1989, 1991; Mages and Mendelsohn 1979).

Furthermore, as Thomae (1990) has observed, accepting the reality of present life circumstances does not necessarily imply passivity. Consistent with Janis's (1958) findings regarding denial and recovery from surgery, when older adults are confronted by a painful present reality that is beyond their control, it may be that the best possible response is to accept the present situation and to rely on memory of the past as consolation. Emphasis on active, problem-centered coping reflects life circumstances more relevant to the young-old than to the old-old. Reminiscence is particularly significant as a coping technique in later life, because it provides a means of solace that fosters adjustment to a reality that is often physically and emotionally painful (Cohler and Galatzer-Levy 1990; Elson 1987; McMahon and Rhudick 1964, 1967).

Time, Memory, and the Course of Adult Life

Across the course of life, there are marked changes in the use of time and memory. For young children, primary focus is on the present, with a growing awareness of the past across the preschool years. The shift from early to middle childhood is marked by a principal concern with the present, while that from childhood to adolescence is marked by changes in sense of time and organization of memory of the past (Cottle 1977; Cottle and Klineberg 1974; Greene 1986, 1990) to include not only past and present but also a connected future. Adolescent use of time shifts from a focus on the present, with an imagined future posed in terms of some idealized person or group, to a more realistic appraisal of what may be attained over time. The adolescent and young adult look forward, planning and anticipating, coping with uncertainty regarding next steps in terms of available opportunities, and the middle-age adult begins to turn to the past as a source of guidance during periods of personal distress (M. Lieberman and Falk 1971). Indeed, across the course of the second half of life, the past may become mythologized, organized in a particular manner to provide meaning for particular present experiences and guidance in coping with problems. There may be a fourth transformation of the course of life as well: that associated with the transformation from middle to later life, sometimes known as the crisis of survivorship. Once again, time and memory become reorganized as, with the death of spouse and friends, reminiscence increasingly replaces time/space relationships as the source of present experience.

The Finitude of Life

One particularly significant feature of the second half of life concerns shared understandings of the finitude of life (Munnichs 1966) and of one's present position in terms of expectable longevity. Neugarten (1979) and Neugarten and Datan (1974b) have portrayed the experience, generally occurring at some point during the fifth decade of life, of realizing that there is less time to be lived than has been lived already. This crisis of finitude is a consequence of the comparison of the trajectory of one's own life with shared expectations concerning the duration of life. Awareness of finitude is heightened by increased acquaintance with mortality through experience of the deaths of parents and other family members and, increasingly, associates (Plath 1980) or members of the same sociohistorical cohort (Jaques 1965, 1980; Pollock 1971a, 1980, 1981). Reading about the death of a movie star or politician who is about the same age or is recalled as playing an important role in remembered earlier life experiences may increase the awareness of finitude.

This heightened awareness of one's own mortality, portrayed by Munnichs (1966) as increased awareness of the finitude of life, and elaborated by Jaques (1965, 1980), Marshall (1975, 1981, 1986), Neugarten (1979), and Sill (1980), results in a transformation in emphasis in temporal orientation from time already lived to time remaining to be lived, and in memory to increased preoccupation with the past and reminiscence. At first, this reminiscence is used actively in the service of coping with life changes associated with career and family (M. Lieberman and Falk 1971; M. Lieberman and Tobin 1983). At some point during the late 40s or early 50s, persons begin looking backward to the past for inspiration and meaning, rather than finding such meaning through anticipation of the future. Cohler and Lieberman (1979) and M. Lieberman and Tobin (1983) have reported findings from a systematic study founded on groups of several hundred adults across gender and ethnicity, showing that men in their early 50s and women in their late 50s are particularly likely to express feelings of lowered morale, increased concerns about health, and increased feelings of anxiety and depression. This sense of disharmony and self-search has been reflected in the popular culture as the "mid-life crisis."

Both men and women, but particularly men, showed marked distress accompanying the transformation to mid-life and increased awareness of finitude. At least in part, these heightened concerns appear to account for first hospitalization for psychiatric illness in the course of life (Gutmann et al. 1979). With advancing age, reminiscence activity becomes increasingly important as a part of taking stock of one's own life, in mourning dreams never realized, and in settling accounts with the past (Butler 1963; Kaminsky 1984a; Moody 1986).

As a consequence of this increased personalization of death and awareness of finitude, persons begin to develop a more inward orientation, earlier portrayed by Jung (1933) as introversion and, more recently, by Neugarten (1973, 1979) as "interiority." This mid-life transformation is characterized by increasing preoccupation with the meaning of life; taking stock of personal accomplishments and disappointments; lessened interest in a wide variety of interdependent ties with kindred, particularly those that are obligatory rather than voluntary (Cohler 1983; Cohler and Grunebaum 1981; Pruchno et al. 1984; Rook 1984); and lessened interest in taking on new challenges. Note that this transformation need not be reflected in changing patterns of social ties, as was earlier suggested in discussions of disengagement (Cumming and Henry 1961; Hochschild 1975; Neugarten 1973). The primary focus of this mid-life transformation is on the impact of a changing sense of time and the use of memory of the past in an effort to maintain a sense of continuity and integrity or coherence of self.

Findings reported by Back (1974), Gutmann (1975, 1977, 1987), Orwoll and Achenbaum (1993), and Sinnott (1982) suggested in addition that there may be gender-related differences across the years of middle and later life in the expression of inferiority, the timing of the transformation to mid-life, the significance of this transformation for continued adjustment, and even gender-related differences in expression of wisdom. Men at mid-life become increasingly concerned with issues of personal comfort and with seeking succor from others, moving away from reliance on active mastery in solving problems at home and at work, whereas women may become somewhat more oriented toward active mastery and "instrumental-executive" activities, moving away from their earlier involvement in caring for others as wife, mother, and kin-keeper (Cohler and Grunebaum 1981; Firth et al. 1970; Gilligan 1982; Gutmann 1987). Findings from Back's (1974) study suggested that, with the advent of mid-life, women begin to see themselves less in terms mediated through such relationships as wife and mother, and more directly in terms of present involvements beyond those of home and family.

As a consequence of increased awareness of the finitude of life, both men and women appear to show increased concern with self and lessened patience for demands on time and energy that, increasingly, are experienced as in "short supply" (Back 1974; Cohler and Lieberman 1980; Cohler and Grunebaum 1981; Erikson 1985; Erikson et al. 1986; Hazan 1980; Kernberg 1980; Lowenthal et al. 1975; Neugarten 1979; Rook 1984). Concern with realization of one's own goals, and with reworking the presently understood story of the course of life to maintain a sense of personal coherence, becomes particularly salient in later middle age, requiring time and energy that is then less available for other pursuits. The ability to mourn goals not attained and to accept the finitude of life without despair provides some evidence of the successful realization of this effort (Pollock 1981).

The sense of a life foreshortened as a result of increasing appreciation of the finitude of life (Munnichs 1966) or personalization of death (Neugarten and Datan 1974b) requires changes in the manner in which time is used in the ordering of this account. As a consequence, there may be a transformation in the experience of time and the use of memory (Cohler and Freeman 1993; M. Lieberman and Falk 1971; M. Lieberman and Tobin 1983) that poses unique problems for the maintenance of a sense of personal integrity. Confronted by an increased awareness of their own mortality, at least some older adults deal with the increased sense of finitude of life by focusing on day-to-day issues rather than worrying about the future. In the words of one man in his 90s, reflecting on the finitude of life: "I take each day as it comes; who can predict the future?" (personal communication). When one relies on the presently experienced past as a source of solace at times of distress and as guidance in resolving problems, the course of daily life is much more structured around the present rather than the future.

Reminiscence in Later Life

Erikson et al. (1986) have well described the significance of reminiscence in later life as a source of the comfort and solace once available through relationships with others. Over time, with the death of friends and relatives and as elderly individuals become survivors of relationships that formerly provided this solace (Horton 1981; Horton et al. 1987; Kohut 1974, 1975, 1977, 1982; Winnicott 1988), memory increasingly serves the functions previously realized through being with others. Reminiscence serves the dual function of providing comfort and serving as a storehouse of memories that are continually reordered over time to preserve a sense of meaning and purpose, even when confronted by adversity and social dislocation. Impairment of memory, which is the consequence of senile dementia, interferes with the ability to foster a sense of a continuing, coherent narrative of the course of life. The depressive affect often observed across the early-to-middle phases of Alzheimer's disease (Lazarus et al. 1987, 1989) may be a reflection of the loss of the narrative capacity essential in preserving meaning that results from the impairment of memory characteristic of Alzheimer's disease.

Across the course of later life, reminiscence is increasingly used in the service of life review (Butler 1963; Kaufman 1986; Tobin 1991), settling accounts with the entire prior course of life, rather than as a guide to present actions, which is more characteristic of middle age (M. Lieberman and

Falk 1971). The life review fosters the increased introspective activity occasioned by the increased awareness of finitude across later life, assisting in the process of maintaining a sense of purpose into oldest age, as long as there is memory accessible regarding the past (Benedek 1959/1973).

Erikson's observation regarding the significance of reminiscence and personal review of the life story points out the importance of the remembered past for the maintenance of morale in later life (Myerhoff 1979, 1992). Butler (1963) has noted the significance of the life review for the reintegration of the remembered past as a part of making sense of life as lived. As Myerhoff (1992) has observed: "the integration with earlier states of being surely provides the sense of continuity and completeness that may be counted as an essential developmental task of old age. It may not yield wisdom . . . it does give what [Erikson] would consider ego integrity, the opposite of disintegration" (p. 239). At the same time, memory itself may be painful, as among those older adults experiencing memory loss, such as patients with early-stage Alzheimer's disease. Forgetting names, dates, and places is personally mortifying and also deprives older adults of the very source of solace and comfort that sustains them when they are confronted by the reality of loss.

Social Ties in Later Life

These reports show the significance of the life story as a source of solace and comfort across the course of life and particularly in later life. Cohler and Galatzer-Levy (1990) have suggested that memories of the past may largely replace interpersonal contact as a source of solace during times of distress. The reality of loss through the death of a spouse and close friends, problems in moving about, and limitations in personal energy all contribute to an increased preference for memories of times spent with others rather than spending time with others in the present. (Although many older persons prefer to take each day as it comes, solace is found in recollection and reminiscence of the past.) Remembering and recounting the life story replaces contact with others as an essential or evoked other and is essential in maintaining a sense of personal integrity and morale. Recalling the past through recounting the presently experienced life story, as in the life of Ingmar Bergman's film (Wild Strawberries 1957) character, Dr. Borg, contributes to personal well-being across the second half of life in ways that may be quite different from the use of the past in either early adulthood or middle age (M. Lieberman and Falk 1971; M. Lieberman and Tobin 1983).

Relations With Family and Friends

This perspective on the intrapsychological significance of social ties differs from perspectives on the significance of attaining interpersonal autonomy rather than maintaining interdependent ties with others as important in realizing personal maturity. Perspectives such as those of the ethological attachment group, portrayed by Bowlby (1982) and extended to the study of adult social relations by Antonucci (1990), Marris (1974/1986), and others, or the separation-individuation paradigm, as formulated by Mahler et al. (1975) and extended in consecutive panels to the study of middle childhood, adolescence and adulthood, and aging (Panel 1973a, 1973b, 1973c) all tend to portray, as a model of adulthood, a degree of interpersonal autonomy that is inconsistent with the reality of social life in adulthood. First, self psychological perspectives emphasize the significance of study of the meaning of social ties over time, as observed through the experience-near context of the psychoanalytic interview (Kohut 1971), rather than observation of time/space relationships as undertaken by Mahler et al. (1975) observing mothers and children together.

Second, experience-near perspectives regarding self emphasize the meaning of others, rather than merely demonstrating that adults maintain significant social ties and reporting on the aggregation of the number and nature of social ties. Much of the literature reporting on the significance of ties with others for adult adjustment has focused on the positive relationship between morale and a larger self-reported social network (Adams 1989; Antonucci 1990). The social network, or convoy of social support, is believed to reduce the otherwise stressful effects of adverse life changes, buffering the individual from mental and physical ill health (Aneshensel and Stone 1982; Antonucci 1990; Caplan and Killilea 1976; Dean and Lin 1977; Eckenroade and Gore 1981; Greenblatt et al. 1979; Kahn and Antonucci 1980; Killilea 1982; Parkes 1972; Schulz and Rau 1985; Turner 1981; Weiss 1982).

Few studies have focused on the manner in which social ties foster morale across the course of life or explored the possibility that the very meaning of the experience of being with others changes across the life course. For example, just as younger adults enjoy being with large numbers of others, older adults prefer a small number of friends and confidantes to offspring for social support (Lee 1979). Across the second half of life, brothers and sisters are likely to play a particularly important role in providing support and assistance and maintaining morale for each other (Cicirelli 1990, 1992). Because of the importance of the offspring relationship across the first half of life, it has been difficult for those studying the family in the second half of life to shift from concern with relations of parents and children to a larger focus on brothers and sisters and other relatives as important for morale and adjustment (Cohler and Altergott 1995).

Much study to date has focused on the receipt of support or care not just outside the experience of receiving such care but also outside the experiencing world of those providing care. As a result of focusing on the recipient of care, much of this study shows the benefits of receiving care among young adults, rather than the costs of providing such care among their middle-aged parents. Cohler (1983), Cohler and Grunebaum (1981), Cohler and Lieberman (1980), Pruchno et al. (1984), and Rook (1984) have all emphasized the interdependent nature of care provided. When a family member experiences adversity, other family members are expected to provide assistance. The impact of adversity and its sequelae radiate outward from the immediate family to a large sphere of relatives like waves radiating out from the point at which a stone hits the water in a pond. Family members are bound together by ties of "invisible loyalty" (Boszormenyi-Nagy and Spark 1973) and do provide assistance for each other in times of distress.

Older family members with a larger number of younger relatives demanding care, rather than older relatives who may be looked to for understanding and solace at time of need, differentially become providers of care. Although such care may have supportive and comforting implications for younger members of the family, it means an increased burden for older family members (Rosenmayr and Kockeis 1963). For example, Cherlin and Furstenberg (1986), Cohler and Grunebaum (1981), Robertson (1977), and Wood and Robertson (1978) all report that grandparents are resentful of the baby-sitting demands placed on them by their young adult offspring. At the same time, particularly among middle-age grandparents, their dependent parents seek care and comfort rather than providing for it. Possibly, care for dependent parents, although often a source of role strain, may be somewhat less a source of distress for the generation in the middle than is caring for young adults and their offspring, as those in middle and late life share a view of the life course explicitly recognizing the finitude of life that is not shared by young adult offspring (Bromberg 1983; Cohler et al. 1988). Young adults find it difficult to view life as foreshortened in ways experienced by their parents.

The "generation in the middle" (Brody 1966, 1970, 1981, 1985), particularly women, are expected to provide care both upward and downward across the generation, often leading to the feelings of dissatisfaction with social ties portrayed by Rook (1984, 1989). Although women have generally been the major caretakers of both older parents and in-laws, Shanas (1979) reported survey findings suggesting that middle-age men are taking a more active role in the care of infirm and cognitively impaired elders. Women have been socialized since early childhood into the roles of kin-keeping and child care (Firth et al. 1970), which has been portrayed by Chodorow (1978), following Komarovsky (1950, 1956, 1962), as "reproduction of mothering." Women in the middle-age generation are particularly likely to report feelings of being overburdened by demands of the social network or convoy and associated feelings of lowered morale. Furthermore, having finished active parenting, middle-age mothers may return to school or start working and feel their children's demands to be an intrusion on their own time and schedule. Indeed, feelings of role strain and overload may be more of a problem than feelings of social isolation among women in late middle age in American society (Dunkel-Schetter and Wortman 1981).

Provision of care for others has different meanings across the second half of life as contrasted with the first half of life, making the middle-age person's response to the increased number of demands additionally difficult. Accompanying the increased interiority across the second half of life is a change in the manner in which others become used as a source of solace for self. In the first place, energy is deployed differently; persons experiencing the mid-life transformation are likely to seek increased time for self and to become increasingly preoccupied with their own experience of aging. Indeed, there is an increased preference for solitude that is too often assumed to reflect social isolation in later life.

Loneliness and Being Alone

Note that studies of older persons find that reports of feelings of loneliness are no more common than earlier in life (Fiske 1980; Lowenthal 1964; Lowenthal and Robinson 1976; Mancini 1979; Mancini et al. 1980; Townsend 1957), although some studies suggest increased loneliness among widowed men (Elwell and Maltbie-Cranwell 1981) and among women who had lived with a spouse for many years, as contrasted with women living alone (Essex and Nam 1987). Bankoff (1983) reported that increased distress is associated with the time immediately following widowhood, whereas, if widowhood happens approximately "on time," in terms of the expectable course of life, much of the loneliness reported in the time immediately following widowhood appears to diminish.

As Fiske (1980) noted in studies of middle and later life, there is a difference between being alone and being lonely. Across the second half of life, with the deaths of family members and friends, there is increasingly diminished access to forms of social support assumed to be available earlier in life. At the same time, with the increased use of reminiscence, first for problem solving in middle age and later in life as a means of providing comforting and maintenance of meaning, being alone both provides time for reminiscence and also requires reminiscence as a means of ensuring meaning. The present, foreshortened with the sense of limited time remaining to be lived, is made meaningful as connected to a remembered past that provides a continued sense of personal integration. Family members and friends may have died or moved away, but continuity with the past is ensured through remembrance of past time. At least part of the terror inspired by cognitive impairment such as that associated with Alzheimer's disease is the associated loss of memory that prevents the use of reminiscence and, ultimately, breakdown in personal integration (Lazarus et al. 1987).

The Experience of Health in Later Life

Health in general is increasingly a concern across the second half of life. Middle age brings a greater sense of physical vulnerability, and "body monitoring" may intensify (Neugarten 1973, 1979). Whitbourne (1985) has discussed the intended and unintended consequences for health of the various strategies that individuals use as they seek to maintain continuity of identity in the face of the mental and physical changes that accompany aging. For adults of all ages, the largest category of fears for the self concern physical condition—health, appearance, and weight. In late life, however, these fears appear to become more vivid and concrete (Cross and Markus 1991). Of the various "feared selves" that older adults report, it is those related to health that they tend to dread most (Hooker 1992).

The focus in studies concerning the impact of health on morale, quality of life, and experience of self in later life has been on health status as subjectively perceived. Older adults' global evaluations of their health are associated with physician ratings and specific health indexes, which have been assumed to be reliable measures (Fillenbaum 1979; La Rue et al. 1979). However, subjective health may be a more sensitive measure predicting mortality (Kaplan et al. 1988; Mossey and Shapiro 1982). Continued physical mobility appears to be central to the older adults' subjective perception of health (Shanas et al. 1968). Illness that does not affect the ability to remain active is less likely to lead to lowered morale or reduced social contact and may be even more important than income level in fostering a sense of personal well-being (Kaufman 1986; Larson 1978; Zautra and Hempel 1984).

Stolar et al. (1991) report that the health problems most clearly affecting morale may be those that cannot be integrated within a coherent life story (Antonovsky 1987). Stolar et al. (1992) found that older adults' overall satisfaction with life was less affected by chronic illnesses such as arthritis and diabetes, which were experienced as understandable and manageable, than by health problems such as bladder trouble, vertigo, or difficulty walking, problems whose causes and treatment were experienced as less clear-cut. The latter problems are likely to be unpredictably disruptive of everyday activities and social contacts.

Despite health worries and ailments, older adults tend to describe their health as good. Indeed, among those ages 65 and older, there does not appear to be an increase with age in the proportion of individuals who regard their health as poor, even though the incidence of health problems does increase (Ferraro 1980; Shanas et al. 1968), and Cockerham et al. (1983) have shown that older adults describe their general health in more positive terms than do younger adults. Older adults' tendency to report that they are in good health may reflect a comparison of self-perceptions with those of age peers, rather than with current objective health status or health earlier in life. Furthermore, as associates begin to die, survival itself may be taken as an indication that one enjoys reasonably good health; with approach of the century mark, the ability to attain this goal becomes particularly salient. During very late life, even though the daily routine becomes less physically demanding, with increased enjoyment of solitude and reminiscence, even somewhat diminished mobility may still be adequate for sustaining morale (Cockerham et al. 1983; Cohler 1993).

Wisdom and Creativity Across the Second Half of Life

The search for a view of aging that challenges the pervasive notion of later life as a time of decline has encouraged attention to issues of wisdom and creativity across the second half of life. Gutmann (1987) noted the respect accorded to elders in traditional society; the greater lived experience that accompanies the passage of years is presumed to lead to 1) a perspective on self and others that is less self-interested than earlier in the course of life, and 2) an enlarged understanding of the nature of life. Following the theoretical perspective initially developed by Gilligan (1982, 1983), Orwoll and Achenbaum (1993) have suggested that older men and women express wisdom in a somewhat different manner. Women may express wisdom principally in the interpersonal realm, evident as communal concerns, whereas men may express wisdom principally within the intrapersonal realm, evident as agentic concerns. However, consistent with Gutmann's (1987) formulation and Achenbaum and Orwoll's (1991) discussion of Job as a wise elder, older men may adopt some of the more communal concerns of women, whereas older women may become somewhat more agentic in the expression of wisdom. However, note that the study of wisdom in later life has become involved in larger contemporary social and political issues, including those concerned with the presence of gender, ethnicity, and age bias across the course of life. Scholarly study has sometimes been designed in an effort to prove the worth of older adults in a society too often preoccupied with the status of masculinity and youth (Kaminsky 1993; Kastenbaum 1993; McCullough 1993; Moody 1986, 1993; Orwoll and Achenbaum 1993).

The Wise Elder as "Ideal Type"

Erikson's (1950/1963, 1960, 1968) epigenetic model of lives from infancy through oldest age portrays wisdom as an attitude of detached concern optimally attained in later life. Faced with finitude, a fragmenting sense of despair—rooted in regrets about the life one has lived, frustration with limitations in the present, and fear and uncertainty about one's future—counters the development of a sense of wholeness, coherence, or integrity brought about through coming to terms with one's life. In successful resolution of the issue of integrity, a sense of despair is transformed into a sense of wholeness (Erikson 1979), rather than being denied through desperate optimism (Erikson et al. 1986), creation of a too-coherent life story (Manheimer 1992), or some other form of what Erikson has called "pseudo-integrity." Tobin (1991) has suggested that over time Erikson has increasingly focused discussions of integrity and wisdom on use of reminiscence, with a sense of wholeness attained through review of one's life. Processes that Erikson (1985) identified with attainment of wisdom have been explored in discussions of reminiscence, life review, and life story (Gohler and Freeman 1993).

The relatively recent increase in attention to wisdom outside the tradition pioneered by Erikson (Sternberg 1990b) can be traced to current concern with successful aging. Viewed from this perspective, wisdom seems especially promising, constituting a gain in functioning that is distinctively associated with attainment of later life. Heckhausen et al. (1989) found that of 100 desirable psychological attributes, "wise" and "dignified" were the only ones expected to emerge in late life.

The initial focus of study was to identify folk notions of wisdom by eliciting characteristics of the prototypic wise person (Chandler and Holliday 1990; Clayton and Birren 1979; Holliday and Chandler 1986; Sternberg 1990a). As Chandler and Holliday (1990) observed, the recurrence of essentially the same set of descriptors across studies suggests that a distinguishable folk concept of wisdom persists despite the presumed loss of the notion of wisdom from discourse in contemporary society (Cole et al. 1993). The wise individual understands self and others; is perceptive, intuitive, empathic, knowledgeable, measured, and experienced; and recognizes essences, contexts, consequences, and multiple perspectives.

In proposing definitions of wisdom, theorists have drawn on these common-sense understandings of wisdom; discussions of wisdom within the philosophical literature; and contemporary conceptions of personality, development, and, especially, cognition (Chandler and Holliday 1990). A thread running through many of these discussions that is consistent with the view of wisdom as coming to terms with mortality and one's life as lived is the notion of recognition of and response to human limitation and doubt about the truth of what one knows (Meacham 1990; Taranto 1989). Baltes et al. (Baltes and Smith 1990; Baltes et al. 1990) and Clayton (1982) view the wise person as possessing high levels of knowledge about life, including awareness of life's uncertainties, social context, and relativity, as well as factual and procedural knowledge about living. Invoking the distinction between fluid intelligence, which may decline in late life, and crystallized intelligence, which does not, they conceptualize wisdom as a form of expertise making possible good judgment, sound advice, and special insight concerning "important but uncertain" life matters. In a series of studies, they have presented a hypothetical person's life dilemma, asked how the person might respond, and evaluated the level of knowledge about life—the wisdom—reflected in the suggested responses.

Although Erikson's portrayal of wisdom as the defining ego strength of old age might imply that it is a normative developmental achievement, Erikson et al. (1986) acknowledged that many of the older adults they interviewed had not been able to gain the perspective that Erikson had identified with wisdom. Consistent with this view, Smith and Baltes (1990) reported that few adults of any age provide commentary reflective of wisdom in response to hypothetical life problems. Wisdom, in other words, appears to be rare. Clayton (1975) has outlined contemporary cultural forces that may work against development or appreciation of wisdom as defined by Erikson, including contemporary preoccupation with youth and mundane, worldly activity.

From the perspective of successful aging, interest in wisdom rests on the assumption that, however rarely attained, it is a late-life accomplishment. Evidence supporting this view is mixed. Older adults believe that their adaptation to the successes and disappointments met in life, and their acceptance of the personal past as "inevitable, appropriate, and meaningful," has increased with age (Ryff and Heinecke 1983). Such acceptance appears to be greater in individuals nominated by others as wise (Orwoll and Perlmutter 1990). Furthermore, both young and middle-age adults project experiencing a greater sense of integrity in late life than they attribute to themselves in the present, suggesting that there is a shared expectation that sense of integrity increases across the life course (Ryff and Heinecke 1983).

The picture is less clear when focusing on wisdom. Adults of various ages tend to nominate older adults when asked to identify someone wise (Orwoll and Perlmutter 1990). There is some evidence that women tend to identify kindred and that men call on experiences at work when nominating those who are wise (Sowarka 1989, cited in Sternberg 1990b), although this may be a cohort-specific pattern reflecting gender-related differences in both meaning and participation within the world of work. In addition, young and middle-age adults associate wisdom with old age (Clayton and Birren 1979). However, older adults associate wisdom less closely with being old than do younger adults and view themselves as no wiser than younger adults see themselves (Clayton and Birren 1979; Orwoll and Perlmutter 1990). From some perspectives (Meacham 1990) this might be viewed as evidence of wisdom (i.e., a knowing that one doesn't know). Alternatively, perhaps wisdom is not a function of age. On life review tasks, theoretically more familiar to older than to younger adults, Baltes and colleagues (Baltes and Smith 1990; Baltes et al. 1990) did not find consistent age differences in wisdom as they defined it that favored older adults, although older adults were represented among those few whose responses were judged to be most indicative of wisdom (Staudinger et al. 1992). Evaluation of responses to life-planning tasks led the research group to propose that wisdom, understood as a form of expert knowledge, may not be global and cumulative; instead, adults may be most "expert" about life matters specific to their place in historical time and in the life course (Smith and Baltes 1990).

For different reasons, Meacham (1990) also rejected a cumulative view of change in wisdom. He argued provocatively that because accumulation of knowledge and power tends to undermine an attitude of doubt concerning what one knows, the expectable course of wisdom is one of decline with age. The young can be wise: He invoked Anne Frank as an example of youthful wisdom. Perhaps the image of the wise elder represents most of all a source of solace and hope for young and middle-age adults (Meacham 1990; Galatzer-Levy and Cohler 1993). The nature of experiences during life that might foster development of wisdom are not well understood. For many current theorists, and perhaps in folk conceptions as well, wisdom is associated with old age because it is seen as something gained through long experience. In contrast, if wisdom connotes a sense of coherence, it is normatively tied to the second half of life when "coherence work" (Moody 1993) intensifies in response to awareness of one's own mortality (Taranto 1989). If wisdom is expertise about life's uncertainties (Baltes and Smith 1990), its acquisition is favored by broad and extensive life experience and nurturance by experts. From this knowledge-acquisition perspective, it is understandable that young adults within present cohorts might be more "expert" than older adults, particularly regarding those problems related to the meaning of work, positive health habits, and quality of life, salient in early adulthood for present cohorts but possibly less salient for older adults.

More recent study has shown little concern with either the inner experience of the wise adult or the experience of engagement with wise others. Erikson et al. (1986) suggested that wisdom provides a source of comfort, understanding, and compassion, shown in Erikson's discussion of Dr. Borg (Erikson 1979; Erikson et al. 1986). Unlike many views of wisdom as a kind of knowledge or mode of cognition, common-sense notions place great emphasis on the web of social relationships within which wisdom exists. These relations have been illustrated by Myerhoff (1992) and others in discussions of late-life reminiscence that suggest how wisdom's potential social obligations and rewards affect the wise person's morale, what meaning and function wise others hold for persons during life (Galatzer-Levy and Cohler 1993), and what role is played by an actual or imagined audience in fostering the experience of gaining wisdom. At least to some extent, during life, we are as wise as we imagine ourselves to be.

Expression of Creativity Across Middle and Later Life

Involvement in creative activity is often assumed to be a means of maintaining vitality into oldest age (Erikson et al. 1986), and interest in late-life creativity has largely been spurred by efforts to counteract the "aging-as-decline" perspective (Cole 1992; Cole et al. 1993). However, older psychometric research on creative potential and the study of changes in creative productivity across the adult years—the two dominant streams of research bearing on late-life creativity—have both been preoccupied with the question of whether creativity diminishes across the second half of life. Although older adults appear to perform less well than younger adults on paper-and-pencil measures of creative ability (Alpaugh and Birren 1977; McCrae et al. 1987), it is not clear whether test performance in any way indexes real-life creativity, or whether group differences of the magnitude found hold real-world significance (Romaniuk and Romaniuk 1981; Schaie 1984, 1990a; Schaie et al. 1973; Simonton 1990c).

Life-course study of creative productivity has largely been concerned with changes in creative production across later life. Historical records of the lifetime output of artists, scientists, and scholars ensure study of real-life creativity among those persons with demonstrated creative ability. Study of aging and creativity becomes more problematic when studying persons who have not demonstrated creativity. The distribution of works produced by individuals at different ages has been charted for numerous disciplines. With some qualifications (Dennis 1956, 1966), the studies suggest that adult output (both of major and of minor works) rises at successive ages until it reaches a peak, with lower output at later ages (Lehman 1953, 1966; Simonton 1990a, 1990b, 1990c). Although attainment of later life is frequently viewed as associated with inevitable and rather early decline in creative achievement, Lehman and Simonton themselves pointed out the many counter examples of artists, scientists, and others whose major creative contributions have occurred late in life. One eminent translator of classical languages has observed that it is impossible to do a decent job of translating classical Greek texts until the eighth or ninth decade of life and attainment of a good working knowledge of Greek. The current era in American society appears to be one in which adults across the adult years experience increasing frustration with the opportunity for personal expression and for attaining an enhanced sense of personal creativity. This sense of frustration regarding individual accomplishment, which is characteristic of mass culture within contemporary bourgeois Western society (Fay 1987; Marcuse 1955), is in marked contrast with Hindu culture, where, as the Indian psychoanalyst Sudhir Kakar (1978, 1979/1992) reported, it is expected that men attaining mid-life will want to withdraw from the world of commerce to seek enhanced vitality through personal creative expression and will be supported in this effort by both family and society.

Much of the study of creativity across the course of life shows that there are important differences in productivity that are closely tied to the nature of the creative work. Simonton (1990c), for example, estimated that peak output for lyric poets and theoretical physicists occurs in their late 20s or early 30s, after which the drop in productivity is marked, whereas among historians and philosophers, the peak occurs in their 50s, with little subsequent decline in productivity. Expectation becomes reality when those working within fields of study such as mathematics or contemporary theoretical physics share the expectation that creative accomplishment must peak early in one's career (Cohen-Shalev 1986; Simonton 1990c). Failure to accomplish important work by a certain age may be viewed fatalistically and is likely to lead to decreased morale.

Whether pursued throughout the adult years or deferred during middle adulthood, artistic activity in later life either may answer a desire for creative expression or constitute a means for warding off boredom or responding to an experienced imperative to "stay active" (L. Lieberman and L. Lieberman 1983). However, in both instances artistic activity fosters morale (Erikson et al. 1986; Lorenzen-Huber 1991). Vaillant (1993) has reported that in two longitudinal studies, both men and women who had been creative as adults expressed higher morale in late life than their less creative counterparts. When the imperative to "keep busy" or "get involved" comes from sources extrinsic to oneself and possibly counter to one's own artistic preferences, however, creative arts, like other extrinsically demanded activities, may be experienced as an unwelcome imposition (Pruyser 1987) and can adversely affect morale. Indeed, busyness may interfere with other less visible creative activity such as life review (Butler 1963; Kastenbaum 1992; Tobin 1991).

Creative activities may be newly and distinctively engaging in late life, as older adults become increasingly concerned with their own experiences and strive to construct accounts of their lives that preserve a sense of coherence (Cohler 1993). Francis (1992) has described a group of retirees whose paintings and sculptures either represented scenes from their work life or incorporated skills and materials drawn from their work world. These older adults, for whom work and retirement held differing meanings, variously evoked, memorialized, reworked, sought to justify, or struggled to come to terms with and integrate the personal past through their work in the arts. Among other older adults, writing appears to provide the medium for life review, understood as an expectable process in which unresolved aspects of the personal past are repeatedly returned to until transformed in a way that provides meaning and a sense of integrity (Kaminsky 1984a, 1984b).

Finally, those adults attaining later life in different historical periods will have had different experiences regarding their own artistic activity. Interviewing the adult children of the 1950s organization men, Leinberger and Tucker (1991) repeatedly heard declarations of a desire for a career in the arts from men and women in early middle age who had grown up in the child- and then youth-centered expressive culture of the mid-20th century. Krantz (1977) and Osherson (1980), who studied career change in mid-life, reported similar concerns among members of the generation of fathers of these youths; men in the older generation sought to leave organizational careers at mid-life to attain increased opportunity for creativity and personal expression.

Conclusion

Study of older adulthood within the context of the course of life as a whole marks an important departure for both psychiatry and the social sciences. With as much as one-third of the life span remaining after retirement in contemporary society, it is essential to reconsider earlier conceptions of the place of the second half of life within the course of life as a whole. It is largely as a consequence of shared understandings of the significance of particular ages that certain chronological ages are imbued with meanings. Understanding of health is also subjectively constructed; regardless of so-called objective indexes of illness, as long as older adults are able to retain independent functioning and manage tasks of daily life, positive morale is maintained, which mitigates against otherwise presumed interference by illness in well-being. With those ages 85 and older the most rapidly growing age group within the population, it is important to reconsider views of personal change and capacity for continued adaptation to social change across later life and also to plan effectively for the social and health needs of this group of older adults throughout the 21st century.

Reconsideration of previous findings has shown the limitations arising from the study of a particular generation or cohort of adults across the second half of life. Older adults, at least until about age 65, are as healthy as younger counterparts and show little of the personal rigidity and decrement in cognitive functioning earlier believed to characterize the later years of life. Improved health across the course of life and greater education and subsequent continued immersion in activities fostering cognitive competence through oldest age have contributed to a generation of particularly effective older adults. Although areas of creative contribution may change over time, there is little evidence of decrement in capacity for creative activity across the years of middle and later life. More than half of persons over age 85 continue to live independently, active and involved in both family and community. Indeed, continued autonomy and capacity for managing everyday life activities characterizes the largest number of older adults and is critically important for maintaining morale and adjustment. Consistent with this portrait of older adults as competent and contributing members of the community, creative and involved in a complex network of relationships with both friends and family, present cohorts of older adults show little of the self-preoccupation earlier assumed to characterize personality in later life.

Implications of this new view of competence and health across the second half of life are important in considering issues of intervention. Although those individuals requiring psychiatric intervention highlight the problems confronted by older adults, to date there has been little consideration regarding issues of primary prevention in older adults that have characterized study of and intervention in childhood and adolescence. Creative reconsideration of issues such as housing, supporting intergenerational living (including that among families of choice), and home-based health care, which fosters positive morale by enabling continued independent living, and increased recognition of the importance of both friends and brothers and sisters as sources of care and support are all important in forestalling the cycle of personal disorganization that ultimately requires psychiatric intervention. Increased attention to issues of quality of life across the course of life remains an issue of highest priority for psychiatry and the social sciences.

References

Achenbaum WA, Orwoll L: Becoming wise: a psycho-gerontological interpretation of the book of Job. Int J Aging Hum Dev 32:21–39, 1991

Adams R: Conceptual and methodological issues in studying friendships of older adults, in Older Adult Friendship: Structure and Process. Edited by Adams R, Blieszner R. Newbury Park, CA, Sage, 1989, pp 17–41

Alpaugh PK, Birren JE: Variables affecting creative contributions across the adult life span. Hum Dev 20:240–248, 1977

Aneshensel C, Stone J: Stress and depression: a test of the buffering model of social support. Arch Gen Psychiatry 39:1392–1396, 1982

Antonovsky A: Unraveling the Mystery of Health: How People Manage Stress and Stay Well. San Francisco, CA, Jossey-Bass, 1987

Antonucci T: Social supports and social relationships, in Handbook of Aging and Social Sciences, 3rd Edition. Edited by Binstock R, George LK. New York, Academic Press, 1990, pp 205–227

Back KW: Transition to aging and the self image, in Normal Aging II. Edited by Palmore E. Durham, NC, Duke University Press, 1974, pp 207–216

Baltes P, Baltes M: Psychological perspectives on successful aging: the model of selective optimization with compensation, in Successful Aging: Perspectives From the Behavioral Sciences. Edited by Baltes P, Baltes M. Cambridge, England, Cambridge University Press, 1990, pp 1–34

Baltes PB, Smith J: Toward a psychology of wisdom and its ontogenesis, in Wisdom: Its Nature, Origins, and Development. Edited by Sternberg R. New York, Cambridge University Press, 1990, pp 87–120

Baltes PB, Smith J, Staudinger UM, et al: Wisdom: one facet of successful aging? in Late Life Potential. Edited by Perlmutter M. Washington, DC, Gerontological Society of America, 1990, pp 63–81

Bankoff E: Social support and adaptation to widowhood. Journal of Marriage and the Family 45:827–839, 1983

Benedek T: Parenthood as a developmental phase: a contribution to the theory of the libido (with discussion), in Contributions to Psychoanalysis. Chicago, IL, Quadrangle Books, 1959/1973, pp 377–407

Bengtson V, Robertson J (eds): Grandparenthood. Newbury Park, CA, Sage, 1985

Bengtson V, Reedy M, Gordon C: Aging and self-conceptions: personality processes and social contexts, in Handbook of the Psychology of Aging. Edited by Birren J, Schaie KW. New York, Van Nostrand Reinhold, 1985, pp 544–593

Birren J, Renner V: Research on the psychology of aging: principles and explanation, in Handbook of the Psychology of Aging. Edited by Birren J, Schaie KW. New York, Van Nostrand Reinhold, 1977, pp 3–38

Borden W: Life review as a therapeutic frame in young adults with AIDS: a developmental perspective. Health Soc Work 4:253–261, 1989

Borden W: Beneficial outcomes in adjustment of HIV seropositivity. Soc Serv Rev 65:434–449, 1991

Bowlby J: Attachment and loss: retrospect and prospect. Am J Orthopsychiatry 52:664–678, 1982

Boszormenyi-Nagy I, Spark C: Invisible Loyalties: Reciprocity in Intergenerational Family Therapy. New York, Harper & Row, 1973

Brim OG Jr, Ryff C: On the properties of life events, in Life-Span Development and Behavior, Vol 3. Edited by Baltes P, Brim OG Jr. New York, Academic Press, 1979, pp 368–388

Brody E: The aging family. Gerontologist 6:201–206, 1966

Brody E: The etiquette of filial behavior. Int J Aging Hum Dev 87–97:1970

Brody E: "Women in the middle" and family help to older people. Gerontologist 21:471– 480, 1981

Brody E: Parent care as a normative family stress. Gerontologist 25:19–29, 1985

Bromberg E: Mother-daughter relationships in later life: the effect of quality of relationship upon mutual aid. Journal of Gerontological Social Work 6:75–79, 1983

Butler R: The life review: an interpretation of reminiscence in the aged. Psychiatry 26:65–76, 1963

Butler R, Lewis M: Aging and Mental Health: Positive Psychosocial Approaches. St. Louis, MO, CV Mosby, 1977

Caplan G, Killilea M (eds): Support Systems and Mutual Help: Multidisciplinary Explorations. New York, Grune & Stratton, 1976

Chandler M, Holliday S: Wisdom in a post apocalyptic age, in Wisdom: Its Nature, Origins, and Development. Edited by Sternberg R. New York, Cambridge University Press, 1990, pp 121–141

Cherlin A, Furstenberg F Jr: The New American Grandparent: A Place in the Family, A Life Apart. New York, Basic Books, 1986

Chodorow N: The Reproduction of Mothering: Psychoanalysis and the Sociology of Gender. Berkeley, The University of California Press, 1978

Cicirelli V: Family support in relation to health problems of the elderly, in Family Relationships in Later Life, Revised Edition. Edited by Brubaker T. Newbury Park, CA, Sage, 1990, pp 212–228

Cicirelli V: Siblings as caregivers in middle and late life, in Gender, Families and Elder Care. Edited by Dwyer J, Coward R. Newbury Park, CA, Sage, 1992, pp 84–104

Clausen J: American Lives: Looking Back at the Children of the Great Depression. New York, The Free Press, 1993

Clayton V: Erikson's theory of human development as it applies to the aged: wisdom as contradictive cognition. Hum Dev 18:119–128, 1975

Clayton V: Wisdom and intelligence: the nature and function of knowledge in the later years. Int J Aging Hum Dev 15:315–321, 1982

Clayton V, Birren J: The development of wisdom across the life-span: a reexamination of an ancient topic, in Life-Span Development Behavior, Vol 3. Edited by Baltes P, Brim OG Jr. New York, Academic Press,

1979, pp 103–135

Cockerham WC, Sharp K, Wilcox JA: Aging and perceived health status. J Gerontol 38:349–355, 1983

Cohen-Shalev A: Artistic creativity across the adult life span: an alternative approach. Interchange 17:1–16, 1986

Cohler B: Autonomy and interdependence in the family of adulthood: a psychological perspective. Gerontologist 23:33–39, 1983

Cohler B: Resilience and the study of lives, in The Invulnerable Child. Edited by Anthony J, Cohler B. New York, Guilford, 1987, pp 363–424

Cohler B: Aging, morale, and meaning: the nexus of narrative, in Voices and Visions of Aging: Toward a Critical Gerontology. Edited by Cole T, Achenbaum WA, Jakobi P, et al. New York, Springer, 1993, pp 107–133

Cohler B, Altergott K: Family theory and the family of the second half of life, in Handbook of Aging and the Family. Edited by Blieszner R, Bedford V. Greenwich, CT, Greenwood Press, 1995, pp 59–94

Cohler B, Freeman M: Psychoanalysis and the developmental narrative, in The Course of Life, Revised Edition, Vol 5: Early Adulthood. Edited by Pollack G, Greenspan S. New York, International Universities Press, 1993, pp 99–177

Cohler B, Galatzer-Levy R: Self, meaning and morale across the second half of life, in New Dimensions in Adult Development. Edited by Nemiroff R, Colarusso C. New York, Basic Books, 1990, pp 214–259

Cohler B, Grunebaum H: Mothers, Grandmothers, and Daughters. New York, Wiley-Interscience, 1981

Cohler B, Lieberman M: Personality change across the second half of life: findings from a study of Irish, Italian and Polish-American men and women, in Ethnicity and Aging. Edited by Gelfand D, Kutznik A. New York, Springer, 1979, pp 227–245

Cohler B, Lieberman M: Social relations and mental health: middle-aged and older men and women from three European ethnic groups. Res Aging 2:454–469, 1980

Cohler B, Stott F: Separation, interdependence, and social relations across the second half of life, in The Psychology of Separation Through the Life-Span. Edited by Bloom-Feshbach J, Bloom-Feshbach S. San Francisco, CA, Jossey-Bass, 1987

Cohler B, Borden W, Groves L, et al: Caring for family members with Alzheimer's disease, in Alzheimer's Disease, Treatment and Family Stress: Directions for Research. Edited by Light E, Lebowitz B. Washington, DC, U.S. Government Printing Office, 1988

Cohler B, Stott F, Musik J: Adversity, vulnerability, and resilience: cultural and developmental perspectives, in Manual of Developmental Psychopathology, II. Edited by Cicchetti D, Cohen D. New York, Wiley, 1995, pp 753–800

Cole T: The Journey of Life: A Cultural History of Aging in America. Cambridge, England, Cambridge University Press, 1992

Cole TR, Achenbaum WA, Jakobi P, Kastenbaum R (eds): Voices and Visions of Aging: Toward a Critical Gerontology. New York, Springer, 1993

Cottle T: Perceiving Time: A Psychological Investigation. New York, Wiley, 1977

Cottle T, Klineberg, S: The Present of Things Future. New York, Free Press, 1974

Cross S, Markus H: Possible selves across the life span. Hum Dev 34:230–255, 1991

Csikszentmihalyi M: Society, culture, and person: a systems view of creativity, in The Nature of Creativity. Edited by Sternberg RJ. New York, Cambridge University Press,1988, pp 325–339

Csikszentmihalyi M, Larson R: Being Adolescent: Conflict and Growth in the Teenage Years. New York, Basic Books, 1984

Cumming E, Henry W: Growing Old: The Process of Disengagement. New York, Basic Books, 1961

Daniels P, Weingarten K: Sooner or Later: The Timing of Parenthood in Adult Lives. New York, Norton, 1982

Datan N, Antonovsky A, Maoz B: A Time to Reap: The Middle Age of Women in Five Israeli Subcultures. Baltimore, MD, The Johns Hopkins University Press, 1981

Datan N, Rodeheaver D, Hughes F: Adult development and aging. Annu Rev Psychol 38:153–180, 1987

Dean A, Lin N: The stress-buffering role of social support. J Nerv Ment Dis 165:403–417, 1977

Dennis W: Age and achievement: a critique. J Gerontol 11:331–333, 1956

Dennis W: Creative productivity between the ages of 20 and 80 years. J Gerontol 21:1–8, 1966

Dunkel-Schetter C, Wortman C: Dilemmas of social support: parallels between victimization and aging, in Aging: Social Change. Edited by Kessler SB, Morgan JN, Oppenheimer VK. New York, Academic Press, 1981, pp 349–381

Durkheim E: The Elementary Forms of the Religious Life (1912). Translated by Swain JW. New York, Free Press/Macmillan, 1963

Eckenroade J, Gore S: Stressful events and social supports: the significance of context, in Social Networks and Social Support. Edited by Gottlieb H. New York, Sage, 1981, pp 43–68

Ekerdt DJ, Bosse E: Change in self-reported health with retirement. Int J Aging Hum Dev 15:213–223, 1982

Elder G: Children of the Great Depression. Chicago, IL, The University of Chicago Press, 1974

Elder G: Historical change in life patterns and personality, in Life-Span Development Behavior, Vol 2. Edited by Baltes P, Brim OG Jr. New York, Academic Press, 1979, pp 117–159

Elder G, Rockwell R: The life-course and human development: an ecological perspective. International Journal of Behavioral Development 2:1–21, 1979

Elwell F, Maltbie-Crannell A: The impact of role losses upon coping resources and life-satisfaction of the elderly. J Gerontol 36:223–232, 1981

Elson M: Self Psychology in Clinical Social Work. New York, Norton, 1987

Erikson E: Childhood and Society, 2nd Edition. New York, Norton, 1950/1963

Erikson E: Human strength and the cycle of generations, in Insight and Responsibility: Lectures on the Ethical Implications of Psychoanalytic Insight. Edited by Erikson E. New York, Norton, 1964, pp 109–158

Erikson E: Identity, Youth and Crisis. New York, Norton, 1968

Erikson E: Reflections on Dr. Borg's life cycle, in Aging, Death and the Completion of Being. Edited by Van Tassel D. Philadelphia, University of Pennsylvania Press, 1979, pp 29–67

Erikson EH: The Life-Cycle Completed: A Review. New York, Norton, 1985

Erikson E, Erikson J, Kivnick H: Vital Involvement in Old Age: The Experience of Old Age in Our Time. New York, Norton, 1986

Essex M, Nam S: Marital status and loneliness among older women: the differential importance of close friends and family. Journal of Marriage and the Family 49:93–106, 1987

Fay B: Critical Social Science. Ithaca, NY, Cornell University Press, 1987

Ferraro KF: Self-ratings of health among the old and old-old. J Health Soc Behav 21:377–383, 1980

Fillenbaum GG: Social context and self-assessments of health among the elderly. J Health Soc Behav 20:45–51, 1979

Firth R, Hubert J, Forge A: Families and Their Relatives: Kinship in a Middle-Class Sector of London. London, Humanities Press, 1970

Fiske M: Tasks and crises of the second half of life: the interrelationship of commitment, coping, and adaptation, in Handbook of Mental Health and Aging. Edited by Birren J, Sloane RB. Englewood Cliffs, NJ, Prentice-Hall, 1980, pp 337–373

Fisseni H-J: Perceived unchangeability of life and some biographical correlates, in Life-Span and Change in Gerontological Perspective. Edited by Munnichs J, Mussen P, Olberich E, et al. New York, Academic Press, 1985, pp 103–132

Folkman S, Lazarus R: An analysis of coping in a middle-aged community sample. J Health Soc Behav 21:219–239, 1980

Francis D: Artistic creations from the work years: the New York world of work, in Workers' Expressions: Beyond Accomodation and Resistance. Edited by Calagione J, Francis D, Nugent D. Albany, NY, State University of New York Press, 1992, pp 48–67

Freud A: The Ego and the Mechanisms of Defense, Revised Edition. New York, International Universities Press, 1936/1966

Galatzer-Levy R, Cohler B: The Essential Other. New York, Basic Books, 1993

George L: Role Transitions in Later Life. Belmont, CA, Wadsworth Publishing Company, 1980

Gilligan C: New maps of development: new visions of maturity. Am J Orthopsychiatry 52:199–212, 1982

Gilligan C: In a Different Voice. Cambridge, MA, Harvard University Press, 1983

Glick I, Weiss R, Parkes C: The First Year of Bereavement. New York, Wiley, 1974

Goldberg E, Comstock G: Epidemiology of life events: frequency in general populations. Am J Epidemiol 111:736–752, 1980

Greenblatt M, Becerra R, Serafetinides E: Social networks and mental health: an overview. Am J Psychiatry 139:977–984, 1979

Greene AL: Future time perspective in adolescence: the present of things future revisited. Journal of Youth and Adolescence 15:99–113, 1986

Greene AL: Great expectations: constructions of the life-course during adolescence. Journal of Youth and Adolescence 19:289–306, 1990

Gutmann D: Parenthood: key to the comparative study of the life-cycle, in Life-Span Developmental Psychology: Normative Life-Crises. Edited by Datan N, Ginsberg L. New York, Academic Press, 1975, pp 167–184

Gutmann D: The cross-cultural perspective: notes toward a comparative psychology of aging, in Handbook of the Psychology of Aging. Edited by Birren J, Schaie KW. New York, Van Nostrand Reinhold, 1977, pp 302–326

Gutmann D: Reclaimed Powers: Toward a Psychology of Men and Women in Later Life. New York, Basic Books, 1987

Gutmann D, Griffin B, Grune J: Developmental contributions to the late-onset affective disorders, in Life-Span Development and Behavior. Edited by Baltes P, Brim OG Jr. New York, Academic Press, 1979, pp 244–263

Haight B: Reminiscing: the state of the art as a basic for practice. Int J Aging Hum Dev 33:1–32, 1991

Hagestad G: Middle Aged Parents and Their Children (Unpublished PhD thesis). Minneapolis, The University of Minnesota, 1974

Hagestad G: Social perspectives on the life course, in Handbook of Aging and the Social Sciences, 3rd Edition. Edited by Binstock R, George LK. New York, Academic Press, 1990, pp 151–168

Hazan H: The Limbo People: A Study of the Constitution of the Time Universe Among the Aged. London, England, Routledge & Kegan Paul, 1980

Heckhausen J, Dixon RA, Baltes PB: Gains and losses in development throughout adulthood as perceived by different adult age groups. Developmental Psychology 25:109–121, 1989

Hochschild A: Disengagement theory: a critique. Am Sociol Rev 40:553–569, 1975

Holliday S, Chandler M: Wisdom: Explorations in Adult Competence. Basel, Switzerland, Karger, 1986

Hooker K: Possible selves and perceived health in older adults and college students. J Gerontol 47:85–95, 1992

Horton P: Solace: The Missing Dimension in Psychiatry. Chicago, IL, The University of Chicago Press, 1981

Horton P, Gewirtz H: Acquisition and termination of first solacing objects in males, females, and in a clinic and nonclinic population: implication for psychological immunity, in The Solace Paradigm: An Eclectic Search for Psychological Immunity. Edited by Horton P, Gewritz H, Kreutter K. Madison, CT, International Universities Press, 1988, pp 159–183

Horton P, Gewirtz H, Kreutter K: The Solace Paradigm: An Eclectic Search for Psychological Immunity. Madison, CT, International Universities Press, 1988

Hultsch D, Plemons J: Life-events and life-span development, in Life-Span Development Behavior, Vol 2. Edited by Baltes P, Brim OG Jr. New York, Academic Press, 1979, pp 1–37

Janis I: Psychological Stress; Psychoanalytic and Behavioral Studies of Surgical Patients. New York, Wiley, 1958

Jaques E: Death and the mid-life crisis. Int J Psychoanal 46:502–514, 1965

Jaques E: The mid-life crisis, in The Course of Life, Vol 3: Adulthood and the Aging Process. Edited by Greenspan S, Pollock G. Washington, DC, U.S. Government Printing Office, 1980, pp 1–23

Jung CG: Modern Man in Search of a Soul. New York, Harcourt, Brace & World, 1933

Kahn R, Antonucci T: Convoys over the life course: attachment, roles, and social support, in Life-Span Development and Behavior, Vol 3. Edited by Baltes P, Brim OG Jr. New York, Academic Press, 1980, pp 253–386

Kakar S: The Inner World: A Psychoanalytic Study of Childhood and Society in India. New Delhi, India, Oxford University Press, 1978

Kakar S (ed): Identity and Adulthood. New Delhi, India, Oxford University Press, 1979/1992

Kaminsky M: The uses of reminiscence: a discussion of the formative literature, in The Uses of Reminiscence: New Ways of Working With Older Adults. Edited by Kaminsky M. New York, Haworth Press, 1984a, pp 137–156 (Also in Journal of Gerontological Social Work 7(1/2):137–156, 1984)

Kaminsky M: Transfiguring life: images of continuity hidden among the fragments. Journal of Gerontological Social Work 7:3–18, 1984b

Kaminsky M: Definitional ceremonies: depoliticizing and reenchanting the culture of age, in Voices and Visions of Aging: Toward a Critical Gerontology. Edited by Cole T, Achenbaum WA, Jakobi P, et al. New York, Springer, 1993, pp 1257–1274

Kaplan G, Barell V, Lusky A: Subjective state of health and survival in elderly adults. J Gerontol 43:114–120, 1988

Kasl S: Stress and health. Annu Rev Public Health 5:319, 1984

Kasl SV, Berkman LF: Some psychosocial influences on the health status of the elderly: the perspective of social epidemiology, in Aging: Biology and Behavior. Edited by McGaugh JL, Keisler SB. New York, Academic Press, 1981, pp 345–377

Kastenbaum R: The creative process: a life-span approach, in Handbook of the Humanities and Aging. Edited by Cole TR, Van-Tassel D, Kastenbaum R. New York, Springer, 1992, pp 285–306

Kastenbaum R: Encrusted elders: Arizona and the political spirit of modern aging, in Voices and Visions of Aging: Toward a Critical Gerontology. Edited by Cole T, Achenbaum WA, Jakobi P, et al. New York, Springer, 1993, pp 160–183

Kaufman S: The Ageless Self: Sources of Meaning in Late Life. Madison, The University of Wisconsin Press, 1986

Kernberg O: Normal narcissism in middle age, in Internal World and External Reality: Object Relations Theory Applied. Edited by Kernberg O. New York, Aronson, 1980, pp 121–153

Killilea M: Interaction of crisis theory, coping strategies, and social support systems, in The Modern Practice of Community Mental Health. Edited by Schulberg HC, Killilea M. San Francisco, CA, Jossey-Bass, 1982, pp 163–214

Kohut H: The Analysis of the Self. New York, International Universities Press, 1971

Kohut H: Remarks about the formation of the self-letter to a student regarding some principles of psychoanalytic research, in The Search for the Self: Selected Writings of Heinz Kohut, 1950–1978, Vol II. Edited by Ornstein P. New York, International Universities Press, 1974/1978, pp 737–770

Kohut H: The self in history, in Self Psychology and the Humanities: Reflections on a New Psychoanalytic Approach by Heinz Kohut. Edited by Strozier C. New York, Norton, 1975, pp 161–170

Kohut H: The Restoration of the Self. Madison, CT, International Universities Press, 1977

Kohut H: Introspection, empathy, and the semi-circle of mental health. Int J Psychoanal 63:395–407, 1982

Kohut H: Self psychology and the sciences of man (1978), in Self Psychology and the Humanities: Reflections on a New Psychoanalytic Approach by Heinz Kohut. Edited by Strozier C. New York, Norton, 1985, pp 73–94

Komarovsky M: Functional analysis of sex roles. Am Sociol Rev 15:508–516, 1950

Komarovsky M: Continuities in family research: a case study. American Journal of Sociology 62:466–469, 1956

Komarovsky M: Blue Collar Marriage. New York, Random House, 1962

Krantz D: The Santa Fe experience, in Work, Aging, and Social Change: Professionals and the One Life-One Career Imperative. Edited by Sarason SB. New York, Free Press, 1977, pp 165–188

Larson R: Thirty years of research on the subjective well-being of older Americans. J Gerontol 33:109–125, 1978

La Rue A, Bank L, Jarvik LF, et al: Health in old age: how do physicians' ratings and self-ratings compare? J Gerontol 34:687–691, 1979

Lazarus R, DeLongis A: Psychological stress and coping in aging. Am Psychol 38:245–254, 1983

Lazarus R, Folkman S: Stress, Appraisal and Coping. New York, Springer, 1984

Lazarus L, Newton N, Cohler B, et al: Frequency and presentation of depressive symptoms in patients with primary degenerative dementia. Am J Psychiatry 144:41–45, 1987

Lazarus L, Cohler B, Lesser J: Dessolution of self in Alzheimer's disease—clinical applications, in Treating Alzheimer's and Other Dementias: Clinical Applications of Recent Research Advances. Edited by Bergener M, Finkel S. New York, Springer, 1995, pp 496–509

Lee G: Children and the elderly: interaction and morale. Res Aging 1:335–359, 1979

Lehman HC: Age and Achievement. Princeton, NJ, Princeton University Press, 1953

Lehman HC: Reply to Dennis's critique of age and achievement. J Gerontol 11:333–337, 1956

Leinberger P, Tucker B: The New Individualists: The Generation After the Organization Man. New York, Harper Collins, 1991

Lieberman L, Lieberman L: Second careers in art and craft fairs. Gerontologist 23:266–272, 1983

Lieberman M, Falk J: The remembered past as a source of data for research on the life-cycle. Hum Dev 14:132–141, 1971

Lieberman M, Peskin H: Adult life crises, in Handbook of Mental Health Aging, 2nd Edition. Edited by Birren J, Sloane RB, Cohen G. New York, Academic Press, 1992, pp 120–146

Lieberman M, Tobin S: The Experience of Old Age: Stress, Coping and Survival. New York, Basic Books, 1983

Lopata H: Women as Widows: Support Systems. New York, Elsevier North-Holland, 1979

Lopata H: Widowhood in an American City. Cambridge, MA, Schenkmann, 1982

Lorenzen-Huber L: Self-perceived creativity in the later years: case studies of older Nebraskans. Educational Gerontology 17:379–390, 1991

Lowenthal MF: Social isolation and mental illness in old age. Am Soc Rev 29: 54–70,1964

Lowenthal MF, Robinson B: Social networks and isolation, in Handbook of Aging and the Social Sciences. Edited by Binstock R, Shanas E. New York, Van Nostrand Reinhold, 1976, pp 432–456

Lowenthal MF, Thurnher M, Chiriboga D, et al: Four States of Life. San Francisco, CA, Jossey-Bass, 1975

Maas H: The development of adult development: recollections and reflections, in Life-Span and Change in Gerontological Perspective. Edited by Munnichs J, Mussen P, Olberich E, Coleman P. New York, Academic Press, 1985, pp 161–176

Mages N, Mendelsohn G: Effects of cancer on patients' lives: a personological approach, in Health Psychology. Edited by Stone GC, Cohen F, Adler N. San Francisco, CA, Jossey-Bass, 1979, pp 255–284

Mahler M, Pine F, Bergman A: The Psychological Birth of the Human Infant. New York, Basic Books, 1975

Mancini J: Family relationships and morale among people 65 years of age and older. Am J Orthopsychiatry 49:292–300, 1979

Mancini J, Quinn W, Gavigan M, et al: Social network interaction among older adults: implications for life satisfaction. Human Relations 33:543–554, 1980

Manheimer RJ: Wisdom and method: philosophical contributions to gerontology, in Handbook of the Humanities and Aging. Edited by Cole TR, Van Tassel D, Kastenbaum R. New York, Springer, 1992, pp 426–440

Marcuse H: Eros and Civilization. Boston, MA, Beacon Press, 1955

Marris P: Loss and Change, Revised Edition. London, England, Routledge & Kegan Paul, 1974/1986

Marshall V: Age and awareness of finitude in developmental gerontology. Omega 6:113–129, 1975

Marshall V: Last Chapters: A Sociology of Death and Dying. Belmont, CA, Wordsworth, 1981

Marshall V: A sociological perspective on aging and dying, in Later Life: The Social Psychology of Aging. Edited by Marshall V. Newbury Park, CA, Sage, 1986, pp 125–146

McCrae R, Costa P: Personality in Adulthood. New York, Guilford, 1990

McCrae RR, Arenberg D, Costa PT: Declines in divergent thinking with age: cross-sectional, longitudinal, and cross-sequential analyses. Psychol Aging 2:130–137, 1987

McCullough L: Arrested aging: the power of the past to make us aged and old, in Voices and Visions of Aging: Toward a Critical Gerontology. Edited by Cole T, Achenbaum WA, Jakobi P, et al. New York, Springer, 1993, pp 184–204

McMahon A, Rhudick P: Reminiscing: adaptational significance in the aged. Arch Gen Psychiatry 10:292–298, 1964

McMahon A, Rhudick P: Reminiscing in the aged: an adaptational response, in Psychodynamic Studies on Aging; Creativity, Reminiscing, and Dying. Edited by Levin S, Kahana R. New York, International Universities Press, 1967, pp 64–78

Meacham JA: The loss of wisdom, in Wisdom: Its Nature, Origins, and Development. Edited by Sternberg RJ. Cambridge, England, Cambridge University Press, 1990, pp 181–211

Moody H: The meaning of life and the meaning of old age, in What Does it Mean to Grow Old? Reflections From the Humanities. Edited by Cole R, Gadow S. Durham, NC, Duke University Press, 1986, pp 11–40

Moody HR: Overview: what is critical gerontology and why is it important, in Voices and Visions of Aging: Toward a Critical Gerontology. Edited by Cole T, Achenbaum WA, Jakobi P, et al. New York, Springer, 1993, xv–xii

Mossey JM, Shapiro E: Self-rated health: a predictor of mortality among the elderly. Am J Public Health 72:800–808, 1982

Munnichs J: Old Age and Finitude: A Contribution to Psychogerontology. New York, Karger, 1966

Myerhoff B: Number Our Days. New York, Dutton, 1979

Myerhoff B: Remembered Lives: The Work of Ritual, Storytelling, and Growing Older. Edited by Kaminsky M. Ann Arbor, The University of Michigan Press, 1992

Neugarten B: Personality in later life: a developmental perspective, in The Psychology of Adult Development. Edited by Eisdorfer C, Lawton MP. Washington, DC, American Psychological Association, 1973, pp 311–338

Neugarten B: Time, age and the life cycle. Am J Psychiatry 136:887–894, 1979

Neugarten B, Datan N: Sociological perspectives on the life cycle, in Life-Span Developmental Psychology: Personality and Socialization. Edited by Baltes P, Schaie K. New York, Academic Press, 1974a, pp 53–69

Neugarten B, Datan N: The middle years, in American Handbook of Psychiatry, Vol 1. Edited by Arieti S. New York, Basic Books, 1974b, pp 596–606

Neugarten B, Hagestad G: Age and the life course, in Handbook of Aging and the Social Sciences. Edited by Binstock R, Shanas E. New York, Van Nostrand Reinhold, 1976, pp 35–55

Offer D, Offer J: From Teenage to Young Manhood. New York, Basic Books, 1975

Offer D, Sabshin M: Adolescence: empirical perspectives, in Normality and the Life Cycle. Edited by Offer D, Sabshin M. New York, Basic Books, 1984

Orwoll L, Achenbaum A: Gender and the development of wisdom. Hum Dev 36:274–296, 1993

Orwoll L, Perlmutter M: The study of wise persons: integrating a personality perspective, in Wisdom: Its Nature, Origins, and Development. Edited by Sternberg RJ. Cambridge, England, Cambridge University Press, 1990, pp 160–177

Osherson S: Holding On or Letting Go: Men and Career Change at Midlife. New York, The Free Press, 1980

Panel (Winestine MC, reporter): The experience of separation-individuation in infancy and its reverberations through the course of life, 1: infancy and childhood. J Am Psychoanal Assoc 21:135–154, 1973a

Panel (Marcus M, reporter): The experience of separation-individuation in infancy and its reverberations through the course of life, 2: adolescence and maturity. J Am Psychoanal Assoc 21:155–167, 1973b

Panel (Sternschein I, reporter): The experience of separation-individuation in infancy and its reverberations through the course of life, 3: maturity, senescence, and sociological implications. J Am Psychoanal Assoc 21:633–645, 1973c

Parkes M: Bereavement: Studies of Grief and Adult Life. New York, International Universities Press, 1972

Perlmutter M: Learning and memory through adulthood, in Aging in Society: Selected Reviews of Recent Research. Edited by Riley M. Hillsdale, NJ, Erlbaum, 1983, pp 219–241

Plath D: Contours of consociation: lessons from a Japanese narrative, in Life-Span Development and Behavior, Vol 3. Edited by Baltes P, Brim OG Jr. New York, Academic Press, 1980, pp 287–305

Pollock G: On time and anniversaries, in The Unconscious Today: Essays in Honor of Max Schur. Edited by Kanzer M. New York, International Universities Press, 1971a, pp 233–257

Pollock G: On time, death and immortality. Psychoanal Q 40:435–446, 1971b

Pollock G: Aging or aged: development or pathology, in The Course of Life, Vol 3: Adulthood and the Aging Process. Edited by Greenspan S, Pollock G. Washington, DC, U.S. Government Printing Office, 1980, pp 549–585

Pollock G: Reminiscence and insight. Psychoanal Study Child 36:278–287, 1981

Pruchno R, Blow F, Smyer M: Life events and interdependent lives. Gerontologist 27:31–41, 1984

Pruyser P: Creativity in aging persons. Bull Menninger Clin 51:425–435, 1987

Robertson J: Grandparenthood: a study of role conceptions. Journal of Marriage and the Family 39:165–174, 1977

Romaniuk JG, Romaniuk M: Creativity across the life span: a measurement perspective. Hum Dev 23:366–381, 1981

Rook K: The negative side of social interaction: the impact of psychological well being. J Pers Soc Psychol 46:1097–1108, 1984

Rook K: Strains in older adults' friendships, in Older Adult Friendship: Structure and Process. Edited by Adams R, Blieszner R. Newbury Park, CA, Sage, 1989, pp 108–128

Rosenmayr L, Kockeis E: Predispositions for a sociological theory of the family. International Social Science Journal 15:410–426, 1963

Rowe J, Kahn R: Human aging: usual and successful. Science 237:143–149, 1987

Ryff C: Successful aging: a developmental approach. Gerontologist 22:209–214, 1982

Ryff C: Personality development from the inside: the subjective experience of change in adulthood and aging, in Life Span Development and Behavior, Vol 6. Edited by Baltes PB, Brim OG Jr. New York, Academic Press, 1984, pp 244–279

Ryff C, Heinecks SG: Subjective organization of personality in adulthood and aging. Journal of Personality and Social Psychology 44:807–816, 1983

Salthouse T: Age-related changes in basic cognitive processes, in The Adult Years: Continuity and Change. Edited by Storandt M, VandenBos G. Washington, DC, American Psychological Association, 1989, pp 5–40

Salthouse T: Cognitive competence and expertise in aging, in Handbook of the Psychology of Aging, 3rd Edition. Edited by Birren J, Schaie KW. New York, Academic Press, 1990, pp 311–319

Schaie KW: Psychological changes from midlife to early old age: implications for the maintenance of mental health. Am J Psychiatry 51:199–218, 1981

Schaie KW: The Seattle longitudinal study: a 2-year exploration of the psychometric intelligence of adulthood, in Longitudinal Studies of Personality. Edited by Schaie KW. New York, Guilford, 1984, pp 64–135

Schaie KW: Intellectual development in adulthood, in Handbook of the Psychology of Aging, 3rd Edition. Edited by Birren J, Schaie KW. New York, Academic Press, 1990a, pp 291–310

Schaie KW: The optimization of cognitive functioning in old age: predictions based on cohort-sequential and longitudinal data, in Successful Aging: Perspectives From the Behavioral Sciences. Edited by Baltes P, Baltes M. Cambridge, England, Cambridge University Press, 1990b, pp 94–117

Schaie KW: The Seattle longitudinal studies of adult intelligence. Current Directions in Psychological Science 2:171–175, 1993

Schaie KW, Labouvie G, Buech B: Generational and cohort-specific differences in adult cognitive behavior: a fourteen-year study of independent samples. Developmental Psychology 9:151–166, 1973

Schulz R, Rau MT: Social support through the life course, in Social Support and Health. Edited by Cohen S, Syme SL. Orlando, FL, Academic Press, 1985, pp 129–149

Shanas E: Social myth as hypothesis: the case of family relations of old people. Gerontologist 19:3–9, 1979

Shanas E, Townsend P, Wedderburn D, et al: Old People in Three Industrial Societies. London, England, Routledge & Kegan Paul, 1968

Sill J: Disengagement reconsidered: awareness of finitude. Gerontologist 37:587–594, 1980

Simonton D: Creativity and wisdom in aging, in Handbook of the Psychology of Aging, 3rd Edition. Edited by Birren J, Schaie KW. New York, Academic Press, 1990a, pp 320–329

Simonton DK: Creativity in the later years: optimistic prospects for achievement. Gerontologist 30:626–631, 1990b

Simonton DK: Does creativity decline in the later years? definition, data, and theory, in Late Life Potential. Edited by Perlmutter M. Washington, DC, Gerontological Society of America, 1990c, pp 83–112

Sinnott J: Correlates of sex roles of older adults. J Gerontol 37:587–594, 1982

Slavney P, McHugh P: Life stories and meaningful connections: reflections on a clinical method in psychiatry and medicine. Perspect Biol Med 27:279–288, 1984

Smith R: Cultural differences in the life cycle and the concept of time, in Aging and Leisure. Edited by Kleemeier R. New York, Oxford University Press, 1961, pp 84–112

Smith J, Baltes PB: Wisdom-related knowledge: age/cohort differences in response to life-planning problems. Development Psychology 26:494–505, 1990

Sorokin P, Merton R: Social time: a methodological and functional analysis. Am J Soc Rev 42:615–629, 1937

Staudinger UM, Smith J, Baltes PB: Wisdom-related knowledge in a life review task: age differences and the role of professional specialization. Psychol Aging 7:271–281, 1992

Sternberg RJ: Wisdom and its relations to intelligence and creativity, in Wisdom: Its Nature, Origins, and Development. Edited by Sternberg

RJ. Cambridge, England, Cambridge University Press, 1990a, pp 142–159

Sternberg RJ (ed): Wisdom: Its Nature, Origins, and Development. Cambridge, England, Cambridge University Press, 1990b

Stolar GE, MacEntee MI, Hill P: Seniors' assessment of their health and life satisfaction: the case for contextual evaluation. Int J Aging Hum Dev 35:305–317, 1992

Taranto MA: Facets of wisdom: a theoretical synthesis. Int J Aging Hum Dev 29:1–21, 1989

Thomae H: Stress, satisfaction, competence—findings from the Bonn longitudinal study on aging, in Clinical and Scientific Psychogeriatrics, I: The Holistic Approaches. Edited by Bergener M, Finkel S. New York, Springer, 1990, pp 117–134

Tobin S: Personhood in Advanced Old Age. New York, Springer, 1991

Tobin S, Lieberman M: Last Home for the Aged. San Francisco, CA, Jossey-Bass, 1976

Townsend P: The Family Life of Old People. London, England, Routledge & Kegan Paul, 1957

Turner J: Social support as a contingency in psychological well-being. J Health Soc Behav 22:357–367, 1981

Uhlenhuth E, Lipman R, Balter M, et al: Symptom intensity and life-stress in the city. Arch Gen Psychiatry 31:759–764, 1974

Vaillant G: Avoiding negative life-outcomes: evidence from a forty-five year study, in Successful Aging: Perspectives From the Behavioral Sciences. Edited by Baltes P, Baltes M. Cambridge, England, Cambridge University Press, 1990, pp 332–358

Vaillant G: The Wisdom of the Ego. Cambridge, MA, Harvard University Press, 1993

Wan TTH: Health consequences of major role losses in later life: a panel study. Res Aging 6:469–489, 1984

Weiss R: Attachment in adult life, in The Place of Attachment in Human Behavior. Edited by Parkes CM, Stevenson-Hinde J. New York, Basic Books, 1982, pp 171–184

Whitbourne S: The psychological construction of the life span, in Handbook of the Psychology of Aging. Edited by Birren J, Schaie KW. New York, Van Nostrand Reinhold, 1985, pp 594–618

Winnicott DW: Human nature. New York: Schockey Books, 1988

Wood V, Robertson J: Friendship and kinship interaction: differential effects on the morale of the elderly. Journal of Marriage and the Family 40:367–375, 1978

Wortman C, Silver R: Coping with irrevocable loss, in Cataclysms, Crises and Catastrophes: Psychology in Action. Edited by VandenBos G, Bryant B. Washington, DC, American Psychological Association, 1987, pp 189–235

Wortman C, Silver R: The myths of coping with loss. J Consult Clin Psychol 57:349–357, 1989

Wortman C, Silver R: Successful mastery of bereavement and widowhood: a life-course perspective, in Successful Aging: Perspectives From the Behavioral Sciences. Edited by Baltes P, Baltes M. Cambridge, England, Cambridge University Press, 1990, pp 225–264

Zoutra A, Hempel A: Subjective well-being and physical health: a narrative literature review with suggestions for future research. Int J Aging Hum Dev 19:95–110, 1984

Zweibel N, Cassel C: Treatment choices at the end of life: a comparison of decision by older patients and their physician-selected proxies. Gerontologist 29:615–621, 1989

Zweibel N, Lydens L: Incongruent perceptions of older adult/caregiver dyads. Family Relations 39:63–67, 1990

SECTION II
Evaluation and Diagnosis

C H A P T E R   7

Kenneth Sakauye, M.D.

Ethnocultural Aspects

> Americans believe in race. Through a set of
> complex, arbitrary and unwritten rules that
> we learn as children, we are trained to
> identify, catalog, and stuff people into
> racial categories. If we can't figure it out,
> we ask. Not knowing what someone is
> often makes us uncomfortable.
> —*The Times-Picayune*, New Orleans, August 15, 1993;
> part of a series on race relations

A lack of understanding of ethnic differences can be the basis for un-der diagnosis, misdiagnosis, insensitivity, or inappropriate or inef-fective treatment of psychiatric disorders in minority populations (Ameri-can Psychiatric Association 1993). The prevalence of these problems is still the subject of debate and study, but little reflection is needed to see that many centers pay no attention to ethnic or cultural differences, and many educators openly espouse the view that cultural discussions are little more than an attempt to force political correctness. Cultural differences are real, even beyond language and communication barriers. Differences in values and beliefs influence the expression of distress, the reason for seeking help, and the credibility of recommendations. Strongly hierarchical family and cultural systems may so influence relationships with authority that they inhibit full disclosure or conversely lead to blind compliance. Racial differences cause different susceptibilities to disease, and to pharmacokinetic and pharmacodynamic variations. The culture of poverty, seen most often in minority populations, creates barriers to access to care and factors that lead to poor compliance. Ethnocentric bias and pseudoscientific racism (like concepts of racial supremacy) lead to stereotyping, which fosters misdiagnosis, undertreatment, and treatment errors (see Table 7–1). Prejudice, which may be bidirectional, leads to hatred, distrust, and poor treatment (American Psychiatric Association 1993; Gaw 1993).

Noting that "a definition of an ethnic group must necessarily be flexible and pragmatic" (p. vi), Thernstrom (1980) catalogued 106 ethnic groups in his edited *Harvard Encyclopedia of American Ethnic Groups*. The large number of ethnic groups and diversity within groups in socioeconomic status, immigrant status, language, genetic phenotypes, and enzymatic polymorphisms often makes consensus difficult regarding the point of comparison to study between groups. Criteria such as language, country of origin, religion, way of life, marriage patterns, leisure time, food preferences, political attitudes, or attitudes for selected issues, often viewed as objective markers for ethnic identity, are often blurred by intermarriage,

Table 7–1.   Role of ethnicity in health care

Variable	Clinical relevance
Language	Often a barrier to treatment
	Implies different cultural values and beliefs
Values and beliefs	Effect credibility of recommendations
	Effect disease presentation and communication
	Effect reason for seeking treatment
	Effect family issues, social networks, habits
Ethnocentric bias	Misdiagnosis
(racial stereotyping)	Undertreatment
	Treatment errors
	Racial pseudoscience
Prejudice	Distrust
(bidirectional)	Overt hostility or mistreatment
	Problems establishing a treatment alliance
Culture of poverty	Barriers to access to care
	Noncompliance and poor health knowledge
	Higher risk factors for illness and mental illness
Biological differences	Risk and prevalence for illness differs
	Pharmacokinetic and pharmacodynamic differences

assimilation, and progressive American-born generational status. The boundary between behaviors caused by socioeconomic stratification and behaviors rooted in out-of-awareness cultural history is not always easy to differentiate. The subjective dimension of ethnicity, or social identity, is often context bound rather than a fixed issue. For example, an African American elderly person may not be aware of race unless interacting with whites. Thus, influences of ethnicity and culture have been difficult to operationally define and simplify for a collective racial group, though they are known to have far-reaching effects on self-esteem, performance, interpersonal relations, and sense of personal control on an individual level (Liebkind 1992; Peterson 1980).

Adding a social definition of minority group membership as a perceived difference and exclusion from the "dominant" reference group allows an extension of minority status to women, groups with different sexual preferences, groups of people who are deaf (deaf culture), or any group who faces the multiple jeopardies of minority status. In this chapter, however, I focus on minorities of color: African Americans, Hispanic Americans, Asian Americans, and Native Americans and Pacific Islanders, where cultural issues are slightly less ambiguous. There is still large variability within these groups and the ethnic groups they represent. This diversity dictated the organization of the chapter around a description of the overriding issues common to the minority populations, rather than descriptions of racial groups per se.

Although there is a growing body of knowledge about these minority populations, there is still a glaring lack of quality research and data on elderly people of color (American Society on Aging 1992). For many numerically small groups, such as Native American tribes, many Indochinese or Pacific Islander groups, and even Hispanic or African American subgroups, little or no information is available. A Medline search from June 1992 through September 1994 revealed no new research papers on categories of "minority and psychiatry and aging," although more than 1,720 citations were listed under "minority or race and psychiatry or psychology." Using a more restrictive search for "minority and psychiatry," only 78 references were indexed. None were indexed under "cross-cultural psychiatry" or "transcultural and psychiatry." Only 55 were indexed under "elderly and minority," and 137 were listed under "ethnic groups and psychiatry." A review of the abstracts led to a smaller number involving new research, and none specifically addressing elderly minorities.

Inferences often have to be drawn from the general adult studies on minority populations and small pilot data. It has only been in the past

5 years that the National Institutes have mandated the inclusion of women and minorities in all federally funded studies and have offered minority supplements to existing grants to establish systematic data on minority populations. This new emphasis may increase the basic knowledge base.

Demographic Profiles (65 or Older)

Ethnic minority populations are growing. Trends over the past decade have shown a trend toward reunification of families for Asian and Hispanic groups and increasing longevity for American-born minority elderly people, with a slight reduction in the excess mortality and shorter life spans that characterized minority populations earlier. African American elderly people, now numbering more than 2 million individuals, include African Americans, African Caribbeans, and individuals of mixed heritage. Hispanics are primarily represented by Mexican Americans (60% of Hispanics), Puerto Ricans (12.2% of Hispanics), Cubans (4%), and South and Central Americans. Black, white, and mixed heritage overlap in the 1990 census (U.S. Bureau of the Census 1990). As shown in Table 7–2, approximately 84% of all Asian Americans residing in the United States are from six ethnic groups: Japanese, Chinese, Filipino, Korean, Vietnamese, and Asian Indian. The percentage of elderly people (over age 62) ranges from higher than the national average for Japanese (19.5%) to much lower than the national average for Vietnamese (4.6%). Native American and native Alaska elderly people comprise several hundred tribal or cultural groups with different languages and degrees of assimilation. Lower education levels and socioeconomic status characterize minority elderly people. Higher rates of immigrant status characterize Asian and Hispanic elderly people, posing special risks for mental health and support (American Psychiatric Association 1993).

Mental health and well-being are strongly related to physical health status and disability (Stewart 1989). A major problem for minority populations has been the experience of greater health problems than the white majority population. More than 50% of older blacks and older Mexican Americans report chronic health conditions, more than 10% greater than the rate for older whites. One-half (50%) of American Indian elderly people have adult-onset diabetes, and American Indians have a 107% higher rate of death from diabetes than the general population. By age 45, American Indians show the same rate of disabilities as non-Indians at age 65, and American Indians have the shortest life expectancy of any racial group (65

Table 7–2. Demographic profiles

Cultural group	Number (% of the total U.S. elderly population)	% of Own ethnic group		% Foreign born	
African American	2,058,100 (8.0)				
Hispanic American	1,161,300 (3.7)				
Mexico		Mexico	4.4		
Puerto Rico		Puerto Rico	4.7		
Central or South America		Cuba	14.8		
		Central or South America	3.0		
Asian American	454,400 (1.4)		6.2	(62 and over)	
		Japanese	19.5	Japanese	37.2
		Chinese	12.5	Chinese	75.9
		Korean	7.2	Korean	80.1
		Filipino	11.3	Filipino	96.3
		Vietnamese	4.6	Vietnamese	100
		Asian Indian	4.3	Asian Indian	19.3
Native American	114,500 (0.8)		5.8		

Note. Minority populations represent 19.7% of the United States population. The total U.S. Census was 248,709,873.
Source. U.S. Bureau of the Census: 1990 Census of Population and Housing Summary, Tape File IC. Washington, DC, 1991.

years). They show a 459% higher rate of death from alcoholism, and a 233% higher rate of death from tuberculosis. The basis for many of these differences lies in socioeconomic disparity, occupations posing higher risks of injury and disability, poor nutrition, and lack of appropriate illness prevention (health promotion) (American Psychiatric Association 1993; American Society on Aging 1992). Health concerns must also be addressed in the provision of mental health to minority elderly people. To many minority elderly people, physical and mental health are not often conceptually separable.

Diagnostic Issues

Prevalence of Mental Illness

Differential rates of psychiatric illness between cultural groups may reflect genetic (racial) differences and differences in risk factors leading to (or protecting against) mental illness. Differential rates may also reflect diagnostic differences or communication barriers. Although the rates of atypical presentations and diagnostic errors are not established, it is important to remain sensitive to the possibility of diagnostic errors with minority elderly people. Insensitivity of existing diagnostic scales (missing a diagnosis when present) as well as poor specificity (failing to distinguish between two somewhat similar disorders like bipolar disorder and psychosis) is well-documented in case examples for minority populations. Examples are as far reaching as the Spanish translations of the Mini-Mental State Exam (MMSE) where linguistic differences even between Hispanic subgroups have required several translation versions (Valle 1989). Differences in social desirability or response sets have led to artifactually higher depression scores on the Center for Epidemiologic Studies—Depression Scale (Radloff 1977) or schizoid traits on the Minnesota Multiphasic Personality Inventory (MMPI) (Hathaway and McKinley, 1989) in Japanese nationals. This is partly a result of cultural (Confucian) values for stoicism and self-sacrifice, which are viewed as part of the depressive continuum in the West (American Psychiatric Association 1993; Robins 1989). Underlying explanations for diagnostic problems with minority populations have included 1) language barriers, 2) different idioms or concepts of illness, 3) lower socioeconomic status and education, and 4) ethnocentric bias of diagnosticians. These factors may be magnified with minority elderly people because of the high proportion of new immigrants of Asian and Hispanic origin and a generally lower socioeconomic status as a result of Jim Crow laws and more subtle forms of discrimination (which unfortunately still persist today). In these groups, there may be a greater adherence to traditional cultural values and beliefs. Translation problems and a lack of validated culture-fair tests quite often exist, leaving the question of diagnostic accuracy in doubt in some studies.

Representativeness of the sample is another central feature that is not easily achieved in minority studies. The Epidemiologic Catchment Area (ECA) survey data (see Table 7–3), which was reanalyzed by race and age for the American Psychiatric Association Task Force on Minority Elderly (American Psychiatric Association 1993), did not include an oversampling

Table 7–3. ECA 6-month prevalence of psychiatric diagnoses by age and race

	White		African American		Hispanic	
Disorder	18–54 y (%)	55 y and over (%)	18–54 y (%)	55 y and over (%)	18–54 y (%)	55 y and over (%)
Bipolar[a]	1.1	—	1.3	—	—	—
Major depression	4.4	1.5	3.7	1.6	4.2	—
Dysthymia[a]	3.7	2.5	2.8	1.8	4.0	—
Alcohol abuse	7.5	2.1	6.3	3.3	8.8	—
Schizophrenia/ schizophreniform illness	1.1	0	1.8	0	—	0
Obsessive-compulsive	2.1	0.9	1.6	1.9	—	0
Phobia	8.9	6.7	15	13.9	8.1	9.1
Somatization	0	0	0	0	0	0
Panic	1.2	—	1.2	—	—	—
Antisocial personality	1.6	—	1.2	—	—	0
Cognitive impairment[b]	0.3	2.3	1.4	9.2	—	—
Any DIS/DSM-III diagnosis	23.6	14.0	27.3	24.7	23.1	18.5

Source. Adapted from Tables 2–2 and 2–3 from American Psychiatric Association (1993). Based on the Diagnostic Interview Schedule (DIS) from the Epidemiologic Catchment Area study, 6-month period, all sides included. Weighted. A dash indicates fewer than 20 unweighted positive cases. Asian and Native Americans were not oversampled; inadequate numbers for analysis.
[a]Lifetime diagnosis. [b]Determined by Mini-Mental State Exam.

of Asians or Native Americans at any site and had less than 20 unweighted positive cases for many diagnostic categories, making it statistically unsound to calculate prevalence estimates. An unexpected finding of an apparently lower rate of depression was found in minority groups despite higher mental health risks, though there was a higher rate for any DSM-III (American Psychiatric Association 1980) diagnosis for African American and Hispanic (largely Mexican American) elderly people, mainly because of much higher rates of phobic disorders and cognitive impairment.

Although differences between elderly immigrants and nonimmigrants were not specifically described, the Los Angeles ECA sample, which oversampled Hispanic Americans, showed Mexico-born Mexican Americans had nearly one-half the lifetime prevalence for most major psychiatric disorders compared with their United States–born counterparts (Escobar 1993). These data were very different from an expected direction of increased psychopathology in the immigrant group. Several possible explanations seem plausible. I am reminded of the complex interaction shown between immigrant status and mental illness in the Midtown Manhattan Study (Srole et al. 1962), the last large National Institute of Mental Health epidemiological study to address the issue of immigration, which showed a strong association between immigrant status, age, time, and mental illness. After ruling out the possibility that mentally ill individuals might be overrepresented in the original immigrant pool, the researchers found that the highest prevalence of mental illness occurred in relatively new immigrants. Elderly immigrants who had been in the United States for many years had a lower prevalence of mental illness than the general population, leading to the widely accepted speculation that because there is a higher rate of early mortality in minority populations, only the strongest and most adaptable immigrants (those in better mental and physical health) are the ones who survive to old age. In addition, because early life experiences may determine vulnerability to some psychiatric disorders, differences in background, birth cohort, and genetic risks are possible. These have not yet been studied.

Suicide rates for African American and Hispanic American elderly people have generally been lower than among whites (Group for the Advancement of Psychiatry 1989). Rates among Japanese, Chinese, and Korean Americans increase with age and seem comparable to whites (about 21 per 100,000), with marginally higher rates of suicide in elderly Chinese and Japanese Americans (McIntosh and Santos 1981). Higher suicide rates can be explained by anomie, poverty, and other social stressors. The lower rates of suicide in elderly minorities have been explained by stronger family ties and extended family networks (social buffers), stronger social importance in the minority family, and strong cultural or religious attitudes against suicide. Japanese Americans have often been assumed to have a higher rate of suicide than whites because of the widely known ritual suicide (*seppuku* or *hara-kiri*), related to an old military code of honor (*Bushido*). However, traditionally this ritual has been reserved for the noble class, and the actual transmission of such attitudes among Japanese immigrants is doubtful. The incidence of suicide in Japanese Americans is generally equivalent to white counterparts, and the pattern of suicide does not appear particularly unusual (Gaw 1993; Group for the Advancement of Psychiatry 1989).

In practice, one must be especially cautious of potential diagnostic errors and minimization of the extent of psychiatric disorders in minority elderly populations given the unexpectedly low rates of psychiatric disorders in existing studies. Recommendations to reduce cultural bias in research settings apply equally well to clinical settings. Rogler (1989) summarized his recommendations: 1) include a period of direct immersion in the culture of the study group, 2) look for unexpected findings (as evidence of cultural influences), 3) adapt to the respondent's cultural context (rather than expect the respondent to behave like everyone else), 4) incorporate ethnic cultural expressions in inquiries, and 5) be aware that cultural factors may influence the psychometric properties of instruments.

Culture-Bound Syndromes and Atypical Presentations

From a medical model for psychiatric classification, biology is viewed as the source of pathogenesis with a putative set of nonoverlapping symptoms characterizing disease states. Under this model, psychological and cultural layers of reality are held to be epiphenomenal, exerting a "pathoplastic effect" on the content of a delusional system or system of thought (Kleinman 1988). On the other extreme, diagnosis from a medical anthropology perspective (cultural psychiatry vantage point) views illness behavior, patterns of help seeking, and treatment responses as distinctive factors rather than symptoms per se. The dichotomy is exemplified by depression experienced entirely as low back pain. The patient might complain that his or her pain is leading to loss of appetite, inability to go out, weakness, and insomnia. Depressive affect and social disinterest are denied. In the absence of explainable medical causes, is this a different phenomenon than depression experienced as existential despair and sadness?

Although major psychiatric disorders, such as psychosis, major depression, bipolar disorder, or dementia, may be less prone to culturally based diagnostic differences, cultural influences seem most evident in diagnosis of personality styles, dysthymia, anxiety, marital or family disorders, and culture-bound syndromes (syndromes that fall outside of conventional diagnostic categories) (Littlewood 1990). It is not difficult to see how a paradigm conflict could cause one to misdiagnose mild psychopathology like dysthymia, make it difficult to engage a patient, or cause a clinician to pejoratively view some behaviors (like somatic expressions) as "primitive defense mechanisms."

One hundred and eighty-five indigenous terms representing "culture-bound" syndromes (see Table 7–4) were investigated in preparation for the DSM-III work group as possible inclusions as new diagnostic categories (Hughes 1985; Simons and Hughes 1993). These disorders are generally rare even within their cultures of origin but, as local diagnostic entities, have a culturally developed theory of causality and cure (often spiritual or herbal). The age distribution of these syndromes is not described, but minority elderly people might be at highest risk to exhibit many culture-bound syndromes because of their foreign-born status or low degree of assimilation.

Dementia

Performance on tests designed to measure cognitive and intellectual function have been particularly vulnerable to influences from language differences (Loewenstein et al. 1993) and education (Valle 1989). Tests that seem most vulnerable to language and cultural effects are digit span (possibly as a result of nonequivalence of phonemes or syllables in a particular digit in different languages), verbal comprehension, and verbal fluency (Loewenstein et al. 1993). Low education has been shown to bias even screening tests such as the Folstein MMSE (Chang et al. 1993) because of deficits in fund of knowledge, learning styles, abstraction, and reading abilities. Correction factors are difficult to develop because of the heterogeneity of minority populations (especially in degrees of language competence and self-education). For example, lowering the cutoff score for the MMSE would reduce false-positive results for poorly educated people or those with poor language skills but would increase false-negative results for others.

An alternative to improve "culture-fair" tests lies in assessing "everyday memory" (Cohen 1989) and instrumental activities of daily living

(IADL) abilities through direct observation of performance on familiar tasks or problems or through naturalistic experiments. This approach remains controversial and has not yet been systematically applied to minority populations. Also, what is "everyday" differs for individuals. For example, rigid gender roles might make household tasks and even household utensils foreign to some men, travel and map-reading foreign to some women. Even memorization of grocery lists might by biased by what is a familiar food to different ethnic populations. Thus, in a clinical setting, caution should be exercised when interpreting mild dysfunction or assessing severity from standard tests in minority elderly persons. Deficits should always be viewed in conjunction with functional correlates and history.

In specific studies designed to minimize the rate of misdiagnosis, lower rates of Alzheimer's dementia (50% less in some series) are present in many ethnic minority groups such as African Americans (Chang et al. 1993), Japanese (with autopsy confirmation) (Homma 1991), and Cree Indians (Hendrie et al. 1993). However, multi-infarct dementia may be present at twice the rate of white counterparts in African Americans and Japanese (American Psychiatric Association 1993). Studies that elucidate the reasons for the differences have broader implications for genetic and environmental risk factors for Alzheimer's dementia.

Biological Differences: Pharmacology of Ethnicity

Although there are no specific data on elderly minority populations, information from a growing body of research on psychobiological differences as a result of ethnicity is emerging and is summarized here because of the importance of the topic despite the absence of age-specific information (see Table 7–5).

Ethnic differences have frequently been noted in response to medications. A World Health Organization cross-cultural study of antidepressants using standardized protocols, found minimal differences in effective dose requirements for Asians, blacks, and whites. However, different rates of side effects and early dropouts from intolerable side effects were noted between groups, especially in Japanese (World Health Organization 1983, 1986). This finding was consistent with the fact that racial groups may have pharmacodynamic differences or enzyme polymorphisms leading to faster or slower metabolism.

Pharmacodynamic differences have not been studied extensively. However, one key example is the slow membrane transport of lithium in many African Americans, which leads to higher intracellular lithium levels,

Table 7–4.   Culture-bound syndromes

Syndrome	Group and location	Description	Possible DSM-IV parallel
Black voodoo	Southern United States	Witchcraft afflictions	Psychosis
Falling out	Southeastern United States Afro-Carribeans	Sudden collapse, cannot see but can understand surrounding events	Posttraumatic stress disorder
Indisposition	Bahamians, Haitians	Sudden collapse, cannot see but can understand surrounding events	Posttraumatic stress disorder
Wind illness (p'a-leng)	Chinese	Morbid fear of the cold, especially of the wind	
Neurasthenia	China, Japan	Weakness or exhaustion of the nervous system	Dysthymia (300.40)
Taijinkyofusho	Japan	Embarrassed of being with others because of blushing, unpleasant body odor, stuttering	Social phobia, body dysmorphic disorder
Shinkeishitsu	Japanese men	Fear of contact with others (obsessions and phobias)	Agoraphobia (but usually in women in the West)
Latah	Malaysia, Indonesia	Hypersensitivity to sudden fright or startle; hypersuggestibility, echopraxia, echolalia, dissociation	Anxiety or panic disorder
Susto	Central and South American	Tiredness, debility attributed to an antecedent fright or startle	Adjustment disorder/dysthymia
Espanto	Spain	Tiredness, debility attributed to an antecedent fright or startle	Adjustment disorder/dysthymia
Ataque de nervios	Puerto Rico	Out of consciousness state caused by malevolent spirits	Psychosis, body dysmorphic disorder

Towatl ye sni	Dakota Sioux	Experience of one's thoughts traveling to the dwelling p	Major depression
Ghost sickness	Navajo	Weakness, loss of appetite, dizziness, fainting, suffocation, dread caused by witches	Panic attack
Wiacinko	Oglala Sioux	Anger, withdrawal, mutism, immobility, suicide caused by disappointments	Major depression

Sources. Kleinman 1989; Golden 1977; Gaw 1993.

Table 7–5. Biological differences

Group	Pharmacogenetics			
	Cytochrome P450 polymorphism	Alcohol and aldehyde dehydrogenase	Acetylation	Conjugation
United States Caucasian	D 8.7% PM S 2.7% PM	0% PM Reference	52%–68% PM	Reference

African American
  United States
  Nigeria
  Bushman
	D 1.9% PM
	D 0%–10% PM
	D 18% PM
		Not reported	Not reported	Not reported

Hispanic Spanish	D 6.6%	0% PM	0% PM	N/A
Asian Japanese	D 0% PM S 18%–23% PM	44% PM 22% PM	10%–15% PM 22% PM	20% slower rate
Chinese	D 0.7% PM S 5.1% PM			
Filipino				Higher COMT activity (faster L-dopa metabolism; more dyskinesia)

North American
  Indians
  Najavo
  Sioux
  Oklahoma
	N/A	2% PM
		5% PM
		16% PM
			43%–54%	N/A

| Group | Pharmacokinetics | | | | Protein binding (varies with medication) |
	Neuroleptics	Tricyclic antidepressants	Benzodiazepines	Lithium	
United States Caucasian	Reference	Reference	Reference	Reference	Reference
African American United States Nigeria Bushman	Not reported	Higher peak plasma concentration (higher delirium rate by age and race)	Increased clearance—higher dose?	Lower membrane countertransport (higher RBC/plasma ratio)—lower therapeutic dose?	N/A
Hispanic Spanish	Same as reference	Same as reference	N/A	N/A	N/A
Asian Japanese Chinese Filipino	Higher peak concentration—lower daily dose? Chinese—PM	Higher peak concentration—lower daily dose?	Slower clearance—lower dose?	Kinetics same—lower therapeutic dose?	TCA—same as reference
North American Indians Najavo Sioux Oklahoma	N/A	N/A	N/A	N/A	N/A

Note. EM = extensive metabolizers; PM = poor metabolizers; D = debrisoquine hydroxylase (cytochrome P450 IID6)—most tricyclics, propranolol, perphenazine; S = S-mephenytoin hydroxylase (cytochrome P450 2C$_{mp}$)—diazepam; COMT = catechol-O-methyltransferase. Alcohol dehydrogenase (ALH) and aldehyde dehydrogenase (ALDS)—ALH and ADLH allelic variations effect ethanol oxidation; acetylation—caffeine, clonazepam, phenelzine, nitrazepam; conjugation—acetaminophen, amobarbital, L-dopa.

Sources. Mendoza et al. 1991; Lin et al. 1993.

explaining efficacy at lower blood levels and increased lithium toxicity for many African Americans (Lin et al. 1993). It is unclear whether this may be related to the presence of hemoglobin S (sickle cell trait or disease) as suggested in some case reports (American Psychiatric Association 1993).

Genetic polymorphisms of the cytochrome P450 system and other enzyme systems help explain pharmacokinetic differences, which lead to marked variation in metabolism of medications (Lin et al. 1993). Most psychopharmacologically active medications are relatively nonpolar and require two metabolic steps, oxidative functionalization and conjugation. The rate-limiting step appears to be hepatic oxidation, predominantly through the P450 isoenzyme system, where a polar group is introduced to increase water solubility. Of greatest interest has been the debrisoquin hydroxylase (cytochrome IID6) and mephenytoin hydroxylase (cytochrome $2C_{mp}$), which metabolize many of the major psychotropic medications. The frequency of poor metabolizer variants of cytochrome P450 IID6 seems higher in whites than minorities, but poor metabolizers of mephenytoin hydroxylase may exceed 20% in some Asians. The variability of enzymes may change with age as well as race. A sizable proportion of Asians show higher sensitivity and toxicity to tricyclic antidepressants and neuroleptic medication. African Americans may show a significant increased sensitivity to lithium at therapeutic blood levels but may have fewer poor metabolizers of other psychotropic medications.

Generational Issues

First-generation immigrants.   The obvious and most widely accepted theme is the problem of "culture shock" or relocation trauma representing adjustment problems for new immigrants (Westermeyer 1993). This relocation trauma is a major problem for many Asian and Hispanic elderly people who move to the United States in late life for family reunification and who are unlikely to work or have language-training opportunities. The problem of isolation is further magnified by the absence of local ethnic neighborhoods, given trends to move to the suburbs and away from "ethnic ghettos." However, utilization of professional help is still rare (American Psychiatric Association 1993).

A particular caution in interpreting low service utilization information is the assumption that minority elderly people have fewer problems or that the family group–oriented (rather than individualistic) minority cultures insist on "taking care of their own." Special strains exist for any immigrant family trying to assimilate that make the older immigrant feel isolated and irrelevant and may actually decrease family intergenerational solidarity (Roberts and Bengston 1990). This isolation is sometimes manifested in shame of the parent or affective distancing. It is especially important to recognize that nonutilization of services may be less related to a preference for family-based care than the existence of barriers to care (finances, language, fear). Problems may not be as severe for long-term immigrants who may have lower psychopathology rates than even the national average (Srole et al. 1962).

American-born immigrants. Much of the minority literature focuses on the special problems of low socioeconomic status in minorities of color. The so-called culture of poverty can exist outside of color, but is often highest in minority populations because of biased treatment from individuals and at times institutionalized barriers to advancement (poor education, lack of mentors, segregation, inequitable resource distribution, and so forth). It becomes a cultural issue, however, when the disparities become entrenched and are concentrated among the minority populations.

The mental health aspect of prejudice is the question of what impact lifelong experiences of racism and poverty have on self-concept, locus of control (that people can shape their own lives), and locus of responsibility (who is to blame for shortcomings . . . them or me). Identification with the negative portrayals of violence, being unintelligent, or being incapable of doing anything have been described. Fitting the stereotype will reinforce a nonminority individual's view that minority individuals are hopeless, apathetic, procrastinating, lazy, depressed, or fearful of trying (Sue and Sue 1990). However, negative self-concept among minority individuals is not universal or even normative despite the privations. Black-identity development models have been proposed that speculate that ethnic identity, like other aspects of the self, follows a developmental continuum. Minority individuals progress from identification with the aggressor (with devaluation of self and one's own ethnic group), to rejection of the dominant culture (and overvaluation of one's own culture), to a balanced and healthy acceptance and tolerance of cultural differences and selective appreciation of attitudes toward the dominant group (Sue and Sue 1990). This identity model has not been empirically tested across the life span (Ponterotto and Wise 1987), but even if most minority elderly persons reach this stage of integrative awareness where they may not show the same degree of anger or rejection, they may still be wary of involvement in a formal care system that had previously excluded them (American Psychiatric Association 1993).

Psychotherapy

> The reasons why minority-group individuals underutilize and prematurely terminate counseling/therapy lie in the biased nature of the services themselves. The services offered are frequently antagonistic or inappropriate to the life experiences of the culturally different client; they lack sensitivity and understanding, and they are oppressive and discriminating toward minority clients. (Sue and Sue 1990, p. 7)

Specific cultural treatment modalities such as acupuncture (in China and Japan), Niakan or Morita therapy (in Japan), herbal healing (throughout Asia), or spiritual healing (e.g., spiritistas, voodoo) are unavailable within the formal care system, but many minority patients use local healers simultaneously, and awareness of this is needed. Elderly patients occasionally go to their local healer for permission to follow the physician's advice.

More germane to psychiatrists, however, is the need to consciously address several generic themes during counseling of minority individuals: 1) culture-bound values (communication patterns, degree of being individually centered, being verbally expressive, being open, or being analytical [believing in cause and effect], and how strong a distinction is made between mental and physical illness), 2) class-bound values (time orientation; need for immediate, short-term goals), 3) language, and 4) the stage of racial and cultural identity development that influences social interactions and view of self (Sue and Sue 1990).

Attitudes toward authority figures often pose initial problems in establishing a therapeutic alliance with a minority patient. Of course, one must bear in mind that there are different responses to authority figures inside the family (parents, grandparents), authorities in the social hierarchy (pastors, community leaders), and outside authorities (physicians, lawyers). Patients might be overly deferential, inhibited, or ashamed of revealing personal feelings or they might alternatively be hostile and suspicious. In addition, strict time consciousness or time pressure may be unimportant if a patient has not worked or is from rural settings. Members of ethnic groups sometimes joke about "ethnic time," where four o'clock actually means 4:15 or 4:30 or even later. These factors are general problems that vary within ethnic populations by gender, by age, by generation level, and by other life experience factors. What is important is that awareness of these issues and open discussion of different expectations often are enough to reduce these attitude differences, which are really external to the central therapeutic themes.

The problems raised also differ for immigrant generations versus American born, by length of residence in the United States and by degree of assimilation and social class (see Figure 7–1). For new immigrants, the primary issues concern adjustment and may involve culture-bound presentations and need for bilingual therapists. Established immigrants may have more social and health-related issues. American-born socioeconomically assimilated elderly people may face problems of racial identity and problems of self-concept. Poorly assimilated elderly people may face problems related to a culture of poverty and face adjustment issues as a result of early health disabilities and language barriers. The impact of prejudice remains a dominant theme for all American-born minority elderly people.

Details about specific groups can be reviewed in general texts such as Gaw (1993), Sue and Sue (1990), and Wilkerson (1986), which elaborate on these issues. Additional abstracts are available in *Ethnic Minority Elderly: A Task Force Report of the American Psychiatric Association* (1993).

Culturally Appropriate Services

To develop culturally appropriate services, the American Society on Aging has outlined several steps based on its 2.5-year Administration on Aging grant to empower elderly people of color (American Society on Aging 1992).

American Society on Aging: Programs for Minorities

Commitment and empowerment.

1. Mission: Agencies must have an explicit commitment to serve older adults from all racial, ethnic, and cultural groups.
2. Governance and Administration: Seek proportional representation of the communities served on governing bodies and administrative staff. Empower persons of color in decisions and have them serve as spokespersons for the agency.
3. Service Approaches and Program: Every effort should be made to make services accessible, understandable, and useful to all sectors of the community.
4. Targeting: Agencies should understand the prevalence of needs among different populations and know that need may exceed expectations based simply on proportional representation of a group within the community.

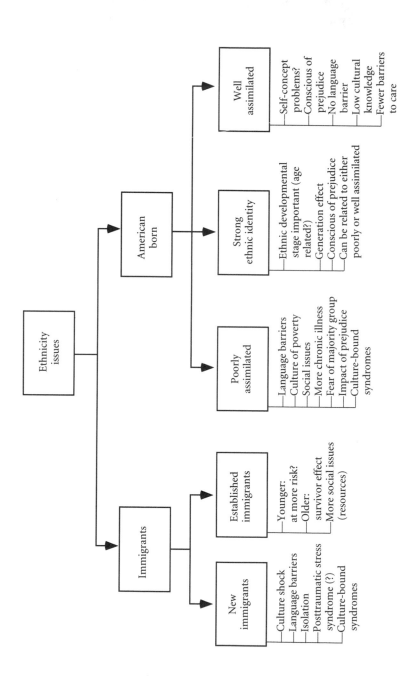

Figure 7–1. Impact of ethnicity on mental health care. The status of immigrant parents and American-born children may be associated with increased "generation gap" and emotional conflicts. Feelings of affection and closeness are different from obligation and affiliation.

5. Outreach and Marketing: The messages and methods of conducting outreach and marketing of services must appreciate cultural diversity and difference.

Considerations for developing a model.

1. Understand the cultural traditions, historical experiences, and social and political networks within the community.
2. Identify and involve community leaders, organizations, grantmakers, and advocates in planning and organizing efforts (planning committee).
3. The planning group and event participants must decide direction and priorities. Encourage the core group to take ownership of the project by coordinating efforts without imposition of a facilitator's point of view.
4. Define goals based on a realistic time line.
5. Work to develop community leaders. (Provide education about aging services and program systems and the skills necessary to affect change.)
6. Design interactive sessions that promote discussion and hands-on activities. (Provide education to validate the experiences and issues affecting elderly people and their families and develop the skills necessary to affect change.)
7. Be available to provide technical assistance.
8. Conduct monthly follow-up with participants.
9. Form relationships between older participants and community professional leadership.
10. Emphasize issues that directly affect the lives of elderly people.

Summary

Research on the mental health of minority elderly populations has received little research attention to date, though this appears to be changing. Minority elderly people are a growing segment of the population, with a large proportion being poor, foreign-born, or both. The reliability of studies on the prevalence of psychiatric disorders in elderly members of minority groups has been questioned because of sampling limitations and instrumentation. Viewing problems from the vantage point of immigrant versus American-born issues is useful in looking at the psychosocial issues and psychotherapy approaches that emerge. The classical problems of culture shock, language and communication barriers, attitude and value differences, and culture-bound syndromes is greatest for new immigrants and the poorly assimilated American-born groups. The impact of prejudice and the culture of poverty remain a dominant problem for other minority elderly people. Biological differences in rates of Alzheimer's dementia in cross-cultural studies have been found that may lead to greater understanding of genetic and environmental risk factors. Pharmacogenetic and pharmacokinetic differences between races explain observed differences in drug response among racial groups (usually less than 5% to 20% are affected). In providing service to minority elderly patients there remains a need for sensitization of mental health professionals to the particular ethnic groups that are being seen and to develop culturally appropriate services. To overcome this need requires conscious attention to the generic themes that affect all ethnic minority elderly people, involvement of the community in program planning and feedback, and immersion into the culture of the group being served.

References

American Psychiatric Association: Diagnostic and Statistical Manual of Mental Disorders, 3rd Edition. Washington, DC, American Psychiatric Association, 1980

American Psychiatric Association: Ethnic Minority Elderly: A Task Force Report of the American Psychiatric Association. Washington, DC, American Psychiatric Association, 1993

American Society on Aging: Serving Elders of Color: Challenges to Providers and the Aging Network. San Francisco, CA, American Society on Aging, 1992

Chang L, Miller BL, Lin KM: Clinical and epidemiologic studies of dementias: cross-ethnic perspectives, in Clinical and Epidemiologic Studies of Dementia: Cross-Ethnic Perspectives, Psychopharmacology and Psychobiology of Ethnicity. Edited by Lin KM, Poland RE, Nakasaki G. Washington, DC, American Psychiatric Press, 1993, pp 223–252

Cohen G: Memory in the Real World. Hillsdale, NJ, Erlbaum, 1989

Escobar JI: Psychiatric epidemiology, in Culture, Ethnicity, and Mental Illness. Edited by Gaw AC. Washington, DC, American Psychiatric Press, 1993, pp 43–74

Gaw AC (ed): Culture, Ethnicity, and Mental Illness. Washington, DC, American Psychiatric Press, 1993

Golden KM: Voodoo in Africa and the United States. Am J Psychiatry 134:1425–1427, 1977

Group for the Advancement of Psychiatry, Committee on Cultural Psychiatry: Suicide Among Ethnic Minorities in the United States (Report No 128). New York, Brunner/Mazel, 1989

Hathaway SR, McKinley JC: Minnesota Multiphasic Personality Inventory—2. Minneapolis, University of Minnesota, 1989

Hendrie HC, Hall KS, Pillay N, et al: Alzheimer's disease is rare in Cree. Int Psychogeriatr 5:5–14, 1993

Homma A: Gerontopsychiatric surveys on age-associated dementia in Japan: recent findings from epidemiological view, in Studies in Alzheimer's Disease: Epidemiology and Risk Factors, Proceedings of the 3rd International Symposium on Dementia. Tokyo, National Center of Neurology and Psychiatry, 1991, pp 31–41

Hughes, CC: Culture bound or construct bound? the syndromes of the DSM-III, in The Culture Bound Syndromes: Folk Illnesses of Psychiatric and Anthropological Interest. Edited by Simons RC, Hughes CC. Bordrecht, Netherlands, D Reidel, 1985, pp 3–24

Jackson JS, Antonnucci TC, Gibson RC: Cultural, racial, and ethnic minority influences on aging, in Handbook of the Psychology of Aging, 3rd Edition. Edited by Birren JE, Schaie KW. San Diego, CA, Academic Press, 1990, pp 103–123

Kleinman A: Rethinking Psychiatry: From Cultural Category to Personal Experience. New York, Free Press, 1988

Liebkind K: Ethnic identity—challenging the boundaries of social psychology, in Social Psychology of Identity and Self-Concept. Edited by Breakwell GM. San Diego, CA, Academic Press, 1992

Lin K-M, Poland RE, Nakasaki G (eds): Psychopharmacology and Psychobiology of Ethnicity. Washington, DC, American Psychiatric Press, 1993

Littlewood R: From categories to contexts: a decade of the new cross-cultural psychiatry. Br J Psychiatry 156:308–327, 1990

Loewenstein DA, Arguelles T, Barker WW, et al: A comparative analysis of neuropsychological test performance of Spanish-speaking and English-speaking patients with Alzheimer's disease. Journals of Gerontology: Psychological Sciences 48:142–149, 1993

McIntosh JL, Santos JF: Suicide among minority elderly: a preliminary investigation. Suicide Life Threat Behav 11:151–166, 1981

Mendoza R, Smith MW, Poland RE, et al: Ethnic psychopharmacology: the Hispanic and Native American perspective. Psychopharmacol Bull 27:449–261, 1991

Peterson W: Concepts of ethnicity, in Harvard Encyclopedia of American Ethnic Groups. Edited by Thernstrom S, Orlov A, Handlin O. Cambridge, MA, Belknap Press/Harvard University Press, 1980, pp 234–242

Ponterotto JG, Wise SL: Construct validity study of the racial identity attitude scale. The Journal of Counseling Psychology 34:218–223, 1987

Radloff LS: The CES-D: a self-report depression scale for research in the general population. Applied Psychological Measurement 3:385–401, 1977

Roberts REL, Bengston VL: Is intergenerational solidarity a unidimensional construct? a second test of a formal model. Journal of Gerontology: Social Sciences 45(1):S12–S20, 1990

Robins LN: Cross cultural differences in psychiatric disorder. Am J Public Health 79:1479–1480, 1989

Rogler LH: The meaning of culturally sensitive research in mental health. Am J Psychiatry 146:296–303, 1989

Sakauye KM: Ethnic variations in family support of the frail elderly, in Family Care of the Frail Elderly. Edited by Goldstein M. Washington, DC, American Psychiatric Press, 1989, pp 63–106

Simons RC, Hughes CC: Culture bound syndromes, in Culture, Ethnicity, and Mental Illness. Edited by Gaw AC. Washington, DC, American Psychiatric Press, 1993, pp 75–93

Srole I, Langer T, Michael S, et al: Mental Health in the Metropolis: The Midtown Manhattan Study. New York, McGraw-Hill, 1962

Stewart AL: Functional status and well being of patients with chronic conditions: results from the medical outcomes study. JAMA 262:907–913, 1989

Sue DW, Sue D: Counseling the Culturally Different: Theory and Practice, 2nd Edition. New York, Wiley, 1990

Thernstrom S, Orlov A, Handlin O (eds): Harvard Encyclopedia of American Ethnic Groups. Cambridge, MA, Belknap Press/Harvard University Press, 1980

U.S. Bureau of the Census: 1990 Census of Population and Housing Summary, Tape File 1C. Washington, DC, 1991

Valle R: Cultural and ethnic issues in Alzheimer's disease family research, in Alzheimer's Disease Treatment and Family Stress: Directions for Research (DHHS Publication No ADM-89-1569). Edited by Light E, Lebowitz BD. Washington, DC, U.S. Government Printing Office, 1989, pp 122–154

Westermeyer JJ: Cross-cultural psychiatric assessment, in Culture, Ethnicity, and Mental Illness. Edited by Gaw AC. Washington, DC, American Psychiatric Press, 1993

Wilkerson CB: Ethnic Psychiatry. New York, Plenum, 1986

World Health Organization: Depressive Disorders in Different Cultures: Report on the WHO Collaborative Study on Standardized Assessment of Depressive Disorders. Geneva, Switzerland, WHO, 1983

World Health Organization: Dose effects of antidepressant medication in different populations: a World Health Organization collaborative study. J Affect Disord 2:S1–S67, 1986

Ivan L. Silver, M.D.
Nathan Herrmann, M.D.

Comprehensive Psychiatric Evaluation

The ability of the geriatric psychiatrist to solve clinical problems is related directly to the comprehensiveness and depth of the data obtained from patients and their families. Historically, little attention has been paid to the psychiatric examination of elderly patients, although recently published comprehensive protocols are now available (Blazer 1989; Oppenheimer and Jacoby 1991). In this chapter, we present a guide for taking the psychiatric history, performing a functional assessment, and examining the mental status of the geriatric patient. Although numerous clinical examples are presented, the specific phenomenology of geriatric mental disorders has yet to be confirmed by careful experimental studies. More specific details about developmental inquiry, special tests, neuroimaging, and medicolegal issues will be found in the relevant sections.

Obtaining a geriatric history and assessing mental status are potentially long and complex tasks because the patient has lived many years and frequently experiences the comorbidity of neurological and medical illness. Emphasis on different aspects of the history will vary depending on the patient's problems. For instance, a corroborative history and a detailed cognitive assessment are priorities in patients with progressive dementing disorders and delirium. The family and past history are important for all patients and are particularly essential in patients with affective or personality disorders.

The goals of the history, functional, and mental status examinations are to 1) establish a provisional diagnosis and differential diagnoses; 2) develop an etiological formulation that traces the biological, psychological, and social factors that have predisposed, precipitated, and now perpetuate the patient's current mental illness; and 3) establish each patient's capacity to function independently.

Characteristics of the Geriatric Psychiatry Assessment

A geriatric psychiatrist must consider the three questions below before the assessment begins:

1. Where should the patient be seen? Geriatric assessments may be undertaken in a variety of settings: at the bedside, in an outpatient office, at home, in an institution, in a day hospital, or in a specialized clinic. Where the clinician sees the patient may be critical because it can determine the quantity and quality of the data collected. For example, generally one cannot expect that completing the assessment in an outpatient office will allow a full assessment of the capacity of a patient with dementia to function at home. This assessment often requires observation and monitoring in the home environment. On the other hand, a workup to rule out reversible causes of dementia requires the facilities of a clinic or hospital setting.
2. Who should participate in the assessment? A basic tenet in geriatric assessment is that, whenever possible, a patient's spouse, caregiver, and family are seen for corroborative information, with appropriate regard for issues of confidentiality. This is critically important in the assessment of patients with cognitive impairment and may be equally important in patients who are cognitively intact. When mental disorders interfere with insight into the nature and quality of the illness, interviewing family members often will provide a truer picture of the person's mental disorder. Historical events are verified and, in many cases, the diagnosis depends on the family members' ability to relate a coherent history. A family member often is the best person to describe the premorbid personality of the patient. This is valuable information because premorbid personality traits may change or

become exaggerated in the context of a variety of geriatric mental illnesses, including dementia, affective disorders, and paranoid disorders.

3. How should the interview be conducted? It is important for each assessment to include an opportunity to talk to the patient alone, particularly when suicidal risk is an issue. All psychiatric interviews should allow for a free exchange of information in an atmosphere of mutual trust that leaves patients with the feeling that they are being understood. Particular attention should be paid to the capacity of the patient to tolerate a psychiatric interview. Severely disturbed or cognitively impaired patients do not tolerate long, detailed interviews well. Brief interviews with active engagement and reassurance facilitate the process.

Consideration must be given to the common sensory impairments seen in some geriatric patients. Patients with poor hearing and vision may require special intervention. When dealing with patients with deafness, it may help to turn on the hearing aid, interview in a quiet room, and speak in a slow, steady, low-pitched voice into the "good ear." A sound amplifying device may be necessary; if one is unavailable the "reverse stethoscope" method may be used: put the stethoscope in the ear of the patient and speak into the diaphragm quietly. For the visually impaired, sitting closer to the patient or ensuring that the patient is wearing corrective lenses is helpful. The appropriate use of touch may reassure the patient and help facilitate the psychiatric interview.

The Organization of the Psychiatric Assessment

A schematic for the geriatric psychiatric assessment is presented in Table 8–1. It is meant only as a tool to organize the data and not as a checklist for the examiner.

The Psychiatric History

Several detailed guides to the assessment of younger adults are available (Ginsberg 1985; Leff and Isaacs 1978; Waldinger 1990). The following discussion is meant as a guide to adapting the traditional psychiatric history to the needs of the geriatric population.

Table 8–1.   Schematic for the geriatric psychiatric assessment

Identifying data
Reliability of informant
Chief complaint
History of presenting illness
Past psychiatric history
Family history
Family psychiatric history
Personal history
Medical history
Current medications
Drug and alcohol history
Physical examination
Functional status
Mental status
Etiological formulation
Provisional diagnosis
Differential diagnoses
Investigations
Comprehensive management plan

Identifying Data

Identifying data can be amended by adding the name of the primary caregiver, whether in or out of the home. If the patient lives in a residential setting, the type of institution is specified.

History of Presenting Illness

The purpose of the history of presenting illness is to document events and arrange them in the order in which they occurred. It is important to record all recent environmental and physical changes in the patient's life. Environmental events and physical illness may precipitate mental illness in elderly patients. For example, recent losses, separations, moves, and changes in support networks may be associated with the onset of affective and paranoid disorders or the exacerbation of cognitive disability. Cognitively impaired, frail elderly patients are particularly predisposed to superimposed delirium when relatively minor toxic, metabolic, or infectious disease intercedes. Certain physical disorders seem to precipitate specific mental disorders. For example, cerebrovascular accidents have been associated with depression and mania (Starkstein and Robinson 1989).

To focus the inquiry, the examiner must be familiar with the natural history and symptomatology of the common mental illnesses in elderly patients. This is important because some mental disorders, particularly affective disorders, may present differently in old age. For example, depression in old age can present in many different ways. Many elderly depressives do not present with the classic sad and tearful demeanor (Post 1962). Common geriatric presentations include the hypochondriacal, agitated depressive who importunes the family in fits of desperation. The patient's frantic pleas for help may look "hysterical" to the observer and feel "manipulative" to the family. Depression may present with negativistic behavior such as a refusal to move, eat, or drink. A suicidal gesture may signal the presence of this disorder. The recent onset in advanced age of phobias, obsessions, or compulsive behavior may signal the beginning of depression.

Vegetative symptoms of depression in elderly patients include sleep, appetite, weight, and energy disturbance; loss of sexual drive; and diurnal variation in mood. The clinician should note abrupt changes in sleep, appetite, and energy because the normal aging process can affect these functions. Weight loss may be quantified by changes in dress or belt size.

Interviewing a family member is essential when a cognitive disorder is suspected. The clinician may have to elicit the entire history of the presenting illness from the family. Cognitive disorders affect memory, language, perception, mood, thinking, personality, and the capacity to function independently in the patient's environment. For example, early in the course of Alzheimer's disease, patients will misplace their belongings, have trouble with the names of familiar people, have trouble remembering new information, and show word-finding difficulties. Personality traits may become exaggerated. Apathy, depressive symptoms, or stealing delusions may coexist. The patient may give up usual household activities, have trouble handling finances, and rely more on the primary caregiver. Impaired executive cognitive function may occur because of depression or brain disease; patients are unable to organize their instrumental activities of daily living, although they remain independent in gross physical function. The primary caregiver is in the best position to provide the clinician with this information.

Past Psychiatric History

The record of past treatment successes and failures can help develop a management plan for the current illness by providing data on the natural history of a patient's mental illness and prognosis.

Family History

Most geriatric patients have deceased parents and may have deceased siblings. The cause of death, age of death, and the health of siblings may give clues about the patient's current problems. Knowing the mental function and living arrangements of the patient's parents or siblings near the end of their lives may be useful. A family psychiatric history provides valuable clues to the patient's diagnosis and may implicate genetic vulnerability.

The past relationship of patients to their parents often determines the quality of family and interpersonal relationships. Because geriatric patients often rely on support for continuous good functioning, it is helpful to know about the quality of their relationships with their spouse or primary caregiver, adult children, grandchildren, and friends.

Personal History

Sometimes it is difficult to decide which events in an elderly patient's past are relevant to current problems and circumstances. Birth, developmental, childhood, and adolescent data are important and may be difficult to verify and corroborate by others. Knowledge of the patient's past sheds light on the vulnerabilities and strengths of each patient and may explain why some patients develop psychiatric symptomatology at particular points in their lives. A review of the life cycle of an individual establishes the premorbid capacity of each patient to adjust to important life's events. These life cycle events may include starting school, leaving home, establishing a career, getting married, the birth of children, the death of parents, children leaving home, the death of siblings, retirement, and the death of a spouse. It is important to inquire whether the patient has had a history of abuse, neglect, or maltreatment at any time. Patients who have been abused by caregivers may be more likely to show paranoid or agitated behavior in institutional care settings or to mistrust formal caregivers.

The personal history should also include an inquiry into the person's activities, religious affiliation, hobbies, and connections with community resources. This information is useful in assessing each individual's social vulnerabilities and strengths.

Documenting a patient's premorbid personality provides a longitudinal view of the patient's characteristic personality function and helps avoid erroneous diagnostic conclusions based on cross-sectional examination. Although this type of information should be elicited from the patient, corroborative history from family or friends is often necessary.

A sexual history is often omitted in elderly patients. This may be caused by the examiner's lack of knowledge or misconceptions about sexuality in old age. A history of sexual orientation and activities and practices and how the mental disorder has affected these functions is essential. For example, some elderly patients are very troubled by the anorgasmic side effects of many psychotropic drugs. Developing a comfortable atmosphere for patients to raise these concerns during the assessment can be extremely therapeutic.

Medical History, Medication Use, and Drug and Alcohol History

The clinician should document carefully all past and current medical problems, dates of onset, and treatment. The comorbidity of physical and mental illness, especially depression, is common in elderly patients (Post 1969). Several physical illnesses, including Parkinson's disease and cerebrovascular disease, can precipitate a mood disorder or paranoid disorder.

A variety of medications can precipitate psychiatric disorders such as delirium, affective disorders, and paranoid disorders (Johnson 1981). A list of all medications, dosages, and date of onset is essential. Over-the-counter medications need to be included in this survey because many, such as bromides, aspirin, and antihistamines, are neurotoxic even in moderate doses.

Drug and alcohol abuse often are underestimated in elderly patients (Brown 1982). Screening for alcoholism can be assisted by asking questions known by the acronym CAGE (Ewing 1984):

1. Have you ever felt you ought to **C**ut down on your drinking?
2. Have people **A**nnoyed you by criticizing your drinking?
3. Have you ever felt bad or **G**uilty about your drinking?

4. Have you ever had a drink first thing in the morning to steady your
    nerves or to get rid of a hangover (**E**ye-opener)?

A careful inquiry into the quantity and frequency of drinking behavior, in addition to the above questions, is helpful.

Functional Assessment

Functional status consists of everyday behaviors that occur in a person's home and community (Rubenstein et al. 1989). The capacity of an elderly person to remain independent often is jeopardized by the coexistence of physical and mental disability (Lawton 1988). This is especially relevant in patients who are cognitively impaired and medically frail. The functional assessment quantifies how well the patient performs important tasks and maintains independence. This assessment ideally employs careful observation of the patient's functioning in the patient's residence. If this is not possible, an interview with the primary caregiver is essential. Lawton and Brody (1969) and Katz et al. (1970) divided the functional assessment into two kinds of activities: physical activities of daily living (ADL) and instrumental activities of daily living (IADL) (see Table 8–2). This assessment 1) documents each patient's functional strengths and vulnerabilities so that appropriate in-home supports for the caregiver and patient can be organized and 2) monitors a patient's progress over time. The functional assessment can provide clues to potentially remediable and underdiagnosed medical and psychiatric conditions. Linking a mental disorder to an impairment in instrumental function often is a way to bring about acceptance of treatment by the patient and family.

Table 8–2. Functional assessment tasks

Activities of daily living	Instrumental activities of daily living
Bathing	Able to use telephone
Ability to transfer	Shopping
Dressing	Food preparation
Going to toilet	Laundry
Grooming	Motor transportation
Ability to feed self	Responsibility for own medication
	Able to handle finances

The Interview With the Informant

Most geriatric psychiatric assessments require taking a history of the patient's problems from a significant other. If this person is the caregiver, specific attention should be given to assessing the caregiver's health, the caregiver's understanding of the patient's illness, a history of the caregiver's relationship with the patient, the stresses in the relationship with the patient, the degree to which the caregiver is providing practical care, and the degree of burden on the caregiver. This information is intended to provide help to the caregiver. The collaborative history may be influenced by the quality of the informant's relationship with the patient, and it may need to be reinterpreted (Oppenheimer and Jacoby 1991).

Mental Status

The mental status examination is a cross-sectional assessment of the mental state of the patient at the time of the psychiatric interview. In an office setting, the examination begins as soon as the clinician meets the patient and family in the waiting room. While greeting the patient, the clinician may note the following: How has the patient greeted the examiner? Does the patient know the reason for the interview? How did the patient arrive for the assessment? Does the patient defer to the family for explanations? These observations often determine whether the clinician sees the patient or the family first. Much of the mental status examination is completed during the history taking. The skilled clinician uses appropriate moments in an interview to explore the phenomenology associated with the mental disorder. One challenge for the clinician examining an impaired elderly patient is to ask about phenomena the patient is experiencing in words the patient can understand. A schematic for the geriatric mental status is presented in Table 8–3.

Appearance and Behavior

Geriatric patients' general appearance and behavior often suggest the underlying psychiatric diagnosis. For example, an elderly patient sitting quietly, looking vacantly into space, dressed in ill-fitting, stained clothes with buttons missing and smelling of urine suggests the possibility of a cognitive disorder. Elderly, depressed patients may lose motivation to take care of their appearance. Meeting a patient who greets the clinician

Table 8–3.   Schematic for geriatric mental status

Appearance and behavior
Speech
Affect
Subjective
Objective
Suicide potential
Thought perception—process/content
Obsessive-compulsive/phobic/anxiety symptoms
Insight and judgment
Competency
Mental
Financial
Cognitive assessment

with hesitation and furtive glances and who does not want the clinician to see the family suggests paranoid symptomatology.

Posture, facial appearance, and movement can reflect mood and thinking disturbances and can be affected by a variety of neurological conditions and psychotropic drugs. For example, the shuffling, tremulous elderly man who does not look at the examiner when he speaks and who will not get out of bed may reflect a person with both Parkinson's disease and depression.

Speech

The rate, quantity, and quality of speech and the presence or absence of speech defects may offer clues to the diagnosis. For example, the spontaneity, volume, and quantity of speech often are reduced in geriatric depression. Speech sounds flat and monotonous when depression affects the person's capacity to express emotion (dysprosodia).

Affect

Clinicians should elicit and describe the subjective affective disturbance of the patient. These subjective complaints potentially may mislead the examiner. For example, as many as 20% of elderly people with depression do not complain about being sad or depressed (Post 1972). Instead, these patients may express their subjective distress as "bad nerves," "funny feelings all over my body," or just feeling "sick."

The examiner notes the predominant affect expressed during the interview and the range, appropriateness, and control of affect. Disturbance in each of these functions may signal a different underlying etiology. For example, incongruous, unrestricted affect may be associated with multi-infarct dementia, a "pained" facial expression may be associated with melancholia or chronic pain, and a blank or flat affect may be associated with Parkinson's disease.

Each geriatric patient requires a careful review of suicide ideation and intent. The accuracy and depth of the inquiry is aided by first asking about suicide ideation and passive death wishes and then, if appropriate, asking about specific intent, methods, and plans. Additional risk factors in elderly patients include poor physical health, past history of suicide attempts, family history of suicide attempts and completions, concurrent alcoholism or depression, the presence of command hallucinations, and social isolation.

Thought

The clinician should note the specific preoccupations of the patient and the presence or absence of delusions. For example, preoccupations in depression include somatic and hypochondriacal concerns, especially with the gastrointestinal, musculoskeletal, and nervous systems. Depressed patients may worry that their health is deteriorating, and these worries may replace the subjective complaint of "depression."

Delusions that are present should be described in detail. Mood-congruent delusions in severe geriatric depression may include delusions of poverty, sin, guilt, nihilism, and hypochondriasis. Hypochondriacal delusions are common and often center on the functions of the bowel and brain. For example, a patient may believe there is a blockage or tumor in the bowel and may subsequently stop eating.

Delusions associated with dementia are common (Drevets and Rubin 1989) and include stealing delusions, delusions of persecution, delusional jealousy (involving the spouse), misidentification syndromes (involving the caregiver or spouse), and reincarnation delusions (involving dead relatives). More complex and systematized delusions of persecution may be present in paranoid patients with apparent intact cognition. Themes seen in these patients include fears about drug dealers, criminals, and prostitutes operating in nearby homes. These patients may fear that they are being monitored and observed constantly. Ideas of reference often are associated.

Thought process abnormalities are less common in elderly patients with intact cognition than in a younger adult psychiatric population (Post

1967). Tangentiality and looseness of associations may be seen in dementias but often are not present in paranoid disorders of old age. Flight of ideas is common in mania of old age. Circumstantiality may be associated with an obsessional personality.

Perception

Perceptual disturbances include illusions, hallucinations, derealization, and depersonalization experiences. Terrifying visual illusions and hallucinations are common to severe delirium in elderly patients. Olfactory and auditory hallucinations are seen in a variety of geriatric disorders including paranoid disorders and affective disorders.

Obsessive-Compulsive, Phobic, or Anxiety Symptoms

There is some evidence that obsessive-compulsive, panic, or phobic symptoms can arise de novo in old age. These symptoms most often appear in the context of a depressive disorder or in the early stages of a dementing disorder. Agoraphobia appears to be the only primary anxiety disorder that appears first in old age to any significant degree (Flint 1994). Posttraumatic stress disorders may occur in later life, particularly in connection with medicosurgical trauma. Patients who present with an apparent late-onset anxiety disorder may have had an unrecognized or an untreated anxiety disorder earlier in life. Such individuals often are described by families as always tense, worried, nervous, or controlling. The significance of anxiety disorders in elderly patients is not well described.

Judgment and Insight

Using information obtained in the history, the clinician determines whether the patient's mental illness interferes with judgment to the extent that it could jeopardize his or her health and safety or that of others. More subtle alterations in judgment include the inability to make and carry out plans and inappropriate behavior in social situations. Traditional tests of judgment that ask the patient what he or she would do in imaginary situations are not very helpful because they are not sensitive to the subtle alterations in judgment seen in many geriatric disorders.

Insight refers to the degree of awareness and understanding the patient has of his or her illness and the need for treatment. It is important to inquire whether the patient realizes that certain events may have predisposed, precipitated, or may be perpetuating his or her illness. Elderly patients' judgment and insight often are affected by the dementias, by paranoid disorders, and by affective disorders with delusions.

Competence

Geriatric psychiatrists often are required to assess a patient's capacity to make decisions. This may involve the patient's ability to make or change a will, give power of attorney, or consent to treatment. The assessment of competence in each area should be tested individually. Competence is best viewed as a task-specific assessment. Therefore, a person might be competent to consent to medical treatment but might not be competent to manage financial affairs or vice versa.

One of the more common competence assessments involves the capacity of the patient to give consent for medical treatment (Applebaum and Grisso 1988). The clinician can use the following questions as a guide: Is the patient aware of experiencing a mental illness? Does the patient understand the nature of the proposed treatment? Does the patient understand the need for treatment and the implications of refusing treatment? Does the mental illness sufficiently interfere with judgment and reasoning that it accounts for refusal of treatment?

Geriatric mental illness may interfere with the capacity of a person to manage his or her finances (Lieff et al. 1984). The following questions may be used to complete this assessment: Does the person have knowledge of his or her current assets? Does the person have knowledge of monthly expenses and bills? Does the person know where assets are located and how they are being managed? Can the person complete simple calculations? Does the person experience delusions (such as delusions of poverty) that interfere with the capacity to manage his or her finances? Is the person experiencing memory impairment sufficient to interfere with his or her capacity to remember recent and past financial transactions? Is the person's judgment so affected (in a manic episode or in dementia, for example) that the patient's finances would be jeopardized?

The Cognitive Assessment

Purpose. The assessment of cognitive function is a crucial component of the geriatric mental status examination. The purpose of this portion of the comprehensive examination is to allow the clinician to answer the following questions:

- Is cognitive impairment present or absent? This question traditionally has been phrased, "Is the illness 'functional' or 'organic?'" In psychogeriatrics, however, the interplay between these two elements often challenges the validity of this diagnostic dichotomy. For example, the patient with depression who presents with what appears to be pseudodementia might be classified as having a "functional" illness, but the patient may be experiencing the earliest symptoms of a bona fide dementing illness (Kral and Emery 1989). Conversely, a patient whose depression follows a left frontal cerebrovascular accident may be classified as having an "organic" illness, but the affective component may respond well to the same somatic modalities as a "functional" illness (Starkstein and Robinson 1989). Awareness of the presence or absence of cognitive impairment is crucial in determining etiology and formulating a treatment plan.

- What is the pattern of the cognitive dysfunction? The pattern of cognitive impairment may reveal important clues about the etiology of the illness. The exact location of a lesion may not be elicited by the screening examination, but the examiner should be able to determine whether the lesion is diffuse or multifocal (as in Alzheimer's disease) or localized (as in a right parietal lobe tumor).

- What is the quantity or severity of the cognitive impairment? When cognitive function examinations are performed longitudinally, the answer to this question helps determine the course and prognosis of the illness. A functional assessment and the assessment of the quality and quantity of cognitive impairment are essential to determine how much care or supervision patients require.

- Is a more elaborate neuropsychological examination necessary? Although much can be learned from a relatively brief screening examination, more detailed testing helps establish a more accurate diagnosis when the findings are extremely subtle or when the clinician suspects an underlying dementia or neurological illness. When the diagnosis of dementia is likely, more detailed testing establishes areas of weakness and strengths in the various cognitive domains for organizing a comprehensive rehabilitation program. The examination should help guide the choice of other investigations, such as electroencephalogram and neuroimaging, required for further diagnosis.

Principles. The cognitive examination begins immediately with history taking. The examiner should comment on aspects such as attention, concentration, memory, and language by listening to how the patient relates the details of the history. These "passive" observations can be supplemented by subtle "in-context" questioning throughout the history (e.g., asking patients the exact date of a wedding anniversary while talking about their marriage, asking patients to name all their grandchildren, or asking what day of the week they were admitted to the hospital).

The cognitive assessment should be documented carefully. A clinician seeing a patient with Alzheimer's disease 2 years after initial diagnosis will be able to compare findings more meaningfully if the first examiner recorded "could recall three out of four objects after 5 minutes," rather than "short-term memory fair."

Another important principle is that the examination must be acceptable to both the patient and the examiner. The examiner should be able to administer the tests easily, with minimal equipment, and in a short period of time. The tests must be nonthreatening to the patient and should not be unduly arduous, particularly if they follow a lengthy history.

The formal assessment always should begin with a short explanation to the patient (e.g., "I would now like to ask you some questions to see how well you can concentrate and remember things"). Elaborate explanations and using the word "test" only serve to heighten the patient's anxiety; being apologetic (e.g., "Some of these questions may seem a little silly . . .") reduces the legitimacy and importance of the exam.

The examination is organized in a hierarchical fashion from basic functions to more complex ones. For example, attention and concentration need to be assessed before any valid testing of memory is done. The examiner will have to demonstrate a degree of flexibility depending on the clinical situation and the degree of impairment demonstrated during the history (e.g., comprehension will need to be tested early in any patient with a suspected aphasia). This hierarchical approach is extended to assess tasks within a given cognitive domain. For example, a patient with suspected concentration impairment might be asked to count backward by 1s from 100 before being asked for serial 7s from 100. The former test is simpler and less threatening; the latter is more likely to demonstrate milder impairment, but it may overwhelm the patient who did not have the opportunity to warm up for the testing procedures. When recording scores on individual tasks, the examiner should note the quality of the responses. "I don't know" responses, confabulations, lack of effort, and perseveration (the pathological repetition of speech or actions) are qualitative comments that provide useful diagnostic information. Table 8–4 outlines an easily administered cognitive assessment that provides the information necessary to answer the questions listed above.

Attention and concentration.   Attention traditionally has been tested using the task of repeating a string of digits forward and backward; concentration has been measured with the serial 7s task. Both tests provide useful information, but elderly persons often feel threatened when confronted with tasks involving numbers or arithmetic. The serial 7s subtraction test, in particular, may depend more on a patient's premorbid intellectual capacity and education than on an underlying impairment of concentration. A simple test to assess attention consists of reading a series of random letters to the patient and asking him or her to indicate (tap or say "yes") every time he or she hears the letter "A." This task can be scored for errors of omission, commission, or perseveration. Simple tests of concentration include asking a patient to state the days of the week backward followed by months of the year backward. If these two tasks are performed well, the patient can be asked to do serial 7s from 100.

Language.   The exact characterization of an aphasia may be beyond the scope of a screening examination of cognition, but the examiner can assess some aspects of a patient's expressive and receptive language function during screening of cognition. After taking the patient's history, the examiner should be able to comment on many aspects of spontaneous speech such as articulation (presence of dysarthria), melody (prosody), the presence of word-finding difficulties, and evidence of specific aphasic errors

Table 8–4.   Format of the cognitive assessment

Attention and concentration
Language
   Spontaneous speech
   Comprehension
   Naming
Orientation
Memory
   Recent
   Remote
Constructional ability
Praxis
Frontal systems

such as paraphasias. Paraphasias include substituting an incorrect word (referred to as verbal or semantic paraphasia; for example, "I cut meat with a 'pen'") or substituting a syllable (called a phonemic or literal paraphasia; for example, "I cut meat with a 'f'ife").

Comprehension can be tested by asking the patient to point to certain objects in the room. The test can be made more difficult by increasing the number of objects in a single command (e.g., "Point to the ceiling, the wall, and then the door") or by proceeding from the concrete (e.g., "Point to the light") to the more abstract (e.g., "Point to the source of illumination"). Alternatively, the examiner may ask a series of questions to which the patient responds "yes" or "no." To detect perseveration, the yes or no responses should vary randomly. This task is made more complex by varying the complexity of the question (e.g., "Is snow white?" versus "Does a stone float on water?" versus "Do you put on your shoes before your socks?"). Comprehension tests involving asking a patient to perform 1-, 2-, or 3-stage commands may be useful but difficult to interpret if the patient has a motor problem or apraxia.

Naming difficulties (anomia) that occur in aphasic patients may be found in patients with dementia such as Alzheimer's disease, toxic metabolic encephalopathies, and raised intracranial pressure (Cummings 1985). Naming referred to as "confrontation naming" is tested by pointing to a series of objects and asking the patient to name each one. The objects should include different categories (colors, body parts, clothing), high-frequency words (blue, red, mouth, hand, shirt, tie), and low-frequency words (purple, knuckles, watch crystal).

Orientation. Orientation is a function of memory and consists of long-term (orientation to person) and short-term (orientation to place and time) components. Orientation to person, place, and time is tested sequentially. Patients are asked their full name, age, and date of birth. Orientation to place is tested by asking where they are and asking which city, state, and country they are in. Patients may be asked their home address and more details of their present location (hospital floor, ward, or room). Orientation to time includes asking the day, date, month, year, and time of day. Patients who respond incorrectly to any of the above can be corrected and retested later in the interview as a test of ability to learn new information.

Memory. Testing memory can be extremely complicated if all its dimensions (immediate, recent, remote, recall, recognition, verbal, and visual) are tested individually. Memory can be assessed quickly and simply for cognitive screen purposes to determine whether more elaborate testing is needed. The examiner begins by telling the patient to remember four words that the patient will be asked to recall in several minutes. Any four unrelated words can be used; the examiner should use the same series of words for every patient to ensure consistency and ease of administration. Immediate recall is tested by asking the patient to repeat the four words immediately after the examiner's first recitation. The patient may require several trials to learn all four words; the number of trials should be recorded. Recent memory is examined by asking the patient to recall the words after 5 minutes. The examiner should record the number of words recalled spontaneously and those recalled with the use of hints. Two kinds of hints or cues are semantic cues (hints related to the category of the object such as "one word was a kind of animal") and phonemic cues (given by progressively reciting the individual sounds or syllables of the word; "B . . . Bl . . . Bla . . . Black," for example).

Remote memory is assessed by noting the patient's knowledge of personal history details and by asking several questions about historical or political facts (names of the president and past president, dates of World War II, what Sputnik was). The performance on this task depends on the patient's premorbid intelligence and education. This task should be modified to account for sociocultural factors (for example, asking a recent immigrant from England the names of prime ministers instead of presidents).

Constructional ability. Constructional ability is assessed by asking the patient to draw or copy two-dimensional and three-dimensional figures. These tasks involve extensive cortical areas and can be quite sensitive to subtle changes in overall cognition; difficulty on these tests may indicate nondominant parietal lobe impairment (Strub and Black 1985).

For proper evaluation of constructional ability the clinician must ensure that adequate light, optimum vision (glasses are worn if necessary), and appropriate motor ability (no gross evidence of weakness or incoordination) are present. Paper should be unlined so that it does not produce interference and the patient should be given a pencil or a pen that writes easily, even at odd angles.

Constructional ability can be tested by asking the patient to draw freehand and to copy figures. The patient can be asked to draw a circle, cross, and a cube (in order of ascending difficulty). If the patient experiences any difficulty, the examiner draws the figure and asks the patient to copy it.

Another simple, useful test of constructional ability is to hand the patient a sheet of paper with a predrawn circle and ask the patient to write in the numbers to make the circle look like the face of a clock. If this is done correctly the patient can be asked to draw in the hands to make the clock read 3 o'clock (a relatively easy task) or 10 minutes past 11 (a relatively difficult task). Clock drawing is a good screening tool that correlates well with overall cognitive functioning (Shulman et al. 1986). It can be used to demonstrate unilateral neglect and perseveration and is useful in following the progression of an illness (for example, relative improvement in a resolving delirium or worsening of a dementia).

Praxis. Ideomotor praxis involves the ability to perform volitional actions on command, in mime, without props (Cummings 1985). Testing involves limb, whole-body, and buccal-lingual commands. To assess limb commands, the patient can be asked "Show me how you would comb your hair with your left hand." Other limb commands may include brushing teeth, turning a key, or using a saw. Both hands should be tested separately. Common errors include performing the actions awkwardly, using the hands as the object instead of pretending to hold the object, needing to use both hands, or verbalizing the task first (Taylor et al. 1987). Whole-body commands include asking the patient to stand like a boxer or to swing a bat like a baseball player. To demonstrate buccal-lingual commands patients can be asked to pretend to lick crumbs off their lips, blow out a candle, or suck through a straw. Impairment of this kind of praxis (i.e., ideomotor apraxia) usually is related to dominant parietal lobe dysfunction.

Frontal systems tasks. Frontal systems tasks are used to screen for dysfunction of the frontal lobes and of their interconnected, subcortical structures. These tests are useful for assessing patients with frontal lobe pathology (such as in Pick's disease) and for assessing the cognitive functioning of patients with extrapyramidal disorders (such as Parkinson's disease). In the latter, dysfunction in the basal ganglia, with its multitude of connections to the frontal lobes, may lead to a pattern of cognitive impairment, referred to as subcortical dementia, that is quantitatively and qualitatively different from cortical dementias (Cummings and Benson 1983). The frontal lobes oversee many cognitive functions, including attention, concentration, verbal fluency, abstraction, insight, and judgment. The following tests have been chosen for use in the cognitive screening because they tend to elicit two important signs associated with frontal lobe dysfunction: perseveration and concrete thinking. (Assessment of attention, concentration, insight, and judgment were described above.)

Perseveration may be obvious from the history and previous testing; it can be assessed further by showing the patient an alternating-sequence diagram or several multiple loops (see Figure 8–1) and asking the patient to copy the diagrams exactly and continue the pattern across the page. Perseverative errors include drawing consecutive squares or triangles with the former and adding extra loops to the latter. Alternatively, the patient can be asked to tap once when the examiner taps twice and twice when the examiner taps once. The examiner, while tapping randomly once or twice, observes whether the patient can learn the correct response, how many errors are committed, and whether the errors are perseverative (e.g., the patient continues to tap twice every time the examiner taps twice). The task can be made more difficult when the examiner asks the patient to tap twice every time the examiner taps once but not to tap at all if the examiner taps twice. Particular attention is paid to whether the patient perseverates on the first series of instructions by continuing to tap once when the examiner taps twice.

Tests to elicit concrete thinking involve testing a patient's ability to think abstractly. The results of these tests need to be interpreted cautiously because they are highly dependent on educational level and cultural background. The patient can be asked to interpret metaphorical speech such as "he's blue," "she's yellow," "a heart of gold," or "heavy-handed." The patient can be asked to interpret some common proverbs such as "don't cry over spilled milk" (low difficulty) or "a stitch in time saves nine" (higher difficulty).

Concrete thinking can be elicited by using a similarities task. The patient is asked to describe how two objects are alike. The task begins with a simple stimulus such as "How are an apple and an orange alike?" The

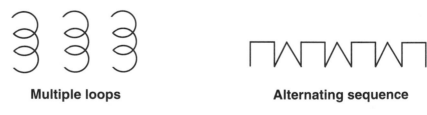

Multiple loops   **Alternating sequence**

Figure 8–1.   Perseveration can be assessed by asking patients to copy the multiple loops drawing or the alternating sequence diagram and continue the pattern across the page.

response "they are both round" may indicate concrete thinking, but the patient should be told the examiner was looking for the response "they are both fruits" before proceeding with the next stimulus. Stimuli are arranged in order of ascending complexity (e.g., orange/apple, shirt/pants, table/chair, airplane/bicycle). Continued responses emphasizing minute individual characteristics (as opposed to the group or category to which the objects belong) are indicative of concrete thinking. This test is less culture-biased than proverbs.

Standardized Assessment Instruments

Standardized assessment instruments are essential tools for clinical investigators, but their utility in every day clinical practice is often underemphasized. These instruments are particularly useful in the circumstances listed below, but they never should take the place of the comprehensive biopsychosocial assessment described above.

For Communicating With Colleagues

Subjective descriptions of symptom severity or degree of impairment can be misleading or unreliable; therefore, scales such as the Mini-Mental State Exam (Folstein et al. 1975) or the Hamilton Depression Rating Scale (Hamilton 1967), which are widely recognized, help standardize communication between physicians.

For Medicolegal and Insurance Purposes

Clinicians may argue the validity and reliability of individual scales or diagnostic tools, but many of these have been embraced by the legal system and insurers because they ostensibly provide systematic standardized descriptions of psychopathology.

To Solve Specific Clinical Problems

Certain rating scales can be used to solve specific clinical problems. For example, the Staff Observation Aggression Scale (Palmstierna and Wistedt 1987) can be used on the ward for documenting antecedents and consequences of aggressive acts. This information is used for designing a behavioral program for aggressive elderly patients.

To Document Change

Recording scores on depression rating scales or cognitive assessment scales effectively can document response to treatment or progression of illness.

For Education Purposes

Standardized assessments often are excellent tools for teaching medical students or allied health professionals. These assessments are taught easily and can elevate awareness of the necessity to consider emotional and cognitive functioning in all elderly patients.

Depression rating scales. Depression rating scales are divided into interviewer-administered and self-report measures. The former generally are more sensitive and specific, whereas the latter generally are easier and quicker to administer (Thompson et al. 1988). The most widely used interviewer-administered measure is the Hamilton Depression Rating Scale (HAM-D) (Hamilton 1967). Its reliability recently has been improved by the development of a structured interview guide (Williams 1988), but its heavy weighting toward somatic symptoms (9 of 17 items) might be problematic for use in an elderly population with a high prevalence of physical illness (Thompson et al. 1988). The Montgomery-Åsberg Depression Rating Scale (MADRS) (Montgomery and Åsberg 1979) places less emphasis on somatic symptoms and may be more suitable in an elderly population (Kearns et al. 1982). This scale is easily administered and very helpful for documenting response to therapy. The most commonly used self-report measures in geriatrics are the Geriatric Depression Scale (GDS) (Yesavage et al. 1983), the Zung self-rating depression scale (Zung 1965), and the Beck Depression Inventory (BDI) (Beck et al. 1961). The GDS, designed specifically for use in elderly patients, is sensitive and specific (Norris et al. 1987). It is easily administered, requiring patients to respond yes or no to a series of 30 statements. A short form (10 items) is available (Sheikh and Yesavage 1986). Self-rated scales are not valid when there is significant cognitive impairment, especially when insight is lost.

Cognitive function and dementia rating scales. There has been a recent proliferation of brief, standardized, easily administered screening examinations for cognitive impairment. Such instruments include the Short Portable Mental Status Questionnaire (Pfeiffer 1975), the Blessed Dementia

Index (Blessed et al. 1968), and the Clifton Assessment Schedule (Pattie and Gilleard 1976). One of the most widely accepted scales is the Mini-Mental State Exam (MMSE) (Folstein et al. 1975). The MMSE provides a measure of cognition that includes tests of orientation, memory, concentration, language, and constructional ability. This examination requires only about 10 minutes and is easy to administer. It is not without weaknesses, but this tool has been used for more than 27 years, has been extensively investigated, and has stood the test of time with acceptable validity and reliability (Tombaugh and McIntyre 1992). Another group of standardized assessments has been designed to complement the MMSE. This group attempts to rate the stage of dementia or the severity of cognitive and noncognitive behavioral impairment. Two such scales are the Global Deterioration Scale (Reisberg et al. 1982) and the Clinical Dementia Rating Scale (Hughes et al. 1982). Another popular scale, the Alzheimer's Disease Assessment Scale (Rosen et al. 1984), combines a cognitive screen with an inventory of noncognitive behaviors to provide an overall measure of illness severity.

Miscellaneous rating instruments.   Scales to measure functional abilities and activities of daily living were discussed above. A number of scales with specific foci can be very useful in clinical practice. The Overt Aggression Scale (OAS) (Yudofsky et al. 1986) and the Staff Observation Aggression Scale (Palmstierna and Wistedt 1987) are useful for evaluating aggressive behavior. The former scale is much more popular. The latter has the advantage of documenting antecedents, aggressive acts, and consequences of aggression; therefore, it aids in developing behavioral management. Simple systematic observation and documentation with this tool has shown a decrease in aggressive behavior in a group of psychogeriatric inpatients (Nilsson et al. 1988). Another useful tool is the Abnormal Involuntary Movement Scale (National Institute of Mental Health 1975). This scale consists of a number of ratings of abnormal movements including a global measure of severity, a rating of incapacity, and a measure of the patient's awareness of the movements. This scale is particularly helpful for monitoring elderly patients on neuroleptic treatment. A popular multidimensional measure of psychopathology is the Brief Psychiatric Rating Scale (Overall and Gorham 1962). This scale consists of 16 measures including anxiety, depression, hostility, hallucinations, and unusual thought content; it has been studied in a psychogeriatric population (Overall and Beller 1984).

Physical and Neurological Examination

All geriatric patients require an appropriate physical examination with special attention directed to the neurological system.

Diagnosis and Formulation

After completing the history and functional, medical, and mental status assessments, the clinician can propose a provisional diagnosis and differential diagnosis, develop an etiological formulation, and establish the capacity of each patient to function independently. The provisional and differential diagnoses will direct the clinician in planning for an orderly series of investigations and tests that will confirm or refute the provisional diagnosis or the specific diagnoses in the differential.

By reorganizing the salient features of the assessment into an etiological formulation, the clinician will develop a working hypothesis of the factors that make this patient vulnerable to developing a mental illness at this particular time. Knowledge of the biopsychosocial vulnerability of each patient is necessary for individualizing the case management. Knowledge of the current capacity of patients to function in their environment will aid in determining what specific social supports must be provided to allow a person to continue living there. A comprehensive management plan, including biological, psychological, and social therapies, logically follows from the results of this assessment.

References

Applebaum PS, Grisso T: Assessing patients' capacities to consent to treatment. N Engl J Med 319:1635–1638, 1988

Beck AT, Ward CH, Mendelson M, et al: An inventory for measuring depression. Arch Gen Psychiatry 4:561–571, 1961

Blazer, DG: The psychiatric interview of the geriatric patient, in Geriatric Psychiatry. Edited by Busse EW, Blazer DG. Washington, DC, American Psychiatric Press, 1989, pp 263–284

Blessed G, Tomlinson BE, Roth M: The association between quantitative measures of dementia and of senile change in the cerebral grey matter of elderly subjects. Br J Psychiatry 114:797–811, 1968

Brown BB: Professionals' perceptions of drug and alcohol abuse among the elderly. Gerontologist 22(6):519–525, 1982

Cummings JL: Clinical Neuropsychiatry. Orlando, FL, Grune & Stratton, 1985

Cummings JL, Benson DF: Dementia: A Clinical Approach. Boston, MA, Butterworth, 1983

Drevets WC, Rubin EH: Psychotic symptoms and the longitudinal course of senile dementia of the Alzheimer type. Biol Psychiatry 25:39–48, 1989

Ewing, JA: Detecting alcoholism: the C.A.G.E. Questionnaire. JAMA 252:1905–1907, 1984

Flint AJ: Epidemiology and cormorbidity of anxiety disorders in the elderly. Am J Psychiatry 151:640–649, 1994

Folstein MF, Folstein SE, McHugh PR: Mini-Mental State: a practical method for grading the cognitive state of patients for the clinician. J Psychiatr Res 12:189–198, 1975

Ginsberg GL: Psychiatry history and mental status examination, in Comprehensive Textbook of Psychiatry. Edited by Kaplan HI, Sadock BJ. Baltimore, MD, Williams & Wilkins, 1985

Hamilton M: Development of a rating scale for primary depressive illness. Soc Clin Psychol 6:278–296, 1967

Hughes CP, Berg L, Danziger WL, et al: A new clinical scale for the staging of dementia. Br J Psychiatry 140:566–572, 1982

Johnson DAW: Drug-induced psychiatric disorders. Drugs 22:57–69, 1981

Katz S, Downs TD, Cash HR, et al: Progress in development of the index of ADL. Gerontologist 10:20–30, 1970

Kearns MP, Cruickshank CA, McGuigan KJ, et al: A comparison of depression rating scales. Br J Psychiatry 141:45–49, 1982

Kral VA, Emery OB: Long term follow-up of depressive pseudodementia of the aged. Can J Psychiatry 34:445–446, 1989

Lawton MP: Scales to measure competence in everyday activities. Psychopharmacol Bull 24:609–614, 1988

Lawton MP, Brody EM: Assessment of older people: self-maintaining and instrumental activities of daily living. Gerontologist 9:179–186, 1969

Leff JP, Isaacs AD: Psychiatric Examination in Clinical Practice. Oxford, England, Blackwell Scientific, 1978

Lieff S, Maindonald K, Shulman K: Issues in determining financial competence in the elderly. Can Med Assoc J 130:1293–1296, 1984

Montgomery SA, Åsberg MA: A new depression scale designed to be sensitive to change. Br J Psychiatry 134:382–389, 1979

National Institute of Mental Health: Development of a dyskinetic movement scale (Publ No 4). Rockville, MD, National Institute of Mental Health, Psychopharmacology Research Branch, 1975

Nilsson K, Palmstierna T, Wistedt B: Aggressive behavior in hospitalized psychogeriatric patients. Acta Psychiatr Scand 78:172–175, 1988

Norris J, Gallagher D, Wilson A, et al: Assessment of depression in geriatric medical out-patients; the validity of two screening measures. J Am Geriatr Soc 35:989–995, 1987

Oppenheimer C, Jacoby R: Psychiatric assessment of the elderly, in Psychiatry in the Elderly. Edited by Jacoby R, Oppenheimer C. Oxford, England, Oxford University Press, 1991, pp 169–198

Overall JE, Beller SA: The brief psychiatric rating scale (BPRS) in geropsychiatric research, I: factor structure on an in-patient unit. J Gerontol 39:187–193, 1984

Overall JE, Gorham DR: The brief psychiatric rating scale. Psychol Rep 10:799–812, 1962

Palmstierna T, Wistedt B: Staff observation aggression scale (SOAS): presentation and evaluation. Acta Psychiatr Scand 76:657–663, 1987

Pattie AH, Gilleard CJ: The Clifton assessment schedule: further validation of a psychogeriatric assessment schedule. Br J Psychiatry 129:68–72, 1976

Pfeiffer E: A short portable mental status questionnaire for the assessment of organic brain deficit in elderly patients. J Am Geriatr Soc 23:433–441, 1975

Post F: The Significance of Affective Symptoms in Old Age. London, England, Oxford University Press, 1962

Post F: Aspects of psychiatry in the elderly. Proc R Soc Med 60:249–254, 1967

Post F: The relationship to physical health of the affective illnesses in the elderly, in Proceedings of the 8th International Congress of Gerontology, Vol 1. Washington, DC: International Association of Gerontology, 1969, pp 198–201

Post F: The management and nature of depressive illness in late life: a follow-through study. Br J Psychiatry 121:393–404, 1972

Reisberg B, Ferris SH, DeLeon J, et al: The global deterioration scale for assessment of primary degenerative dementia. Am J Psychiatry 139:1136–1139, 1982

Rosen WG, Mohs RC, Davis KL: A new rating scale for Alzheimer's disease. Am J Psychiatry 141:1356–1364, 1984

Rubenstein LV, Calkins DR, Greenfield A, et al: Health status assessment for elderly patients. J Am Geriatr Soc 37:562–569, 1989

Sheikh JI, Yesavage JA: Geriatric depression scale: recent evidence and development of a shorter version. Clin Gerontol 5:165–173, 1986

Shulman KI, Shedletsky R, Silver IL: The challenge of time: clock-drawing and cognitive function in the elderly. International Journal of Geriatric Psychiatry 1:135–140, 1986

Starkstein SE, Robinson RG: Affective disorders and cerebrovascular disease. Br J Psychiatry 154:170–182, 1989

Strub RL, Black FW: The Mental Status Examination in Neurology. Philadelphia, PA, FA Davis, 1985

Taylor MA, Sierles FS, Abrams R: The neuropsychiatric evaluation, in The Textbook of Neuropsychiatry. Edited by Hales RE, Yudofsky SC. Washington, DC, American Psychiatric Press, 1987

Thompson LW, Futterman A, Gallagher D: Assessment of late life depression. Psychopharmacol Bull 24:577–586, 1988

Tombaugh TN, McIntyre NJ: The Mini-Mental State Examination: a comprehensive review. J Am Geriatr Soc 40:922–935, 1992

Waldinger RJ: Psychiatry for Medical Students, 2nd Edition. Washington, DC, American Psychiatric Press, 1990

Williams JBW: A structured interview guide for the Hamilton Depression Rating Scale. Arch Gen Psychiatry 45:742–747, 1988

Yesavage J, Brink TL: Development and validation of a geriatric depression screening scale: a preliminary report. J Psychiatry Res 17:37–49, 1983

Yudofsky SC, Silver JM, Jackson W, et al: The Overt Aggression Scale for the objective rating of verbal and physical aggression. Am J Psychiatry 143:35–39, 1986

Zung WWK: A self rating depression scale. Arch Gen Psychiatry 12:63–70, 1965

Cathy A. Alessi, M.D.
Christine K. Cassel, M.D.

Medical Evaluation and Common Medical Problems

M edical illness is common in older patients, and geriatric psychia-trists should be aware of medical problems that may be affecting their patients. Many medical illnesses may present with psychiatric mani-festations. The older psychiatric patient often will benefit from a careful medical evaluation to identify physical problems that may be contributing to psychiatric disease or that may be having a significant impact on the older person's quality of life. Certain medical illnesses and geriatric syndromes are quite common in older people and can be managed by the psychiatrist, with referral when appropriate. The geriatric psychiatrist can play a key role in identifying signs and symptoms that signal physical deterioration or missed diagnoses in the older patient. Several laboratory tests routinely are obtained in older psychiatric patients, and the psychiatrist should be skilled in the initial interpretation and appropriate referral based on these results. The geriatric psychiatrist should be aware of the major issues involved in two common indications for referral for medical evaluation: medical clearance for electroconvulsive therapy and medical aspects of antidepressant therapy. Medical illness may present with subtle or nonspecific findings in the older patient and, therefore, may go unrecognized or may be erroneously ascribed

We wish to acknowledge the excellent secretarial help of Marci Stahl.

to "normal aging." A large body of literature describes the distinction between physiological change caused by normal aging and change caused by disease. An awareness of both types of change is important in the care of the older patient. Changes with normal aging impair the body's homeostatic mechanisms and may result in decreased ability of the older person to deal with acute insult. Changes caused by disease are quite common: Approximately 80% of people older than 65 have at least one chronic disease or disability (Soldo and Manton 1985). The geriatric psychiatrist should be aware of these distinctions when making decisions about the management of the older patient.

Psychiatric Manifestations of Medical Illness in the Older Patient

Psychiatric symptoms can occur with practically any physical illness that has systemic involvement, that can cause metabolic disturbance, or that has direct central nervous system (CNS) effects. A variety of drugs can cause psychiatric symptoms at toxic doses, at normal therapeutic levels, or during periods of withdrawal (Abramowicz 1986). Older patients may have several coexisting conditions or may be taking several medications that potentially could explain or contribute to their psychiatric symptoms.

Physical illness is extremely common in psychiatric patients. In a large study of outpatients and inpatients ages 18 years or older in the California public mental health system, 39% of study patients had an active, important physical disease and 9% had physical disease judged to exacerbate their mental disorders (Koran et al. 1989). Likewise, comorbid psychiatric disorders are extremely common in elderly medical patients. For example, major affective disorder has been identified in up to one-third of geriatric medical outpatients and 45% of geriatric medical inpatients (Kitchell et al 1982; Okimoto et al. 1982).

A more recent study of elderly hospitalized medical inpatients found that 27% of patients had at least one research diagnostic criteria (RDC) psychiatric diagnosis; depression was most common (16% of subjects). One year later, only one-third of subjects had received mental health treatment, and 65% of the subjects with depression remained depressed (Rapp et al. 1991).

Physical illness in older patients may present as any of several psychiatric syndromes such as dementia, delirium, depression (see Table 9–1),

Table 9–1. Physical disorders associated with depression in the older patient

Neurological	**Endocrine and metabolic**
Parkinson's disease	Hyperthyroidism, hypothyroidism
Stroke	Hyperparathyroidism, hypoparathyroidism
Alzheimer's disease	Cushing's disease
Subdural hematoma	Addison's disease
Temporal lobe epilepsy	Hyperkalemia, hypokalemia
Amyotrophic lateral sclerosis	Hypernatremia, hyponatremia
Multiple sclerosis	Hypercalcemia, hypocalcemia
Normal pressure hydrocephalus	Hyperglycemia, hypoglycemia
Malignancy	Hypomagnesemia
Brain tumor	Hypoxemia
Leukemia	Vitamin B_{12} deficiency
Pancreatic	**Drugs**
Lung (particularly oat cell)	CNS drugs (e.g., benzodiazepines, alcohol,
Bone metastasis with	levodopa, major tranquilizers)
hypercalcemia	Antihypertensives (e.g., β-blockers, clonidine,
Organ failure	reserpine, methyldopa, prazocin,
Renal failure	guanethidine)
Liver failure	Steroids (e.g., prednisone, estrogen)
Congestive heart failure	Chemotherapy (e.g., vincristine, L-asparaginase,
Infections	interferon)
Viral illness	Cimetidine
Chronic CNS infections	Digoxin
	Other
	Chronic pain
	Anemia
	Sleep disorders (e.g., sleep apnea)

Note. CNS = central nervous system.

or anxiety (see Table 9–2). Each of these syndromes has multiple potential physical etiologies (Alexopoulos et al. 1988; Consensus Conference 1987; Cummings 1985; Cummings et al. 1984; Lipowski 1989; Ouslander 1982; U'Ren 1989; Woodcock 1983). Dementia and delirium are discussed in other chapters. Physical disorders associated with depression and anxiety are listed in Tables 9–1 and 9–2, respectively.

Several important clinical clues can alert the geriatric psychiatrist to the possibility of an underlying physical disorder in the patient with psychiatric illness (Ouslander 1982; Vickers 1988; Woodcock 1983). These clues include

Table 9–2.   Physical disorders associated with anxiety in the older patient

Neurological	**Cardiac**
Early dementia	Coronary artery disease
Transient ischemic attack and stroke	Cardiac arrhythmias
Seizure disorder	Mitral valve prolapse
Endocrine	**Pulmonary**
Hypoglycemia emboli	Recurrent pulmonary
Hyperthyroidism	Chronic lung disease
Hypoparathyroidism	**Other**
Cushing's disease	Chronic pain
Drugs	Anemia
Thyroid replacement	Sleep disorders (e.g., sleep apnea)
Barbiturates	
Steroids	
Stimulants	
Vasodilators	
Caffeine	
Withdrawal from benzodiazepines, alcohol, barbiturates, neuroleptics, antidepressants	

- Abnormal level of consciousness
- Atypical age at onset of symptoms
- Lack of expected family history
- Symptoms more severe than expected
- Coexisting physical illnesses that can cause psychiatric symptoms
- Poor response to psychiatric treatment
- Abrupt personality change followed by psychopathology

Medical Evaluation of the Older Psychiatric Patient

The medical evaluation of the older psychiatric patient includes a thorough history and physical examination, cognitive screening, mental status examination, functional assessment, and appropriate screening laboratory tests. The initial history and physical examination of the older patient usually is a lengthy process, particularly for patients with an extensive past medical history, several current physical complaints, or physical limitations that interfere with the examination. This initial evaluation frequently requires more than one visit, particularly for frail patients who are easily fatigued by the examination process. For a review of history

Table 9–3. Laboratory screening tests in older psychiatric patients

Complete blood count	Syphilis serology
Blood glucose	Vitamin B_{12} and folate assays
Serum electrolytes	Urinalysis
Blood urea nitrogen and creatinine	Electrocardiogram
Liver enzymes	Chest X ray
Thyroid function text (thyroxine level, free thyroxine index, thyroid-stimulating hormone level)	

taking and the initial physical examination, refer to a geriatric medicine text (e.g., Calkins et al. 1986; Cassel et al. 1989; Kane et al. 1989; Rossman 1986; Rowe and Besdine 1988). Psychiatric evaluation of the older patient, which is essential, is discussed elsewhere in this text.

Screening laboratory tests (see Table 9–3) commonly are ordered for older psychiatric patients to rule out physical illness, particularly in patients with psychiatric symptoms that are of recent onset, are severe, or are resistant to therapy. Which screening tests are ordered is determined by the patient's clinical presentation. One study of older patients admitted to a psychiatric unit found only the following screening tests useful in detecting and treating an illness: midstream urine collection, chest X ray, vitamin B_{12} assay, electrocardiogram, and blood urea nitrogen (Kolman 1984).

Common Medical Problems

The geriatric psychiatrist should be aware of the more common medical conditions of older people. Some aspects of initial diagnosis and therapy of these common conditions can be appropriately managed by the psychiatrist, and the psychiatrist can play a major role in identifying features that signal deterioration or missed diagnoses.

Arthritis

The most common chronic condition among persons ages 65 years and older is arthritis; it affects nearly 50% (Soldo and Manton 1985) of persons in this age group. One study suggested the prevalence is even higher in older inpatients, with more than 75% of patients admitted to an acute geriatric unit having evidence of arthritis (Jenkinson 1989). Painful or stiff joints in older patients usually are caused by osteoarthritis, which involves deterioration and abrasion of the articular cartilage. One-third of older patients have significant symptoms of joint discomfort, and approximately 10% have significant limitation caused by osteoarthritis. The joints usually involved include the hands (proximal and distal interphalangeal joints), hips, knees, feet (first metatarsal-phalangeal joints), the cervical spine, and the lower lumbar spine. The diagnosis is suggested by symptoms in one or more of these joints combined with evidence of degenerative changes on plain X rays. X-ray evidence of degenerative disease does not necessarily correlate with symptom severity, however. There are no diagnostic blood tests for osteoarthritis. An elevated erythrocyte sedimentation rate, weight loss, or constitutional symptoms suggest another disease process. Treatment of osteoarthritis is symptomatic; acetaminophen taken on a regular basis several times per day, physical therapy, and exercise can improve comfort and mobility. If these measures are inadequate, aspirin or nonsteroidal anti-inflammatory drugs (NSAIDs) can be helpful, but these agents can cause severe gastric mucosal injury (to the point of life-threatening gastric ulceration) or renal insufficiency in susceptible patients. Elderly patients, particularly women, are at increased risk of major gastrointestinal complications from NSAIDs; the majority of these patients are asymptomatic on these drugs prior to the complication. Alternative analgesics, such as nonacetylated salicylates (e.g., salsalate) should be considered in older patients. Additional measures to prevent gastrointestinal complications when older patients, particularly women, must be treated with NSAIDs include discontinuation of cigarettes and alcohol, use of the lowest effective dose of NSAID, administration of enteric-coated preparations or administration with antacids or food, and discontinuation of NSAID when the agent is no longer necessary. Administration of misoprostol can be considered, especially during the first few months of NSAID therapy and in patients with risk factors for gastrointestinal complications of NSAIDs (Jones and Schubert 1991). Small doses of codeine may be useful in patients with severe symptoms who cannot tolerate other agents, but the risks of sedating side effects are a major concern. Joint replacement should be considered in older patients with severe limiting symptoms or limitation of an important or meaningful activity that cannot be corrected through optimal conservative therapy. The other major rheumatic diseases in older patients with joint discomfort include gout, pseudogout, polymyalgia rheumatica (with or without temporal arthritis), rheumatoid arthritis, and infectious arthritis (Moskowitz 1987; Sorenson 1989).

Hypertension

The second most common chronic condition in older people is hypertension. Hypertension affects 40% to 69% of persons over age 65 years (Soldo and Manton 1985; Working Groups on Hypertension in the Elderly 1986). Patients may have "classic" diastolic hypertension (diastolic blood pressure greater than 90 mm Hg) or isolated systolic hypertension (systolic blood pressure greater than 160 mm Hg and diastolic blood pressure less than 90 mm Hg). One situation to be aware of is the falsely elevated cuff blood pressure that may be seen in some older patients ("pseudohypertension"). This probably is caused by calcification of the brachial artery, and it may be accompanied by a positive "Osler's sign" (a palpable, pulseless brachial or radial artery after blood pressure cuff occlusion) (Messerli et al. 1985). Secondary causes of hypertension are considered in patients with onset of hypertension after age 55 years or with accelerated hypertension after age 65. Refractory hypertension associated with progressive renal insufficiency suggests possible renovascular disease such as renal artery stenosis. Other clinical clues to this surgically correctable lesion include an abdominal bruit and/or severe retinopathy. A clue to another surgically correctable secondary cause of hypertension, an aldosterone-producing adenoma, is hypokalemia less than 3.6 mEq/L. An extensive workup for secondary causes of hypertension is generally recommended in older patients only when hypertension cannot be controlled medically.

Three major trials of antihypertensive treatment in elderly patients have been published recently: the American Systolic Hypertension in the Elderly Program (SHEP), the Swedish Trial in Old Patients With Hypertension (STOP-Hypertension), and the British Medical Research Council (MRC) Trial of Treatment of Hypertension in Older Adults. These trials all compared diuretic and/or β-blocking agents with placebo. All three trials showed that treatment of hypertension in elderly patients reduces the risk of stroke and cardiovascular events; in the STOP-Hypertension trial there was also a decrease in total mortality with treatment (Dahlof et al. 1991; Hansson 1993; MRC Working Party 1992; SHEP Cooperative Research Group 1991).

Recommendations vary on how aggressively to treat hypertension in older patients because of concerns about complications of antihypertensive therapy. However, results of the trials mentioned above highlight the importance of antihypertensive treatment in elderly patients. Most authors currently recommend that a systolic blood pressure of 160 mm Hg or greater or a diastolic blood pressure of 90 mm Hg or greater in an older person should be treated. Nonpharmacological treatment should include weight reduction in obese patients, moderate sodium restriction, moderation of alcohol, and regular aerobic isotonic exercise. Drug therapy should be started if nonpharmacological therapy does not reduce blood pressure adequately or if the blood pressure is high enough to mandate immediate drug therapy. The following guidelines have been suggested when treating older patients with antihypertensive medications:

- Start with a low dose of one drug
- Increase dose slowly
- Minimize the number of pills and doses
- Monitor for side effects
- Encourage home blood pressure monitoring
- Choose drugs based on coexisting conditions that may interact with drug treatment

The goal of therapy should be a systolic blood pressure less than 160 mm Hg and a diastolic blood pressure less than 90 mm Hg (Tjoa and Kaplan 1990).

When thiazide diuretics are used in older patients they generally are started at lower doses than for younger patients (e.g., 12.5 mg of hydrochlorothiazide per day). Limiting side effects of diuretics include frequent urination, orthostasis, dehydration, sodium and potassium depletion, and azotemia. Hyperglycemia, hyperuricemia, and increased lipid levels also may occur. The dehydration that diuretics may cause can be a particular problem in patients receiving tricyclic antidepressants because of aggravation of orthostatic hypotension. In general, psychiatric symptoms caused by diuretic therapy are seen only in patients who develop metabolic abnormalities.

β-Blockers can be used in older patients, but with careful attention to the appearance of bradycardia, heart block, bronchospasm, and congestive heart failure. Advantages of β-blockers include antianginal effects, possible cardioprotective effects, and low incidence of orthostatic hypotension. Disadvantages include the important risk of depression and the less serious but troublesome side effects of restless sleep and somnolence. These agents also may alter lipid metabolism. Calcium channel blockers may be used and may be slightly more effective in elderly patients. Important potential side effects include risk of heart block in susceptible patients, potential decreased cardiac contractility, reflex tachycardia, flushing, headache, and peripheral edema. These agents generally do not cause significant orthostatic hypotension or CNS side effects. Angiotensin-converting enzyme (ACE) inhibitors are generally well tolerated; potential side effects include hyperkalemia, nonproductive cough, and worsening of renal function in patients with congestive heart failure, hyponatremia, or bilateral renal artery stenosis. ACE inhibitors may be the drugs of choice in patients with congestive heart failure because of evidence of increased survival and in patients with diabetes where there is evidence of a renal protective effect with these agents. CNS side effects generally are not a problem. Centrally acting agents such as clonidine, guanethidine, and methyldopa can produce sedation and depression. Reserpine has been associated with depression. α-Blockers can be effective and should be considered in patients who have symptoms of prostatism; these agents may cause significant orthostasis (Applegate 1989; Tjoa and Kaplan 1990; Tuck et al. 1988).

Care should be taken when choosing psychiatric medications in patients who are taking antihypertensives with CNS or orthostatic side effects. It may be desirable to discuss a change in antihypertensive medication with the primary care physician.

Diabetes Mellitus

Glucose intolerance increases with age; approximately one-third of patients older than age 65 have an abnormal glucose tolerance test. It is unclear whether all these patients require therapy. An abnormal fasting blood sugar is the preferable method of diagnosing diabetes in the older population. Between 10% to 20% of older patients have diabetes; it has been estimated that 50% of people with diabetes in the United States are older than 65 years. The rates in men and women are virtually equal (Harris 1990). The majority of older patients with diabetes have type II (non-insulin-dependent diabetes mellitus), although some of these patients may require insulin therapy. Patients typically are overweight and had onset of diabetes after age 40 years. The required treatment varies considerably and may include diet, weight loss, oral hypoglycemic agents, or insulin; some patients will require a combination of these modalities. Doses of oral agents or insulin are started low and are increased slowly to avoid hypoglycemia, which is a major risk in older patients. Hypoglycemia may present with psychiatric symptoms ranging from subtle dullness to coma, and nocturnal hypoglycemia may be a cause of insomnia in treated diabetic patients.

Acute hyperglycemia in older diabetic patients generally presents not as diabetic ketoacidosis but as hyperglycemic hyperosmolar nonketotic coma (HHNKC). These patients may present with mental status changes and with weakness, polyuria, and polydipsia. Mortality is as high as 25% to 50%. Acute hyperglycemia without HHNKC can cause psychiatric symptoms ranging from subtle personality changes to delirium. The mental status changes of hyperglycemia with or without HHNKC may resolve slowly, particularly in patients with underlying CNS disease (Cooppan 1987; Riesenberg 1989).

Complications of chronic diabetes involve multiorgan disease and generally reflect microvascular and macrovascular disease or neurological involvement. Three-fourths of deaths in older diabetic patients are caused by cardiovascular disease, primarily ischemic heart disease and stroke (Harris 1990). It has been established that intensive blood sugar control decreases the risk of these complications in patients with type I (insulin-dependent) diabetes. This point has not been established in older patients with type II diabetes, but most experts suggest that good blood sugar control in these patients decreases risk of chronic complications. Nonspecific complaints such as fatigue may be caused by chronic hyperglycemia and may improve with good blood sugar control. Mental efficiency is frequently impaired in older persons with diabetes (U'Ren et al. 1990). In the older patient, attempts at tight control must be balanced with the risks of hypoglycemia. In the management of diabetes, glycosylated hemoglobin levels can help evaluate overall control. Cigarette smoking increases the risk of complications with diabetes, and the psychiatrist can play a key role in assisting patients, particularly those with diabetes, with smoking cessation.

Constipation

Most healthy older outpatients have a bowel frequency within the same range as their younger counterparts (three times per day to three times per week), but older patients complain of constipation more often and use laxatives more often (Connell et al. 1965; Donald et al. 1985). In one large study, 26% of women and 16% of men over 65 years reported recurrent constipation. Risk factors for constipation were increased age, female gender, use of multiple drugs, pain in the abdomen, and hemorrhoids (Stewart et al. 1992). Additional factors that may contribute to constipa-

Table 9–4.   Common causes of constipation in the older patient

Intrinsic bowel lesions	Endocrine and metabolic
Colorectal carcinoma	Hypothyroidism
Anorectal disease (e.g., hemorrhoids, fissures)	Adrenal and pituitary hypofunction
Diverticular disease	Hypokalemia
Inflammatory bowel disease	Hypercalcemia
Ischemic bowel disease	Uremia
Irritable bowel disease	**Drugs**
Hypomotility disorders (e.g., idiopathic slow transit, idiopathic megacolon)	Analgesics
Neurological	Antacids (e.g., calcium carbonate, aluminum hydroxide)
Dementia	Anticholinergics (e.g., antihistamines, tricyclic antiparkinsonian agents, antidepressants, neuroleptics)
Stroke	
Autonomic neuropathy (e.g., diabetes, pernicious anemia)	
Psychiatric	Antihypertensives, diuretics
Depression	Laxative abuse
Chronic psychosis	Other (e.g., iron, phenytoin, barium, bismuth)

tion in older patients include decreased fluid and dietary fiber intake, decreased activity, intrinsic bowel lesions, endocrine and metabolic disorders, and constipating drugs. Constipation can be a significant problem in psychiatric patients, particularly those on medications with anticholinergic effects. Common causes of constipation in older patients are listed in Table 9–4.

The older patient with constipation should have a rectal examination to rule out fecal impaction or anorectal disease such as hemorrhoids or rectal fissure. Those who present with new or worsened constipation without obvious etiology should have a study to view their colon. Colonoscopy should be considered early in particular patient groups, such as those with a family history of colon cancer. Older patients with weight loss and hemoccult-positive stools should have colonoscopy. Screening blood tests, particularly a complete blood count and thyroid function tests, may aid diagnosis.

The first step in treating constipation is to discontinue unnecessary constipating drugs and treat any contributing diseases. Patients should be encouraged to increase physical activity, fluid intake, and dietary fiber. Bulk-forming agents such as methylcellulose or psyllium may be added to the diet. Patients with hard stools may benefit from a stool softener such as docusate preparations. Other agents to consider are lactulose, enemas, and suppositories. Lactulose can be given at a starting dose of 15 ml to 30 ml at bedtime and increased if necessary. Sorbitol is less expensive than lactulose and evidence suggests it is just as effective (Lederle et al. 1990). Prepackaged enemas are simple and usually safe. Bisacodyl suppositories usually are more effective than glycerin suppositories.

Some agents require special precautions in older patients. Oral mineral oil is not recommended because of the risks of impaired absorption of fat-soluble vitamins and of aspiration with consequent lipoid pneumonia. Stimulant laxatives (cascara, senna, bisacodyl, and castor oil) are recommended only for short-term use because of cramping and fluid and electrolyte loss. Chronic use of stimulant laxatives can cause colonic smooth muscle changes resulting in severe, resistant constipation (cathartic colon). Saline laxatives such as magnesium and sodium salts carry a risk of fluid loss with chronic use but can be used for short-term therapy. Soap-suds or hydrogen peroxide enemas should not be used because of mucosal irritation.

Fecal impaction should be suspected and a rectal examination performed in patients with severe or chronic constipation and in patients who develop fecal incontinence or paradoxical diarrhea (i.e., diarrhea in the presence of a fecal impaction). High fecal impaction beyond the range of digital rectal examination may be viewed on plain X rays of the abdomen. If enemas are not successful, careful manual disimpaction may be necessary but can be quite uncomfortable for the patient. A fecal impaction must be removed prior to therapy with stimulant laxatives because of the risk of severe cramping or obstruction (Alessi and Henderson 1988). High fecal impaction may be difficult to relieve, but repeated enemas and suppositories can be successful. Whole gut irrigation (by nasogastric tube) or oral treatment with polyethylene glycol-saline solution also have been suggested (Puxty and Fox 1986; R.G. Smith et al. 1978).

Weight Loss and Malnutrition

Weight loss is a common symptom in older patients with psychiatric or medical illness. Unintentional weight loss of 5% of body weight in 6 months or 10% in 1 year is significant and should be evaluated for an organic cause. A medical cause is not found in about one-fourth to one-third of patients with weight loss. The most common medical causes found are malignancy and gastrointestinal disease. Depression was the most common cause in one recent study of elderly outpatients with weight loss (Thompson and Morris 1991). Another study found the best predictor of involuntary weight loss in elderly patients on a geriatric rehabilitation unit was the number of general oral health problems such as poor oral hygiene or the inability to chew; other important predictors were household income, age, smoking, nutritional intake, and education (Sullivan et al. 1993).

The extent of laboratory testing in the older patient with psychiatric symptoms and weight loss depends on clinical clues to an underlying medical illness, degree of weight loss, and overall status of the patient. Typical screening tests include complete blood count, electrolytes, blood urea nitrogen, creatinine, liver function tests, glucose, serum protein and albumin, calcium, thyroid function tests, erythrocyte sedimentation rate, stools for occult blood, urinalysis, and chest X ray. Further testing is guided by the history, physical examination, and results of screening laboratory tests (Marton et al. 1981; Morley et al. 1986).

The prevalence of malnutrition in older patients varies with the population studied. Malnutrition is reported in less than 5% of ambulatory outpatients but occurs in up to two-thirds of hospitalized and institutionalized older persons. This diagnosis often is missed; one study found that physicians did not record malnutrition or weight loss as a problem in nearly 50% of older outpatients with these problems, and the physicians prescribed nutritional supplements in only one-fourth of those affected (Manson and Shea 1991). Malnourished patients can present with weight loss, weakness, skin problems, and changes in mental status. Laboratory tests to identify malnutrition include serum albumin (a value less than 3 g/dl to 3.5 g/dl is significant), total lymphocyte count (values less than 1,500/cm^3 are significant), and the presence of anergy on skin testing. However, albumin may not be reliable and anergy may occur without malnutrition in older patients. Anthropometric measures such as age-adjusted weight and height, skinfold thickness, and arm muscle circumference can be used. Another commonly used measure is the body mass index, which is the body weight in kilograms divided by the square of height in meters. Calorie counts can determine whether the patient's energy intake is adequate. Treatment of malnutrition includes making food accessible, treating underlying causes, and using nutritional supplements (orally or by tube feedings) when appropriate (Morley 1986; Morley et al. 1986).

Anemia

Although mild anemia is common in older people and frequently no obvious etiology can be found, most authors recommend that the anemic older patient be evaluated for etiology. Healthy older people should maintain a normal hemoglobin value. The World Health Organization criterion for anemia is a hemoglobin less than 13 g/dl for men and 12 g/dl for women. Surveys suggest the incidence of anemia is 6% to 30% for elderly men and 10% to 22% for elderly women (Mansouri and Lipschitz 1992). The classic signs of anemia are pallor, weakness, and fatigue. The older anemic patient may present with behavioral changes or confusion. If the anemia is recognized and treated, the symptoms can respond dramatically to relatively small improvements in hemoglobin. Evaluation of the anemic patient should be approached systematically. A coexisting low platelet count and low white blood cell count suggests pancytopenia. An elevated reticulocyte count suggests that the patient's bone marrow is responding appropriately to some insult such as hemolysis, blood loss, or a toxin. A normal or low reticulocyte count (reticulocyte index less than two) in the face of anemia suggests that the bone marrow is not responding appropriately. Further identification of the anemia (based on the red blood cell size) as microcytic, macrocytic, or normocytic can be made by reviewing the peripheral smear. Multiple causes of anemia can coexist in the older patient.

The patient with a microcytic anemia (defined as a mean corpuscular volume [MCV] of less than 84 fl) should have serum iron studies and stool examination for occult blood. A low serum ferritin indicates iron deficiency and serum ferritin is the best predictor of bone marrow iron stores, but ferritin can be raised falsely into the normal range by liver disease or inflammatory disorders. Low serum iron and raised total iron-binding capacity (TIBC) can be seen in iron-deficiency anemia, but these tests may not be reliable in older patients because the presence of a chronic disease can lead to a normal or low total iron-binding capacity even in the presence of an iron-deficiency anemia. Authors vary in recommendations for serum testing for iron-deficiency anemia in elderly patients; bone marrow aspiration is needed to assess iron stores in some cases. Results from one study of iron deficiency in older persons suggest that older patients with a serum ferritin greater than 100 µg/L can be treated as not having iron deficiency, patients with serum ferritin less than 18 µg/L can be treated as having iron deficiency, and patients with values between 18 and 100 should have a bone marrow aspiration to evaluate iron stores (Guyatt et al. 1990). To avoid bone marrow aspiration until absolutely necessary, it may be assumed that the older patient has an iron-deficiency anemia if the serum ferritin level is less than or equal to 50 µg/L or if the serum ferritin level is less than or equal to 75 µg/L and the transferrin saturation (serum iron/TIBC) is less than or equal to .08. Intermediate results should be followed by bone marrow aspiration. The primary concern in the older patient with iron deficiency is gastrointestinal blood loss. Stool examination for occult blood is important; however, negative stool exams should not preclude bowel studies when an iron-deficiency anemia is present. Many geriatric physicians avoid barium studies and evaluate the iron-deficient patient with colonoscopy as the initial test to increase diagnostic accuracy and to avoid subjecting the older patient to two bowel preparation procedures.

Anemia of chronic disease is a diagnosis of exclusion made only in patients who have a documented chronic disease and otherwise normal hematological evaluation. Iron studies typically show decreased iron and TIBC.

Macrocytic anemia (defined as an MCV of more than 100 fl) from megaloblastic red blood cell changes in older patients can be caused by deficiency of folate or vitamin B_{12}. Red cell folate levels are more reliable than serum folate levels but are not available in all laboratories. If there is no malabsorption, folate deficiency can be corrected with folic acid (1 mg/day orally). The most frequent cause of vitamin B_{12} deficiency in the older patient is pernicious anemia. The normal lower limit of serum vitamin B_{12} level is uncertain in the older patient, and the necessity for a Schilling test to document pernicious anemia in every older patient with a low B_{12} has been debated. The Schilling test may be useful in patients with borderline B_{12} levels. Other measures of vitamin B_{12} deficiency that may help clarify the diagnosis include increased levels of methylmalonic acid in the urine and elevated serum methylmalonic acid or total homocystine level. Vitamin B_{12} deficiency is associated with a variety of neurological symptoms including paresthesias, dysesthesias, abnormal proprioception, and dementia. Psychiatric symptoms described include delirium, hallucinations, personality changes, delusions, depression, acute psychoses, and mania. Neurological changes of B_{12} deficiency can occur prior to hematological changes. Patients with vitamin B_{12} deficiency generally require lifelong monthly intramuscular B_{12} injections. Oral treatment usually is not effective. It has been debated whether folate deficiency alone can cause neurological symptoms. Correction of folate deficiency in the face of undiagnosed vitamin B_{12} deficiency can precipitate progression of neurological symptoms.

Normocytic anemia should be evaluated with stool examination for occult blood, a reticulocyte count, and examination of the peripheral smear for evidence of hemolysis. Testing for iron-deficiency anemia, folate deficiency, and B_{12} deficiency often are recommended in the older anemic patient because of the possibility of early or mixed disease (Cohen and Crawford 1986; Freedman 1985).

Thyroid Disease

Estimates of the prevalence of thyroid disease in elderly patients vary from less than 2% to as much as 14%. Higher rates are noted in hospital settings. In one study of hospitalized older patients, only 27% of patients had normal values for all thyroid function studies (Simons et al. 1990). The presentation of thyroid disease in the older patient may be subtle or atypical. Symptoms—such as fatigue, constipation, and functional decline—that are erroneously attributed by some to "old age" may be seen with thyroid disease. Screening for thyroid disease in older patients with psychiatric symptoms is recommended because thyroid disease in older patients is common and the symptoms can mimic or exacerbate psychiatric illness.

The immunoradiometric methods of thyroid-stimulating hormone assay (the so-called supersensitive thyroid-stimulating hormone measures) allow the distinction between normal (euthyroid) and low (hyperthyroid) levels of thyroid-stimulating hormone; therefore, this supersensitive thyroid-stimulating hormone assay may be used as a single screening test of thyroid function (Caldwell et al. 1985; Feit 1988). The thyroid-stimulating hormone response to exogenous thyrotropin-releasing hormone is used less commonly clinically but has been studied in older psychiatric patients. For example, patients with major depression have a blunted thyroid-stimulating hormone response; studies have varied on whether patients with Alzheimer's disease have a blunted thyroid-stimulating hormone response. Different etiologies have been suggested to explain these findings in terms of the pathophysiology of these psychiatric disorders (Molchan et al. 1991).

Older patients with hyperthyroidism may present with the classic signs and symptoms such as heat intolerance, weight loss, tremor, and palpitations. They may also present with single-organ-system symptoms (such as atrial fibrillation) or with "apathetic hyperthyroidism" (characterized by anorexia, fatigue, weight loss, and general decline) without the hypermetabolic symptoms of hyperthyroidism. Laboratory testing in hyperthyroidism reveals a high serum T_4; high free thyroxine index (FTI); and a low, generally undetectable thyroid-stimulating hormone. "T_3 thyrotoxicosis" is a hyperthyroid state with elevated serum T_3 but normal serum T_4. The initial test for hyperthyroidism should be a thyroid-stimulating hormone level. If the level is low, the serum free T_4 index or serum free T_4 concentration should be measured; a high value for either confirms the diagnosis of hyperthyroidism (Woeber 1992). Free T_3 level should be obtained if thyroid-stimulating hormone is low and T_4 is normal. Initial therapy for hyperthyroidism in the older patient generally involves a β-blocker such as propranolol and an antithyroid medication such as propylthiouracil. Definitive treatment in older patients usually is accomplished with radioactive iodine therapy, after which up to one-third of patients become hypothyroid.

The major symptoms of hypothyroidism in older patients are lassitude, constipation, cold intolerance, fatigue, and decreased mentation. The symptoms may develop slowly and be attributed to "aging," depression, or dementia. Patients with myxedema have the features of hypothyroidism with soft tissue accumulation of mucopolysaccharides. Laboratory testing in hypothyroidism reveals low serum T_4 and FTI with elevated levels of thyroid-stimulating hormone. In frail older patients, or those with cardiac disease, thyroid hormone replacement starts at low doses, such as 0.025 mg of L-thyroxine per day, and is gradually increased by 0.025 mg at monthly intervals; patients are monitored for side effects and normalization of serum thyroid-stimulating hormone levels. Overreplacement should be avoided, so thyroid hormone dose should be increased until the thyroid-stimulating hormone level is within but not below the normal range. Myxedema coma is a life-threatening presentation of hypothyroidism that occurs almost exclusively in patients older than age 50. It generally occurs in patients with chronic myxedema who experience some additional insult such as sedating medications or an acute illness. Myxedema coma is a medical emergency that requires intravenous L-thyroxine therapy (Robuschi et al. 1987).

Three additional patterns of TFT abnormality are euthyroid hyperthyroxinemia, euthyroid sick syndrome, and subclinical hypothyroidism. Euthyroid hyperthyroxinemia is characterized by an elevated T_4 with normal thyroid-stimulating hormone. These patients are clinically euthyroid, and the elevated serum T_4 level generally resolves spontaneously. Euthyroid sick syndrome, which is recognized by low serum T_3 or T_4 with normal serum thyroid-stimulating hormone, has been described in hospitalized patients with serious systemic illness of various etiologies. The reverse T_3 level usually is high in euthyroid sick syndrome. Subclinical (compensated) hypothyroidism is a very common pattern of abnormal TFTs in older patients characterized by elevated thyroid-stimulating hormone with normal T_4 and FTI. It may progress to overt hypothyroidism, especially in patients with thyroid-stimulating hormone values greater than 20 μU/ml or with high-titer positive thyroid microsomal antibodies (Rosenthal et al. 1987). The hypothyroidism should be treated in patients with high thyroid-stimulating hormone, normal T_4, and depression if the clinician believes the depression is caused by decreased thyroid function.

A significant percentage of newly admitted psychiatric patients who are clinically euthyroid have some abnormality in initial TFTs, particularly an elevated T_4 or FTI, that reverts to normal after approximately 2 weeks. In patients with an acute psychiatric illness, without signs or symptoms of thyroid disease and with mild or nonspecific abnormalities on initial TFTs, it is reasonable simply to observe the patients and repeat the TFTs after approximately 2 weeks (Feit 1988).

Geriatric Syndromes

Certain medical problems that are common in older patients may go untreated if they are not specifically addressed. They are singled out here to alert the psychiatrist to recognize these "geriatric syndromes" and to refer patients for evaluation when appropriate.

Hearing and Visual Impairment

Hearing impairment occurs in 25% to 45% of persons older than 65 and 90% of those older than 80. The normal ear is most sensitive to frequencies between 500 Hz and 4,000 Hz, the approximate range of human speech (Lavizzo-Mourey and Siegler 1992). Hearing loss in older people usually is in the high-frequency range, which is important in conversation. Although there are various definitions of hearing impairment, at least one author reports that hearing is abnormal in older people if pure tones softer than 40 dB in more than one frequency are not heard in one or both ears (Lavizzo-Mourey 1991).

Hearing impairment can be associated with significant emotional, social, and communication dysfunction—all of which can affect the quality of life of the older person (Mulrow et al. 1990). However, fewer than 20% of those impaired receive any form of hearing aid. Screening guidelines have not been established; however, annual screening of older persons with a hand-held audioscope and use of a screening questionnaire has been recommended (Mulrow and Lichtenstein 1991). When there is a question of hearing impairment, the first step is to examine the ear for cerumen occluding the external ear canal. If the ear is clear of cerumen, patients can be tested with a hand-held audioscope or referred to an audiologist for testing. There are several questionnaires available to evaluate the significance of hearing impairment (American Speech, Language, and Hearing Association 1989; Lichtenstein et al. 1988; Mader 1984). Individuals with hearing impairment should be referred to an audiologist for assessment and prescription of an appropriate hearing device. Older patients who are initially reluctant to accept a hearing aid may, with encouragement, benefit markedly from the correction of their hearing impairment.

Visual impairment is present in almost 15% of persons ages 65 and older and in almost 30% of those over 85 years. The most frequent causes of blindness in older patients are cataracts and macular degeneration. Other important causes are glaucoma and diabetic retinopathy. Patients can be screened by testing visual acuity, performing an ophthalmoscopic examination, and checking intraocular pressure (Straatsma et al. 1985). Treatment of vision impairment in older people has a positive impact on their quality of life; one recent large study found that within 1 year of treatment for vision problems older people had better driving skills, participated in more activities, had better mental health, and reported more life satisfaction (Brenner et al. 1993).

Urinary Incontinence

Urinary incontinence is a problem in up to one-third of community-dwelling older patients and in even higher numbers of those acutely hospitalized. The majority of patients with incontinence have some relief of symptoms if the incontinence is recognized by the clinician, properly evaluated, and treated. However, the patient may not mention the incontinence unless specifically asked. Incontinence can be an acute or chronic problem. Common causes of acute incontinence are urinary tract infection, restricted mobility, altered mental status, drugs (particularly diuretics and those with anticholinergic or sedating properties), polyuria, and fecal impaction. Patients who suddenly develop urinary incontinence should have some procedure (straight catheterization or bladder ultrasound) to rule out urinary retention with overflow incontinence. A postvoid residual of more than 100 ml is considered significant (Ouslander 1986).

There are various classifications of chronic urinary incontinence. One commonly used system classifies chronic incontinence as stress, urge, overflow, or functional incontinence. The initial evaluation of chronic incontinence includes a focused history and physical examination including pelvic examination in women, a urinalysis, and postvoid residual determination. It is not clear whether treating asymptomatic bacteriuria in the patient with chronic incontinence is of any benefit; however, most authors recommend a course of antibiotic in this situation (Ouslander 1986).

Symptoms of stress incontinence include loss of small amounts of urine with increases in intra-abdominal pressure such as a cough or laugh. The presence of stress incontinence can be documented by the "pad test" where the female patient with a full bladder is asked to cough while holding a pad between her legs; involuntary loss of urine establishes the diagnosis. Common treatments of stress incontinence include Kegel exercises or an α-adrenergic agonist (such as phenylpropanolamine) and perhaps estrogen.

The patient with urge incontinence usually describes an uncontrollable urge to void, with loss of large amounts of urine. Simple bedside cystometry (which involves filling the bladder via a urethral catheter to capacity or until an involuntary detrusor contraction occurs) may identify the involuntary bladder contractions of urge incontinence. Referral for formal cystometry may be indicated. Urge incontinence is commonly treated with an agent such as oxybutynin.

Overflow incontinence is the loss of small amounts of urine associated with an overdistended bladder. Patients with overflow incontinence and a significant postvoid residual should have urologic evaluation. Functional incontinence is loss of urine associated with an inability to get to the toilet because of immobility or other functional problems. Several measures to improve access to the toilet may improve functional incontinence. It is essential to realize that a patient may have multiple causes of incontinence. Referral to a specialist is recommended for patients with chronic urinary incontinence that is difficult to diagnose or is present in a patient with other findings such as severe pelvic prolapse in women, an enlarged prostate in men, or hematuria or prior urologic procedure in either gender.

Falls

Falls occur in one-third of community-dwelling persons older than age 65 and in more than one-half of nursing home residents each year. Falls increase with age and are more common in women until age 75, after which the frequency is similar in both sexes (Tinetti and Speechley 1989). Researchers have found that 5% of falls result in a fracture, and up to 10% of falls result in other serious injury. The wide range of etiologies for falls in older persons includes neurological disorders (such as Parkinson's disease) with gait and postural abnormalities, environmental hazards (such as loose rugs or electric cords), drugs that cause orthostatic hypotension, and mental status changes. Falls have multiple causes in most cases. The psychiatrist should question the older person about falls, particularly when medications are added or when dosage changes are made (Tinetti et al. 1988). At least one recent study suggests that falls are a marker for serious underlying illnesses and disabilities that can be identified and potentially treated. The majority of these underlying problems can be identified from a careful history and physical examination (Rubenstein et al. 1990).

Immobility

Immobility can have serious consequences in older patients. These consequences include contractures (which can develop in days or weeks), deep venous thrombosis and embolization, osteopenia, orthostasis, atelectasis and pneumonia, constipation, urinary retention, and pressure sores. Common conditions that lead to immobility in older patients are arthritis, hip fracture, stroke, generalized weakness, and pain. Patients confined to bed should be mobilized as quickly as possible. Bedridden patients should have range-of-motion exercises to prevent contractures and subcutaneous heparin therapy to prevent thrombosis; they should be turned frequently to avoid skin breakdown (Harper and Lyles 1988).

Pressure Sores

The majority of pressure sores occur in older patients, with a prevalence of up to 30% in older hospitalized patients. More than 90% of pressure sores occur over one of the following sites: sacrum, ischial tuberosity, greater trochanter, calcaneus, and lateral malleolus. Factors that lead to pressure sores include pressure to one area for more than 2 hours, shearing forces, friction on the skin surface, and moisture (Allman 1989). Methods of preventing pressure sores include mobilizing patients, relieving pressure in bedridden patients (by repositioning the body at a 30° angle every 2 hours), keeping skin clean and dry, and maintaining adequate nutrition. Pressure sores that are limited to the dermis (grade I) or subcutaneous fat (grade II) are treated by being kept clean and dry. Pressures sores that involve, but are limited by, the deep fascia (grade III) or are extensive in depth and penetrate the deep fascia (grade IV) can be treated with debridement and loosely packed saline-soaked gauze dressing changes. Surgical repair may be more appropriate, however. The clinician should be aware of closed pressure sores, which are extensive deep fascia wounds that appear benign on the surface (Shea 1975). Many different skin preparations and dressings are available for the treatment of pressure sores; no consensus has yet been reached on the most appropriate treatments to use for particular types of pressure sores (D. M. Smith et al. 1991).

Common Laboratory Abnormalities

Various screening laboratory tests often are obtained in older patients who present with psychiatric symptoms (see Table 9–3). The psychiatrist should be familiar with the initial approach to abnormalities of these tests and obtain referral when appropriate. The approach to anemia, glucose abnormalities, abnormal thyroid function test, vitamin B_{12} deficiency, and folate deficiency already have been addressed.

Serum Electrolytes

Serum sodium level reflects body water balance. Hypernatremia usually is the result of fluid loss (e.g., from diarrhea, osmotic diuresis, sensible losses, and diabetes insipidus from lithium therapy); patients with hypernatremia (who have increased plasma osmolality) should develop thirst. However, older patients have been shown to have a decrease in thirst sensation (hypodipsia) and are at risk for dehydration. Patients with hypernatremia can present with confusion.

Hyponatremia can result from a variety of etiologies. Treatment of hyponatremia requires clinical assessment of volume status. This assessment is critical because patients with volume excess and edema, and those with the syndrome of inappropriate antidiuretic hormone secretion, are treated with water restriction; those with decreased volume status are treated with saline (Narins et al. 1982). Symptoms depend on the severity of hyponatremia and how rapidly the change in sodium level has occurred. CNS symptoms such as confusion, lethargy, coma, and seizures are associated with sodium levels below 120 to 125 mEq/L.

Blood Urea Nitrogen and Creatinine

Glomerular filtration rate declines with age and places older patients at increased risk for developing acute renal failure when exposed to insults such as nephrotoxic drugs and dyes or episodes of low renal perfusion. Blood urea nitrogen and creatinine may overestimate renal function in older patients because of decreased protein intake and decreased muscle mass. Therefore, serum levels of blood urea nitrogen and creatinine may be within normal limits despite decreased renal function, and minor elevations of these tests may represent significant renal impairment. Equations designed to calculate estimated creatinine clearance often are erroneous in older people. Timed collection of urine to estimate creatinine clearance is recommended (Malmrose et al. 1993). Medications with renal excretion (e.g., penicillin and some other antibiotics, aspirin, and bronchodilators) should be prescribed initially in low doses in older patients, and drug levels should be monitored (if available).

Liver Function Tests

Liver function remains adequate throughout life in normal older patients. There is evidence, however, that hepatic metabolism of some drugs decreases with age, and caution should be taken with these agents.

Commonly ordered screening tests that reflect liver disease include bilirubin, transaminases, and alkaline phosphatase. These tests may be abnormal in a variety of disorders such as viral hepatitis, drug-induced hepatitis, cirrhosis, biliary tract obstruction, malignancy, hemolysis, and prolonged fasting. Some psychiatric medications may cause hepatitis. Drug-induced hepatitis can present with a cholestatic, a hepatitic, or a mixed pattern. Phenothiazines can cause a cholestatic-type drug-induced hepatitis with marked bilirubin elevation (primarily direct bilirubin), marked alkaline phosphatase elevation, and only mild to moderate transaminase elevations. Monoamine oxidase inhibitors can cause a predominantly hepatitic picture with marked transaminase elevation and lesser increase in alkaline phosphatase.

Syphilis Serology

There has been a dramatic increase in the number of cases of primary and secondary syphilis reported in the United States. One recent study suggested an increase in early (recently acquired) syphilis in elderly patients

(Berinstein and DeHertogh 1992). There are two basic types of serological tests for syphilis. The first is nonspecific reagin antibody testing (e.g., Venereal Disease Research Laboratories test [VDRL] and Rapid Plasma Reagin [RPR] test). The second is specific antitreponemal antibody testing (e.g., Fluorescent Treponemal Antibody-Absorption Test for Syphilis [FTA-ABS] and the Microhemagglutinations-Treponema pallidum [MHA-TP] immobilization test). The VDRL and RPR tests have a high false-positive rate; therefore, positive results should be followed by an FTA-ABS or MHA-TP test. A false-negative VDRL test may occur in patients with primary syphilis who have not yet developed reactivity. In one-third of patients with latent or tertiary syphilis, the VDRL titer may spontaneously decline over time. One recent study in an acute care setting found that many older patients with positive syphilis serology did not have adequate evaluation (Naughton and Moran 1992).

Asymptomatic neurosyphilis develops in approximately one-third of patients after 1 year or more of untreated syphilis. Symptomatic neurosyphilis can be meningovascular, parenchymal, or mixed disease. Meningovascular neurosyphilis presents as subacute or chronic meningitis. Parenchymal neurosyphilis may present as general paresis or tabes dorsalis. General paresis is characterized by progressive dementia, alterations in speech, and generalized weakness with hyperreflexia. Irritability, grandiose delusions, and hallucinations may occur. Tabes dorsalis is characterized by progressive ataxia, paresthesias, sharp pains, and sensory dysfunction. The Argyll-Robertson pupil (reacts to accommodation but not to light) may be seen in general paresis and in tabes dorsalis.

The diagnosis of neurosyphilis is based on cerebrospinal fluid findings of an elevated protein level and/or mononuclear pleocytosis. A positive cerebrospinal fluid VDRL test is diagnostic but not present in all cases. Older patients with positive serology and neurological symptoms should have a lumbar puncture.

Penicillin is the treatment of choice for all stages of syphilis. Specific treatment recommendations vary. Primary, secondary, and latent syphilis of less than 1 year's duration should be treated with 2.4 million units of benzathine penicillin intramuscularly as a single dose. The classic treatment for neurosyphilis is a 10-day course of intravenous penicillin followed by three weekly doses of benzathine penicillin.

After therapy for syphilis, the results of VDRL testing should be followed for evidence of decline in titer or conversion to seronegative status (which may take months). The results of FTA-ABS testing remain positive with or without therapy. Lumbar puncture should be repeated in patients with neurosyphilis to determine adequacy of treatment (Ward and Szebenyi 1986).

Urinalysis

Urinary tract infection is the most common cause of gram-negative sepsis in older patients. Symptoms of urinary tract infection in older patients may include changes in mental status; functional decline; abdominal pain or nausea and vomiting in addition to, or instead of, dysuria; and urinary frequency. Older patients with serious infection may lack a febrile response. Urinalysis usually reveals bacteriuria and, commonly, enteric rods. Some older patients may not have significant pyuria. Diagnosis of urinary tract infection is made based on urine culture and sensitivity. Mild symptomatic urinary tract infection in older patients should be treated with a 7- to 10-day course of oral antibiotics rather than the single-dose therapy recommended for younger patients. Intravenous antibiotic treatment is recommended for serious infection. Men with urinary tract infections (not related to recent catheterization) and women with recurrent urinary tract infections should have a urologic referral (Zweig 1987).

Asymptomatic bacteriuria is common in older patients, especially women, and increases in frequency with age, hospitalization, and institutionalization. Its significance is unclear. Treatment of asymptomatic bacteriuria has not been shown to affect subsequent morbidity or mortality and probably should not be undertaken (Nordenstam et al. 1986). However, patients with incontinence and asymptomatic bacteriuria probably deserve a trial of antibiotic therapy. Almost all patients with chronic indwelling urinary catheters will have bacteriuria and pyuria. These patients should not be treated with antibiotics if asymptomatic (Ouslander 1986).

Medical Clearance for Electroconvulsive Therapy

Electroconvulsive therapy (ECT) is an effective and safe form of treatment for depression in elderly patients. Patients who fail to respond to chemical antidepressant therapy may respond to ECT at a rate as high as 80% to 85%. However, subjects over age 80 years may have more cardiovascular complications and falls with ECT therapy compared to subjects ages 65–80 (Cattan et al. 1990). Maintenance ECT has been found to be safe and effective for patients over age 75 years, even in the presence of medical disease (Dubin et al. 1992).

Pretreatment evaluation of the older patient prior to ECT should focus on neurological and cardiovascular status. A contraindication to ECT is the presence of increased intracranial pressure. ECT can be given safely in stroke patients after neurological status has stabilized or even in patients with brain tumors who are carefully monitored during treatments.

Cardiac events are the major cause of mortality reported from ECT. Patients with cardiac disease have a higher rate of cardiac complications during ECT, but with close monitoring (for arrhythmias and ischemic episodes), ECT can be given with relative safety even to patients with severe cardiovascular disease (Zielinski et al. 1993). All older patients should have cardiac monitoring during ECT treatments. ECT causes a diffuse autonomic discharge that can lead to severe bradycardia or even asystole if patients are not given atropine for cholinergic blockade. Heart rate, blood pressure, and plasma catecholamines increase immediately after ECT in patients who are given atropine. Pretreatment evaluation of cardiac status should focus on the presence of hypertension, angina, heart failure, and arrhythmias. If these problems are controlled, the patient may have ECT (Pearlman 1991). Patients with hypertension who develop extreme blood pressure rise after ECT may need to have a prophylactic β-blocker. Calcium channel blockers and nitroprusside have been used to reduce the blood pressure rise after ECT. β-Blockade also may be necessary in patients with angina. Intravenous lidocaine may be used in patients with a history of ventricular arrhythmia; however, it is best given after the electrically induced convulsion because lidocaine can interfere with seizure induction. Pacemaker patients can receive ECT after pacer function has been documented. Demand pacemakers should be converted to fixed mode with an external magnet immediately prior to ECT, and the patient should be appropriately grounded. ECT has been done in the immediate postmyocardial infarction period in severe cases of depression, generally with a resuscitation team present. However, if possible, it is recommended to wait at least 6 weeks after myocardial infarction to allow cardiac status to stabilize.

Patients with respiratory diseases may be at increased risk from ECT, particularly those patients with ventilatory compromise and/or carbon dioxide retaining patients with compromised hypoxic drive who may not tolerate the brief period of apnea with ECT. Prolonged apnea has been reported in patients taking the drug echothiophate in eyedrop form to prevent glaucoma when succinylcholine is administered for ECT (Packman 1978). This drug should be discontinued before ECT therapy is instituted.

Many of the potential risks of ECT therapy can be prevented with careful technique. In selected patients, pretreatment oxygen therapy may decrease the risk of memory deficits and cardiac arrhythmias. Succinylcholine is given for muscle relaxation to decrease cardiovascular strain and decrease the risk of fractures; this is particularly important in patients with osteoporosis. Cardiac monitoring is required as previously noted. Atropine can prevent the risk of bradycardia and asystole; it should be decreased in dosage or avoided in patients with pacemakers, arrhythmias, or hypertension. Patients with glaucoma should have adequate topical treatment prior to pretreatment atropine (Elliot et al. 1982; Salzman 1982; Woodcock 1983).

Several psychotropic medications may interact with ECT therapy. Concomitant use of ECT and lithium should be avoided because of the reported risks of developing delirium (sometimes with seizure) and prolongation of neuromuscular blocking drugs used during ECT. Most experts recommend stopping antidepressants prior to ECT, primarily because of concerns over adverse cardiovascular effects. However, there is evidence that the combination of ECT and antidepressant therapy may be beneficial in some cases. The abrupt discontinuation of certain psychotropic drugs, especially those with strong anticholinergic effects, can be problematic. There is some evidence that benzodiazepines may reduce the therapeutic effect of ECT. Neuroleptics are believed to be safe with ECT; some data suggest a beneficial effect of the combination of neuroleptics and ECT (Kellner et al. 1991).

Cognitive effects of ECT are another important consideration. Transient memory loss (retrograde and anterograde) is well documented. These cognitive effects may be lessened by attention to electrode placement and stimulus dosage. Animal studies and limited human trials suggest that treatment with drugs with antiamnestic properties (e.g., opioid antagonists, vasopressin, and adrenocorticotropic hormone) may lessen cognitive effects; usefulness of these agents is not clear, however (Krueger et al. 1992). The most promising drug therapy for attenuating cognitive effects of ECT may be administration of T_3; a controlled trial is under way to test the effectiveness of this therapy.

Medical Aspects of Antidepressant Therapy

The major adverse side effects of the tricyclic and tetracyclic antidepressant medications include sedation and anticholinergic, adrenergic, and cardiovascular effects. The sedative effects of some antidepressants can pose a major problem in older patients. Nighttime dosing of sedating antidepressants (such as tertiary amines) or use of less-sedating drugs (such as secondary amines) can help prevent this problem. Anticholinergic effects can occur with nearly all tricyclic and tetracyclic antidepressants. Newer heterocyclic compounds (e.g., trazodone and fluoxetine) avoid anticholinergic effects. Typical anticholinergic effects include delirium, dry mouth, constipation, tachycardia, blurred vision, and urinary retention. An increase in heart rate may not be tolerated in patients with unstable angina, and patients with chronic atrial fibrillation should be carefully observed. Patients should be questioned about these anticholinergic symptoms and about signs of adrenergic hyperactivity such as tremors and sweating. Some clinicians suggest using bethanechol to reduce anticholinergic side effects in patients who otherwise do well on tricyclics; however, availability of newer antidepressants with little or no anticholinergic side effects may make this practice unnecessary. Usually it is best to treat drug side effects by decreasing or eliminating the offending agent rather than adding another drug. Clinically significant orthostatic hypotension is common with antidepressant therapy in older patients and is presumably caused by antagonism of peripheral α_1-adrenergic receptors. The best predictor of postural hypotension with antidepressant therapy is preexisting orthostatic hypotension. Orthostatic hypotension is more likely to develop in patients with left ventricular impairment and/or in patients taking other drugs like diuretics or vasodilators (Glassman and Preud'homme 1993). Careful monitoring of orthostatic blood pressure and symptoms of hypotension is required before and during treatment. The occurrence of orthostatic hypotension may be reduced with low doses, divided doses, and slowly increasing doses. Paradoxically, pretreatment orthostatic hypotension was shown in a study to predict favorable treatment response (Jarvik et al. 1983). Bupropion and serotonin selective reuptake inhibitors do not appear to cause orthostatic hypotension. Monoamine oxidase inhibitors, on the other hand, may lead to orthostatic hypotension, supine hypotension, and hypertensive reactions.

A quinidine-like effect has been demonstrated by a reduced frequency of premature ventricular contractions in patients receiving imipramine, nortriptyline, or maprotiline. These agents may prolong intracardiac conduction. Caution is recommended in patients with preexisting conduction disturbances and those receiving class IA antiarrhythmic drugs such as quinidine. The antiarrhythmic agent may need to be reduced or discontinued while the patient is receiving an antidepressant. In vitro studies have demonstrated that these drugs do not lower cardiac output even in patients with impaired ventricular function. Agents such as bupropion, trazodone, and serotonin selective reuptake inhibitors do not appear to prolong cardiac conduction and appear to be safe in patients with conduction disease. Bupropion has some antiarrhythmic properties and trazodone has been show to be arrhythmogenic (Glassman and Preud'homme 1993). Monoamine oxidase inhibitors do not seem to have significant cardiac conduction, rhythm, or left ventricular function effects.

An electrocardiogram should be taken prior to initiating antidepressant therapy in older patients. It has been suggested that tricyclic antidepressants should not be started if bifascicular block, second-degree heart block, or Q-T prolongation is present, unless the patient is under careful observation in a hospital setting. Simple first-degree arteriovenous block or hemiblock increases the risk of complications to a small, but probably insignificant, degree. A repeat electrocardiogram after treatment has begun is necessary in all patients with heart disease to monitor prolongation of the PR, QT, and QRS duration (which most patients develop); worsening of arteriovenous block; and ventricular arrhythmias (Dietch and Fine 1990; Thompson et al. 1983; Veith 1982). ECT generally is preferred in patients with significant heart disease and severe depression. If there are no contraindications, other antidepressants, such as monoamine oxidase inhibitors, may be useful.

Conclusions

Medical illness is common in older patients, and geriatric psychiatrists should be aware of physical problems that may be affecting their patients. Older patients frequently have causative or coexistent medical illness that can affect their psychiatric care significantly. The psychiatrist should be able to recognize medical problems, initiate treatment, and refer to other clinicians when appropriate.

References

Abramowicz M: Drugs that can cause psychiatric symptoms. Med Lett Drugs Ther 28:81–86, 1986

Alessi CA, Henderson CT: Constipation and fecal impaction in the longterm care patient. Clin Geriatr Med 4:571–588, 1988

Alexopoulos GS, Young RC, Meyers BS, et al: Late-onset depression.

Psychiatr Clin North Am 11:101–112, 1988

Allman RM: Pressure ulcers among the elderly. N Engl J Med 320:850–853, 1989

American Speech, Language, and Hearing Association: Guidelines for the identification of hearing impairment/handicap in adult/elderly persons. American Speech, Language, Hearing Association Journal 31:59–63, 1989

Applegate WB: Hypertension in elderly patients. Ann Intern Med 110:901–915, 1989

Berinstein D, DeHertogh D: Recently acquired syphilis in the elderly population. Arch Intern Med 152:330–332, 1992

Brenner MH, Curbow B, Javitt JC, et al: Vision change and quality of life in the elderly: response to cataract surgery and treatment of other chronic ocular conditions. Arch Ophthalmol 111:680–685, 1993

Caldwell G, Gow SM, Sweeting VM, et al: A new strategy for thyroid function testing. Lancet 1:1117–1119, 1985

Calkins E, Davis PT, Ford AB (eds): The Practice of Geriatrics. Philadelphia, PA, WB Saunders, 1986

Cassel CK, Walsh JR, Shepard M: Clinical evaluation of the patient, in Geriatric Medicine, 2nd Edition. Edited by Cassel CK, Reisenberg D, Sorenson LB, et al. New York, Springer-Verlag, 1989, pp 102–110

Cattan R, Barry PP, Mead G, et al: Electroconvulsive therapy in octogenarians. J Am Geriatr Soc 38:753–758, 1990

Cohen HJ, Crawford J: Hematologic problems, in The Practice of Geriatrics. Edited by Calkins E, Davis PJ, Ford AB. Philadelphia, PA, WB Saunders, 1986, pp 519–531

Connell AM, Hilton C, Irvine G, et al: Variation of bowel habits in two population samples. Br Med J 2:1095–1099, 1965

Consensus Conference: Differential diagnosis of dementing diseases. JAMA 258:3411–3416, 1987

Cooppan R: Determining the most appropriate treatment for patients with non-insulin dependent diabetes mellitus. Metabolism 365:17–21, 1987

Cummings JL: Acute confusional states, in Clinical Neuropsychiatry. New York, Grune & Stratton, 1985, pp 68–74

Cummings JL, Benson DF: Dementia: A Clinical Approach. Boston, MA, Butterworth, 1984

Dahlof B, Lindholm LH, Hansson L, et al: Morbidity and mortality in the Swedish Trial in old patients with hypertension (STOP-Hypertension). Lancet 338:1281–1285, 1991

Dietch JT, Fine M: The effect of nortriptyline in elderly patients with cardiac conduction disease. J Clin Psychiatry 51:65–67, 1990

Donald IP, Smith RG, Cruikshank JG, et al: A study of constipation in the elderly living at home. Gerontology 31:112, 1985

Dubin WR, Jaffe R, Roemer R, et al: The efficacy and safety of maintenance ECT in geriatric patients. J Am Geriatr Soc 40:706–709, 1992

Elliot DL, Linz DH, Kane JA: Electroconvulsive therapy: pretreatment medical evaluation. Arch Intern Med 142:979–981, 1982

Feit H: Thyroid function in the elderly. Clin Geriatr Med 4:151–161, 1988

Freedman ML (ed): Clinical disorders of iron metabolism in the elderly. Clin Geriatr Med 4(1):729–745, 1985

Glassman AH, Preud'homme XA: Review of the cardiovascular effects of heterocyclic antidepressants. J Clin Psychiatry 54 (suppl):16–22, 1993

Guyatt GH, Patterson C, Ali M, et al: Diagnosis of iron-deficiency anemia in the elderly. Am J Med 88:205–209, 1990

Hansson L: Future goals for the treatment of hypertension in the elderly with reference to STOP-Hypertension, SHEP, and the MRC trial in older adults. Am J Hypertens 6:405–435, 1993

Harper CM, Lyles YM: Physiology and complications of bedrest. J Am Geriatr Soc 36:1047–1054, 1988

Harris MI: Epidemiology of diabetes mellitus among the elderly in the United States. Clin Geriatr Med 6:703–719, 1990

Jarvik LF, Read SL, Mintz J, et al: Pretreatment orthostatic hypotension in geriatric depression: predictor of response to imipramine and doxepine. J Clin Psychopharmacol 3:368–372, 1983

Jenkinson ML, Bliss MR, Brain AT, et al: Peripheral arthritis in the elderly: a hospital study. Ann Rheum Dis 48:227–231, 1989

Jones MP, Schubert ML: What do you recommend for prophylaxis in an elderly woman with arthritis requiring NSAIDS for control? Am J Gastroenterol 86:264–268, 1991

Kane RL, Ouslander JB, Abrass IB: Essentials of Clinical Geriatrics, 2nd Edition. New York, McGraw-Hill, 1989

Kellner CH, Nixon DW, Bernstein HJ: ECT—drug interaction: a review. Psychopharmacol Bull 27:595–609, 1991

Kitchell MA, Barnes RF, Veith RC, et al: Screening for depression in hospitalized geriatric medical patients. J Am Geriatr Soc 30:174–177, 1982

Kolman PBR: The value of laboratory investigation of elderly psychiatric patients. J Clin Psychiatry 45:112–116, 1984

Koran LM, Sox HC, Marton KI, et al: Medical evaluation of psychiatric patients, I: results in a state mental health system. Arch Gen Psychiatry 46:733–740, 1989

Krueger RB, Sackeim ITA, Gamzu ER: Pharmacologic treatment of the cognitive side effects of ECT: a review. Psychopharmacol Bull 28:409–424, 1992

Lavizzo-Mourey RJ, Siegler EL: Hearing impairment in the elderly. J Gen Intern Med 7:191–198, 1992

Lederle FA, Busch DL, Mattox KM, et al: Cost-effective treatment of constipation in the elderly: a randomized double-blind comparison of sorbitol and lactulose. Am J Med 89:597–601, 1990

Lichtenstein MJ, Bess FH, Logan SA: Validation of screening tools for identifying hearing-impaired elderly in primary care. JAMA 259:2875–2878, 1988

Lipowski ZJ: Delirium in the elderly patient. N Engl J Med 320:578–581, 1989

Mader S: Hearing impairment in elderly persons. J Am Geriatr Soc 32:548–553, 1984

Malmrose LC, Gray SL, Pieper CF, et al: Measured versus estimated creatinine clearance in a high-functioning elderly sample: MacArthur Foundation study of healthy aging. J Am Geriatr Soc 41:715–721, 1993

Manson A, Shea S: Malnutrition in elderly ambulatory medical patients. Am J Public Health 81:1195–1197, 1991

Mansouri A, Lipschitz DA: Anemia in the elderly patient. Med Clin North Am 76:619–630, 1992

Marton KI, Sox HC Jr, Krupp JR: Involuntary weight loss: diagnostic and prognostic significance. Ann Intern Med 95:568–574, 1981

Messerli FH, Ventura HO, Amodea C: Osler's maneuver and pseudohypertension. N Engl J Med 312:1548–1551, 1985

Molchan SE, Lawlor BA, Hill JL, et al: The TRH stimulation test in Alzheimer's disease and major depression: relationship to clinical and CSF measures. Biol Psychiatry 30:567–576, 1991

Morley JE: Nutritional status of the elderly. Am J Med 81:679–695, 1986

Morley JE, Silver AJ, Fiatarone M, et al: Geriatric grand rounds: nutrition and the elderly. J Am Geriatr Soc 34:823–832, 1986

Moskowitz RW: Primary osteoarthritis: epidemiology, clinical aspects, and general management. Am J Med 83:5–10, 1987

MRC Working Party: Medical research council trial of treatment of hypertension in older adults: principal results. Br Med J 304:405–412, 1992

Mulrow CD, Aguilar C, Endicott JE, et al: Association between hearing impairment and the quality of life of elderly individuals. J Am Geriatr Soc 38:45–50, 1990

Mulrow CD, Lichtenstein MJ: Screening for hearing impairment in the

elderly: rationale and strategy. J Gen Intern Med 6:249–258, 1991

Narins RG, Jones ER, Stom MC, et al: Diagnostic strategies in disorders of fluid, electrolyte, and acid-base homeostasis. Am J Med 72:496–520, 1982

Naughton BJ, Moran MB: Patterns of syphilis testing in the elderly. J Gen Intern Med 7:273–275, 1992

Nordenstam GR, Brandenberg CA, Oden AS, et al: Bacteriuria and mortality in an elderly population. N Engl J Med 314:1152–1156, 1986

Okimoto JT, Barnes RF, Veith RC, et al: Screening for depression in geriatric medical patients. Am J Psychiatry 139:799, 1982

Ouslander JG: Illness and psychopathology in the elderly. Psychiatr Clin North Am 5:145–157, 1982

Ouslander JG (ed): Diagnostic evaluation of geriatric urinary incontinence. Clin Geriatr Med 2(4):715–730, 1986

Packman PM, Meyer DA, Verdum RM: Hazards of succinylcholine administration during electrotherapy. Arch Gen Psychiatry 35:1137–1141, 1978

Pearlman C: Electroconvulsive therapy: current concepts. Gen Hosp Psychiatry 13:128–137, 1991

Puxty JAH, Fox RA: Golytely : a new approach to fecal impaction in old age. Age Aging 15:182–184, 1986

Rapp SR, Parisi SA, Wallace CE: Comorbid psychiatric disorders in elderly medical patients: a 1-year prospective study. J Am Geriatr Soc 39:124–131, 1991

Riesenberg D: Diabetes mellitus, in Geriatric Medicine, 2nd Edition. Edited by Cecil CK, Riesenberg D, Sorenson LB, et al. New York, Springer-Verlag, 1989, pp 228–238

Robuschi G, Safran M, Braverman LE, et al: Hypothyroidism in the elderly. Endocr Rev 8:142–153, 1987

Rosenthal MJ, Hunt WC, Garry PJ, et al: Thyroid failure in the elderly: microsomal antibodies as discriminant for therapy. JAMA 258:209–213, 1987

Rossman I (ed): Clinical Geriatrics, 3rd Edition. Philadelphia, PA, JB Lippincott, 1986

Rowe JW, Besdine RW (eds): Geriatric Medicine, 2nd Edition. Boston, MA, Little, Brown, 1988

Rubenstein LZ, Josephson KR, Schulman BL, et al: The value of assessing falls in an elderly population: a randomized clinical trial. Ann Intern Med 113:308–316, 1990

Salzman C: Electroconvulsive therapy in the elderly patient. Psychiatr Clin

North Am 5:191–197, 1982

Shea JD: Pressure sores: classification and management. Clin Orthop 112:89–100, 1975

SHEP Cooperative Research Group: Prevention of stroke by antihypertensive drug treatment in older persons with isolated systolic hypertension. JAMA 265:3255–3264, 1991

Simons RJ, Simon JM, Demers LM, et al: Thyroid dysfunction in elderly hospitalized patients: effect of age and severity of illness. Arch Intern Med 150:1249–1253, 1990

Smith DM, Winsemius DK, Besdine RW: Pressure sores in the elderly: can this outcome be improved? J Gen Intern Med 6:81–93, 1991

Smith RG, Currie JEJ, Walls ADF: Whole gut irrigation: a new treatment for constipation. Br Med J (Clin Res Ed) 2:396–397, 1978

Soldo BJ, Manton KG: Health status and service needs of the oldest old: current patterns and future trends. Milbank Mem Fund Q Health Soc 63:286–319, 1985

Sorenson LB: Rheumatology, in Geriatric Medicine, 2nd Edition. Edited by Cecil CK, Reisenberg D, Sorenson LB, et al. New York, Springer-Verlag, 1989, pp 184–211

Stewart RB, Moore MT, Marks RG, et al: Correlates of constipation in an ambulatory elderly population. Am J Gastroenterol 87:859–864, 1992

Straatsma BR, Foos RY, Horwitz J, et al: Aging-related cataract: laboratory investigation and clinical management. Ann Intern Med 102:82–92, 1985

Sullivan DH, Martin W, Flaxman N, et al: Oral health problems and involuntary weight loss in a population of frail elderly. J Am Geriatr Soc 41:725–731, 1993

Thompson MP, Morris LK: Unexplained weight loss in the ambulatory elderly. J Am Geriatr Soc 39:497–500, 1991

Thompson TL, Moran MG, Nies AS: Psychotropic drug use in the elderly. N Engl J Med 308:194–199, 1983

Tinetti ME, Speechley M: Prevention of falls among the elderly. N Engl J Med 320:1055–1059, 1989

Tinetti ME, Speechley M, Ginter SF: Risk factors for falls among elderly persons living in the community. N Engl J Med 319:1701–1707, 1988

Tjoa HI, Kaplan NM: Treatment of hypertension in the elderly. JAMA 264:1015–1018, 1990

Tuck ML, Griffiths RF, Johnson LE, et al: Hypertension in the elderly. J Am Geriatr Soc 36:630–643, 1988

U'Ren RC: Anxiety, paranoia, and personality disorders, in Geriatric Medicine, 2nd Edition. Edited by Cecil CK, Reisenberg D, Sorenson LB, et al. New York, Springer-Verlag, 1989, pp 491–500

U'Ren RC, Riddle MC, Lezak MD, et al: The mental efficiency of the elderly person with type II diabetes mellitus. J Am Geriatr Soc 38:505–510, 1990

Veith RC: Depression in the elderly: pharmacologic considerations in treatment. J Am Geriatr Soc 30:581–586, 1982

Vickers R: Medical aspects of aging, in Essentials of Geriatric Psychiatry. Edited by Lazarus LW, Jarvik LF, Foster JR, et al. New York, Springer-Verlag, 1988

Ward TT, Szebenyi SE: Sexually transmitted diseases: syphilis, in A Practical Guide to Infectious Diseases, 2nd Edition. Edited by Reese RE, Douglas RG. Toronto, Little, Brown, 1986

Woeber KA: Thyrotoxicosis and the heart. N Engl J Med 327:94–98, 1992

Woodcock J: Psychiatry, in Medical Consultation: Role of the Internist on Surgical, Obstetric, and Psychiatric Services. Edited by Kammerer WS, Gross RJ. Baltimore, MD, William & Wilkins, 1983

Working Group on Hypertension in the Elderly: Statement on hypertension in the elderly. JAMA 256:70–74, 1986

Zielinski RJ, Roose SP, Devanand DP, et al: Cardiovascular complication of ECT in depressed patients with cardiac disease. Am J Psychiatry 150:904–909, 1993

Zweig S: Urinary tract infections in the elderly. Am Fam Physician 35:123–130, 1987

Jeff Victoroff, M.D.

The Neurological Evaluation

The primary goal of the neurological evaluation in geriatric psychiatry is to identify evidence of nervous-system dysfunction that may relate to psychiatric status. Traditionally, this is viewed as the opportunity to discover "organic" causes of psychiatric disturbance. However, our expanding knowledge of the biology of behavior compels us to reconsider this traditional view. Because we accept that all behavior is based in brain function, the distinction between "organic" and "nonorganic" or "functional" disturbances represents a false dichotomy. We are now trying to understand the way in which neurobiological factors interact with environmental/psychological factors to produce behavior. Therefore, our goal is to evaluate the role of the geriatric nervous system in mediating both the homeostasis of the internal biopsychological milieu and the patient's responsiveness to his or her environment and to attempt to identify changes in this nervous system/environment interaction that ultimately may be expressed as changes in behavior. In practical terms, we use the

This work is supported by National Institute on Aging Grant T32 AG001172-02 and by the French Foundation for Alzheimer's Research Grant L890608. I thank Drs. D. Frank Benson and Jeffrey L. Cummings for valuable editorial review and comment.

neurological evaluation—in concert with the history, mental status examination, medical examination, and selected laboratory tests—as one component of the integrated neurobehavioral approach to the geriatric psychiatric patient.

There are two kinds of changes in the geriatric nervous system that may be reflected as changes in behavior: 1) there are the changes related to normal aging and 2) there are pathological changes—many of which increase in incidence and prevalence among the elderly. After a review of the neurology of normal aging, I describe the common neurodegenerative disorders of elderly people. I conclude with a discussion of the neurological evaluation and its role in the comprehensive assessment of disorders of behavior in geriatric patients.

The Neurology of Normal Aging

Changes attributed to aging of the nervous system are usually regarded as negative and inevitable. However, three factors bear consideration. 1) It is often difficult to distinguish normal aging from pathological change. Some investigators argue that the role of aging has been overemphasized and that many age-associated decrements in function can actually be accounted for by a wide array of environmental factors (Rowe and Kahn 1987). 2) Although there are measurable decrements in some functions, we cannot presume that all of these changes are maladaptive. 3) There is considerable individual variation, with some individuals exhibiting substantial preservation of function. Nonetheless, the average aging nervous system undergoes several important changes that may have an impact on behavior, both by directly affecting function and by changing the way in which the patient perceives the environment.

The peripheral nervous system and the muscular system—the pathway of communication from the central nervous system to the motor system and the final motor effectors themselves—both exhibit a progressive and measurable decrement in function with advancing age. In many cases this represents a combination of age-related factors, diseases of the nervous system, and systemic diseases, including endocrine, nutritional, and vascular causes (Baker 1989). Primary sensory receptors change in structure and decline in number with age, and neurons exhibit 1) demyelination and remyelination, 2) distal greater than proximal axonal degeneration, 3) loss of fast-conducting peripheral axons, and 4) lipofuscin accumulation (Spencer and Ochoa 1981). There are age-related declines in the number of anterior horn cells and motor cranial nerve nuclei as well as demyelination and remyelination of motor roots. The result is a progressive decrease in the number of functioning motor units after age 60. Muscle fiber atrophy is common, particularly among the type II fibers, with a prolongation in isometric twitch properties, and total muscle mass may decrease by 25%–43%; remaining fibers exhibit signs of denervation, with the presence of target cells as well as ragged red fibers, ring fibers, lipofuscin accumulation, and increased interstitial connective tissue and fat (Hubbard and Squier 1989; Munsat 1984). Electrophysiology shows decreased amplitude of sensory action potentials, decline in both sensory and motor nerve conduction velocities, increased duration of motor units, and reduced somatosensory evoked potentials with age (Smith 1989). There is evidence that exercise may attenuate some of these age-related changes in skeletal muscle structure and function (Thompson 1994).

Most pertinent to the neuropsychiatric evaluation are the age-related changes in the brain. There have been estimates of loss of cortical neurons with aging as high as 30%–60%, corresponding to roughly 1% loss per annum above age 60, with the greatest losses among large neurons (Anderson et al. 1983; Henderson et al. 1980). Questions have been raised about the techniques used to make these estimates, but the bulk of evidence favors decreases in number of cortical neurons, in neuronal density, and in dendritic arborizations as well as a relative increase in glial cells (Coleman and Flood 1987). There are comparable losses of certain subcortical and brain stem neurons, especially in putamen, nucleus basalis of Meynert, substantia nigra, and locus ceruleus, with relative preservation of cells in the inferior oliva (Riederer and Krusik 1987). These neuronal losses represent population averages, and individuals may experience varying degrees of loss. There are age-related declines in both synapse density and reactive synaptogenesis (a marker of plasticity), although certain neuronal pools retain the capacity for synaptic sculpting throughout life, suggesting continued adaptability of the brain in older people (Cotman 1990; Masliah et al. 1993; Perry et al. 1993). There are age-related decreases in cerebral blood flow, independent of cerebral vascular disease (Takeda et al. 1988). It is less clear whether there is also a decline in cerebral metabolic rate, with some investigators finding clear age-related declines, particularly in frontal cortex (e.g., Chawluk et al. 1985) and others finding no decline with age (e.g., Rapoport 1986). This variability of findings may relate to selection bias in different studies or to the existence of regional declines in cerebral metabolism with age.

There are age-related changes in function that may relate to the physiological changes reviewed above, and these should be taken into account in the neurological examination of the elderly patient. Both special and general sensory systems decline in function. Motor performance exhibits an overall decline, more for maximal performance tasks than for habitual tasks (Stones and Kozma 1985). Strength, balance, postural reflexes, and hand steadiness all decline with age (Stelmach et al. 1989; Teravainen and Calne 1983). There is a drop-off in reaction time after the 20s, more marked after age 50 (Welford 1988). Note that both endurance and resistive exercise may significantly improve muscle strength and function in the elderly (Rogers and Evans 1993), suggesting that ongoing physical activity might ameliorate some of these observed age-related deficits. Aging may also have an impact on cognition, although it is difficult to determine whether such declines represent normal aging or reflect the earliest signs of progressive dementing processes. These cognitive declines appear in aspects of attention, memory, language, and spatial performance (Binks 1989; Kirasic and Allen 1985; Plude and Hoyer 1985).

In summary, the aging nervous system declines in structure and function, both centrally and peripherally. There may also be cognitive decline independent of the pathology of recognized dementing diseases. For both physical and cognitive function, it remains uncertain how much decline is inevitably age-related and how these changes may be modified by activity. A familiarity with these changes may offer perspective to the neurological evaluation of the elderly psychiatric patient, both by helping distinguish normal from pathological processes and by orienting the examination toward vulnerable systems that may affect behavior.

Common Neurological Disorders

Neurological disorders, including dementias, may be the most common cause of geriatric disability, outpacing respiratory, cardiovascular, and orthopedic/rheumatic disorders (Broe and Creasey 1989; Drachman and Long 1984). In addition to their direct impact on function, neurological disorders may interact with other disorders to produce disability, as for instance when weakness or sensory loss increase the risk of orthopedic disability. With the aging of the population and the advancement of medical treatment for nonneurological conditions, this disproportionate prevalence of neurological disorders will probably increase in the coming decades. Just as we face the challenge of determining whether age-related changes in the nervous system are "normal" or "pathological," we also face the challenge of determining whether late-onset neurological disorders represent exaggerations of normal aging or pathophysiologically distinct conditions. There is even some uncertainty regarding whether these clinically distinct disorders are actually separate diseases. Pending further advances in our knowledge of the biological causes of these disorders, it remains important to discriminate between these clinically distinguishable conditions. Nervous system disorders may result from a variety of insults, including trauma, neoplasia, metabolic disorders, infection, demyelinating disease, vascular disease, and neurodegeneration. Although the primary dementing conditions are described in other chapters, a brief discussion is offered here summarizing the clinical features, epidemiology, pathology, and treatment of the most common central nervous system disorders of the elderly.

Cerebrovascular disease (CVD) is a single term that encompasses a complex, multifaceted disorder. The brain may be injured by acute, subacute, or chronic vascular changes from the intracranial or extracranial circulatory system. Although CVD may refer to the steady-state condition of abnormal vasculature, in practice it usually refers to a spectrum of clinical events, and sequelae, related to altered blood flow in the brain: transient ischemic attack (TIA), reversible ischemic neurological deficit (RIND), ischemic and hemorrhagic infarction (stroke), and subarachnoid hemorrhage. By convention, TIAs refer to sudden focal neurological deficits attributed to cerebral ischemia, with complete clinical resolution within 24 hours, and RINDs refer to deficits persisting beyond 24 hours but resolving within 2 weeks. However, 35% of RINDs are associated with changes detected with the use of computed tomography (CT) (Koudstaal et al. 1992), suggesting that these categorical distinctions may not represent pathophysiological differences as much as clinically detectable reference points along a continuum. Stroke is the most common neurological disorder of the elderly and the third leading cause of death in the United States. Stroke rates are age-related, doubling with each decade from the fifth through the ninth. After an apparent decline in the rate of stroke during the 1960s and 1970s, attributed to increasingly successful management of hypertension, there is evidence of a leveling off of the rate of decline or possibly even an increase in stroke rate since the early 1980s.

TIAs can occur in the anterior (carotid) or posterior (vertebrobasilar) circulation. Common symptoms of carotid TIAs are transient monocular blindness (or amaurosis fugax), and transient hemispheric syndromes that often produce motor or sensory changes of a limb. Vertebrobasilar TIAs usually manifest as diplopia, vertigo, dysarthria, or ataxia. Although transient cerebral ischemia may also cause syncope or seizures, these clinical events themselves are not usually referred to as TIAs.

Stroke refers to the syndrome of a lasting change in central function attributed to CVD. The causes of stroke are manifold, but the most common categories include stroke caused by thrombosis within the intracranial vessel; stroke caused by embolus from the extracranial carotid artery; stroke as a result of cardiogenic embolus; stroke caused by global hypoperfusion; or stroke caused by hematological changes such as hypercoagulable states. The symptoms of stroke are extremely variable. Carotid territory hemispheric strokes often present with contralateral motor or sensory deficits, visual field deficits, or impairment of higher cortical functions such as aphasias, apraxias, or confusion. Vertebrobasilar territory strokes often present with dizziness or vertigo, ataxia or staggering gait, diplopia, occipital visual field deficits, or motor and/or sensory syndromes attributable to ischemia of the brain stem nuclei and tracts.

Intracranial hemorrhage may occur because of primary hypertensive hemorrhage, rupture of aneurysm or arteriovenous malformation, or trauma. Primary hypertensive hemorrhage, usually associated with long-standing chronic hypertension, has a rapid or sudden onset of focal neurological deficit, often progressing over several hours, sometimes accompanied by impairment of consciousness. The most common sites of primary hypertensive hemorrhage are the putamen and adjacent internal capsule, the thalamus, the cerebellum, and the pons. Subarachnoid hemorrhage, most often as a result of rupture of a saccular aneurysm, usually presents with the sudden onset of severe headache, often associated with nausea, vomiting, and impairment or loss of consciousness. Focal neurological deficits are less common. The outcome of subarachnoid bleeding is related to the relative preservation of consciousness after the bleeding. Minor head trauma may cause subdural hematoma in elderly individuals, which may present as headache, focal neurological deficits, lethargy, or simply as a change in behavior that is sometimes mistakenly attributed to neurodegenerative dementia or functional psychiatric disorder.

Treatment of stroke can be divided into primary prevention (before the first episode), secondary prevention (after the first episode), and acute intervention. Primary and secondary prevention of stroke focuses on control of known risk factors including hypertension, smoking, alcohol use, and obesity. Chronic antiplatelet therapy with aspirin or ticlopidine has been shown to reduce the risk of stroke among patients who have experienced a TIA or stroke. Some patients with symptomatic high-grade carotid stenosis (greater than 50%–75%) will benefit from carotid endarterectomy, although uncertainty remains regarding the best strategy for patient selection. The management of acute stroke is changing as new approaches and agents are developed. Although chronic hypertension may lead to stroke, there is evidence that blood pressure should not be lowered rapidly in the setting of an acute stroke since this may exacerbate cerebral hypoperfusion. Anticoagulation appears to be beneficial when the stroke is small, nonhemorrhagic, and progressing, and novel antithrombotic heparinoid agents may prove more efficacious than heparin. Other approaches to acute intervention under investigation include several reperfusion strategies such as hemodilution to reduce viscosity and improve cerebral blood flow, thrombolysis with agents such as streptokinase and tissue plasminogen activator, and thrombolysis via percutaneous transluminal intracranial angioplasty. Reports of the efficacy of the various reperfusion methods are mixed and involve possible increased risks of hemorrhage and edema. Recent findings regarding the cellular pathophysiological sequence of acute ischemic infarction suggest possible benefits of neuroprotective agents that may interrupt this sequence. Neurotoxicity as a result of postsynaptic reception of excitatory amino acid (EAA) neurotransmitters such as N-methyl-D-aspartate may be ameliorated by EAA receptor blockers or by agents that prevent EAA release, although receptor blockade may cause unacceptable behavioral side effects. Excessive calcium influx may contribute to cell death and may be inhibited by dihydropyridine calcium channel blockers. Free radical production may play a role in ischemic cell death, suggesting possible benefits of antioxidants or free radical scavengers such as the 21 amino steroids (lazaroids). Even a high dose of conventional glucocorticosteroids may prove beneficial if introduced early enough. Despite the promise of these new methods, most studies suggest a brief window for intervention with neuroprotective agents, perhaps limited to as little as 60–120 minutes after a stroke. Treatment of subarachnoid hemorrhage is focused on limiting further bleeding by management of blood pressure and surgical clipping of the aneurysm. Surgery has the best outcome in patients who have retained normal consciousness. Treatment of subdural hematoma depends on the size and the evidence of increased intracranial pressure or shift of intracranial structures. Large hematomas require surgical evacuation.

Temporal arteritis is a perivascular inflammatory condition of the temporal branches of the external carotid artery. The condition occurs almost exclusively in the elderly, most often affecting those ages 60 to 80. The patient presents with unilateral temporal region headache, ipsilateral visual impairment, as well as systemic signs of illness such as fever, anorexia, malaise or depression, increased white count, and elevated sedimentation rate. The involved temporal artery may be tender and prominent. There is an overlap between temporal arteritis and the syndrome of polymyalgia rheumatica, in which diffuse myalgia without focal weakness occurs, sometimes combined with the cranial symptoms and pathological changes of temporal arteritis (DiBartolomeo and Brick 1992). Because it is possible for temporal arteritis to occur in the presence of a normal sedimentation rate, psychiatrists may conceivably encounter depressed patients in whom this diagnosis has not previously been suspected. Prompt recognition is important, because intervention with corticosteroids may preserve vision.

Brain tumors occur throughout life, and primary intracranial tumors occur in roughly 10 per 100,000 adults, exhibiting an age-related increase in prevalence. The most common cell type first diagnosed among the elderly is the glioma, which accounts for nearly 50% of brain tumors. About half of gliomas are the slower-growing low-grade astrocytomas, whereas the other half are the fast-growing glioblastoma multiforme. Meningiomas account for about 15% of adult brain tumors; metastatic tumors, pituitary tumors, and acoustic neuromas each account for about 10% of tumors. The most common sources of adult brain metastases are the lung, breast, and gastrointestinal tract.

The clinical presentation of intracranial tumors depends greatly on both location and rate of growth. Slow-growing tumors may cause focal neurological signs, personality change, or seizures long before there is any symptomatic increase in intracranial pressure. Pituitary tumors may occur either with visual field defects related to pressure on the optic chiasm or endocrine dysfunctions related to the changes in the secretion of gonadotropins, prolactin, adrenocorticotropin, or thyroid-stimulating hormone. Tumors in the cerebellopontine angle, most often acoustic neuromas, may cause unilateral hearing loss and sometimes facial weakness or numbness. Rapidly growing tumors, either in the cerebellum or the cerebral hemispheres, may show signs and symptoms of increased intracranial pressure, including lethargy, confusion, ataxia, nausea, and vomiting. Tumors sometimes appear suddenly, like a stroke, either because they reach a critical threshold of size or because they hemorrhage. The clinical outcome of intracranial tumors also varies significantly depending on cell type, location, and rate of growth. Slow-growing meningiomas may be essentially cured by surgical removal. Fast-growing glioblastomas are notoriously difficult to treat and often lead to death within 1 year of diagnosis regardless of therapy.

Treatment of intracranial tumors is directed at decreasing intracranial pressure, unblocking flow of cerebrospinal fluid, removing the bulk of the tumor, and killing neoplastic cells. Depending again on the type and location of the tumor, treatment may involve several modalities, alone or in combination. Corticosteroids are used to control the vasogenic edema associated with many tumors. Neurosurgery may be used to biopsy the tumor to identify cell type, to remove the entire tumor, to reduce the size of the lesion without complete removal, or to shunt fluid from the ventricles. Conventional chemotherapy has been of limited value in the treatment of gliomas, the most common tumors of adulthood. Radiotherapy has been a mainstay of intracranial tumor treatment, and new techniques make it increasingly possible to deliver focused doses of irradiation via particle beams, high-energy stereotactic radiosurgery, or focused gamma rays. Promising new treatment avenues include immunotherapy, selective opening of the blood-tumor barrier to enhance chemotherapy, and gene therapy.

Subacute combined degeneration refers to the neurological disorder caused by vitamin B_{12} deficiency, most often related to pernicious anemia. There is loss of both myelin and axons in the white matter of the spinal cord, as well as peripheral neuropathy. This combination of lesions leads to the characteristic mix of upper and lower motor neuron signs, including absent ankle jerks and positive Babinski signs. Patients present with numbness and sometimes tingling of the feet, decreased position sense causing sensory ataxia, and spastic paraparesis. Cognitive changes and psychiatric symptoms are attributed to cerebral demyelination. Monthly vitamin B_{12} injections may restore some function and prevent further deterioration.

Parkinson's disease is a progressive disabling neurological condition. Parkinson's disease should be distinguished from parkinsonism, the associated clinical syndrome marked by motor slowing (bradykinesia or akinesia), rigidity, resting tremor, and disorders of gait and postural stability. While parkinsonism occurs in Parkinson's disease, this syndrome is not diagnostic of Parkinson's disease since it may also occur in other conditions involving damage to the nigrostriatal dopamine system. Parkinson's disease was first described by James Parkinson in 1817 (Tyler 1987), and seems to be one of the most common neurodegenerative disorders, although it is difficult to accurately measure the prevalence of Parkinson's disease because of variations in diagnostic threshold and access to expert neurological evaluation. It is clear, however, that the prevalence of Parkinson's disease is age related. Parkinson's disease is rare before age 40, with an age-related increase in prevalence rising rapidly with each decade, affecting roughly 1% of those over age 65 (Jankovic and Calne 1987). Many patients developed Parkinson's disease after the epidemic of encephalitis lethargica of 1917–1926, but this cannot be regarded as the principal cause of Parkinson's disease since the age-related incidence of Parkinson's disease is about the same in the population born after that epidemic. There may be a slightly higher prevalence among men than among women. Idiopathic Parkinson's disease is progressive, with or without treatment.

The cause of Parkinson's disease is unknown, but the pathology is well documented, with degeneration of the pigmented brain stem nuclei most severe in the dopaminergic neurons in the pars compacta of the midbrain's substantia nigra, which is the origin of the nigrostriatal dopamine pathway to the basal ganglia. Lewy bodies (eosinophilic intraneuronal cytoplasmic inclusions) are also associated with idiopathic Parkinson's disease. As noted above, a variety of conditions may damage the nigrostriatal dopamine system or the basal ganglia and produce parkinsonism. Idiopathic Parkinson's disease may be the most common of these, but research into the causes of Parkinson's disease has been advanced by the study of such causes of parkinsonism as the amyotrophic lateral sclerosis/parkinsonism/dementia complex that occurs in the Chamorro indians of Guam, and the syndrome produced by the toxic compound 1-methyl-D4-phenyl-1,2,5,6-tetrahydropyridine (MPTP). There is little evidence of a pattern of inheritance suggesting a genetic cause of idiopathic Parkinson's disease, and to date no environmental agent has been conclusively associated with the disease.

Clinically, the core syndrome is marked by an insidious onset of motor slowing, associated with a regular rhythmic resting tremor of about 4–7 Hz, most apparent in one or both hands, and a characteristic "cogwheel" rigidity of the limbs consisting of tremulous resistance to passive movement throughout the range of motion around large joints. In patients who have little or no tremor, the rigidity may have a smoother feel than classic cogwheeling. Facial expression is diminished (the "masklike" facies) and gait is usually abnormal, with a stooped posture, hesitation, shuffling, small steps, and a loss of postural righting reflexes that puts the patient at risk for falls. Behavior change in Parkinson's disease may affect up to 77% (Mortimer 1988), thus Parkinson's disease may be an important cause of psychiatric disability among the elderly. Identification of even subtle signs of Parkinson's disease on examination is important because there may be a long subclinical prodrome (Ward 1987) during which the patient may be at risk for behavioral complications such as depression and dementia with little overt evidence of the disease. Patients with prodromal Parkinson's disease exhibit increased sensitivity to neuroleptics. Depression in Parkinson's disease appears to be more frequent than can be accounted for by a reaction to disability. The clinical features of Parkinson's disease may vary considerably between patients, with asymmetric presentation or with relative predominance of tremor, rigidity, or postural instability. There is also considerable heterogeneity in age at onset, rate of progression, and responsiveness to medications (Koller 1992). The differential diagnosis of parkinsonism includes idiopathic Parkinson's disease, neuroleptic-induced parkinsonism, progressive supranuclear palsy, striatonigral degeneration or olivopontocerebellar atrophy, and parkinsonism associated with stroke. Certain clinical features may help to distinguish Parkinson's disease from the motor slowing of depression and from neuroleptic effects: the bradykinesia of Parkinson's disease, unlike that of depression, will usually be associated with rigidity. Neuroleptic-induced parkinsonism may present with cogwheel rigidity but is associated with resting tremor less often than is idiopathic Parkinson's disease.

The main treatment strategy for idiopathic Parkinson's disease has been to replete the dopamine deficit with the precursor L-dopa. To increase delivery of L-dopa to the brain, it is usually administered with carbidopa, which decreases the peripheral metabolism of L-dopa by inhibiting the enzyme dopa-decarboxylase. Alternative treatment strategies include agents such as pergolide mesylate and bromocriptine mesylate (direct dopamine receptor agonists), benztropine mesylate and trihexyphenidyl hydrochloride (anticholinergics), and the monoamine oxidase-B inhibitor L-deprenyl. These agents have been used alone or in combination with L-dopa-carbidopa. Anticholinergic agents may be particularly helpful for ameliorating tremor. Although most patients with idiopathic Parkinson's disease will benefit from these anti-Parkinson's treatments, patients with related disorders causing rigidity, such as stroke-induced parkinsonism, Wilson's disease, or multiple system atrophy, are less likely to respond. There is some evidence that L-deprenyl may delay the progression of Parkinson's disease. Interest is currently rapidly increasing regarding the potential benefits of transplanting fetal or recombinant cells into the brain to substitute for the loss of dopaminergic neurons, although this approach is in the early stages of development.

Multiple system atrophy (MSA) refers to a group of primary neurodegenerative conditions that have in common idiopathic neuronal loss in several central sites or systems. These conditions are probably best classified as variations on the theme of combined degeneration. MSA exhibits a predilection for damage to the basal ganglia (especially the posterior putamen and pars externa of the globus pallidus), the brain stem (especially the pontine nuclei and inferior olivas), the spinal cord (especially the intermediolateral cell columns), and the cerebellar Purkinje cells. Although the term MSA might well apply to most of the neurodegenerative conditions, including Parkinson's disease, Huntington's Disease, Friedreich's ataxia, and progressive supranuclear palsy, it is usually used to refer to 1) degeneration of the pons and cerebellum (olivopontocerebellar atrophy), 2) degeneration of the nigra and striatum (striatonigral degeneration), or 3) combinations of these two forms of degeneration. In general, MSA has earlier onset than idiopathic Parkinson's disease and a variety of neurological symptoms affecting muscle tone and movement. It is often associated with the autonomic symptoms of the Shy-Drager syndrome, particularly postural hypotension.

Olivopontocerebellar atrophy is a multiple system atrophy associated with degeneration of the inferior oliva and pontine nuclei of the brain stem and cerebellar atrophy most prominent in the middle cerebellar peduncles. The disorder is infrequent but not rare. Most cases may be inherited dominantly. Cerebellar ataxia is the outstanding clinical feature, but other clinical characteristics include parkinsonism, motor neuron syndrome, spasticity, and autonomic dysfunction with sometimes disabling postural hypotension. Olivopontocerebellar atrophy has been shown to be associated with cognitive deficits (Kish et al. 1988) and with depression. The autonomic dysfunction is associated with cell loss in the lateral horns and intermediolateral columns of the spinal cord. The parkinsonism may be associated with a loss of striatal dopamine (Kish et al. 1992). L-Dopa therapy is usually ineffective.

Striatonigral degeneration is a rarely diagnosed multiple system atrophy, clinically similar to Parkinson's disease, but with a different pathological picture. As in Parkinson's disease, there is progressive rigidity, bradykinesia, and postural instability. As in olivopontocerebellar atrophy, postural hypotension may occur in many cases. Pathologically, as in Parkinson's disease, there is cell loss in the pars compacta of the substantia nigra. Unlike Parkinson's disease, there is also degeneration in the putamen and caudate nuclei of the basal ganglia. These patients may initially be diagnosed with Parkinson's disease but tend to respond poorly to anti-Parkinson's agents.

Progressive supranuclear palsy is another progressive neurodegenerative condition that shares some clinical features with Parkinson's disease. The precise prevalence is unclear, but progressive supranuclear palsy is not a rare condition. Onset is typically between ages 50 and 70, with imbalance, visual complaints, and difficulty swallowing. As in Parkinson's disease, there is rigidity, most apparent in the trunk but also in the limbs. Unlike Parkinson's disease, there is a characteristic disorder of extraocular movements consisting of a supranuclear ophthalmoplegia, which first restricts downgaze, later upgaze, and later still may paralyze all voluntary eye movements. Reflex eye movements, induced by rapid passive head movement, are preserved, demonstrating that the pathway from the nuclei to the extraocular muscles is intact and that the dysfunction must be superior to these brain stem nuclei (hence, supranuclear). Patients also develop a pseudobulbar palsy consisting of slurred speech, masked facies, and dysphagia. Cognitive deficits are common as the disorder progresses. Pathological degeneration is found in several upper brain stem and diencephalic areas, including the vestibular nuclei, pretectal nuclei, superior colliculi, red nuclei, subthalamic nucleus, and globus pallidus. Treatment with anti-Parkinson's agents may be somewhat helpful for the rigidity.

Amyotrophic lateral sclerosis (ALS or Lou Gehrig's disease) is a motor neuron disorder with a prevalence of 4–6 per 100,000. Onset usually occurs after age 40, with a rapid rise in incidence over the subsequent three decades of life. The pathology of ALS involves loss of the anterior motor horn cells of the spinal cord and the motor nuclei of the brain stem (sparing the ocular motor nuclei), as well as corticospinal tract degeneration. The clinical presentation may reflect the spastic weakness of upper motor neuron damage, the flaccid/atrophic weakness of lower motor neuron involvement, or both. Typically patients present with weakness of one or more limbs, gait disorder, dysarthria, dysphagia, and muscle atrophy. The neurological examination reveals variable degrees of weakness and muscle atrophy with fasciculations, often including characteristic atrophy and fasciculations of the tongue. Deep tendon reflexes may be increased or decreased. Sensation and mentation are typically preserved, unfortunately leaving patients with clear insight into their inevitable deterioration. The principal differential diagnosis is cervical spondylosis, which can mimic most of the clinical syndrome of ALS but is much more likely to be treatable. ALS is progressively disabling, ultimately affecting essentially all the major axial muscle groups, including respiratory muscles, with death usually occurring 2 to 5 years after onset. About 10% of cases are familial. It has recently been shown that familial ALS is associated with mutations of the gene on chromosome 21q encoding Cu/Zn-binding superoxide dismutase (Rosen et al. 1993), suggesting that the pathophysiology of ALS is related to toxicity by the superoxide anion. This finding has generated hope that antioxidant therapy, for instance with vitamin E, may have a neuroprotective effect in ALS. Excitatory neurotoxicity associated with glutamate may also play a role in the pathophysiology of ALS. There is recent promising evidence that riluzole (2-amino-6-[trifluoromethoxy]benzothiazole), which modulates glutaminergic neurotransmission, may slow progression and improve survival of patients with ALS (Bensimon et al. 1994).

Huntington's disease is an hereditary, autosomal dominant disorder characterized by movement disorder, dementia, and changes in personality. Huntington's disease affects about 4–8 per 100,000 (Mayeux 1984). Although there is a range of age at onset, and childhood-onset cases occur, most cases first exhibit symptoms at ages 40 to 50. Pathologically, Huntington's disease produces loss of neurons in the striatum, especially the caudate nucleus and putamen, with less damage to the cortex, thalamus, and brain stem. Clinically, patients may present with an insidious onset of any of the three cardinal features 1) a hyperkinetic movement disorder that is usually choreic, with abrupt involuntary jerking or writhing of the muscles of the face, trunk, and limbs; 2) dementia, with a progressive deterioration in cognitive function; and 3) psychiatric changes marked by irritability, disinhibition, variably progressing to frank psychosis. On neurological examination, the involuntary limb movements produce a dancing type of gait, and patients are unable to hold the tongue protruded. Neuroleptic therapy may decrease both the dyskinetic motor movements and the psychiatric symptoms. The gene responsible for Huntington's disease has recently been found on chromosome 4p. This finding should strengthen the role of genetic counseling, and may lead to new avenues of treatment.

Creutzfeldt-Jakob disease and *Gerstmann-Sträussler-Scheinker syndrome* are both rare transmissible degenerative disorders associated with brain accumulation of a protease-resistant prion protein. Almost all cases of Gerstmann-Sträussler-Scheinker syndrome and about 10%–15% of cases of Creutzfeldt-Jakob disease are familial. The pathology of Creutzfeldt-Jakob disease is notable for cytoplasmic vacuoles in neurons and glia, giving the brain a characteristic spongiform microscopic appearance. Clinically, Creutzfeldt-Jakob disease manifests with the gradual onset of dementia, which comes to be accompanied by weakness, spasticity, extrapyramidal-type rigidity, and myoclonic jerks. These jerks are more lightning-like than the choreic jerks of Huntington's disease and may be evoked by stimuli such as loud noises or tapping the reflexes. Creutzfeldt-Jakob disease is rapidly progressive, with death usually occurring within 1 year of diagnosis. Gerstmann-Sträussler-Scheinker syndrome is a related transmissible encephalopathy, with the pathological appearance of both amyloid plaques, as in Alzheimer's disease, and spongiform change, as in Creutzfeldt-Jakob disease. Clinically, Gerstmann-Sträussler-Scheinker syndrome is a rare condition presenting with dementia and ataxia. No treatments are currently available for either Creutzfeldt-Jakob disease or Gerstmann-Sträussler-Scheinker syndrome.

Neurological Assessment: Potential Relationship to Psychopathology

There are a number of ways to regard the relationship between neurological abnormalities and behavioral changes: 1) the neurological condition might be considered the proximate biological cause of the psychiatric condition, such as dementia as a result of neurosyphilis; 2) the neurological condition and psychiatric condition may be two manifestations of a shared neurobiological change, such as right hemiparesis and depression caused by left frontal lobe infarction (Robinson et al. 1984); 3) the neurological condition may represent a psychological stressor that lowers the threshold for appearance of the psychiatric condition, such as an adjustment reaction with depressed mood related to lumbar spondylosis (Love 1987); 4) a psychiatric condition may serve as a stress under which a previously covert neurological impairment becomes apparent (e.g., the emergence of an underlying dementia during an episode of depression) (Kral 1983); 5) the treatment for the neurological condition may produce or exacerbate psychopathology, such as psychosis related to L-dopa therapy in Parkinson's disease (Klawans 1982); 6) treatment of a psychiatric condition may produce or exacerbate a neurological problem (e.g., the wide range of neuroleptic-induced extrapyramidal disorders) (Marsden and Jenner 1980); 7) a somatoform psychiatric disorder may mimic or embellish a neurological disorder, as in hysterical paralysis (Strub and Black 1988); 8) a psychological factor may lead to elaboration of an underlying neurological disorder (e.g., the co-occurrence of seizures and pseudoseizures); and 9) these two conditions may be independent but coincident in time. To determine the causal relationship between co-occurring neurological and psychiatric conditions is valuable, although in many cases present knowledge does not permit precise determination of causality in behavioral dysfunction. Therefore, in the discussion that follows, the emphasis is on practical strategies to integrate the neurological assessment into the neuropsychiatric evaluation.

Neurological History

Given the behavioral significance of neurological disease, the geriatric psychiatric evaluation must always include a careful neurological history. In addition, because of the possibilities of denial, somatization, or failing memory, it is important to seek independent confirmation of neurological complaints or experiences, usually from a spouse or other close relative. Furthermore, because even remote or seemingly unrelated neurological events may be important in the genesis of a behavioral problem (e.g., the minor "bump on the head" that led to an undetected subdural hemorrhage and gradual personality change), it is important to press for any neurological experiences or symptoms of possible relevance. The focus and depth of this exploration will depend on individual circumstances; however, a good general neurological review should consider the following signs and symptoms.

Cognitive Change

A neurological disorder may produce both cognitive and noncognitive dysfunction (e.g., dementia and paranoia in Alzheimer's disease). Therefore, the interview should include a careful review of subtle new intellectual deficits such as forgetfulness, verbal symptoms such as word-finding difficulty, or visuospatial symptoms such as difficulty navigating through town.

Head Trauma

Approximately 200–300 per 100,000 of the population are admitted to hospitals for head trauma each year, and there are probably many more nonhospitalized cases (Jennett and Teasdale 1981). Although the likelihood of behavioral sequelae may increase in cases with loss of consciousness or scalp laceration, even minor head trauma deserves consideration as a possible precipitant of postconcussion syndrome, subdural hematoma, or posttraumatic epilepsy. Moreover, injuries without direct trauma to the occiput—such as whiplash—can produce cognitive and affective changes (Yarnell and Rossie 1988). The recovery from head trauma is likely to be slower and less complete in older patients (Fogel and Duffy 1994; Wrightson 1989).

Acute Decline in Function

Any acute change in function raises the question of stroke or transient ischemic attack. Small strokes may escape recognition or medical evaluation until the secondary behavioral problems emerge—such as dementia or affective change—because they fail to produce overt focal symptoms or signs. A slowly progressive process may reach a critical stage and then present with acute symptoms suggestive of stroke (e.g., an expanding tumor mass, which finally produces observable dysfunction). On the other hand, a nonacute process may present in a "pseudo-acute" way when other factors lower the patient's reserve; an example is the appearance of the first signs of primary degenerative dementia during a stressful time such as a move, a loss, or a medical problem.

Transient or Paroxysmal Neurological Symptoms

Syncopal episodes often suggest a cardiac arrhythmia with increased stroke risk (and possible association with anxiety disorders). However, transient ischemic attacks or partial seizures may go unrecognized because of a vague or atypical history. Inquiring about any faints or "funny turns" may elicit this history.

Dizziness

As noted above, peripheral vestibulopathy is common in the elderly and may produce both subjective symptoms and gait unsteadiness. In the patient complaining of "dizziness," it is important to distinguish light-headedness—a near fainting sensation that can be a result of postural hypotension, vasovagal responses, or presyncopal symptoms of cardiac arrhythmia—from vertigo—a sense of movement with respect to the surroundings that may be produced by a wide range of central or peripheral vestibular pathology including behaviorally relevant conditions such as migraine, vertebrobasilar insufficiency, or posterior fossa tumors (Baloh 1984).

Progressive Focal Motor or Sensory Dysfunction

Weakness, numbness, or discoordination of any part of the body requires neurological evaluation. Although symptoms confined to a single extremity may initially suggest a peripheral process without relevance to behavior, many disorders with potential behavioral associations (e.g., multi-infarct dementia, idiopathic Parkinson's disease, or ALS may show asymmetric or focal symptoms).

Alteration in Special Senses

Changes in hearing or vision, in particular, may relate to psychiatric dysfunction in three ways: primary sensory disorders may produce sensory deprivation that is associated with hallucinations in the affected sensory modality (Benson 1989; Cummings 1985); sensory disorders may create misperceptions of the environment, which potentially lead to such problems as the paranoia of the hearing impaired (Cooper and Curry 1976); sensory disorders may be symptomatic of a central dysfunction (stroke, tumor, or demyelinating disease), which itself may alter behavior.

New Headache

Although a lifetime history of vascular or muscle-tension headaches is probably not relevant to a new behavioral disorder, the recent onset of headaches in an elderly patient, or a significant change in previous headache symptoms, suggests the possibility of intracranial mass lesion or increased intracranial pressure, chronic meningitis, or temporal arteritis (in addition to more common problems such as hypertension, cervical spondylosis, sinusitis, or glaucoma).

Gait Disturbance

Gait disorders have been reported to produce disability in 13% of elderly people, even excluding those gait disturbances caused by specific medical diseases (Larish et al. 1988). Although geriatric gait disorders are often multifactorial, complaints of new dysfunction can be suggestive of behaviorally relevant disorders (e.g., multi-infarct dementia, increased intracranial pressure, normal pressure hydrocephalus, or Parkinson's disease).

Sleep Disturbance

Aging is associated with decreased slow wave sleep and increased nocturnal wakefulness. One-third of the elderly experience frequent sleep interruptions caused by apnea or hypopnea, even in the absence of complaints about sleep. Snoring is increasingly common with age, usually indicates some degree of upper airway obstruction, and is associated with hypertension and cardiovascular disease (Dement et al. 1985). Therefore, nocturnal respiratory status may be compromised not only in patients with sleep complaints such as daytime sleepiness, choking attacks, or morning headache but also in those who simply snore. A history of snoring or other sleep disturbance may be relevant to the presenting psychiatric problem, since there is evidence that sleep apnea may be associated with psychopatholgy or cognitive deficits (Kales et al. 1985; Telakivi et al. 1988).

Exposure to Centrally Acting Substances

Substance use or abuse can result in neurological and psychiatric symptoms, sometimes combined. A history of alcohol abuse, even if remote, must be taken into account as a possible cause of cognitive decline. Occupational exposure to toxins such as solvents or heavy metals should be queried. Because the elderly are both exposed to more prescription medications and may be more sensitive to behavioral side effects than younger patients, it is important to document recent drug use.

Neurological Examination

The neurological examination requires experience, practice, and sophistication in neuroanatomy to yield the most fruitful results; for this reason, nonneurologists sometimes hesitate to perform a complete examination. However, the elderly psychiatric patient often has combined medical, neurological, and psychiatric symptoms. Proficiency and confidence in the techniques of the neurological examination puts the geriatric psychiatrist in a position to offer a unique synthesis of biological and behavioral knowledge in the assessment of the patient, making the development of these examination skills an extremely valuable asset. Excellent general reviews of the neurological examination are available in standard neurology texts such as that of Adams and Victor (1989) or in specialized references (e.g., Brazis et al. 1985; DeJong 1979). However, the examination of the elderly patient requires special knowledge of the neurology of aging. The following discussion focuses on both the distinctive features of the geriatric neurological examination and the behavioral significance of neurological signs.

In this examination, there are three goals: 1) to objectively assess physical signs and to distinguish the signs of normal aging from pathological abnormalities; 2) to assess the neurological significance of abnormal signs, both by determining the anatomy of the responsible lesion and generating testable hypotheses regarding the differential diagnosis of the abnormality; and 3) to assess the potential behavioral significance of abnormal signs. In performing the examination, the geriatric psychiatrist may be faced with a frightened, confused, distracted, uncooperative, or even combative patient. Establishing rapport and maintaining flexibility can mitigate these factors; however, even the most challenging patients can be assessed in some detail by careful observation of their spontaneous activity and responses to events in the environment.

Observation

The neurological examination begins at the first moment the examiner catches sight of the patient. Throughout the historical interview, important information can be gathered regarding the posture, gait, coordination; excesses or deficiencies of movement or the symmetry of facial, truncal, and appendicular activity; attention to or neglect of extrapersonal space; eye movements; and the response to visual, auditory, and somatosensory stimuli in the environment. By the time the formal examination begins, the examiner will have formulated questions about apparent dysfunction that can be tested in depth.

Mental Status Examination

The mental status examination is described in Chapter 8, entitled "Comprehensive Psychiatric Evaluation." As above, the performance of the patient during the course of both the psychiatric interview and mental status examination will provide clues to focus the detailed neurological examination. For example, mental slowness may be a sign of subcortical pathology, particularly of the basal ganglia, and will therefore mandate a careful search for abnormalities of tone, posture, gait, or the presence of resting tremor. Idiosyncratic speech or paraphasias may be signs of left hemisphere dysfunction and require investigation for evidence of right corticospinal or sensory system pathology.

Cranial Nerves

Taste and olfaction both show age-related decline in sensitivity, especially after the age of 50, with women exhibiting superior olfactory abilities throughout life. Of those ages 65 to 80, 60% show olfactory impairment; nearly 25% are anosmic (Doty et al. 1984; Verillo and Verillo 1985). Deficiency of the first cranial nerve is most likely to be behaviorally significant when it is unilateral, suggesting possible basal frontal or mesial temporal pathology on the affected side. Olfaction may be tested by exposure to pungent but nonvolatile smells such as cloves or soap, although the availability of "scratch and sniff" cards may improve standardization.

Elderly patients lose visual acuity as a result of presbyopia and are increasingly vulnerable to ophthalmological disorders, which may be apparent on fundoscopy, including cataracts, glaucoma, age-related macular degeneration, anterior ischemic optic neuropathy, and retinal vascular disease (Chisholm 1989; Kasper 1989). Visual acuity can be tested with a hand-held Snellen eye chart at 14 inches, with and without corrective lenses, but presbyopia may make vision at distance the better measure. Visual fields can be roughly assessed by confrontation, testing each eye separately, and overcoming the patient's urge to look directly toward the stimulus by brief, unilateral finger movements. More subtle deficits may be identified in cooperative patients with small test objects such as colored pinheads. Pupils become smaller with aging (senile miosis) and the pupillary light reflex is often diminished or even absent (Chisholm 1989; Loewenfield 1979), although asymmetry of response represents an afferent pupillary defect. The presence of papilledema is an important sign of increased intracranial pressure; however, the absence of papilledema cannot be taken as evidence of normalcy because even massive hemispheric tumors may not produce this sign, and papilledema does not usually occur in space-occupying intracranial lesions in the elderly (Caird 1982; Fetell and Stein 1989). The loss of previously observed spontaneous venous pulsations in the optic disc may be a more sensitive sign of increased intracranial pressure.

Eye movements change with age; there are increased saccadic latencies (the speed of shifting gaze to fixate upon a target) and breakdown of smooth pursuit movements, and such disruptions of normal movement may themselves impair vision (Hutton and Morris 1989). Normal aging is also associated with limitation of upward gaze and less so of downward gaze (Chamberlain 1971). This normal restriction must be distinguished from two patterns of eye movements with potential relevance to behavioral disorders: 1) the Parinaud syndrome (upgaze paralysis, retraction nystagmus, and pupillary light-near dissociation), which may be associated with pineal region masses; and 2) marked restriction of vertical gaze with preservation of oculocephalic reflexes, which suggests progressive supranuclear palsy. Any other paresis of eye movement, nonconjugate movement or nystagmus requires further investigation of brain stem, cerebellar, and vestibular function.

Facial asymmetry can be a normal variant or a sign of unilateral facial weakness. Because residual weakness from an old Bell's palsy may be misleading, the examiner should inquire about this past condition, and examine the patient's driver's license to determine whether an asymmetry is new. Excessive bucco-oral facial movements are sometimes attributable to ill-fitting dentures or chewing of gum; these confounding variables should be ruled out by examining the patient with his or her mouth empty. Dyskinetic lingual-facial-buccal movements are common in elderly patients with no history of neuroleptic exposure (Weiner and Klawans 1973), and, in particular, the edentulous state may predispose the patient to oral dyskinesias (Koller 1983), although neuroleptic-induced tardive dyskinesia must be strongly suspected in older psychiatric patients.

Hearing declines with age, primarily caused by presbycusis, a multifactorial condition that can involve sensorineural hearing loss caused by a declining population of cochlear ganglion cells, conductive loss, and possible changes in the central auditory pathway (Mackenzie 1989). The accumulated effect of noise injury, as well as possible effects of toxins, infections, Meniere's disease, and, rarely, acoustic neuroma can contribute to hearing impairment. The vestibular system declines in function, with up to 40% loss of myelinated fibers in the aged vestibule (Yoder 1989). Standard eighth nerve examination should include simple hearing tests, such as assessing the patient's awareness of rubbed fingertips near the ear, a ticking wristwatch, a tuning fork, or whispered words. Because speech perception is probably the most clinically important hearing ability, it is especially useful to document the patient's ability to hear words spoken at conversational levels at different distances. The Weber and Rinne tests should supplement these bedside hearing tests to distinguish conductive from sensorineural deficits. Given the potential for hearing defects to produce emotional distress in the elderly, particularly paranoia, a noticeable deficit on bedside testing justifies formal audiometric evaluation.

Speech may roughen slightly with age, and dysarthria may occur from causes as benign as loose dentures, but progressive hoarseness or nasality may signal more serious problems such as laryngeal neoplasia, myasthenia, or motor neuron disease. Soft, hypophonic speech can be a sign of pathology in subcortical regions, and patients with Parkinson's disease with dementia will typically have softer speech with impaired melody when compared with patients with Alzheimer's disease (Cummings et al. 1988). Excessive movement of the tongue may be a sensitive indicator of tardive dyskinesia, particularly if the patient fails to keep the tongue extended on command. However, fasciculations (a marker of motor neuron disease) can best be observed with the tongue relaxed in the floor of the mouth.

Motor Examination

The initial observation of the patient, as remarked above, is a rich source of information about the function of the motor system. Particular emphasis should be placed on the degree and character of spontaneous movement. Movement disorders in the geriatric psychiatry patient constitute a special diagnostic challenge, because they may represent: normal aging effects; idiopathic movement disorders that increase in prevalence among the aged; medication side effects, especially those of neuroleptics; or the consequences of the psychiatric illness. Furthermore, because movement disorders have been associated with depression and dementia (Girotti et al. 1988; Mayeux 1984), the co-occurrence of movement disorder and psychiatric disturbance raises the question of the degree of interdependence of these diagnoses. To distinguish psychogenic alterations in movement from neurological movement disorders it is important to supplement observation with examination of resting tone, muscle bulk, power, and deep tendon reflexes.

Resting tone increases with age, both for limbs and axial muscles, with paratonia or gegenhalten—the tendency to increase tone in response to rapid displacements of the limb by the examiner—occurring in 10%–12% of those ages 70 to 79 and in 21% of those over 80 years old. It remains unclear whether paratonia represents a normal finding or a sign of diffuse cerebral dysfunction (George 1989; Jenkyn et al. 1985). However, marked rigidity reflects pathology, particularly when accompanied by either a spastic catch suggesting upper motor neuron disease or with cogwheeling suggestive of basal ganglia disease. Reduction of movement or hypokinesis may represent psychomotor retardation, which can signal depression, but also is called *bradykinesia* and is seen in metabolic disorders such as hypothyroidism or basal ganglia disorders including parkinsonism. The combination of bradykinesia, resting tremor, cogwheel rigidity, and loss of postural reflexes should be familiar as the syndrome of parkinsonism, which can either occur as the result of degenerative nervous system disease such as Parkinson's disease, striatonigral degeneration, and progressive supranuclear palsy, or as an extrapyramidal side effect of psychotropic medications, most frequently neuroleptics (Adams and Victor 1989; Klawans and Tanner 1984).

Excessive movements or hyperkinesias may be normal in form—such as the hyperactivity of the agitated, manic, stimulant-affected or akathetic patient—or abnormal in form—as seen in the neuroleptic-induced dyskinesias, or with tremors, tics, and choreoathetosis. Hyperactivity with abnormal form is usually a result of basal ganglia pathology; hyperactivity with normal form possibly relates to dysfunction of a limbic-mesencephalic psychomotor activity circuit (Victoroff 1989). In the presence of generalized hyperactivity with normal form, or motor restlessness, clinical features may help to distinguish psychogenic hyperactivity from neuroleptic-induced akathisia. Subjective restlessness occurs in both, but patients with akathisia may show more inability to remain still, more shifting from foot to foot, and may exhibit a coarse tremor (Braude et al. 1983).

Truncal or appendicular choreic, athetotic, or otherwise dyskinetic movements may be reduced when the patient is seated and so are better examined with the patient standing at rest, walking, and during activating procedures such as touching the thumb with each finger or standing with arms outstretched and eyes closed (Simpson and Singh 1988). Such dyskinetic movements have a differential diagnosis that includes Huntington's disease, Wilson's disease, acquired hepatocerebral degeneration, senile chorea, and tardive dyskinesia (Klawans and Tanner 1984). Because the degenerative causes of dyskinesia are rare and because the incidence of tardive dyskinesia is 5% per year, or even greater among the elderly exposed to neuroleptics (Baldessarini 1988), it is probable that neuroleptic-induced tardive dyskinesia is overwhelmingly the most common pathological cause of dyskinesia in geriatric psychiatric patients. However, as many as 32% of nonneuroleptic-exposed elderly may exhibit spontaneous dyskinesias (Blowers et al. 1981), suggesting that the nervous system in older adults is susceptible to producing these movements, which may explain the age-associated increased vulnerability to neuroleptic effects.

Muscle bulk, as noted above, declines with age. On examination, atrophy of the interosseous muscles of the hands may be particularly evident, and the most common cause of such focal atrophy is probably arthritic joint disease (Baker 1989). However, focal wasting can also occur with limb disuse, either from altered activity, trauma, or a cortical insult such as stroke. Neurologically, wasting is important as a sign of lower motor neuron dysfunction, which can be focal, as in spondylosis or spinal mass lesions, or diffuse as in motor neuron disease. Observation of the resting muscle may reveal fasciculations, which are pathognomonic of lower motor neuron dysfunction as occurs in ALS. Measurement of homologous parts on opposite sides of the body will aid in confirming an impression of asymmetry. Diffuse wasting may also signal the anorexia of depression or medical problems including metabolic, infectious, and neoplastic disorders. The wasting syndrome of human immunodeficiency virus is emerging as another possible diagnosis.

Examination of strength in each major muscle group requires consideration of the patient's willingness to generate a maximal effort. Elderly patients may—for good reason—fear excessive exertion, and even their best efforts cannot be compared with those of younger patients. Instead, it is better to use each muscle as the control for the contralateral muscle. For most screening purposes, bedside testing of the upper extremities should include the deltoids, biceps, triceps, flexors, extensors of the wrists and fingers, and intrinsic hand muscles. Testing in the lower extremities should include the iliopsoas, gluteus, quadriceps, hamstrings, anterior tibialis, and soleus/gastrocnemius. Patterns of weakness may have both localizing and diagnostic value. For example, unilateral weakness prompts the search for other localizing signs to discriminate upper from lower motor neuron dysfunction and to delineate the extent of the focal lesion. Disproportionate proximal weakness is common in myopathies or metabolic disorders such as hypothyroidism, whereas distal weakness may predominate in neuropathies. Disproportionate loss of extensor strength in the arms with relative preservation of flexors is common in upper motor neuron disorders. Diffuse weakness is difficult to interpret and may represent psychogenic enervation or a wide range of medical conditions, including the neuropathic and myopathic disorders.

Hand tremor has been observed in 2%–43% of healthy elderly people (Hobson and Pemberton 1955; Prakash and Stern 1973). This condition is usually a fine rapid distal tremor, present on maintaining an antigravity posture, and should be distinguished from the 5- to 7-Hz resting tremor of parkinsonism. Essential tremor is a heredofamilial postural tremor of 6–11 Hz, which sometimes first appears in old age (Koller 1984). A rapid distal tremor can also occur either as the effect of medication (including stimulants, antidepressants, or lithium) or drug withdrawal syndromes. Asymmetric or unilateral tremor may be caused by asymmetric nervous system dysfunction; however, tremors often appear asymmetrically in parkinsonism, essential tremor, or normal aging.

Coordination

Coordination testing does not assess a single system in isolation, but instead evaluates the orchestration of motor activities as a result of the harmonious interaction of the pyramidal system, basal ganglia, and cerebellum. Observing fine finger movements such as rapid, successive opposition of the thumb and other digits may elicit defects of corticospinal tract function. The finger-to-nose test may exhibit abnormalities with dysfunction of different systems: corticospinal tract pathology may produce smooth but weak or ineffectual reaching; basal ganglia pathology may produce bradykinesia and tremor, which does not increase with arm extension; cerebellar pathology may produce overshooting, lateral dysmetria, or tremor that increases with arm extension. The classic intention tremor, or dysmetric performance on the finger-to-nose test, appears in 20% of healthy elderly people (Howell 1949). For this reason, it is sometimes difficult to distinguish between relatively benign age-related incoordination and an important diagnostic clue to cerebellar system pathology. Significant overshoot on attempted rapid movement to a target, whether with saccadic eye movements or limb movements, may distinguish clinically important cerebellar-system dysfunction. Cerebellar dysfunction may also produce disorganized or erratic rapid-alternating movements (dysdiadochokinesis, which is often tested by instructing the patient to alternately slap a surface with the pronated or supinated hand), awkward heel-to-shin performance, and failure to check recoil when the examiner suddenly releases the flexed arm.

Disorders that produce these appendicular signs of cerebellar dysfunction may include lesions intrinsic to or compressing the cerebellum but can also occur with lesions of cerebellar connections (e.g., in the vestibular system, red nucleus, inferior oliva, ventral lateral thalamus, or frontal lobe). Causes of this cerebellar type of appendicular incoordination include posterior fossa neoplasm, cerebrovascular disease, demyelinating disease, or, less often, one of several degenerative conditions including olivopontocerebellar atrophy, dentatorubral degeneration, or Azorean disease—a familial condition of cerebellar dysfunction and parkinsonian features in patients of Portugese-Azorean descent. Alcoholic cerebellar degeneration may also produce these appendicular cerebellar signs, but more often produces truncal ataxia caused by midline cerebellar degeneration, with relative preservation of appendicular function.

Reflexes

Deep-tendon reflexes are reduced with age, most often at the ankle, but also, in some studies, at the biceps, triceps, and patella (Howell 1949; Prakash and Stern 1973). Because reflexes may be reduced and anxiety may make relaxation difficult for the elderly patient, reinforcing maneuvers are sometimes required to elicit the reflexes, such as asking the patient to clench his or her teeth while testing the upper extremities, or using the Jendrassik maneuver, asking patients to hook their hands in front of their chest and pull them in opposite directions as the examiner taps the patellae.

Diffuse hyporeflexia disproportionate to age may commonly be a sign of peripheral neuropathy, less commonly of myopathy. In hypothyroidism the reflexes may be slow both to respond and to relax.

Unilateral or focal loss of a reflex may represent peripheral or lower motor neuron damage, commonly as the result of cervical or lumbar spondylosis, less commonly as the result of tabes dorsalis, syringomyelia, or spinal tumor.

Diffuse hyperreflexia occurs in bilateral lesions of the pyramidal system above the midcervical level, in states of neuromuscular irritability such as tetany, and in hyperthyroidism.

Focally increased reflexes, particularly when combined with pathological signs such as the Babinski or Hoffman, alert the examiner to unilateral pathology affecting the descending pyramidal system; however, it is possible for pathology in cortical regions outside of the motor cortex to produce unilateral hyperreflexia (e.g., prefrontal or temporal lesions), possibly by remote effects on the motor strip.

Two patterns of special relevance to behavior are 1) the combination of absent reflexes and positive Babinski signs seen in subacute combined degeneration resulting from vitamin B_{12} deficiency, which is a cause of reversible dementia, and 2) the combination of hyperreflexia and atrophy with fasciculations seen in amyotrophic lateral sclerosis, which may be associated with both depression and dementia (Davis 1987; Montgomery and Erickson 1987).

Frontal Release Signs

A group of reflexes has been referred to as frontal release signs or primitive reflexes. They represent the exaggeration of normal reflexes or reappearance of reflexes seen in infancy, thereby indicating an impairment of nervous-system function. However, it is important to consider the presence of such reflexes in light of their prevalence among healthy older individuals. The palmomental reflex (contraction of the mentalis muscle of the face on stroking the palm) has been found in 41%–60% of the healthy elderly individuals, with increasing frequency for each decade from the sixth through the ninth (Jacobs and Gossman 1980). The snout reflex (puckering or pursing of the lips in response to light pressure above the upper lip) has been found in 26%–33% of the healthy elderly individuals (Jacobs and Gossman 1980; Jenkyn et al. 1985). The glabellar tap response (inability to inhibit blinking during a series of finger taps to the glabellar region) has been found in 37% of healthy older persons (Jenkyn et al. 1985). In addition, Jensen et al. (1983) found no difference in the prevalence of the palmomental or glabellar reflexes between healthy subjects and patients with cerebral disease, with the exception that patients with basal ganglia disorders more frequently had a positive glabellar tap. Jenkyn et al. (1985) found that 95% of subjects over age 70 had five to seven abnormal signs on examination. Further, patients may have substantial frontal lobe damage yet have no grasp, snout, suck, rooting, hyperactive jaw jerk, or palmomental reflexes (Benson et al. 1981). Hence, the presence of these reflexes may reveal evidence of nervous-system degeneration but cannot be taken as proof of behaviorally significant frontal lobe pathology, nor can their absence be used to rule out such pathology.

Sensation

There is a well-established decline in vibratory sensation beginning by ages 50 to 60, and there are lesser declines in thermal, touch, and pain discrimination (Olney 1989; Pearson 1928). These changes probably relate to combined functional declines of sensory receptors, peripheral nerves, roots, and tracts (Baker 1989). Although decreased detection of vibratory stimuli may be a result of normal aging, marked vibratory insensitivity combined with poor proprioception and/or a positive Romberg sign (swaying on standing that markedly increases when the eyes are closed), will alert the examiner to peripheral neuropathy or posterior column dysfunction as in subacute combined degeneration. There has also been observed an age-related decline in discrimination of competing tactile stimuli presented to different locations (Kokmen et al. 1977; Levin and Benton 1973). This insensitivity to double simultaneous stimulation may complicate diagnosis of sensory neglect, unless there is a notable asymmetry.

Gait

Critchley and others have noted that the gait of the healthy elderly people shares many of the features of Parkinson's disease, with short steps, rigidity, and flexion posture (Coffey 1989; Critchley 1931). Stoplight photography of walking, healthy, elderly men reveals shortened steps, diminished arm swing, and anteroflexion of the upper torso (Murray et al. 1969). However, these findings are confounded by the fact that elderly patients may walk slowly for a variety of reasons, and a decrease in freely-chosen walking rate will naturally produce a decreased length of stride (Larish et al. 1988). Thus, in the older patient with gait disturbance, it is often difficult to distinguish pathology from normal aging and to sort out the contribution of multiple potential contributing factors, including 1) decreased proprioception; 2) decreased vision; 3) impaired postural reflexes; 4) weakness; 5) rigidity; 6) extrapyramidal dysfunction; 7) vestibulopathy; 8) cerebellar ataxia; 9) diffuse frontal lobe pathology; 10) cervical or lumbar spondylosis; 11) joint restriction; 12) pain; 13) postural hypotension; 14) medication effect; 15) fear of falling based on prior mishaps; and 16) a wide range of focal and diffuse central disorders including stroke, tumor, and hydrocephalus (Adams 1984; Manchester et al. 1989; Stelmach et al. 1989; Tinetti 1989).

To best observe gait impairment, the patient should be examined standing in place, walking, walking on heels and toes, and tandem walking (feet in line). The examiner should observe the rate, length, and width of stride; stability of turns; arm swing; and foot strike for any atypical features. Postural reflexes can be assessed both on the Romberg test and by observing the response to displacement (lightly pushing the standing patient in different directions). Table 10–1 summarizes common gait abnormalities seen in a typical neurological referral population. There are several patterns of gait that may have specific diagnostic significance:

Frontal gait "apraxia" with poor initiation, halting steps, and an impression of magnetic attachment to the floor, can be associated with bilateral frontal lobe dysfunction, which may occur as a result of multiple strokes, Binswanger's disease, or idiopathic frontal lobe degeneration. Normal pressure hydrocephalus can produce the triad of dementia, incontinence, and a gait disturbance of the frontal type.

Parkinsonian gait will be distinguished from normal aging by the degree of the slowing, rigidity, and shortening of steps; by the presence of festination (acceleration as if chasing the center of gravity); and by the association with resting tremor. Again, depression may produce bradykinesia

Table 10–1.   Causes of gait disorders in a neurological referral practice

Disorder	Frequency (%)	Causes
Frontal gait disorder	20	Normal pressure hydrocephalus
		Multiple strokes
		Binswanger's disease
Sensory imbalance	18	Neuropathy
		Multiple sensory deficits
Myelopathy	16	Cervical spondylosis
		Vitamin B_{12} deficiency
Parkinsonism	10	Idiopathic Parkinson's disease
		Drug-induced parkinsonism
		Progressive supranuclear palsy
Cerebellar degeneration	8	Neurodegenerative disease
		Alcohol
Toxic or metabolic	6	Hepatic encephalopathy, encephalopathy
		uremia, hypoglycemia
Undetermined	14	

Source.   Adapted from Sudarsky 1990.

but should not produce rigidity or tremor. Parkinsonian gait may occur with idiopathic Parkinson's disease, progressive supranuclear palsy, striatal infarction, or neuroleptic medication exposure.

Broad-based gait occurs with 1) cerebellar or vestibular dysfunction, as in chronic alcoholism causing midline cerebellar atrophy, 2) loss of proprioception, as in tabes dorsalis resulting from syphilis or subacute combined degeneration because of vitamin B_{12} deficiency; 3) toxic or metabolic encephalopathy (e.g., hepatic encephalopathy); or 4) multiple sensory deficits. Patients with these disorders also often exhibit unsteadiness on the Romberg test.

Spastic gait occurs with myelopathy, most often caused by cervical spondylosis. The gait is typically stiff-legged, with plantar flexion at the ankle causing the toes to drag.

Hemiparetic gait occurs with any unilateral upper-motor-neuron disorder, most commonly following a stroke, and typically appears as a limp with unilateral spasticity, foot drop, and circumduction of the affected leg.

Orthopedic gait is a general term for the wide range of alterations in gait occuring in association with focal joint and limb disorders, most often arthritic conditions. In one community study, these disorders were more common than neurological disorders as causes of abnormal gait (Lundgren-Lindquist et al. 1983).

The careful neurological examination of an elderly patient may yield multiple findings that suggest abnormal function. The examiner is sometimes faced with subtle, equivocal findings, findings that do not clearly fit a pattern or even seem contradictory. In part, this may be a result of the simultaneous effects of multiple common pathologies, such as cervical or lumbar spondylosis, metabolic or vascular neuropathies, or remote injuries that make it more challenging to identify pertinent new changes. Experience helps in developing a sense for the critical threshold at which a given finding is likely to indicate clinically important dysfunction, and expert examiners may shift their estimate of probability of a certain disorder when certain groups of signs seem more prominent than others. Nonetheless, the neurological examination can be difficult and somewhat subjective even for experienced clinicians. When the examination yields equivocal positive findings, a reasonable approach may be to err on the side of suspecting meaningful dysfunction and to pursue the issue by consultation and appropriate laboratory testing.

Integrated Neurobehavioral Evaluation

Significant changes occur with age in the structure and function of both the central and peripheral nervous system. In addition, the incidence and prevalence of many neurological disorders increases with age. The neurological evaluation should be considered as one component of an integrated neurobehavioral assessment that includes the psychiatric interview and examination, cognitive testing, neurological examination, and laboratory testing. Because there is an increased probability of organic medical problems with age, there should be a low threshold for supplementing the neurological examination with laboratory tests. Although this is particularly true when the examination suggests a specific central nervous system disorder, we should be modest about the limits of physical diagnosis: even when no focal or localizing signs are identified, laboratory testing may reveal a specific factor that plays a significant role in the genesis of the behavioral disturbance. Although it is often difficult to render a cost-benefit analysis of such testing, the opportunity to discover potentially treatable causes of behavioral disorder is a compelling mandate. As our sophistication in neurobiology grows, so will these opportunities.

The aging of the population will confront the medical community with a large increase in the number of elderly patients who have both psychiatric disturbances and neurological problems. At the same time, the disciplines of neurology and psychiatry are evolving in concert toward an integrated understanding of the neuropsychiatry of behavioral disturbance. The geriatric psychiatrist is in a unique position, drawing on a broad base of knowledge in gerontology, neurology, and psychiatry, to offer a synthesis of disciplinary approaches in the evaluation and treatment of the behavioral distress among the elderly.

References

Adams RD: Aging and human locomotion, in Clinical Neurology of Aging. Edited by Albert ML. New York, Oxford University Press, 1984, pp 381–386

Adams RD, Victor M: Principles of Neurology, 4th Edition. New York, McGraw-Hill, 1989

Anderson JM, Hubbard BM, Coghill GR, et al: The effect of advanced old age on the neuron content of the cerebral cortex. J Neurol Sci 58:235–244, 1983

Baker PCH: The aging neuromuscular system. Semin Neurol 9:50–59, 1989

Baldessarini RJ: A summary of current knowledge of tardive dyskinesia. Encephale 14:263–268, 1988

Baloh RW: Dizziness, Hearing Loss and Tinnitus: The Essentials of Neurotology. Philadelphia, PA, FA Davis, 1984

Bensimon G, Lacomblez L, Meininger V, the ALS/Riluzole study group: A controlled trial of riluzole in amyotrophic lateral sclerosis. N Engl J Med 330:585–591, 1994

Benson DF: Disorders of visual gnosis, in Neuropsychology of Visual Perception. Edited by Brown JW. Hillsdale, NJ, Lawrence Erlbaum, 1989, pp 59–78

Benson DF: Psychomotor retardation. Neuropsychiatry, Neuropsychology, and Behavioral Neurology 3:36–47, 1990

Benson DF, Stuss DT, Naeser MA, et al: The long-term effects of prefrontal leukotomy. Arch Neurol 38:165–189, 1981

Binks M: Changes in mental functioning associated with normal aging, in The Clinical Neurology of Old Age. Edited by Tallis R. Chichester, Wiley, 1989, pp 27–39

Blowers AJ, Borison RL, Blowers CM, et al: Abnormal involuntary movements in the elderly (letter). Br J Psychiatry 139:363–364, 1981

Braude WM, Barnes TRE, Gore SM: Clinical characteristics of akathisia, a systematic investigation of acute psychiatric inpatient admissions.

Br J Psychiatry 143:139–150, 1983

Broe GA, Creasey H: The neuroepidemiology of old age, in The Clinical Neurology of Old Age. Edited by Tallis R. Chichester, England, Wiley, 1989, pp 51–65

Brazis PW, Masdea JC, Biller J: Localization in Clinical Neurology. Boston, MA, Little, Brown, 1985

Caird FI: Examination of the nervous system, in Neurological Disorders in the Elderly. Edited by Caird FI. Bristol, Wright PSG, 1982, pp 44–51

Chamberlain W: Restriction in upward gaze with advancing age. Am J Ophthalmol 71:341, 1971

Chawluk J, Alavi A, Hurtig H, et al: Altered pattern of cerebral glucose metabolism in aging and dementia. J Cerebral Blood Metal 5(suppl 1):S121–S122, 1985

Chisholm I: Visual failure, in The Clinical Neurology of Old Age. Edited by Tallis R. Chichester, England, Wiley, 1989, pp 335–346

Coffey DJ: Disorders of movement in aging. Semin Neurol 9:46–49, 1989

Coleman PD, Flood DG: Neuron numbers and dendritic extent in normal aging and Alzheimer's disease. Neurobiol Aging 8:521–545, 1987

Cooper AF, Curry AR: The pathology of deafness in the paranoid and affective psychoses of later life. J Psychosom Res 20:97–105, 1976

Cotman CW: Synaptic plasticity, neurotrophic factors, and transplantation in the aged brain, in Handbook of the Biology of Aging, 3rd Edition. Edited by Schneider EL, Rowe JW. New York, Academic Press, 1990, pp 255–274

Critchley M: The neurology of old age. Lancet 1:1221–1230, 1931

Critchley M: Neurologic changes in the aged. J Chronic Dis 3:459–477, 1956

Cummings JL: Clinical Neuropsychiatry. Orlando, FL, Grune & Stratton, 1985, pp 221–233

Cummings JL, Darkins A, Mendez M, et al: Alzheimer's disease and Parkinson's disease: comparison of speech and language alterations. Neurology 38:680–684, 1988

Davis AS: Neuropsychological measures in patients with amyotrophic lateral sclerosis (letter). Acta Neurol Scand 75:284, 1987

DeJong RN: The Neurologic Examination. Hagerstown, MD, Harper & Row, 1979

Dement W, Richardson G, Prinz P, et al: Changes of sleep and wakefulness with age, in Handbook of the Biology of Aging, 2nd Edition. Edited by Finch CE, Schneider EL. New York, Van Nostrand Reinhold, 1985, pp 692–717

DiBartolomeo AG, Brick JE: Giant cell arteritis and polymyalgia rheumatica. Postgrad Med 91:107–191, 1992

Doty RL, Shaman P, Applebaum SL, et al: Smell identification ability: changes with age. Science 226:1441–1443, 1984

Drachman DA, Long RR: Neurological evaluation of the elderly patient, in Clinical Neurology of Aging. Edited by Albert ML. New York, Oxford University Press, 1984, pp 97–113

Fetell MR, Stein BM: General considerations, in Merritt's Textbook of Neurology. Edited by Rowland LP. Philadelphia, PA, Lea & Febiger, 1989, pp 275–285

Fogel BS, Duffy J: Elderly patients, in Neuropsychiatry of Traumatic Brain Injury. Edited by Silver JM, Yudofsky SC, Hales RE. Washington, DC, American Psychiatric Press, 1994, pp 413–441

George J: The neurological examination of the elderly patient, in The Clinical Neurology of Old Age. Edited by Tallis R. Chichester, England, Wiley, 1989, pp 67–75

Girotti F, Soliveri P, Carella F, et al: Dementia and cognitive impairment in Parkinson's disease. J Neurol Neurosurg Psychiatry 51:1498–1502, 1988

Henderson G, Tomlinson BE, Gibson PH: Cell counts in human cerebral cortex in normal adults throughout life using an image analyzing computer. J Neurol Sci 46:113–136, 1980

Hobson W, Pemberton J: The Health of the Elderly at Home. London, England, Butterworth, 1955

Howell TH: Senile deterioration of the central nervous system. Br Med J 1:56–58, 1949

Hubbard BM, Squier MV: The physical aging of the neuromuscular system, in The Clinical Neurology of Old Age. Edited by Tallis R. Chichester, England, Wiley, 1989, pp 3–26

Hutton JT, Morris JL: Looking and seeing with age related neurologic illness and normal aging. Semin Neurol 9:31–38, 1989

Jacobs L, Gossman MD: Three primitive reflexes in normal adults. Neurol 30:184–188, 1980

Jankovic J, Calne DB: Parkinson's disease: etiology and treatment. Current Neurol 7:193–234, 1987

Jenkyn LR, Reeves AG, Warren T, et al: Neurologic signs in senescence. Arch Neurol 42:1154–1157, 1985

Jennett B, Teasdale G: Prognosis after severe head injury, in Management of Head Injuries. Edited by Jennett B, Teasdale G. Philadelphia, PA, FA Davis, 1981, pp 317–332

Jensen JPA, Gron U, Pakkenberg H: Comparison of three primitive reflexes in neurological patients and in normal individuals. J Neurol Neurosurg Psychiatry 46:162–167, 1983

Kales A, Caldwell AB, Cadieux RJ, et al: Severe obstructive sleep apnea, II: associated psychopathology and psychosocial consequences. J Chronic Dis 38:427–434, 1985

Kasper RL: Eye problems of the aged, in Clinical Aspects of Aging. Edited by Reichel W. Baltimore, MD, Williams & Wilkins, 1989, pp 445–453

Kirasic KC, Allen GL: Aging, spatial performance and spatial competence, in Aging and Human Performance. Edited by Charness N. Chichester, England, Wiley, 1985, pp 191–224

Kish SJ, El-Awar M, Schut L, et al: Cognitive deficits in olivopontocerebellar atrophy: implications for the cholinergic hypothesis of Alzheimer's dementia. Ann Neurol 24:200–206, 1988

Kish SJ, Robitaile Y, El-Awar M, et al: Striatal monoamine neurotransmitters and metabolites in dominantly inherited olivopontocerebellar atrophy. Neurology 42:1573–1577, 1992

Klawans H: Behavioral alterations and the therapy of parkinsonism. Clin Neuropharmacol 5:S29–S37, 1982

Klawans H, Tanner CM: Movement disorders in the elderly, in Clinical Neurology of Aging. Edited by Albert ML. New York, Oxford University Press, 1984, pp 387–403

Kokmen E, Bossemeyer RW, Barney J, et al: Neurological manifestations of aging. J Gerontol 32:411–419, 1977

Koller WC: Edentulous orodyskinesia. Ann Neurol 13:97–99, 1983

Koller WC: Diagnosis and treatment of tremors. Neurol Clin 2:499–514, 1984

Koller WC: How accurately can Parkinson's disease be diagnosed? Neurology 42:6–16, 1992

Koudstaal PJ, van-Gijn J, Frenken CW, et al: RIND, minor stroke: a continuum, or different subgroups? J Neurol Neurosurg Psychiatry 55:95–97, 1992

Kral VA: The relationship between senile dementia (Alzheimer type) and depression. Can J Psychiatry 28:304–306, 1983

Larish DD, Martin PE, Mungiole M: Characteristic patterns of gait in the healthy old. Ann NY Acad Sci 515:18–32, 1988

Levin HS, Benton AL: Age and susceptibility to tactile masking effects. Gerontol Clin 15:1–9, 1973

Levin HS, Benton AL, Grossman RG: Neurobehavioral Consequences of Closed Head Injury. New York, Oxford University Press, 1982

Loewenfield IE: Pupillary changes related to age, in Topics in Neuro-Opthalmology. Edited by Thompson HS. Baltimore, MD, Williams & Wilkins, 1979

Love AW: Depression in chronic low back pain patients: diagnostic efficiency of three self-report questionnaires. J Clin Psychol 43:84–89, 1987

Lundgren-Lindquist B, Aniansson A, Rundgren A: Functional studies in 79-year-olds, III: walking performance and climbing capacity. Scand J Rehab Med 15:125–131, 1983

Mackenzie I: Disturbances of hearing and balance, in The Clinical Neurology of Old Age. Edited by Tallis R. Chichester, England, Wiley, 1989, pp 363–375

Manchester D, Woollacott M, Zederbauer-Hylton N, et al: Visual, vestibular and somatosensory contributions to balance control in the older adult. Journal of Gerontology: Medical Sciences 44:M118–M127, 1989

Marsden CD, Jenner P: The pathophysiology of extrapyramidal side-effects of neuroleptic drugs. Psychol Med 10:55–72, 1980

Masliah E, Mallory M, Hansen L, et al: Quantitative synaptic alterations in the human neocortex during normal aging. Neurology 43:192–197, 1993

Mayeux R: Behavioral manifestations of movement disorders. Neurol Clin 2:527–540, 1984

Montgomery GK, Erickson LM: Neuropsychological perspectives in amyotrophic lateral sclerosis. Neurol Clin 5:61–81, 1987

Mortimer JA: The dementia of Parkinson's disease. Clin Geriatr Med 4:785–797, 1988

Munsat TL: Aging of the neuromuscular system, in Clinical Neurology of Aging. Edited by Albert ML. New York, Oxford University Press, 1984, pp 404–423

Murray MP, Kory RC, Clarkson BH: Walking patterns in healthy old men. J Gerontol 24:169–178, 1969

Olney RK: Diseases of peripheral nerves, in The Clinical Neurology of Old Age. Edited by Tallis R. Chichester, England, Wiley, 1989, pp 171–189

Pearson GHJ: Effect of age on vibratory sensibility. Archives of Neurology and Psychiatry 20:482–496, 1928

Perry EK, Piggott MA, Court JA, et al: Transmitters in the developing and senescent human brain. Ann NY Acad Sci 695:69–72, 1993

Plude DJ, Hoyer WJ: Attention and performance: identifying and localizing age deficits, in Aging and Human Performance. Edited by Charness N. Chichester, England, Wiley, 1985, pp 47–99

Prakash C, Stern G: Neurological signs in the elderly. Age Aging 2:24–27, 1973

Rapoport SI: Positron emission tomography in normal aging and Alzheimer's disease. Gerontology 32:6–13, 1986

Riederer P, Krusik P: Biochemical and morphological changes in the aging brain, in The London Symposia (EEG Suppl 39). Edited by Ellingson RJ, Murray NMF, Halliday AM. Elsevier, 1987, pp 389–395

Robinson RG, Kubos KL, Starr LB, et al: Mood disorders in stroke patients: importance of location of lesion. Brain 107:81–93, 1984

Rogers J, Bloom FE: Neurotransmitter metabolism and function in the aging central nervous system, in Handbook of the Biology of Aging, 2nd Edition. Edited by Finch CE, Schneider EL. New York, Van Nostrand Reinhold, 1985, pp 645–691

Rogers MA, Evans WJ: Changes in skeletal muscle with aging: effects of exercise training. Exerc Sport Sci Rev 21:65–102, 1993

Rosen DR, Siddique T, Patterson D, et al: Mutations in Cu/Zn superoxide dismutase gene are associated with familial amyotrophic lateral sclerosis. Nature 362:59–62, 1993

Rowe JW, Kahn RL: Human aging: usual and successful. Science 237:143–149, 1987

Simpson GM, Singh H: Tardive dyskinesia rating scales. Encephale 14:175–182, 1988

Smith J: Clinical neurophysiology in the elderly, in The Clinical Neurology of Old Age. Edited by Tallis R. Chichester, England, Wiley, 1989, pp 89–97

Spencer PS, Ochoa J: The mammalian peripheral nervous system in old age, in Aging and Cell Structure. Edited by Johnson J. New York, Plenum, 1981, pp 35–103

Stelmach GE, Phillips J, DiFabio RP, et al: Age, functional postural reflexes and voluntary sway. Journal of Gerontology: Biological Sciences 44:B100–B106, 1989

Stones MJ, Kozma A: Physical performance, in Aging and Human Performance. Edited by Charness N. Chichester, Wiley, 1985, pp 261–292

Strub RL, Black FW: Neurobehavioral Disorders: A Clinical Approach. Philadelphia, PA, FA Davis, 1988, pp 451–475

Sudarsky L: Geriatrics: Gait disorders in the elderly. N Engl J Med 322:1441–1446, 1990

Takeda S, Matsuzawa T, Matsui H: Age-related changes in cerebral blood flow and brain volume in healthy subjects. J Am Geriatr Soc 36:293–297, 1988

Telakivi T, Kajaste S, Partinen M, et al: Cognitive function in middle age
    snorers and controls: role of excessive daytime somnolence and sleep-
    related hypoxic events. Sleep 454–462, 1988

Teravainen H, Calne DB: Motor system in normal aging and Parkinson's
    disease, in The Neurology of Aging. Edited by Katzman R, Terry R.
    Philadelphia, PA, FA Davis, 1983, pp 85–109

Thompson LV: Effects of age and training on skeletal muscle physiology
    and performance. Phys Ther 74:71–81, 1994

Tinetti ME: Instability and falling in elderly patients. Semin Neurol 9:39–
    45, 1989

Tyler KL: A history of Parkinson's disease, in Handbook of Parkinson's
    Disease. Edited by Koller WC. New York, Marcel Dekker, 1987

Verillo RT, Verillo V: Sensory and perceptual performance, in Aging and
    Human Performance. Edited by Charness N. Chichester, England,
    Wiley, 1985, pp 1–46

Victoroff JI: Hyperactivity syndrome of Alzheimer's disease. Bull Clan
    Neurosci 54:34–42, 1989

Ward C: The genetics and epidemiology of Parkinson's disease, in Degen-
    erative Neurological Disease in the Elderly. Edited by Griffiths RA,
    McCarthy ST. Bristol, England, Wright, 1987, pp 20–28

Weiner WJ, Klawans HL: Lingual-facial-buccal movements in the elderly,
    II: pathogenesis and relationship to senile chorea. J Am Geriatr Soc
    21:318–320, 1973

Welford AT: Reaction time, speed of performance, and age. Ann NY Acad
    Sci 515:1–17, 1988

Wrightson P: Management of disability and rehabilitation services after
    minor head injury, in Mild Head Injury. Edited by Levin HS, Eisenberg
    HM, Benton AL. New York, Oxford University Press, 1989

Yarnell PR, Rossie GV: Minor whiplash head injury with major debilita-
    tion. Brain Inj 2:255–258, 1988

Yoder MG: Geriatric ear, nose, and throat problems, in Clinical Aspects of
    Aging. Edited by Reichel W. Baltimore, MD, Williams & Wilkins, 1989,
    pp 454–463

Marilyn S. Albert, Ph.D.

Neuropsychological Testing

A variety of cognitive disorders occur with increasing frequency as people age, including progressive disorders of dementia and cognitive disorders secondary to psychiatric syndromes. These cognitive disorders produce considerable morbidity and mortality, and although only some of them can be completely reversed with treatment, appropriate management can substantially improve quality of life and reduce the development of secondary disorders. Thus, it is in the best interest of the patient for health professionals to become attuned to the possible presence of cognitive dysfunction in older patients and to be familiar with appropriate procedures for evaluation and referral. This chapter focuses on the role of neuropsychological testing in the assessment of cognitive dysfunction in elderly individuals, because there is much that a physician, especially a psychiatrist, can do to identify the presence of cognitive dysfunction and to ensure that it is properly assessed.

Neuropsychological Test Batteries

At least two basic approaches exist to the selection of a neuropsychological test protocol. Some individuals use a predetermined test battery, such as the Halstead-Reitan Neuropsychological Test Battery (Reitan 1979) or the

Luria-Nebraska Battery (Goldin 1981). Others select from tests relevant to the diagnostic question. However, even in the latter case, certain core tests tend to be relied on more heavily than others.

If the neuropsychologist is not using the same standard battery in every testing situation, the selection is determined by a number of factors among which the diagnostic issue at hand is of primary importance. If, for example, language abnormalities are prominent and one is trying to determine whether they are the result of strokes or a primary progressive dementia such as Alzheimer's disease, the neuropsychologist may examine reading, writing, comprehension, repetition, naming, and spontaneous speech in some detail, using a standardized aphasia battery such as the Boston Diagnostic Exam (Goodglass and Kaplan 1972) or the Western Aphasia Battery (Kertesz 1980). If language abnormalities are minimal but memory deficits are prominent and the differential diagnosis is among several primary progressive dementias, then the clinician might choose to limit the language assessment to an evaluation of naming, using a task such as the Boston Naming Test (Kaplan et al. 1983), and examine memory from a variety of perspectives, including immediate and delayed recall and recognition in both the verbal and nonverbal domains.

In selecting tests it is important to consider the patient's level of impairment. If difficult tests are chosen, moderately and severely impaired patients are likely to become fatigued, feel overwhelmed, and either fail to perform at their best or refuse to continue with the evaluation. Thus, reduced versions of lengthier tests (e.g., the reduced Wechsler Adult Intelligence Scale—Revised [WAIS-R; Wechsler 1981]) or tests designed for impaired patients (e.g., the Mattis Dementia Rating Scale [Mattis 1976]) would be wise choices rather than a lengthy and complex battery of tests such as the entire WAIS-R or the Halstead-Reitan battery.

Regardless of approach, it is useful to organize the neuropsychological report into broad areas of function such as attention, language, memory, visuospatial ability, conceptualization, and general intelligence. In this way, the physician's understanding of the test result is enhanced.

Attention

Attention is important for the clinician to consider because simple attentional abilities must be preserved for any other task to be performed adequately. If the patient has difficulty keeping his or her mind on the task for 1 to 3 minutes at a time, it will not be possible to assess other areas of function. For this reason, attention is often assessed before other cognitive domains have been evaluated. Auditory and visual attention can be assessed easily by means of digit span and letter cancellation. Several continuous performance tasks are also available for this purpose. Many of these have been adapted for computer administration so that both accuracy and latency can be recorded.

Language

Language testing for aphasia should, of course, include an evaluation of comprehension, repetition, reading, writing, and naming. Several standardized batteries are available for this purpose (Goodglass and Kaplan 1972; Kertesz 1980). Some include brief aphasia screening tests that are useful for identifying the existence of a problem without giving a detailed analysis (Halstead and Wepman 1949). If aphasia has been ruled out or is not suspected, confrontation naming (Kaplan et al. 1983) should almost always be part of the assessment of an older individual, because decreases in naming ability occur with age and are also a prominent symptom of a number of disorders common among elderly individuals (e.g., Alzheimer's disease).

Memory

A detailed evaluation of memory is essential in the assessment of the elderly patient. Memory dysfunction occurs in almost all of the cognitive disorders common in elderly individuals, and the nature and severity of the memory impairment can serve as one of the major guidelines to the diagnosis. The assessment of memory is complicated because changes in memory capacity occur as people age. Therefore, careful testing is often necessary to differentiate normal from pathological memory performance. Fortunately, many memory tests are available from which to choose. The ones used commonly today are the California Verbal Learning Test (Delis et al. 1986); Wechsler Memory Scale—Revised (WMS-R; Wechsler 1987); Rey Auditory Verbal Learning Test (Rey 1964); Selective Reminding Test (Buschke and Fuld 1974); Randt Memory Test (Randt et al. 1980); and the memory task on the CERAD Battery (Morris et al. 1989). Although some of these tests were developed for use with elderly individuals, most were designed for younger populations and are now being applied to older individuals.

Visuospatial Ability

The assessment of visuospatial ability is more difficult in elderly than in young individuals because of the prevalence of visual sensory deficits in this age range. In all of the cognitive domains previously discussed, function can be evaluated either orally or visually. However, it is not so for visuospatial ability, and alternate means of administration are more difficult to develop. It is, for example, difficult to enlarge test stimuli such as blocks or sticks. Therefore, figure copying is the method of assessment that is most likely to be successful. Figures can be chosen to span a great range of difficulty and, as mentioned earlier, can be adapted (by using photographic enlargement or a felt-tipped pen) for individuals with moderate sensory impairments. Even then it may be necessary to allow for a greater margin of error.

Perception

In addition to constructional ability, the clinician should assess perceptual capacity. Figure-matching tasks are a good analogue for figure copying. They have the added advantage that they can be administered to patients with severe cognitive deficits—patients in whom it is otherwise difficult to assess spatial function.

Executive Function

The interrelated group of abilities known as executive function include abilities responsible for cognitive flexibility, concept formation, and self-monitoring. A partial list of available tests includes the Trail Making Test (Reitan 1958), the Modified Card Sorting Test (Nelson 1976), the Visual-Verbal Test (Feldman and Drasgow 1951), the similarities subtest of WAIS-R (Wechsler 1981), and the Proverbs Test (Gorham 1956).

Many of these tests are lengthy, and shortened versions are better for clinical assessment; for example, the Modified Card Sorting Test (Nelson 1976) is the shortened version of the Wisconsin Card Sorting Test (Heaton 1985). The advantage of tasks from the WAIS-R such as proverb interpretation or similarities is that they are generally arranged in order of difficulty. Thus, the harder items can be omitted if the individual fails on easier items. In addition, tasks have been designed to assess abstraction in patients with moderate to severe cognitive impairments who fail the standard tests (Mattis 1976).

General Intelligence

An assessment of general intelligence will allow the clinician to determine whether the individual has access to previously acquired knowledge. The vocabulary subtest of the WAIS-R is well known as the best quick estimate of intelligence quotient (IQ). To interpret the results, the clinician must have a general sense of the individual's premorbid level of ability. Because tests that are purported to assess premorbid ability, such as the vocabulary subtest of the WAIS-R and the Nelson Adult Reading Test (Nelson and O'Connell 1978), often show declines even in mildly impaired patients, information regarding education and occupation is important in assessing premorbid cognitive status. Considerable data exist to suggest that elderly people with a poor educational background (i.e., 0–8 years) perform worse on a broad range of cognitive tasks than elderly people with a good educational background (i.e., 10–16 years) (Anthony et al. 1982). Therefore the clinician must be extremely cautious in interpreting the test results of an elderly individual with limited formal education.

Overall Cognitive Function

Physicians often need a screening test to get quick notion of the patient's level of cognitive function. These tests include the Mini-Mental State Exam (Folstein et al. 1975), the Short Portable Mental Status Questionnaire (Pfeiffer 1975), the Mental Status Questionnaire (Kahn et al. 1960), the Blessed Dementia Index (Blessed et al. 1968), and the East Boston Memory Test (Scherr et al. 1988).

Limitations of Tests

Although administering such tests is an excellent idea, it is important to know that they are prone to the confounding effects of education. Individuals with high premorbid ability can score in the unimpaired range despite having experienced a substantial amount of cognitive decline. Conversely, individuals with low educational achievement may be misidentified as impaired. In addition, the cutoff points on many of the existing screening tests are designed to identify moderately to severely impaired individuals to minimize false-positive assessments. Thus, individuals in the early stages of a disorder of dementia such as Alzheimer's disease may still perform in the unimpaired range on a short screening test. Note that such tests were not designed to measure subtle aspects of behavior. Thus, they may show little or no decline over time in a patient who can be shown by other measures to have declined substantially.

Administration of Cognitive Tests

The manner in which the neuropsychological assessment of an older person is conducted can contribute greatly to its success. As in any cognitive evaluation, the testing environment should be quiet and well lit. A window should be at the patient's back, because glare can be a problem for an older person. Although standard testing stimuli should be used whenever possible, versions that have been adapted for elderly individuals with sensory or other impairments should be available. Visual stimuli can often be enlarged on a photocopy machine if the lines on the original are too thin. Otherwise, it may be necessary to redraw the stimuli with a felt-tipped pen to increase visibility. If the clinician presents visual stimuli on a computer screen, it is important for the stimuli to be pretested to ensure they are large enough and have sufficient light-dark contrast for the elderly person to view them easily. It should be possible to adjust the volume on a tape machine for most older people to hear. Despite these adjustments, the presence of sensory limitations should always be noted and factored into the evaluation.

With elderly individuals probably more than with any other group, it is important to establish a friendly and nonthreatening environment. As a group, elderly people have less education than the young and are more intimidated by the testing situation. If they are experiencing cognitive deficits, they may be aware of them and be embarrassed, afraid, or anxious.

The order in which tests are given also can serve to reduce tension in the test situation. The clinician should begin with tasks that are unlikely to be stressful so that there is time for the patient to become acclimated to the test situation and for the tester to establish rapport with the patient. Tasks that are stressful should be followed, whenever possible, with tasks that are not. Remember that success on a task need not be equated with an absence of stress. Timed tasks or tasks in which items are repeated over and over again (as in word list learning) are often stressful, even if the patient ultimately performs with some degree of accuracy.

Older individuals tend to take more time and fatigue more easily than younger people. The danger exists of fatigue causing artificially lower scores on later tasks. The psychiatrist must, therefore, be especially attentive to a patient's tiring and be prepared to stop a test session to continue on another day.

Differential Diagnosis of Common Disorders in Elderly People

A number of disorders that affect cognition are increasingly common as people get older. Dementia is the most common syndrome of chronic progressive cognitive decline seen in elderly individuals. Dementia is a general term used to describe a chronic and substantial decline in two or more areas of cognitive function. It is unlike amnesia, which causes a severe and striking deficit in only one area of cognitive function (i.e., memory). Some dementias are nonprogressive (e.g., alcoholic dementia), but most are progressive. Although all dementias are accompanied by a memory impairment, the nature of the impairment differs substantially among patients. For example, Alzheimer's disease patients demonstrate a rapid rate of forgetting during brief delays (Hart et al. 1988; Moss et al. 1986; Welsh et al. 1991), whereas Pick's disease patients do not (Moss and Albert 1988). Patients with Huntington's disease show relative preservation of verbal recognition memory versus nonverbal recognition memory (Butters et al. 1983). The other cognitive deficits that accompany memory impairments also vary widely among patient groups.

The nature of the onset and progression of the cognitive deficits also differs greatly among the major disorders of dementia. A carefully collected cognitive history is, therefore, an essential adjunct to a dementia workup and often makes the difference between an accurate diagnosis and an inaccurate one. Most of the dementias have an insidious onset and develop slowly and gradually. These include Alzheimer's disease, Pick's disease, Parkinson's dementia, and progressive supranuclear palsy. Creutzfeldt-Jakob disease, the most virulent disorder of dementia, develops insidiously too but is known for a rapid rate of progression from onset to death (often within 1 year). Personality change or psychiatric syndromes, such as depression, also are seen in disorders of dementia, and whether they precede or follow the onset of cognitive decline is critical for an accurate diagnosis. The initial symptoms of a multi-infarct dementia develop acutely, but because multiple large or small cerebral infarcts are the cause of the cognitive decline, the ultimate clinical picture can take many years to develop, although in a stepwise and stuttering fashion.

Thus, each disorder of dementia has a unique cognitive history and a unique pattern of spared and impaired function that can help the clinician identify it. The most common disorders of dementia seen in elderly individuals and the cognitive profile associated with depression are discussed below.

Alzheimer's Disease

The first and most noticeable symptom generally observed in patients with Alzheimer's disease is a severe anterograde memory deficit. Early in the course of disease, this deficit is confined mainly to an impairment of secondary memory, but as the disease progresses, primary memory deficits develop. The striking aspect of this difficulty in acquiring new information is the rapid rate at which information is forgotten in secondary memory. Comparisons of dementias of differing etiologies suggest that Alzheimer's disease patients lose more information over a brief delay than patients with Huntington's disease (Moss et al. 1986), Pick's disease (Moss and Albert 1988), or progressive supranuclear palsy (Milberg and Albert 1989). With the use of a continuous recognition paradigm, this rapid rate of forgetting was demonstrated to be evident chiefly during the initial 10 minutes after exposure to new material (Hart et al. 1988). Therefore, retention intervals falling within this period are diagnostically the most useful. Recall paradigms with brief intervals between exposure to information and its immediate and delayed recall (e.g., 15 seconds versus 2 minutes, respectively) are thus best in accentuating differences among patients. Many standard memory tests can be readily adapted to these constraints.

The rapid rate of forgetting in Alzheimer's disease is probably the result of the striking damage to the hippocampal complex. A high density of neurofibrillary tangles and neuritic plaques in the medial temporal lobe has been noted, particularly the afferent neurons of the entorhinal cortex and the efferent neurons of the subiculum (Hyman et al. 1984). This condition appears to functionally disconnect the hippocampal formation from the rest of the cerebral cortex. The large declines in choline acetyltransferase seen in Alzheimer's disease (Davies and Maloney 1976) probably contribute to this memory impairment of Alzheimer's disease patients. However, because the alteration in acetylcholine levels is thought to result from neuronal loss in the basal forebrain (Whitehouse et al. 1981) and basal forebrain damage is seen in other disorders of dementia with less severe memory impairment early in the course of disease (Tagliavini and Pilleri 1983), it is unlikely that the cholinergic deficit alone is responsible for the

Alzheimer's disease patient's particularly severe pattern of memory impairment.

Recent data suggest that, in addition to a memory impairment, the other cognitive deficits most commonly seen in the early stages of Alzheimer's disease are difficulty with concept formation, cognitive flexibility, and self-monitoring (Grady et al. 1989; Lafleche and Albert in press; Morris and Fulling 1983). As indicated above, these abilities are collectively known as executive function, and significant impairments in this area have a substantial impact on daily function. Even early in the course of disease, tasks that require cognitive flexibility and monitoring are commonly impaired (e.g., preparing meals, paying bills, or balancing a checkbook). These difficulties in executive function probably cannot be attributed to pathology in the frontal lobes. There is little evidence to suggest that the frontal lobes have extensive pathology early in the course of the disease (Brun and Gustafson 1976). Moreover, positron-emission tomography (PET) scan data uniformly demonstrate that frontal declines in glucose metabolism are a late phenomenon in Alzheimer's disease (Chase et al. 1984; Haxby et al. 1988). Probably, abnormalities in executive function result from a loss of neocortical synapses (DeKosky and Scheff 1990; Masliah et al. 1993; Terry et al. 1991). The partial degeneration of an intracortical projection system early in the course of disease could produce difficulties in tasks that require rapid and simultaneous integration of multiple types of information. Alternatively, these difficulties may arise from pathological changes in subcortical structures, such as the basal forebrain, that modulate cortical function (Whitehouse et al. 1981). The basal forebrain projects to numerous cortical and subcortical regions; thus it can serve as a source of integrated information to the cortex.

In the most typical presentation of Alzheimer's disease, language deficits (e.g., difficulty with confrontation naming) and spatial deficits (e.g., difficulty with figure copying) develop after the onset of memory dysfunction (Bayles and Kaszniak 1987; Rosen 1983). These deficits have been attributed to neurofibrillary tangle and neuritic plaque formation in multimodal association cortices (Kemper 1984; Pearson et al. 1985).

The initial symptoms of a patient with Alzheimer's disease typically provide subtle evidence of memory difficulty. Patients may begin by repeating themselves, forgetting names, or forgetting appointments. Patients are often aware of these difficulties but tend to minimize them. On neuropsychological testing, patients early in the course of Alzheimer's disease often have IQs in the normal range (i.e., 110) but have substantial difficulty with memory, set shifting, and conceptualization and slight difficulty with naming. For example, a patient with an IQ of 110 may have a memory quotient (based on the WMS-R) of 90—a 20-point discrepancy (a person's memory quotient should be approximately equal to the IQ).

Delayed-recall performance on a memory test, such as the word list learning test on the CERAD battery, also would be impaired. Although a patient may learn as many as 6 of the 10 words on the list learning task, only 1 or 2 will be recalled after a brief delay. Impairments in set shifting and sequencing are often revealed by performance on the Trail Making Test. This task requires an individual to first connect a series of numbers in order, and then connect alternating numbers and letters in order (i.e., 1 with A, 2 with B, and so on). Mildly impaired Alzheimer's disease patients are generally slow on both tasks and make errors on the second. Impairments on the similarities subtest of the WAIS-R also are common. Responses are likely to be concrete (e.g., an apple and an orange are alike because they both have peels). Performance on the Mattis Dementia Rating Scale (DRS) also reflects these difficulties. A mildly impaired Alzheimer's disease patient may score 121 of a possible 144 on the DRS (with losses primarily on the memory and conceptualization subtests). Difficulty in naming also may be apparent on items from the Boston Naming Test (e.g., there are 15 such items included in the CERAD battery, the task consists of a series of line drawings that patients are asked to name). Patients may fail to spontaneously name some of the drawings, giving either category descriptions or semantic associates of the target word (e.g., "ladle" for "funnel," "musical instrument" for "accordion," and "not plier" for "tongs"). Despite these obvious difficulties, performance on the Mini-Mental State Exam may be good in a well-educated, mildly impaired patient (e.g., 28 of 30). In such a patient, errors invariably occur on the recall portion of the test.

Dementia of the Frontal Lobe Type

Several pathological entities have been associated with a progressive process of dementia that involves the frontal lobes. Recently these disorders have been called dementia of the frontal lobe type (Neary et al. 1988) to differentiate them from dementia of the Alzheimer's type. To date, three different pathological entities have been described (Lund and Manchester Groups 1994). These include classic Pick's disease (Pick 1892); so-called Pick's type II (Neumann and Cohn 1967); and nonspecific abnormalities primarily consisting of spongiosis, gliosis, and atrophy (Knopman et al. 1990). These disorders begin as one of two types of presentations:

1) changes in personality, such as lack of impulse control, stereotyped behavior, and inappropriate affect; or 2) gradually progressive abnormalities in language (Neary et al. 1988).

Although memory function is abnormal early in the course of disease, it is less severely affected than in Alzheimer's disease. Dementia of the frontal lobe type patients remember less than unaffected individuals immediately after being exposed to the material, but thereafter they do not forget as rapidly as they did initially (Moss and Albert 1988). Note that the hippocampus has been reported as spared in some patients with dementia of the frontal lobe type patients (Constantinidis et al. 1974). Spatial ability is typically reported as relatively intact, even in advanced disease (Neary et al. 1988), congruent with the relative absence of pathological changes in the parietal cortex. Of note, the electroencephalogram remains normal until late in the course of frontal lobe syndromes (Neary et al. 1988).

The accurate identification of this group of syndromes is important for good patient management. Early in the course of disease, dementia of the frontal lobe type patients give the appearance of having well-preserved abilities because of relatively mild memory deficit. However, their inappropriate behavior makes them severe management problems, and unprepared families can became distraught (Gustafson 1987). Dementia of the frontal lobe type patients profit from being treated like psychiatric patients, with whom they are sometimes confused (Neary et al. 1988). Enabling families to understand that the cause of the disorder is a brain disease generally helps them to adapt to the cognitive and personality changes and the extremes of behavior dementia of the frontal lobe type patients display. The initial episodes that raise concern are generally related to inappropriate behavior that is uncharacteristic of the patient (e.g., leaving the scene of an accident, making sexually explicit statements in public, developing obsessions with food, or compulsively carrying out certain routines). Some patients become emotionally labile and irritable.

With regard to neuropsychological testing early in the course of disease, the dementia of the frontal lobe type patient may appear normal in many respects (e.g., reveal an estimated verbal IQ of 104, a memory quotient of 118, and a score of 29 on the Mini-Mental State Exam). Despite the apparent normality of the scores, however, patients typically have clear cognitive deficits in domains associated with frontal lobe function. They have difficulty with proverb interpretation. For example, when asked to explain the proverb "barking dogs seldom bite," they may say "They try to act fiercer to cover up the fact that they're really gentle." Set-shifting abilities also are compromised. They are generally slow on the Trail Making Test and, more importantly, make errors. Naming may be impaired; the patient may score 49 out of 60 on the Boston Naming Test. Errors consist primarily of semantic associates of the target word (e.g., "fancy fish" for "seahorse" or "harmonica" for "accordion"). Although the score on the WMS-R may be within normal range, memory typically varies. For example, on the Delayed Recognition Span Test, verbal recognition span may be 11 (which is normal), but after both the 15-second and the 2-minute delay, the patient may recall only four words (considerably less than one would have predicted given a good recognition span). The items missed on the Mini-Mental State Exam may also be related to recall. Variability, both within and across test sessions, suggests that the patients' memory deficit may be at least partially the result of declines in concentration.

As indicated above, patients with dementia of the frontal lobe type also can have a gradually progressive language deficit (Cole et al. 1979; Wechsler et al. 1982). Therefore, a gradually progressive language deficit is not restricted to the pathological diagnosis of Alzheimer's disease. Because the early symptoms of dementia of the frontal lobe type mimic a gradually progressive aphasia, these patients benefit from nonverbal communication strategies rather than the mnemonic aids often recommended for Alzheimer's disease patients.

Parkinson's Dementia

A significant number of patients with Parkinson's disease develop a dementia syndrome. Prevalence rates vary from 25% to 40% (Brown et al. 1984), but they appear to be higher than would be explained by the co-occurrence of Alzheimer's disease and Parkinson's disease. Indeed, some Parkinson's disease patients with dementia have neuritic plaques and neurofibrillary tangles that are found at autopsy (the pathological hallmarks of Alzheimer's disease), although others do not (Jellinger 1987).

Given this complex pathological picture, it is not surprising that the neuropsychological deficits associated with Parkinson's disease patients with dementia are varied and heterogeneous. Most have the cognitive deficits associated with Parkinson's disease, namely, visuospatial dysfunction and difficulty with concept formation and set shifting (Boller et al. 1984; Hovestadt et al. 1987; Taylor et al. 1986). These deficits have been most commonly ascribed to cell loss in the basal ganglia (with projections to the prefrontal cortex) and to the declines in dopamine, which accompany the neuronal loss (Divac 1972).

When dementia develops in Parkinson's disease patients, it generally includes substantial difficulty with memory (El-Awar et al. 1987) and occasionally with linguistic skills such as confrontation naming. Recently, implicit memory problems, both in motor-skill learning (i.e., pursuit rotor) and in verbal priming have been reported in patients with Parkinson's disease dementia (Heindel et al. 1989). Because patients with Alzheimer's disease have preserved motor-skill learning but impaired verbal priming (Heindel et al. 1989), it may be that a subgroup of patients with Parkinson's disease dementia with preserved motor-skill learning and impaired verbal priming identifies the subgroup of patients with Parkinson's disease dementia and coexistent Alzheimer's disease.

Progressive Supranuclear Palsy

Although progressive supranuclear palsy is a rare disorder, it is being studied with increasing frequency because it is a dementia in which damage is restricted almost entirely to subcortical areas (Steele et al. 1964). Patients with Huntington's disease ultimately develop neocortical damage (Bruyn et al. 1979), as do demented patients with Parkinson's disease (Divac 1972), leaving progressive supranuclear palsy as the classic subcortical dementia. Pathological damage in progressive supranuclear palsy appears to be limited to the basal ganglia, brain stem, and cerebellar nuclei. It is therefore striking that memory function in the early stages of progressive supranuclear palsy is near normal levels, even when tasks requiring initiation and sequencing, such as verbal fluency, are devastated (Milberg and Albert 1989). Patients with progressive supranuclear palsy also have difficulty with so-called frontal tasks such as card sorting, which is thought to result from a disconnection of the frontal lobes from subcortical structures (Pillon et al. 1986). This hypothesis has received some recent support from single-photon emission computed tomography (SPECT) data showing frontal metabolic declines in patients with progressive supranuclear palsy (Goffinet et al. 1988). Although the matter has not been examined, memory may remain intact in patients with progressive supranuclear palsy until late in the course of disease if it is assessed in a manner that minimizes the profound initiation and conceptualization deficit of progressive supranuclear palsy patients.

The neurological deficits of progressive supranuclear palsy (e.g., ophthalmoplegia or gait disturbance) are generally diagnostic of the disorder so that memory testing may not be needed for establishing the diagnosis. However, a demonstration of preserved memory in the face of profound initiation and conceptualization deficits will greatly assist care-givers in patient management.

In a typical progressive supranuclear palsy patient, the neurological examination is strikingly abnormal. The patient often has a masked face, reduced spontaneous blinking, a positive snout and glabellar reflex, hypokinesia, bradykinesia, abnormal gait, and markedly abnormal eye movements. Lack of vertical eye movements and limited horizontal eye movements are common.

Neuropsychological testing often shows marked impairments in abstraction, response initiation, and motoric set-shifting tasks. Naming and memory may also be deficient but less so. Estimated IQ may be reduced (Henry et al. 1973), primarily because of difficulty with the similarities and vocabulary subtests of the WAIS-R. For example, a mildly impaired progressive supranuclear palsy patient may be unable to say how "north" and "west" are alike but know that the distance from New York to Paris is about 3,000 miles. Proverb interpretation is also generally concrete. Difficulty with response initiation is often most dramatic on verbal tasks. Spontaneous speech shows immense latencies. During critical points in a narrative, usually over sub-stantive words or action verbs, a patient may stop for as long as 2 minutes before continuing. This greatly reduced initiation is reflected in a markedly impaired performance on word list generation. For example, when asked to name all the words beginning with the letter S, a mildly impaired patient with progressive supranuclear palsy may produce only three in 1 minute, which is the 0 percentile of performance. On the other hand, on verbal tasks—in which the stimulus for the response is provided, such as on confrontation naming—a patient may be less impaired. Thus, a patient who is in the 0 percentile in word list generation may score 67 out of 85 on the Boston Naming Test. Memory may be abnormal but irregularly so. For example, a patient may fail to recall all three of the words on the Mini-Mental State Exam but recall both sentences on the Mattis Dementia Rating Scale. The score on the WMS-R may not be substantially worse than immediate recall, suggesting that patients with progressive supranuclear palsy do not have a particularly rapid rate of forgetting.

Huntington's Disease

Huntington's disease is another disorder that causes dementia and that is generally diagnosed by the presence of a characteristic neurological ab-normality (i.e., chorea) (Caine 1986). A history of Huntington's disease in other family members is also sought, because Huntington's disease is a genetic disorder (Weingartner et al. 1981). Occasionally, however, there is no family history of Huntington's disease (e.g., because of illegitimacy, broken family, or unknown adoption) and the choreic movements are atypical. In these instances neuropsychological testing can be helpful.

Patients with Huntington's disease have poor verbal and nonverbal recall and poor nonverbal recognition. However, as mentioned earlier, verbal recognition is well preserved early in the course of disease (Butters et al. 1983; Moss et al. 1986) and so is verbal priming compared with motor skill learning, as mentioned earlier (Heindel et al. 1989). Patients with early Huntington's disease also have good confrontation-naming ability and relative preservation of many of the verbal tasks on the WAIS-R, such as information, vocabulary, and similarities (Josiassen et al. 1982), while showing impairment in many of the WAIS-R subtests that deal with spatial and arithmetic ability, such as arithmetic, digit span, picture arrangement, and digit-symbol (Butters et al. 1978; Josiassen et al. 1982). A combination of this pattern of preserved and impaired function should be diagnostic. Huntington's disease patients typically have a history of motor and cognitive dysfunction. Patients may report hand spasms and increasing problems with tripping, even on smooth surfaces, along with mild difficulty with memory that is less evident to others than it is to the patients themselves. The neurological examination, of course, reveals the characteristic choreic movements of Huntington's disease.

Neuropsychological testing in a mildly impaired patient may yield an estimated verbal IQ of 99 (100 being the average for the population), with a memory quotient (WMS-R) of 90, the 9-point differential between the two being suggestive of memory difficulties. However, verbal recognition span tends to be selectively preserved in a mildly impaired patient (e.g., Wechsler 1981) compared with recognition span for faces (Buschke and Fuld 1974) or spatial positions (Rey 1964). Tasks that require speed, sequential planning, and set formation also are generally deficient. The Trail Making Test may also be performed poorly, for example, in the 10th percentile on the first portion (Trails A) and the 25th percentile on the second (Trails B). Verbal fluency is also typically impaired (e.g., 27th percentile). Spatial tasks such as figure copying are generally accurate but demonstrate slight difficulty with planning. Naming is often within normal limits.

Multi-Infarct Dementia

Cerebrovascular disease most commonly appears clinically as the "stroke syndrome" (Mohr et al. 1980). Although not all forms of vascular disease in the central nervous system involve stroke (e.g., cardiac arrest or prolonged hypotension), the disorders that produce dementia are generally the result of multiple strokes over time. These have been labeled multi-infarct dementia (Hachinski et al. 1974) to emphasize that the deficits result from actual infarcts and not from diffuse narrowing of blood vessels.

These dementias are characterized by at least two clinical pictures. When large-vessel disease produces multiple cerebral emboli, large discrete cerebral infarcts typically occur. The focal cognitive deficits that result include aphasia, apraxia, agnosia, and amnesia, depending on the anatomic distribution of the lesion. Repeated strokes lead to a stepwise development of multiple cognitive deficits.

Medium- or small-vessel disease, secondary to atherosclerosis of the small vessels that penetrate subcortical white matter, produces more incomplete, diffuse infarction of brain tissue. Defined in this manner, the latter encompasses the syndrome known as state lacunair, or lacunar state, (Marie 1901) and Binswanger's disease (Fisher 1982). These disorders produce a more insidious decline and are harder to differentiate from progressive primary dementias such as Alzheimer's disease than those produced by large-vessel disease. Because the cognitive deficits depend on the location and size of the tissue damage, it has been difficult to identify a consistent cognitive profile (Cummings et al. 1987; Perez et al. 1975). Neuroimaging procedures, such as magnetic resonance imaging, also can be inconclusive because multiple regions of high signal intensity do not always reflect infarction (Johnson et al. 1987) and are often seen in individuals of high cognitive abilities as well as in those with dementia. The most useful information in the diagnosis of lacunar disease and other associated disorders tends to be provided by a careful cognitive history and neurological examination, in combination with neuroimaging procedures.

Neuropsychological testing in a mildly impaired patient with a lacunar disease (i.e., a patient with a score of 19 on the Mini-Mental State Exam) may show cognitive deficits reflective of aphasia. For example, patients may be unable to write single words (e.g., they write "squar" for "square" and "scoss" for "cross"). A sentence on the Mini-Mental State Exam may show a similar linguistic impairment (e.g., "I came your by automobile"). Difficulty reading simple sentences and misnaming of letters of the alphabet may also occur. Repetition may be impaired. Naming may be below normal but less impaired than reading, writing, and repetition. Consistent with these deficits would be a severe impairment in word list generation. When asked to name in 1 minute all the things one can buy in a supermarket, a mildly impaired patient may produce only three items. Such patients also may show difficulty with even simple alternating movements (e.g., they may not be able to perform even alternate taps with the index finger of each hand). Drawings that involve alternation also may be impaired. Only the simplest verbal and visual abstractions are performed correctly by such patients. Memory impairment may, however, be variable. Orientation may be only mildly impaired; patients may know the month, the year, and the names of the president, the governor, the hospital, and the city. They may recall a simple sentence after 10 minutes, but they may not recall any of the three words on the Mini-Mental State Exam.

Depression

Some depressed patients show a variety of cognitive deficits. The differential diagnosis between depression and the primary progressive dementias such as Alzheimer's disease and Pick's disease is, therefore, often difficult. The best method for differentiating these two populations is, unfortunately, unknown. Patients with depression have been reported to show deficits in vigilance (Byrne 1977; Frith et al. 1983), memory (Breslow et al. 1980; Caine 1986; Cronholm and Ottosson 1961; Henry et al. 1973; Neville and Folstein 1979; Raskin et al. 1982; Silbermann et al. 1983; Sternberg and Jarvik 1976), and conceptualization (Caine 1986; Raskin et al. 1982), all abilities that are impaired in Alzheimer's disease and that in some studies were said not to differentiate patients with depression from those with primary progressive dementia. Contradictions in the results of various studies probably occurred because the age of the subjects and the severity and type of depression varied widely. For example, tests that differentiate 55-year-old patients with depression and dementia may not discriminate from 70-year-old patients because of the added alterations in test performance introduced by age-related changes in cognition. Seventy-five-year-old patients with multiple treated episodes of depression throughout their lives are likely to be systematically different from 75-year-old patients with a first depressive episode. Patients with atypical depressions and cognitive deficits may differ from patients with a more typical depressive profile. Differences among patient populations along these dimensions are likely to be the cause of some of the differences between published reports.

Nevertheless, some general statements can be made. First, it is essential to clarify the order in which the cognitive deficits occurred relative to the depression. Furthermore, because the order of events must be reconstituted retrospectively, the psychiatrist must attempt to determine whether the patient was truly depressed at the relevant time. This determination can often be difficult because many disorders of dementia, particularly Alzheimer's disease, produce an apathy and withdrawal from activities that families often interpret as depression. In an elderly individual, there are likely to be many real-life events that can reasonably be considered causally related to a depression (e.g., retirement, the death of a close friend or spouse). Therefore, considerable skill is needed to reconstruct these past events from an interview with the patient and the family.

Second, the clinician should attempt to give several different tests within the same cognitive domain to examine intertest variability. Depressed patients often show large differences in performance among tests of a similar nature (e.g., tests of delayed recall), whereas patients with dementia do not. These fluctuations by the depressed patient are thought to be secondary to changes in attention, motivation, and mood.

Finally, the literature indicates that some aspects of cognition are unimpaired in depression. These include recognition of high-imagery words (Silbermann et al. 1983), recall of related words that have previously been sorted (Weingartner et al. 1981), paired associate learning (Breslow et al. 1980), and rate of forgetting over time (Cronholm and Ottosson 1961). Naming and arithmetic ability also are reported to be unimpaired in comparison to individuals without depression (Caine 1986).

Delirium

A delirium, also known as an acute confusional state, is by definition, a cognitive disorder of acute onset, usually of hours or days. Although delirium is a well-known clinical phenomenon (Lipowski 1985), few systematic studies exist. Epidemiological investigations have been hampered by the lack of precise diagnostic criteria and the inconsistent use of terms. Cognitive studies have been mostly anecdotal. Despite these limitations in knowledge, it is important to discuss acute confusion in some detail because it is believed to be one of the most highly prevalent disturbances of mental function in elderly individuals. Because the clinical symptoms are similar to dementia and psychosis, delirium is frequently misdiagnosed. Misdiagnosis can lead to increased morbidity and mortality, because it often is the only presenting symptom of a severe illness, which if left untreated, can have serious consequences. This chapter reviews the clinical presentation of acute confusion, its prevalence among elderly individuals, its cognitive hallmarks, possible causes, and management.

The DSM-IV (American Psychiatric Association 1994) criteria of delirium state that the patient must show 1) clinical features that develop rapidly and that tend to fluctuate during the course of the day; 2) disturbance of consciousness (i.e., reduced clarity of awareness) with reduced ability to focus; 3) a change in cognition (such as a memory deficit, disorientation, language disturbance, or the development of a perceptual disturbance that is not better accounted for by a pre-existing established or evolving dementia; and 4) evidence from the history, physical exam, or laboratory findings that the disturbance is caused by the direct physical consequences of a general medical condition.

As these criteria suggest, the symptoms of a delirium span a spectrum of clinical signs and symptoms. Patients who develop acute confusion vary from those who have previously shown no evidence of cognitive dysfunction to those who have been moderately to severely impaired. Likewise, the symptoms can vary from acute agitation, which may require restraints and medication, to a quiet confusion that goes unobserved but can be equally disabling in terms of the patient's ability for self-care.

As these examples suggest, the overt symptoms of acute confusional state patients have little in common, aside from the acute change in behavior. The disturbance of consciousness that is thought to be an essential feature of acute confusional state may not result in grossly inattentive behavior. Although the inattentive behavior may consist of the patient staring into space and being unaware of his or her environment or being mildly inattentive (e.g., failing to follow simple directions), it also may be reflected in the patient being tangential (e.g., changing the subject suddenly or telling a story unrelated to the question asked), distractible (e.g., responding to questions that are asked of someone walking in the hall), hypervigilant (e.g., examining an object in the room over and over), or focused on a persistent thought (e.g., looking for a possession that is not there).

In addition to its variability across patients, acute confusional state can fluctuate dramatically within individuals over the course of an episode. Therefore, the patient with acute confusional state may appear perfectly attentive at some points during the day but be distractible or hypervigilant at others. Changes in psychomotor activity, another common manifestation of acute confusional state, also may fluctuate greatly, with the patient being sluggish at times and restless at others. Similarly, the hallucinations and delusions that can occur in acute confusional state are rarely constant over the course of the day. Reports suggest that they are most common when the patients are either just falling asleep or just waking up (Lipowski 1980). It is clinical lore that acute confusional state patients frequently exhibit "sundowning" (i.e., display an exacerbation of symptoms after sundown). Although acute confusional state is a cognitive disorder, the variability in its clinical signs and symptoms and the absence of well-controlled prospective studies make it difficult to describe its cognitive hallmarks.

A disturbance in attention probably is the most consistent symptom (Mesulam and Geschwind 1976). Tasks such as digit span and crossing out a repeating letter have therefore been suggested for use in a screening battery for acute confusional state. However, for patients who are not overtly confused at the time of assessment, these measures may be insensitive to an underlying disturbance. For example, a study of acute confusional state in patients undergoing cataract extraction showed that a manual continuous performance test, in which the subject was asked to cross out as many letter *e*'s as possible on a single sheet of prose during 1 minute, was not affected when other cognitive tasks were (Burrows et al. 1985).

The assessment of a patient with a possible acute confusional state presents a challenge to the clinician. The limitations in knowledge and the consequent ambiguities in the diagnostic process should not dissuade the psychiatrist from trying to make as careful an evaluation as possible because acute confusional state leads to considerable morbidity and mortality in elderly individuals.

Summary

Numerous common conditions occur in elderly individuals that affect cognitive function. The clinician who sees elderly patients with great frequency must become familiar with the hallmarks of these conditions, as well as current management and treatment possibilities, to provide optimal care.

References

American Psychiatric Association: Diagnostic and Statistical Manual of Mental Disorders, 4th Edition. Washington, DC, American Psychiatric Association, 1994

Anthony JC, LeResche L, Niaz U, et al: Limits of the Mini-Mental State as a screening test for dementia and delirium among hospital patients.

Psychol Med 12:397–408, 1982

Bayles KA, Kaszniak AW: Communication and Cognition in Normal Aging and Dementia. Boston, MA, Little, Brown, 1987

Blessed G, Tomlinson BE, Roth M: The association between quantitative measures of dementia and of senile changes in the cerebral gray matter of elderly subjects. Br J Psychiatry 114:797–811, 1968

Boller F, Passafiume D, Keefe NC, et al: Visuospatial impairment in Parkinson's Disease. Arch Neurol 41:485–490, 1984

Breslow R, Kocsis J, Belkin B: Memory deficits in depression: evidence utilizing the Wechsler Memory Scale. Percept Mot Skills 51:541–542, 1980

Brown RG, Marsden CD, Quinn N, et al: Alterations in cognitive performance and affect arousal during fluctuations in motor function in Parkinson's disease. J Neurol Neurosurg Psychiatry 47:454–465, 1984

Brun A, Gustafson L: Distribution of cerebral degeneration in Alzheimer's disease: a clinico-pathological study. Arch Psychiatr Nervenkr 223:15–33, 1976

Bruyn GW, Bots G, Dom R: Huntington's chorea: current neuropathological status, in Advances in Neurology, Vol 23: Huntington's Disease. Edited by Chase T, Wexter N, Barbeau A. New York, Raven, 1979, pp 83–94

Burrows J, Briggs RS, Elkington AR: Cataract extraction and confusion in elderly patients. Clinical and Experimental Gerontology 7:51–70, 1985

Buschke H, Fuld PA: Evaluating storage, retention, and retrieval in disordered memory and learning. Neurology 11:1019–1025, 1974

Butters N, Albert MS, Sax DS, et al: The effect of verbal mediators on the pictorial memory of brain-damaged patients. Neuropsychologia 21:307–323, 1983

Butters N, Sax D, Tarlow S: Comparison of the neuropsychological deficits associated with early and advanced Huntington's disease. Arch Neurol 35:585–589, 1978

Byrne DC: Affect and vigilance performance in depressive illness. J Psychiatr Res 13:185–191, 1977

Caine E: The neuropsychology of depression: the pseudodementia syndrome, Neuropsychological Assessment of Neuropsychiatric Disorders. Edited by Grant I, Adams KM. New York, Oxford University Press, 1986, pp 221–243

Chase T, Foster N, Fedio P, et al: Regional cortical dysfunction in Alzheimer's disease as determined by positron emission tomography. Ann Neurol 15:5170–5174, 1984

Cole M, Wright D, Banker BQ: Familial aphasia due to Pick's disease. Ann Neurol 6:158, 1979

Constantinidis J, Richard J, Tissot R: Pick's disease: histological and clinical correlation. Eur Neurol 11:208–217, 1974

Cronholm B, Ottosson J: Memory functions in endogenous depression. Arch Gen Psychiatry 5:193–197, 1961

Cummings JL, Miller B, Hill MA: Neuropsychiatric aspects of multi-infarct dementia and dementia of the Alzheimer type. Arch Neurol 44:389–393, 1987

Davies P, Maloney AJR: Selective loss of central cholinergic neurons in Alzheimer's disease (letter). Lancet 2:1403, 1976

Delis DC, Kramer JH, Fridlund A, et al: California Verbal Learning Test. San Antonio, TX, Psychological Corp, 1986

DeKosky S, Scheff S: Synapse loss in frontal cortex biopsies in Alzheimer's disease: correlation with cognitive severity. Ann Neurol 27:457–464, 1990

Divac I: Neostriatum and functions of the prefrontal cortex. Acta Neurobiol Exp 32:461–477, 1972

El-Awar M, Becker JT, Hammond KM, et al: Learning deficit in Parkinson's disease: comparison with Alzheimer's disease and normal aging. Arch Neurol 44:180–184, 1987

Feldman MJ, Drasgow JA: A visual-verbal test for schizophrenia. Psychiatr Q Suppl 25:55–64, 1951

Fisher CM: Lacunar strokes and infarcts: a review. Neurology 32:871–876, 1982

Folstein MF, Folstein SE, McHugh PR: "Mini-Mental State": a practical method for grading cognitive state of patients for the clinician. J Psychiatr Res 12:189–198, 1975

Frith CD, Stevens M, Johnstone EC, et al: Effects of ECT and depression on various aspects of memory. Br J Psychiatry 142:610–617, 1983

Goffinet AM, Devolder AG, Gillain C, et al: Positron tomography demonstrates frontal lobe hypometabolism in progressive supranuclear palsy. Ann Neurol 25:131–139, 1988

Goldin CJ: A standardized version of Luria Nebraska neuropsychological tests, in Handbook of Clinical Neuropsychology. Edited by Filskov S, Voll TJ. New York, Wiley-Interscience, 1981

Goodglass H, Kaplan E: The Assessment of Aphasia and Related Disorders. Philadelphia, PA, Lea & Febiger, 1972

Gorham DR: A proverbs test for clinical and experimental use. Psychol Rep 1:1–12, 1956

Grady GL, Haxby JV, Horwitz B, et al: Longitudinal study of the early neuropsychological changes in dementia of the Alzheimer type. J Clin Exp Neuropsychol 10:576–596, 1989

Gustafson L: Frontal lobe degeneration of non-Alzheimer type, II: clinical picture and differential diagnosis. Arch Gerontol Geriatr 6:209–223, 1987

Hachinski VC, Lassen NA, Marshall J: Multi infarct dementia, a cause of mental deterioration in the elderly. Lancet 2:207–210, 1974

Halstead WC, Wepman JM: The Halstead-Wepman aphasia screening test. J Speech Hear Disord 14:9–15, 1949

Hart RP, Kwentus JA, Harkins SW, et al: Rate of forgetting in mild Alzheimer's type dementia. Brain Cogn 7:31–38, 1988

Haxby J, Grady C, Koss E, et al: Heterogeneous anterior-posterior metabolic patterns in dementia of the Alzheimer type. Neurology 18:1853–1863, 1988

Heaton R: Wisconsin Card Sorting Test. Odessa, TX, Psychological Assessment Resources, 1985

Henry GM, Weingartner H, Murphy DL: Influence of affective states and psychoactive drugs on verbal learning and memory. Am J Psychiatry 130:219–224, 1973

Heindel WC, Salmon DP, Shults CW, et al: Neuropsychological evidence for multiple implicit memory systems: a comparison of Alzheimer's, Huntington's, and Parkinson's disease patients. J Neurosci 9:582–587, 1989

Hovestadt A, deJong GJ, Meerwaldt JD: Spatial disorientation as an early symptom of Parkinson's disease. Neurology 37:485–487, 1987

Hyman BT, Van Hoesen GW, Damasio AR, et al: Alzheimer's disease: cell-specific pathology isolates the hippocampal formation. Science 225:1168–1170, 1985

Jellinger K: Neuropathological substrates of Alzheimer's disease and Parkinson's disease. J Neural Transm 24:109–129, 1987

Johnson KA, Davis KR, Buonanno FS, et al: Comparison of magnetic resonance and roentgen ray computed tomography in dementia. Arch Neurol 44:1075–1080, 1987

Josiassen RC, Curry L, Roemer RA, et al: Patterns of intellectual deficit in Huntington's disease. J Clin Neuropsychol 4:173–183, 1982

Kahn RL, Goldfarb AL, Pollack M, et al: Brief objective measures for the determination of mental status in the aged. Am J Psychiatry 111:326–328, 1960

Kaplan E, Goodglass H, Weintraub S: Boston Naming Test. Philadelphia,

PA, Lea & Febiger, 1983

Kemper T: Neuroanatomical and neuropathological changes in normal aging and dementia, in Clinical Neurology of Aging. Edited by Albert ML. New York, Oxford University Press, 1984, pp 9–52

Kertesz A: Western Aphasia Battery. London, Ontario, University of Western Ontario, 1980

Knopman D, Mastri A, Frey W, et al: Dementia lacking distinctive histologic features: a common non-Alzheimer degenerative dementia. Neurology 40:251–256, 1990

Lafleche G, Albert M: Executive function deficits in mild Alzheimer's disease. Neuropsychology 9:313–320, 1995

Lipowski ZJ: Delirium: Acute Brain Failure in Man. Springfield, IL: Charles C Thomas, 1980

Lipowski ZJ: Delirium (acute confusional state), in Handbook of Clinical Neurology. Edited by Vinken PJ, Bruyn GW, Klawans HL. New York, Elsevier, 1985, pp 523–559

Lund and Manchester Groups: Clinical and neuropathological criteria for frontotemporal dementia. J Neurol Neurosurg Psychiatry 57:416–418, 1994

Marie P: Des foyers lacunaires de desintegration et de differents autres etats cavetaures du cerveau. Rev Med 21:281–298, 1901

Masliah E, Mallory B, Hanson L, et al: Quantitative synaptic alterations in the human cortex during normal aging. Neurology 43:192–197, 1993

Mattis S: Dementia rating scale, in Geriatric Psychiatry. Edited by Bellack R, Karasu B. New York, Grune & Stratton, 1976, pp 77–121

Mesulam M, Geschwind N: Mental status in the postoperative period. Urol Clin North Am 3:199–215, 1976

Milberg W, Albert MS: Cognitive differences between patients with Alzheimer's disease and supranuclear palsy. J Clin Exp Neuropsychol 11:605–614, 1989

Mohr JP, Fisher CM, Adams RD: Cerebrovascular diseases, in Harrison's Principles of Internal Medicine. Edited by Isselbacher K, Adams RD. New York, McGraw-Hill, 1980, pp 1922–1941

Morris JC, Fulling K: Early Alzheimer's disease: diagnostic considerations. Arch Neurol 45:345–356, 1983

Morris JC, Heyman A, Mohs R, et al: The Consortium to Establish a Registry for Alzheimer's Disease (CERAD), I: clinical and neuropsychological assessment of Alzheimer's disease. Neurology 39:1159–1165, 1989

Moss MD, Albert MS: Alzheimer's disease and other dementing disorders, in Geriatric Neuropsychology. Edited by Albert MS, Moss MB. New York, Guilford, 1988, pp 145–178

Moss M, Albert M, Butters N, et al: Differential patterns of memory loss among patients with Alzheimer's disease, Huntington's disease and alcoholic Korsakoff's syndrome. Arch Neurol 43:239–246, 1986

Neary D, Snowden JS, Northen B, et al: Dementia of frontal lobe type. J Neurol Neurosurg Psychiatry 51:353–361, 1988

Nelson HE: A modified card sorting test sensitive to frontal lobe defects. Cortex 12:313–324, 1976

Nelson HE, O'Connell A: Dementia: the estimation of premorbid intelligence levels using the new adult reading test. Cortex 14:234–244, 1978

Neumann MA, Cohn R: Progressive subcortical gliosis, a rare form of presenile dementia. Brain 90:405–417, 1967

Neville HJ, Folstein MF: Performance on three cognitive tasks by patients with dementia, depression, or Korsakoff's syndrome. Gerontology 25:285–290, 1979

Pearson R, Esiri MM, Hiorns RW, et al: Anatomical correlate of the distribution of the pathologic changes in the neocortex in Alzheimer's disease. Proc Natl Acad Sci USA 82:4531–4534, 1985

Perez FI, Gay J, Taylor R: WAIS performance of neurologically impaired aged. Psychol Rep 37:1043–1047, 1975

Pfeiffer E: A short portable mental status questionnaire for the assessment of organic brain deficit in elderly patients. J Am Geriatr Soc 23:433–441, 1975

Pick A: On the relation between aphasia and senile atrophy of the brain, in Classics in Modern Translation. Edited by Rottenberg DA, Hochberg FH. New York, Hasner Press, 1892, pp 35–40

Pillon B, Dubois B, Lhermitte F, et al: Heterogeneity of cognitive impairment in progressive supranuclear palsy, Parkinson's disease, and Alzheimer's disease. Neurology 36:1179–1185, 1986

Randt CT, Brown ER, Osborne DJ: A memory test for longitudinal measurement of mild to moderate deficits. Clin Neuropsychol 2:184–194, 1980

Raskin A, Friedman AS, DiMascio A: Cognitive and performance deficits in depression. Psychopharmacol Bull 18:196–202, 1982

Reitan RM: Validity of the Trail Making Test as an indication of organic brain damage. Percept Mot Skills 8:271–276, 1958

Reitan RM: Halstead-Reitan Neuropsychological Test Battery. Tucson, Neuropsychology Laboratory, University of Arizona, 1979

Rey A: L'examen clinique en psychologie. Paris, Presses Universitaires de

France, 1964

Rosen WG: Neuropsychological investigation of memory, visuoconstructional, visuoperceptual, and language abilities in senile dementia of the Alzheimer type, in The Dementias. Edited by Mayeux R, Rosen WG. New York, Raven, 1983, pp 66–74

Scherr PA, Albert MS, Funkenstein HH, et al: Correlates of cognitive function in an elderly community population. J Epidemiol 128:1084–1091, 1988

Silbermann EK, Weingartner H, Laraia M, et al: Processing of emotional properties of stimuli by depressed and normal subjects. J Neurol Ment Dis 171:10–14, 1983

Steele JC, Richardson JC, Olszewiski J: Progressive supranuclear palsy. Arch Neurol 10:333–359, 1964

Sternberg DE, Jarvik ME: Memory functions in depression. Arch Gen Psychiatry 33:219–224, 1976

Tagliavini F, Pilleri I: Basal nucleus of Meynert: a neuropathological study in Alzheimer's disease, simple senile dementia, Pick's disease, Huntington's chorea. J Neurol Sci 62:243–260, 1983

Taylor AE, Saint-Cyr JA, Lang AE: Frontal lobe dysfunction in Parkinson's disease. Brain 109:845–883, 1986

Terry R, Masliah E, Salmon D, et al: Physical basis of cognitive alterations in Alzheimer's disease: synapse loss is the major correlate of cognitive impairment. Ann Neurol 30:572–580, 1991

Wechsler D: The Wechsler Adult Intelligence Scale—Revised. San Antonio, TX, Psychological Corp, 1981

Wechsler D: Wechler Memory Scale—Revised. San Antonio, TX, Psychological Corp, 1987

Wechsler AF, Verity MA, Rosenschein S, et al: Pick's disease: a clinical, computed tomographic, and histologic study with golgi impregnation observations. Arch Neurol 39:287–290, 1982

Weingartner H, Gold P, Ballenger JD, et al: Effects of vasopressin on human memory function. Science 211:601–603, 1981

Welsh K, Butters N, Hughes J, et al: Detection of abnormal memory decline in mild cases of Alzheimer's disease using CERAD neuropsychological measures. Arch Neurol 48:278–281, 1991

Whitehouse PJ, Price DL, Clark AW, et al: Alzheimer disease: evidence for selective loss of cholinergic neurons in the nucleus basalis. Ann Neurol 10:122–126, 1981

Richard Margolin, M.D.
Peter Moran, M.B., L.R.C.P., S.I.

Neuroimaging

P sychiatric diagnosis in the elderly is often difficult. Traditionally, the process has involved interview, general physical and neurological examinations, and laboratory tests. In more recent years, these methods have been increasingly complemented by a set of procedures known as *neuroimaging*. This term denotes several methods for creating images of various facets of brain structure or function. Although some neuroimaging techniques were introduced decades ago, the field has become much more sophisticated with the introduction since the 1970s of powerful computerized methods. The more important and widely utilized of these newer methods include X-ray computed tomography (CT), magnetic resonance imaging (MRI), positron-emission tomography (PET), single photon emission computed tomography (SPECT), and computerized electroencephalography. In this chapter we present an overview of these techniques, including methodology and appropriate use in geriatric mental disorders. Because it is impossible to discuss the individual techniques comprehensively in this chapter, the reader desiring more information is referred to detailed reviews on CT (Hounsfield 1980), MRI (Partain et al. 1988), PET (Phelps and Mazziotta 1985), and SPECT (Proceedings 1987, 1988). Comprehensive reviews of the major modalities, with particular reference to geriatric psychiatry, have also been published (Coffey and Cummings 1994; Margolin and Daniel 1990; Pietrini and Rapoport 1994).

Methodology

Although there are many ways to consider the various imaging methods, several key concepts deserve special attention. Perhaps the most important is the distinction between structural and functional imaging. Structural imaging techniques delineate facets of cerebral anatomy such as the size, location, and shape of brain regions. Functional imaging techniques reveal elements of cerebral physiology such as blood flow, metabolism, and parameters of neurotransmission. CT and MRI are structural imaging modalities, whereas PET and SPECT are functional imaging methods.

Another important concept is the spatial nature of the data produced. Earlier brain imaging techniques such as pneumoencephalography—as well as some techniques still being used (e.g., multiprobe cerebral blood flow [CBF] systems)—were essentially planar, collapsing the inherently three-dimensional shape of the brain into two dimensions. The newer methods, by contrast, are all tomographic in that they produce several parallel, thin, slicelike images of the brain, called *tomograms*. A tomogram literally means a picture of a slice. Tomographic methods are a major advance over planar techniques because they provide markedly increased detail (information density).

A final concept common to all the tomographic techniques is the manner in which their data are collected and displayed. Several standard orientations for data acquisition exist. These are called the *transverse, sagittal,* and *coronal* planes. The transverse orientation, although not universally defined in exactly the same way, generally refers to a plane that passes through the orbits and the internal auditory meati. The sagittal plane is roughly perpendicular to the transverse plane and cleaves the midline through the interhemispheric fissure. The coronal plane is vertically oriented and perpendicular to the sagittal plane.

With regard to data display, sets of images are usually presented using a shades-of-gray scale. The particular meaning of the scale varies with each modality. Color display scales are also used, but in such schemes individual colors have no special meaning in themselves. Images can be recorded on film or displayed on computer monitors. Currently images are interpreted by a trained radiologist, usually a neuroradiologist, or for some modalities a nuclear medicine specialist. Advances in computer technology and image analysis methods portend semiautomatic interpretation of images in the future.

Computed Tomography

Developed in the 1970s, CT quickly became widely used in neuropsychiatry. The ability to obtain tomographic images of brain structure noninvasively was perceived by clinicians as a tremendous development. In CT images, gray- and white-matter zones as well as the cerebrospinal fluid (CSF) compartment can be individually visualized. Both normal anatomy and pathological structural alterations can be appreciated. The method uses a thin X-ray beam that is passed through the head; intervening tissues absorb the beam according to their relative densities. The residual beam is recorded by a detector apparatus. Each image is produced sequentially by slightly advancing the bed on which the patient lies and repeating the data acquisition process. Separately, a computer converts the absorption patterns into images in a procedure called *reconstruction.* CT can readily distinguish tissues of quite different density but cannot do as well with tissues of marginally different density, such as gray and white matter.

CT is relatively easy for patients to tolerate. Although head-dedicated CT scanners exist, the procedure is generally performed on a device able to admit the torso. Thus, the aperture of the scanner is not confining, and a standard examination requires less than an hour. A practical consideration for CT and all the other techniques is that stabilization and immobilization of the patient's head and body during the data acquisition period are essential for high-quality images. The advent of helical CT, also known as *spiral* or *volume acquisition CT,* has decreased imaging times. In this technique there is a continuous spiral motion of the X-ray tube detector through the area being scanned, allowing a head CT scan to be completed in 10 seconds. Usually about 15 to 20 slices are obtained in a clinical study; their customary orientation is transverse. In the usual gray-scale display scheme, white represents structures of highest density, and black, those of least density.

CT can be performed with or without *contrast media.* This term denotes substances, usually containing iodine, that absorb X rays well. It has been recognized for almost a decade that intracranial blood vessels can be outlined by performing CT after intravenous delivery of contrast media. A CT scan so performed is called a *contrast-enhanced scan.* Unfortunately, although some abnormalities are definitely better seen with contrast, a small but significant percentage of patients are allergic to contrast media. Patients at risk cannot always be identified before the procedure is performed. Nonionic or low osmolar contrast media with low allergy potential are currently available, and as a result, contrast reactions have decreased in frequency.

Magnetic Resonance Imaging

MRI has become widely used in clinical practice since the 1980s. During that time its growth has been phenomenal. In contrast to CT, which measures only tissue density, MRI is actually a set of distinct procedures that as a whole reveal details about various facets of the physicochemical composition of the brain. The term *magnetic resonance* denotes the property of nuclei of certain elements to spin about an axis when exposed to a magnetic field. The most common element possessing this property is hydrogen, and consequently hydrogen (or proton) imaging is the basis of almost all current MRI systems. A magnetic resonance scanner is a device that applies a steady magnetic field together with pulses of radio frequency energy to an area of a patient's body. The scanner also incorporates a receiver that records the response to the applied energy of nuclei in the cells of the body region being scanned.

Two key parameters have been described in MRI that reflect distinct tissue responses to magnetic perturbation. These parameters are called the *T1* and *T2 relaxation times*. Images reflecting either T1 or T2 may be created by varying details of the data acquisition process. The T1-weighted image is somewhat similar to a non–contrast-enhanced CT image of the brain in that it generally represents anatomy and faithfully depicts spatial relationships among structures in the brain. It provides excellent, even extraordinary, visualization of contrast between gray and white matter. T1-weighted MRI is distinctly superior to CT in this regard. The T2-weighted image, on the other hand, is markedly influenced by tissue water content and does not closely correspond to anatomic detail. It is proving very useful, however, in revealing localized pathological abnormality that is not evident on images obtained with other techniques.

A clinical magnetic resonance scan typically includes 15 to 20 images per acquisition. Usually a complete examination requires two to four sequences, giving a total of 40 to 80 images. A number of data acquisition schemes, called *pulse sequences,* are currently being explored in cranial MRI, and there is no consensus as to which is the most efficient or useful in neuropsychiatric indications. Probably the most commonly used scheme, however, is the spin echo sequence. In this approach, a proton density image and a T2-weighted image are produced essentially simultaneously at each scanning plane. A proton density image is intermediate in appearance between T1- and T2-weighted images. The process is repeated multiple times to image the entire brain. The relatively recent advent of fast spin echo techniques has shortened scanning times, allowing increased accessibility and diminished patient discomfort. Nevertheless, MRI is still probably the most stressful neuroimaging procedure for patients, as a head scan can take up to 30 minutes, and the apparatus can be experienced as confining. In many centers, a screening questionnaire is given to patients prior to the day of their scan; this includes a query about previous claustrophobic symptoms. Patients who respond positively are asked to be accompanied to their scan by a friend or family member and are usually sedated prophylactically, with diazepam being the drug of choice in most centers.

As in CT, a gray-scale image display scheme is customary; however, the term *signal intensity* is used instead of density, reflecting the heterogeneity of the MRI modality. In this scheme, white represents areas of highest signal intensity, and black, the areas of lowest signal intensity. It is important to realize that a given brain structure can appear very different on proton density, T1-weighted, and T2-weighted images; for example, the lateral ventricles are generally seen as black on T1-weighted images and white on T2-weighted images.

In contrast to CT, the patient is not moved between image acquisitions. MRI is somewhat more challenging for patients than CT because the scanner aperture is smaller; thus, there is often a feeling of confinement, and an MRI examination can sometimes take more than an hour. A significant advantage of MRI is its ability to produce images in any plane, not just the transverse plane. In routine clinical practice, several sagittal views and a complete set of transverse images are obtained. However, more extensive sagittal or coronal views are very helpful in certain clinical situations. For example, sagittal views image the pituitary gland very well. Contrast media have also been developed for MRI; the most widely used clinically is a gadolinium salt (gadodiamide, or GdDTPA-BMA).

Positron-Emission Tomography

PET is the most advanced functional neuroimaging modality developed to date. It is a nuclear medicine technique that depends on certain properties of positrons (subatomic particles belonging to the class called *antimatter*). They have the mass and charge of electrons and are thus also known as *antielectrons*. Positron-emitting elements for PET do not occur naturally in any quantity but can be produced artificially with a medical cyclotron. Such radioactive elements are then chemically bonded to a molecule of interest in a process known as *radiochemistry*. Molecules so produced are called *radiotracers*. In PET, a radiotracer is injected intravenously or inhaled while the patient lies with part of the body inside the PET scanner's aperture. The PET scanner detects the radiation produced when a positron emitted by a radiotracer collides with an unbound electron in tissue. Because the two particles have opposite charge, they annihilate each other and, following the law of conservation of energy, emit two photons of 511 keV energy at 180° to each other (Coffey and Cummings 1994). The PET scanner uses this property to localize the source of the energy, thus allowing images of the distribution of tracer presence to be reconstructed.

Many investigators believe that PET has considerable potential in psychiatry. The basis for this viewpoint is twofold. First, positron-emitting isotopes of the key component elements of biologically important molecules exist, including oxygen, carbon, and nitrogen. As a result, among the PET radiotracers that have been created are some very interesting molecules for the study of psychiatric disorders. Second, PET is in principle a quantitative method. On introduction to the body, the fate of the PET radiotracer depends on the way the various cellular systems and organs it encounters "see" it. For example, some tracers are extensively metabolized, whereas others are not; some are trapped by the brain, but others remain in the vascular compartment. Although the PET scanner detects only total radioactivity in an organ, a mathematical model can be applied to such uptake data. Such a procedure, called *tracer kinetic modeling*, enables creation of images that precisely reflect a physiological process.

Although PET brain research began in the 1970s, its applications in psychiatry, and certainly in geriatric psychiatry, are still emerging. With PET several important physiological processes can be imaged, of which regional cerebral blood flow (CBF), regional cerebral metabolic rate for glucose (CMR_{glu}), and regional cerebral metabolic rate for oxygen (CMR_{O_2}) have been the most thoroughly studied so far. However, work with neurotransmission (e.g., dopamine, acetylcholine, and serotonin systems) and protein synthesis is also promising. As newer ligands are being synthesized, more and more receptors and neurotransmitters are becoming accessible to in vivo measurement (Kapur et al. 1994).

Like CT and MRI, PET also generates tomographic images, with the exact number dependent on the particular scanner type. The most current PET scanners produce between 15 and 31 parallel slices simultaneously.

For some applications this number is sufficient; if additional detail is desired, the acquisition can be repeated after moving the patient slightly. From the patient's perspective, PET's tolerability is between that of CT and MRI. Although obtaining a single set of slices can take very little time, a complete brain survey (multiple sets of slices) might require from 10 to 90 minutes, depending on the physiological process being studied. An intravenous line is usually necessary, and some types of PET study require arterial catheterization.

Single Photon Emission Computed Tomography

SPECT is a derivation of PET that uses relatively standard nuclear medicine cameras instead of specially developed scanners. The SPECT tracers that have been synthesized for neuropsychiatric applications have incorporated isotopes of technetium, iodine, or xenon, although tracer agents for benzodiazepine and dopamine receptors are to be released soon for clinical use. Three tracers of CBF are currently commercially available: iofetamine hydrochloride I 123 (Spectamine) and technetium Tc 99m exametazime (Ceretec), and technetium Tc 99m bicisate (Neurolite), which was approved and made widely available for clinical use in 1995. Technetium Tc 99m exametazime has superior imaging characteristics, as it is very stable. Brain uptake is rapid, and clearance from the brain is very slow. One application for this is in sleep research, where technetium Tc 99m exametazime can be injected during a specific sleep stage and the patient scanned in the morning. Although SPECT CBF measurements have been approved for clinical use only in stroke patients, research results imply that they are valuable in a variety of neuropsychiatric conditions, including dementia, seizure disorders, traumatic brain injury, drug abuse, acquired immunodeficiency syndrome (AIDS), and depression (Holman and Devous 1992; Juni 1994). Fully satisfactory quantitative models for SPECT imaging of CBF are not yet available for any tracer but are under development. "While it initially appeared that brain SPECT would suffer from a number of limitations relative to PET, recent improvements in instrumentation and radiopharmaceuticals as well as increasingly compelling clinical evaluations suggest a primary role for SPECT in the diagnosis of a number of highly prevalent neurological diseases" (Holman and Devous 1992, p. 188).

SPECT also produces tomograms, usually about 60. The procedure is quite tolerable for patients. In the most widely implemented system, the patient lies on an open bed while a large flat gamma camera orbits the head.

Practical Consideration in the Use of Neuroimaging in Geriatric Psychiatry

From the perspectives of the geriatric psychiatrist, radiologist, and patient, there are many practical distinctions among these methods. Some, such as the length of time for data acquisition and the extent of discomfort, confinement, and invasiveness, are especially important considerations for frail elderly patients and have been discussed. Other factors important in understanding neuroimaging methods include resolution, hazards, accessibility, and cost. Resolution refers to the detail that can be visualized in an image. Technically it is defined by the smallest objects that can be discriminated within an image. Data concerning these parameters are summarized in Table 12–1.

It is fair to say that each technique has its strengths and weaknesses. In terms of resolution, CT and MRI are clearly superior, but considerable progress in this respect has been made in PET; in fact, PET is approaching a theoretical maximum resolution of approximately 3 mm. The resolution achieved so far with SPECT is quite inferior to that of PET and definitely limits its clinical value; it is still unclear whether technological advances will significantly improve SPECT's resolution.

CT, PET, and SPECT all require the use of ionizing radiation, which is well recognized to carry certain risks. The doses, however, are generally modest and compare favorably with those of traditional radiological procedures. MRI is alone in not involving radiation exposure. In fact, with the exception of patients with certain types of cardiac pacemaker or surgical clips, its known risks are not significant. As with any new medical procedure or drug, it is possible that long-term risks will become apparent with experience.

Table 12–1.   Practical considerations in the use of neuroimaging techniques in geriatric psychiatry

Technique	Resolution (mm)	Radiation	Accessibility	Cost per study ($)[a]
CT	1–2	Yes	Wide	500
MRI	1–2	No	Fairly wide	750–1,000
PET	3–5	Yes	Limited	1,200–2,500
SPECT	6–8	Yes	Increasing	750

[a]Prices do not reflect regional variations unless a range is given and are representative of an average United States city market in early 1994. These prices are typical of a "routine" study. Some studies have higher costs if additional optional components are performed.

Use of Neuroimaging Methods in Geriatric Psychiatry

Although neuroimaging has already become useful clinically in some mental disorders of late life (notably the organic dementias), a larger number of conditions have been investigated in research studies. These include organic nondementia syndromes, as well as the psychoses, affective disorders, and anxiety disorders. Only in the areas of dementia and normal aging have elderly populations been the specific focus of neuroimaging research programs; in the other disorders, patients and controls of young, middle-age, and elderly groups have been mixed together. This mixing clearly limits the conclusions that can be drawn about the ultimate value of these imaging techniques in geriatric psychiatry.

In turning to the use of the various imaging methods in geriatric psychiatry, it is reasonable to ask, "What is the primary value of the structural and functional imaging techniques?" Anatomic abnormalities in the brain, at the level resolvable with current imaging methods, are "macroscopic." CT and MRI can detect pathological abnormalities such as atrophy, edema, infarction, and tumor. These disturbances regularly occur in major neuropsychiatric disorders such as dementia, delirium, and poststroke depression. In these conditions such disturbances affect brain structures subserving key psychological processes (e.g., cognition, language, mood, and affect). Knowledge of the brain regions affected by such tissue-disruptive processes can enhance the geriatric psychiatrist's understanding of symptomatology.

Potentially much more valuable in appreciating brain-behavior relationships in psychiatric disease are the functional imaging techniques. Details of several neurophysiological processes have been demonstrated with imaging techniques, including CBF, metabolism, and parameters of neurotransmitter function. It is reasonable to suppose that abnormalities in these physiological processes may occur in psychiatric disease before their anatomic correlates can be identified. Furthermore, in most psychiatric diseases, anatomic abnormalities are not known. Thus, the functional imaging techniques are regarded by many as promising more sensitive and specific data about neural disturbance in mental disorders than the structural imaging methods can provide.

Aging

Before reviewing neuroimaging findings in individual disorders, it is important to consider briefly some information that has emerged from studies of normal aging. Knowledge of age-specific changes in human neuroanatomy and physiology is developing rapidly. It is already clear that definite structural and physiological changes occur with aging in many brain regions and systems (Coffey and Cummings 1994; Veith and Raskind 1988; Waller and London 1987). Some familiarity with the major findings in the neurobiology of aging is crucial because aging-related processes and disease-related processes interact in subtle ways in geriatric psychiatric syndromes. Certain disorders, most notably the dementias, are strongly associated with age. Imaging studies inevitably reflect a mixture of age- and disease-related phenomena.

The primary macroscopic morphological change known to occur with aging is brain atrophy, noted as an increase in the volume of the CSF space and a decrease in brain volume (Schwartz et al. 1985). Ventricular enlargement may provide a more sensitive index of brain aging than does cortical atrophy (Coffey and Cummings 1994). The CSF space in humans is composed of the third, fourth, and lateral ventricles and the subarachnoid space. The ventricles are easily identified on CT or MRI scans in the depths of the brain, whereas the subarachnoid space is visualized as the sulci adjacent to cortical gyri. Besides atrophy, both gray- and white-matter densities have also been reported to decrease. Finally, white-matter abnormalities of uncertain significance are seen occasionally with CT and regularly with MRI in otherwise healthy elderly persons; these abnormalities are discussed in this chapter.

Age-related changes have also been identified in functional measures. CMR_{glu} and CMR_{O_2} seem stable, at least in studies of very healthy individuals, but CBF declines (Duara et al. 1983; Pantano et al. 1984). However, data remain somewhat contradictory. Marshal (1992) found a significant decline in regional CBF (rCBF) only in two frontal gyri, whereas CMR_{O_2} was reduced throughout the cerebral cortex except for the orbitofrontal gyrus, hippocampal, and lateral occipital regions. The regional pattern of these metabolic parameters may change with aging. Ingvar (1979) proposed the term *hyperfrontality* to refer to the normal pattern of frontal CBF being greater than parietal CBF. This pattern is lost with aging. Age-related neurotransmitter physiology changes have also been found with PET. For example, Wong and associates (1984) found age-related decrements in dopamine D_2-receptor binding in various cortical regions and the basal ganglia.

Some of the same structural and functional abnormalities that occur in aging have been revealed by neuroimaging methods to also occur in various psychiatric diseases in young and middle-age persons; for example, ventricular and sulcal enlargement as well as hypofrontality have been found in subpopulations of schizophrenic patients. When patients with such diseases are studied for the first time with imaging procedures in late life, it may be impossible to separate the effects of age from those of disease. The possibility of dual contributions to imaging findings must therefore be borne in mind.

Dementia

Among geriatric psychiatric disorders, dementia is the most common setting for the application of neuroimaging techniques. Two factors have led to this development. The first is the valuable data about cerebral morphology and function that the techniques provide. The second is the current lack of a reliable, biologically based nonimaging method for positive diagnosis of the major dementing disorders. Nevertheless, although the technological advances made in these techniques since the 1970s have been spectacular and the likelihood of further progress is substantial, neuroradiological tools have still not replaced the traditional clinical evaluation used in diagnosing dementia and the complementary techniques (e.g., lumbar puncture, electroencephalography, and analysis of blood chemistries) that help identify specific etiologies.

Numerous structural and functional imaging studies of patients with Alzheimer's disease, multi-infarct dementia, and other types of dementia have been published. In this work CT, MRI, PET, and SPECT have all been used. A number of well-conducted studies have either focused on individual types of dementia or compared control subjects with patients with dementia who had mixed diagnoses. In this section we first describe the key findings in the several major etiologies and then comment on the clinician's use of the techniques in differential diagnosis.

Alzheimer's disease. Although presenile-onset and senile-onset dementias of the Alzheimer type have in the past been considered by some to be separate diseases, they are considered in this chapter as one condition, called Alzheimer's disease. Because Alzheimer's disease is the major cause of dementia in developed countries, it is not surprising that this condition has been the dementing disorder most studied by neuroimaging. McGeer (1986) comprehensively reviewed the major neuroimaging studies performed in Alzheimer's disease. Modern structural imaging in Alzheimer's disease began with the use of CT. Huckman and colleagues (1975) first found ventriculomegaly with CT in the mid-1970s in virtually all members of a group of elderly dementia patients. Although the severity of brain atrophy has varied, many studies subsequently confirmed the finding in both young (Brinkman et al. 1981) and old (Gado et al. 1982) Alzheimer's disease patients.

Because macroscopic cerebral atrophy is generalized in advanced Alzheimer's disease, the most common pattern on CT or MRI is matched sulcal and ventricular enlargement. Sulcal enlargement has been less consistently seen than ventriculomegaly, at least in CT studies (Albert et al. 1984a). Atrophy on CT or MRI scans cannot be used to make a presumptive diagnosis of Alzheimer's disease. However, quantitative analyses using MRI distinguish most patients with Alzheimer's disease from healthy, elderly control subjects by showing reductions in brain size and increases in CSF in the Alzheimer's disease group (DeCarli et al. 1990). In addition to global atrophy, various patterns of regional atrophy have also been reported, and the absence of atrophy is commonly encountered, especially in early Alzheimer's disease. Thus, Alzheimer's disease patients are separable from controls on the basis of CT or MRI findings only statistically in group analyses, not individually.

In addition to atrophy, decrements in tissue density (especially in white matter) have also been reported (Albert et al. 1984b; Bondareff et al. 1981; Naeser et al. 1980). These decrements can be either diffuse and detectable only with quantitative analysis, or focal and identifiable by visual inspection of scans.

Serious efforts have been made to translate findings of atrophy or hypodensity into clinically useful tools for diagnosing Alzheimer's disease. Unfortunately, primarily because of the great overlap with findings in healthy elderly persons, it has not been possible to develop either manual or automated schemes for this purpose.

The advent of MRI has occasioned several studies of Alzheimer's disease (Besson et al. 1983, 1985; Brant-Zawadzki et al. 1985; Erkinjuntti et al. 1984; Fazekas et al. 1987). DeCarli et al. (1990) and McGeer (1986) confirmed that brain atrophy could be identified with MRI. Besson and associates (1983) found increased T1 values in gray and white matter of many cortical regions; they also found increased white-matter proton density values (Besson et al. 1985). MRI has produced some intriguing findings, not previously seen clearly with CT, with respect to the status of the white matter in Alzheimer's disease. These data are discussed in detail in this chapter.

It is not surprising that Alzheimer's disease has been one of the disorders most actively explored by PET investigators. CBF, CMR_{O_2}, and CMR_{glu} changes have all been investigated. Frackowiak (1987) reviewed these studies comprehensively; two key findings have emerged. The first is that all three parameters of brain metabolism are significantly decreased in advanced Alzheimer's disease, on the order of 20% to 30% (Frackowiak et al. 1981). Despite the reductions in blood flow, evidence suggests that occult hypoperfusion is not directly involved in the pathogenesis of Alzheimer's disease. Second, a pattern seemingly unique to Alzheimer's disease has been noted in imaging of CMR_{glu}; this pattern has been replicated by several groups (Benson et al. 1983; Chase et al. 1984; Duara et al. 1986; Ferris et al. 1983; Friedland et al. 1983) and has been reviewed by Kapur et al. (1994). The pattern consists of a bilateral localized metabolic deficiency in the posterior parietal and temporal lobes (Chase et al. 1983). With advancing disease the frontal lobes are also affected, and the severity of the metabolic dysfunction increases, particularly in the parietal lobes (Jagust et al. 1987). Foster et al. (1983) also demonstrated that the site of focal hypometabolism in Alzheimer's disease sometimes parallels predominant features of the clinical presentation. For example, some Alzheimer's disease patients with prominent aphasia had focal defects in the left temporal cortex, whereas patients with marked visuospatial incoordination had such abnormalities in the superior right parietal lobe. It is not yet apparent how often these nonparietal or unilateral parietal focal deficits occur.

Two focal points of PET work in Alzheimer's disease are noteworthy. The first concerns the manifestations of Alzheimer's disease early in its course. Haxby and associates (1985) have identified parietal lobe metabolic defects, even in patients with minimal dementia who could not be distinguished from controls in neuropsychological tests thought to be mediated by parietal systems. There also seems to be an inverse correlation between overall symptoms and regional metabolism (Coffey and Cummings 1994). Another theme of PET research is the comparison of patients with early-onset versus late-onset Alzheimer's disease. Small and colleagues (1989) have shown that early-onset Alzheimer's disease patients show parietal hypometabolic defects more significantly than late-onset Alzheimer's disease patients. A number of SPECT studies of Alzheimer's disease have also now been conducted; the results confirm PET findings of biparietal hypoperfusion (Holman 1986; Holman and Devous 1992; Testa et al. 1988).

Multi-infarct dementia. The classic CT signature of multi-infarct dementia is the presence of multiple nonenhancing infarcts, which can be of variable size and can be located in the cortex, white matter, or subcortical nuclei. There are several variants of multi-infarct dementia, and the terminology needs improvement. One variant of multi-infarct dementia, subcortical arteriosclerotic encephalopathy (SAE)—Binswanger's disease—appears on CT as multiple infarcts in the periventricular white matter (Roman 1987). On MRI scans white matter demyelination is seen pathologically as hyperintensities on T2-weighted images in the periventricular and deep white matter regions (Coffey and Cummings 1994). Infarcts caused by occlusion of perforating arteries in the subcortical nuclei and white matter are called lacunes. Thus, another variant of multi-infarct dementia, in which multiple lacunes exist, is known as the lacunar state. Lacunes are usually less than 1 cm in size and may be round or slit-like. They account for up to 20% of strokes (Mohr 1983), and lacunar dementia often features prominent frontal system dysfunction (Wolfe et al. 1990). Unfortunately, the absence of visible stroke-affected tissue on CT scans of patients with dementia does not entirely rule out multi-infarct dementia, because some stroke tissue is isodense with surrounding parenchyma (Harsch et al. 1988) and because some affected areas may be very small (Cummings 1987; Knopman and Rubens 1986; Kohlmeyer 1979). CT more commonly misses brain stem strokes, but in practice its sensitivity in chronic supratentorial stroke is very high (Aichner and Gerstenbrand 1989).

The MRI features of stroke and multi-infarct dementia have been the subject of several careful reviews (Ford et al. 1989; Kessler 1988). Characteristic findings exist for both early and completed stroke. The geriatric psychiatrist generally does not evaluate patients with multi-infarct dementia in close proximity to acute strokes; thus, the pattern in completed stroke is more relevant. The majority of strokes are thrombotic in origin; a minority are hemorrhagic. Completed thrombotic infarctions typically demonstrate a pattern of decreased signal intensity on T1-weighted images and increased signal on T2-weighted images. Chronic hemorrhagic infarctions display a core of hyperintense signal on T1- and T2-weighted images, surrounded by a rim of hypointense signal, especially on T2-weighted images (Ford et al. 1989). Although the resolution is similar in MRI and CT, MRI is superior in detecting small infarctions, especially lacunes (Brown et al. 1988), and brain stem strokes.

An important and still imperfectly clarified issue in the application of neuroimaging in dementia is the significance of the white-matter lesions (WMLs) revealed by MRI. Not long after the introduction of MRI into general clinical use, WMLs, particularly in T2-weighted images, were reported in scans of both healthy elderly patients and patients with dementia (Bradley et al. 1984; Brant-Zawadzki et al. 1985). A number of groups have investigated this subject in detail (Fazekas et al. 1987; George et al. 1986) and have identified several distinct patterns, including periventricular lesions, ventricular pole lesions, and focal (punctate) or diffuse (confluent) abnormalities in the deep white matter.

The several patterns previously described have varying significance. Frontal horn capping is not necessarily pathological (Zimmerman et al. 1988). It may represent an age-accentuated pattern of CSF transudation from the interstitial space into the ventricles. Uniform periventricular hyperintensity is of similarly uncertain diagnostic significance, occurring commonly in elderly individuals both with and without dementia (Fazekas et al. 1987). Discrete, deep WMLs may have a variety of causes, ranging from frank infarction to chronic vascular insufficiency (Braffman et al. 1988). Vasculitis and multiple sclerosis, known causes in younger persons, must also be considered if the clinical data so indicate. Overall these lesions have different pathological correlates and may be of variable clinical significance (Chimowitz et al. 1992).

Considerable variation exists in the frequency of WMLs reported (Erkinjuntti et al. 1984; George et al. 1986), but a rate of about 30% in unselected elderly patients is credible (Braffman et al. 1988). Although these lesions are clearly found in some healthy individuals (Fazekas 1989), they are more frequently encountered in dementia than in normal aging (Fazekas et al. 1987). They occur in both Alzheimer's disease and multi-infarct dementia patients at a rate higher than that seen in control subjects; a rate approaching 100% is reported in multi-infarct dementia. Their frequency increases with cardiovascular risk factors, including hypertension and diabetes mellitus (Gerard and Weisberg 1986), which is suggestive of a vascular etiology. However, even in patients with such risk factors, extrapolation from the finding of WMLs to a diagnosis of SAE is a temptation not supported by present knowledge. Many more patients with dementia have WMLs than meet strict criteria for SAE (Caplan and Schoene 1978). Furthermore, not even prominent WMLs rule out Alzheimer's disease.

PET findings in multi-infarct dementia are based on the results of stroke research performed with this technique. Several studies have noted the metabolic and blood flow patterns in acute and completed strokes. The examination of CBF, CMR_{glu}, CMR_{O_2}, and the oxygen extraction fraction (OEF) in stroke is useful. Normally these parameters are tightly coupled and blood supply is not limiting. OEF is an indicator of the reserve capacity of blood flow. Although the changes in these parameters during the evolution of a stroke are complex, a completed stroke classically produces a region of matched hypometabolism and decreased blood flow (Frackowiak 1987). OEF is not increased. The zone of hypometabolism is often substantially larger than would be predicted from examining CT or MRI scans. Abnormalities in distant sites are seen that reflect the impact of a stroke on neural connectivity. The larger functional than structural zone of impairment indicates that tissue surrounding the infarct may be damaged but still alive and reflects biochemical processes initiated by the stroke in surrounding tissue. On PET scans multi-infarct dementia presents as focal areas of decreased metabolism and blood flow in the areas of known infarcts (Frackowiak 1985). There is no specific regional pattern in multi-infarct dementia as there is in Alzheimer's disease. Only very incomplete comparison studies of the diagnostic value of PET and CT/MRI in stroke have been executed; the work done so far supports the idea that they could have complementary roles. SPECT studies of multi-infarct dementia are still fragmentary, but as with Alzheimer's disease, they generally confirm the PET findings. Technetium Tc 99m bicisate SPECT appears reasonably accurate for distinguishing vascular dementia from Alzheimer's disease when bilateral temporoparietal defects are present (Holman and Devous 1992).

Other dementias. A multitude of etiologic entities in addition to Alzheimer's disease and multi-infarct dementia can cause dementia. These include neurodegenerative dementias such as Pick's disease, progressive supranuclear palsy, Huntington's disease, and the dementia associated with Parkinson's disease; normal pressure hydrocephalus–induced dementia; Creutzfeldt-Jakob disease and other infectious disorders; posttraumatic dementia; dementia induced by hypoxia; alcoholic and other metabolic dementias; and endocrine-related dementias. Recently added to this list is dementia caused by human immunodeficiency virus (HIV) infection. The neuroimaging findings in all of these dementias cannot be individually reviewed here, but a few comments may be helpful.

Some of these dementias have specific associated neuroimaging findings. In Pick's disease, for example, the diagnosis is supported by the finding of focal frontotemporal atrophy and reductions in CBF and CMR. In progressive supranuclear palsy, retention of a rim of cortical metabolism/ flow surrounding a generalized frontal reduction has been claimed. In normal pressure hydrocephalus, ventriculomegaly out of proportion to sulcal atrophy may be seen with either CT or MRI. Periventricular hyperintensity may also be seen on MRI in patients with this condition. Dementia caused by HIV infection is frequently associated with the finding of focal areas of white-matter hypodensity on CT scans or similar zones of increased T2 signal on MRI scans. PET studies show diminished metabolism in the same areas. Brain perfusion SPECT is highly sensitive for the detection of AIDS dementia complex. Early disease is easily separated from healthy subjects and non-HIV psychoses (Holman and Devous 1992).

Other Organic Mental Disorders

Parkinson's disease and Huntington's disease have also been studied by neuroimaging. CT and MRI scans are not often abnormal in patients with Parkinson's disease, but CT findings suggesting subcortical atrophy or frontal atrophy have been associated with cognitive impairment in Parkinson's disease (Starkstein and Leiguarda 1993). Imaging of dopamine receptors in the basal ganglia is being investigated, and PET has been shown to detect asymptomatic dopaminergic lesions that may be a preclinical indicator for the development of Parkinson's disease (Karbe et al. 1992). Psychiatric complications of Parkinson's disease, including dementia, and L-dopa–induced psychosis are common, but studies of subgroups of Parkinson's disease patients with and without these complications have been inconclusive.

Huntington's disease is commonly associated with psychiatric symptoms. In advanced disease, caudate head atrophy can be seen with structural imaging. PET has demonstrated a characteristic metabolic signature earlier in the course of the disease (Phelps et al. 1982)—namely, a marked reduction in basal ganglia CMR_{glu}. The concept has been advanced that this phenomenon may be detectable even preclinically (Mazziotta et al. 1987).

Psychoses

Considerable neuroimaging research has been conducted in schizophrenia. Shelton and Weinberger (1986) and Coffman and Nasrallah (1986) summarized the structural studies using CT and MRI, respectively. As these reviews indicate, many studies using CT and several using MRI have replicated the original finding of ventriculomegaly in schizophrenia (Johnstone et al. 1978) or found sulcal enlargement. Coffman and Nasrallah (1986) have suggested that these phenomena may be related to fetal or peripartum events with prolonged or delayed neurodevelopmental expression. Because increase of CSF space is also associated with aging, prudence is advised in the interpretation of scans from elderly patients with schizophrenia.

Several groups have studied schizophrenia with PET. The major finding in these studies has been frontal hypometabolism hyperfrontality of CBF and CMR (Buchsbaum et al. 1984; Wolkin et al. 1988). However, initial onset may be associated with frontal hypermetabolism (Cleghorn et al. 1989), but with chronicity of symptoms and neuroleptic treatment, the picture may change to one of frontal hypometabolism (Kapur et al. 1994). A correlation with chronicity and negative symptoms has been suggested. Few of these studies included many elderly patients. With regard to late-onset psychoses, studies demonstrate that altered brain structure and/or function is a predisposing factor. Reported changes fall into three broad categories; global structural change, white-matter hyperintensities on MRI, and CBF changes documented on SPECT scans (Coffey and Cummings 1994). The appropriate clinical use of neuroimaging in elderly schizophrenia patients is currently limited to the setting of a change in psychopathologic symptoms suggestive of the onset of another condition, particularly an organic brain disorder.

Affective Disorders

Relatively few structural imaging studies in affective disorders have focused specifically on elderly patients. Jaskiw and colleagues (1987) and Schlegel and Kretzschmar (1987a, 1987b) reviewed many of these. Most CT studies have concluded that ventricular brain ratio increases in depression but not to the degree found in Alzheimer's disease (Pearlson et al. 1989). In adult patients of diverse ages, several investigators noted relative ventricular enlargement as well as associations between ventriculomegaly and the presence of various indices of severity, including delusions, chronicity, and number of hospitalizations. The results overall did not reveal consistent anatomic abnormalities in such conditions as major depression, bipolar disorder, or dysthymia. Changes noted on MRI scans of depressed versus nondepressed elderly subjects include increased lateral and third ventricle size, greater cortical sulcal atrophy (Coffey et al. 1993; Rabins et al. 1991), enlarged Sylvian fissures, increased temporal horn size (Rabins et al. 1991), and smaller frontal lobe volumes (Coffey et al. 1993).

Because there are few anatomical correlates of affective disorders, and because of their cyclic nature, the functional neuroimaging techniques are best fitted for investigating them. The first such studies of affective disorders actually used a nonimaging technique—namely, the multiple-probe xenon Xe 133 techniques (both intra-arterial and inhalational) of regional CBF. These studies had predictably complex results (Margolin and Daniel 1990), with both the presence of differences (Mathew et al. 1980) and the absence of differences (Gur et al. 1983; Silfverskiold and Risberg 1989) being reported between unipolar depressed, bipolar depressed, and bipolar mania patients and controls studied at rest.

Although xenon probe techniques are still being used, methodological complexities and limitation of the data produced from cortical structures are factors favoring the replacement of these methods by PET and SPECT. Again, few if any studies specifically focusing on elderly patients have been reported. PET studies have explored CMR_{glu} differences between various mood disorder groups and controls. In two early studies (Baxter et al. 1985; Buchsbaum et al. 1984), no difference in whole brain metabolism was found between unipolar depressive patients and controls. Baxter et al.'s study found relatively reduced values in a bipolar depressed subgroup, however, and the Buchsbaum study reported hypofrontality— again, especially in the bipolar depressed subgroup. A more recent study by Baxter and associates (1989) reported a localized deficiency in left anterolateral prefrontal cortex in both unipolar and bipolar depressive patients compared with healthy or bipolar mania patients. With medication, and especially response to medication, this abnormality normalized. It is interesting that the location of this abnormality is the same as the predominant location of cortical damage in stroke patients who become depressed (Robinson et al. 1984). In addition to frontal hypometabolism on PET, studies have reported involvement of the candate-putamen, as well as of limbic structures, in depression (Kapur et al. 1994).

Neuroimaging and Differential Diagnosis

From the geriatric psychiatrist's perspective, perhaps the most important use of neuroimaging is in differential diagnosis, because a variety of distinct neurological and psychiatric disorders present in late life with a common set of psychopathological features. Thus far the primary differential diagnostic use of neuroimaging in geriatric psychiatry has been in the evaluation of dementia. Not only can various neurological and systemic conditions cause dementia, but functional psychiatric conditions, usually severe depression, can also imitate it (i.e., depressive pseudodementia) (Wells 1979).

Both structural and functional neuroimaging methods have potential roles in the differential diagnosis of dementia. CT and MRI are useful in the exclusion of a number of structural brain diseases that can cause dementia. CT's value as a screening tool in this process is indisputable; its relatively limited cost is a particular asset.

When pulse sequences are used to produce both T1- and T2-weighted images, MRI is superior to CT for detecting cerebral atrophy and structural abnormalities. Virtually all the disorders that can be detected by CT can be appreciated at least as well by MRI. Whether MRI will replace CT as the primary neuroimaging screening tool depends primarily on economic factors (MRI is still moderately more expensive) and other practical factors. Table 12–2 shows a number of disorders that entail associated cognitive, affective, or personality changes, the diagnosis of which can be facilitated by CT or MRI. Figure 12–1 shows images typical of some of these conditions.

In addition to positively identifying specific dementia-producing etiologies, structural imaging can be used for true differential diagnosis by subgrouping patients on the basis of their imaging findings. For example, Naeser and colleagues (1980), using CT attenuation values as an indicator of brain density, were able to differentiate patients with presenile dementia from patients with pseudodementia.

Because cerebral dysfunction is likely to occur earlier than structural abnormality in most geriatric psychiatric disorders, PET and SPECT should enable advances in differential diagnostic capabilities. Their use for this purpose has been documented in dementia. Kuhl (1984) demonstrated that PET can distinguish dementia of the Alzheimer's type, multi-infarct dementia, and depressive pseudodementia (Figure 12–2). It should be remembered that in the absence of postmortem histopathologic examination, no "gold standard" exists against which imaging findings must be compared.

Table 12–2. Common geriatric psychiatric disorders that can be evaluated by structural neuroimaging

Alzheimer's disease
Stroke and multi-infarct dementia
Tumors (both benign and malignant)
Hydrocephalus, including normal pressure hydrocephalus
Brain trauma and hemorrhage
Subdural hematoma
Abscess
Encephalitis, HIV-induced neuropathology

Source.   Adapted from Margolin and Daniel 1990.

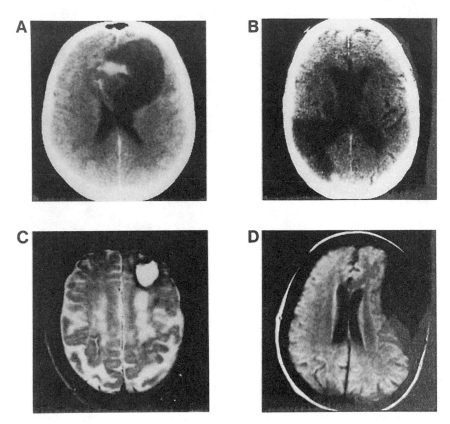

Figure 12–1. *A:* CT image of a low-grade astrocytoma presenting clinically as insidiously progressive dementia without localizing signs. *B:* CT image of a right parietal lobe (nondominant hemisphere) stroke, presenting with behavior change out of proportion to focal neurological findings. *C:* MRI image of extensive white-matter abnormalities in an elderly patient with clinically mixed dementia, Alzheimer type, and multi-infarct dementia. *D:* MRI image of an arachnoid cyst; chemical characteristics of the cyst fluid distinguished it from subdural hematoma, obviating a diagnostic trephination.

Serial scans can be helpful in distinguishing etiologies, and specialized neuroimaging modalities are occasionally appropriate. An example of a specialized procedure is radionuclide cisternography, which can help to distinguish normal pressure hydrocephalus dementia from Alzheimer's disease. Sluggish CSF dynamics, as demonstrated by prolonged lateral ventricle retention of a radiotracer injected into the lumbar CSF space, correlates with normal pressure hydrocephalus dementia. Similarly, angiography may be helpful in suspected cerebral vasculitis.

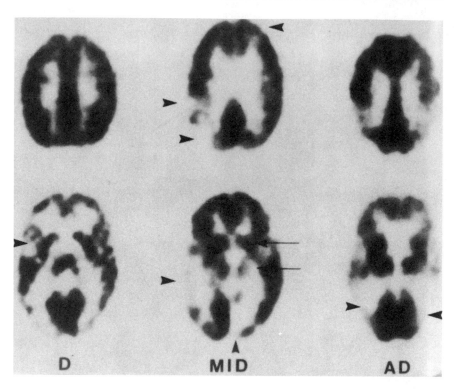

Figure 12–2. Three clinical entities (left, right, and middle image sets) studied by PET. For each case the upper image represents a higher brain slice, and the lower image, a lower brain slice. The left image set demonstrates the left anterior prefrontal lobe metabolic defect noted in depression. The center image set displays irregular zones of reduced metabolism compatible with areas of infarction seen on CT and with anatomic defects seen later on postmortem examination. This pattern is seen in multi-infarct dementia. The right image set demonstrates the bilateral parietal defect characteristic of Alzheimer's disease. *Source.*   Kuhl 1984.

Future Prospects

Structural neuroimaging will remain essential for detecting several key neurological disorders of late life associated with significant mental symptoms, at least until definitive biological tests become available for specific disorders. CT's long-term future in this area is uncertain because MRI is likely to assume an increasingly routine role. In MRI, postmortem correlations are urgently needed to clarify the issue of the significance of the pathological white-matter changes that are frequently found (Braffman et al. 1988).

Although structural imaging tools will remain valuable, the arrival of functional neuroimaging techniques (PET and SPECT) may genuinely alter the diagnostic strategy in geriatric psychiatry. This change will come about if the promise of these techniques in such areas as the imaging of neurotransmitter physiology and the brain correlates of mental or emotional activity can be realized and made practical in clinical situations. For example, it is possible that studies of cholinergic systems in Alzheimer's disease (Coyle et al. 1983), norepinephrine and serotonin in mood disorders, and dopamine in schizophrenia and late-onset psychosis will become regular components of future diagnostic evaluations. Such studies might be performed at baseline and after administration of a potentially effective course of pharmacotherapy. Alternatively, future metabolic or blood flow investigations in depression or dementia might employ cognitive tasks during imaging to differentially activate specific brain regions. For PET to fulfill its potential, cost and access obstacles must be removed; for SPECT to achieve recognized clinical status, quantitative models must be developed for the physiological processes being imaged. Whatever the details, however, reasoned speculation suggests that neuroimaging has a substantial future in geriatric psychiatry.

References

Aichner F, Gerstenbrand F: Computed tomography in cerebrovascular disease, in Handbook of Clinical Neurology, Vol 10: Vascular Diseases Series, Part II. Edited by Toole JF. Amsterdam, The Netherlands, Elsevier Science, 1989

Albert M, Naeser MA, Levine HL, et al: Ventricular size in patients with presenile dementia of the Alzheimer's type. Arch Neurol 41:1258–1263, 1984a

Albert M, Naeser MA, Levine HL, et al: CT density numbers in patients with senile dementia of the Alzheimer's type. Arch Neurol 41:1264–1269, 1984b

Baxter LR, Phelps ME, Mazziotta JC, et al: Cerebral metabolic rates for glucose in mood disorders. Arch Gen Psychiatry 42:441–447, 1985

Baxter LR, Schwartz JM, Phelps ME, et al: Reduction of prefrontal cortex glucose metabolism common to three types of depression. Arch Gen Psychiatry 46:243–250, 1989

Benson DF, Kuhl DE, Hawkins RA, et al: The fluorodeoxyglucose ^{18}F scan in Alzheimer's disease and multi-infarct dementia. Arch Neurol

40:711–714, 1983

Besson JA, Corrigan FM, Foreman EI, et al: Differentiating senile dementia of Alzheimer type and multi-infarct dementia by proton NMR imaging. Lancet 2:789, 1983

Besson JA, Corrigan FM, Foreman EI, et al: Nuclear magnetic resonance (NMR), II: imaging in dementia. Br J Psychiatry 146:31–35, 1985

Bondareff W, Baldy R, Levy R: Quantitative computed tomography in senile dementia. Arch Gen Psychiatry 38:1365–1368, 1981

Bradley WG, Waluch V, Brant-Zawadzki M, et al: Patchy periventricular white matter lesions in the elderly: a common observation during NMR imaging. Noninvasive Medical Imaging 1:35–41, 1984

Braffman BH, Zimmerman RA, Trojanowski JQ, et al: Brain MR: pathologic correlation with gross and histopathology, II: hyperintense white-matter foci in the elderly. Am J Roentgenol 151:559–566, 1988

Brant-Zawadzki M, Fein G, Van Dyke C, et al: MR imaging of the aging brain: patchy white-matter lesions and dementia. Am J Neuroradiol 6:675–682, 1985

Brinkman SD, Sarwar M, Levin HS, et al: Quantitative indexes of computed tomography in dementia and normal aging. Radiology 138:89–92, 1981

Brown JJ, Hesselink JR, Rothrock JF: MR and CT of lacunar infarcts. Am J Roentgenol 151:367–372, 1988

Buchsbaum MS, DeLisi LE, Holcomb HH, et al: Anteroposterior gradients in cerebral glucose use in schizophrenia and affective disorders. Arch Gen Psychiatry 41:1159–1166, 1984

Caplan LR, Schoene WC: Clinical features of subcortical arteriosclerotic encephalopathy (Binswanger disease). Neurology 28:1206–1215, 1978

Chase TN, Foster NL, Mansi L: Alzheimer's disease and the parietal lobe. Lancet 2:225, 1983

Chase TN, Foster NL, Fedio P, et al: Regional cortical dysfunction in Alzheimer's disease as determined by positron emission tomography. Ann Neurol 15 (suppl):S170–S174, 1984

Chimowitz MI, Estes ML, Furlan AJ, et al: Further observations on the pathology of subcortical lesions identified on magnetic resonance imaging. Arch Neurol 49:747–752, 1992

Cleghorn JM, Garnett ES, Nahmias C, et al: Increased frontal and reduced parietal glucose metabolism in acute untreated schizophrenia. Psychiatry Res 28:119–133, 1989

Cleghorn JM, Franco S, Szechtman B, et al: Toward a brain map of auditory hallucinations. Am J Psychiatry 85:224–227, 1992

Coffey CE, Cummings JL (eds): The American Psychiatric Press Textbook of Geriatric Neuropsychiatry. Washington, DC, American Psychiatric Press, 1994

Coffey CE, Wilkinson WE, Weiner RD, et al: Quantitative cerebral anatomy in depression: a controlled magnetic resonance imaging study. Arch Gen Psychiatry 50:7–16, 1993

Coffman JA, Nasrallah HA: Magnetic resonance imaging in schizophrenia, in The Neurology of Schizophrenia. Edited by Nasrallah HA, Weinberger DR. Amsterdam, The Netherlands, Elsevier, 1986

Coyle JT, Price DL, DeLong MR: Alzheimer's disease: a disorder of cortical cholinergic innervation. Science 219:1184–1190, 1983

Cummings JL: Multi-infarct dementia: diagnosis and management. Psychosomatics 28:117–125, 1987

DeCarli C, Kaye JE, Rapoport SI: Critical analysis of the use of computer assisted transverse axial tomography to study human brain in aging and dementia of the Alzheimer type. Neurology 40:884–886, 1990

Duara R, Margolin RA, Robertson-Tchabo EA, et al: Resting cerebral glucose utilisation as measured with positron emission tomography in 21 healthy men between the ages of 21 and 83 years. Brain 106:761–775, 1983

Duara R, Grady C, Haxby J, et al: Positron emission tomography in Alzheimer's disease. Neurology 36:879–887, 1986

Erkinjuntti T, Sipponen JT, Iivanainen M, et al: Cerebral NMR and CT imaging in dementia. J Comput Assist Tomogr 8:614–618, 1984

Fazekas F: Magnetic resonance signal abnormalities in asymptomatic individuals: their incidence and functional correlates. Eur Neurol 29:164–168, 1989

Fazekas F, Chawluk JB, Alavi A, et al: MR signal abnormalities at 1.5 T in Alzheimer's dementia and normal aging. Am J Roentgenol 149:351–356, 1987

Ferris SH, de Leon MJ, Wolf AP, et al: Positron emission tomography in dementia, in The Dementias. Edited by Mayeux R, Rosen WG. New York, Raven, 1983, pp 123–129

Ford CS, Buonanno FS, Kistler PJ: Magnetic resonance imaging in cerebrovascular disease, in Handbook of Clinical Neurology, Vol 10: Vascular Diseases Series, Part II. Edited by Toole JF. Amsterdam, The Netherlands, Elsevier, 1989

Foster NL, Chase TN, Fedio P, et al: Alzheimer's disease: focal cortical changes shown by positron emission tomography. Neurology 33:961–965, 1983

Frackowiak RS: The pathophysiology of human cerebral ischaemia: a new perspective obtained with positron tomography. Q J Med 57:713–727, 1985

Frackowiak RS: Energy metabolism and neurotransmitter function in ageing and the dementias, in Clinical Efficacy of Positron Emission Tomography. Edited by Heiss W-D, Pawlik G, Herholz K, et al. Amsterdam, The Netherlands, Martinus Nijhoff, 1987

Frackowiak RS, Pozzilli C, Legg NJ: Regional cerebral oxygen supply and utilisation in dementia: a clinical and physiological study with oxygen-15 and positron tomography. Brain 104:753–778, 1981

Friedland RP, Budinger TF, Ganz E: Regional cerebral metabolic alterations in dementia of the Alzheimer type: positron emission tomography with (18-F)-2-fluorodeoxyglucose. J Comput Assist Tomogr 7:590–598, 1983

Gado M, Hughes CP, Danziger W, et al: Volumetric measurements of the cerebrospinal fluid spaces in demented subjects and controls. Radiology 144:535–538, 1982

George AE, de Leon MJ, Kalnin A, et al: Leukoencephalopathy in normal and pathologic aging, II: MRI of brain lucencies. Am J Neuroradiol 7:567–570, 1986

Gerard G, Weisberg LA: MRI periventricular lesions in adults. Neurology 36:998–1001, 1986

Gur RE, Skolnick BE, Gur RC: Brain function in psychiatric disorders, II: regional cerebral blood flow in medicated unipolar depressives. Arch Gen Psychiatry 41:695–699, 1983

Harsch HH, Tikofsky RS, Collier BD: Single photon emission computed tomography imaging in vascular stroke. Arch Neurol 45:375–376, 1988

Haxby JV, Duara R, Grady CL, et al: Relations between neurophysiological and cerebral metabolic asymmetries in early Alzheimer's disease. J Cereb Blood Flow Metab 5:193–200, 1985

Holman LB: Perfusion and receptor SPECT in the dementias—George Taplin memorial lecture. J Nucl Med 27:855–860, 1986

Holman LB, Devous MD: Functional brain SPECT: the emergence of a powerful clinical method. J Nucl Med 33:1888–1904, 1992

Hounsfield GN: Computed medical imaging. J Comput Assist Tomogr 4:665–674, 1980

Huckman MS, Fox JH, Topel JL: The validity of criteria for the evaluation of cerebral atrophy by computerized tomography. Radiology 116:85–92, 1975

Ingvar D: Hyperfrontal distribution of the cerebral grey matter flow in resting wakefulness: on the functional anatomy of the conscious state. Acta Neurol Scand 60:12–25, 1979

Jagust WJ, Budinger TF, Reed BR: The diagnosis of dementia with single photon emission computed tomography. Arch Neurol 44:258–262, 1987

Jaskiw GE, Andreasen NC, Weinberger DR: X-ray computed tomography and magnetic resonance imaging in psychiatry, in Psychiatry Update: American Psychiatric Association Annual Review, Vol 6. Edited by Hales RE, Frances AJ. Washington, DC, American Psychiatric Press, 1987, pp 260–299

Johnstone EC, Crow TJ, Frith CD: The dementia of dementia praecox. Acta Psychiatr Scand 57:305–324, 1978

Juni JE: Taking brain SPECT seriously: reflections on recent clinical reports in the *Journal of Nuclear Medicine.* J Nucl Med 35:1891–1895, 1994

Kapur S, Houle S, Brown G: Positron emission tomography in psychiatry: new sights, new insights. Jefferson Journal of Psychiatry 12:58–74, 1994

Karbe N, Holthoff V, Rudolf J, et al: Positron emission tomography in degenerative disorders of the dopaminergic system. Journal of Neurological Transmission 4:121–130, 1992

Kessler RM: NMR imaging of ischemic cerebrovascular disease, in Magnetic Resonance Imaging, 2nd Edition. Edited by Partain CL, Price RR, Patton JA, et al. Philadelphia, PA, WB Saunders, 1988

Knopman DS, Rubens AB: The validity of computed tomographic scan findings for the localization of cerebral functions: the relationship between computed tomography and hemiparesis. Arch Neurol 43:328–332, 1986

Kohlmeyer K: A comparison of cerebral angiography and computer tomography in patients with stroke. Fortschr Geb Roentgenstrahlen Nuklearmed Erganzungsbd 131:361–368, 1979

Kuhl DE: Imaging local brain function with emission computed tomography. Radiology 150:625–631, 1984

Margolin RA, Daniel DG: Neuroimaging in geropsychiatry, in Clinical and Scientific Psychogeriatrics, Vol 2. Edited by Bergener M, Finkel SI. New York, Springer, 1990, pp 162–186

Marshal G: Regional cerebral oxygen consumption, blood flow, and blood volume in healthy human aging. Arch Neural 49:1013–1020, 1992

Mathew RJ, Meyer JS, Francis DJ: Cerebral blood flow in depression. Am J Psychiatry 137:1449–1450, 1980

Mazziotta JC, Phelps ME, Pahl JJ, et al: Reduced cerebral glucose metabolism in asymptomatic subjects at risk for Huntington's disease. N Engl

J Med 316:357–362, 1987

McGeer PL: Brain imaging in Alzheimer's disease. Br Med Bull 42:24–28, 1986

Mohr JP: Lacunes. Neurol Clin 1:201–221, 1983

Naeser MA, Gebhardt C, Levine HL: Decreased computerized tomography numbers in patients with presenile dementia. Arch Neurol 37:401–409, 1980

Pantano P, Baron JC, Lebrun-Grandie P: Regional cerebral blood flow and oxygen consumption in human ageing. Stroke 15:635–641, 1984

Partain CL, Price RR, Patton JA, et al (eds): Magnetic Resonance Imaging, 2nd Edition. Philadelphia, PA, WB Saunders, 1988

Pearlson PD, Rabins PV, Kim WS, et al: Structural brain changes and cognitive deficits in elderly depressives with and without reversible dementia ("pseudodementia"). Psychol Med 19:573–584, 1989

Phelps ME, Mazziotta JC: Positron emission tomography: human brain function and biochemistry. Science 228:799–809, 1985

Phelps ME, Mazziotta JC, Huang S-C: Study of cerebral function with positron computed tomography. J Cereb Blood Flow Metab 2:113–162, 1982

Pietrini P, Rapoport SI: Functional neuroimaging: positron-emission tomography in the study of cerebral blood flow and glucose utilization in human subjects at different ages, in The American Psychiatric Press Textbook of Geriatric Neuropsychiatry. Edited by Coffey CE, Cummings JL. Washington, DC, American Psychiatric Press, 1994, pp 195–213

Proceedings of the clinical SPECT symposium. Am J Physiol Imaging 2:127–166, 1987

Proceedings of the hexamethyl-propylene amine oxime (HM-PAO) symposium. J Cereb Blood Flow Metab 8 (suppl):S95–S123, 1988

Rabins PV, et al: Corticol magnetic resonance imaging changes in elderly inpatients with major depression. Am J Psychiatry 148:617–620, 1991

Robinson RG, Kubos KL, Starr LB, et al: Mood disorders in stroke patients: importance of location of lesion. Brain 107:81–93, 1984

Roman GC: Senile dementia of the Binswanger type: a vascular form of dementia in the elderly. JAMA 258:1782–1788, 1987

Schlegel S, Kretzschmar K: Computed tomography in affective disorders, I: ventricular and sulcal measurements. Biol Psychiatry 22:4–14, 1987a

Schlegel S, Kretzschmar K: Computed tomography in affective disorders, II: brain density. Biol Psychiatry 22:15–23, 1987b

Schwartz M, Creasey H, Grady CL, et al: Computed tomographic analysis of brain morphometrics in 30 healthy men, aged 21 to 81 years. Ann Neurol 17:146–157, 1985

Shelton RC, Weinberger DR: X-ray computed tomography studies in schizophrenia: a review and synthesis, in Handbook of Schizophrenia, Vol 1. Edited by Nasrallah HA, Weinberger DR. Amsterdam, The Netherlands, Elsevier, 1986

Silfverskiold P, Risberg J: Regional cerebral blood flow in depression and mania. Arch Gen Psychiatry 46:253–259, 1989

Small GW, Kuhl DE, Riege WH, et al: Cerebral glucose metabolic patterns in Alzheimer's disease: effect of gender and age at dementia onset. Arch Gen Psychiatry 46:527–532, 1989

Starkstein SE, Leiguarda R: Neuropsychological correlates of brain atrophy in Parkinson's disease: a CT-scan study. Mov Disord 1:51–55, 1993

Testa HJ, Snowden JS, Neary D, et al: The use of [99mTc]-HM-PAO in the diagnosis of primary degenerative dementia. J Cereb Blood Flow Metab 8 (suppl):S123–S126, 1988

Veith RC, Raskind MA: The neurobiology of aging: does it predispose to depression? Neurobiol Aging 9:101–117, 1988

Waller SB, London ED: Noninvasive diagnostic techniques to study age-related cerebral disorders, in Psychogeriatrics: An International Handbook. Edited by Bergener M. New York, Springer, 1987

Wells CE: Pseudodementia. Am J Psychiatry 136:895–900, 1979

Wolfe N, Linn R, Babikian VL, et al: Frontal systems impairment following multiple lacunar infarcts. Arch Neurol 47:129–132, 1990

Wolkin A, Angrist B, Wolf A, et al: Low frontal glucose utilization in chronic schizophrenia: a replication study. Am J Psychiatry 145:251–253, 1988

Wong DF, Wagner HN, Dannals RF, et al: Effects of age on dopamine and serotonin receptors measured by positron tomography in the living human brain. Science 226:1393–1396, 1984

Zimmerman RD, Fleming CA, Lee BC, et al: Periventricular hyperintensity as seen by magnetic resonance: prevalence and significance. Am J Neuroradiol 7:13–20, 1988

Andrew Leuchter, M.D.
Daniel Holschneider, M.D.

Electroencephalography

The electroencephalogram (EEG) was developed as a clinical test in the 1930s by Dr. Hans Berger, a psychiatrist. Ironically, in the more than five decades since its introduction into clinical practice, the EEG has become a technique most commonly performed under the supervision of, and interpreted by, neurologists. In fact, neurologists have made the greatest use of this test, most commonly using it to help corroborate the diagnosis of seizure disorders.

Since its introduction, however, it has been clear that the EEG has a special role in the assessment of older adults. Berger (1937) himself reported that the EEG changes with aging and is abnormal in a high proportion of individuals with dementia. To date, the EEG remains the single most cost-effective physiological test to indicate the presence of an encephalopathy. It therefore is necessary that the geriatric psychiatrist understand the fundamentals of EEG interpretation.

Despite the frequency with which an EEG is ordered, the specific indications for this test as well as the guidelines for interpreting its results remain unclear. This chapter reviews the major clinical uses of the EEG, its role in evaluating common clinical syndromes, and the usefulness of EEG results.

Indications for Electroencephalography

There are two primary reasons to perform an EEG in geriatric psychiatry: 1) to evaluate a possible dementia, delirium, or mental disorder caused by a general medical condition; and 2) to evaluate a possible seizure disorder. Although the test is commonly ordered to "rule out" one of these conditions, normal EEG results cannot rule out brain disease; they simply establish that the presence of such disease is less likely.

An EEG is not indicated whenever brain disease is known or suspected to exist. Rather, in psychiatry the test is useful primarily in four situations: 1) the presence of brain disease is suspected, but there is no clear etiology or the presentation is unusual; 2) the presence of brain disease is possible, but it is difficult to differentiate from some other psychiatric illness (e.g., depression); 3) the course of a psychiatric illness is unusual or the illness is refractory to treatment; and 4) a structural imaging study would be advisable but is unavailable.

Electroencephalogram Findings of Normal Aging

Any discussion of the application of electroencephalography must consider that the normal EEG in older adults may differ significantly from that seen in young adults. The EEG cannot fully exclude a diagnosis of brain disease in elderly patients because many of the findings of normal aging may mimic brain disease.

Although there is considerable variation in the normal EEG at any age, a typical EEG in a young adult (ages 20 to 60 years), who is awake and resting with eyes closed, shows a pattern of moderate-amplitude, sinusoidal electrical activity in the back of the head at a frequency of 8–12 Hz (the so-called posterior dominant or α rhythm), with a mean frequency for young adults of 10 Hz. Visual inspection of the EEG shows negligible slow-wave activity in the 0–4 Hz range (δ) and little detectable in the 4–8 Hz range (θ) except when the patient is drowsy. Low-amplitude fast activity (greater than 12 Hz, or β rhythms) predominates in the anterior and central head regions.

In adults over age 60, increased slowing occurs as a normal finding. This slowing may be of two types. First, there commonly is slowing of the posterior dominant rhythm. This rhythm remains in the α range, but the mean for a group of elderly subjects reportedly slows to 9 Hz by age 90.

Some healthy elderly subjects have been reported to have α rhythms as slow as 8 Hz, but a posterior dominant rhythm below the α range in the waking and alert state always is considered pathological (Obrist 1976; Obrist et al. 1966).

The second type of normal slowing is intermittent θ slowing seen over the temporal regions. This slow activity, which is intermixed with the normal background rhythms, commonly occurs at a frequency of 6–8 Hz and may occur in brief runs. It has been reported to occur in up to 40% of healthy volunteers (Busse et al. 1954; Torres et al. 1983). Some investigators believe that this pattern of mild, intermixed slowing is indicative of subclinical cerebrovascular disease and they have shown that in carefully screened control subjects the prevalence drops tenfold. For current clinical standards, however, this finding is still considered within normal limits (Niedermeyer 1987a).

Slowing may be accentuated by drowsiness in either young or old subjects, but it is particularly likely to emerge early in drowsiness among elderly subjects. This slowing is most often seen in the frontal regions, where trains of semirhythmic δ activity may be seen. This δ slowing may occasionally be mistaken for frontal intermittent rhythmic δ activity (FIRDA), a pathological rhythm often associated with metabolic encephalopathy and sometimes deep midline lesions (Zurek et al. 1985). Because of sensory losses and other factors, elderly patients are more likely to become drowsy during EEG recordings, so it is vital that they be alerted often during the procedure and that their state of arousal be noted in the report.

Other EEG changes are also commonly seen with aging. Amplitude of the signal generally decreases, as does the response to photic stimulation (Niedermeyer 1987a). In some individuals, there is an increase in the amount of sharp-wave activity seen in the temporal regions intermixed with slowing, but this activity should be readily distinguishable from true epileptiform activity. The changes in β activity with aging are less clear, with equal numbers of studies finding either increases or decreases in fast activity (Niedermeyer 1987a; Spehlmann 1981).

Electroencephalogram in the Evaluation of Specific Disorders

Various clinical situations that may prompt the geriatric psychiatrist to order an EEG are discussed in the following sections.

Primary Degenerative Dementia of the Alzheimer's Type

The finding that first generated clinical interest in the EEG was that institutionalized patients with dementia demonstrated excessive, diffuse slowing of background rhythms, as well as slowing of the posterior dominant rhythm. This finding proved to be nonspecific, seen primarily in more advanced cases of dementia as well as in a variety of organic conditions.

Five decades of clinical experience, however, have demonstrated that the EEG has clear uses in patients with possible or definite dementia, delirium, or mental disorder caused by a general medical condition. The most common use is in the initial evaluation of possible Alzheimer's disease. Experts differ as to the indications for an EEG in the initial evaluation. Whereas some believe that it should be ordered in all cases, a National Institutes of Health consensus conference concluded that the test should be ordered only when the etiology of the dementia is unclear or the presentation is unusual (Group for the Advancement of Psychiatry 1988). Because the etiology of dementia is usually unclear and presentations frequently are unusual, an EEG is ordered in most cases in clinical practice.

The EEG frequently is not ordered in the initial evaluation of a patient with possible Alzheimer's disease because it is generally believed that the EEG is normal in cases of mild dementia (Cummings and Benson 1992). However, a recent study found that, among 104 patients who were to be evaluated for possible dementia and whose testing had previously shown normal or equivocal mental status, the EEG was abnormal in nearly 50% of these cases (Leuchter et al. 1993a). These findings suggest that the standard EEG is highly sensitive to the presence of even mild encephalopathy. EEG abnormalities are nonspecific, however, and also may be seen in patients with depression.

When a baseline tracing from the patient's premorbid state is available, the EEG may be particularly helpful in the evaluation of subsequent dementia. Even when a patient's EEG remains within normal limits overall, it may show slowing that is excessive for that individual. Baseline tracings, however, are seldom available.

Other Causes of Dementia

The EEG does have some utility in the differential diagnosis of dementia, and it may help to distinguish Alzheimer's disease from other dementing illnesses. Vascular dementia commonly shows focal or lateralizing abnormalities in contrast to the diffuse and symmetric pattern of slowing seen in Alzheimer's disease. Focal abnormalities frequently are absent in cases of vascular dementia; diffuse deep white-matter ischemic disease (e.g., Binswanger's disease), where there are no cortical infarcts or lesions undercutting the cortex, may show a pattern indistinguishable from that of Alzheimer's disease. Structural imaging studies of the brain (computed tomography [CT] or magnetic resonance imaging [MRI]) clearly are most useful in corroborating the diagnosis of vascular dementia.

In Creutzfeldt-Jakob disease, an uncommon cause of dementia in elderly patients, the EEG reveals frontally predominant triphasic waves, paroxysmal lateralizing epileptiform discharges, or some other pseudoperiodic sharp-wave complex within 12 weeks of onset of clinical symptoms in more than 90% of cases (Spehlmann 1981). As the disease progresses, these sharp-wave complexes attenuate and disappear into a background of slow-wave activity. Although it is not pathognomonic of the illness, the presence of pseudoperiodic discharges in the presence of a rapidly progressive dementia is highly suggestive of the diagnosis. The absence of these periodic discharges after 10 weeks of clinical symptoms makes the diagnosis suspect (Chiappa and Young 1978).

Huntington's chorea frequently presents with a progressive loss of amplitude of the EEG, with or without slowing. The dementia that accompanies thyroid disease may have dramatic attenuation of EEG amplitude. Other forms of dementia, such as Pick's disease, the dementia accompanying Parkinson's disease, and progressive supranuclear palsy, do not have characteristic EEG presentations that help distinguish them from Alzheimer's disease (Niedermeyer 1987b; Spehlmann 1981). Even in the forms of dementia that do have particular EEG presentations, the EEG is primarily used as a tool for confirming the diagnosis; clinical history and physical examination are likely to be more useful in establishing the diagnosis.

Depression

The EEG may be useful in cases in which there is a suspicion that cognitive impairment is caused by depression. Neuropsychological tests, commonly used in such cases, are liable to be adversely affected by motivational or attention problems. The EEG, however, is a clinically available measure of brain function that can help distinguish between these two illnesses. Abnormal EEG results may be seen in depressed elderly patients (Leuchter et al. 1993a), but these abnormalities are usually mild. Furthermore, these abnormalities may be caused by subclinical brain disease distinct from dementia (Leuchter and Holschneider 1994; Oken and Kaye

1992). Another limitation is that EEG results may be normal early in the course of a dementia, so that follow-up testing may be necessary to detect an encephalopathy.

Toxic and Metabolic Conditions

Because it is a sensitive (albeit nonspecific) screen for encephalopathic conditions, the EEG is useful for detecting excess morbidity attributable to reversible toxic or metabolic conditions. For example, a patient with mild cognitive impairment, but severe slowing on EEG, may have another disease process instead of, or in addition to, Alzheimer's disease (Cummings and Benson 1992).

A common finding in elderly patients is that one or more medications that a patient is receiving are causing a toxic encephalopathy. Such an encephalopathic process would be expected to present electrographically with increased slow-wave activity as well as slowing of the posterior dominant rhythm. It may be difficult to determine when medications are causing or contributing to an encephalopathy because, even in therapeutic dosages, many psychoactive and nonpsychoactive drugs may cause EEG changes. Antidepressants or neuroleptics commonly cause slowing of the posterior dominant rhythm and an increased amount of slow-wave activity (Fink 1968). Lithium similarly may cause increased slowing, and, at toxic levels, it may cause focal abnormalities or spike discharges (Law 1979). In therapeutic doses, benzodiazepines and other sedative-hypnotics usually cause increased 20- to 25-Hz β activity (Fink 1968), most commonly in a frontocentral pattern. In high doses, these drugs may cause increased slowing as well.

One of the most common causes of drug-induced cognitive dysfunction in elderly patients is drugs with anticholinergic effects. These drugs routinely cause increased amounts of slowing in the EEG (Pfefferbaum et al. 1979). If increased slowing is detected in the EEG of a patient taking a drug known to cause cognitive dysfunction, it may be prudent to discontinue or replace the drug with a nonoffending agent.

The EEG may help to detect unsuspected metabolic derangements, because blood chemistry panels cannot screen for all possible endocrinopathies, electrolyte imbalances, and toxic substances. Apart from increased slowing, other patterns that may be seen in metabolic encephalopathy include FIRDA, triphasic waves, and sharp waves. Depending on the distribution and the frequency of occurrence of these waveforms, a specific etiology of metabolic encephalopathy may be suggested. For example, the most common cause of 2–3 per second frontally predominant triphasic waves is hepatic encephalopathy. Such waveforms also may be seen, however, in patients with chronic renal failure (Hughes 1982). The clinical history and other laboratory tests are clearly necessary to interpret these nonspecific findings.

Delirium and Changes in Mental Status

Although the EEG is most often ordered in elderly patients for evaluating possible dementia, the most justifiable use is in the evaluation of delirium. It first was established in the 1940s that the degree of slowing in the EEG among patients with delirium is directly related to the level of confusion and that improvements in the EEG reflect improvements in mental status (Engel and Romano 1944; Romano and Engel 1944). The EEG, therefore, is an important confirmatory tool, and it is difficult to make the diagnosis of delirium in the absence of EEG slowing (Lipowski 1987). The EEG may also be useful in evaluating the course of delirium. In cases where the mental status exam is equivocal or difficult to perform, as in a patient on a ventilator or one with aphasia, the EEG may be useful for monitoring resolution of the encephalopathy. Interventions to improve the patient's condition should diminish EEG slowing, and persistent severe slowing suggests either that the cause of the delirium has not been corrected or that another illness (e.g., dementia) exists. It is unclear how long EEG slowing may persist after the resolution of a delirium.

When a patient's mental status has declined acutely and a stroke is suspected, the EEG commonly shows focal slowing very early, whereas the CT scan may not show changes for several days (Niedermeyer 1987c). In situations where a structural imaging study of the brain is desirable but unavailable, the EEG may be used. There may, however, be a significant mass lesion (particularly in the deep white matter) without any EEG changes.

Finally, the EEG may be useful in following the course of dementia. As a patient's mental status declines, the EEG is marked by concomitant increases in slowing, loss of the posterior dominant rhythm, and, occasionally, the emergence of spike foci. If the patient has had a baseline EEG and later has an abrupt decline in function, a repeat tracing may be useful in determining the cause of the loss in functional status. For example, a significant decline in function with no change in EEG patterns would be unusual and might suggest the development of superimposed depression.

Seizure Disorders

Most patients who develop seizure disorders do so in the first two decades of life. Thereafter, the incidence of new-onset seizure disorders drops, only to rise again after age 60 years. The elderly have been estimated to account for approximately 24% of new-onset cases of epilepsy (Sander et al. 1990). The most common causes of late-onset seizures are stroke, trauma, and mass lesions (Ettinger and Shinnar 1993; Lühdorf et al. 1986; Sung and Chu 1990). Among these individuals, the EEG is useful to confirm the diagnosis, to help establish the type of seizure, and to define the area of origin of the epileptic discharge. The geriatric psychiatrist generally does not establish the diagnosis of epilepsy or initiate treatment for seizures; these tasks usually are performed by a consulting neurologist. This section, therefore, focuses primarily on clinical guidelines for the ordering and interpretation of EEG in patients with possible seizures.

Seizures in older adults most commonly present with periodic alterations in level of consciousness or behavior. In most cases, the diagnosis is straightforward, with frank lapses of consciousness that may be associated with loss of motor tone or abnormal movements, incontinence, and postictal confusion. In such cases, the EEG provides confirmatory evidence and may help guide treatment.

In some cases—such as patients with possible loss of consciousness, episodic confusion, waxing and waning mental status, refractory depression, or panic attacks—a seizure disorder enters the differential diagnosis. The discovery of a seizure focus in these patients may be clinically significant because there are reports in the literature of individuals with seizure foci whose refractory depressions or panic disorders are responsive to anticonvulsants. The index of suspicion for seizures usually is not high in such cases and the EEG is typically ordered for atypical cases, such as a patient with panic attacks who is briefly unresponsive. It is not routinely recommended for evaluation of patients with panic disorder. The test is usually requested to rule out seizures. The EEG, however, cannot rule out a seizure disorder; it has been estimated in studies of late-onset epilepsy that 10%–47% of patients with seizure disorders have normal EEGs (Ahuja and Mohanta 1982; Carney et al. 1969; Hyllested and Pakkenberg 1963; Lühdorf et al. 1986; Shigemoto 1981; Woodcock and Cosgrove 1964), a rate somewhat lower than that estimated for middle aged adults. The false-negative rate is dependent in part on the etiology of the seizure, with lower false-negative rates reported in patients with brain tumors and higher false-negative rates in patients with seizures of unknown etiology (Carney et al. 1969; Lühdorf et al. 1986).

To perform an adequate electroencephalographic screen for a seizure disorder, a recording of at least 30 minutes should be performed using several different electrode montages. Furthermore, if the patient's physical health and mental state permit, activation procedures such as hyperventilation, photic stimulation, stage II sleep, and sleep deprivation may be useful to activate an underlying seizure focus.

In cases in which epileptiform abnormalities (i.e., spikes or spike-and-wave complexes) are detected, a diagnosis of a seizure disorder is not certain. Depending on the location and nature of the abnormality, epileptiform abnormalities predict the existence of a clinical seizure disorder with differing degrees of reliability. For example, frequent spike-and-wave complexes in the anterior temporal region are correlated with clinical seizures in more than 90% of otherwise healthy adults, whereas isolated occipital spikes have less than a 40% correlation with seizures (Niedermeyer 1987d). The surest method to establish a link between an observed epileptiform abnormality and a possible seizure disorder is to perform a prolonged (possibly ambulatory) EEG recording and to observe changes in the state or behavior of the patient that are linked to electroencephalographic changes.

In interpreting the significance of epileptiform abnormalities, the clinical history and condition of the patient must be considered. Some chronic illnesses (such as renal failure) or degenerative diseases of the brain (such as Alzheimer's disease) may lead to the development of generalized sharp waves or spike foci that have a low association with clinical seizures. In the final analysis, seizures are diagnosed on the basis of clinical presentation (Pinkus and Tucker 1985).

Quantitative Electroencephalography

Several factors limit the application of conventional EEG in psychiatric practice. These include the need for specialized training to interpret an EEG record and problems of interrater reliability. Perhaps the most difficult problem has been defining a gold standard by which to differentiate normal from abnormal cerebral activity across individuals of different ages and genders. In geriatric psychiatry specifically, the value of the EEG to evaluate a possible encephalopathy is limited by difficulties in quantifying normal amounts of slowing in the elderly.

Quantitative electroencephalography (QEEG) overcomes several of the limitations of conventional EEG. With the use of computer-based techniques, QEEG can quantify the amount of cerebral energy in an individual EEG and the amount concentrated in slow wave bands (a measure that may indicate disease) (Figure 13–1). The amount of slowing can be compared to age- and gender-based norms. Statistically significant regional differences are displayed as topographical maps in each frequency band. Quantitative analysis does not eliminate the problem that the EEG changes resulting from normal aging are qualitatively similar to the features of organic brain disease. QEEG yields more reliable and reproducible measurements of brain activity, however, and increases the sensitivity to subtle focal or generalized alterations in brain function (Figure 13–2).

A variety of QEEG parameters, such as absolute power, relative power, and spectral ratios, also provide information that is not accessible from the visual inspection of the conventional recording. These parameters appear to be complementary in that they are additive in the detection of abnormality and yield different regional information regarding abnormality (Leuchter et al. 1993b).

QEEG is also useful for the detection of a dementing illness (Duffy et al. 1984; Nuwer 1988; Prichep et al. 1983). A number of investigators have

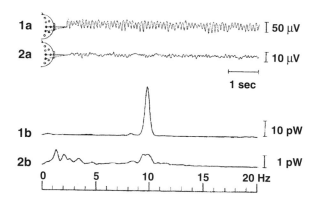

Figure 13–1.   Samples of a normal posterior dominant rhythm *(1a)* and an abnormal rhythm with excessive intermixed slowing such as that seen in patients with dementia *(2a)*. The computer-generated frequency spectra show that the normal rhythm consists of power concentrated at 10 Hz *(1b)*, whereas the abnormal rhythm *(2b)* contains considerable power at lower frequencies.

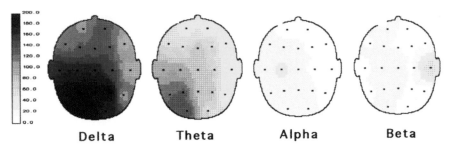

Figure 13–2. Quantitative EEG maps of absolute power in the δ, θ, α, and β frequency bands. The maps show excess generalized δ and θ power, with maximum focal intensity in the left parietal-occipital region. This patient with vascular dementia had a discrete left parietal infarct, with maximal θ and δ slowing in the area of the lesion. Maps represent the head as viewed from above, with frontal regions at the top of each map. Colors represent the absolute EEG power in each frequency band measured in microvolts squared and displayed according to the color scale on the left.

demonstrated that patients with dementia have increased δ and θ power, decreased α and β power, and decreased mean frequency (Leuchter and Holschneider 1994). Although researchers correctly identify up to 90%–95% of subjects with dementia, the issue of how early in the course of a dementia QEEG may be useful as a screening tool remains uncertain. Using differing QEEG measures in a variety of scalp locations, different groups have reported sensitivities and specificities in early dementia in the range of 20%–70% and 70%–100%, respectively (Brenner et al. 1986; Coben et al. 1990; John et al. 1988; Leuchter et al. 1987; Prichep et al. 1983).

New QEEG measures of fiber tract damage have been shown to be useful in the diagnosis and assessment of dementia and its treatment. Coherence, a measure of the synchronization of electrical activity from different regions within an individual, has proved useful in distinguishing dementia of the Alzheimer's type (DAT) and multi-infarct dementia (MID) subjects and in detecting fiber tract dysfunction associated with periventricular white matter changes on MRI (Leuchter et al. 1987, 1992, 1994a). Furthermore, low baseline coherence is an indicator of poorer functional status at 2-year follow-up in patients with dementia (Leuchter et al. 1994b) and poorer outcome and increased mortality in patients with depression (Leuchter et al. 1994c). QEEG measures may reveal normalization of neocortical activity in DAT patients treated with tacrine (Alhainen et al. 1991). Furthermore, QEEG has been shown to be useful in selecting optimal drug dose in DAT patients with intraventricularly administered bethanechol, with supraoptimal doses leading to increased slow-wave power (Leuchter et al. 1991).

QEEG has shown distinctive advantages over conventional EEG for assessing the diagnosis, course, and prognosis of subjects with delirium. Grossly excessive slowing in the face of relatively mild cognitive impairment suggests the presence of delirium instead of, or in addition to, dementia (Figure 13–3). This severity of slowing is better estimated by quantitative rather than visual analysis (Brenner 1991) and may help differentiate delirium from dementia subjects (Jacobson et al. 1993a, 1993b; Koponen et al. 1989). More-

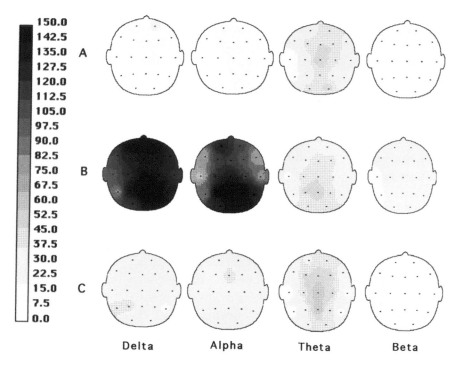

Figure 13–3. Quantitative EEG maps of absolute power for a patient at baseline *(A),* during acute lithium intoxication *(B),* and 2 weeks after the lithium was discontinued *(C).* Slow-wave power greatly increased during this episode of delirium and resolved afterward. Each row shows four maps representing (from the left) the δ, θ, α, and β bands of EEG frequencies. Maps represent the head as viewed from above with frontal regions at the top of each map. Colors represent the absolute EEG power in each brain region in each frequency band measured in microvolts squared and displayed according to the color scale to the left.

over, decreases in slow-wave power may actually precede improvements in mental status (Leuchter and Jacobson 1991).

A new QEEG measure that may prove useful for the study of dementia, depression, and other psychiatric illnesses is called cordance. Cordance is a measure of brain electrical activity that is sensitive to damage to afferent fiber tracts supplying the cortex. Cortical deafferentation, as might result from a focal lesion, produces regional attenuation of perfusion and QEEG power. Although such cortex produces low power, it is concentrated in pathological (i.e., slow-wave) bands. Cordance combines both absolute and relative power (percentage of total power in a given frequency band) to yield a measure that has a stronger association with perfusion than other QEEG measures. Additionally, cordance maps have been shown in the research setting to show a striking similarity to PET or SPECT scans (Leuchter et al. 1994d, 1994e).

The role of QEEG in the assessment of depression is unclear. Pollock and Schneider (1990) reviewed studies performed over the preceding decade that attempted to distinguish depression from dementia and found that no single feature appears to be robust for the diagnosis of depression. Several investigators have used a multivariate statistical approach to the diagnosis of depression (John et al. 1977; Shagass et al. 1984) and have reported overall accuracy in classification of 60%–90%. The stability of these multivariate methods for diagnosis remains to be verified.

QEEG is on the verge of being useful for a broad number of routine clinical settings. Quantitative analysis is more sensitive to the proportion of energy in any frequency band and, therefore, may find greater application in the assessment of global brain function or detecting focal brain dysfunction. QEEG is less sensitive in the detection of very fast (milliseconds) transient EEG activity and in the recognition of specific wave morphologies. Thus, conventional EEG remains preferable to QEEG for detecting epileptiform abnormalities. At present, QEEG remains an adjunct to conventional EEG in the study of psychiatric illnesses (American Psychiatric Association Task Force on Quantitative Electrophysiological Assessment 1991), and it should not be considered part of a routine evaluation. Currently, its main usefulness is in selected clinical situations in which mild degrees of encephalopathy may better be detected by QEEG. These include 1) evaluations of mild head trauma, toxic metabolic states, and early dementia; 2) serial evaluations of the progression or resolution of a delirium; 3) evaluations of pseudodementia versus early dementia; and 4) detection of subtle focal abnormality and the differential diagnosis of dementia.

Conclusion

The EEG plays a prominent role in the evaluation of brain disease among geriatric psychiatry patients, and it generally is quite sensitive to the presence of encephalopathic conditions as well as seizure disorders. The EEG tracing generally does not yield results that are diagnostic of any illness; rather, its findings are either consistent with (e.g., slowing in Alzheimer's disease), supportive of (e.g., triphasic waves in Creutzfeldt-Jakob disease), or highly suggestive of the presence of a particular illness (e.g., anterior temporal spike-and-wave foci in a seizure disorder).

EEG is a noninvasive, inexpensive, and portable technology. Its cost-effectiveness is likely to be increased further by computer analysis that will require less physician time. As computer prices decline, QEEG systems will become a more available means of imaging pathophysiological changes in brain function. Clinical correlation and development of new QEEG measures such as coherence and cordance hold great promise for improving diagnostic accuracy in the future.

References

Ahuja GK, Mohanta A: Late onset epilepsy. Acta Neurol Scand 66:216–226, 1982

Alhainen K, Partanen J, Reinikainen K, et al: Discrimination of tetrahydroaminoacridine responders by a single dose pharmaco-EEG in patients with Alzheimer's disease. Neurosci Lett 127:113–116, 1991

American Psychiatric Association Task Force on Quantitative Electrophysiological Assessment: Quantitative electroencephalography: a report on the present state of computerized EEG techniques. Am J Psychiatry 148:961–964, 1991

Berger H: On the electroencephalogram of man: 12th report. Arch Psychiatr Nervenkr 106:165–187, 1937

Brenner R: Utility of electroencephalography in delirium: past views and current practice. International Psychogeriatrics 3:211–229, 1991

Brenner R, Ulrich R, Spiker D, et al: Computerized EEG spectral analysis in elderly normal, demented, and depressed subjects. Electroencephalogr Clin Neurophysiol 64:482–492, 1986

Busse EW, Barnes RH, Silverman AJ, et al: Studies of the process of aging: factors that influence the psyche of elderly persons. Am J Psychiatry 110:897–903, 1954

Carney LR, Hudgins RL, Espinosa RE, et al: Seizures beginning after the age of 60. Arch Intern Med 124:707–709, 1969

Chiappa K, Young R: The EEG as a definitive diagnostic tool early in the course of Creutzfeldt-Jacob disease. Electroencephalogr Clin Neurophysiol 45:26, 1978

Coben LA, Chi D, Snyder AZ, et al: Replication of a study of frequency analysis of the resting awake EEG in mild probable Alzheimer's disease. Electroencephalogr Clin Neurophysiol 75:148–154, 1990

Cummings J, Benson D: Dementia: A Clinical Approach. Boston, MA, Butterworth, 1992

Duffy FH, Albert MS, McAnulty G: Brain electrical activity in patients with presenile and senile dementia of the Alzheimer type. Ann Neurol 16:439–448, 1984

Engel G, Romano J: Delirium, II: reversibility of the electroencephalogram with experimental procedures. Arch Neurol Psychiatr 51:378–392, 1944

Ettinger AB, Shinnar S: New-onset seizures in an elderly hospitalized population. Neurology 43:489–492, 1993

Fink M: EEG classification of psychoactive compounds in man: a review and theory of behavioral associations, in Psychopharmacology: A Review of Progress 1957–1967. Edited by Effron DH. Washington, DC, U.S. Government Printing Office, l968, pp 497–507

Group for the Advancement of Psychiatry: The Psychiatric Treatment of Alzheimer's Disease. New York, Brunner/Mazel, 1988

Hughes JR: EEG in Clinical Practice. Boston, MA, Butterworth, 1982

Hyllested K, Pakkenberg H: Prognosis in epilepsy of late onset. Neurology 13:651–654, 1963

Jacobson S, Leuchter AF, Walter DO: Conventional and quantitative EEG in the diagnosis of delirium among the elderly. J Neurol Neurosurg Psychiatry 56:153–158, 1993a

Jacobson S, Leuchter AF, Walter DO, et al: Serial quantitative EEG among elderly subjects with delirium. Biol Psychiatry 34:135–140, 1993b

John E, Karmel B, Corning W, et al: Neurometrics: numerical taxonomy identifies different profiles of brain functions within groups of behaviorally similar people. Science 196:1393–1410, 1977

John ER, Prichep LS, Fridman J, et al: Neurometrics: computer-assisted differential diagnosis of brain dysfunctions. Science 239:162–169, 1988

Koponen H, Partanen J, Paakkonnen A, et al: EEG spectral analysis in delirium. J Neurol Neurosurg Psychiatry 52:980–985, 1989

Law MD: Evaluation of psychiatric disorders and the effects of psychotherapeutic and psychomimetic agents, in Current Practice of Clinical

Electroencephalography. Edited by Klass DW, Daly DD. New York, Raven, 1979, pp 395–419

Leuchter A, Jacobson S: Quantitative measurement of brain electrical activity in delirium. International Psychogeriatrics 3:231–247, 1991

Leuchter A, Spar J, Walter D, et al: Electroencephalographic spectra and coherence in the diagnosis of Alzheimer's-type and multi-infarct dementia. Arch Gen Psychiatry 44:993–998, 1987

Leuchter A, Read S, Walter DO, et al: Stable bimodal response to cholinomimetic drugs in Alzheimer's disease: brain mapping correlates. Neuropsychopharmacology 4:165–173, 1991

Leuchter A, Newton TF, Cook IA, et al: Changes in brain functional connectivity in Alzheimer-type and multi-infarct dementia. Brain 115:1543–1561, 1992

Leuchter AF, Daly KA, Rosenberg-Thompson S, et al: The prevalence of electroencephalographic abnormalities among patients with possible organic mental syndromes. J Am Geriatr Soc 41:605–611, 1993a

Leuchter A, Cook IA, Newton TF, et al: Regional differences in brain electrical activity in dementia: use of spectral power and spectral ratio measures. Electroencephalogr Clin Neurophysiol 87:385–393, 1993b

Leuchter AF, Holschneider D: Quantitative electroencephalography: neurophysiological alterations in normal aging and geriatric neuropsychiatric disorders, in Textbook of Geriatric Neuropsychiatry. Edited by Coffey E, Cummings J. Washington, DC, American Psychiatric Press, 1994, pp 215–240

Leuchter AF, Dunkin J, Lufkin R, et al: The effects of white-matter disease on functional connections in the aging brain. J Neurol Neurosurg Psychiatry 57:1347–1354, 1994a

Leuchter AF, Simon SL, Daly KA, et al: Quantitative EEG correlates of outcome in elderly pstchiatric patients, I: cross-sectional and longitudinal assessment of patients with dementia. Am J Geriatr Psychiatry 2:200–209, 1994b

Leuchter AF, Simon SL, Daly KA, et al: Quantitative correlates of outcome in elderly psychiatric patients, II: two-year follow-up of patients with depression. Am J Geriatr Psychiatry 2:290–299, 1994c

Leuchter AF, Cook IA, Lufkin RB, et al: A new method for assessment of cerebral perfusion and metabolism using quantitative electroencephalography. Neuroimage 1:208–219, 1994d

Leuchter AF, Cook IA, Mena I, et al: Assessing cerebral perfusion using quantitative EEG cordance. Psychiatry Res 55:141–152, 1994e

Lipowski Z: Delirium (acute confusional states). JAMA 258:1789–1792, 1987

Lühdorf K, Jensen LK, Plesner AM: Etiology of seizures in the elderly. Epilepsia 27:458–463, 1986

Niedermeyer E: EEG and old age, in Electroencephalography: Basic Principles, Clinical Applications, and Related Fields, 2nd Edition. Edited by Niedermeyer E, Lopes da Silva F. Baltimore, MD, Urban and Schwarzenberg, 1987a, pp 301–308

Niedermeyer E: EEG and dementia, in Electroencephalography: Basic Principles, Clinical Applications, and Related Fields, 2nd Edition. Edited by Niedermeyer E, Lopes da Silva F. Baltimore, MD, Urban and Schwarzenberg, 1987b, pp 309–315

Niedermeyer E: Cerebrovascular disorders and EEG, in Electroencephalography: Basic Principles, Clinical Applications and Related Fields, 2nd Edition. Edited by Niedermeyer E, Lopes da Silva F. Baltimore, MD, Urban and Schwarzenberg, 1987c, pp 275–299

Niedermeyer E: Epileptic seizure disorders, in Electroencephalography: Basic Principles, Clinical Applications, and Related Fields, 2nd Edition. Edited by Niedermeyer E, Lopes da Silva F. Baltimore, MD, Urban and Schwarzenberg, 1987d, pp 405–510

Nuwer MR: Quantitative EEG, II: frequency analysis and topographic mapping in clinical settings. J Clin Neurophysiol 5:45–85, 1988

Obrist WD: Problems of aging, in Handbook of Electroencephalography and Clinical Neurophysiology, Vol 6A. Edited by Remond A. Amsterdam, Elsevier, 1976, pp 207–229

Obrist WD, Henry CE, Justiss WA: Longitudinal changes in the senescent EEG: a 15-year study. Proceedings of the Seventh International Congress of Gerontology. Vienna, International Association of Gerontology, 1966

Oken BS, Kaye JA: Electrophysiologic function in the healthy, extremely old. Neurology 42:519–526, 1992

Pfefferbaum A, David KL, Coulter CL, et al: EEG effects of physostigmine and choline chloride in humans. Psychopharmacology 62:225–233, 1979

Pinkus J, Tucker G: Behavioral Neurology. New York, Oxford University Press, 1985

Pollock VE, Schneider LS: Quantitative, waking EEG research on depression. Biol Psychiatry 27:757–780, 1990

Prichep L, Gomez MF, Johns ER, et al: Neurometric electroencephalographic characteristics of dementia, in Alzheimer's Disease: The Standard Reference. Edited by Reisberg B. New York, Macmillan, 1983, pp 252–257

Romano J, Engel G: Delirium, I: electroencephalographic data. Archives of Neurology and Psychiatry 51:356–377, 1944

Sander JWAS, Hart UM, Johnson AL, et al: National general practice study of epilepsy: newly diagnosed epileptic seizures in general population. Lancet 336:1267–1271, 1990

Shagass C, Romer RA, Straumanis JJ, et al: Psychiatric diagnostic discriminations with combinations of quantitative EEG variables. Br J Psychol 144:581–592, 1984

Shigemoto T: Epilepsy in middle age or advanced age. Folia Psychiatr Neurol Jpn 35:287–293, 1981

Spehlmann R: EEG Primer. Amsterdam, Elsevier, 1981

Sung C-Y, Chu N-S: Epileptic seizures in elderly people: aetiology and seizure type. Age Aging 19:25–30, 1990

Torres F, Faoro A, Loewenson R, et al: The electroencephalogram of elderly subjects revisited. Electroencephalogr Clin Neurophysiol 56:391–398, 1983

Woodcock S, Cosgrove JBR: Epilepsy after the age of 50. Neurology 14:34–40, 1964

Zurek R, Schiemann Delgado J, Froescher W, et al: Frontal intermittent rhythmic δ activity and anterior bradyrhythmia. Clin Electroencephalogr 16:1–10, 1985

Psychiatric Disorders of the Elderly

Barry Reisberg, M.D.

Alzheimer's Disease

Epidemiology

Alzheimer's disease is a major illness of the modern era. Prevalence varies, in part with the age of the population; however, approximately 0.5% to 1% of the population of most modern industrialized nations are probably afflicted by overt manifestations of Alzheimer's disease. Livingston (1994) recently reviewed the literature concerning prevalence studies. Findings in these studies differ depending in part on the definitions and methodologies used, whether institutionalized populations were surveyed, and other factors in case ascertainment. However, Livingston concluded that most studies find that nearly 5% of people ages 65 years or older have dementia, of which Alzheimer's disease is the most common cause. In the United States, community population surveys have indicated that up to 10%–15% of elderly community residents have Alzheimer's disease or closely related dementias of late life (Evans et al. 1989; Katzman 1986). Because 30 million people in the United States are older than 65 years, it is frequently estimated that approximately 3 to 4 million persons in the United States have Alzheimer's disease.

Alzheimer's disease is the major cause of institutionalization in the United States. More than 1.5 million persons in the United States reside in nursing homes. Note by comparison that under 1 million people are institutionalized in United States hospitals at any time. About three-fourths of the 1.5 million United States nursing home residents have dementia (Chandler and Chandler 1988; Rovner et al. 1986). Most of these nursing home residents with dementia have Alzheimer's disease as a major underlying cause or contributing factor to their cognitive disturbance. Consequently, Alzheimer's disease is estimated to be a significant source of morbidity and reason for institutionalization in 800,000–900,000 United States nursing home residents, approximately the same number of persons as in all United States hospitals at any time.

Alzheimer's disease is also a major cause of death, particularly in industrialized nations with elderly populations. Dementia and Alzheimer's disease in particular have long been known to be a source of increased mortality in comparison with comparably elderly cohort populations (Barclay et al. 1985; Go et al. 1978; Goldfarb 1969; Jarvik and Falek 1963; Kaszniak et al. 1978; Kral 1962; Molsa et al. 1986; Reding et al. 1984; Reimanis and Green 1971; Roth 1955; Thompson and Eastwood 1981). The morbidity and mortality associated with Alzheimer's disease make this single major illness the fourth leading cause of death in the United States and other industrialized nations after all forms of heart disease combined, all forms of cancer combined, and all forms of stroke (Eagles et al. 1990; Weiler 1987). These mortality statistics are likely to become increasingly disturbing because the incidence and mortality associated with stroke have been decreasing over the course of this century and the incidence of Alzheimer's disease has been increasing as the population ages; Alzheimer's disease is soon likely to replace stroke as the third leading cause of death in the United States and other industrialized nations.

Diagnosis and Symptoms

Introduction

The diagnosis of Alzheimer's disease is arrived at on the basis of clinical observations of the onset, course, and characteristic signs and symptoms of this common condition (American Psychiatric Association 1994). The presence of dementia is generally established initially. This may be accomplished by documenting deterioration in both cognitive and functional symptomatic domains. A mental status screening instrument such as the Mini-Mental State Exam (MMSE) (Folstein et al. 1975), the Information-Memory-Concentration test (IMC) (Blessed et al. 1968), or similar instruments (Kahn et al. 1960; Pfeiffer 1975) can be useful in documenting the magnitude of cognitive capacity. However, the clinician must be aware of the limitations of such screening instruments.

Low education is one well-known cause of a reduction of scores on mental status assessment (Crum et al. 1993; Murden et al. 1991; Uhlmann and Larson 1991). Other illnesses and conditions also will produce a lower score on various mental status assessments. These include conditions that interfere with the ability to write (e.g., severe arthritis, severe Parkinson's disease, or paralysis secondary to a stroke), conditions that interfere with concentration (e.g., mania and maniform states, depression, acute intoxication, or delusions associated with any of numerous medical disorders), and conditions that interfere with speech (e.g., severe depression or a stroke).

Once dementia is suspected, a dementia workup is performed. This includes serum enzyme studies, corpuscular blood counts and differentials, urinalysis, serum vitamin B_{12} and serum folate studies, thyroid studies, and a computed tomography (CT) or magnetic resonance imaging (MRI) brain scan. Salient conditions that may produce or contribute to dementia that are revealed by these studies include electrolyte disturbances, hypoglycemia, severe hepatic or renal disease, anemia, vitamin B_{12} or folate deficiency, thyroid disease, space-occupying brain lesions, and hydrocephalus. If considered appropriate, other studies such as a venereal disease research laboratory or human immunodeficiency virus (HIV) testing should be performed.

With the suspected presence of dementia and the possible primary or secondary role of identifiable contributory factors, the clinician then determines the evidence for a decline in cognitive and functional capacities and whether the nature of the decline and the clinical presentation are consistent with that of dementia of the Alzheimer's type. Because the signs and symptoms and history of decline in Alzheimer's disease vary markedly depending on the stage of the illness and other factors, diagnosis ultimately depends on a knowledge of the symptomatology of Alzheimer's disease. Clearly, differential diagnosis ultimately depends on an adequate knowledge of AD symptomatology and the symptomatology of other similar and related conditions.

Symptomatology of Alzheimer's Disease: An Overview

The clinical symptomatology of Alzheimer's disease consists most notably of cognitive, functional, and behavioral concomitants. Each of these symptomatic domains can be described on a continuum with the corresponding symptoms in normal aging. Table 14–1 provides a summary of the cognitive, functional, and behavioral concomitants of aging and progressive dementia of the Alzheimer's type as outlined in the Global Deterioration Scale (GDS) (Reisberg et al. 1982). Approximate mean scores on the MMSE at each of the global stages also are shown in Table 14–1. In addition to the GDS staging system, other similar procedures for describing the continuum of clinical change in aging and progressive dementia have been published (Cummings and Benson 1986; Hughes et al. 1982; Pfeffer et al. 1982). The most widely used of these alternative staging systems is the Clinical Dementia Rating (CDR) scale (Berg 1988; Hughes et al. 1982). Figure 14–1 shows the CDR stages approximately corresponding to each of the GDS stage levels outlined. Table 14–2 provides a more specific and detailed description of the specific functional losses that occur in association with aging and Alzheimer's disease and their approximate relationship to the GDS stages. Table 14–3 outlines the major behavioral changes that commonly occur in Alzheimer's disease and that appear to be amenable to

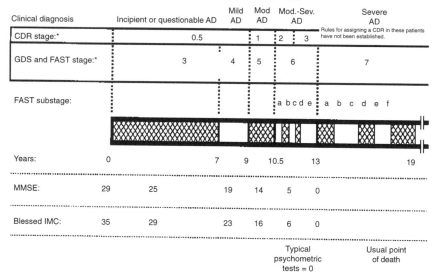

Figure 14–1. Typical time course of Alzheimer's disease (AD). *Stage range comparisons shown between the CDR and GDS/FAST stages are based on published functioning and self-care descriptions. CDR = Clinical Dementia Rating; FAST = Functional Assessment Staging; GDS = Global Deterioration Scale; IMC = Information–Memory–Concentration test; MMSE = Mini-Mental State Exam.

neurotransmitter psychopharmacological intervention, and Figure 14–2 provides a general outline of the frequency of occurrence of these symptoms with the advance of Alzheimer's disease.

Stages of Illness Development

Normal (stage 1).   Many elderly people are free of both subjective complaints of cognitive decrement and objective clinically manifest evidence of cognitive or functional decline. On the GDS given in Table 14–1, such individuals are referred to as being in stage 1 (normal). Current epidemiological data indicate that only a minority of elderly individuals fall within this category (Lane and Snowdon 1989; Lowenthal et al. 1967; Sluss et al. 1980).

Normal aged forgetfulness (stage 2).   Most elderly people, when queried, maintain the conviction that they can no longer remember such things as personal names as well as they could 5 or 10 years previously. Convictions of decrements in recalling where objects have been placed, in the ability to concentrate, and in recalling words from one's vocabulary also are common. In most cases, these subjective symptoms occur in the absence of overt, clinically manifest decrements in cognitive or functional capacity. The diagnostic terminology "age-associated memory impairment" (AAMI) also has been suggested for persons with these age-related subjective deficits (Crook et al. 1986). The similar diagnostic category "age-related cognitive decline" has been added to the DSM-IV (American Psychiatric Association 1994).

To many elderly people, these subjective complaints of cognitive decrement are so troubling that they are the single major reason that persons take medications in many nations in the world today. The specific kinds of treatment or medication taken for these symptoms vary with nationality and culture. In various European nations today, medications commonly taken for these subjective complaints of cognitive decrement include ginkgo biloba plant derivatives, piracetam, ergoloid mesylates, and nimodipine. In the United States and Canada, these medications are either unavailable, unknown, not believed to be indicated for these symptoms, or considered nonefficacious. Substances taken often in North America for these subjective complaints of cognitive impairment include multivitamins, lecithin, choline preparations, and various nonprescription mixtures of these and other substances.

Despite the troubling nature of these common subjective complaints of cognitive decrement in elderly people, longitudinal studies indicate that

Table 14–1. Global Deterioration Scale for age-associated cognitive decline and Alzheimer's disease[a]

GDS stage	Clinical characteristics	Diagnosis	Approximate mean MMSE[b,c]
1	No subjective complaints of memory deficit. No memory deficit evident on clinical interview.	Normal	29–30
2	Subjective complaints of memory deficit, most frequently in following areas: (a) forgetting where one has placed familiar objects. (b) forgetting names one formerly knew well. No objective evidence of memory deficit on clinical interview. No objective deficit in employment or social situations. Appropriate concern with respect to symptomatology.	Normal aged forgetfulness	29
3	Earliest clear-cut deficits. Manifestations in more than one of the following areas: (a) patient may have gotten lost when traveling to an unfamiliar location. (b) co-workers become aware of patients' relatively poor performance. (c) word and/or name finding deficit become evident to intimates. (d) patient may read a passage or book and retain relatively little material. (e) patient may demonstrate decreased facility remembering names upon introduction to new people. (f) patient may have lost or misplaced an object of value. (g) concentration deficit may be evident on clinical testing.	Mild neurocognitive disorder	25

4	Objective evidence of memory deficit obtained only with an intensive interview. Decreased performance in demanding employment and social settings. Denial begins to become manifest in patient. Mild to moderate anxiety frequently accompanies symptoms.	Mild Alzheimer's disease	20
5	Clear-cut deficit on careful clinical interview. Deficit manifest in following areas: (a) decreased knowledge of current and recent events. (b) may exhibit some deficit in memory of personal history. (c) concentration deficit elicited on serial subtractions. (d) decreased ability to travel, handle finances, etc. Frequently no deficit in following areas: (a) orientation to time and place. (b) recognition of familar persons and faces. (c) ability to travel to familiar locations. Inability to perform complex tasks. Denial is dominant defense mechanism. Flattening of affect and withdrawal from challenging situations. Patient can no longer survive without some assistance. Patient is unable during interview to recall a major relevant aspect of current life, e.g.,	Moderate Alzheimer's disease	14

(continued)

Table 14–1. Global Deterioration Scale for age-associated cognitive decline and Alzheimer's disease[a] (*continued*)

GDS stage	Clinical characteristics	Diagnosis	Approximate mean MMSE[b,c]
5 (*continued*)	(a) his or her address or telephone number of many years. (b) the names of close family members (such as grandchildren). (c) the name of the high school or college from which he or she graduated. Frequently some disorientation to time (date, day of the week, season, etc.) or to place. An educated person may have difficulty counting backward from 40 by 4s or from 20 by 2s. Persons at this stage retain knowledge of many major facts regarding themselves and others. They invariably know their own names and generally know their spouse's and children's names. They require no assistance with toileting or eating but may have difficulty choosing the proper clothing to wear.		
6	May occasionally forget the name of the spouse upon whom they are entirely dependent for survival. Will be largely unaware of all recent events and experiences in their lives. Retain some knowledge of their surroundings; the year, the season, etc. May have difficulty counting by 1s from 10, both backward and sometimes forward.	Moderately severe Alzheimer's disease	5

Will require some assistance with activities of daily living:
 (a) may become incontinent.
 (b) will require travel assistance but occasionally will be able to travel to familiar locations.
Diurnal rhythm frequently disturbed.
Almost always recalls own name.
Frequently continues to be able to distinguish familiar from unfamiliar persons.
Personality and emotional changes occur. These are variable and include
 (a) delusional behavior, e.g., patient may accuse spouse of being an impostor; may talk to imaginary figures in the environment or to own reflection in the mirror.
 (b) obsessive symptoms, e.g., person may continually repeat simple cleaning activities.
 (c) anxiety symptoms, agitation, and even previously nonexistent violent behavior may occur.
 (d) cognitive abulia, e.g., loss of willpower because an individual cannot carry a thought long enough to determine a purposeful course of action.

7

All verbal abilities are lost over the course of this stage.
Early in this stage words and phrases are spoken, but speech is very circumscribed.

0

Severe Alzheimer's disease

(continued)

Table 14–1. Global Deterioration Scale for age-associated cognitive decline and Alzheimer's disease[a] (*continued*)

GDS stage	Clinical characteristics	Diagnosis	Approximate mean MMSE[b,c]
7 (*continued*)	Later there is no speech at all—only grunting. Incontinent; requires assistance toileting and feeding. Basic psychomotor skills (e.g., ability to walk) are lost with the progression of this stage. The brain appears to no longer be able to tell the body what to do. Generalized and cortical neurological signs and symptoms are frequently present.		

Note. MMSE = Mini-Mental State Exam.

[a]*Source.* Reisberg et al. 1982.

[b]*Source.* Folstein et al. 1975.

[c]*Source.* Reisberg et al. 1988.

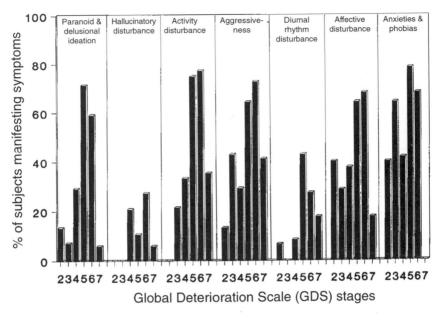

Figure 14–2.   Incidence of behavioral neuropsychiatric symptoms in age-associated memory impairment, mild neurocognitive disorder, and progressive Alzheimer's disease.

most elderly people with these complaints do not decline when followed over intervals of a few to many years (Flicker et al. 1993a; Reisberg et al. 1986b). However, it is not clear whether elderly people with these common complaints of cognitive deficit, in the absence of overtly manifest deficits, are more likely to develop Alzheimer's disease years later than individuals of equivalent age who do not have these subjective complaints. Similarly, the etiology of these subjective deficits is unclear. They may be the result of generalized brain changes commonly observed in elderly people including generalized brain atrophy, increased quantities of senile plaques and neurofibrillary tangles, and decreased cholinergic and other neurotransmitter system functioning. Alternatively, these common subjective complaints of cognitive decrement in elderly people may be the result of other factors such as the sensory losses and motoric slowing accompanying the aging process.

Research in this area is proceeding. This research indicates that although elderly people with these subjective complaints do perform well within the normal range on many neuropsychological tests, those who subsequently deteriorate perform poorly on some test measures that

Table 14–2. Functional Assessment Staging (FAST) in aging and progressive Alzheimer's disease(AD)[a] and time course of functional loss[b] (choose highest consecutive level of disability)

FAST stage	Clinical characteristics	Level of functional incapacity	Clinical diagnosis	Estimated duration of FAST stage or substage in AD[c]
1	No difficulty, either subjectively or objectively.	No deficit	Normal adult	
2	Complains of forgetting location of objects. Subjective work difficulties.	Subjective forgetting	Age-associated memory impairment	
3	Decreased job functioning evident to co-workers. Difficulty in traveling to new locations. Decreased organizational capacity.[d]	Complex occupational performance	Mild neurocognitive disorder	7 years
4	Decreased ability to perform complex tasks (e.g., planning dinner for guests), handling personal finances (e.g., forgetting to pay bills), difficulty marketing, etc.[d]	Instrumental ADL	Mild Alzheimer's disease	2 years
5	Requires assistance in choosing proper clothing to wear for the day, season, or occasion (e.g., patient may wear the same clothing repeatedly, unless supervised).[d]	Incipient ADL	Moderate Alzheimer's disease	18 months
6	(a) Improperly putting on clothes without assistance or cuing (e.g., may put street clothes on over night clothes, or put shoes on wrong feet, or have difficulty buttoning clothing) occasionally or more frequently over the past weeks.[d]	Deficient ADL	Moderately severe Alzheimer's disease	5 months

(b) Unable to bathe properly (e.g., difficulty adjusting bathwater temperature), occasionally or more frequently over the past weeks.[d]	Deficient ADL		5 months
(c) Inability to handle mechanics of toileting (e.g., forgets to flush the toilet, does not wipe properly or properly dispose of toilet tissue) occasionally or more frequently over the past weeks.[d]	Deficient ADL		5 months
(d) Urinary incontinence (occasionally or more frequently over the past weeks).[d]	Incipient incontinence		4 months
(e) Fecal incontinence (occasionally or more frequently over the past weeks).[d]	Incipient incontinence		10 months
7 (a) Ability to speak limited to approximately a half a dozen intelligible different words or fewer in the course of an average day or in response to queries in the course of an interview.	Semiverbal	Severe Alzheimer's disease	12 months
(b) Speech ability limited to the use of a single intelligible word in an average day or in response to queries in the course of an interview (the person may repeat the word over and over).	Semiverbal		18 months
(c) Ambulatory ability lost (cannot walk without personal assistance).	Nonambulatory		12 months

(continued)

Table 14–2. Functional Assessment Staging (FAST) in aging and progressive Alzheimer's disease(AD)[a] and time course of functional loss[b] (choose highest consecutive level of disability) (*continued*)

FAST stage	Clinical characteristics	Level of functional incapacity	Clinical diagnosis	Estimated duration of FAST stage or substage in AD[c]
7 (*continued*)				
	(d) Cannot sit up without assistance (e.g., the individual will fall over if there are no armrests on the chair).	Immobile		12 months
	(e) Loss of the ability to smile.	Immobile		18 months
	(f) Loss of the ability to hold up head independently.	Immobile		12 months or longer

Note. ADL = activities of daily living.
[a]*Source.* Reisberg 1988.
[b]*Source.* Adapted from Reisberg 1986.
[c]In subjects without other complicating illnesses who survive and progress to the subsequent deterioration stage.
[d]Scored primarily on the basis of information obtained from a knowledgeable informant and/or caregiver.

involve more complex cognitive processing or multimodality cognitive processing (Flicker et al. 1993b). Examples of tests that appear to be useful in discriminating subjects who subsequently deteriorate from those who do not include the digit symbol substitution test from the Wechsler Adult Intelligence Scale (WAIS) (Wechsler 1955), a test of symbolic memory and memory performance; a shopping list test (McCarthy et al. 1981) involving selective reminding and recall procedures (Buschke and Fuld 1974); a delayed spatial recall task (Flicker et al. 1984); a facial recognition memory task (Ferris et al. 1980a); and a remote memory questionnaire (Squire 1974). Other measures, such as neuroimaging of hippocampal atrophy, may prove useful to discriminate benign from malignant outcome subgroups in these ostensibly healthy subjects (de Leon et al. 1993b).

Mild neurocognitive disorder (stage 3). Clinicians also can identify a stage in which deficits become manifest but are only subtly manifest in the context of a detailed clinical interview. People at this stage (stage 3, in Tables 14–1 and 14–2) can generally carry out all simple and complex activities of daily life in which they formerly engaged, including marketing, meal preparation, and management of personal finances. Furthermore, their performance of these activities of daily life is approximately at the same level as in previous years. However, people at this stage who engage in complex occupational and social activities may begin to manifest performance deficits that become evident to intimates and co-workers. For example, a professional at this stage may find that he or she, seemingly for the first time, is unable to complete a report. Similarly, decreased memory for names of co-workers, clients, students, or employees may become evident as may a general decline in organizational capacity.

Clinical examination at this stage may reveal evidence of decreased capacities in various areas. For example, concentration and calculation deficits may be noted on serial subtraction. Memory deficits may become suspect on detailed questioning or when the patient repeats queries or phrases in the course of a conversation. Decreased performance on queries related to the patient's orientation may be evident or suspect. Clinicians also may detect deficits in performance on a variety of cognitive tasks reflecting the ability to copy designs, to perform simple arithmetic calculations, or in other areas. However, in all instances the deficits are subtle and perhaps only evident to the clinician who is familiar either with the patient's previous performance capacity or with the general performance of elderly patients on the particular task.

Formal testing of cohorts of patients at this stage reveals significantly decreased performance on many psychological tests (Reisberg et al. 1988). The greater the amount of cognition processing required and the greater the memory delay interval, the greater the difference in performance of persons at this stage from the performance of cohorts at previous stages (Flicker et al. 1993b). Although the mean score on the MMSE for persons at this stage is approximately 25, clinicians occasionally will note patients at this stage who score perfectly on the MMSE but show overt deficits such as repeating themselves or having major recall deficits.

Many of these subjects manifest deterioration when followed over intervals of a few to several years. However, a substantial minority do not manifest deterioration even when followed for a decade or longer. In this benign minority, the etiology of the subtly observed deficits is not always clear. Presumably, in many cases these deficits may be associated with subtle brain trauma, medical problems, or psychiatric conditions.

In most patients with these subtle deficits, longitudinal study indicates that these deficits are a harbinger of subsequent clearly manifested Alzheimer's disease. Longitudinal study also indicates that symptoms in this stage may persist for as long as 7 years (Reisberg et al. 1989a). Alternatively, these symptoms might not be clinically notable at all even in retrospect, particularly in elderly people who are not called on to perform complex occupational or social tasks. Methodologies for distinguishing which of these subjects will subsequently manifest deterioration are presently being described (de Leon et al. 1993b; Flicker et al. 1993b). However, until clinically useful methodologies become widely available that can reliably determine which of these subjects will subsequently manifest clear symptoms of Alzheimer's disease and which subjects will not, a diagnostic terminology such as "mild neurocognitive disorder" or "symptoms compatible with incipient Alzheimer's disease" is probably most accurately and usefully applied to subjects in this third global deterioration stage.

Mild Alzheimer's disease (stage 4).   Clinicians also can distinguish a stage in which deficits become readily manifest in the course of a detailed clinical interview but in which persons can still potentially maintain themselves independently in community settings. On the global deterioration scale in Table 14–1, these persons are at stage 4.

Functionally, persons at this stage frequently manifest deficits in such complex activities of daily life as managing their personal finances, meal preparation, or marketing skills. For example, persons at this stage sometimes may come to professional attention because of difficulties in paying their rent properly. In other cases, spouses begin to assume increasing financial responsibility. Frequently, at this stage family members may note that their mother or grandmother no longer prepares the holiday meal with accustomed facility. Sometimes the patient will avoid such activities entirely saying that they are now "too old for that" or that they "no longer have the energy they used to," hence avoiding having to expose their decreased capacities. Other functional deficits that may become evident at this stage include decreased ability to order food from a menu in a restaurant, the patient instead turning to the spouse or family member and asking "why don't you pick something for me?" Despite these deficits, persons at this stage can still generally perform basic activities of daily life including independent dressing and bathing.

Cognitive deficits become overtly manifest. Concentration and calculation deficits are frequently so marked that an educated person has difficulty subtracting serial 7s from 100 and even serial 4s from 40. Overt deficits in recent memory are frequently apparent such that major recent events are sometimes not recalled. For example, patients may have gone away on a recent holiday and have forgotten where they were or whom they visited. Remote memory also may be overtly impaired to such an extent that the spouse's memory of the patient's past becomes better than the patient's memory. Orientation is also frequently impaired at this stage, with marked deficit in recalling the date and/or the month and/or the season.

Other clinically manifest changes also become evident at this stage. For example, spouses and family members frequently note that the patient seems quieter, is more withdrawn, or walks more slowly than formerly. Family members frequently interpret these symptoms as signs of depression, and community physicians may treat these patients with antidepressants. However, in most cases the psychiatrist will note the absence of overtly dysphoric mood, suicidal ideation, initial or terminal insomnia, and appetite disturbance seen in depressive disorder and recognize these symptoms as common manifestations of mild Alzheimer's disease.

Longitudinal studies indicate that a diagnosis of Alzheimer's disease can be reliably determined in most cases at this stage when other causes of cognitive and functional decrements have been excluded or taken into consideration (Flicker et al. 1993b; McKhann et al. 1984; Reisberg et al. 1986b). The mean duration of this stage has been estimated to be 2 years (Reisberg et al. 1989a).

Moderate Alzheimer's disease (stage 5). At this stage, deficits are of sufficient magnitude to preclude independent community survival (Table 14–1, stage 5). Functionally, in addition to increasing incapacity in handling complex activities of daily life (finances, marketing, or meal preparation), patients begin to lose the ability to choose the proper clothing to wear for the season and the activities of the day. Frequently, for the first time the spouse will begin to suggest to the patient the clothes he or she should put on. Many patients will begin to wear the same clothes day after day unless they are provided with direction. Over the course of this stage, the ability to drive an automobile is lost.

Patients generally have concentration and calculation deficits of sufficient magnitude that errors are evident on subtracting serial 2s from 20. Recent memory deficits characteristically are such that major current aspects of personal and public life are frequently not recalled. The patient may not recall his or her address, weather conditions, or the name of the current United States president. Generally, the patient will recall some major aspects of current life but not others. Remote memory deficits are not overt unless the clinician queries in detail. If specific questions are asked regarding childhood and early life experiences, the clinician will generally find that the patient no longer recalls the names of some of the schools attended and from which he or she may have graduated. Orientation is often impaired sufficiently that the patient may not recall the current year. If the patient knows the year, he or she generally errs in recalling the month or season of the year.

Mood disturbances are most overtly an exaggeration of those that were manifest in the previous stage. Slowing of gait and withdrawal frequently become more evident. Other symptoms such as tearfulness, delusions, and agitation may become increasingly evident although the magnitude of these symptoms, collectively, is invariably greatest in the next disease stage. The mean duration of this fifth global deterioration stage is 1.5 years (Reisberg et al. 1989a).

Moderately severe Alzheimer's disease (stage 6).   Deficits become sufficiently severe at this stage that patients begin to require assistance with basic activities of daily life. In addition to not being able to choose their clothing, patients lose the ability to dress and bathe themselves without assistance. In the latter portion of this stage, increasing difficulties with toileting and continence are noted. Without supervision, patients throw the toilet tissue in the wrong place or fail to clean themselves properly. Urinary incontinence generally precedes fecal incontinence.

Cognitive impairment in this stage is manifest by deficits of sufficient magnitude that patients often will have difficulty counting backward from 10 by 1s; will state only a portion of their current address; and be unable to recall any of the schools that they attended, their mother's or father's name, or their state, town, or country of origin, although they generally can still recall their own names. Occasionally, patients at this stage may misidentify or not recall the name of their spouse. In the latter part of this stage, the spouse is frequently confused with a dead parent. Cognitive and symbolic explanations are recognized for this confusion because the spouse is generally assisting the patient with activities with which his or her parents assisted in childhood.

Behavioral changes become overtly manifest in this stage. Agitation and activity disturbances replace the previously noted withdrawal. In most patients the behavioral disturbances are sufficiently great to necessitate treatment with psychotropic agents. Nonpharmacological management also becomes a major concern. In most cases, a caregiver is required to assist the spouse in maintaining and managing the patient in a community setting. Ambulation is frequently compromised to the extent that the patient takes small steps while walking. Medication or concomitant medical illness may further compromise ambulatory abilities, and there may be a tendency to fall.

At the end of this stage, speech ability declines, manifest for example in the patient repeating words or phrases (verbigeration), interspersing genuine words with neologisms, or in paucity of speech. The total duration of stage 6 is approximately 2.5 years.

Severe Alzheimer's disease (stage 7).   This stage may last for many years. Patients require continuous assistance with basic activities of daily life including dressing, bathing, and toileting. A third of United States nursing home population, approximately 500,000 Americans, appear to be in this stage (German et al. 1985; Gurland et al. 1992; Mayeux et al. 1992; Teresi et al. 1994).

Patients in this final stage have severely limited speech abilities. Generally, repeated queries directed at the patient collectively produce responses of no more than six intelligible words. Later, even this severely limited vocabulary is further compromised, and the clinician can frequently identify a single word substage. The specific final word varies (e.g., "yes," "no," or "OK"). Subsequently, the Alzheimer's disease patient loses the ability to utter even a single intelligible word in response to forceful queries. After this, the patient is functionally nonverbal, although spontaneous words are occasionally uttered in response to pain or other internal or external stimuli.

Early in this stage, ambulatory abilities remain intact in most patients; however, patients are susceptible to insults (e.g., medication) or injuries (e.g., a hip fracture) that may compromise ambulatory ability. After speech ability is lost, ambulatory ability is invariably lost. This loss may occur in various ways. Some patients begin to lean over to one side. Other patients begin to lean forward or backward or develop a twisted gait before full loss of ambulating capacity. After ambulatory ability is lost, the patient with Alzheimer's disease is capable of walking only with personal assistance. The patient does not have the cognitive capacity to use a walker or to manipulate a wheelchair. Subsequently, the patient also loses the ability to sit up independently in a chair. Unless armrests are present, the patient will fall over.

Many patients with Alzheimer's disease die at about the point when they lose the ability to walk or to sit up. Common sources of morbidity and mortality in these patients include decubiti, which may become infected, and pneumonia, frequently associated with aspiration. Patients with Alzheimer's disease who survive lose the ability to smile. Facial expressions become limited to grimaces. Subsequently, patients lose the ability to hold up their head without assistance. A few patients with Alzheimer's disease survive for years even beyond this point. The most striking observation in such patients is increasing contractures of all four extremities.

Early in this final stage, behavioral problems often decrease. Consequently, physicians who have placed patients on medication for control of behavioral problems will find that the patient requires less and less medication as this stage evolves. An exception is screaming, which may appear in stage 7, especially in patients who have lost ambulatory ability prematurely but who maintain robust verbal capacities. Although uncommon, when it occurs, this screaming is a dramatic symptom of early stage 7, and such patients can be severely disruptive in chronic care or other settings.

Patients with Alzheimer's disease generally die approximately 2 years after the onset of this final stage. However, six separate substages can be identified as this final stage evolves, each of which may last a year or longer. Consequently, some patients survive in this final stage for 7 years or longer. Patients in stage 7 generally achieve only 0 or bottom scores on traditional cognitive, mental status, and psychometric tests (Mohs et al. 1986; Wilson and Kaszniak 1986). Recently, more sensitive tests have been developed for these severe patients who demonstrate continual loss of cognition as Alzheimer's disease evolves (Sclan et al. 1990).

Symptomatology: Neurobehavioral

Behavioral symptoms are characteristic concomitants of Alzheimer's disease (American Psychiatric Association 1994; Baker et al. 1991; Burns et al. 1990a, 1990b; Cummings et al. 1987; Drevets and Rubin 1989; Merriam et al. 1988; Reisberg et al. 1986a, 1987b, 1989b; Rubin et al. 1987; Steele et al. 1990; Teri et al. 1988, 1992; Wragg and Jeste 1989). Seven major categories of potentially remediable behavioral symptoms in Alzheimer's disease are readily identified. The categories are as follows: A) paranoid and delusional ideation; B) hallucinatory disturbances; C) activity disturbances; D) aggressivity; E) sleep disturbances; F) affective disturbances; and G) anxieties and phobias. Although these general symptomatic categories are not specific for Alzheimer's disease, the specific symptomatic manifestations in each of these categories are characteristic of Alzheimer's disease and related dementias.

The behavioral symptoms in Alzheimer's disease appear to be the characteristic result of two interacting processes: 1) the neurobehavioral changes occurring in the brain of the patient with Alzheimer's disease and 2) the cognitive changes occurring with the progression of Alzheimer's disease. The common specific symptoms in each of these major categories that occur in Alzheimer's disease are listed in Table 14–3. The general occurrence of symptoms in each of the major categories with the advance of Alzheimer's disease can be seen in Figure 14–2.

Paranoid and Delusional Ideation

In moderate Alzheimer's disease (stage 5), about 40% of patients have suspicions that spouses or caregivers are hiding or stealing objects from them, and about 25% have suspicions regarding the nature of their domicile (e.g., saying, "take me home," when they are home) or the identity of those around them (e.g., saying, "who are you?" to their spouse and mistrusting the response, "I'm your husband, dear"). Most patients also manifest other suspicions or false beliefs such as that they are still working or that dead relatives are alive. Although the occurrence of these symptoms appears to peak in stage 5, the disturbances associated with these symptoms (e.g., violence because of false beliefs and suspicions) probably peaks in stage 6.

Hallucinatory Disturbances

These occur in a minority of patients at various points throughout the evolution of Alzheimer's disease. Visual hallucinations are the most common type. Although these experiences (e.g., the patient sees dead relatives or hears intruders coming into the home) can be dramatic in terms of the

Table 14–3.   Behavioral symptomatology in Alzheimer's disease

A.   Paranoid and delusional ideation

1. *The "people are stealing things" delusion.*   Alzheimer's disease patients can no longer recall the precise whereabouts of household objects. This is probably the psychological explanation for what apparently is the most common delusion of Alzheimer's disease patients—that someone is hiding or stealing objects. More severe manifestations of this delusion include the belief that persons are actually coming into the home to hide or steal objects; the patient may actually speak with or listen to the intruders.

2. *The "house is not one's home" delusion.*   As a result of their cognitive deficits, Alzheimer's disease patients may no longer recognize their home. This appears to account, in part, for the common conviction of the Alzheimer's disease patient that the place in which they are residing is not their home. Consequently, while actually at home, Alzheimer's disease patients commonly request that their caregiver "take me home." Of potential danger to the patient are actual attempts to go home.

3. *The "spouse (or other caregiver) is an impostor" delusion.*   As cognitive deficit progresses, Alzheimer's disease patients recognize their caregivers less well, and a frequent delusion of the Alzheimer's disease patient is that persons are impostors. In some instances anger and even violence may result from this conviction.

4. *The delusion of "abandonment."*   With the progression of intellectual deficit in Alzheimer's disease, patients retain a degree of insight into their condition and they may be aware of the burden they impose. These insights are probably related to common delusions and fears of abandonment, institutionalization, or a conspiracy to institutionalize them.

5. *The delusion of "infidelity."*   The insecurities described above are also related to the Alzheimer's disease patient's occasional conviction that the spouse or other caregiver is unfaithful, sexually or otherwise.

6. *Other suspicions, paranoid ideation, or delusions.*   Less commonly expressed delusions are phantom boarder (strangers are living in the home); delusions that one still carries on activities in which one actually no longer participates (e.g., working, traveling); delusions about former family members or the present status of family members (e.g., father is still alive; daughter is still a child); delusion of doubles (e.g., there are two of the same person); and paranoid ideation about strangers (people staring or plotting to do harm).

B.   Hallucinatory disturbances

1. *Visual hallucinations.*   These can be vague or clearly defined. Commonly, for example, Alzheimer's disease patients see intruders or dead relatives at home.

Table 14–3. Behavioral symptomatology in Alzheimer's disease *(continued)*

 2. *Auditory hallucinations.* Occasionally, in the presence or absence of visual hallucinations, Alzheimer's disease patients may hear dead relatives, intruders, or others whispering or speaking to them; sometimes the voices are only heard when caregivers are not present.

 3. *Other hallucinations.* Less commonly, other forms of hallucinations may be observed in Alzheimer's disease patients (e.g., smelling a fire or something burning; patients perceiving imaginary objects, such as a piece of paper, which they may offer the caregiver).

C. Activity disturbances

The decreased cognitive capacity of Alzheimer's disease patients renders them less capable of channeling their energies in socially productive ways. Because motor abilities are not severely compromised until the final stage of the illness, patients may develop various psychological/motoric solutions for the need to channel their energies. A few of the most common examples are the following:

 1. *Wandering.* For a variety of reasons including inability to channel energies, anxieties, and delusions such as those described above and the decreased cognitive abilities per se, Alzheimer's disease patients frequently wander away from the home or caregiver. Restraint may be necessary and this, in turn, may provoke anger or violence in patients.

 2. *Purposeless activity (cognitive abulia).* Alzheimer's disease patients may not be able to carry a thought long enough to complete a purposeful movement. This results in a variety of purposeless, frequently repetitive activities, including opening and closing a purse or pocketbook, packing and unpacking clothing, repeatedly putting on and removing clothing, opening and closing drawers, incessant repetition of demands or questions, or simply pacing. Among the most severe manifestations of this syndrome is repetitive self-abrading.

 3. *Inappropriate activities.* These occur primarily as a result of decreased cognitive capacities, increased anxieties and suspiciousness, and excess physical energies. They include storing and hiding objects in inappropriate places (e.g., throwing clothing in the wastebasket, putting empty plates in the oven). Attempts by the caregiver to prevent these inappropriate activities may be met by anger or even violence.

D. Aggressivity

 1. *Verbal outbursts.* As already noted, these may occur in association with many of the behavioral symptoms already described. They can also occur as isolated phenomena. For example, an Alzheimer's disease patient may begin to use unaccustomed foul or abusive language with intimates and/or with strangers.

 2. *Physical outbursts.* These also may occur as part of the aforementioned syndromes or as an isolated manifestation. The

(continued)

Table 14–3.   Behavioral symptomatology in Alzheimer's disease *(continued)*

Alzheimer's disease patient may, in response to frustration or seemingly without cause, strike out at the spouse or caregiver.

3. *Other agitation.*   This includes anger that is expressed nonverbally, for example, the patient's stewing. Also common is negativity manifested by the patient's resistance to bathing, dressing, toileting, walking, or participating in other activities. Agitation may also be expressed as continuous and seemingly incessant talking (i.e., pressured speech), by panting (hyperventilation), banging, or in other ways.

E. **Sleep disturbances**

Sleep problems are a frequent and significant part of the behavioral syndrome of Alzheimer's disease. They may, in part, be the result of decreased cognition (which upsets habitual and other diurnal cues), the energy and motoric changes occurring in the illness, and the neurochemical processes predisposing to agitation and psychosis.

1. *Day/night disturbance.*   The most common sleep problem in Alzheimer's disease patients is multiple awakenings in the course of the night. These can occur in the context of an overall decrease in sleep or in association with increased daytime napping.

F. **Affective disturbances**

The depressive syndrome of Alzheimer's disease is primarily reactive in nature; it tends to frequently become manifest somewhat earlier in the course of Alzheimer's disease than many of the other symptoms described above and may be related to the pattern of insight and denial in the patient.

1. *Tearfulness.*   This predominant depressive manifestation generally occurs in brief periods. If queried as to the reason for tearfulness, patients might respond that they are crying because "the person I once was is gone," or because "of what is happening to me," or "I forget the reason." This tearfulness frequently may be a precursor of more severe behavioral symptomatology.

2. *Other depressive manifestations.*   A depressive syndrome may coexist with early Alzheimer's disease just as other illnesses may coexist with Alzheimer's disease. The most common affective symptom in Alzheimer's disease is the patient saying "I wish I were dead" or uttering a similar phrase, frequently in a repetitive and manneristic fashion. These pessimistic commentaries of the patient are not accompanied by any more-overt suicidal ideation or gestures.

G. **Anxieties and phobias**

These either may be related to the previously described behavioral manifestations of Alzheimer's disease or may occur independently.

1. *Anxiety regarding upcoming events (Godot syndrome).*   This common syndrome appears to result from decreased cognitive and, more specifically, memory abilities in the Alzheimer's disease patient and

Table 14–3. Behavioral symptomatology in Alzheimer's disease *(continued)*

from the inability to channel remaining thinking capacities productively. Consequently, the patient will repeatedly query with respect to an upcoming event. These queries may be so incessant and persistent as to become intolerable to family and caregivers.

2. *Other anxieties.* Patients commonly express previously nonmanifest anxieties regarding their finances, their future, and their health (including their memory), and regarding previously nonstressful activities, such as being away from home.

3. *Fear of being left alone.* This is the most commonly observed phobia in Alzheimer's disease, but as a phobic phenomenon, it is out of proportion to any real danger. For example, the anxieties may become apparent as soon as the spouse goes into another room. Less dramatically, the patient may simply request of the spouse or caregiver, "Don't leave me alone."

4. *Other phobias.* Patients with Alzheimer's disease sometimes develop a fear of crowds, of travel, of the dark, or of activities such as bathing.

Source. Adapted from Reisberg et al. 1987a, 1987b.

impression that these symptoms leave with relatives or other caregivers, they generally do not by themselves require treatment apart from reorientation and reassurance.

Activity Disturbances

Activity disturbances are among the most common and the most troubling behavioral symptoms in Alzheimer's disease. All disturbances in this category peak in both occurrence and in magnitude of disturbance in the sixth global deterioration stage.

Although all of these symptoms can be disturbing when they occur, the most commonly disturbing activity in Alzheimer's disease is probably verbal repetitive behavior. The patient's repeated queries, in particular, are both difficult to ignore and difficult for the spouse or caregiver to respond to. These repetitious statements or queries may be disturbing throughout most of the course of Alzheimer's disease. In some patients, repetition is an early clinical manifestation of mild neurocognitive disorder, whereas in others insistent questioning is most disturbing in stage 6. Pacing, wandering, and moving or hiding objects are common symptoms, especially in stage 6, although they also commonly occur earlier in the course of Alzheimer's disease.

Aggressivity.   Aggressive symptoms include verbal outbursts, anger, and resistance to participation in daily activities. They probably occur as a complex psychological response to both circumstances and neurochemical changes. Patients sometimes try to conceal their deficits by adopting an aggressive posture, strike out as a result of frustrations associated with their cognitive deficits, or resist activities that they no longer comprehend well. The patient's aggression, in part, is a response to the frustrations engendered by the caregiver's inability to tolerate the patient's condition and the patient's perception of those frustrations.

Aggressive symptoms appear to peak in frequency and intensity in stage 6, although most patients in stage 5 also manifest one or more of these symptoms. Fortunately, threats and violence occur in only a minority of patients at any point in the course of the illness. In stage 6, about 25% of patients exhibit threatening or violent behavior (Reisberg et al. 1989b).

Sleep disturbances.   The nature of the sleep disturbance in Alzheimer's disease is different from that observed in other psychiatric entities. The sleep disturbance of Alzheimer's disease is marked by fragmented sleep (i.e., frequent awakenings in the course of the night, apart from for purposes of urination) in contrast to the initial or terminal insomnia seen in depression. When sleep is markedly disturbed, caregivers may consider this sleep disturbance the most troubling symptom associated with the patient's disease.

Affective disturbances.   True depressive disorder (i.e., major depression) may occur in association with mild neurocognitive disorder or mild Alzheimer's disease. Classic affective disorder virtually never occurs in association with moderately severe or severe Alzheimer's disease. The affective symptoms that are commonly seen in association with Alzheimer's disease include an increase in tearfulness. The patient may attribute this tearfulness to the more general symptoms of Alzheimer's disease. Another notable affective symptom of Alzheimer's disease is reflected in the patient saying, "I wish I were dead," or uttering a similar phrase, often in a repetitive manner. These statements are not accompanied by true dysphoric ideation. Neither are these utterances accompanied by other overt suicidal ideation. "I wish I were dead" appears to be a manneristic and pessimistic commentary on their overall situation. Such utterances can be received as poignant commentaries by concerned family members who may be pained by the patient's insight into the situation.

Anxieties and phobias.   Anxieties and phobias are common symptoms that occur throughout the course of Alzheimer's disease. A frequent anxiety occurs regarding upcoming appointments or other events that the patient can no longer organize as well as previously. Consequently, keeping track of appointments and associated activities becomes a constant preoccupation. This preoccupation, because it appears to fill the void in the patient's increasingly empty life, has been termed the "Godot syndrome" (Reisberg et al. 1986a). The patient repeatedly queries the spouse and others about forthcoming events. About 40% of patients with mild neurocognitive disorder appear to manifest this symptom, which is also commonly seen in more severely impaired patients (Reisberg et al. 1989b). An effective approach to these symptoms is simply not to inform patients about forthcoming appointments.

Other anxieties that are common in Alzheimer's disease sometimes occur on a stage-specific basis. For example, patients with mild Alzheimer's disease (stage 4) may develop new anxieties about personal finances or income taxes that in fact they are less capable of managing. Later in the course of Alzheimer's disease, in the moderately severe stage (stage 6), shortly before the development of urinary incontinence, some patients become anxious about toileting, going to the toilet repeatedly and seemingly constantly. It would appear that the patient is aware of increasingly limited cognitive capacity to maintain continence and responds accordingly. Later, sometime after the development of actual incontinence, this anxiety disappears.

The most common phobia associated with Alzheimer's disease is fear of being left alone that often develops at about the same time the Alzheimer's disease patient loses the ability to manage independently (i.e., moderate Alzheimer's disease [stage 5]). About 40% of Alzheimer's disease patients in stage 5 and 6 have this symptom. Management concomitants of this common fear in Alzheimer's disease are readily identifiable. For example, patients may resist outside caregivers as an "invasion of their home" until the advent of this symptom. Once this fear develops and patients genuinely require assistance, they usually will accept the additional assistance that is necessary.

Another common phobia that develops in stage 5 or later is a fear of bathing. Strategies for management include hand-held showers, sponge bathing, and the spouse "modeling" by getting into the bath with the patient.

Symptomatology: Neurological

Alzheimer's disease is a degenerative brain disease, and it is accompanied by physically manifest neurological symptoms, apart from the cognitive, functional, and neurobehavioral changes that have been outlined above.

Subtle increased activity of the deep tendon reflexes is detectable even in many patients with mild neurocognitive disorder (Franssen et al. 1991). Primitive reflexes thought to be reactions to noxious and painful stimuli and therefore termed nociceptive reflexes (e.g., the glabellar, snout, and palmomental reflexes) are present in many patients with mild neurocognitive disorder or mild Alzheimer's disease. Other neurological reflexes become clearly manifest only with the advance of severe Alzheimer's disease (e.g., grasp, sucking, and rooting reflexes, and an abnormal plantar response [Basavaraju et al. 1981; Franssen et al. 1991, 1993; Huff et al. 1987; Paulson and Gottlieb 1968]). Perhaps the most striking neurological concomitant of Alzheimer's disease in the latter stages is an increase in rigidity (Franssen et al. 1991, 1993; Huff and Growdon 1986). This increase in rigidity appears to be associated with a stooped posture before the loss of ambulation and with the development of contractures in the immobile Alzheimer's disease patient.

Symptomatology: Neuroradiological

Cortical brain atrophy and cerebral ventricular dilation have long been recognized as concomitants of aging in general and the dementia of Alzheimer's disease in particular (Baillie 1795; Wilks 1864). The advent of CT scanning permitted the clear visualization of these changes. Cerebral ventricular dilation and, to a lesser extent, cerebral cortical atrophy as evidenced by increased sulcal size have been shown to occur in Alzheimer's disease to a greater extent than in elderly control subjects (de Leon et al. 1979; Huckman et al. 1975; Roberts et al. 1976). The magnitude of these relationships, however, is not large, and considerable overlap occurs between cognitively normal elderly subjects and Alzheimer's disease patients with dementia in terms of the magnitude of both cerebral ventricular dilation and cerebral cortical atrophy. For example, studies using CT imaging have found only a .3 Pearson correlation coefficient between global dementia severity in Alzheimer's disease and cerebral ventricular dilation magnitude (Reisberg et al. 1988). Similar results have been obtained in MRI studies of the relationship between cerebral ventricular dilation and mental status scores or other measures of cognitive severity (Kumar et al. 1994; Murphy et al. 1993).

The essential clinical message that clearly emerges from these studies is that atrophic changes on neuroimaging alone are never a reason for a dementia diagnosis. Such changes, however, may be cause for a comprehensive clinical assessment. Additionally, generalized atrophic changes seen on neuroimaging may be associated not only with aging and Alzheimer's disease but also with various non-Alzheimer's disease–related neuropsychiatric and medical conditions such as alcohol abuse or schizophrenia (Burns 1994; Rabins et al. 1987).

Another neuroimaging change commonly seen in Alzheimer's disease patients, particularly through the use of MRI imaging, is cerebral white-matter disease known as leukoaraiosis or Binswanger's changes. These commonly observed findings have been shown to be associated with hypertension, age, and cerebral infarctions. They also may have some association with the magnitude of dementia; however, this association is not strong. White-matter changes are not diagnostic either of dementia or of cerebral infarction (Besson 1994; Erkinjuntti et al. 1994).

With the use of sensitive procedures and appropriate angulation, the magnitude of hippocampal atrophy visualized with MRI or similar techniques appears to be useful in distinguishing healthy elderly individuals from early Alzheimer's disease patient groups (de Leon et al. 1993a). However, these techniques have not come into general clinical usage.

Symptomatology: Electrophysiological

Progressive increments in slow-wave activity have long been recognized as concomitants of progressive dementia in Alzheimer's disease (Hughes et al. 1989; Kaszniak et al. 1979; McAdam and Robinson 1957). More recent studies using quantitative analysis of the electroencephalogram (EEG) have elucidated these relationships more clearly (Breslau et al. 1989; Coben et al. 1990; Prichep et al. 1994; Sterletz et al. 1990; Williamson et al. 1990). A progressive increase is noted in θ-wave EEG activity that appears to accompany even the earliest cognitive changes in Alzheimer's disease. With increasing cognitive impairment, increments in δ-wave EEG activity also become evident. However, the magnitude of the relationship between cognitive or other aspects of deterioration in Alzheimer's disease and progressive EEG slowing does not exceed approximately a .5 Pearson correlation coefficient (Prichep et al. 1994). Moreover, EEG slowing is seen in non-Alzheimer's disease dementias and in many other physiological states. Hence, although electrophysiological slowing on the EEG can be indicative of Alzheimer's disease, these measures are not diagnostic of Alzheimer's disease unless used in conjunction with other clinical procedures. Evoked potential measures and other electrophysiological parameters that also have been studied in patients with Alzheimer's disease do not yet have convincing clinical utility.

Symptomatology: Neurometabolic

Cerebral blood flow has long been recognized as diminished in normal aging (Kety and Schmidt 1948) and, to a greater extent, in dementia (Obrist et al. 1970). The advent of positron emission tomography (PET) in the 1980s permitted an examination of cerebral metabolism in Alzheimer's disease. Initial studies showed cerebral metabolism to be decreased in Alzheimer's disease (Ferris et al. 1980a), and these decrements have been confirmed in numerous studies. Although cerebral metabolic decrements occur in Alzheimer's disease, studies have indicated that the decrements are greatest in the parietotemporal regions and frontal cortex. Decrements are generally less notable in the motor cortical regions, occipital regions, and cerebellum. Neither the magnitude of the relationship between decreased cerebral metabolism and Alzheimer's disease nor the specificity of these decrements, either globally or regionally, have rendered PET a diagnostic or severity measure for Alzheimer's disease in the absence of a comprehensive clinical evaluation. PET has shown promise, however, as an early marker of preclinical, but subsequently manifest, Alzheimer's disease (Haxby et al. 1986).

Single photon emission computerized tomography (SPECT) is another neuroimaging tool that has come into usage in Alzheimer's disease assessment. PET results are considered a standard against which SPECT procedures and results should be compared; however, SPECT is more widely available. Results of SPECT studies indicate blood flow decrements in Alzheimer's disease (Gemmell et al. 1987; Hurwitz et al. 1991; Neary et al. 1987; Podreka et al. 1987). Clinical correlation is a necessity in interpreting these SPECT findings.

Pathology, Pathogenesis, and Etiology

The salient pathological brain changes of Alzheimer's disease are the presence of senile plaques and neurofibrillary tangles (Alzheimer 1907; Blessed et al. 1968; Braak and Braak 1991; Khachaturian 1985; Mirra et al. 1991; Redlich 1898). Recent studies have elucidated the nature of these pathological features of Alzheimer's disease and their possible relationship to etiopathogenesis. However, the primary versus secondary roles of these pathological features and their essential presence in late-life Alzheimer's disease continue to require elucidation.

Classic neuritic senile plaques are composed of a central core of homogeneous-appearing material, termed *amyloid*, surrounded by cellular debris, referred to as the *neurite.* The amyloid consists of the β-amyloid peptide, a 42–43 amino acid peptide. This peptide fragment is derived from the amyloid protein precursor (APP), which has been shown to be encoded in the long arm of chromosome 21 (Goldgaber et al. 1987; Kang et al. 1987; Tanzi et al. 1987). At least two naturally occurring cleavage mechanisms for the breakdown of APP have been demonstrated, one of which results in β-amyloid deposition (Esch et al. 1990; Golde et al. 1992; Haass et al. 1992; Sisodia et al. 1990). Evidence suggests that the β-amyloid peptide is widely distributed in the body as well as being present in increased quantities in the brain in elderly individuals and especially patients with Alzheimer's disease (Seubert et al. 1992).

The neurofibrillary tangles are composed of paired helical filaments (Kidd 1963). The major constituent of these paired helical filaments is the tau protein (Kondo et al. 1988; Wischik et al., 1988a, 1988b). In addition, other constituents have been identified, notably including ubiquitin, a widely distributed protein (Mori et al. 1987; Perry et al. 1987).

These hallmark neuropathological features of Alzheimer's disease, the amyloid-containing senile plaques and the neurofibrillary tangles containing paired helical filaments, are found in healthy elderly subjects and are age-associated phenomena. These neuropathological features also are associated with the magnitude of dementia in Alzheimer's disease. They also are found in non-Alzheimer's disease pathological conditions. For example, amyloid deposits in the brain have been noted to be a feature of hereditary cerebral hemorrhage with amyloidosis-Dutch type (HCHWA-D) (Levy et al. 1990), and neurofibrillary tangles similar or identical to those in Alzheimer's disease may be seen in such diverse conditions as myotonic dystrophy and progressive supranuclear palsy (Bancher et al. 1987; Kiuchi et al. 1991).

The possible role of these neuropathological features of Alzheimer's disease in the etiopathogenesis of the disease has been strengthened by two groups of observations. One is that persons with Down's syndrome (i.e., trisomy of chromosome 21) develop the neuropathological features of Alzheimer's disease early in life and also are prone to the development of dementia in midlife. Even more striking evidence of the possible pathogenic role of amyloid has emerged from the findings that some families with early onset of Alzheimer's disease have mutations in the APP gene (Goate et al. 1991; Mullan et al. 1992). However, APP mutations have not been shown to occur in the common, late-life form of Alzheimer's disease and do not occur in many familial forms of Alzheimer's disease.

A genetic factor in the etiology of Alzheimer's disease also is supported by the finding of mutations on chromosome 14 associated with familial early-onset Alzheimer's disease (Schellenberg et al. 1992) and mutations on chromosome 19 associated with familial late-onset Alzheimer's disease (Pericak-Vance et al. 1991).

A possible role for a different kind of genetic factor in the etiopathogenesis of Alzheimer's disease has been suggested by findings that persons with a genetic marker that codes for an apolipoprotein (a molecule primarily responsible for lipid transport in various organs) are prone to the development of Alzheimer's disease. Three different subtypes of the apolipoprotein type E allele are inherited: $Apo\ E_2$, $Apo\ E_3$, and $Apo\ E_4$. Persons may be homozygous or heterozygous for any of these alleles. Studies have shown that persons who are homozygous for the Apo E_4 allele have as much as an eightfold increase in the risk of developing Alzheimer's disease (Corder et al. 1993; Poirier et al. 1993). Persons with Apo E_4 in heterozygous form also are at increased risk for the development of Alzheimer's disease.

Because a majority of patients with Alzheimer's disease may have at least one copy of the Apo E_4 gene, this inherited predisposition to Alzheimer's disease appears to be a significant factor in many persons with late-onset Alzheimer's disease. Persons who are homozygous for the E_4 allele are a small minority of the elderly and Alzheimer's disease population. The precise role of the apolipoprotein genes in Alzheimer's disease etiopathogenesis is a subject of considerable current speculation and investigation.

Many other factors have been implicated or considered in the etiopathogenesis of Alzheimer's disease. Nerve growth factor, hormonal factors, and neuroimmunological mechanisms are among the mechanisms under investigation. Neurotrophic factors can protect brain cells against insults of various kinds, including many of the injuries that have been implicated in Alzheimer's disease. Stress is known to be associated with brain damage through corticosteroid-related mechanisms that have been considered of possible relevance in Alzheimer's disease. Neuronal damage in Alzheimer's disease has been associated with an inflammatory cascade that may be of primary or secondary relevance in terms of continuing neurodegeneration. One of the most intriguing recent theories concerns a possible role of apoptosis or programmed cell death in the etiopathogenesis of Alzheimer's disease and of the interaction of this phenomenon with trophic factors (Johnson 1994). Oxidative damage and a possible role for antioxidants have been considered as possibly fundamental in pathogenesis, and clear evidence exists for neurometabolic and mitochondrial changes in Alzheimer's disease (Beal 1994). Evidence also exists that disorders in calcium homeostasis may contribute to neurodegeneration in Alzheimer's disease (Mattson 1994).

Aluminum is one of the most prominent toxic agents that has been studied in the etiopathogenesis of Alzheimer's disease. The major bases for the aluminum hypothesis are as follows: 1) aluminum has been known to cause neurotoxicity when introduced into mammalian brains (Crapper and Dalton 1973); 2) aluminum has been associated with dialysis encephalopathy in humans (Alfrey et al. 1976); 3) aluminum has been associated with neurofibrillary tangle–associated neurons and aluminasilicate of senile plaques (Candy et al. 1986; Perl and Brody 1980); and 4) epidemiological studies have shown higher proportions of Alzheimer's disease cases in communities with higher aluminum concentrations in drinking water (Martyn et al. 1989), and increased exposure to aluminum-containing products has sometimes been associated with Alzheimer's disease occurrence (Graves et al. 1990). However, all studies do not support the association of aluminum (Wisniewski 1986) or the association of aluminum concentration in drinking water (Wettstein et al. 1991; Wood et al. 1988) with neurofibrillary pathology. Most studies examining the relationship of aluminum-containing products to Alzheimer's disease occurrence have been negative. Consequently, it is unlikely that aluminum is a primary agent in Alzheimer's disease etiopathogenesis (Lord Walton 1991). In addition to aluminum, other toxic agents are being investigated in the etiopathogenesis of Alzheimer's disease. Notable among these theories is the possible role of zinc in amyloid formation (Bush et al. 1994). Current knowledge of the etiology of Alzheimer's disease can be summarized as follows: 1) the etiology is unknown, and 2) age, genetic mutations, chromosome 21 trisomy, and the presence of an apolipoprotein E_4 allele have been convincingly implicated as major risk factors.

Differential Diagnosis

Alzheimer's disease remains a clinical diagnosis. Consequently, the differential diagnosis of Alzheimer's disease is based on a recognition of the characteristic clinical features and course. Laboratory procedures, neuroimaging, electrophysiological studies, and other investigations may assist the clinician in arriving at a proper diagnosis. Differential diagnosis in Alzheimer's disease encompasses two kinds of decisions: 1) establishing the primary etiology of cognitive impairment, and 2) establishing the nature and relevance of excess morbidity in the patient with Alzheimer's disease. A complete discussion of differential diagnostic issues is potentially broad and requires a detailed knowledge of diverse relevant diagnostic entities. However, some salient elements, particularly relevant for the geriatric psychiatrist, are reviewed here.

Geriatric Depression

Early Alzheimer's disease has certain clinical features that are similar to those in depressive disorder. Both early Alzheimer's disease (i.e., stage 4 [mild Alzheimer's disease] and stage 5 [moderate Alzheimer's disease]) and depressive disorder are marked by symptoms that include flattening of affect, decreased verbalization, slowing of gait, and, to a lesser extent, generalized psychomotor slowing. Consequently, family members of patients with Alzheimer's disease during the first Alzheimer's disease-related visit to the clinician commonly complain that the patient "is depressed." Although the symptoms of Alzheimer's disease and depression (Table 14–4, first column) are superficially similar, their etiology differs.

In mild and moderate Alzheimer's disease, the observed emotional withdrawal and decreased verbalizations appear to be a response to decreased cognitive capacities that result in impaired ability to respond appropriately and with a full range of emotions. The slowed gait and generalized motoric slowing of the patient with Alzheimer's disease are on a continuum that begins early in the course of the disease and that ultimately results in complete loss of ambulatory and other motor capacities.

In depressive disorder, these same symptoms (i.e., flattened affect, paucity of speech, slowed gait, and psychomotor retardation) appear to be associated primarily with reversible neurochemical disturbances rather than cognitive or progressive brain changes. Evidence for this latter statement includes 1) the occurrence of these symptoms in depression in the absence of any concomitant clearly manifest cognitive changes and 2) the response of these symptoms in depressive disorder to pharmacological agents that affect neurotransmitter and related neurochemical disturbances.

Cognitive assessment helps distinguish the overlapping clinical symptoms of Alzheimer's disease and depressive disorder. In depressive disorder, the above-mentioned symptoms frequently occur in the absence of coexisting manifest cognitive disturbance, whereas in Alzheimer's disease these symptoms almost always emerge at a point in the evolution of the disease at which cognitive disturbances are overtly manifest. However, differential diagnosis is enormously complicated by the frequent presentation of cognitive disturbance as a manifestation of geriatric depression. In addition, it is occasionally difficult to elicit clearly manifest cognitive losses in mild Alzheimer's disease.

Table 14–4. Symptomatology associated with Alzheimer's disease and depressive affective disorder: similarities and differences

Symptoms shared by Alzheimer's disease and depressive disorder secondary to the cognitive (not mood) disturbance in Alzheimer's disease	Symptoms occurring in Alzheimer's disease and depressive disorder that are superficially similar[a]	Symptoms primarily associated with depressive disorder
Flattened affect	Paranoid and delusional ideation	Pervasive dysphoria
Paucity of speech	Hallucinations	Feelings of guilt
Slowed gait	Activity disturbances	True suicidal ideation
Generalized psychomotor slowing	Aggressivity	
	Diurnal rhythm disturbance (i.e., sleep disturbance)	
	Affective disturbance	
	Anxieties and phobias	

Source. Adapted from Reisberg 1992.

[a]Although categorically similar, the specific symptoms in these broad categories of behavioral disturbance differ in Alzheimer's disease and depressive affective disorder. The nature and incidence of specific symptoms in the behavioral pathologic syndrome of Alzheimer's disease is outlined in Table 14–3 and Figures 14–1 and 14–2.

Pervasive dysphoria and true suicidal ideation are common features of depressive disorders. When these symptoms occur in the geriatric patient, with or without associated cognitive disturbance, they may respond to antidepressant treatments. However, patients with Alzheimer's disease commonly manifest depressive-type symptoms including episodes of tearfulness and manneristic statements such as "I wish I were dead." These common clinical symptoms in Alzheimer's disease, reminiscent of depressive disorder, are to be distinguished from the pervasive dysphoria and true suicidal ideation observed in depressive disorder.

Many behavioral symptoms that are superficially similar in Alzheimer's disease and depressive disorder differ in their specific manifestations (Table 14–4, second column). In Alzheimer's disease, common delusions are that people are stealing things or the spouse is an impostor (see Table 14–3). In depressive disorder, the nature and content of delusional ideation differs, and delusions commonly are of a self-deprecating nature. Both Alzheimer's disease and depressive disorder are characterized by sleep disturbance.

However, in Alzheimer's disease the sleep disturbance is characterized by fragmented sleep, whereas in depressive disorder, sleep disturbance is classically manifest as initial or terminal insomnia or both. Anxieties and phobias are notable features both in Alzheimer's disease and in depressive disorder. However, in Alzheimer's disease anxieties are expressed, for example, as repetitive queries regarding upcoming events, and the most common phobia is a fear of being left alone, whereas in depression other kinds of anxieties and phobias are more common.

As noted above, cognitive disturbances can be a manifestation of geriatric depressive disorder. Although older adults with depression may have more difficulties with cognition, interestingly they are no more likely than persons at midlife to report cognitive problems (Blazer 1989).

At times this cognitive disturbance is subjective only (i.e., the patient complains of cognitive impairment). However, objective assessment (e.g., with mental status assessment) does not reveal evidence of impairment, and consequently the complaints of disturbance are out of proportion to the magnitude of cognitive deficit. In these cases a diagnosis of "pure" affective disturbance may be arrived at and treatment plans and prognosis formulated accordingly.

In contrast, the cognitive impairment accompanying geriatric depression may be objectively and subjectively manifest (LaRue et al. 1986). With treatment of depression, the cognitive disturbance may remit in association with the remittance of the affective disturbance and in some of these cases does not return. However, follow-up studies have shown that, in a substantial number of these cases, cognitive disturbance may become manifest over the subsequent 2- to 4-year interval and the depressive disorder will, in retrospect, be identifiable as a harbinger of subsequently manifest Alzheimer's disease (Agbayewa 1986; Baker et al. 1991; Kral 1982). For example, in a study of 44 subjects whose mean age was greater than 75 years who were assessed as having "depressive pseudodementia" (i.e., both depression and cognitive disturbance) at baseline and whose cognitive disturbances remitted initially, 39 patients (89%) developed dementia consistent with Alzheimer's disease at follow-up (Kral and Emery 1989) over 4 to 18 years. The proportion of patients who advance to dementia varies in different studies, probably depending on the population, follow-up interval, criteria for dementia, and other factors. For example, Pearlson et al. (1989) found only 1 of 11 patients manifested overt dementia after a 2-year follow-up.

In some patients the depression remits while the cognitive disturbance continues despite successful treatment of the affective symptoms. The cognitive disturbance nevertheless may remit in the subsequent weeks or months after the affective symptoms have been successfully treated. If the cognitive disturbance does remit, it may return in succeeding months and years.

Another possible clinical scenario is that the affective symptoms are successfully treated, but the cognitive disturbance persists. In retrospect it will be clear in these cases that the depressive symptoms were occurring in the context of an underlying dementia, most commonly Alzheimer's disease.

Clearly, depression and Alzheimer's disease have many areas of symptom similarity and overlap. This situation is not surprising because many of the neurotransmitter changes in depressive disorder and in Alzheimer's disease are similar and to some extent overlapping (Forstl et al. 1992; Whitehouse 1987; Zubenko et al. 1990). For example, noradrenergic deficits (Bondareff et al. 1982), dopaminergic decrements (Cross et al. 1984a), and serotonergic changes (Bowen et al. 1983; Cross et al. 1984b) have been reported in both disorders, although all of these changes appear to be more consistently reported in depressive disorder.

Cerebrovascular Dementia

Classic neuropathological studies indicated that cerebrovascular factors, specifically loose soft tissue and blood (also termed *cerebral softening*) presumably resulting from cerebral ischemia, appeared to be the major contributor to dementia etiopathogenesis in about 10%–15% of patients at autopsy (Tomlinson et al. 1970). At autopsy an additional 25% of patients in these classic studies manifested marked cerebrovascular changes in association with neuropathological brain changes of Alzheimer's disease (i.e., senile plaques and neurofibrillary tangles).

Building on these findings, Hachinski and associates (1974) coined the term *multi-infarct dementia* to encompass those cases in which cerebrovascular factors are primary features in dementia etiopathogenesis. As conceptualized by Hachinski, multi-infarct dementia was characterized by an abrupt onset, a stepwise course, evidence of strokes including focal neurological signs and symptoms, and associated stroke risk factors, such as hypertension (Hachinski 1983). A modified version of a multi-infarct scale designed by Hachinski for the assessment of infarct risk has come into wide usage (Rosen et al. 1980). In clinical practice, this classic conception of a dementia with both an abrupt onset and a stepwise course is infrequently observed. On those occasions when a fluctuating, stepwise course is seen in association with dementia, the clinician will frequently trace the source of fluctuation to a low serum vitamin B_{12} level, severe arteriosclerotic narrowing, or some other, nonmultiple infarct, pathological origin.

Current understanding of the role of cerebrovascular factors in dementia etiology includes the salient observation that strokes that are clinically or radiologically manifest can produce a pathology that may include cognitive impairment. To the extent that the strokes are bilateral and injure the cortex, hippocampi, or other relevant brain regions, they may result in generalized cognitive disturbances (i.e., dementia). However, as focal neurological lesions, strokes also can produce a variety of signs and symptoms that are not seen in Alzheimer's disease, such as unilateral deficits in motoric function or cranial nerve findings.

Strokes also can produce other pathologies that are seen in the course of Alzheimer's disease but that occur out of sequence with the temporal and ordinal emergence of pathology in the course of Alzheimer's disease. For example, strokes can produce urinary incontinence with or without any accompanying cognitive or cognition-related functional disturbance. Urinary incontinence does occur in Alzheimer's disease patients; however, in uncomplicated Alzheimer's disease, the urinary incontinence occurs after patients have acquired serious functional disturbance (see Table 14–2). A cerebral infarction also can produce a loss of ambulatory capacity. This ambulatory loss may be accompanied by associated cognitive and functional disturbances secondary to the stroke. Even if the stroke does produce associated cognitive and functional losses, these losses will not necessarily follow or mimic the patterns of disturbance seen in Alzheimer's disease (summarized in Tables 14–1 and 14–2). In general, the damage produced by the stroke and the degree to which the infarct lesions produce bilateral deficits will determine the extent to which the clinical picture of the dementia secondary to the infarction mimics or resembles that seen in Alzheimer's disease.

Although the stepwise pattern of loss described by Hachinski is rarely observed, infarct-related dementia is frequently accompanied by an abrupt onset or a temporal pattern of deficit and loss that is distinct from that observed in Alzheimer's disease. Functionally, the temporal pattern of loss in Alzheimer's disease can be retrospectively reconstructed. The approximate temporal sequence of functional loss in Alzheimer's disease is shown in Table 14–2. Studies have supported the ordinal and temporal sequence of emergence of functional loss shown in Table 14–2 (Sclan and Reisberg 1992). For example, in a study of patients with probable Alzheimer's disease free of non-Alzheimer's disease–related central nervous system pathology, about 90% of patients followed the ordinal sequence of deficit shown in Table 14–2. In the remaining 10% of patients, the order of functional loss differed from that shown in Table 14–2 only slightly (Sclan and Reisberg 1992). Consequently, the ordinal and temporal patterns of functional losses shown in Table 14–2 can assist clinicians in making judgments of the extent to which the etiology of deficits observed is inconsistent with those anticipated in Alzheimer's disease and therefore possibly attributable to infarction-related pathology.

Other Dementia Etiologies

Several conditions that affect cerebral function can produce generalized cognitive disturbances and either dementia or a clinical syndrome similar to dementia. These diverse conditions include head trauma, cerebral primary or secondary neoplasms, encephalitis caused by infectious agents, fungal agents or other organisms producing diffuse cerebral trauma, prion or "slow virus infection" such as Creutzfeldt-Jakob disease, metabolic or electrolyte disturbances, endocrine disturbances, nutritional disturbances including vitamin B_{12} and folate deficiencies, hereditary conditions such as Huntington's disease, cerebral toxins such as heavy metal poisoning, various pharmacological agents, normal pressure hydrocephalus, progressive supranuclear palsy, Pick's disease, and frontal lobe dementias—in addition to Alzheimer's disease, depression, and cerebral infarction. A standard clinical workup will assist in determining the possible relevance of these diverse pathological etiologies. This workup should include a complete corpuscular blood count and differential, serum electrolytes, and serum enzyme studies; a urinalysis; serum vitamin B_{12} and folate studies; thyroid studies; and a CT or MRI brain scan. When appropriate, other studies including an EEG, cerebral spinal fluid examination, a VDRL test, and HIV testing may be performed. The clinician should treat any elucidated remediable pathology.

Knowledge of the clinical symptomatology and course of Alzheimer's disease also will assist in the differential diagnosis of these diverse conditions. For example, normal pressure hydrocephalus commonly presents with gait disturbance. This is generally followed by urinary incontinence and subsequently by cognitive and cognition-related functional disturbances, such as decreased ability to manage instrumental activities of daily life. With Alzheimer's disease the temporal order of cognitive and functional losses is very different. Patients with Alzheimer's disease first manifest decreased ability to manage instrumental activities of daily life, then urinary incontinence develops, and later severe gait disturbance occurs (Tables 14–1 and 14–2).

Excess Morbidity

Physical pathology, apart from central nervous system pathology, also may have an impact on morbidity in the patient with Alzheimer's disease. For example, arthritis, a history of hip fracture, scoliosis associated with osteoporosis, peripheral vascular disease, and loss of vision associated with cataracts or other ocular pathology commonly occur in elderly individuals and may interfere with ambulation in the patient with Alzheimer's disease. When Alzheimer's disease and these sources of comorbidity coexist they frequently increase specific morbidity in a synergistic manner.

The clinician must assess the relevance of any additional pathology for the patient with Alzheimer's disease. Again, the temporal and ordinal sequence of functional losses in Alzheimer's disease (Table 14–2) can be useful in assisting the clinician in these differential diagnostic assessments. For example, if a clinician is treating a GDS and Functional Assessment Staging (FAST) stage 6 patient with haloperidol and the patient loses ambulatory capacity, the clinician must determine whether this ambulatory loss is the result of an extrapyramidal side effect from the haloperidol or the result of the progression of Alzheimer's disease. If the patient with Alzheimer's disease is still capable of speaking in sentences then the ambulatory loss is likely to be associated with excess morbidity, such as extrapyramidal side effects of the haloperidol treatment. The clinician will need to adjust pharmacological treatment accordingly.

Treatment

The treatment of Alzheimer's disease consists of proper clinical management and pharmacological intervention. Although no treatment has convincingly been demonstrated to halt or even retard the fundamental pathological process of Alzheimer's disease, appropriate management and pharmacological intervention can decrease stress and burden for the patient and the caregiver, postpone institutionalization, and minimize excess morbidity.

Management

Management needs in aging and Alzheimer's disease vary depending on the stage of the condition (Reisberg 1984). Special management strategies that should be considered in the patient with Alzheimer's disease include support groups and day care centers. Recently, support groups have become available for patients in the incipient and early stages (mainly GDS stages 3 and 4) of the disease and appear to be useful. Support groups for spouses and family members have long been available and are an important and useful resource. Day care centers are particularly useful for stage 5 and less-agitated stage 6 patients. The Alzheimer's Association (Chicago, IL) is an important resource and can help families get appropriate legal and financial planning advice.

Pharmacological Treatment

The primary purpose of pharmacological treatment in Alzheimer's disease is the remediation of the commonly occurring behavioral symptoms shown in Table 14–3 (Reisberg et al. 1986a). As already noted, these behavioral symptoms are common in patients with Alzheimer's disease (Figure 14–2), although their occurrence varies markedly with the stage of Alzheimer's disease. In general, these symptoms should only be treated if they are troubling or burdensome for the caregivers or a source of distress or danger for the patient.

The behavioral symptoms generally respond well to a low dosage of neuroleptic when they occur in the stage 4 or 5 patient (Reisberg et al. 1987b). In one study of thioridazine treatment, the mean dosage at which patients responded was about 50 mg (Reisberg et al. 1987b). However, the dose range at which patients responded was variable, and the dose of any medication should be individualized to the particular patient.

Depressive symptoms also are common in patients with mild to moderate Alzheimer's disease (GDS stages 4 and 5), and a fully manifest major depressive disorder may occur. Depressive symptoms such as dysphoric mood with associated anxieties or sleep disturbance may respond to antidepressant pharmacological treatment.

Behavioral symptoms peak in terms of magnitude of disturbance in stage 6. Treatment of these symptoms in this stage also becomes particularly difficult. There is a paucity of well-controlled clinical research in this area (Coccaro et al. 1990; Maletta 1990; Schneider and Sobin 1991; Schneider et al. 1990). This is compounded by the recent introduction of new categories of potentially relevant pharmacotherapeutic agents. Clinical experience is probably the best guide to treatment. Occasionally, behavioral symptoms in the stage 6 patient do respond satisfactorily to low-dose neuroleptic treatment. More commonly, however, neuroleptic treatment is insufficient unless the clinician raises the dose to the point at which generally intolerable side effects occur (e.g., falling in the case of thioridazine treatment and akathisia or rigidity in the case of treatment with haloperidol). It appears that the side effects can be avoided and the patient satisfactorily treated with a multiple neurotransmitter intervention strategy. The combination of a low-dose neuroleptic with a serotonergic agent such as trazadone or selective serotonin reuptake inhibitor such as sertraline is frequently useful. Trazodone has the added advantage of a sedative effect that assists in the normalization of sleep patterns.

Behavioral problems and agitation wax and wane throughout the course of moderately severe Alzheimer's disease (GDS stage 6), a stage that lasts, as noted above, an average of 2.5 years. Control of these symptoms is a major problem at this point. Although a specific approach to control of symptomatology has been recommended herein, clinicians have considered other approaches for control as well. Medications that have been advocated or studied include (in addition to the neuroleptics and antidepressant medications) propranolol, carbamazepine, lithium carbonate, sodium valproate, and buspirone (Billig et al. 1991; Colenda 1988; Maletta 1990; Mellow et al. 1993; Schneider and Sobin 1991; Schneider et al. 1990; Tiller et al. 1988). The superiority of particular pharmacological approaches over others is not clear from the present literature.

In stage 7 Alzheimer's disease, behavioral symptoms abate and continue to decline as this stage advances over the course of years. A symptom that sometimes becomes dramatic, although infrequent, at this point is screaming (Teri et al. 1992). Although uncommon, when screaming occurs, it can be a major problem. Treatment for this symptom and other behavioral symptoms in stage 7 is similar to the treatments recommended in stage 6. In general the dosages of medication can be gradually reduced over the course of stage 7.

Recently, an alternative pharmacological treatment approach has become available with the advent of tacrine, a reversible cholinesterase inhibitor. This treatment is based on the remediation of cholinergic neurotransmitter decrements, one of the most consistent changes accompanying the evolution of Alzheimer's disease. Studies of tacrine treatment in Alzheimer's disease have shown mixed results. Initial positive reports (Summers et al. 1981, 1986) were criticized (Division of Neuropharmacological Drug Products, Food and Drug Administration 1991) and followed by generally negative studies (Chatelier et al. 1990; Gauthier et al. 1990). More recent studies of tacrine have been positive (Davis et al. 1992; Farlow et al. 1992). The hope is that tacrine or other cholinergic treatments might mitigate some of the cognitive disturbances in Alzheimer's disease; however, evidence exists that the primary effect of cholinergic agents might be on the mood and behavioral disturbances accompanying Alzheimer's disease (Cummings et al. 1993). On the basis of the encouraging results from studies reviewed by the U.S. Food and Drug Administration, tacrine has received approval for marketing in the United States for the treatment of mild to moderate dementia of the Alzheimer type. Note that approval has been based on studies that have demonstrated statistically significant improvement in comparison with placebo on both performance-based assessment of cognition and a clinician's global assessment of change. Clinicians who consider prescribing this medication also should be aware of potential side effects. These include both classic cholinergic side effects and hepatotoxicity. The potential for the latter necessitates frequent (weekly) monitoring of serum transaminase levels in patients receiving this treatment.

Nonpharmacological Treatment of Behavioral Disturbances

Pharmacological approaches alone are inadequate for the treatment of behavioral disturbances in Alzheimer's disease. These disturbances are related to various factors including 1) the patient's inability to channel energies in useful directions; 2) the patient's anger and fear regarding his or her reduced capacities; 3) the spouse's anger at the disastrous turn of events that the illness has imposed upon them and the patient's response to the spouse's anger; 4) the patient's anxieties and discomfort regarding being bathed, dressed, and the advent of incontinence; and 5) in institutional settings, the patient's reaction to institutional constraints. The clinician should be prepared to arrange for the mitigation of all of these psychological aspects of the treatment of Alzheimer's disease (Jarvik and Small 1988; Mace and Rabins 1981; Rabins et al. 1982; Teri et al. 1992).

For example, in terms of the patient's inability to channel energies in useful directions, an activity planning approach has been advocated for patients cared for in community settings (Tanner and Shaw 1985). Additionally, day care centers for patients with Alzheimer's disease are available in most communities; these centers provide various kinds of structured activities for patients and simultaneously provide respite for spouses.

Another treatment approach has been developed for mitigating the cycle of anger and resultant behavioral disturbance that frequently occurs between Alzheimer's disease patients and their caregivers. This cycle may be severe between the spouse, who is understandably frustrated and disturbed by the patient's illness, and the patient, who is also frustrated and disturbed by his or her cognitive and other difficulties and losses. The psychological treatment entails a behavioral approach that examines the antecedents of the disturbing behaviors, the nature of the disturbing behaviors themselves, and the consequences of the behavioral disturbance. Having identified these "ABCs" (antecedents, behaviors, and consequences), efforts are devoted to breaking the cycle of disturbance by appropriate interventions (Teri and Logsdon 1990).

The clinician also should be prepared to intervene to mitigate disturbances associated with the functional losses that occur with the progression of Alzheimer's disease. For example, incontinence can be mitigated by a schedule of regular toileting. Nighttime incontinence may be less avoidable. If this occurs, the clinician should be prepared to suggest absorbent bedding and proper procedures for maintaining optimal cleanliness and skin care.

With the progression of Alzheimer's disease, patients become less steady on their feet and more fearful regarding the activities of daily life that they no longer fully comprehend. The clinician can assist by suggesting aids such as bath rails, bath mats, hand-held showers, or toilet railing. When patients become immobile, the clinician should recommend appropriate frequent movement schedules to prevent the occurrence and development of pressure ulcerations (decubiti). Ulcerated skin or soiled clothing from incontinence may result in increased agitation in the patient. As part of a comprehensive program of treatment of agitation, the clinician should counsel appropriately regarding the prevention and treatment of these conditions.

Prognosis and Outcome

The prognosis of Alzheimer's disease is an integral feature of the disease and has been discussed earlier in this chapter. As already noted, subjective complaints of cognitive impairment are common in elderly individuals but are generally benign. Similarly, the earliest subtly manifest clinical symptoms do not necessarily presage an inevitable deteriorating course. However, these subtle symptoms, or mild neurocognitive disorder (stage 3), are frequent harbingers of the degenerative dementia of Alzheimer's disease.

Figure 14–1 provides a synopsis of current understanding regarding the prognosis of Alzheimer's disease. Shown in Figure 14–1 is duration in terms of global, functional, and mental status assessments previously reviewed in this chapter (i.e., the GDS, FAST, and MMSE). Also shown is course in terms of other global and mental status assessments that are commonly used, the clinical dementia rating (CDR) (Berg 1988; Hughes et al. 1982), and the information and memory concentration test of Blessed et al. (1988).

A few salient features of the course of Alzheimer's disease should be noted: 1) The "border stage" of mild neurocognitive disorder is frequently not noted clinically or noted only retrospectively. However, when detected at the earliest possible point, generally in a patient who is called on to perform complex occupational tasks, fully one-third of the time course of Alzheimer's disease may be in this stage. 2) Clinicians can often reliably diagnose degenerative Alzheimer's disease from the beginning of stage 4, corresponding to an MMSE score of about 23. The mean duration of Alzheimer's disease from an MMSE score of 23 to an MMSE score of 0 (corresponding to the end of stage 6) is about 6 years. Therefore, patients lose about 3 to 4 points on the MMSE per year. 3) Most patients die after they have become nonverbal, at approximately the point when ambulatory ability and the ability to sit up are lost. Consequently, patients generally survive about 2 to 3 years after the bottoming out of traditional mental status assessments such as the MMSE. However, some patients survive for 6 or more years in this final, 7th GDS and FAST stage.

The total duration of Alzheimer's disease depends on how soon it is detected and how quickly the patient dies, among other factors. The mean time from diagnosis to death is about 6 to 8 years; however, the potential duration of Alzheimer's disease from the earliest clinical manifestation to death is about 20 years (Figure 14–1). Age and gender have not been shown to influence the course of Alzheimer's disease. Excess morbidity, such as the occurrence of cerebral infarctions (mixed dementia) appears to result in a more rapid clinical deterioration. The influence of other factors (such as Apo E genotype) on Alzheimer's disease course is unknown, although some familial forms of Alzheimer's disease appear to manifest a more rapid deteriorating course.

The most common cause of death in patients with Alzheimer's disease is pneumonia. Commonly this occurs in association with aspiration. Patients in the 7th stage have decreased capacity to masticate and swallow food. Consequently, a soft food or liquid diet becomes necessary, and proper time must be devoted to feeding. Even with proper care, aspiration may occur. Psychotropic medication may further interfere with swallowing and increase the tendency to aspiration as a result of extrapyramidal and other side effects. In addition to the danger of aspiration, progressive immobility also predisposes to pneumonia.

A second major cause of morbidity and mortality in the final stage of Alzheimer's disease is decubital ulceration. Proper positioning and management of incontinence are necessary to prevent this common complication. If not prevented, ulcerations can serve as a locus of infection with resultant sepsis, fever, and frequently death. Patients with Alzheimer's disease also are prone to death from stroke, cancer, and other common causes of death in elderly individuals, although some patients appear to die of no cause other than progressive Alzheimer's disease.

References

Agbayewa O: Earlier psychiatric morbidity in patients with Alzheimer's disease. J Am Geriatr Soc 34:561–564, 1986

Alfrey AC, Le Gendre GR, Kaehay WD: The dialysis encephalopathy syndrome: possible aluminum intoxication. N Engl J Med 294:184–188, 1976

Alzheimer A: Uber eine eigenartige Erkrankung der Hirnrinde. Allgemeine Zeitschrift fur Psychiatrie und Psychisch-Gerichtlich Medicin 64:146–148, 1907

American Psychiatric Association: Diagnostic and Statistical Manual of Mental Disorders, 4th Edition. Washington, DC, American Psychiatric Association, 1994

Baillie M: The morbid anatomy of some of the most important parts of the human body (1795). Oceanside, NY, Dabo, 1977 edition

Baker FM, Kokmen E, Chandra V, et al: Psychiatric symptoms in cases of clinically diagnosed Alzheimer's disease. J Geriat Psychiatry Neurol 4:71–78, 1991

Bancher C, Lassmann H, Budka H, et al: Neurofibrillary tangles in Alzheimer's disease and progressive supranuclear palsy: antigenic similarities and differences. Acta Neuropathol 74:39–46, 1987

Barclay LL, Zemcov A, Blass JP, et al: Factors associated with duration of survival in Alzheimer's disease. Biol Psychiatry 20:86–93, 1985

Basavaraju NG, Silverstone F, Libow L, et al: Primitive reflexes and perceptual sensory tests in the elderly—their usefulness in dementia. J Chronic Dis 34:367–377, 1981

Beal MF: Energy, oxidative damage, and Alzheimer's disease: clues to the underlying puzzle. Neurobiol Aging 15(suppl):S171–S174, 1994

Berg L: Clinical Dementia Rating (CDR). Psychopharmacol Bull 24:637–639, 1988

Besson JAO: Magnetic resonance imaging and spectroscopy in dementia, in Dementia. Edited by Burns A, Levy R. London, Chapman & Hall, 1994, pp 427–436

Billig N, Cohen-Mansfield J, Lipson S: Pharmacological treatment of agitation in a nursing home. J Am Geriatr Soc 39:1002–1005, 1991

Blazer D: Current concepts: depression in the elderly. N Engl J Med 320:164–166, 1989

Blessed G, Tomlinson BE, Roth M: The association between quantitative measures of dementia and senile change in the cerebral gray matter of elderly subjects. Br J Psychiatry 114:797–811, 1968

Blessed G, Tomlinson BE, Roth M: Blessed-Roth dementia scale (DS). Psychopharmacol Bull 24:705–708, 1988

Bondareff W, Mountjoy CQ, Roth M: Loss of neurons of origin of the adrenergic projection to cerebral cortex (nucleus locus ceruleus) in senile dementia. Neurology 32:164–168, 1982

Bowen DM, Allen SJ, Benton JS, et al: Biochemical assessment of serotonergic and cholinergic dysfunction and cerebral atrophy in Alzheimer's disease. J Neurochem 41:266–272, 1983

Braak H, Braak E: Neuropathological staging of Alzheimer related changes. Acta Neuropathol 82:239–259, 1991

Breslau J, Starr A, Sicotte N, et al: Topographic EEG changes with normal aging and SDAT. Electroencephalogr Clin Neurophysiol 72:281–289, 1989

Burns A: Computed tomography, in Principles and Practice of Geriatric Psychiatry. Edited by Copeland JRM, Abou-Saleh MT, Blazer DG. Chichester, England, Wiley, 1994, pp 467–471

Burns A, Jacoby R, Levy R: Psychiatric phenomena in Alzheimer's disease, I: disorders of thought content. Br J Psychiatry 157:72–76, 1990a

Burns A, Jacoby R, Levy R: Psychiatric phenomena in Alzheimer's disease, II: Disorders of perception. Br J Psychiatry 157:76–81, 1990b

Buschke H, Fuld PA: Evaluating storage, retention and retrieval in disordered memory and learning. Neurology 11:1019–1025, 1974

Bush AI, Pettingell WH, Multhaup G, et al: Rapid induction of Alzheimer A beta amyloid formation by zinc. Science 265:1464–1467, 1994

Candy JM, Oakley AE, Klinowski J, et al: Aluminosilicates and senile plaque formation in Alzheimer's disease. Lancet 1:354–357, 1986

Chandler JD, Chandler JE: The prevalence of neuropsychiatric disorder in a nursing home population. J Geriat Psychiatry Neurol 1:71–76, 1988

Chatelier G, Lacomblez L, on behalf of Group Francaise d'Etude de la Tetrahydroaminoacridine: Tacrine (tetrahydroaminoacridine; THA)

and lecithin in senile dementia of the Alzheimer type: a multicentre trial. Br Med J 300:495–499, 1990

Coben LA, Chi D, Snyder AZ, et al: Replication of a study of frequency of the resting awake EEG in mild probable Alzheimer's disease. Electroencephalogr Clin Neurophysiol 75:148–154, 1990

Coccaro EF, Kramer E, Zemishlany Z, et al: Pharmacologic treatment of noncognitive behavioral disturbances in elderly demented patients. Am J Psychiatry 147:1640–1645, 1990

Colenda CC: Buspirone in treatment of agitated demented patient (letter). Lancet 1:1169, 1988

Corder EH, Saunders AM, Strittmatter WJ, et al: Gene dose of apolipoprotein E type 4 allele and the risk of Alzheimer's disease in late onset families. Science 261:921–923, 1993

Crapper DR, Dalton A: Alterations in short-term retention, conditioned avoidance response, acquisition and motivation following aluminum induced neurofibrillary degeneration. Physiol Behav 10:925–933, 1973

Crook T, Bartus RT, Ferris SH, et al: Age-associated memory impairment: proposed diagnostic criteria and measures of clinical change—report of a NIMH work group. Dev Neuropsychol 2:261–276, 1986

Cross AJ, Crow TJ, Ferrier IN, et al: Serotonin receptor changes in dementia of the Alzheimer type. J Neurochem 43:1574–1581, 1984a

Cross AJ, Crow TJ, Johnson JA, et al: Studies on neurotransmitter receptor systems in neocortex and hippocampus in senile dementia of the Alzheimer-type. J Neurol Sci 64:109–117, 1984b

Crum RM, Anthony JC, Bassett SS, et al: Population-based norms for the Mini-Mental State Examination by age and educational level. JAMA 269:2386–2391, 1993

Cummings J, Miller B, Hill M, et al: Neuropsychiatric aspects of multi-infarct dementia and dementia of the Alzheimer type. Arch Neurol 44:389–393, 1987

Cummings JL, Benson DF: Dementia of the Alzheimer type: an inventory of diagnostic clinical features. J Am Geriatr Soc 34:12–19, 1986

Cummings JL, Gorman DG, Shapira J: Physostigmine ameliorates the delusions of Alzheimer's disease. Biol Psychiatry 33:536–541, 1993

Davis KL, Thal LJ, Gamzu ER, et al: A double-blind, placebo-controlled multicenter study of tacrine for Alzheimer's disease. N Engl J Med 327:1253–1259, 1992

de Leon MJ, Ferris SH, Blau I, et al: Correlations between CT changes and behavioral deficits in senile dementia. Lancet 2:859–860, 1979

de Leon MJ, Golomb J, George AE, et al: Hippocampal formation atrophy: prognostic significance for Alzheimer's disease, in Alzheimer's Disease: Advances in Clinical and Basic Research. Edited by Corain B, Iqbal K, Nicolini M, et al. Chichester, England, Wiley, 1993a, pp 35–46

de Leon MJ, Golomb J, George AE, et al: The radiologic prediction of Alzheimer's disease: the atrophic hippocampal formation. American Journal of Neuroradiology 14:897–906, 1993b

Division of Neuropharmacological Drug Products, Food and Drug Administration: Tacrine as a treatment for Alzheimer's dementia: an interim report from the FDA. N Engl J Med 324:349–352, 1991

Drevets W, Rubin E: Psychotic symptoms and the longitudinal course of senile dementia of the Alzheimer type. Biol Psychiatry 25:39–48, 1989

Eagles JM, Beattie JAG, Restall DB, et al: Relation between cognitive impairment and early death in the elderly. Br Med J 300:239–240, 1990

Erkinjuntti T, Gao F, Lee DH, et al: Lack of difference in brain hyperintensities between patients with early Alzheimer's disease and control subjects. Arch Neurol 51:260–268, 1994

Esch FS, Keim PS, Beattie EC, et al: Cleavage of amyloid beta peptide during constitutive processing of its precursor. Science 248:1122–1124, 1990

Evans DA, Funkenstein HH, Albert MS, et al: Prevalence of Alzheimer's disease in a community population of older persons: higher than previously reported. JAMA 262:2551–2556, 1989

Farlow M, Gracon S, Hershey L, et al: A controlled trial of tacrine in Alzheimer's disease. JAMA 268:2523–2529, 1992

Ferris SH, Crook T, Clark E, et al: Facial recognition memory deficits in normal aging and senile dementia. J Gerontol 35:707–714, 1980a

Ferris SH, de Leon MJ, Wolf AP, et al: Positron emission tomography in the study of aging and senile dementia. Neurobiol Aging 1:127–131, 1980b

Flicker C, Bartus RT, Crook T, et al: Effects of aging and dementia upon recent visuospatial memory. Neurobiol Aging 5:275–283, 1984

Flicker C, Ferris SH, Reisberg B: A longitudinal study of cognitive function in elderly persons with subjective memory complaints. J Am Geriatr Soc 41:1029–1032, 1993a

Flicker C, Ferris SH, Reisberg B: A two-year longitudinal study of cognitive function in normal aging and Alzheimer's disease. J Geriat Psychiat Neurol 6:84–96, 1993b

Folstein MF, Folstein SE, McHugh PR: Mini-Mental State: a practical method for grading the cognitive state of patients for the clinician. J Psychiatr Res 12:189–198, 1975

Forstl H, Burns A, Luthert P, et al: Clinical and neuropathological correlates of depression in Alzheimer's disease. Psychol Med 22:877–884,
1992

Franssen EH, Reisberg B, Kluger A, et al: Cognition-independent neurologic symptoms in normal aging and probable Alzheimer's disease.
Arch Neurol 48:148–154, 1991

Franssen EH, Kluger A, Torossian CL, et al: The neurologic syndrome of
severe Alzheimer's disease: relationship to functional decline. Arch
Neurol 50:1029–1039, 1993

Gauthier S, Bouchard R, Lamontagne A: Tetrahydroaminoacridine-
lecithin combination treatment in patients with intermediate-stage
Alzheimer's disease: Results of a Canadian double-blind, crossover,
multicenter study. N Engl J Med 322:1272–1276, 1990

Gemmell HG, Sharp PF, Besson JA, et al: Differential diagnosis in dementia using the cerebral blood flow agent 99m-Tc-HMPAO: a SPECT
study. J Comput Assist Tomogr 11:398–402, 1987

German PS, Shapiro S, Kramer M: Nursing home study of the Eastern
Baltimore epidemiological catchment area study, in Mental Illness in
Nursing Homes: Agenda for Research. Edited by Harper MS, Lebowitz
B. Washington, DC, National Institute of Mental Health, 1985

Go RCP, Todorov AB, Elston RC, et al: The malignancy of dementias. Ann
Neurol 3:559–561, 1978

Goate A, Chartier-Harlin M-C, Mullan M, et al: Segregation of a missense
mutation in the amyloid precursor protein gene with familial
Alzheimer's disease. Nature 349:704–706, 1991

Golde TE, Estus S, Younkin LH, et al: Processing of the amyloid protein
precursor to potentially amyloidogenic fragments. Science 255:728–
730, 1992

Goldfarb A: Predicting mortality in the institutionalized aged. Arch Gen
Psychiatry 21:172–176, 1969

Goldgaber D, Lerman MI, McBride OW, et al: Characterization and chromosomal localization of a cDNA encoding brain amyloid of
Alzheimer's disease. Science 235:877–880, 1987

Graves AB, White E, Koepsell TD, et al: The association between aluminum-containing products and Alzheimer's disease. J Clin Epidemiol
43:35–44, 1990

Gurland BJ, Wilder DE, Cross P, et al: Screening scales for dementia: toward reconciliation of conflicting cross-cultural findings. Int J Geriatr
Psychiatry 7:105–113, 1992

Haass C, Koo E, Mellon A, et al: Targeting of cell-surface beta-amyloid precursor protein to lysosomes: alternative processing into amyloid-bearing fragments. Nature 357:500–503, 1992

Hachinski VC: Differential diagnosis of Alzheimer's dementia: multi-infarct dementia, in Alzheimers Disease. Edited by Reisberg B. New York, Free Press, 1983, pp 188–192

Hachinski VC, Lassen NA, Marshall J: Multi-infarct dementia: a cause of mental deterioration in the elderly. Lancet 2:207–210, 1974

Haxby JV, Grady CL, Duara R, et al: Neocortical metabolic abnormalities precede nonmemory cognitive defects in early Alzheimer's-type dementia. Arch Neurol 43:882–885, 1986

Huckman MS, Fox J, Topel J: The validity of criteria for the evaluation of cerebral atrophy by computed tomography. Radiology 116:85–92, 1975

Huff FJ, Growdon JH: Neurological abnormalities associated with severity of dementia in Alzheimer's disease. Can J Neurol Sci 13:403–405, 1986

Huff FJ, Boller F, Luchelli F, et al: The neurologic examination in patient's with probable Alzheimer's disease. Arch Neurol 44:929–932, 1987

Hughes CP, Berg L, Danziger WL, et al: A new clinical scale for the staging of dementia. Br J Psychiatry 140:566–572, 1982

Hughes JR, Shanmugham S, Wetzel LC, et al: The relationship between EEG changes and cognitive functions in dementia: a study in a VA population. Clin Electroencephalogr 202:77–85, 1989

Hurwitz T, Ammann W, Chu D, et al: Single photon emission computed tomography using 99m-Tc-HM-PAO in the routine evaluation of Alzheimer's disease. Journal Canadien Des Sciences Neurologiques 18:59–62, 1991

Jarvik LF, Falek A: Intellectual stability and survival in the aged. J Gerontol 18:173–176, 1963

Jarvik L, Small G: Parentcare: A Commonsense Guide for Adult Children. New York, Crown, 1988

Johnson EM Jr: Possible role of neuronal apoptosis in Alzheimer's disease. Neurobiol Aging 15:S187–S189, 1994

Kahn RL, Goldfarb AI, Pollack M, et al: Brief objective measures for the determination of mental status in the aged. Am J Psychiatry 117:326–328, 1960

Kang J, Lemaire HG, Unterbeck A, et al: The precursor of Alzheimer's disease amyloid βA4 protein resembles a cell-surface receptor. Nature 325:733–736, 1987

Kaszniak AW, Fox J, Gandell DL, et al: Predictors of mortality in presenile and senile dementia. Ann Neurol 3:246–252, 1978

Kaszniak AW, Garron DC, Fox JC, et al: Cerebral atrophy, EEG slowing, age, education and cognitive functioning in suspected dementia. Neurology 29:1273–1279, 1979

Katzman R: Alzheimer's disease. N Engl J Med 314:964–973, 1986

Kety S, Schmidt C: The nitrous oxide method for quantitative determination of cerebral blood flow in man: theory, procedure and normal values. J Clin Invest 27:475–483, 1948

Khachaturian ZS: Diagnosis of Alzheimer's disease. Arch Neurol 42:1097–1105, 1985

Kidd M: Paired helical filaments in electron microscopy in Alzheimer's disease. Nature 197:192–193, 1963

Kiuchi A, Otsuka N, Namba Y, et al: Presenile appearance of abundant Alzheimer's neurofibrillary tangles without senile plaques in the brain in myotonic dystrophy. Acta Neuropathol 82:1–5, 1991

Kondo J, Honda T, Mori H, et al: The carboxyl third of tau is tightly bound to paired helical filaments. Neuron 1:827–834, 1988

Kral VA: Senescent forgetfulness: benign and malignant. Can Med Assoc J 86:257–260, 1962

Kral VA: Depressiv pseudodemenz und senile demenz von Alzheimer-type: eine pilot-studie. Nervenarzt 53:284–288, 1982

Kral VA, Emery OB: Long-term follow-up of depressive pseudodementia of the aged. Can J Psychiatry 34:445–446, 1989

Kumar A, Newberg A, Alavi A, et al: MRI volumetric studies in Alzheimer's disease. Am J Geriat Psychiatry 2:21–31, 1994

Lane F, Snowdon J: Memory and dementia: a longitudinal survey of suburban elderly, in Clinical and Abnormal Psychology. Edited by Lovibond P, Wilson P. New York, Elsevier North-Holland, 1989, pp 365–376

LaRue A, D'Elia LF, Clark EO, et al: Clinical tests of memory in dementia, depression, and healthy aging. J Psychol Aging 1:69–77, 1986

Levy E, Carman MD, Fernandez-Madrid IJ, et al: Mutation of the Alzheimer's disease amyloid gene in hereditary cerebral haemorrhage, Dutch type. Science 248:1124–1126, 1990

Livingston G: The scale of the problem, in Dementia. Edited by Burns A, Levy R. London, Chapman & Hall, 1994, pp 21–35

Lord Walton: Alzheimer's Disease and the Environment. Oxford, Alden Press, 1991

Lowenthal PM, Berkman PL, Buehler JA, et al: Aging and Mental Disorder in San Francisco: A Social Psychiatric Study. San Francisco, CA, Jossey-Bass, 1967

Mace N, Rabins PV: The 36-Hour Day. Baltimore, MD, Johns Hopkins University Press, 1981

Maletta GJ: Pharmacologic treatment and management of the aggressive demented patient. Psychiatric Annals 20:446–455, 1990

Martyn CN, Barker DJ, Osmond C, et al: Geographical relation between Alzheimer's disease and aluminum in drinking water. Lancet 1:59–62, 1989

Mattson MP: Mechanism of neuronal degeneration and preventative approaches: quickening the pace of AD research. Neurobiol Aging 15 (suppl):S121–S125, 1994

Mayeux R, Denaro J, Hemenegildo N, et al: A population-based investigation of Parkinson's disease with and without dementia: relationship to age and gender. Arch Neurol 49:492–497, 1992

McAdam W, Robinson RA: Prognosis in senile deterioration. J Ment Sci 103:821–823, 1957

McCarthy M, Ferris SH, Clark E, et al: Acquisition and retention of categorized material in normal aging and senile dementia. Exp Aging Res 7:127–135, 1981

McKhann G, Drachman D, Folstein M, et al: Clinical diagnosis of Alzheimer's disease: report of the NINCDS-ADRDA work group under the auspices of Department of Health and Human Services Task Force on Alzheimer's disease. Neurology 34:939–944, 1984

Mellow AM, Solano-Lopez C, Davis S: Sodium valproate in the treatment of behavioral disturbance in dementia. J Geriat Psychiatry Neurol 6:205–209, 1993

Merriam AE, Aronson M, Gaston P, et al: The psychiatric symptoms of Alzheimer's disease. J Am Geriatr Soc 36:7–12, 1988

Mirra SS, Heyman A, McKeel D, et al: The Consortium to Establish a Registry for Alzheimer's Disease (CERAD), II: standardization of the neuropathologic assessment of Alzheimer's disease. Neurology 41:479–486, 1991

Mohs R, Kim G, Johns C, et al: Assessing changes in Alzheimer's disease: memory and language, in Handbook for Clinical Memory Assessment. Edited by Poon LW. Washington, DC, American Psychological Association, 1986, pp 149–155

Molsa PK, Marttila RJ, Rinne UK: Survival and cause of death in Alzheimer's disease and multi-infarct dementia. Acta Neurol Scand 74:103–107, 1986

Mori H, Kondo J, Ihara Y: Ubiquitin is a component of paired helical filaments in Alzheimer's disease. Science 235:1641–1644, 1987

Mullan M, Crawford F, Axelman K, et al: A pathogenic mutation for probable Alzheimer's disease in the APP gene at the N-terminus of β-amyloid. Nature Genetics 1:345–347, 1992

Murden RA, McRae TD, Kaner S, et al: Mini-Mental State Exam scores vary with education in blacks and whites. J Am Geriatr Soc 39:149–155, 1991

Murphy DGM, DeCarli CD, Daly E, et al: Volumetric magnetic resonance imaging in men with dementia of the Alzheimer type: correlations with disease severity. Biol Psychiatry 34:612–621, 1993

Neary D, Snowden JS, Shields RA, et al: Single photon emission tomography using 99m-Tc-HMPAO in the investigation of dementia. J Neurol Neurosurg Psychiatry 50:1101–1109, 1987

Obrist WD, Chivian E, Cronquist S, et al: Regional cerebral blood flow in senile and presenile dementia. Neurology 20:315–322, 1970

Paulson G, Gottlieb G: Developmental reflexes: the reappearance of foetal and neonatal reflexes in aged patients. Brain 91:37–52, 1968

Pearlson GD, Rabins PV, Kim WS, et al: Structural brain CT changes and cognitive deficits in elderly depressives with and without reversible dementia ("pseudodementia"). Psychol Med 19:573–584, 1989

Pericak-Vance MA, Bebout JL, Gaskell Jr, et al: Linkage studies in familial Alzheimer's disease: evidence for chromosome 19 linkage. Am J Hum Genet 48:1034–1050, 1991

Perl DP, Brody J: Alzheimer's disease: x-ray spectrometric evidence of aluminum accumulation in the neurofibrillary tangle bearing neurons. Science 208:297–299, 1980

Perry G, Friedman R, Shaw G, et al: Ubiquitin is detected in neurofibrillary tangles and senile plaque neurites of Alzheimer disease brains. Proc Natl Acad Sci USA 84:3033–3036, 1987

Pfeffer RI, Kurosaki TT, Harrah CH, et al: Measurement of functional activities in older adults in the community. J Gerontol 37:323–329, 1982

Pfeiffer EA: Short portable mental status questionnaire for the assessment of organic brain deficit in the elderly. J Am Geriatr Soc 23:433–441, 1975

Podreka I, Suess E, Goldenberg G, et al: Initial experience with technetium-99m HMPAO brain SPECT. J Nucl Med 28:1657–1666, 1987

Poirier J, Davignon J, Bouthillier D, et al: Apolipoprotein E polymorphism and Alzheimer's disease. Lancet 342:697–699, 1993

Prichep LS, John ER, Ferris SH, et al: Quantitative EEG correlates of cognitive deterioration in the elderly. Neurobiol Aging 15:85–90, 1994

Rabins P, Mace N, Lucas M: The impact of dementia on the family. JAMA

248:333–335, 1982

Rabins PV, Pearlson GD, Jayaram G, et al: Elevated ventricle-to-brain ratio in late-onset schizophrenia. Am J Psychiatry 144:1216–1218, 1987

Reding AJ, Haycox J, Wigforss K, et al: Follow-up of patients referred to a dementia service. J Am Geriatr Soc 32:265–268, 1984

Redlich E: Uber miliare sklerosen der Hirnrinde bei seniler Atrophie. Jahrbuchfuer Psychiatric und Neurologic 17:208–216, 1898

Reimanis G, Green RF: Imminence of death and intellectual decrement in the aging. Dev Psychol 5:270–272, 1971

Reisberg B: Stages of cognitive decline. Am J Nurs 84:225–228, 1984

Reisberg B: Dementia: a systematic approach to identifying reversible causes. Geriatrics 41(4):30–46, 1986

Reisberg B: Functional assessment staging (FAST). Psychopharmacol Bull 24:653–659, 1988

Reisberg B: Memory dusfunction and dementia: diagnostic considerations, in Clinical Geriatric Psychopharmacology, 2nd Edition. Edited by Salzman C. Baltimore, MD, Williams & Wilkins, 1992, pp 255–276

Reisberg B, Ferris SH, de Leon MJ, et al: The Global Deterioration Scale for assessment of primary degenerative dementia. Am J Psychiatry 139:1136–1139, 1982

Reisberg B, Borenstein J, Franssen E, et al: Remediable behavioral symptomatology in Alzheimer's disease. Hosp Community Psychiatry 37:1199–1201, 1986a

Reisberg B, Ferris SH, Shulman E, et al: Longitudinal course of normal aging and progressive dementia of the Alzheimer's type: a prospective study of 106 subjects over a 3.6 year mean interval. Prog Neuropsychopharmacol Biol Psychiatry 10:571–578, 1986b

Reisberg B, Borenstein J, Franssen E, et al: BEHAVE-AD: a clinical rating scale for the assessment of pharmacologically remediable behavioral symptomatology in Alzheimer's disease, in Alzheimer's Disease: Problems, Prospects, and Perspectives. Edited by Altman HJ. New York, Plenum, 1987a, pp 1–16

Reisberg B, Borenstein J, Salob SP, et al: Behavioral symptoms in Alzheimer's disease: phenomenology and treatment. J Clin Psychiatry 48 (suppl):9–15, 1987b

Reisberg B, Ferris SH, de Leon MJ, et al: Stage-specific behavioral, cognitive, and in vivo changes in community residing subjects with age-associated memory impairment (AAMI) and primary degenerative dementia of the Alzheimer type. Drug Development Research 15:101–114, 1988

Reisberg B, Ferris SH, de Leon MJ, et al: The stage specific temporal course of Alzheimer's disease: functional and behavioral concomitants based upon cross-sectional and longitudinal observation. Prog Clin Biol Res 317:23–41, 1989a

Reisberg B, Franssen E, Sclan SG, et al: Stage specific incidence of potentially remediable behavioral symptoms in aging and Alzheimer's disease: a study of 120 patients using the BEHAVE-AD. Bull Clin Neurosci 54:95–112, 1989b

Roberts MA, Caird FI, Grossart KW, et al: Computerized tomography in the diagnosis of cerebral atrophy. J Neurol Neurosurg Psychiatry 39:905–915, 1976

Rosen WG, Terry RD, Fuld PA, et al: Pathological verification of ischemia score in differentiation of dementias. Ann Neurol 7:486–488, 1980

Roth M: The natural history of mental disorders arising in the senium. J Ment Sci 101:281–301, 1955

Rovner BW, Kafonek S, Filipp L, et al: Prevalence of mental illness in a community nursing home. Am J Psychiatry 143:1446–1449, 1986

Rubin E, Morris J, Storandt M, et al: Behavioral changes in patients with mild senile dementia of the Alzheimer's type. Psychiatry Res 21:55–61, 1987

Schellenberg GD, Bird TD, Wijsman EM, et al: Genetic linkage evidence for a familial Alzheimer's disease locus on chromosome 14. Science 258:668–671, 1992

Schneider LS, Sobin PB: Non-neuroleptic medications in the management of agitation in Alzheimer's disease and other dementia: a selective review. Int J Geriatr Psychiatry 6:691–708, 1991

Schneider LS, Pollack VE, Lyness SA: A meta-analysis of controlled trials of neuroleptic treatment in dementia. J Am Geriatr Soc 38:553–563, 1990

Sclan SG, Reisberg B: Functional assessment staging (FAST) in Alzheimer's disease: reliability, validity and ordinality. Int Psychogeriat 4 (suppl 1): 55–69, 1992

Sclan SG, Foster JR, Reisberg B, et al: Application of Piagetian measures of cognition in severe Alzheimer's disease. Psychiatr J Univ Ott 15:221–226, 1990

Seubert P, Vigo-Pelfrey C, Esch F, et al: Isolation and quantification of soluble Alzheimer's β-peptide from biological fluids. Nature 359:325, 1992

Sisodia S, Koo E, Beyreuther K, et al: Evidence that beta-amyloid protein in Alzheimer's disease is not derived by normal processing. Science 248:492–495, 1990

Sluss TK, Rabins P, Gruenberg EM: Memory complaints in community residing men (abstract). Gerontologist (part II) 20:201, 1980

Squire LR: Remote memory as affected by aging. Neuropsychologia 12:429–435, 1974

Steele C, Rovner B, Chase GA, et al: Psychiatric symptoms and nursing home placement of patients with Alzheimer's disease. Am J Psychiatry 147:1049–1051, 1990

Sterletz LJ, Reyes PF, Zolewska M, et al: Computer analysis of EEG activity in dementia of the Alzheimer type and Huntington's disease. Neurobiol Aging 11:15–20, 1990

Summers WK, Viesselman JO, Marsh GM, et al: Use of THA in treatment of Alzheimer-like dementia: pilot study in twelve patients. Biol Psychiatry 16:145–153, 1981

Summers WK, Majovski LV, Marsh GM, et al: Oral tetrahydroaminoacridine in long-term treatment of senile dementia, Alzheimer type. N Engl J Med 315:1241–1245, 1986

Tanner F, Shaw S: Caring: A Family Guide to Managing the Alzheimer's Patient at Home. East Hanover, NJ, Sandoz Pharmaceuticals, 1985

Tanzi RE, Gusella JF, Watkins PC, et al: Amyloid beta protein gene: cDNA, mRNA distribution, and genetic linkage near the Alzheimer locus. Science 235:880–884, 1987

Teresi J, Lawton MP, Ory M, et al: Measurement issues in chronic care populations: dementia special care. Alzheimer Dis Assoc Disord 8(suppl 1):S144–S183, 1994

Teri L, Logsdon R: Assessment and management of behavioral disturbances in Alzheimer's disease. Compr Ther 6:36–42, 1990

Teri L, Larson E, Reifler B: Behavioral disturbance in dementia of the Alzheimer's type. J Am Geriatr Soc 36:1–6, 1988

Teri L, Rabins P, Whitehouse P, et al: Management of behavior disturbance in Alzheimer's disease: current knowledge and future directions. Alzheimer Dis Assoc Disord 6:77–88, 1992

Thompson EG, Eastwood MR: Survivorship and senile dementia. Age Aging 10:29–32, 1981

Tiller JWG, Dakis JA, Shaw JM: Short-term buspirone treatment in disinhibition with dementia (letter). Lancet 2:510, 1988

Tomlinson BE, Blessed G, Roth M: Observations on the brains of demented old people. J Neurol Sci 11:205–242, 1970

Uhlmann RF, Larson EB: Effect of education on the Mini-Mental State Examination as a screening test for dementia. J Am Geriatr Soc 39:876–880, 1991

Wechsler D: Wechsler Adult Intelligence Scale. New York, Psychological

Corporation, 1955

Weiler P: The public health impact of Alzheimer's disease. Am J Public Health 77:1157–1158, 1987

Wettstein A, Aeppli J, Gautschi K, et al: Failure to find a relationship between mnestic skills of octogenarians and aluminum in drinking water. Int Arch Occup Environ Health 63:97–103, 1991

Whitehouse PJ: Neurotransmitter receptor alterations in Alzheimer disease: a review. Alzheimer Dis Assoc Dis 1:9–18, 1987

Wilks S: Clinical notes on atrophy of the brain. J Ment Sci 10:383, 1864

Williamson PC, Merskey H, Morrison S, et al: Quantitative electrophysiologic correlates of cognitive decline in normal elderly subjects. Arch Neurol 47:1185–1188, 1990

Wilson R, Kaszniak A: Longitudinal changes: progressive idiopathic dementia, in Handbook for Clinical Memory Assessment. Edited by Poon LW. Washington, DC, American Psychological Association, 1986, pp 285–293

Wischik CM, Novak M, Edwards PC, et al: Structural characterization of the core of the paired helical filament of Alzheimer disease. Proc Natl Acad Sci USA 85:4884–4888, 1988a

Wischik CM, Novak M, Thogersen HC, et al: Isolation of a fragment of tau derived from the core of the paired helical filament of Alzheimer disease. Proc Natl Acad Sci USA 85:4506–4510, 1988b

Wisniewski HM: No evidence for aluminum in etiology and pathogenesis of Alzheimer's disease. Neurobiol Aging 7:532–535, 1986

Wood DJ, Cooper C, Stevens J, et al: Bone mass and dementia in hip fracture patients from areas with different aluminum concentrations in water supplies. Age Aging 17:415–419, 1988

Wragg R, Jeste D: Overview of depression and psychosis in Alzheimer's disease. Am J Psychiatry 146:577–587, 1989

Zubenko GS, Mossy J, Koop U: Neurochemical correlates of major depression in primary dementia. Arch Neurol 47:209–214, 1990

Stephen Read, M.D.

Vascular Dementias

V ascular dementia in DSM-IV (American Psychiatric Association 1993) supplants multi-infarct dementia in DSM-III-R (American Psychiatric Association 1987); this change reflects the continuing evolution of our understanding of cerebrovascular injury. Vascular dementia patients display a diversity of clinical syndromes depending on the location and type of cerebrovascular disease. Therefore, vascular dementia offers a rich array of opportunities to analyze relationships between Axis I syndromes and Axis III disorders. Concepts of vascular dementia have been expanded as a result of technological developments, especially in neuroimaging, but this has increased rather than reduced controversy in many areas (see, for example, Brust 1988 versus O'Brien 1988).

Epidemiology

Tomlinson, Blessed, and Roth (1970) found cerebral infarction to be the second most common cause of dementia. Most subsequent studies concur, although methodological problems mandate caution in drawing firm conclusions (Brayne 1993; Jorm et al. 1987). Different criteria for inclusion account for reported rates of vascular dementia varying from 4.5%

to 39%. Recent studies using careful case definition in community samples suggest that the incidence of vascular dementia is less than 10%; another 10% to 20% of dementia patients show cerebrovascular and degenerative (especially Alzheimer-type) pathology (Kase 1991).

As in Alzheimer's disease, the incidence of dementia with evidence of cerebral infarcts increases with age: rates below age 60 are 1.0 per 100,000, rising to 20.7, 105.2, and 213.2 in each succeeding decade. Overall incidence appears to be declining, consistent with the declining incidence of stroke (Kokmen et al. 1988), but the incidence of vascular dementia may approach or even surpass Alzheimer's disease in the oldest-old patients (Skoog et al. 1993).

Comparing rates of dementia among different geographic locations may provide clues to possible relationships among genetic and environmental factors, but the existing data are rudimentary. In an extensive review, Jorm (1991) concluded that studies from the United States, Canada, Britain, and Australia show a consistent preponderance of Alzheimer's disease over vascular dementia. Prevalence rates are closer in Scandinavian studies: some show equivalent numbers of Alzheimer's disease and vascular dementia patients. Studies from Japan and the single available Chinese study show a preponderance of vascular dementia. There are no studies from other countries.

Diagnosis and Symptomatology

Various elements of clinical and laboratory examination are discussed elsewhere. In this chapter, I address points of special relevance in detecting cerebrovascular disease and assessing its role in the dementia patient.

History

The circumstances of any acute change in the course of a patient's dementia should be examined for evidence of possible cerebrovascular disease. Familiarity with the features of stroke syndromes will increase the clinician's confidence in evaluating the likelihood of cerebrovascular insult. Subtle motor, sensory, or mental status changes commonly are overlooked, especially if they improve, but even a clearcut stroke may not be mentioned by the patient or caregiver who is focussed on the dementia that is "obviously" Alzheimer's disease. Table 15–1 presents the most common risk factors for cerebrovascular disease (Wolf 1985). The presence of these factors is not

Table 15–1. Risk factors for cerebrovascular disease

Hypertension	Major predisposing factor in multiple forms of cardiac and cerebrovascular disease, especially stroke and white-matter lesions.
Arrhythmia	Frequent in patients with vascular dementia (Bucht et al. 1984), especially atrial fibrillation (Wolf et al. 1978) and sick sinus syndrome with bradycardia (Simonsen et al. 1980); often associated with episodic hypotension and cardiogenic embolism.
Diabetes mellitus	Confers risk for cognitive impairment (Perlmuter et al. 1984) plus a relative risk of 2–3:1 for stroke and of 2–5:1 for myocardial infarction compared with people without diabetes (Nathan 1993).
Vasculitis	Inflammatory disease (e.g., temporal arteritis)
Pulmonary disease	Neuropsychologic deficits are associated with chronic hypoxemia (Grant et al. 1987).
Substance abuse	Cigarette smoking and alcohol use predispose to vascular disease and hypertension.
Hyperlipidemia	Debate continues over dietary factors and vascular disease; the interpretation of lipid levels in elderly patients is particularly uncertain (Ulbricht and Southgate 1991).

diagnostic, but increases the suspicion of cerebrovascular disease and may provide clues to specific pathology or pathogenetic mechanisms.

Examination

Evidence of focal brain injury should be sought from mental status and physical examination. The study of stroke victims has contributed to the understanding of focal brain disease from the time of Broca's 1860s description of aphasia with left frontal lobe infarction, the rich literature available increases sensitivity to identifying stroke syndromes, which may provide strong clinical support for a diagnosis of vascular dementia. Other sources include Absher and Benson 1993; Chui 1989; Cummings 1993; Fisher 1982; and Strub and Black 1985. Gait abnormality or focal motor or sensory findings may be the residuum of a clinical event significant to the dementia. Similarly, the presence of cardiovascular pathology may provide clues to pathogenetic mechanism. Special attention may be placed on orthostatic blood pressure, which should be determined in patients with syncope and parkinsonian syndromes who are on medications that can block baroreceptor responses.

Laboratory Studies

Several studies recommended for routine dementia evaluation by the National Institutes of Health Consensus Development Conference (1987) are particularly relevant to assessing the role of cerebrovascular disease in dementia: complete blood count for anemia and hemolysis, and fasting and 2-hour postprandial blood glucose for diabetes mellitus. Overall glucose control in known diabetic patients can be assessed with hemoglobin A_{1c} level. Hypothyroidism or hyperthyroidism may underlie or complicate cardiovascular disease and may cause delirium directly. Elevated sedimentation rate screens for inflammatory disease. Electrocardiogram (ECG) may reveal arrhythmia or ischemic cardiac disease. Twenty-four-hour ambulatory ECG should be considered for episodic syncope. More detailed tests of cardiopulmonary function may be required for each individual.

Neuroimaging

Neuroimaging techniques are discussed in Chapter 12; aspects of structural and functional brain imaging relevant to vascular dementia are discussed here. Electroencephalography (EEG) (see Chapter 13) may reveal nonspecific abnormalities or focal slowing caused by stroke. Recent studies have identified features of quantitative EEG that may be specific to vascular dementia (Leuchter et al. 1992). Structural brain imaging with X-ray computed tomography (CT) or magnetic resonance imaging (MRI) is recommended for evaluation of vascular dementia. MRI has supplanted CT to evaluate cerebrovascular disease because of MRI's superior definition and sensitivity (especially to gray-matter lesions) and its ability to image deep brain tissue adjacent to bony structures. Lacunae, white-matter lesions, or stroke requires review for clinical correlation. The following may be found in healthy elderly patients (Drayer 1988a, 1988b): 1) enlargement of the ventricles (especially the third ventricle), cortical sulci, and the spaces around the vermis of the cerebellum in the sixth or seventh decade; and 2) areas of white-matter hyperintensity in 30%–80% of elderly patients. Areas of hyperintensity in the basal ganglia and hypointensity on T2-weighted images of the putamen are common and of uncertain significance.

Extensive literature reflects the controversy over the significance of subcortical white matter abnormalities, which may be referred to as subcortical arteriosclerotic encephalopathy, unidentified bright objects, or leukoaraiosis (Hachinski et al. 1987). Leukoaraiosis may be seen in normal elderly patients, Alzheimer's disease patients, and vascular dementia patients. Fein et al. (1990) found normal neuropsychological test patterns in patients with leukoaraiosis even when severe white-matter changes of up to 7 years' duration were present. Other studies, however, support a reluctance to consider findings of leukoaraiosis as inconsequential: Boone et al. (1992) found more severe leukoaraiosis associated with impaired neuropsychological performance; measures of attention and frontal lobe function were the most sensitive markers. Ylikoski et al. (1993) found that leukoaraiosis correlated with decreased speed of mental processing. The proposal by Kawabata et al. (1993) that functional brain imaging studies can help resolve the significance of structural lesions has been helpful. For example, Sultzer et al. (1995) have recently linked PET-defined hypometabolism of structurally normal cerebral cortex to subcortical lesions seen on MRI scan.

Cerebral blood flow (CBF) is regulated closely to maintain stable cerebral metabolic oxygen rate (CMR_{O_2}). At rest, gray-matter CMR_{O_2} is approximately four times that of white matter. CBF is maintained by mechanisms that are poorly defined but are independent of systemic factors until the extremes of cardiovascular decompensation are reached. This is true in elderly patients, except for slight decreases in oxygen and glucose utilization (Brown and Frackowiak 1991; Drayer 1988a). Positron-emission tomography (PET) with glucose analogues or oxygen provides direct measures of metabolic activity but remains more available as a research tool than for clinical studies. Single photon emission computed tomography (SPECT) is a measure of CBF that correlates closely with metabolic activity in most situations. SPECT is more readily available, but techniques are less standardized and resolution of images is less exact than PET (see Chapter 12).

Although overall oxygen utilization decreases proportionally with the severity of dementia, PET studies have failed to show areas of chronic ischemia in dementia; that is, reduced tracer uptake is caused by decreased neuronal activity rather than substrate insufficiency or gross limitation of CBF. Areas of decreased CBF correlate with previous ischemic insults. For example, PET and SPECT both reveal multiple defects in cases of multiple strokes. Case reports suggest that PET and SPECT can reveal 1) clinically important vascular lesions not visible on CT or MRI and 2) findings suggestive of "incomplete cerebral infarction" referred to by Lassen (1982). Full definition of the role of functional neuroimaging awaits carefully designed studies, however.

Neuropsychology

Delineation of focal or "patchy" deficits supports the diagnosis of vascular dementia, but the definitive neuropsychological profile to distinguish vascular dementia from Alzheimer's disease remains elusive (Liston and La Rue 1983a). For example, Fuld (1984) developed a Wechsler Adult Intelligence Scale profile to distinguish Alzheimer's disease from normal aging, but it does not discriminate Alzheimer's disease from vascular dementia reliably (Brinkman et al. 1986). Gainotti et al. (1989) found differences in the overall pattern of memory impairment: Alzheimer's disease patients had an absent primacy effect compared with vascular dementia patients. On the Halstead-Reitan Neuropsychological Test Battery (Reitan 1979), vascular dementia patients tend to have earlier impairment of motor function in relation to cognitive deficits compared with Alzheimer's disease patients (Barth and Macciocchi 1986; Storrie and Doerr 1981).

Defining a "signature" neuropsychological profile for Alzheimer's disease has been difficult; therefore, it may be optimistic to expect a definitive profile for vascular dementia, which is pathologically diverse. Observations made in other patient groups may be relevant to vascular dementia. Delaney et al. (1980) and Russell and Polakoff (1993) found that patients had significant deficits persisting after a "transient" ischemic attack. Sotaniemi et al. (1981) found impaired Stroop performance preoperatively predictive of postcardiac surgery impairments in neuropsychological performance. Correlations with functional neuroimaging can be expected to provide clarification of these important issues.

Rating Scales

The 13-item ischemia scale in Table 15–2 was derived from observations by Slater and Roth (1963) of clinical features more common in patients with vascular dementia than in those with degenerative disease. Originally validated against clinical diagnosis and brain scans (Hachinski et al. 1975), the ischemia scale remains the most frequently used rating scale for vascular dementia.

Numerous criticisms and amendments have been offered for the ischemia scale. For example, Rosen et al. (1980) found support for only 8 of the 13 ischemia scale items in a study with pathological correlation using only a small number of subjects. Loeb and Gandolfo (1983) proposed using four ischemia scale items plus CT evidence of stroke; their sample was larger, but validation was by clinical evaluation rather than

Table 15–2. Ischemia scale

Feature	Point value
Abrupt onset[a]	2
Stepwise deterioration[a]	1
Fluctuating course	2
Nocturnal confusion	1
Relative preservation of personality	1
Depression	1
Somatic complaints[a]	1
Emotional incontinence[a]	1
History or presence of hypertension[a]	1
History of strokes[a]	2
Evidence of associated atherosclerosis	1
Focal neurological symptoms[a]	2
Focal neurological signs[a]	2

Note. Total scores of 4 or less are considered consistent with a degenerative process such as Alzheimer's disease; scores of 7 or greater are found in patients with cerebrovascular insult, who are often presumed to have vascular dementia (Hachinski et al. 1975).
[a]Items supported by Rosen et al. 1980.

autopsy. Small (1985) suggested further grading the severity of ischemia scale features and weighting observer confidence. Other criticisms of the ischemia scale include the omission of risk factors for cerebrovascular disease other than hypertension and atherosclerosis and arbitrary weighting of items. Although the ischemia scale cannot be regarded as definitive for identifying vascular dementia, its use may improve the clinician's diagnostic sensitivity pending more detailed study.

Diagnostic Criteria

The DSM-IV criteria for vascular dementia (American Psychiatric Association 1994) are listed in Table 15–3. These criteria consist of the definition of dementia and an assessment of vascular etiology, leaving substantial discretion to the clinician. Criteria for dementia may present some difficulty because of the variability of cerebrovascular disease. For example, memory impairment (criterion A1) is not as uniform in vascular dementia as in Alzheimer's disease; for example, patients with Balint's syndrome or an aphasia do not have true amnestic deficits. An alternative diagnosis (such as Cognitive Disorder Not Otherwise Specified—294.9) creates a distinction based on a difference of uncertain significance.

Table 15–3.   DSM-IV diagnostic criteria for vascular dementia

A.   The development of multiple cognitive deficits manifested by both
    (1)   memory impairment (impaired ability to learn new information or to
        recall previously learned information)
    (2)   one or more of the following cognitive disturbances:
        (a)   aphasia (language disturbance)
        (b)   apraxia (impaired ability to carry out motor activities despite
            intact motor function)
        (c)   agnosia (failure to recognize or identify objects despite intact
            sensory function)
        (d)   disturbance in executive functioning (i.e., planning, organizing,
            sequencing, abstracting)
B.   The cognitive deficits in criteria A1 and A2 each cause significant
    impairment in social or occupational functioning and represent a
    significant decline from a previous level of functioning.
C.   Focal neurological signs and symptoms (e.g., exaggeration of deep tendon
    reflexes, extensor plantar response, pseudobulbar palsy, gait abnormalities,
    weakness of an extremity) or laboratory evidence indicative of
    cerebrovascular disease (e.g., multiple infarctions involving cortex and
    underlying white matter) that are judged to be etiologically related to the
    disturbance.
D.   The deficits do not occur exclusively during the course of a delirium.

Code based on predominant features:
    290.41   with delirium
    290.42   with delusions
    290.43   with depressed mood
    290.40   uncomplicated
    Specify if (can be applied to any of the above subtypes):
    With behavioral disturbance
Coding note: Also code cerebrovascular condition on Axis III.

Source.   Reprinted from DSM-IV. Used with permission.

    Criterion C specifies the basis for classifying the dementia as vascular. Diagnosis of multi-infarct dementia in DSM-III-R required stepwise course, "patchy" deficits, focal neurological signs and symptoms, and evidence of significant and related cerebrovascular disease. DSM-IV criteria accept vascular dementia with slowly and relentlessly progressive course but leave significant room for clinician judgment about the relationship of cerebrovascular disease to the dementia. No specific guidelines are given for neuroimaging or for neuropsychology. Consequently, clinicians wanting to evaluate future studies of vascular dementia must continue to attend to the details of case selection to assess the comparability of samples.

Other diagnostic systems have emerged in the absence of criteria supported by careful clinical/pathological studies (Liston and La Rue 1983a, 1983b). Renewed interest in vascular dementia has led to reconsideration of diagnosis (Chui et al. 1992; Loeb 1988). Research based on recent consensus criteria (Roman et al. 1993) that use probable, possible, and definite to grade certainty of diagnosis can be expected to yield progress in delimiting the proper role of clinical, laboratory, imaging, and pathological studies in vascular dementia.

Etiology and Pathogenesis

With multiple mechanisms of cerebrovascular injury resulting in heterogeneous pathological findings, vascular dementia is paradigmatic for a "final common pathway" syndrome. Classification may be based on mechanisms of cerebrovascular injury, on anatomic site of brain injury, or on mixed clinical/pathological findings (reviewed in Garcia and Brown 1992). Brun et al. (1992) found that the overwhelming majority of vascular dementia cases fell into several discrete pathological syndromes; these classifications (Table 15–4) from the Lund Longitudinal Dementia Study will be used as the basis for this discussion.

Multiple cerebral infarctions was the most common cause of vascular dementia in the Lund study, accounting for one-third of vascular dementia cases. Tomlinson et al. (1970) described a volumetric effect of infarction: dementia was common with a volume of infarcted tissue greater than 50 ml and was expected with a volume greater than 100 ml. In the Lund series, infarcts affected cerebral cortex more than white matter. These strokes most commonly were related to large arteries, especially the middle cerebrals; thrombosis was the most common stroke mechanism followed (more rarely) by embolism and hemorrhage. A zone of incomplete infarction attributed to a penumbra of ischemia surrounding the infarct was also common.

The relationship between the amount of tissue destruction and dementia can be oversimplified, however. On the one hand, dementia follows stroke in only 1%–7% of patients (Kotila et al. 1986), supporting Drachman's (1993) caution against considering dementia a result of simply adding stroke deficits. On the other hand are the unfortunate patients in whom a small amount of tissue loss results in grievous functional loss

Table 15–4.   Pathological classification of vascular dementia

---

   I.   Multi-infarct dementia
       A.   Large cortical infarctions
       B.   Diffuse microcortical infarcts
       C.   Strategic infarct dementia
  II.   Subcortical ischemic lesions
       A.   Multiple lacunes
       B.   Binswanger's disease
 III.   Posthypoperfusion injury
 IV.   Other
       A.   Venous thrombosis
       B.   Posthemorrhagic dementia
       C.   Diffuse small vessel disease
           (1) Vasculitis
           (2) Multiple small vessel thromboses

---

and dementia because of strategic location. This loss most often affects either the thalamus or angular gyrus, usually bilaterally.

The second most common pathology in the Lund series was subcortical disease, characterized by the presence of multiple lacunae and/or progressive white-matter encephalopathy. Lacunar state is defined by the presence of multiple small (0.5- to 15-mm diameter) infarcts. These typically are found in the basal ganglia, thalamus, pons, and cerebral white matter in association with penetrating branches of large arteries damaged by hypertensive arteriosclerosis. Tomlinson et al. (1970) and Fisher (1982) discount the contribution of lacunae to dementia, but other studies (Ishii et al. 1986; Munoz 1991; Sourander and Walinder 1987) support this connection.

Binswanger's disease refers to degeneration of cerebral white matter characterized by demyelination, axonal loss, and gliosis. Binswanger's disease occurred alone in 14% of the Lund sample and accompanied other lesions in additional patients. Brain imaging studies, especially MRI, have revived interest in Binswanger's disease, which was largely neglected following Binswanger's original 1894 description (Roman 1987). Chronic hypertension and episodic hypoperfusion and hypoxic episodes have been implicated in the pathogenesis of Binswanger's disease, but the role of each remains unclear. Dementia in Binswanger's disease may develop in a progressive or stepwise course and there may be concomitant lacunar and/or cortical stroke.

Cerebral hypoperfusion from low cardiac output and/or hypotension of multiple etiologies can result in posthypoperfusion dementia with or without borderzone infarction. Hypoxia may accompany many of these episodes; the relative contribution of each factor cannot be delineated at this time. Posthypoperfusion dementia was found alone in 6% of the Lund cases and was an additional finding in other vascular dementia and Alzheimer's disease cases. Older persons in general, and especially those with other pre-existing vascular disease, may be at increased risk for posthypoperfusion injury.

Care and Treatment

Pending the ability to reverse neuronal injury, treatment for vascular dementia must be discussed in terms of the general management of dementia, medical care issues, and accompanying psychiatric syndromes. The geriatric psychiatrist may serve as consultant to another clinician or treatment team and often is in a crucial position to coordinate overall management, particularly when behavioral issues predominate.

Care and Management

Recommendations are most effective when they derive from the specifics of the patient's situation. A comprehensive evaluation should address basic needs and capacities such as gait stability, hygiene, and nutrition. Safety considerations include the potential for wandering, household security, managing appliances, use of drugs and alcohol, smoking, driving, and access to weapons. Referral for advice on legal and financial matters may be indicated. Cultural and individual values must be weighed to balance dignity, autonomy, safety, and supervision. Caring for dementia patients can be stressful and may provide the potential for physical and/or emotional abuse of the patient. Emotional and practical support for the caregiver may be vital. Ascertaining the patient's values in terms of intensity of care may alleviate later decision-making difficulties for the caregivers; physician assessment of condition and prognosis facilitates realistic discussion of advanced directives.

The optimal treatment setting depends on community options, family resources, and the patient's condition. Mild dementia usually is compatible with remaining at home; moderate dementia requires closer supervision and community programs such as adult day care; severe dementia mandates full-time, often institutional, care (Read 1990). Referral to social service, home health, or community agencies may be necessary depending on family resources. Referral to the local chapter of the Alzheimer's Association or to stroke support programs may be helpful.

Many dementia patients benefit from structured group settings, and institutions provide care that is increasingly cost effective as severity increases (Weinberger et al. 1993). Respite for caregivers (in-home by family, neighbors, or paid caregivers, or in a skilled nursing facility or board-and-care facility) may delay the permanent transition to institutional care and may ease the decision when it becomes inevitable. Straightforward discussion of these issues can alleviate guilt on the part of caregivers who may dread this eventuality.

Medical Management

Axis III disorders in the vascular dementia patient can be expected to include at least some risk factors (Table 15–1) or etiologic elements (Table 15–4). Other medical disorders, such as renal impairment, often will be present and will affect overall management. Meyer et al. (1986) reported limited improvement with attention to risk factors in vascular dementia patients: cognition was optimal in hypertensive patients if systolic blood pressure was maintained between 135 mm Hg and 150 mm Hg, and cessation of smoking benefited nonhypertensive patients. Medications for other somatic disorders may have less predictable effects in the vascular dementia patient compared with elderly or younger dementia patients.

Prevention of vascular dementia, or at least a reduction in incidence, may be attainable if appropriate attention is paid to cardiovascular disease before overt cerebral insult. The apparently reduced prevalence of vascular dementia in the past 20 years may be a result of the reduced incidence of stroke. Careful attention to cerebral function in studies of cardiovascular therapeutics (in patients considering pacemakers or carotid endarterectomy, for instance) would help guide future treatment recommendations.

Psychiatric Management

Problems such as paranoia, suspicion, hostility, anxiety, depression, and abnormal activity cause the most severe burden among dementia caregivers (Rabins et al. 1982). Attention to psychiatric diagnosis and treatment, therefore, has the potential to improve the quality of life for the disturbed patient and to alleviate caregiver distress. These problems affect the patient's adaptability to programs such as adult day care. These complications are formally recognized in the fifth digit of the diagnostic code; the expanded options offered in DSM-IV are listed in Table 15–3. (If more than one abnormality is present, the dominant one should be coded.)

Inattention and confusion are the hallmarks of delirium. The vascular dementia patient, known to have cardiovascular disease and most likely taking several medications, especially is prone to delirium. Caregivers familiar with the patient and those trained in mental status monitoring are more likely to report acute mental status changes accurately. Management is confounded by the fact that many psychotropic medications may cause confusion directly or through effects on the cardiovascular system (Greenberg 1989; Signer and Read 1989).

Delusions and hallucinations are coded separately, although they often co-exist. Paranoia is common, and the quality of delusions varies from vague, shifting references to elaborate, florid constructions; complex delusions are more characteristic of vascular dementia than Alzheimer's disease (Cummings 1985). Hallucinations are most commonly visual and may underlie delusions. For example, belief in a phantom boarder may derive from hallucinations or from failure to recognize one's own mirror image. Improving lighting or removing provocatively patterned materials may reduce visual misperception. Reassurance may be appropriate and medication avoidable if there is no sense of threat and no fear, anger, or other affective component. Neuroleptics are most likely to be beneficial in more severe cases. Inpatient psychiatric care may be required if a serious threat is present; institutionalization may be required if psychosis disrupts home living.

Mood disorders in vascular dementia may adversely affect cognitive and social function. Clinically, depression has been considered more characteristic of vascular dementia than of Alzheimer's disease, but confirmation has not been consistent. Wragg and Jeste (1989) report incidences of depression complicating dementia of between 10% and 80% in different series; at least part of this wide variation is attributable to problem biases, such as referral biases, and differing diagnostic criteria. The impairments of awareness and communication of the vascular dementia patient can cause uncertainty in applying diagnostic criteria for mood disorders, but the series of studies by Robinson's group (Signer and Read 1989) demonstrated strong similarity between poststroke depression and idiopathic major depressive disorder. Treatment studies have focussed on nortriptyline, and rates of response are equivalent to primary major depression (Lipsey et al. 1984). Anecdotal reports support the use of nontricyclic agents with reduced potential for cardiovascular side effects.

Disruptive behavior may not be associated with a well-defined psychiatric syndrome but may require clinical attention. Evaluation may delineate a relationship between the behavior and a particular neuropsychiatric deficit such as aphasia, prosopagnosia, or environmental disorientation; practical management ideas may follow. Evaluation for speech or occupational therapy may be indicated in some patients. Pharmacological interventions have not been evaluated adequately; recommendations are essentially empirical and based, at best, on case reports. The useful addition of subcategory diagnoses of perceptual, behavioral, and communication disturbance in DSM-IV may foster more systematic studies of these common and difficult problems.

Prognosis

Mortality in vascular dementia is increased compared with age- and sex-matched control subjects, although prognostic studies are limited by the same factors as epidemiological studies. Variability in prognosis is expected on the basis of differences in underlying cardiovascular disease and other disease. Two studies reported higher mortality in patients with vascular dementia. Molsa et al. (1986) found a relative mortality ratio of 1.6:1 for vascular disease compared with Alzheimer-type dementia in Finland. Three-year mortality in a community-based study of 85-year-old subjects in Sweden was 23% without dementia, 42.2% with Alzheimer's disease, and 66.7% with vascular dementia (Skoog et al. 1993).

Conclusion

Although cerebrovascular disease is recognized widely as the second most common cause of dementia, few aspects—including fundamental questions concerning validation of clinical, imaging, neuropsychological, and pathological features—remain without controversy. Careful attention to defining case samples more precisely will provide a greater understanding of the true role of cerebrovascular disease in dementia. Study of those at risk for cerebrovascular injury may advance knowledge of the pathogenesis of vascular dementia even as there is reason to hope this potentially preventable disorder will become rare.

References

Absher JR, Benson DF: Disconnection syndromes: an overview of Geschwind's contributions. Neurology 43:862–867, 1993

American Psychiatric Association: Diagnostic and Statistical Manual of Mental Disorders, 3rd Edition, Revised. Washington, DC, American Psychiatric Association, 1987

American Psychiatric Association: Diagnostic and Statistical Manual of Mental Disorders, 4th Edition. Washington, DC, American Psychiatric Association, 1994

Barth JT, Macciocchi SN: Dementia: implications for clinical practice and research, in Handbook of Clinical Neuropsychology, Vol 2. Edited by Filskov SB, Boll TJ. New York, Wiley, 1986, pp 398–425

Boone KB, Miller BL, Lesser IM, et al: Neuropsychological correlates of white-matter lesions in healthy elderly subjects. Arch Neurol 49:549–554, 1992

Brayne C: Clinicopathological studies of the dementias from an epidemiological viewpoint. Br J Psychiatry 162:439–446, 1993

Brinkman SD, Largen JW, Cushman L, et al: Clinical validators: Alzheimer's disease and multi-infarct dementia, in Clinical Memory Assessment of Older Adults. Edited by Poon LW. Washington, DC, American Psychological Association, 1986, pp 307–313

Brown WD, Frackowiak RSJ: Cerebral blood flow and metabolism studies in multi-infarct dementia. Alzheimer Dis Assoc Disord 5:131–143, 1991

Brun A, Gustafson L, Samuelson SM, et al: Neuropathology of late life. Dementia 3:125–130, 1992

Brust JCM: Vascular dementia is overdiagnosed. Arch Neurol 45:799–801, 1988

Bucht G, Adolfsson R, Winblad B: Dementia of the Alzheimer type and multi-infarct dementia: a clinical description and diagnostic problems. J Am Geriatr Soc 32:491–498, 1984

Chui HC: Dementia: a review emphasizing clinicopathologic correlation and brain-behavior relationships. Arch Neurol 46:806–814, 1989

Chui HC, Victoroff JI, Margolin D, et al: Criteria for the diagnosis of ischemic vascular dementia proposed by the State of California Alzheimer's Disease Diagnostic and Treatment Centers. Neurology 42:473–480, 1992

Cummings JL: Organic delusions: phenomenology, anatomical correlations, and review. Br J Psychiatry 146:184–197, 1985

Cummings JL: Frontal-subcortical circuits and human behavior. Arch Neurol 50:873–880, 1993

Delaney RC, Wallace JD, Egelko S: Transient cerebral ischemic attacks and neuropsychological deficit. J Clin Neuropsychol 2:107–114, 1980

Drachman DA: New criteria for the diagnosis of vascular dementia: do we know enough yet? Neurology 43:243–245, 1993

Drayer BP: Imaging of the aging brain, I: normal findings. Radiology 166:785–796, 1988a

Drayer BP: Imaging of the aging brain, II: pathologic conditions. Radiology 166:797–806, 1988b

Fein G, Van Dyke C, Davenport L, et al: Preservation of normal cognitive functioning in elderly subjects with extensive white-matter lesions of long duration. Arch Gen Psychiatry 47:220–223, 1990

Fisher CM: Lacunar strokes and infarcts: a review. Neurology 32:871–876, 1982

Fuld PA: Test profile of cholinergic dysfunction and of Alzheimer-type dementia. J Clin Neuropsychol 6:380–392, 1984

Gainotti G, Monteleone D, Parlato E, et al: Verbal memory disorders in Alzheimer's disease and multi-infarct dementia. J Neurolinguistics 4:327–345, 1989

Garcia JH, Brown GG: Vascular dementia: neuropathologic alterations and metabolic brain changes. J Neurol Sci 109:121–131, 1992

Grant I, Prigatano GP, Heaton RK, et al: Progressive neuropsychologic impairment and hypoxemia. Arch Gen Psychiatry 44:999–1006, 1987

Greenberg R: The patient with cardiovascular disease, in Treatments of Psychiatric Disorders: A Task Force Report of the American Psychiatric Association. Washington, DC, American Psychiatric Association, 1989

Hachinski VC, Iliff LD, Zilhka E, et al: Cerebral blood flow in dementia. Arch Neurol 32:632–637, 1975

Hachinski VC, Potter P, Merskey H: Leuoko-araiosis. Arch Neurol 44:21–23, 1987

Ishii N, Nichihara Y, Imamura T: Why do frontal lobe symptoms predominate in vascular dementia with lacunes? Neurology 36:340–345, 1986

Jorm AF: Cross-national comparisons of the occurrence of Alzheimer's and vascular dementias. Eur Arch Psychiatry Clin Neurosci 240:218–222, 1991

Jorm AF, Korten AE, Henderson AS: The prevalence of dementia: a quantitative integration of the literature. Acta Psychiatr Scand 76:465–479, 1987

Kase CS: Epidemiology of multi-infarct dementia. Alzheimer Dis Assoc Disord 5:71–76, 1991

Kawabata K, Tachibana H, Sugita M, et al: A comparative I-123 IMP SPECT study in Binswanger's disease and Alzheimer's disease. Clin Nucl Med 18:329–336, 1993

Kokmen E, Chandra VJ, Schoenberg BS: Trends in incidence of dementing illness in Rochester, Minnesota, in three quinquennial periods, 1960–1974. Neurology 38:975–980, 1988

Kotila M, Waltimo O, Niemi ML, et al: Dementia after stroke. Eur Neurol 25:134–140, 1986

Lassen NA: Incomplete cerebral infarction. Stroke 13:522–523, 1982

Leuchter AF, Newton TF, Cook IA, et al: Changes in brain functional connectivity in Alzheimer-type and multi-infarct dementia. Brain 115: 1543–1561, 1992

Lipsey JR, Robinson RG, Pearlson GD, et al: Nortriptyline treatment of post-stroke depression: a double-blind study. Lancet 1:297–300,1984

Liston EH, La Rue A: Clinical differentiation of primary degenerative and multi-infarct dementia: a critical review of the evidence, I: clinical studies. Biol Psychiatry 18:1451–1465, 1983a

Liston EH, La Rue A: Clinical differentiation of primary degenerative and multi-infarct dementia: a critical review of the evidence, II: pathological studies. Biol Psychiatry 18:1467–1484, 1983b

Loeb C: Clinical criteria for the diagnosis of vascular dementia. Eur Neurol 28:87–92, 1988

Loeb C, Gandolfo C: Diagnostic evaluation of degenerative and vascular dementia. Stroke 14:399–401, 1983

Meyer JS, Judd BW, Tawaklna T, et al: Improved cognition after control of risk factors for multi-infarct dementia. JAMA 256:2203–2209, 1986

Molsa PK, Marttilla RJ, Rinne UK: Survival and cause of death in Alzheimer's disease and multi-infarct dementia. Acta Neurol Scand 74:103–107, 1986

Munoz DM: The pathological basis of multi-infarct dementia. Alzheimer's Disease and Related Disorders 5:77–90, 1991

Nathan DM: Long-term complications of diabetes mellitus. N Engl J Med 328:1676–1685, 1993

National Institutes of Health Consensus: Development Conference Statement—Differential diagnosis of dementing diseases, Vol 6, No 11. Bethesda, MD, U.S. Department of Health and Human Services, July 6–8, 1987

O'Brien MD: Vascular dementia is underdiagnosed. Arch Neurol 45:797–798, 1988

Perlmuter LC, Hakami MK, Hodgson-Harrington C, et al: Decreased cognitive function in aging non-insulin-dependent diabetic patients. Am J Med 77:1043–1048, 1984

Rabins PV, Mace NL, Lucas MJ: The impact of dementia on the family. JAMA 248:333–335, 1982

Read S: Community resources, in Alzheimer's Disease: Treatment and Long-Term Management. Edited by Cummings JL, Miller BL. New York, Marcel Dekker, 1990, pp 235–244

Reitan RM: Halstead-Reitan Neuropsychological Test Battery. Tucson: Neuropsychology Laboratory, University of Arizona, 1979

Roman GC: Senile dementia of the Binswanger type. JAMA 258:1782–1788, 1987

Roman GC, Tatemichi TK, Erkinjuntti T, et al: Vascular dementia: diagnostic criteria for research studies (Report of the NINDS-AIREN International Workshop). Neurology 43:250–260, 1993

Rosen WG, Terry RD, Fuld PA, et al: Pathological verification of ischemic score in differentiation of dementias. Ann Neurol 7:486–488, 1980

Russell EW, Polakoff D: Neuropsychological test patterns in men for Alzheimer's and multi-infarct dementia. Arch Clin Neuropsychol 8:327–343, 1993

Signer SF, Read SL: The patient with stroke, in Treatments of Psychiatric Disorders: A Task Force Report of the American Psychiatric Association. Washington, DC, American Psychiatric Association, 1989

Simonsen E, Nielson JS, Neilson BL: Sinus node dysfunction in 128 patients: a retrospective study with follow-up. Acta Med Scand 20:8–34, 1980

Skoog I, Nilsson L, Palmertz B, et al: A population-based study of dementia in 85-year-olds. New Engl J Med 328:153–158, 1993

Slater E, Roth M: Clinical Psychiatry, 3rd Edition. Baltimore, MD, Williams & Wilkins, 1963, pp 593–596

Small GW: Revised ischemic score for diagnosing multi-infarct dementia. J Clin Psychiatry 46:514–517, 1985

Sotaniemi KA, Juolasmaa A, Hokkanen ET: Neuropsychologic outcome after open-heart surgery. Arch Neurol 38:2–8, 1981

Sourander P, Walinder J: Hereditary multi-infarct dementia: morphological and clinical studies of a new disease. Acta Neuropathol (London) 39:247–254, 1987

Storrie M, Doerr H: Characterization of Alzheimer type dementia utilizing an abbreviated Halstead-Reitan Battery. Clin Neuropsychol 2:78–82, 1981

Strub RL, Black FW: The Mental Status Examination in Neurology. Philadelphia, PA, FA Davis, 1985

Sultzer DL, Mahler ME, Cummings JL, et al: Cortical abnormalities associated with subcortical lesions in vascular dementia. Arch Neurol 52:773–780, 1995

Tomlinson BE, Blessed G, Roth M: Observations on the brains of demented old people. J Neurol Sci 11:205–242, 1970

Ulbricht TLV, Southgate DAT: Coronary heart disease: seven dietary factors. Lancet 338:985–992, 1991

Weinberger M, Gold DT, Divine GW, et al: Expenditures in caring for patients with dementia who live alone. Am J Public Health 83:338–341, 1993

Wolf PA: Risk factors for stroke. Stroke 16:359–360, 1985

Wolf PA, Dauber TR, Thomas HE, et al: Epidemiologic assessment of chronic atrial fibrillation and risk of stroke: the Framingham study. Neurology 28:973–977, 1978

Wragg RE, Jeste DV: Overview of depression and psychosis in Alzheimer's Disease. Am J Psychiatry 146:577–587, 1989

Ylikoski R, Ylikoski A, Erkinjuntti T, et al: White matter changes in healthy elderly persons with attention and speed of mental processing. Arch Neurol 50:818–824, 1993

Benjamin Liptzin, M.D.

Delirium

Delirium has been recognized as a global disturbance of brain function for several thousand years. It is important for geriatric psychiatrists because it is common (particularly in elderly patients in general hospitals), it is frequently overlooked, it may be associated with high morbidity (e.g., institutionalization) or mortality, and it is often induced inadvertently by treatment. A number of published papers have reviewed the diagnosis, evaluation of associated medical conditions, and clinical management of patients with delirium (Beresin 1988; Lipowski 1983, 1987, 1989; Liston 1982, 1989). Lipowski (1990) provided a comprehensive review of these studies and summarized the published literature on delirium through 1989. Until recently, however, there was little systematic research to clarify the diagnostic criteria, document the epidemiology, identify associated abnormalities in brain function, and document the course and outcomes of patients diagnosed with delirium. In this review, I will describe the current thinking in these areas, as well as in the evaluation and management of patients with delirium.

Diagnosis and Symptomatology

The term *delirium* has become accepted among psychiatrists in the last 10 years as the term to describe transient global cognitive disorders that may occur at any age and that are judged to be caused by an organic etiology (Lipowski 1983). Previously, poorly defined terms such as acute confusional states or acute brain syndromes were used. Until the publication of DSM-III (American Psychiatric Association 1980), little attention was paid to the need for explicit criteria to facilitate communication among psychiatric researchers and clinicians. In a recent review, Liptzin et al. (1993) described some of the controversies regarding the diagnostic criteria in DSM-III and DSM-III-R (American Psychiatric Association 1987) and proposed new criteria for delirium in DSM-IV (American Psychiatric Association 1994) (see Table 16–1).

The new criteria focus on the core features that define the syndrome of delirium. These features are impairment of consciousness with an attentional disturbance; change in cognition (e.g., memory deficit, disorientation, or language disturbance) or a perceptual disturbance (e.g., misinterpretation, illusion, or hallucination) that is not better accounted for by a preexisting, established, or evolving dementia; and a disturbance that develops over a short period and tends to fluctuate over the course of the day. In addition to these core features, delirium is often associated with a disturbance in the sleep-wake cycle, with a reversal in the usual pattern so that the person may sleep during the day and be up all night. The person may at times become agitated or be lethargic. In the DSM-IV criteria, delirium can be subclassified as caused by a general medical condition, to multiple etiologies, or as substance-induced. Although not specifically subclassified in DSM-IV, several subtypes of delirium have been described (Lipowski 1990). The hyperactive form that is usually associated with the image of a delirious patient is characterized by psychomotor

Table 16–1.   DSM-IV diagnostic criteria for delirium due to a general medical condition

---

A.   Disturbance of consciousness (i.e., reduced clarity of awareness of the environment) with reduced ability to focus, sustain, or shift attention.

B.   A change in cognition (such as memory deficit, disorientation, language disturbance) or the development of a perceptual disturbance that is not better accounted for by a preexisting, established, or evolving dementia.

C.   The disturbance develops over a short period of time (usually hours to days) and tends to fluctuate during the course of the day.

D.   There is evidence from the history, physical examination, or laboratory findings that the disturbance is caused by the direct physiological consequences of a general medical condition.

Source.   Reprinted from DSM-IV. Used with permission.

overactivity, hyperalertness, restlessness, excitability, and hyper- vigilance. The patient may have loud or pressured speech. In contrast, the hypoactive patient shows a reduced level of psychomotor activity and alertness, and he or she is generally quiet and listless. Such a patient speaks little and may drift off into sleep even in the course of an interview. These patients formerly were labeled as having acute confusion and frequently were not identified by nursing staff. Liptzin and Levkoff (1992) reported that in elderly hospitalized patients, most patients have symptoms of both subtypes at various times and should be called mixed type. Ross et al. (1991) also described phenomenological subtypes of delirium defined on the basis of alertness. They suggested that the subtypes may have different pathophysiology and thus potentially different treatments.

Epidemiology

The study of the epidemiology of delirium was hampered until recently by the absence of agreed on criteria for diagnosis. Levkoff et al. (1991a) reviewed a variety of screening instruments used to detect the possible presence of delirium. The publication of explicit criteria in DSM-III, however, allowed investigators to operationalize and standardize the case finding methods (Albert et al. 1992; Johnson et al. 1990). Levkoff et al. (1991a) reviewed studies published through 1990 and concluded that in medical inpatients the prevalence of delirium defined by DSM-III criteria ranges from 11% to 16% and the incidence ranges from 4% to 10%. Similarly, recent studies of postoperative delirium using DSM-III criteria report a rate of 28%–44% in elderly patients with a hip fracture, 26% in patients undergoing elective joint replacement, and 6.8% in a somewhat younger group undergoing myocardial revascularization (Levkoff et al. 1991a). Using DSM-III criteria and a standardized Delirium Symptom Interview, Liptzin et al. (1991) studied a large group of elderly patients admitted to a general hospital and found that 38.5% met criteria for delirium. Levkoff et al. (1991a) showed that the rate was quite different for patients admitted from a long-term care facility (64.9%) compared with patients admitted from the community (24.2%). A more recent study of elderly patients admitted with acute illness to a geriatric unit found that 22% met DSM-III-R criteria for delirium (Jitapunkul et al. 1992).

All the above studies were done with hospitalized populations, in part because patients sick enough to develop delirium usually require hospitalization. However, in a community survey, the prevalence of delirium in persons over 55 was estimated to be 1.1% (Folstein et al. 1991).

Risk Factors

The major risk factors for developing delirium appear to be pre-existing cognitive impairment, advanced age, and severity of comorbid medical illness. In the past 10 years, epidemiological studies have attempted to identify more specific risk factors for the development of delirium though not all have used DSM-III criteria or standardized case-finding techniques.

Trzepacz et al. (1985) analyzed 133 cases or organic mental disorders from a total of 771 patients referred for psychiatric consultation from a general hospital. They concluded that there was a trend toward an increasing incidence of delirium as the number of medical diagnoses or etiological factors increased. Etiological factors most commonly associated with delirium were the general categories of drugs (48%), metabolic disorders (30%), specific neurological disorders (20%), infections (17%), and hypoxia (14%). In this selected sample, the group of elderly patients referred did not have a greater representation of delirium than the younger group despite being twice as likely to have dementia. The delirious elderly patients had more medical problems than the younger group and were more likely to have pulmonary, renal, endocrine, or cardiovascular illnesses. Younger delirious patients were more likely to have alcohol intoxication or withdrawal.

Levkoff et al. (1988) analyzed the factors associated with a discharge diagnosis of delirium among 1,285 patients admitted to a large teaching hospital. Although chart diagnoses are clearly an underestimate of the true prevalence of delirium, the study using multivariate analyses identified four factors that distinguished 80% of all cases of delirium: 1) a urinary tract infection at any time during the hospital stay; 2) no urinary tract infection, but low serum albumin on admission; 3) neither urinary tract infection nor lower serum albumin but elevated white blood cell count on admission; or 4) none of these risk factors but proteinuria on admission.

Foreman (1989) studied 71 nonsurgical patients over age 60 and found that 27 developed "confusion" during hospitalization. In this study, confused patients were either hypernatremic, hypokalemic, hyperglycemic, hypotensive, had elevated creatinine and blood urea nitrogen (BUN), or received more medications. Rockwood (1989) studied 80 elderly patients admitted to a general medical service. He found that confused patients tended to be older, more ill, and more likely to have chronic cognitive impairment. Trzepacz et al. (1989a) reported on 247 liver transplantation candidates. They found that, although both delirious and nondelirious subjects had high levels of overall stress, those with delirium had significantly poorer adaptive functioning and lower occupational, family, and social scale ratings. Bowman (1992) studied the relationships among anxiety, the unexpected nature of an unplanned surgical event, and the development of postoperative delirium. She found that subjects responded with greater anxiety and a higher incidence of delirium when surgery was unexpected than when it was planned.

Francis et al. (1990) studied 229 elderly patients and found that abnormal sodium levels, illness severity, dementia, fever or hypothermia, psychoactive drug use (defined as narcotic analgesics, sedative-hypnotics, and minor tranquilizers), and azotemia were associated with an increased risk of delirium. Patients with three or more risk factors had a 60% rate of delirium. Schor et al. (1992) used multivariate techniques to determine risk factors for delirium in 325 elderly hospitalized patients. The independent risk factors for in-hospital delirium included prior cognitive impairment, age over 80 years, fracture on admission, symptomatic infection, and being male. Among medication groups, only neuroleptic use and narcotic use were independently associated with delirium; anticholinergic drug use was not associated with delirium. Using data from this same study, Levkoff et al. (1992) reported that preexisting cognitive impairment and advanced age were associated with increased risk of developing delirium in patients admitted from the community (but not from an institution). Patients admitted from an institution were more likely to experience delirium than those from the community. Jitapunkul et al. (1992) studied 184 patients admitted with acute illness to a geriatric medical unit. The conditions most commonly associated with DSM-III-R delirium were infection and stroke. Onset of acute illness of less than 15 days, a reported history of dementia or recent confusion, and presence of a definite site of infection were more likely in patients with delirium. Delirious patients had more serious preexisting diseases than nondelirious patients and a higher number of admissions during the 2 years prior to the index admission.

Course and Outcomes

Delirium generally presents on admission or early in a hospitalization. Levkoff et al. (1994) report that almost half the patients who develop delirium in the hospital meet criteria by the third day of hospitalization. Many patients experience a prodromal period with some symptoms of delirium prior to the onset of the full syndrome. Of all patients who met DSM-III criteria for delirium, 50% met them the same day that they experienced a new onset of any one individual symptom and 86% met criteria within two days of the appearance of their first new symptom (Levkoff et al. 1992). Bowman (1992) in a study of surgical patients noted that the greatest incidence of delirium occurred on the third postoperative day.

Other studies have looked at the acute and long-term outcomes in patients with delirium. Rabins and Folstein (1982) reported that medically ill delirious patients had higher fatality rates than dementia, cognitively intact, or depressed patients. Thomas et al. (1988) studied 133 hospitalized patients and found that the mean length of hospitalization was significantly longer in delirious compared with nondelirious patients. The mortality rate was also much higher in the delirious patients. Similarly, Francis et al. (1990) found that delirious patients stayed in the hospital longer, and were more likely to die or be institutionalized than patients who did not develop delirium. Six months after discharge, illness severity predicted mortality but delirium was not an independent risk factor. At 2-year follow-up, cases of delirium had a higher mortality rate and loss of independent community living (Francis et al. 1992). Patients with "quiet" presentations of acute confusion who often were not recognized by physicians as having delirium also had a poor prognosis.

Levkoff et al. (1992) reported that delirium was not associated with an increased risk of mortality in 6 months of follow-up when age, sex, preexisting cognitive impairment, and illness severity were controlled for. Delirium was associated with a prolonged hospital stay and an increased risk of institutional placement among community-dwelling elderly people. During the hospital stay, only 4% of delirious patients experienced resolution of all new symptoms of delirium before hospital discharge and only 20.8% and 17.7%, respectively, had resolution of all new symptoms by 3 and 6 months after hospital discharge. These data suggested that delirium may not be as acute or transient as previously believed.

Etiologies

Case reports of delirium and systematic studies suggest that it can be caused by almost any serious medical illness or drug intoxication in a vulnerable individual (Table 16–2). These possible etiologies should be considered in the evaluation of delirious patients (see "Evaluation" section in this chapter). The search for etiologies is essential so that the underlying illness can be treated. However, in many cases, there is no single cause.

Table 16–2. Causes of delirium

Drug intoxication
> Psychotropic drugs: Antidepressants, sedative-hypnotics, anxiolytics, neuroleptics, lithium
> Other prescribed medications: Cardiac: digitalis, antiarrhythmics, antihypertensives; GI: cimetidine, ranitidine; anti-inflammatory agents; narcotic analgesics
> Over-the-counter drugs: Alcohol, antihistamines/anticholinergics

Drug withdrawal
> Alcohol, sedative-hypnotics/anxiolytics

Metabolic disorders
> Hypoxia, hypoglycemia and hyperglycemia, electrolyte imbalance, acid-base imbalance, kidney failure, hepatic failure, anemia, vitamin deficiencies, endocrinopathies

Cardiovascular disorders
> Congestive heart failure, myocardial infarction, cardiac arrhythmia, shock

CNS disorders
> Head trauma, seizures, cerebrovascular diseases, infections, space-occupying lesions (tumor, subdural hematoma, abscess)

Infections

Sleep deprivation

Postoperative states

Koponen et al. (1989a) studied 70 elderly patients who met DSM-III criteria for delirium and found the most common etiologies were stroke, infections, and metabolic disorders. A clear organic triggering factor could be found for 87% of the patients. Francis et al. (1990) reported the most common etiologies of delirium as fluid and electrolyte disturbances, infection, drug toxicity, metabolic disturbances, and sensory or environmental disturbances. Drugs associated with delirium included narcotics, benzodiazepines, anticholinergic medications, methyldopa, and nonsteroidal anti-inflammatory agents. An intracerebral process was implicated in only two cases. Alcohol or sedative drug withdrawal was a possible cause for comorbid condition in five cases. In only 36% of the cases could a single definite etiology be established. In another 20%, a single medical condition was believed to be a probable cause of delirium. For the remainder of the patients, multiple possible etiologies were assigned.

Jitapunkul et al. (1992) reported that stroke was the major associated condition in their population. They noted, however, that this association may be explained by the tendency in the United Kingdom to admit elderly stroke patients to geriatric rather than medical or neurological wards. In any study, therefore, the associations found are highly dependent on the kind of patients admitted to the particular unit. Thus, hip fracture is more likely to be associated with delirium in an orthopedic ward than in a general medical ward.

Pathogenesis

In studying the underlying brain mechanisms that may be related to the development of delirium, one hypothesis is that delirium results from altered cholinergic states in the brain (Blass and Plum 1983). For many years it has been known that anticholinergic drugs could cause delirium. This phenomenon was systematically studied by Itil and Fink (1966) using an experimental situation. Tune and Bylsma (1991) reported significant correlations between elevated serum concentrations of anticholinergic medications measured by a radioreceptor assay and the development of cognitive impairment, including delirium. In summarizing other studies, they point out that elderly patients are particularly vulnerable to the effects of these medications because of age-related declines in cholinergic neurotransmission. Koponen et al. (1991) measured acetylcholinesterase in cerebrospinal fluid and did not find that this cholinergic marker was reduced in delirious patients compared with control subjects. However, they suggested that more elaborate methods are needed to separate striatal from cortical activity. Trzepacz et al. (1992) described an animal model for delirium using rats treated with atropine. They reported that electroencephalogram (EEG) changes, as well as difficulty with attention and memory, sleepwake cycle reversal, and changes in behavior (lack of focused direction, irritability, fluctuating levels of activity, and excessive random sniffing), appeared consistent with signs and symptoms seen in human delirium.

Other neurotransmitters that have been studied include somatostatin and β-endorphin. Koponen et al. (1989c) reported that delirious patients showed significant reductions of cerebrospinal fluid somatostatinlike immunoreactivity compared with control subjects. At 1-year follow-up, there was a further reduction in these levels and significant correlations with Mini-Mental State Exam (MMSE) scores (Koponen et al. 1990). The same group found that cerebrospinal fluid β-endorphin-like immunoreactivity was significantly lower in the delirious patient group than in control subjects while in the hospital (Koponen et al. 1989d) and at 1-year follow-up

(Koponen and Riekkinen 1990). This measure did not correlate with age or neuroleptic drug dosage but did correlate with MMSE scores. Ross (1991) reviewed the role of various neurotransmitters in delirium and hypothesized that the cholinergic, GABAergic, histaminergic, and serotonergic systems may be important in different aspects of delirium.

The EEG has been used to study abnormal brain function in delirious patients for many years. (For further information on the use of EEGs see Chapter 13.) Romano and Engel (1944) found that decreased background EEG frequency and disorganization of the EEG correlated with reduced arousal. Brenner (1991) reviewed the usefulness of EEGs in the evaluation of delirium. He noted that, in most patients with delirium, the EEGs will show diffuse slowing and the degree of the EEG changes correlates with the severity of the encephalopathy. Leuchter et al. (1993) suggest that the EEG is a moderately sensitive but nonspecific indicator of brain dysfunction in elderly people. Leuchter and Jacobson (1991) suggested that quantitative EEG is a clinically useful supplement to the conventional EEG for the assessment of elderly patients with delirium. Using more sophisticated computerized spectral analysis of the EEG, Trzepacz et al. (1989b) found that mean peak activity was lower in delirious than in nondelirious patients with chronic liver disease. Koponen et al. (1989b), using quantitative EEG techniques, found that reductions in the proportion of α activity and in mean frequency were associated with declining cognitive function as measured by the MMSE (Folstein et al. 1975) and that increases in the proportion of δ activity were associated with increased length of delirium and hospital stay. They also observed that delirious patients with coexisting dementia consistently showed the most abnormal EEGs. Jacobson et al. (1993) used quantitative EEG techniques to assist in the differential diagnosis of encephalopathy in elderly subjects with delirium, dementia, and delirium with dementia. The variables that were most useful in distinguishing delirium from dementia were amount of θ activity, relative power in the δ frequency band, and the brain map of absolute power with the scale maximum of 103 μV^2. The θ alone was able to classify nearly 89% of cases correctly with only 6% of delirium cases misclassified as dementia.

Another approach to the study of delirium involves brain imaging techniques to try to localize areas of brain damage. (For further information on neuroimaging see Chapter 12.) Figiel and collaborators, using magnetic resonance imaging (MRI) or computed tomography (CT) scans, have identified lesions of the basal ganglia in patients who develop delirium during antidepressant drug treatment (Figiel et al. 1989). The same group identified abnormalities of the basal ganglia and moderate-to-severe subcortical white-matter lesions in patients who developed delirium during a course of electroconvulsive therapy (Figiel et al. 1990a, 1990b). They also cited other published reports of agitated delirium following acute cerebral infarctions that involve the basal ganglia and subcortical white matter (Caplan et al. 1988; Mori and Yamaddri 1987). They suggest that lesions in these areas may predispose patients to the development of delirium. Koponen et al. (1989a) did CT scans on patients with delirium. Patients differed from control subjects significantly in ventricular dilation and cortical atrophy. Focal changes were also more common in the delirious patients, and these changes tended to concentrate in the high-order association areas of the right hemisphere. They suggested that structural brain disease plays a marked predisposing role in the development of delirium in elderly patients.

Differential Diagnosis

The most common differential diagnostic question when evaluating a patient with delirium is whether the person has dementia rather than delirium, from delirium alone, or from dementia and delirium. Memory impairment or disorientation can be seen in both delirium and dementia, but the person with dementia is usually alert, whereas the patient with delirium will have fluctuating alertness. In the presence of symptoms of delirium, it is essential to have information from family members, caretakers, or medical records to determine if symptoms of dementia were preexisting. Even if a person has a clear history of dementia, an acute change in mental status accompanied by the full-blown syndrome of delirium can be diagnosed and in this case both diagnoses should be given. If the prior history is unclear, it is best to make a provisional diagnosis of delirium. Doing so will lead to a more active diagnostic and therapeutic approach to the patient.

Delirium characterized by delusions, disordered thinking, and agitation must be distinguished from schizophrenia, schizophreniform disorder, or mania. The symptoms of mania overlap with those of delirium and sometimes occur secondary to a general medical condition (Krauthammer and Klerman 1978). In delirium, the symptoms tend to fluctuate over the course of the day, and delusions are fragmented and unsystematized in contrast to schizophrenia or mania. It is also unusual for schizophrenia to appear in late life for the first time. Mania may appear in late life, but there are usually antecedent depressions. In delirium there is also usually impairment in orientation or memory in contrast to the other disorders. The EEG is also more likely to be abnormal in delirium than in the other disorders.

Some patients may have some but not all symptoms of delirium. Such subsyndromal presentations need to be carefully assessed because they may be harbingers of a full-blown delirium and may signal an underlying medical disorder.

Evaluation

The patient suspected of having delirium must be carefully observed and examined. A careful mental status examination is essential. (See Chapter 8 for more detail on the mental status examination.) If patients are not asked specific mental status questions, one may miss patients who have had a change in mental status and are not sure where they are or why they are in a hospital. In addition to formal tests of orientation, memory, and attention, the patient should be observed for behavioral symptoms of delirium. These include restlessness, suspiciousness, somnolence, hyperalertness, unstable mood, belligerence, or distractibility. Because patients fluctuate, it is not unusual for a patient to seem pleasant and cooperative on rounds in the morning but agitated and disoriented at night. Even if a patient seems completely intact, it is important to review any notes written in the medical record over the past 48 hours and ask the nursing staff on the unit about abnormal behavior. Any abnormalities in cognition, perception, or behavior should be checked with family members, caretakers, or previous medical records to determine if they were present before the acute illness that led to the hospitalization.

Delirium is caused by many different disorders, and these disorders need to be systematically investigated through history taking, physical examination, and laboratory evaluation. Prescription and nonprescription medications (including alcohol) can lead to delirium in an older person who has reduced metabolism of the drug or increased sensitivity to its effects because of age or drug-disease or drug-drug interactions. If there is no obvious medication causing the delirium, it is necessary to carefully evaluate each organ system. Often, multiple abnormalities will be uncovered; it will not be clear which one is the specific cause of the delirium. In addition to a standard laboratory assessment that includes a complete blood count, chemistry profile, and urinalysis, the clinical history may suggest a possible infection and other sources sought. An electrocardiogram (ECG) may be important if a cardiac etiology is suspected. If a central nervous system disorder is suspected, an EEG, CT or MRI scan, and a lumbar puncture should be considered. As discussed above, the EEG, particularly with newer quantitative techniques, may be a useful adjunct though the diagnosis is generally made on clinical grounds. Obrecht et al. (1979) suggested that the EEG was a helpful investigation in patients with an acute confusional state, particularly in identifying patients with intracranial pathology. Similarly, Roberts and Caird (1990) suggested that CT scans can identify potentially treatable lesions such as brain tumors or subdural hematomas in a significant number of patients with a recent onset of confusion.

Treatment

The most important treatment for patients who are recognized as having delirium is to discover the underlying medical cause and reverse the abnormality if possible. Until the patient's medical condition stabilizes, however, the patient will generally need to be observed in a safe environment, usually a hospital. Whatever the underlying etiology, general supportive measures can be helpful. Considerable attention has been paid to nursing interventions in general medical patients (Morency 1990), postoperative patients (Neelon 1990), cancer patients (Rando 1990), and hip fracture patients (Brannstrom et al. 1989; Williams et al. 1985). The patient should be kept in a quiet room with lights on in the daytime and a night light after bedtime. Stimulation should not be excessive, but some gentle music or a television program may be soothing. Orientation cues such as a calendar or a clock should be visible. Sensory impairments should be corrected with eyeglasses or a hearing aid. Family members should be encouraged to spend time with the patient for reassurance and orientation. Staff interventions should be carefully explained in a firm but caring manner. Physical restraints should be used only if the patient is unsupervised and at risk of falling or pulling out intravenous lines, urinary catheters, or other tubes.

In the quiet, confused patient, the above interventions along with careful monitoring may be sufficient to support the patient until the delirium clears. The highly agitated or psychotic patient may need pharmacological intervention, and often a psychiatric consultation is requested (Liptzin 1991). In a delirium resulting from withdrawal from alcohol or other central nervous system depressants such as sedative-hypnotic drugs, a standard approach to detoxification should be used. Generally, this involves the use of a benzodiazepine such as chlordiazepoxide. In other agitated patients, a short-acting benzodiazepine such as lorazepam 0.25 mg to 2 mg, depending on the patient's size or frailty, can be given every 4 hours if needed up to a maximum of 8 mg per day. The use of benzodiazepines is controversial because too high a dose can increase confusion and daytime somnolence and some patients may have paradoxical agitation even on low doses. In psychotic patients or if the above-mentioned medications do not provide the needed control, a neuroleptic drug can be used. The butyrophenones are generally preferable to low-potency sedating phenothiazines (chlorpromazine or thioridazine) because the latter have strong anticholinergic effects that can aggravate the delirium. Haloperidol 0.5 mg to 5 mg can be given orally or intramuscularly every 4 hours up to a maximum of 20 mg per day and titrated to the patient's response and tolerance. The patient needs to be carefully observed for extrapyramidal side effects and the dose reduced if necessary. The intravenous use of haloperidol has been reported by Moulaert (1989) and Gelfand et al. (1992), who stated that intravenous haloperidol is the treatment of choice for patients suffering from delirium.

Summary

Delirium is a common condition in general hospital psychiatry but is often missed by other medical specialists or nurses. It can be associated with high morbidity and mortality. Symptoms usually are transient but can persist for months in some patients. Prior cognitive impairment is the major risk factor but severity of medical illness and number of medications also can contribute. Almost any general medical condition can cause delirium. Therefore, the history should be comprehensive and a thorough medical work-up carried out. Supportive nursing care is essential. In highly agitated patients, sedation with a short-acting benzodiazepine or neuroleptic may be necessary.

References

Albert MS, Levkoff SE, Reilly CH, et al: The Delirium Symptom Interview: an interview for the detection of delirium in hospitalized patients. J Geriatr Psychiatry Neurol 5:14–21, 1992

American Psychiatric Association: Diagnostic and Statistical Manual of Mental Disorders, 3rd Edition. Washington, DC, American Psychiatric Association, 1980

American Psychiatric Association: Diagnostic and Statistical Manual of Mental Disorders, 3rd Edition, Revised. Washington, DC, American Psychiatric Association, 1987

American Psychiatric Association: Diagnostic and Statistical Manual of Mental Disorders, 4th Edition. Washington, DC, American Psychiatric Association, 1994

Beresin EV: Delirium in the elderly. J Geriatr Psychiatry Neurol 1:127–143, 1988

Blass JP, Plum F: Metabolic encephalopathies in older adults, in The Neurology of Aging. Edited by Katzman R, Terry RD. Philadelphia, PA, FA Davis, 1983, pp 189–220

Bowman AM: The relationship of anxiety to development of postoperative delirium. J Gerontol Nurs 1:24–30, 1992

Brannstrom B, Gustafson Y, Norberg A, et al: Problems of basic nursing care in acutely confused and non-confused hip-fracture patients. Scand J Caring Sci 1:27–34, 1989

Brenner RP: Utility of EEG in delirium: past views and current practice. International Psychogeriatrics 3:211–229, 1991

Caplan LR, Schmahmann GD, Raquis CS, et al: Caudate infarcts. Neurology 38:262, 1988

Figiel GS, Krishnan KRR, Breitner JC, et al: Radiologic correlates of antidepressant-induced delirium: the possible significance of basal-ganglia lesions. J Neuropsychiatry Clin Neurosci 2:188–190, 1989

Figiel GS, Coffey CE, Djang WT, et al: Brain magnetic resonance imaging findings in ECT- induced delirium. J Neuropsychiatry 1:53–58, 1990a

Figiel GS, Krishnan KRR, Doraiswamy PM: Subcortical structural changes in ECT-induced delirium. J Geriatr Psychiatry Neurol 3:172–176, 1990b

Folstein MF, Folstein SE, McHugh PR: Mini-Mental State: a practical method for grading the cognitive state of patients for the clinician. J Psychiatr Res 12:189–198, 1975

Folstein MF, Bassett SS, Romanoski AJ, et al: The epidemiology of delirium in the community: the Eastern Baltimore Mental Health Survey. International Psychogeriatrics 3:169–176, 1991

Foreman MD: Confusion in the hospitalized elderly: incidence, onset and associated factors. Res Nurs Health 12:21–29, 1989

Francis J, Kapoor WN: Prognosis after hospital discharge of older medical patients with delirium. J Am Geriatr Soc 40:601–606, 1992

Francis J, Martin D, Kapoor WN: A prospective study of delirium in hospitalized elderly. JAMA 8:1097–1101, 1990

Gelfand SB, Indelicato J, Benjamin J: Using intravenous haloperidol to control delirium. Hosp Community Psychiatry 43:215, 1992

Itil T, Fink M: Anticholinergic drug-induced delirium: experimental modification, quantitative EEG and behavioral correlations. J Nerv Ment Dis 6:492–507, 1966

Jacobson SA, Leuchter AF, Walter DO: Conventional and quantitative EEG in the diagnosis of delirium among the elderly. J Neurol Neurosurg Psychiatry 56:153–158, 1993

Jitapunkul S, Pillay I, Ebrahim S: Delirium in newly admitted elderly patients: a prospective study. Q J Med 83:307–314, 1992

Johnson JC, Gottlieb GL, Sullivan E, et al: Using DSM-III criteria to diagnose delirium in elderly general medical patients. J Gerontol 45:113–119, 1990

Koponen H, Riekkinen P: A longitudinal study of cerebrospinal fluid beta-endorphin-like immunoreactivity in delirium: changes at the acute stage and at one-year follow-up. Acta Psychiatr Scand 82:323–326, 1990

Koponen H, Hurri L, Stenback U, et al: Computed tomography findings in delirium. J Nerv Ment Dis 4:226–231, 1989a

Koponen H, Partanen J, Paakonen A, et al: EEG spectral analysis in delirium. J Neurol Neurosurg Psychiatry 52:980–985, 1989b

Koponen H, Stenback U, Mattila E, et al: Cerebrospinal fluid somatostatin in delirium. Psychol Med 19:605–609, 1989c

Koponen H, Stenback U, Mattila E, et al: CSF beta-endorphin-like immunoreactivity in delirium. Biol Psychiatry 25:938–944, 1989d

Koponen H, Stenback U, Mattila E, et al: Delirium among elderly persons a2dmitted to a psychiatric hospital: clinical course during the acute stage and one-year follow-up. Acta Psychiatr Scand 79:579–585, 1989e

Kopenen H, Reinikainen K, Riekkinen PJ: Cerebrospinal fluid somatostatin in delirium, II. changes at the acute stage and at one year follow-up. Psychol Med 20:501–505, 1990

Koponen H, Sirvio J, Reinikainen KJ, et al: A longitudinal study of cerebrospinal fluid acetylcholinesterase in delirium: changes at the acute stage and at one-year follow-up. Psychiatry Res 38:135–142, 1991

Krauthammer C, Klerman GL: Secondary mania. Arch Gen Psychiatry 35:1333–1338, 1978

Leuchter AF, Jacobson SA: Quantitative measurement of brain electrical activity in delirium. Psychogeriatr 3:231–247, 1991

Leuchter AF, Daly KA, Rosenberg-Thompson S, et al: Prevalence and significance of electroencephalographic abnormalities in patients with suspected organic mental syndromes. J Am Geriatr Soc 41:605–611, 1993

Levkoff SE, Safran C, Cleary PD, et al: Identification of factors associated with the diagnosis of delirium in elderly hospitalized patients. J Am Geriatr Soc 36:1099–1104, 1988

Levkoff SE, Cleary PD, Liptzin B, et al: Epidemiology of delirium: an overview of research issues and findings. International Psychogeriatrics 3:149–167, 1991a

Levkoff SE, Liptzin B, Cleary P, et al: Review of research instruments and techniques used to detect delirium. International Psychogeriatrics 3:253–271, 1991b

Levkoff SE, Evans DA, Liptzin B, et al: Delirium, the occurrence and persistence of symptoms among elderly hospitalized patients. Arch Intern Med 152:334–340, 1992

Levkoff SE, Liptzin B, Evans DA, et al: Progression and resolution of delirium in elderly patients hospitalized for acute care. Am J Geriatric Psychiatry 2:230–238, 1994

Lipowski ZJ: Transient cognitive disorders (delirium, acute confusional states) in the elderly. Am J Psychiatry 140:1426–1436, 1983

Lipowski ZJ: Delirium (acute confusional states). JAMA 258:1789–1792, 1987

Lipowski ZJ: Delirium in the elderly patient. N Engl J Med 320:578–582, 1989

Lipowski ZJ: Delirium: Acute Confusional States. New York, Oxford University Press, 1990

Liptzin B: Delirium, in Conn's Current Therapy. Edited by Rakel RE. Philadelphia, PA, WB Saunders, 1991

Liptzin B, Levkoff SE: An empirical study of delirium subtypes. Br J Psychiatry 161:843–845, 1992

Liptzin B, Levkoff SE, Cleary PD, et al: An empirical study of diagnostic criteria for delirium. Am J Psychiatry 148:454–457, 1991

Liptzin B, Levkoff SE, Gottlieb G, et al: Delirium. J Neuropsychiatry Clin Neurosci 5:154–160, 1993

Liston EH: Delirium in the aged. Psychiatr Clin North Am 5:49–66, 1982

Liston EH: Delirium, in Treatment of Psychiatric Disorders: A Task Force Report of the American Psychiatric Association. Washington, DC, American Psychiatric Association, 1989, pp 804–815

Morency CR: Mental status change in the elderly: recognizing and treating delirium. J Prof Nursing 6:356–365, 1990

Mori E, Yamaddri A: Acute confusional state and acute agitated delirium. Arch Neurol 44:139–143, 1987

Moulaert P: Treatment of acute nonspecific delirium with I.V. haloperidol in surgical intensive care patients. Acta Anaesth Belg 40:183–186, 1989

Neelon VJ: Postoperative confusion. Crit Care Nurs Clin N Am 4:579–587, 1990

Obrecht R, Okhomina FOA, Scott DF: Value of EEG in acute confusional states. J Neurol Neurosurg Psychiatry 42:75–77, 1979

Rabins PV, Folstein MF: Delirium and dementia: diagnostic criteria and fatality rates. Br J Psychiatry 140:149–153, 1982

Rando EV: Delirium in elderly cancer patients: nursing management. Dimens Oncol Nurs 2:5–8, 1990

Roberts MA, Caird FI: The contribution of computerized tomography to the differential diagnosis of confusion in elderly patients. Age Aging 19:50–56, 1990

Rockwood K: Acute confusion in elderly medical patients. J Am Geriatr Soc 37:150–154, 1989

Romano J, Engel GL: Studies of delirium, I: electroencephalographic data. Arch Neurol Psychiatry 51:356–377, 1944

Ross CA: CNS arousal systems: possible role in delirium. International Psychogeriatrics 3:353–371, 1991

Schor JD, Levkoff SE, Lipsitz LA, et al: Risk factors for delirium in hospitalized elderly. JAMA 6:827–831, 1992

Thomas RI, Cameron DJ, Fahs MC: A prospective study of delirium and prolonged hospital stay. Arch Gen Psychiatry 45:937–940, 1988

Trzepacz PT, Teague GB, Lipowski ZJ: Delirium and other organic mental disorders in a general hospital. Gen Hosp Psychiatry 7:101–106, 1985

Trzepacz PT, Brenner R, VanThiel DH: A psychiatric study of 247 liver transplantation candidates. Psychosomatics 2:147–153, 1989a

Trzepacz PT, Sclabassi RJ, VanThiel DH: Delirium: a subcortical phenomenon? J Neuropsychol Clin Neurosci 3:283–290, 1989b

Trzepacz PT, Leavitt M, Ciongoli K: An animal model for delirium. Psychosomatics 4:404–415, 1992

Tune LE, Bylsma FW: Benzodiazepine-induced and anticholinergic-induced delirium. International Psychogeriatrics 3:397–408, 1991

Williams MA, Campbell EB, Raynor WJ, et al: Reducing acute confusional states in elderly patients with hip fractures. Research in Nursing Health 8:329–337, 1985

C H A P T E R   1 7

David K. Conn, M.B., F.R.C.P.C.

Other Dementias and Mental Disorders Due to General Medical Conditions

The most common causes of dementia are Alzheimer's disease and the vascular dementias. The first half of this chapter discusses other forms of dementia that always should be considered in the differential diagnosis of progressive cognitive impairment. The second half of this chapter describes the secondary mental disorders referred to as "organic mental disorders" in DSM-III-R; they include amnestic syndrome, organic mood syndrome, organic anxiety syndrome, organic delusional syndrome, organic hallucinosis, and organic personality syndrome. The term "organic" has been deleted in DSM-IV; the actual physical disorder or responsible substance must be specified (e.g., mood disorder due to stroke) (American Psychiatric Association 1994).

Other Dementias

In DSM-IV, the requirement for a diagnosis of dementia includes the development of multiple cognitive deficits manifested by 1) memory impairment and 2) at least one of the following: aphasia, apraxia, agnosia, or a disturbance in executive functioning. The deficits must cause significant impairment in social or occupational functioning and must represent a significant decline from a previous level of functioning (American Psychiatric Association 1994). A large number of disorders are known to cause dementia. Katzman (1991) lists approximately 70 diseases; an abbreviated list of important causes can be found in Table 17–1. In a review of nine published studies, Katzman (1991) found that 65.9% of patients had Alzheimer's disease, 17.1% had other progressive dementias (most commonly multi-infarct dementia), 10.5% had dementias for which specific treatment was indicated (most commonly hydrocephalus or dementias associated with alcohol dependence or tumors), 4.7% had dementias suitable for specific interventions (most commonly caused by drug toxicity or metabolic disturbances), and 1.8% had dementias of uncertain etiology. Clarfield (1988), in a review of 42 published studies of 2,889 subjects, investigated the "reversibility" of dementia and found that 56.8% of cases had Alzheimer's disease, 13.3% had multi-infarct dementia, depression accounted for 4.5%, alcohol abuse for 4.2%, and drug abuse for 1.5%.

Table 17–1.   Diseases that may present as dementia

Alzheimer's disease	Toxic dementia
Other degenerative diseases	Alcoholic dementia
Pick's disease	Metallic poisons
Frontal lobe degeneration	Organic poisons (e.g., solvents)
Huntington's disease	Dementia following head injury
Parkinson's disease	Dementia syndrome of depression
Diffuse Lewy body disease	Drugs
Amyotrophic lateral sclerosis	Psychotropic medications
Progressive supranuclear palsy	Antihypertensives
Wilson's disease	Anticonvulsants
Vascular dementias	Digitalis
Multi-infarct dementia	Anticholinergic agents
Lacunar dementia	Nutritional disorders
Binswanger's disease	Vitamin B_{12} deficiency
Infections	Folate deficiency
Creutzfeldt-Jakob disease	Pellagra (vitamin B_6 deficiency)
AIDS	Thiamine deficiency
Postencephalitic dementia	Metabolic disorders
Neurosyphilis	Hyperthyroidism
Normal pressure hydrocephalus	Hypothyroidism
Space-occupying lesions	Hypercalcemia
Subdural hematoma	Renal failure
Brain tumor	Hepatic encephalopathy
Multiple sclerosis	Cushing's syndrome
Vasculitis	Addison's disease

Follow-up, described in 11 studies, revealed that 8% of the patients improved, at least partially, and 3% fully returned to premorbid levels of functioning. These etiologies most commonly included depression (26%), drugs (28%), and metabolic conditions (15.5%).

Maletta (1990) has criticized the use of the term "reversible" dementia and notes that the concept creates misunderstanding. He suggests the alternative of labeling dementias whose continuing decline responds to treatment as "remediable," "remittable," or "arrestable."

Focal Cortical Dementias

Pick's Disease

In 1892, Arnold Pick described a 71-year-old man with a 3-year history of dementia. An autopsy revealed distinct atrophy of the frontal and temporal lobes. The disorder usually begins between 40 and 60 years, and most patients survive for 6–12 years. Alzheimer's disease is at least 10 times as common as Pick's disease. About 20% of cases are familial with an autosomal dominant pattern of inheritance (Cummings and Benson 1992; Groen and Endtz 1982).

From a clinical standpoint, a number of features help differentiate Pick's disease from Alzheimer's disease (Table 17–2). In Pick's disease the earliest changes usually are related to personality. These changes are typical of a frontal lobe syndrome with disinhibited and socially inappropriate behavior. The speech language disturbances include slow, deliberate speech with long pauses, anomia, echolalia, perseveration, and mutism (Jung and Solomon 1993). Klüver-Bucy syndrome may occur during the early course of the illness, but there is sparing of memory, visuospatial abilities, and the ability to calculate. The potential features of Klüver-Bucy syndrome in patients with Pick's disease include hyperphagia, gluttony, hypermetamorphosis, emotional blunting, hypersexuality, and visual or auditory agnosia. Increased food intake with weight gain and affective changes are common to a significant degree (Cummings and Duchen 1981).

The computed tomography (CT) scan may be normal during the early stages of Pick's disease, but focal atrophy of the frontal or temporal lobes often is seen subsequently. The magnetic resonance imaging (MRI) scan may reveal lobar atrophy, and the positron-emission tomography (PET) scan may reveal diminished glucose metabolism in the frontal and temporal lobes (Kamo et al. 1987). Single-photon emission computed

Table 17–2. Distinguishing features of Pick's disease versus Alzheimer's disease

	Pick's disease	Alzheimer's disease
Personality change	Early	Late
Amnesia	Late	Early
Language disturbance	Early	Late
Stereotypies	Early	Mid or late
Apraxia, agnosia, alexia	Late	Variable
Klüver-Bucy syndrome	Early	Late
Visuospatial disorientation	Rare	Common
Age of risk	Mean 50s, up to 80	Risk increases with age
Length of illness	2–11 years	5–25 years
CT scan	Temporal/frontal atrophy	Widespread atrophy
Gross pathology	Anterior hemispheric atrophy	Posterior hemispheric atrophy
Histopathology	Pick bodies	Neurofibrillary tangles
	Inflated cells	Senile plaques
	White matter gliosis	Granulovacuolar degeneration
	Loss of dendritic spines	

Source. Cummings and Benson 1992; Jung and Solomon 1993.

tomography (SPECT) studies have shown hypoperfusion of the frontal lobes. The histology demonstrates Pick bodies (which consist of an intracytoplasmic mass composed of neurofilaments and neurotubules), inflated cells, white matter gliosis, and loss of dendritic spines.

The etiology of Pick's disease is unknown; therefore, there is no specific treatment available and management consists primarily of supportive and symptomatic treatment.

Other Dementias With Frontal Lobe Involvement

Several other degenerative disorders can affect frontal lobe function:

1. Frontal lobe degeneration without Pick's pathology and with nonspecific histological changes (neuronal loss and gliosis) has been described by Brun (1987).

2. Amyotrophic lateral sclerosis can be associated with a degenerative dementia with frontal lobe features that may predate the motor neuron findings.
3. Neuronal intranuclear hyalin inclusion disease is a rare degenerative disorder that can affect frontal lobes. The disease may occur early in life. It exhibits extrapyramidal syndrome and other motor problems such as chorea or ataxia in addition to the dementia. Patients may become aggressive and belligerent.
4. Progressive subcortical gliosis can affect frontal and temporal lobes.

Other disorders that can lead to a frontal lobe syndrome with dementia include stroke (particularly involving the anterior cerebral artery), multiple sclerosis, hydrocephalus, and syphilis. Depression may be associated with features of a frontal lobe type dementia (dementia syndrome of depression) with evidence of reduced frontal lobe metabolic activity.

Subcortical Dementias

The concept of "subcortical dementia" was first described by Albert and colleagues in 1974. Four cardinal features were proposed as characteristic of subcortical dementia in describing the cognitive deficits found in progressive supranuclear palsy. These included forgetfulness, slowness of mental processes, affective changes (particularly depression), and intellectual deficits characterized by an impaired ability to manipulate acquired knowledge. Aphasia, agnosia, and apraxia, which are common in cortical dementia, are absent in patients with pure subcortical dementia.

Huntington's Disease

Huntington's disease is an idiopathic degenerative disease characterized by dementia and chorea. It was first described by George Huntington in 1872. The disease is inherited as an autosomal dominant trait with approximately 50% of offspring affected; the gene for the illness is located on chromosome 4. Recent isolation of the gene will permit more accurate presymptomatic testing (Huntington's Disease Collaborative Research Group 1993). When requested by family members, such testing must take place within a carefully designed genetic counseling program. The average length of time from onset to death is 14 years. The average age at onset is 35 to 40 years, although more than 20% of those affected develop the illness after age 50.

Dementia is a consistent component of the disorder. Affective illness occurs in more than 50% of patients, and a considerable number develop psychotic features or a schizophrenia-like disorder (Caine and Shoulson 1983; Lieberman et al. 1979). There is evidence to suggest that suicide accounts for the death of as many as 7% of these patients (Reed et al. 1958).

The first mental status changes usually are irritability, untidiness, loss of interest, and other personality changes. Dewhurst and colleagues (1969) reported that 57 of 102 patients presented with psychiatric disturbances. The dementia primarily is subcortical in nature and consists of slowing of cognition and memory disturbance that become apparent soon after the chorea begins. Language problems include mild word-finding difficulties, impaired verbal fluency, and dysarthria. The memory disturbance, which is prominent, is characterized by equal difficulty in recalling remote information compared with recently learned material. Subjects perform poorly on frontal systems tasks, and concentration and judgment are impaired.

The CT scan often shows atrophy of the caudate nuclei. The PET scan may show decreased metabolic activity before caudate atrophy is visible on the CT scan (Hayden et al. 1986), and the cerebral spinal fluid (CSF) may show decreased levels of γ-aminobutyric acid (GABA) (Bala Manyam et al. 1978). Levels of GABA and glutamic acid decarboxylase are reduced by up to 90% in the basal ganglia.

There is no specific treatment for this illness. However, the associated psychiatric disorders often respond to treatment. The depression may improve with antidepressants, lithium, or electroconvulsive therapy (ECT) (Leonard et al. 1974; McHugh and Folstein 1975), and psychosis or severe irritability may improve with neuroleptic medication. During the early course of the illness, chorea can also be treated with low-dose neuroleptic drugs.

Dementia in Parkinson's Disease

Most studies of large numbers of patients with Parkinson's disease estimate that dementia is present in 35%–55% (Cummings and Benson 1992). Neuropsychological testing tends to demonstrate preservation of recognition memory but impairment of spontaneous recall and of temporal ordering of learned information. Abnormalities are present on tests of frontal-subcortical systems. Although some individuals may have both Alzheimer's disease and Parkinson's disease, the dementia of Parkinson's does not appear generally to derive from associated Alzheimer's disease. A number of studies demonstrate that Parkinson's patients with dementia have severe neuronal loss in subcortical nuclei but do not have the characteristic pathology of Alzheimer's disease.

Lewy bodies (hyaline inclusion bodies) may accompany neuronal loss in involved nuclei (e.g., nucleus basalis of Meynert and brain stem nuclei). Cummings (1988) has suggested that marked dopamine deficiency may result in cognitive deterioration and that cholinergic deficiency contributes. Many patients receiving dopaminergic agents develop psychotic symptoms; this presents a treatment dilemma because neuroleptic medications are likely to worsen motor symptoms of Parkinson's disease. Newer neuroleptic drugs such as clozapine or risperidone may be useful in this situation (Friedman and Lannon 1989). The clinician should consider a diagnosis of depression in patients with Parkinson's disease, because depression may worsen cognitive performance and often responds well to treatment.

Progressive Supranuclear Palsy

Progressive supranuclear palsy (PSP) was described by Steele et al. (1964). It is an extrapyramidal syndrome characterized by pseudobulbar palsy, axial rigidity, supranuclear gaze paresis, and dementia. The onset of the illness is most common in the sixth or seventh decade; the average length of time until death is 5 to 10 years. The illness is more common in men than women.

Apathy and slowness often are part of the initial presentation of PSP. Memory consolidation and retrieval of information are impaired, and performance of frontal system tasks is abnormal. Clinical characteristics include more rigidity of midline structures than of the limbs. In contrast to individuals with Parkinson's disease, patients with PSP have an erect posture often with extension of the neck. The associated ophthalmoplegia is manifested by an initial loss of downward gaze. Upward gaze is impaired subsequently. Sleep disturbance and depression occur frequently (Aldrich et al. 1989).

The areas most affected include the subthalamic nucleus, red nucleus, globus pallidus, substantia nigra, and dentate nucleus. The pathology consists of cell loss, neurofibrillary tangles, and granulovacuolar degeneration.

A variety of treatments, including dopaminergic agents, have been tried. Akinesia may improve with L-dopa (Mendell et al. 1970), although response usually is disappointing. Some improvement has been noted with amantadine, and other reports indicate that benztropine and amitriptyline have been helpful for some patients (Haldeman et al. 1981; Newman 1985). Aggressive behavior in PSP has been treated effectively with trazodone (Schneider et al. 1989).

Normal Pressure Hydrocephalus

The syndrome of normal pressure hydrocephalus was first described by Adams et al. (1965). The clinical presentation includes a triad of dementia, gait disturbance, and urinary incontinence. These features are associated with evidence of ventricular dilation in the absence of significantly elevated intracranial pressure. The etiology of normal pressure hydrocephalus generally is idiopathic, although about one-third of patients have a history of subarachnoid bleeding, most commonly caused by a ruptured aneurysm (Katzman 1977). Depressive symptoms and apathy are not uncommon (Price and Tucker 1977), but psychosis is rare (Dewan and Bick 1985).

Common radiological findings include enlarged ventricles with a ballooned appearance on CT scan and with disproportionate enlargement of frontal horns and temporal horns compared with posterior horns of the lateral ventricles. Isotope cisternography can be helpful, although the results do not predict treatment outcome reliably. After injection of an isotope into the lumbar region, there is rapid diffusion into the ventricles and a subsequent failure of the isotope to rise into the sagittal region over the next 48 to 72 hours. There is some evidence that CSF drainage tests may predict response to treatment. The possibility that a progressively dementing illness can be reversed by a surgical procedure is appealing. The surgical shunt may have been used excessively in the past, but with careful selection of appropriate patients, it appears that about 50%–60% of surgical patients improve to some degree. A study by Thomsen et al. (1986), in which 40% of 40 patients improved cognitively after ventricular atrial shunt, suggested that a better postoperative outcome was associated with a known cause of normal pressure hydrocephalus, a short history, and absence of gyral atrophy. Some serious complications can occur including infection, hemorrhage, or blockage of the shunt. Note that the literature on surgery for normal pressure hydrocephalus consists primarily of case series rather than controlled trials. Patients with significant depression may respond to antidepressants, and there is one report of a patient with a shunt who was treated with ECT (Tsuang et al. 1979).

Dementias Caused by Infectious Disease

Creutzfeldt-Jakob Disease

This form of dementia was first described by Creutzfeldt in 1920 and by Jakob in 1921. It is a rare illness with a rapid onset of dementia (incidence of about 1 per 1 million). Onset of the illness usually is in the sixth or seventh decade of life. The disease is rapidly progressive with 50% of the patients dying in 6–9 months. Three disease stages have been identified. Initially, the person has vague symptoms that may include fatigue, insomnia, depression, anxiety, mental slowness, or unpredictable behavior. In the second stage, there is evidence of widespread disease of the central nervous system with the development of dementia and numerous neurological disturbances including cerebellar ataxia, aphasia, blindness, brain stem involvement, and myoclonic jerks. In the final stage of the illness, the person enters a vegetative state and coma leading to death. This illness is believed to be caused by a transmissible agent; namely, a slow virus or prion. The term *prion* describes an unconventional agent consisting of small glycoprotein particles that are resistant to inactivation and that produce spongiform changes in the brain. Human-to-human transmission has occurred after corneal transplantation, after the use of depth electrodes, and after the use of human growth hormone from pituitary glands.

Patients who may have this illness do not need to be isolated. Special care must be taken with blood or CSF: objects contaminated by infected tissue should be autoclaved and tissues and disposable equipment should be incinerated. Stool, urine, saliva, or other secretions are not believed to be infectious (Cummings and Benson 1992).

The CT scan may show cortical atrophy or may show no significant change. The EEG may show slowing or synchronous triphasic sharp wave complexes. Neuropathological findings include neuronal degeneration, proliferation of astrocytes, and sponginess of the gray matter. Neuronal loss is found throughout the cortex, thalamus, brain stem, and spinal cord. There is no recognized specific treatment so patients primarily require supportive care.

HIV Encephalopathy

Older patients can have acquired immunodeficiency syndrome (AIDS), although this disease usually occurs in the younger age groups. When the human immunodeficiency virus (HIV) produces dementia, the disorder is referred to as HIV encephalopathy or AIDS dementia complex. It is believed that HIV invades the brain shortly after systemic infection and remains latent for long periods (Resnick et al. 1988). The HIV virus tends to affect subcortical structures with relative sparing of the cortex (Navia et al. 1986). Early complaints include forgetfulness and poor concentration with slowed thinking. Apathy and social withdrawal may occur and psychotic symptoms may be present occasionally. Patients do not develop disturbances of language ability. The term *AIDS dementia complex* refers to a combination of advanced intellectual deficits and a complex of motor and behavioral abnormalities. The term has been criticized because not all components of the complex are always present.

A study of 132 patients with equivocal or subclinical AIDS reported that approximately 25% developed clinically significant dementia within 9 months and another 25% within 1 year (Sidtis et al. 1989). However, a longitudinal study found no decline in neuropsychological profile among 238 patients with Centers for Disease Control (CDC) stages II and III for 1 year (Selnes et al. 1990). Fifty subjects who developed AIDS during the study were excluded. It is important to consider that individuals with AIDS may have systemic illness, infections, or central nervous system malignancies that could account for their cognitive impairment. Azidothymidine (AZT) may lead to improved cognitive functioning in individuals with HIV encephalopathy (Yarchoan et al. 1987). Apathy, poor motivation, and attention deficits may respond to methylphenidate or dextroamphetamine (Fernandez et al. 1988).

Dementia Associated With Metabolic Disorders

Metabolic disorders and toxic states often result in a disturbance of cognitive and intellectual functioning. When this occurs abruptly and the course is limited, a diagnosis of delirium or acute confusional state is made. When onset is gradual and the course progresses insidiously, the disorder may represent a dementia. Because of the high rates of chronic illness and the relatively high rates of drug consumption in elderly patients, those individuals over 65 are more likely to experience toxic or metabolic dementias (Warshaw et al. 1982). Recognition of these causes of dementia is vital as they are often reversible. The causes of metabolic dementia include endocrine disorders such as thyroid, adrenal, and parathyroid disorders; hypoxia; hepatic encephalopathy; renal failure; vitamin deficiencies; and electrolyte disturbances.

Hypothyroidism can lead to dementia with or without psychosis. Hyperthyroidism may present as a dementia without the classic features of an overactive thyroid. Cushing's disease and Addison's disease may lead to features of dementia; hyperparathyroidism should be suspected if serum calcium levels are elevated in a patient with dementia. The most common cause of basal ganglia calcification with dementia is hypoparathyroidism.

Dementia After Head Injury

Approximately 500,000 individuals per year in the United States experience a head injury that is serious enough for hospitalization. Between 70,000 and 90,000 of these will develop a lifelong disability (Goldstein 1990). The majority of these injuries result from motor vehicle accidents. Significant posttraumatic amnesia and residual cognitive impairment are now known to follow head injuries in which there was no obvious loss of consciousness (Cummings and Benson 1992). Dementia after head trauma may result from three different forms of neuropathological injury: 1) diffuse axonal injury as a result of shearing forces; 2) focal contusions, hemorrhages, and lacerations; and 3) hypoxic ischemic insults. Diffuse axonal injury primarily affects subcortical white matter, the mesencephalon, and the diencephalon. Brain injury may occur at the point of injury (coup injury) or on the opposite side of the brain (contracoup). Traumatic contusions are especially common in the anterior temporal and inferior frontal lobes.

Cognitive difficulties include retrograde and anterograde amnesia with deficits in encoding and retrieval of new information, disorganized thinking, and poor concentration. Language disturbances, especially fluent aphasias, occur in approximately 30% of individuals with severe head injury. The post–head injury syndrome may include symptoms of depression, apathy, withdrawal, or anxiety; the full syndrome of posttraumatic stress disorder may coexist.

After severe injuries, the CT scan may show contusions and atrophy. The MRI scan may reveal white matter abnormalities. CT and MRI scans may be normal in some patients with permanent disability, although SPECT and PET studies may demonstrate abnormalities.

Dementia pugilistica is a syndrome of dementia and ataxia that may develop as a result of repeated head trauma. This is demonstrated in the study of former boxers. Neuropathological findings include diffuse brain atrophy, ventricular dilation, and deep pigmentation of the substantia nigra. Patients require intensive neurorehabilitation programs because continued recovery may take place for several years. Treatment of depression often is necessary.

Dementia Associated With Toxic Substances

Consistently heavy alcohol intake for a prolonged period (10–20 years) may result in dementia. Individuals who abuse alcohol are vulnerable to the development of deficiency syndromes such as Korsakoff's psychosis or pellagra. The high risk of subdural hematoma or hepatic encephalopathy can further complicate the presentation. Alcoholic dementia generally is mild and slowly progressive. Many persons with chronic alcoholism show enlarged lateral ventricles and widening of the cortical sulci; remarkably, these abnormalities may reverse if the individual refrains from further alcohol intake (Carlen et al. 1978). There is some evidence that alcohol primarily causes white matter atrophy because of its toxic effect on myelin (de la Monte 1988).

Exposure to some metals (e.g., lead, arsenic, mercury, manganese, nickel, bismuth, and tin) can result in dementia. Exposure to a variety of industrial compounds such as organic solvents and insecticides also can result in the development of dementia. Aluminum has been implicated as a cause of dialysis dementia and may have a role in the development of Alzheimer's disease. Dialysis dementia is a serious, often fatal, syndrome that occurs primarily in patients receiving long-term hemodialysis (Mach et al. 1988). The development of this dementia appears to be related to the amount, source, and duration of aluminum exposure, although undefined cofactors may exist. Antacids containing aluminum have been implicated in some cases. The development of dialysis dementia is not related to a patient's age, sex, or race. Clinical features include personality change, myoclonus, and seizures. Management includes reducing exposure to aluminum and treatment with the chelating agent deferoxamine.

Dementia Associated With Brain Tumors

Symptoms and signs of brain tumors depend on the location and speed of growth of the tumor and on the presence or absence of increased intracranial pressure or local edema. The onset often is insidious, although persistent headache is not uncommon. Some patients may develop localizing signs such as focal weakness, sensory disturbance, or visual field defects. The clinician needs to be aware that some tumors (usually frontal, temporal, or midline tumors) may present with only cognitive difficulties or personality changes. Dementia occurs in up to 70% of patients with frontal lobe tumors (commonly meningiomas, gliomas, or metastatic tumors) (Avery 1971; Cummings and Benson 1992). Dementia or delirium can occur with tumors of other brain regions. Tumors that invade the hypothalamus can cause somnolence, hyperphagia, and rage attacks. Basal ganglia tumors can present with memory impairment, poor concentration, depression, and personality changes. Tumors of the brain stem can result in lethargy, personality changes, and mutism. The possibility that a tumor can present with features that are identical to Alzheimer's disease or vascular dementia strongly supports the practice of getting a routine CT scan during the early stages of a dementing illness.

Mental Disorders Due to General Medical Conditions

In DSM-IV, the secondary organic mental disorders are renamed "mental disorders due to a general medical condition" (American Psychiatric Association 1994). The medical condition should be listed on Axis I and on Axis III when judged to be etiologically related to the mental disorder.

The classification of organic mental disorders, new in DSM-III, represented a radical departure from previous classification systems (American Psychiatric Association 1980). In discussing the approach of DSM-III, Lipowski (1984) noted that the essential feature of the newly described syndromes no longer was cognitive impairment but "psychological or behavioral abnormality associated with transient or permanent dysfunction of the brain." The concept of organicity no longer was synonymous with the presence of cognitive impairment. The division of organic syndromes into acute and chronic subtypes was abandoned in DSM-III because it forced the clinician to classify the patient's condition as either reversible or not on the basis of a purely cross-sectional assessment. Criticisms were leveled against the new classification system (Spitzer et al. 1983): it was described as overinclusive and overcomplex, possibly hindering case finding for epidemiological studies, imposing premature closure on the issue of cause, and leaving too much to the clinician's judgment. Note that the organic mental syndromes and disorders constituted the only section in DSM-III-R in which the clinician must make an etiologic diagnosis.

The clinician using the DSM-III-R diagnostic system may have encountered difficulties. Using history, physical examination, or laboratory tests, the clinician had to judge whether a specific factor is etiologically relevant to particular psychopathology. Note that the same challenge exists with DSM-IV because the clinician must determine that the disturbance is the direct physiological consequence of a particular medical condition. When a patient has a past psychiatric history or strong family psychiatric history with significant medical disease, it may be impossible to determine which of these factors is most relevant. Patients often have features of several organic syndromes, and in DSM-III-R it was necessary to use the residual category of organic mixed syndrome. Patients with mild symptoms of depression, an organic labile (pseudobulbar) affect, or localized cognitive impairment did not always fulfill diagnostic criteria and, therefore, were difficult to classify. A similar residual category (cognitive disorder not otherwise specified) is available in DSM-IV, with examples such as postconcussion disorder noted as appropriate (American Psychiatric Association 1994).

One particular clinical concern relates to the consequences of establishing a definitive biological etiology. For example, if a patient's depression is attributed entirely to stroke, then other etiologic factors such as early life experiences, family history of depression, medications, and other recent losses may be overlooked. It is vitally important, therefore, that the clinician continue to search for other contributing factors and consider the full array of potential interventions (Conn 1989), despite having established an etiologic factor.

Spitzer and colleagues (1992) noted that the term *organic* implies a functional/structural, psychological/biological, and mind/body dualism. They suggested that in DSM-IV the term *organic mental disorders* should be renamed either "secondary disorders" (if they are caused by physical disorders) or "substance-induced disorders." Although acknowledging that the original dichotomies may have been valuable when there was little understanding of how the CNS functions, they argued that these terms are at variance with the growing body of evidence of the importance of biological factors in the etiology of major "nonorganic" mental disorders. There have been several criticisms of this proposal. Lipowski (1990, 1991) argued that the term *organic* serves a useful function and that its abolition will create confusion, impede communication, and be at odds with ICD-10. Goldman (1991) argued that loss of the term will have a negative impact on consultation-liaison psychiatry. It is clear that the disorders themselves remain the same whether using the term *organic mental disorder* or *secondary mental disorder,* or naming the specific medical condition, is preferred.

Amnestic Disorder

The DSM-III-R diagnostic criteria for amnestic syndrome included 1) evidence of short-term memory impairment and long-term memory impairment and 2) no evidence of delirium or dementia (American Psychiatric Association 1987). The first criterion in DSM-IV is "the development of memory impairment as manifested by the inability to learn new information or the inability to recall previously learned information" (American Psychiatric Association 1994). Clinically, three types of memory are recognized: 1) *immediate memory* (e.g., measured by digit span), which is highly dependent on attention capacity; 2) *short-term memory,* defined as recall after a short period of distraction; there are differences of opinion about the length of this period, but most clinicians use a period of 2–5 minutes; and 3) *long-term memory* (e.g., measured by recall of early life events or historical figures).

The central feature of the amnestic syndrome is the inability to store, retain, and reproduce new information; this leads to anterograde amnesia (i.e., an impairment in the ability to lay down new memories during the period following the onset of an illness). The ability to immediately recall information is preserved, however. Defects in long-term memory are usually present although they may be less severe than the loss of short-term memory. The result is retrograde amnesia: an impaired ability to recall information that existed prior to the onset of an illness. Neuropsychologists divide the deficits in anterograde amnesia into 1) faulty encoding, 2) faulty consolidation, 3) accelerated forgetting, and 4) faulty retrieval (Kopelman 1987). Confabulation (the production of inaccurate, erroneous answers to straightforward questions) may occur in the amnestic patient. Patients may provide incorrect answers based on personal or past experiences, in which case the responses are coherent and reasonable, or they may give impossible, inappropriate, adventuresome, or gruesome responses ("fantastic" confabulation).

The most common cause of amnestic syndrome is Wernicke's encephalopathy, which is believed to be caused by thiamine deficiency (Adams and Victor 1985). It is most often seen in persons with chronic alcoholism, but it also may occur in isolated elderly patients (who may have a primary psychiatric diagnosis such as depression or paranoid disorder producing nutritional deficiencies).

Prompt treatment with parenteral thiamine is critical. The majority of patients will develop Korsakoff's syndrome (Reuler et al. 1985), which is chronic and characterized by severe anterograde and moderate retrograde amnesia. Patients with Korsakoff's syndrome often have severely compromised insight, and only 25% of patients make a full recovery (Victor et al. 1971).

Disease processes that affect the diencephalic and medial temporal structures (mamillary bodies, fornix, and hippocampus) can cause the amnestic syndrome. The symptoms appear to be related to bilateral sclerosis of the mamillary bodies and degenerative changes in the dorsal medial nucleus of the thalamus in patients with thiamine deficiency (Horvath 1988; Stoudemire 1987).

Differential Diagnosis

Transient global amnesia is a syndrome characterized by development of anterograde amnesia, which may last for several hours, and a short period of retrograde amnesia. Patients are bewildered but have no other clinical or neurological deficits. The syndrome may be related to decreased blood flow in the posterior hemispheric or inferior temporal regions. Transient global amnesia can be precipitated by emotional stressors and Merriam (1988) has suggested that this disorder may result from a disturbance in the brain's intrinsic benzodiazepine ligand system.

Psychogenic amnesia is characterized by inability to recall vital personal information such as the patient's name. There may be a loss of specific, emotionally charged information such as of a recent loss. Major depression also may be present, and patients may display "la belle indifférence." Postictal states should also be considered in the differential diagnosis.

Treatment

Medical treatment of the primary etiologic factor is the first consideration. Rehabilitation may involve specific therapies (cognitive and behavioral) to maximize the individual's level of functioning. Strategies useful at any age to help patients increase memory function include reorientation therapy; the programmed use of diaries, notebooks, or other aids; and specific memory training programs.

Mood Disorder Due to a General Medical Condition

The category "mood disorder due to a general medical condition" has replaced organic mood syndrome in DSM-IV (American Psychiatric Association 1994). Mood disorders are listed also in the substance-related disorders category.

Psychiatrists frequently are consulted to rule out depression in the medically ill, and a number of diagnostic difficulties may emerge. Many physical illnesses and drugs may cause symptoms (e.g., fatigue, decreased energy, insomnia, weakness, poor concentration, and anorexia) that facilitate a diagnosis of depression in healthy patients. It may be difficult for the clinician to decide whether or not to attribute these symptoms to depression. The rate of depression in medical populations appears to be between 12% and 32% (Stoudemire 1988). Approximately 20% of nursing home residents and 35% of elderly patients in chronic care hospitals have symptoms suggesting the presence of major depression (Katz et al. 1989; Sadavoy et al. 1990).

Many patients with neurological disease display evidence of aprosodia or organic emotional lability. Prosody is the affective and inflectional coloring of speech, including syllable and word stress, rhythm, cadence, and pitch. Together with gesture and mimicry, prosody provides the emotional element to speech. Prosody can be disturbed by right-hemisphere lesions and by disorders of the basal ganglia, cerebellum, and brain stem. As a result, the patient may present with a flat, monotonous voice; this can lead to underestimation or overestimation of the severity of an emotional disorder such as depression. The flat, emotionless voice may be mistaken for depression or, conversely, genuine feelings of sadness and distress may be unconvincingly presented. Patients with brain disease may have organic emotional lability; that is, they cry (or occasionally laugh) frequently and intensely with decreased control, often in response to a question or other interaction that produces emotional change. This behavior may give the clinician the false impression of depression. However, organic labile affect may be a signal of an underlying depressive illness (Ross and Rush 1981) and may improve with antidepressants (Schiffer et al. 1985).

Many illnesses and drugs are reputed to cause depression; however, a more accurate characterization is that many of these conditions are associated with depression. Stoudemire (1987) cautioned that the attribution of "medication or disease as the cause of depression should be approached with some degree of caution and skepticism and case reports and lists of such should be approached and evaluated critically."

Stroke and Parkinson's disease are associated with depression in elderly patients. At least one-fourth of stroke victims appear to develop a major depression, and depressive symptoms may occur in more than one-half of all patients following stroke (Robinson et al. 1984). However, in a recent study of all strokes occurring in an English health district, House and colleagues (1991) found much lower rates of depression. Their results showed only 9% of patients had a major depression 6 months poststroke, with an additional 11% diagnosed as dysthymic disorder or adjustment disorder with depressed mood. Follow-up studies report that the high-risk period for poststroke depression lasts for approximately 2 years (Robinson and Price 1982). According to Robinson and colleagues (1983), patients with left-hemisphere strokes are more vulnerable to depressive symptoms, especially when the lesion is close to the frontal pole. Other studies, however, have failed to show a consistent association between side of lesion and presence of depression (House 1987). There is evidence from animal studies that poststroke depression may be related to widespread depletion of norepinephrine following a localized lesion of the cortex. Mayberg and colleagues (1988) reported a PET study showing alterations in serotonin receptor binding following stroke that correlated with the severity of depression.

Studies of the frequency of depression in Parkinson's disease vary considerably. They suggest that 25%–70% of patients with Parkinson's disease experience depression (Cummings 1992). Depressed patients with Parkinson's disease have lower levels of the serotonin metabolite 5-hydroxyindoleacetic acid in their cerebrospinal fluid than do nondepressed patients with Parkinson's disease (Mayeux et al. 1984). The degree of physical disability and the duration of the disease do not seem to correlate with the severity of the depression. Parkinson's disease can present with depression (Kearney 1964), but this relation has not been studied well.

Other disorders clearly associated with depression include endocrine disorders (particularly hypothyroidism, Addison's disease, and Cushing's syndrome). Hyperthyroidism, also, may present with depressive symptoms in elderly patients ("apathetic hyperthyroidism"). Other important conditions include occult carcinomas (particularly of the pancreas), viral illnesses, pernicious anemia, and collagen-vascular diseases.

Medications associated with depression include antihypertensives, especially reserpine and methyldopa. The evidence that other antihypertensives (such as propranolol) cause depression is much weaker (Paykel et al. 1982). Some clinicians believe that β-blockers such as atenolol, which are less likely to cross the blood-brain barrier than others such as propranolol, are consequently less likely to cause depression. Steroids appear to cause depression, although a labile emotional state with features of euphoria and anxiety commonly is associated with use of steroids.

Factors that alter the major neurotransmitter systems implicated in primary mood disorders (norepinephrine and serotonin) or limbic-hypothalamic functions probably precipitate the development of organic mood disorders (Cummings 1985a).

The manic state is rarer than depressive symptoms (which are very common) in elderly, medically ill patients. The presentation includes pressure of speech, flight of ideas, hyperactivity, insomnia, distractibility, grandiosity, and poor judgment. A variety of conditions, such as agitated delirium or the disinhibited subtype of frontal lobe syndrome, can mimic mania, which might account for some of the conditions that are said to be associated with secondary mania. Table 17–3 lists common diseases and drugs associated with secondary mania in elderly patients. There is a preponderance of cerebral organic disorders, particularly among men (Shulman and Post 1980), and in elderly patients who develop mania for the first time at age 60 or older. Cummings (1985a) suggested that the localized neurological conditions linked to mania appear to include right-hemisphere lesions or lesions close to the third ventricle and hypothalamus.

There is evidence that antidepressants and ECT can be effective in the treatment of mood disorder accompanying stroke or Parkinson's disease (Harvey 1986; Lipsey et al. 1984; Murray et al. 1986). Treatment of the acute manic state generally requires neuroleptic medication. Lithium may be effective in treating secondary mania occurring in conjunction with brain

Table 17–3. Common diseases and drugs associated with secondary mania in elderly patients

Medical illnesses	Medications
Central nervous system	Corticosteroids
Stroke	Thyroxin
Cerebral neoplasms (especially	Levodopa
right hemisphere)	Bromocriptine
Multiple sclerosis	Sympathomimetics
Encephalitis	Amphetamines
Syphilis	Cimetidine
Head injury	
Hyperthyroidism	
Uremia	
Hemodialysis	

disease, although frequent blood levels must be taken to avoid toxicity (Rosenbaum and Barry 1975; Young et al. 1977). Patients with a primary mood disorder may benefit from a combination of psychopharmacological agents and psychotherapy and patients with secondary depression may also benefit greatly from a variety of psychiatric treatments. Individual supportive therapy and group therapy may provide great benefit. The families of elderly patients experiencing physical illness and an associated mood disturbance often require a great deal of support.

Anxiety Disorder Due to a General Medical Condition

The essential feature of organic anxiety syndrome according to DSM-III-R was recurrent or persisting anxiety and/or panic due to a specific organic factor (American Psychiatric Association 1987). The new DSM-IV term is *anxiety disorder due to a general medical condition* (American Psychiatric Association 1994). Anxiety disorders also are listed in the substance-related disorders category. Obsessions and compulsions are included in DSM-IV. Common symptoms include feelings of apprehension, tension, dread, or panic; autonomic and visceral symptoms including tachycardia, hyperventilation, increased sweating, dizziness, numbness and tingling, diarrhea, and urinary frequency also occur. Other symptoms include decreased concentration, tremor, restlessness, and, occasionally, perceptual changes such as derealization, depersonalization, or even hallucinations.

Anxiety may be a learned response or may reflect a neurotransmitter abnormality. Factors predisposing an individual to anxiety (e.g., genetic and psychodynamic factors) probably play a role in the development of organic anxiety syndrome. The most common etiologies of this disorder include hyperthyroidism, hypercortisolism, hypoglycemia, and some potentially toxic agents such as amphetamines and other psychostimulants, caffeine, and sympathomimetic agents (Cummings 1985a; Stoudemire 1987). Rare etiologies include pheochromocytoma, carcinoid syndrome, brain tumors, and epilepsy (especially complex partial seizures). Any condition that causes hypoxia is likely to cause anxiety. Alcohol and drug withdrawal syndromes produce an anxiety syndrome but are separately classified.

Management should focus on identifying and treating the primary cause. While this process is under way, benzodiazepines or buspirone may be helpful in controlling the symptoms of anxiety. β-Blockers may have a role in managing anxiety, especially when symptoms are primarily of a somatic nature, but their use in this capacity has not been well studied in elderly patients. Psychotherapy, relaxation techniques, and hypnosis may help the patient.

Psychotic Disorder Due to a General Medical Condition, With Delusions

Organic delusional syndrome was characterized in DSM-III-R by the occurrence of prominent delusions that can be attributed to an organic factor. Exclusion criteria included dementia and delirium. The new term in DSM-IV is *psychotic disorder due to a general medical condition with delusions* (American Psychiatric Association 1994). Psychotic disorders are also listed in the substance-related disorders category. The delusions may be simple and persecutory in nature, or they may be complex, systematized beliefs. The delusions may be related to specific neurological deficits such as anosagnosia, denial of blindness (Anton's syndrome), or reduplicative paramnesia (in which a patient claims to be present simultaneously in two locations). Specific delusions such as Capgras's syndrome (the delusion that significant people have been replaced by identically appearing impostors), delusional jealousy, delusions of infestation, and De Clerambault's syndrome (erotomania) all have been linked to specific organic causes as discussed in Cummings's (1985b) extensive review of organic delusions.

Cummings documented approximately 70 medical causes, drugs, and toxic agents implicated in producing delusions. He noted that many of these appear to occur in the setting of an acute confusional state, and others appear to be linked to dementia. These conditions, therefore, would not qualify for a diagnosis of organic delusional syndrome. Because most of the literature in this area predated the diagnostic concept of organic delusional syndrome, it is difficult, in retrospect, to define which of these disorders may cause a delusional state specifically. Table 17–4 lists some of the possible causes of organic delusional syndrome in elderly patients (Cummings 1985b; Stoudemire 1987).

Certain conditions and medications clearly have been linked to the development of delusions. These include CNS disorders such as Huntington's disease, Parkinson's disease, idiopathic calcification of the basal ganglia, and spinocerebellar degenerations. Disorders affecting the temporal-limbic regions (e.g., epilepsy and herpes encephalitis) and

Table 17–4. Possible causes of organic delusional syndrome in elderly
patients

Medical illnesses	Drugs and toxins
Central nervous system	L-Dopa
Stroke	Bromocriptine
Parkinson's disease	Amantadine
Epilepsy	Isoniazid
Idiopathic basal ganglia calcification	Corticosteroids
Spinocerebellar degeneration	Digitalis
Herpes encephalitis	Amphetamines
Huntington's disease	Methylphenidate
Thyroid and adrenal disorders	Lidocaine
Vitamin B_{12} deficiency	Procainamide
Folate deficiency	Ephedrine
Systemic lupus erythematosus	Phenytoin

tumors or strokes involving the temporal lobe or subcortical regions all
are implicated in the development of delusions. Certain medications such
as L-dopa and corticosteroids appear to be frequent culprits among medications and toxic agents linked to the development of psychosis. Psychosis
may be related to delirium in some cases, however. Prospective studies to
investigate the relationship to delirium would be useful.

Cummings (1985b) suggested a relationship among organic delusional
syndrome, cortical function, and the limbic system. He proposed that limbic or basal ganglia dysfunction predisposes to abnormal emotional experiences that are interpreted by the intact cortex and lead to complex,
intricately structured delusions. Subcortical and limbic lesions may disrupt ascending dopaminergic pathways, which have been implicated in
schizophrenia. He noted that predisposing factors include genetic constitution, early life experiences, personality characteristics, the location and
extent of lesions, and the age at onset of the primary illness.

In conjunction with treating the primary condition, neuroleptic medications may be indicated in treating organic delusional syndrome.
Cummings's (1985b) prospective study of 20 consecutive patients with organic delusions suggested that response to treatment was variable. Simple
delusions, which are more common in patients with dementia, responded
best to treatment with neuroleptic drugs, whereas complex delusions were
more resistant. Note that, even without treatment, simple delusions tend
to have a better prognosis. Goldman (1992) reported a positive response to
haloperidol in a small series of patients with organic delusional disorder

on a consultation-liaison psychiatry service. Delusions, especially complex delusions, can lead to misguided actions that may be highly disruptive to family or nursing home routines. As a result, staff or families may need a considerable degree of support and education in managing patients with persisting delusions. Because paranoid thinking may be linked to cognitive impairment and misinterpretation of the environment, the gradual development of a trusting relationship with staff and ongoing reorientation and reassurance may be beneficial. Although the mainstay of treatment is psychopharmacological, other approaches (e.g., behavioral management and psychotherapy) may play an important role (Proulx 1989; Sadavoy and Robinson 1989).

Psychotic Disorders Due to a General Medical Condition, With Hallucinations

The essential feature of organic hallucinosis in DSM-III-R was the presence of prominent, persistent, or recurrent hallucinations caused by a specific organic factor. The hallucination must not occur during the course of delirium or dementia (American Psychiatric Association 1987). The new term in DSM-IV is *psychotic disorder due to a general medical condition with hallucinations* (American Psychiatric Association 1994). Hallucinations can occur in any sensory modality (auditory, visual, tactile, olfactory, or gustatory) and can vary from simple and unformed to highly complex and organized. The individual may be aware that the hallucinations are imaginary or may be convinced of their reality.

Sensory deprivation related to loss of vision or hearing is a frequent cause of hallucinations in elderly patients. In a study of visual hallucinations in elderly patients, 29% of 150 successive referrals to a geriatric psychiatrist reported visual perceptual disturbances. There was a significant correlation between the presence of hallucinations and eye pathology (Berrios and Brook 1984). Visual hallucinations have been subdivided into "release" and "irritable" types (Brust and Behrens 1977). Release hallucinations are usually formed images and tend to occur in the area of a field deficit. They are associated with any focal lesion in the visual pathway. Irritable (ictal) hallucinations are brief, stereotyped visual experiences. With primary eye disease hallucinations may be simple or complex; for example, following eye surgery (especially if the eyes are patched).

Other causes of hallucinations include alcoholic hallucinosis (auditory), delirium tremens (visual and tactile), complex partial seizures, and lesions (especially of temporal-limbic structures). The differential diagnosis includes schizophrenia, especially when auditory hallucinations occur.

Medications and toxic agents responsible for hallucinations include hallucinogens, amphetamines, antiparkinsonian agents, thyroxin, steroids, antibiotics (especially intravenous penicillin), digoxin, sympathomimetics, cimetidine, narcotics, and heavy metals.

Tactile hallucinations occur most commonly in toxic and metabolic disturbances or drug withdrawal states (Berrios 1982). Olfactory and gustatory hallucinations are caused most commonly by complex partial seizures.

Mechanisms suggested in the pathophysiology of hallucinations include a "perceptual release theory" (i.e., decreased sensory input results in the release of spontaneous central nervous system activity); the intrusion of dreams into the waking state (narcolepsy, hypnogogic hallucinations); serotonin antagonism (hallucinogens); and the role of hemispheric specialization (more commonly right-hemisphere lesions or seizure foci) (Cummings 1985a).

Management includes ensuring maximum sensory input by treating underlying disorders or through use of improved hearing or visual aids. Anticonvulsants such as carbamazepine are indicated for treating seizures. The use of neuroleptic medications may be helpful but has not been well studied. Neuroleptic medications may help to decrease anxiety or fear associated with the hallucinations.

Personality Change Due to a General Medical Condition

The cardinal feature of this disorder, which was previously termed organic personality syndrome, is a personality disturbance caused by a specific medical condition. The personality disturbance represents a change from the individual's previous characteristic personality pattern. Exclusion criteria include delirium and dementia. The subtypes in DSM-IV include labile, disinhibited, aggressive, apathetic, and paranoid types (American Psychiatric Association 1994).

Any disease that damages frontal lobes may lead to a "frontal lobe personality syndrome." Neoplasms, head trauma, cerebrovascular accidents, multiple sclerosis, and Huntington's disease all are associated with this syndrome. An insidious presentation of personality change may herald the onset of a more global dementia. This applies particularly to patients with

Pick's disease, which primarily affects the frontal lobes; the same may be true of other dementias such as Alzheimer's disease.

Cummings (1985a) has described three separate frontal lobe syndromes that, in practice, tend to overlap. The syndromes described are 1) orbitofrontal syndrome characterized by disinhibition and impulsive behavior ("pseudopsychopathic"); 2) frontal convexity syndrome (in which apathy predominates); and 3) medial-frontal syndrome (which is associated with akinesia). Disinhibited behavior may cause dramatic behavioral change, and there may be totally uncharacteristic behavior incorporating loss of social tact; rude, tasteless, or inappropriate language; and antisocial behavior. The emotions may be labile with episodic euphoria, inappropriate jocularity, and hyperactivity. There may be inappropriate sexual behavior. Individuals often are easily distracted and lack the ability to monitor and evaluate their own behavior and performance. Insight and judgment often are impaired significantly. On examination, patients may display some of these behaviors or, conversely, may be apathetic. Patients' inability to program new motor tasks (e.g., the fist-cut-slap test) may lead to motor perseveration or impersistence. There may be decreased word fluency, impaired abstraction and categorization skills, and difficulty shifting set (e.g., Wisconsin Card Sorting Test).

Another personality syndrome is described in some patients with long-standing seizure disorders, particularly complex partial seizures. The essential features consist of emotional "viscosity" (pedantic and overinclusive thinking), hyperreligiosity, hypergraphia, intense emotional reactions, humorlessness, hypermoralism, and changes in sexual behavior (most frequently hyposexuality) (Bear and Fedio 1977). There are no specific data for elderly patients.

Frontal lobe syndrome may cause dramatic problems for the patient and the family. Behavior may be frightening to others and may necessitate calling the police or outside agencies. It may be difficult to involve the individual in a treatment program because of decreased insight. Patients with disinhibited behavior may require a combined behavioral and pharmacological approach. Various medications have been used in an attempt to control disinhibited and aggressive behavior. The first line of treatment generally is a neuroleptic drug. Other drugs reported anecdotally to improve this behavior include propranolol, lithium, trazodone, and carbamazepine. Behavior management programs may be of benefit but require the cooperation of families or caregivers living with the patient (Haley 1983; Proulx 1989).

Conclusion

Clearly a need exists for further research to aid understanding of the complex relationships between behavior and neuropsychiatric disorders. Although the emphasis from an etiologic standpoint is on "organic factors," it is important to consider factors predisposing to the development of these disorders. These predisposing factors—such as premorbid personality style, previous life experiences, family psychodynamics, and environmental-cultural influences—may be important in developing a formulation and management plan. Optimal care of these patients, whether in the institution or in the community, requires an integrated and multidisciplinary approach. Primary interventions often involve treating the underlying organic factors and using psychopharmacological agents. However, other interventions such as individual and family psychotherapy, behavioral management programs, and environmental manipulations may be important adjuncts in the care of these patients.

References

Adams RD, Fisher CM, Hakim S, et al: Symptomatic occult hydrocephalus with "normal" cerebrospinal fluid pressure: a treatable syndrome. N Engl J Med 273:117–126, 1965

Adams RD, Victor M: Principles of Neurology, 3rd Edition. New York, McGraw-Hill, 1985

Albert M, Feldman RG, Wills AL: The "subcortical dementia" of progressive supranuclear palsy. J Neurol Neurosurg Psychiatry 37:121–130, 1974

Aldrich MS, Foster NL, White RF, et al: Sleep abnormalities in progressive supranuclear palsy. Ann Neurol 25:477–581, 1989

American Psychiatric Association: Diagnostic and Statistical Manual of Mental Disorders, 3rd Edition. Washington, DC, American Psychiatric Association, 1980

American Psychiatric Association: Diagnostic and Statistical Manual of Mental Disorders, 3rd Edition, Revised. Washington, DC, American Psychiatric Association, 1987

American Psychiatric Association: Diagnostic and Statistical Manual of Mental Disorders, 4th Edition. Washington, DC, American Psychiatric Association, 1994

Avery TL: Seven cases of frontal tumour with psychiatric presentation. Br J Psychiatry 119:19–23, 1971

Bala Manyam NV, Hare TA, Katz L, et al: Huntington's disease: cerebrospinal fluid GABA levels in at-risk individuals. Arch Neurol 35:728–730, 1978

Baringer JR, Gajdusek C, Gibbs CS Jr, et al: Transmissible dementias: current problems in tissue handling. Neurology 30:302–303,1980

Bear DM, Fedio P: Quantitative analysis of interictal behaviour in temporal lobe epilepsy. Arch Neurol 34:454–467, 1977

Berrios GE: Tactile hallucinations: conceptual and historical aspects. J Neurol Neurosurg Psychiatry 45:285–293, 1982

Berrios GE, Brook P: Visual hallucinations and sensory delusions in the elderly. Br J Psychiatry 144:662–664, 1984

Brun A: Frontal lobe degeneration of the non-Alzheimer type, I: neuropathology. Arch Gerontol Geriatr 6:193–208, 1987

Brust JCH, Behrens MM: "Release hallucinations" as the major symptom of posterior cerebral artery occlusion: a report of 2 cases. Ann Neurol 2:432–436, 1977

Caine ED, Shoulson I: Psychiatric syndromes in Huntington's disease. Am J Psychiatry 140:728–733, 1983

Carlen PL, Wortzman G, Holgate RC, et al: Reversible atrophy in recently abstinent chronic alcoholics measured by computed tomography scans. Science 200:1076–1078, 1978

Clarfield AM: The reversible dementias: do they reverse? Ann Intern Med 109:476–486, 1988

Conn DK: Neuropsychiatric syndromes in the elderly: an overview, in Psychiatric Consequences of Brain Disease in the Elderly—A Focus on Management. Edited by Conn DK, Grek A, Sadavoy J. New York, Plenum, 1989

Cummings JL: Clinical Neuropsychiatry. New York, Grune & Stratton, 1985a

Cummings JL: Organic delusions: phenomenology, anatomical correlations, and review. Br J Psychiatry 146:184–197, 1985b

Cummings JL: Intellectual impairment in Parkinson's disease: clinical, pathologic, and biochemical correlates. J Geriatr Psychiatry Neurol 1:24–36, 1988

Cummings JL: Depression and Parkinson's disease: a review. Am J Psychiatry 149:443–454, 1992

Cummings JL, Benson DF: Dementia—A Clinical Approach. Boston, MA, Butterworth-Heinemann, 1992

Cummings JL, Duchen LW: The Kluver-Bucy syndrome in Pick disease. Neurology 31:1415–1422, 1981

Dewan MJ, Bick A: Normal pressure hydrocephalus and psychiatric patients. Biol Psychiatry 20:1127–1131, 1985

Dewhurst K, Oliver J, Trick KLK, et al: Neuro-psychiatric aspects of Huntington's disease. Confin Neurol 31:258–268, 1969

Fernandez F, Adams F, Levy JK, et al: Cognitive impairment due to AIDS-related complex and its response to psychostimulants. Psychosomatics 29:38–46, 1988

Friedman JH, Lannon MC: Clozapine in the treatment of psychosis in Parkinson's disease. Neurology 39:1219–1221, 1989

Goldman SA: Concerns and issues of the diagnostic category of organic mental disorders in the DSM-IV (letter). Psychosomatics 32:112, 1991

Goldman SA: Organic delusional disorder on a consultation-liaison psychiatry service. Psychosomatics 33:343–352, 1992

Goldstein M: Traumatic brain injury: a silent epidemic. Ann Neurol 27:327, 1990

Groen JJ, Endtz LJ: Hereditary Pick's disease: second re-examination of a large family and discussion of other hereditary cases, with particular reference to electroencephalography and computed tomography. Brain 105:443–459, 1982

Haldeman S, Goldman JW, Hyde J, et al: Progressive supranuclear palsy, computed tomography, and response to antiparkinsonian drugs. Neurology 31:442–445, 1981

Haley WE: A family behavioural approach to the treatment of the cognitively impaired elderly. Gerontologist 23:18–20, 1983

Harvey NS: Psychiatric disorders in parkinsonism, I: functional illness and personality. Psychosomatics 27:91–103, 1986

Hayden MR, Martin AJ, Stoessl AJ, et al: Positron emission tomography in the early diagnosis of Huntington's disease. Neurology 36:888–894, 1986

Horvath TB: Organic brain syndromes, in Psychiatry, Revised Edition. Edited by Michels R, Cooper AM, Guze SB, et al. Philadelphia, PA, JB Lippincott, 1988

House A: Mood disorders after stroke: review of the evidence. International Journal of Geriatric Psychiatry 2:211–221, 1987

House A, Dennis M, Mogridge L, et al: Mood disorders in the year after first stroke. Br J Psychiatry 158:83–92, 1991

Huntington's Disease Collaborative Research Group: A novel gene containing a trinucleotide repeat that is expanded and unstable on Huntington's disease chromosomes. Cell 72:971–983, 1993

Jung R, Solomon K: Psychiatric manifestations of Pick's disease. International Psychogeriatrics 5:187–202, 1993

Kamo H, McGeer PL, Harrop R, et al: Positron emission tomography and histopathology in Pick's disease. Neurology 37:439–445, 1987

Katz IR, Lesher E, Kleban M, et al: Clinical features of depression in the nursing home. International Psychogeriatrics 1:5–15, 1989

Katzman R: Normal pressure hydrocephalus, in Dementia, 2nd Edition. Edited by Wells CE. Philadelphia, PA, FA Davis, 1977, pp 69–92

Katzman R: Diagnosis and management of dementia, in Principles of Geriatric Neurology. Edited by Katzman R, Rowe JW. Philadelphia, PA, FA Davis, 1991

Kearney TR: Parkinson's disease presenting as a depressive illness. J Irish Med Assoc 54:117–119, 1964

Kopelman MD: Amnesia: organic and psychogenic. Br J Psychiatry 150:428–442, 1987

Leonard DP, Kidson MA, Shaunon PJ, et al: Double-blind trial of lithium carbonate and haloperidol in Huntington's chorea. Lancet 2:1208–1209, 1974

Lieberman A, Dziatolowski M, Neophytides A, et al: Dementias of Huntington's and Parkinson's disease. Adv Neurol 23:273–280, 1979

Lipowski ZJ: Organic mental disorders—an American perspective. Br J Psychiatry 144:542–546, 1984

Lipowski ZJ: Is "organic" obsolete? Psychosomatics 31:342–344, 1990

Lipowski ZJ: Reply to R.L. Spitzer, M. First, G. Tucker: Organic mental disorders and DSM-IV (letter). Am J Psychiatry 148:396, 1991

Lipsey JR, Robinson RG, Pearlson GD, et al: Nortriptyline treatment of post-stroke depression: a double-blind treatment trial. Lancet 1:297–300, 1984

Mach J, Korchik W, Mahowald M: Dialysis dementia, in Treatment Considerations for Alzheimer's Disease and Related Dementing Illnesses (Clinics in Geriatric Medicine). Edited by Maletta G. Philadelphia, PA, WB Saunders, 1988, pp 853–868

Maletta GJ: The concept of "reversible" dementia—how nonreliable terminology may impair effective treatment. J Am Geriatr Soc 38:136–140, 1990

Mayberg HS, Robinson RG, Wond DF, et al: PET imaging of cortical S_2 serotonin receptors after stroke—lateralised changes and relationship to depression. Am J Psychiatry 145:937–943, 1988

Mayeux R, Stern Y, Cote L, et al: Altered serotonin metabolism in depressed patients with Parkinson's disease. Neurology 34:642–646, 1984

McHugh PR, Folstein MF: Psychiatric syndromes of Huntington's chorea:

a clinical and phenomenologic study, in Psychiatric aspects of neurologic disease. Edited by Benson DF, Blumer D. New York, Grune & Stratton, 1975, pp 267–285

Mendell JR, Chase TN, Engel WK: Modification by l-dopa of a case of progressive supranuclear palsy. Lancet 1:593–594, 1970

Merriam AE: Emotional arousal-induced transient global amnesia: case report, differentiation from hysterical amnesia, and an etiologic hypothesis. Neuropsychiatry, Neuropsychology and Behavioral Neurology 1:73–78, 1988

de la Monte SM: Disproportionate atrophy of cerebral white matter in chronic alcoholics. Arch Neurol 45:990–992, 1988

Murray GB, Shea VA, Conn DK: Electroconvulsive therapy for post-stroke depression. J Clin Psychiatry 47:258–260, 1986

Navia BA, Jordan BD, Price RW: The AIDS dementia complex, I: clinical features. Ann Neurol 19:517–524, 1986

Newman GC: Treatment of progressive supranuclear palsy with tricyclic antidepressants. Neurology 35:1189–1193, 1985

Paykel ES, Fleminger R, Watson JP: Psychiatric side effects of antihypertensive drugs other than reserpine. J Clin Pharmacol 2:14–39, 1982

Price TRP, Tucker GJ: Psychiatric and behavioral manifestations of normal pressure hydrocephalus. J Nerv Ment Dis 164:51–55, 1977

Proulx GB: Management of disruptive behaviours in the cognitively impaired elderly: integrating neuropsychological and behavioural approaches, in Psychiatric Consequences of Brain Disease in the Elderly: A Focus on Management. Edited by Conn DK, Grek A, Sadavoy J. New York, Plenum, 1989

Reed TE, Chandler JH, Hughes EM, et al: Huntington's chorea in Michigan, I: demography and genetics. Am J Hum Genet 10:201–225, 1958

Resnick L, Berger JR, Shapshak P, et al: Early penetration of the blood-brain barrier by HIV. Neurology 38:9–14, 1988

Reuler JB, Girard DE, Cooney TG: Wernicke's encephalopathy. N Engl J Med 312:1035–1039, 1985

Robinson RG, Price TR: Post-stroke depressive disorders: a follow-up study of 103 outpatients. Stroke 13:635–641, 1982

Robinson RG, Kubos KL, Starr LB, et al: Mood changes in stroke patients: relationship to lesion location. Compr Psychiatry 24:555–566, 1983

Robinson RG, Starr LB, Price TR: A two-year longitudinal study of mood disorders following stroke: prevalence and duration at six months follow-up. Br J Psychiatry 144:256–262, 1984

Rosenbaum AH, Barry MJ Jr: Positive therapeutic response to lithium in hypomania secondary to organic brain syndrome. Am J Psychiatry 132:1072–1073, 1975

Ross ED, Rush J: Diagnosis and neuroanatomical correlates of depression in brain-damaged patients. Arch Gen Psychiatry 38:1344–1354, 1981

Sadavoy J, Robinson A: Psychotherapy and the cognitively impaired elderly, in Psychiatric Consequences of Brain Disease in the Elderly. Edited by Conn DK, Grek A, Sadavoy J. New York, Plenum, 1989

Sadavoy J, Smith I, Conn DK, et al: Depression in geriatric patients with chronic medical illness. International Journal of Geriatric Psychiatry 5:187–192, 1990

Schiffer RB, Herndon RM, Rudick RA: Treatment of pathological laughing and weeping with amitriptyline. N Engl J Med 312:1480–1482, 1985

Schneider LS, Gleason RP, Chui HC: Progressive supranuclear palsy with agitation: response to trazodone but not to thiothixine or carbamazepine. J Geriatr Psychiatry Neurol 2:109–112, 1989

Selnes OA, Miller E, McArthur J, et al: HIV-1 infection: no evidence of cognitive decline during the asymptomatic stages. Neurology 40:204–208, 1990

Shulman K, Post F: Bipolar affective disorder in old age. Br J Psychiatry 136:26–32, 1980

Sidtis JJ, Thaler H, Brew BJ, et al: The interval between equivocal and definite neurological signs and symptoms in the AIDS dementia complex, in Abstracts of the Fifth International Conference on AIDS. International Development Research Centre, Montreal, 1989

Spitzer RL, Williams JBW, Skodol AE: International Perspectives on DSM-III. Washington, DC, American Psychiatric Association, 1983

Spitzer RL, First MB, Williams JBW, et al: Now is the time to retire the term "organic mental disorders." Am J Psychiatry 149:240–244, 1992

Steele JC, Richardson JC, Olszewski J: Progressive supranuclear palsy. Arch Neurol 10:333–359, 1964

Stoudemire A: Depression in the medically ill, in Psychiatry, Revised Edition. Edited by Michels R, Cooper AM, Guze SB, et al. Philadelphia, PA, JB Lippincott, 1988

Stoudemire GA: Selected organic mental disorders, in Textbook of Neuropsychiatry. Edited by Hales RE, Yudofsky SC. Washington, DC, American Psychiatric Press, 1987, pp 125–139

Thomsen AM, Borgeson SE, Bruhn P, et al: Prognosis of dementia in normal pressure hydrocephalus after a shunt operation. Ann Neurol 20:304–310, 1986

Tsuang MT, Tidball JS, Geller D: ECT in a depressed patient with shunt in place for normal pressure hydrocephalus. Am J Psychiatry 136:1205–1206, 1979

Victor M, Adams RD, Collins GH: The Wernicke-Korsakoff Syndrome. Oxford, Blackwell Scientific Publications, 1971

Warshaw GA, Moore JT, Friedman SW, et al: Functional disability in the hospitalized elderly. JAMA 248:847–850, 1982

Yarchoan R, Berg G, Brouwers P, et al: Response of human immunodeficiency-virus-associated neurological disease to 3-azido-3-deoxythymidine. Lancet 1:132–135, 1987

Young LD, Taylor I, Holmstrom V: Lithium treatment of patients with affective illness associated with organic brain symptoms. Am J Psychiatry 134:1405–1407, 1977

Sidney Zisook, M.D.
Stephen R. Shuchter, M.D.

Grief and Bereavement

This chapter describes the grief and bereavement of elderly persons: it outlines "normal" grief reactions, discusses complications and risk factors, and reviews information on treatment interventions. According to the 1990 census, more than 2 million people can be expected to die each year in the United States (Information Please Almanac 1993). Each death leaves, on average, approximately five relatives or close friends behind (Cleiren 1991); therefore, more than 10 million people experience bereavement each year. Bereavement, a ubiquitous event that may occur at any point during the lifecycle, is particularly prevalent in the elderly population. Deleterious effects of bereavement may be compounded in this group by other challenges and losses associated with aging (declining health, mobility, cognitive abilities, income, and function; loss of social and occupational roles; diminished personal independence; and loss of friends and relatives). It is a testimony to the adaptive capacities of elderly persons that most bereaved individuals in late life ultimately are able to grieve for their loss, to reengage, and to function adequately in their daily lives. A minority, however, recover marginally, or not at all, and continue to be debilitated in physical, psychological, and/or social functioning for years. Health practitioners working with elderly patients need to have a comprehensive knowledge of normal grief, common complications, and

risk factors to understand the experiences that bereaved individuals encounter, to avert complications that may be preventable, and to manage
most effectively those that are not.

Although elderly persons are vulnerable to a myriad of losses (e.g.,
spouses, siblings, adult children, grandchildren, friends, and pets) this
chapter focuses primarily on the effects of spousal bereavement. The death
of a spouse is by far the most studied form of bereavement in late life. In
the United States, there are more than 800,000 new widows and widowers
each year. The approximately 11 million widows and 2 million widowers
make up more than 7% of the population in the United States. Most of
these men and women are elderly: the mean age at widowhood is 69 years
for men and 66 years for women in the United States. Among people ages
65 or over, more than 50% of all women and 13% of men have been widowed at least once (U.S. Bureau of the Census 1984).

Spousal bereavement, which often is considered the prototypical severe life stressor (Holmes and Rahe 1967), has been associated with prolonged personal suffering, declining mental and physical health (Klerman
and Izen 1977; Osterweis et al. 1984; Stroebe and Stroebe 1993a), an elevated risk for suicide (MacMahon and Pugh 1965), and an increased risk
of death for reasons other than suicide (Kaprio et al. 1987). The fact that
widowed persons, especially women, have much of their lives before them
adds to the burden (the mean duration of widowed life is 4 years for widowers and 7 years for widows); therefore, most widows are faced with living alone on a reduced income into old age. They are challenged by the
tasks of establishing a life independent of their deceased spouses; dealing
with evolving family relationships and support networks; and meeting emotional, health, and practical needs over the long term (Hansson et al. 1993).

Normal Grief

Stages of Grief

Several investigators have proposed stages of emotional response through
which bereaved individuals pass as they attempt to come to terms with
the loss of a loved one (Bowlby 1980/1981; Devaul et al. 1979; Horowitz
1986). Most of these stage models include an initial period of shock, disbelief, and denial; an intermediate mourning period of acute somatic
emotional discomfort and social withdrawal; and a culminating period
of reorganization and recovery. However, examination of the existing data

on bereavement suggests that there is considerable variability in the specific kinds of emotions, their sequence, and intensity that are experienced (Lund 1989; Silver and Wortmann 1980). Clinicians should view such "stages" of grief not literally but as general, flexible guidelines that may describe, but not prescribe, where an individual ought to be in the normal grieving process. Grief is not a linear process with concrete boundaries; it is a composite of overlapping, fluid phases that vary from person to person (Shuchter and Zisook 1993).

The Duration of Grief

There is little agreement about the time course of normal grief and bereavement. Several investigators have found that symptoms of depression frequently remain as long as 1 year (Bornstein et al. 1973; Zisook and Shuchter 1991a) or 2 years (Lund et al. 1985; Harlow et al. 1991; Zisook and Shuchter 1993b) after the death of a loved one. Parkes (1971) found that only a minority of widows could recall the past with pleasure or anticipate the future with optimism 13 months after the death of their husbands. Most widows described themselves as sad, poorly adjusted, depressed, thinking often of their deceased husbands, having clear visual memories of them, and still grieving a great deal of the time. Parkes concluded that the process of grieving often continued for more than 13 months, and that the question of how long grief lasts was still unanswered. Other findings (Zisook 1987) are in agreement with those of Goin (1979) who suggested that "you don't get over it—you get used to it." Some aspects of working out the grieving process may never end for a significant proportion of otherwise normally bereaved individuals.

Multidimensional Assessment of Grief

Grief is a highly individualized process. There are many ways to grieve and an individual's grief may vary from moment to moment. A multidimensional approach seems best suited to understanding grief and bereavement. Table 18–1 presents six overlapping dimensions of grief including affective states, coping strategies, continued relationships with the deceased, new relationships, functioning, and an evolving new identity (Shuchter 1986).

Dimension 1: Emotional and cognitive experiences.   Most men and women experience some form of initial shock and denial when confronted by the news that a loved one is dead; there is an interval during which the

Table 18–1.   Dimensions of grief

Emotional and cognitive experiences
Coping strategies
The continuing relationship with the deceased
Health, occupational, and social functioning
Relationships
Identity, self-esteem, and worldview

impact of the loss does not register fully. Varying degrees of numbness and detachment often are present during this time. The emotional pangs and anguish of grief soon emerge. These are painful, often total, body experiences of autonomic explosion: a wrenching of the gut, shortness of breath, chest pain, lightheadedness, weakness, rapid welling-up of tears, and uncontrollable crying. These responses often erupt suddenly and un-expectedly in the first days and weeks. They are more apt to be precipi-tated over time by reminders of the deceased. For some bereaved persons, everything is a reminder of their loss, and their pain remains unremitting for an extended period. The frequency and intensity of such pain gener-ally subsides as time passes, although it may reemerge in response to re-minders of the loss.

Closely associated with the emotional pain is a sense of loss, yearning, pining, and searching behaviors (Bowlby 1973). It is not only the person that is lost, but also intimacy, companionship, security, life-style, roles, a sense of meaning, and visions of the future. Disruption of attachment bonds, intense forms of insecurity, fear, and anxiety emerge. The anxiety may be felt as free-floating waves or time-limited panic. Vivid and de-tailed intrusive images of the deceased often arise, particularly at times when the individual's mind is not actively engaged, such as when home alone or before falling sleep. These intrusive images may be more com-mon when the death was sudden and unexpected (Horowitz 1986; Jacobs 1993; Rynearson 1990).

Clinical experience shows that feelings such as anger, guilt, or regret may plague the bereaved person intermittently. After the loss of a loved one, bereaved persons normally, although not universally, experience feel-ings of anger that may be felt as irritability, hatred, resentment, envy, or a sense of unfairness. The anger may be directed at the deceased, family, friends, God, physicians, or self. Guilt is common and variable. The most intense and lasting forms of guilt often are associated with the perception that the bereaved person may have contributed to the death or suffering of the deceased by improper feeding, by inadequate support, by failing to prevent unhealthy attitudes or life-styles, or by not pushing physicians hard enough to detect the disorder. Survival guilt may be particularly intense and tenacious when the bereaved person may, in fact, be responsible for this loss (e.g., having been the driver in a fatal vehicular accident). Often, after a long life together, the bereaved person is disturbed by a sense of unfinished business or unfulfilled wishes. The ultimate regret, however, is that the loved one was not able to continue to live a healthy and happy life.

Mental disorganization may be manifested by varying degrees of distractibility, poor concentration, confusion, forgetfulness, and lack of clarity, particularly in the early weeks of bereavement. The cumulative effect of the numerous upheavals in the mental, emotional, and cognitive lives of the bereaved person often lead to a sense of being overwhelmed, out of control, helpless, and powerless. The prospect of facing the myriad tasks of daily living and survival alone, of being battered by recurrent pain, and of being cognitively impaired may be perceived as a set of unmanageable forces. Even individuals who previously considered themselves to be strong emotionally may feel unable to cope.

The reality of being alone and the intensity of loneliness emerge over time. This loneliness often becomes more severe or it may initially manifest itself after the first several months of bereavement when family and friends begin to pull back and lessen their support. Loneliness can be one of the most painful and persistent aspects of bereavement for older bereaved spouses, and is may be felt even when the bereaved person is not alone (Lund et al. 1986a).

Not all of a bereaved person's affective experiences are negative and painful. Relief may be felt, occasionally at the expense of increased guilt feelings, especially after a prolonged illness. Bereaved persons often are surprised at their capacity to feel joy, peace, or happiness at the same time they are feeling sorrowful.

Dimension 2: Coping.   Facing reality initiates pain, which sets off a variety of protective mechanisms. Ideally, bereaved persons are able to regulate the amount of pain they can bear at one time and divert the rest using the most adaptive coping strategies possible. Examples of coping methods used to protect against the pain of grief include numbness and disbelief; emotional control and suppression; altered perspectives such as intellectualization, rationalization, and humor; faith; avoidance or exposure; activity; involvement with others; passive distraction such as listening to the radio or watching television; and indulgence in food or drink. Individuals generally use similar coping strategies to help them through the stress of bereavement that they use to manage other stress in their lives. However, it is possible that frail, elderly patients—who often are limited by fewer supports, resources, and coping capacities—may be at a disadvantage for making use of coping skills.

Dimension 3: The continuing relationship with the deceased. The fundamental dilemma facing the bereaved person may be that reality demands they accept life without their loved one at the same time that (equally important) inner psychological forces dictate that they maintain their attachment and that they retrieve what has been lost (Bowlby 1969). Freud (1917/1957) originally conceptualized the work of grief to be the gradual detachment of the libido from the deceased: "Reality-testing has shown that the loved object no longer exists, and it proceeds to demand that all libido shall be withdrawn from its attachment to it." In modifying Freud's original libidinal theory, contemporary theorists postulate that the task of grief is to realign attachment bonds rather than giving them up (Bowlby 1961; Glick et al. 1974; Parkes 1972; Rubin 1990; Shuchter and Zisook 1987; Worden 1991). In one sense, the person is dead and a major aspect of a living and breathing relationship has been lost; in another sense, the deceased person lives on indefinitely. There are many ways that bereaved individuals have found to maintain important aspects of the relationship. For example, many bereaved persons perceive that the deceased continues to have an existence either in a spiritual form, such as in heaven, or in a material form, such as being at the burial site or where ashes have been scattered. The bereaved person frequently maintains contact during the early weeks and months by an intermittent sense of anticipation that the deceased will suddenly appear: searching in crowds; hearing approaching footsteps or voices; seeing an image of the deceased; feeling the deceased hovering and watching out for or protecting the bereaved person. The bereaved individual frequently may communicate with the deceased, asking for advice or summarizing the day's events. Note that all these "unusual" experiences occur in the context of normal reality testing. Other ways of maintaining contact with the deceased include symbolic representations such as maintaining the deceased's clothing, writings, favored possessions, jewelry, or pets and through living legacies such as identification phenomena (e.g., identifying with the illness, mannerisms, or goals of the deceased), carrying out the deceased's mission, memorial donations, or seeing the deceased live on in descendants. Bereaved individuals often dream of the deceased, sometimes experiencing vivid visions of the individual returning or explaining why they have been away. Periodic visitations to the cemetery or lighting candles at a place of worship may keep memories alive. Ultimately, memories become the most powerful means of continuing the relationship with the deceased. These memories often are bittersweet: on one hand, they provide comfort in bringing the spouse back to life; on the other hand, they stimulate pain as a reminder of loss.

Dimension 4: Functioning. Bereavement has an impact on health, occupational functioning, and social functioning. Health may be compromised after the death of a loved one (Caserta et al. 1990); bereaved persons are at risk for increased drinking, abuse of drugs, major depression, anxiety disorders, and disorders similar to posttraumatic stress (Horowitz 1986; Klerman 1977; Osterweis 1984; Zisook and Shuchter 1991b). (The "Complications of Grief" section of this chapter discusses this further.) Other forms of dysfunction include impaired work performance, social inhibition, and isolation. The challenges of new roles or new demands, such as filing insurance claims or obtaining social security benefits, may appear overwhelming to bereaved persons. Older men may have to learn to take care of themselves for the first time: cooking, shopping, and keeping house. Women may be challenged by the requirements of home repairs, servicing the car, or maintaining legal and financial records (Lund et al. 1986a). Help with some of these mundane but troublesome difficulties may obviate turmoil and complications.

Dimension 5: Relationships. Bereavement alters the dynamics of many relationships (Lund et al. 1990). There may be changes in relationships' needs, in levels of closeness or support, or in the nature of roles or meanings. Some relationships may end and others may begin, but all are affected. Complex changes occur within the family. For example, there may be conflicts in the expectations of the children and surviving parent over issues of emotional support, finances, decision making, and future directions in a family where a spouse dies and where there are grown children. The survivor may have to contend with the grief of surviving parents, children, inlaws, siblings, and with their efforts to enlist support for themselves. There is an opportunity for achieving greater intimacy, repairing old wounds, and sharing grief; conversely, conflict and disruption may be exacerbated.

Friends may be a major source of support for the bereaved person, especially when empathy and sympathy are freely given and when friends are accepting of the enormous fluctuations of feelings, moods, and needs of a bereaved person. Friends can share the pain and allow its free expression. This may be true especially in elderly people when many friends of the bereaved person may have had similar experiences and can form an informal support group. Enduring and supportive friendships may evolve with those people whose life experiences are similar to the survivor's loss and pain. Generally, people who have experienced grief can offer greater acceptance and comfort to bereaved persons; but there are times when friends may feel threatened or overwhelmed by the intensity of a bereaved person's neediness and suffering.

Eventually, most widows and widowers must deal with the intricacies of single life. When they attempt to begin a new romance they may be challenged by continued devotion to the spouse, societal sanctions, fears of recurring loss, and perceived disloyalty of the children (Lund et al. 1993). This may be particularly difficult for an older individual who has not dated for many years and who may be somewhat frightened and perplexed by contemporary social and dating customs.

Dimension 6: Identity.   Persons living through the profoundly disruptive experience of bereavement are subject to dramatic changes in the way they view themselves and their world. Bereaved individuals initially feel helpless and overwhelmed; these feelings eventually give way to more positive self-images as bereaved individuals find themselves able to tolerate their grief, carry out tasks, and learn new ways of dealing with the world. There is an evolving sense of strength, autonomy, independence, assertiveness, and maturity (Pollock 1987). Bereaved individuals frequently become more appreciative of daily living and (perhaps) more patient, accepting, and giving; people unable to meet these challenges stagnate and do not experience personal growth. Therapy or support groups may be necessary in such cases to facilitate growth and to help the bereaved person achieve an integrated, healthy self-concept and a stable worldview.

Complications of Grief

Grief is a complex, multidimensional process involving physical, psychological, and sociological reactions and responses. Although the majority of people do not become seriously ill or die immediately following a significant loss, prevailing evidence suggests that bereaved persons are at high risk for a number of complications. Sanders (1993) pointed out that "grief affects everyone, but unequally." Some bereaved individuals have relatively uncomplicated grief reactions; others may experience multiple complications. Some people are affected so severely that they die; others seem to take grief in stride, painfully acknowledging the loss while managing to go on with their lives (Cleiren 1991). The two major categories of complications are 1) those that arise from the process of grief itself (too little, too much, or too long) and 2) medical and psychiatric disorders that often occur or worsen following a significant loss.

There is no one-to-one correlation between known risk factors and the specific complications of grief. However, several risk factors have been identified as seriously debilitating and as potentially leading to a number of possible complications (Sanders 1993). These include multiple, sudden, or unexpected deaths such as suicide and murder; catastrophic circumstances; and stigmatized deaths such as from abortion or AIDS (Parkes 1993; Rynearson and McCreery 1993); preexisting personality in the bereaved person marked by insecurity, low self-esteem, dependence, and characteristic difficulties coping with stress (Parkes 1990); a relationship with the deceased marked by ambivalence or undue dependency (Parkes 1975); loss of a child (Osterweis et al. 1984; Sanders 1980); poor health, depression, or prior substance abuse (Zisook and Shuchter 1993b); multiple concurrent life stresses or other crises (Parkes 1971; Raphael 1983); and perceived lack of social support (Gallagher et al. 1981; Vachon 1982). In a study of the course and predictors of spousal bereavement in late life, Lund et al. (1993) found that those widows/widowers who remarried, had supportive relationships with others, or who were active in their religion were somewhat more likely to be doing well at follow-up than were individuals with more problematic social relationships. The strongest predictors of adjustment to bereavement, however, were the personal resources unique to each person: positive self-esteem and personal competencies in managing the tasks of daily life.

The idea of gender and age as substantial risk factors are somewhat controversial. Some studies have found that men are more likely than women to experience a number of complications of bereavement, but no fully consistent story has yet emerged (Osterweis et al. 1984; Sanders 1993). Several studies have suggested that youth is a relative risk factor for many bereavement complications and that elderly people tend to adjust better than young adults to the stress of bereavement (Jacobs 1993; Osterweis 1984; Sanders 1993; Stroebe and Stroebe 1993b). It may be that the pacing of grief is affected more by age than are the occurrences of complications. Zisook et al. (1994) and Sanders (1981) found that the observed increased intensities of grief and depression found in young compared with old individuals during the first year of bereavement diminish or even reverse during the second year.

Complications in the Process of Grief

Absent, delayed, or inhibited grief (too little).   Absent, delayed, or inhibited grief reactions are relatively common in children under the age of 5 and in elderly persons (Parkes 1965). Stern et al. (1951) was struck by the absence of apparent grief in middle-aged to elderly bereaved individuals. Because many of the individuals in this study experienced somatic illnesses, Stern suggested that the affective disturbance of grief was channeled somehow into somatic symptoms. Cumming and Henry (1961), on the other hand, believed that a process of "disengagement" takes place at approximately age 65 and that "with age occurs a mutual severing of ties between a person and others in his society" so that events such as loss of a spouse are less traumatic than in younger age groups. Parkes (1965) concludes that an inhibition of grief may be a characteristic of the old and that the long-term effects of this inhibition are unknown.

Although it is widely held that an overt expression of grief is healthy and essential whereas its absence is pathological (Deutsch 1937), recent empirically based studies on grief outcomes have not confirmed this association (Wortman and Silver 1989). Despite the data, we often are consulted by concerned friends or relatives of bereaved individuals (particularly elderly ones) who worry that insufficient grief is being displayed, fearing that the bereaved person is keeping everything inside and will ultimately burst. Often, however, individuals do not burst, but rather grieve in their own way and in their own time. Such attenuated grief reactions are most likely to occur when the relationship with the deceased had been unduly dependent and/or ambivalent (Parkes and Weiss 1983; Raphael and Maddison 1976), the prebereavement relationship did not have a deep quality of attachment (if, for example, the bereaved individual has an intensely narcissistic personality disorder), or the grief is inhibited by the presence of a major psychiatric disorder (Raphael et al. 1993).

Hypertrophic grief (too much).   Overly intense grief has not been described fully or studied comprehensively. Grief is considered one of the most intensely painful emotions ever experienced; therefore, it is difficult to state when its intensity might be considered exaggerated. Usually, the frequency and intensity of the acute pangs of grief begin to lessen by the third to fourth month after the loss. Several investigators have found that early intense grief reactions correlate significantly with later distress and sometimes with major depression (Clayton 1990; Parkes 1972; Zisook and Shuchter 1991a). Although no known risk factors have been identified, it appears that hypertrophic grief reactions generally are uncommon (Parkes 1983), particularly in older individuals (Zisook et al. 1990b). When grief responses and preoccupation with the deceased are so intense that they interfere with function and are not substantially lessened within the first few months of bereavement, careful consideration should be given to whether symptoms of a major depression, anxiety disorder, or a posttraumatic stress disorder have evolved to complicate the bereavement and impede its progress. Treatment should be directed at the psychiatric disorder if criteria for one or more of these syndromes are met.

Chronic grief (too long). According to Parkes (1965), chronic grief may be the most common form of complication. Chronic grief frequently is reported in young and middle-age adults, most often in women and in adolescents. The reaction in chronic grief is prolonged and the general impression is of deep, pressing, and unrelenting sorrow. Individuals are repeatedly overwhelmed by their yearning and despair, and they are unable to give up their intense preoccupation and idealization of the deceased. There is no consensus regarding how long grief lasts before it should be termed chronic. It is the unmodulated intense preoccupation with the deceased, rather than the length of grieving and its interference with other relationships or functioning, that define pathological grief. Most investigators would not consider periodic preoccupation with the deceased (such as on or around holidays or anniversaries) to be evidence of chronic grief. However, persistent and pervasive preoccupation accompanied by dysphoria and/or other complications of grief lasting beyond the first year after the loss is considered too long and requires clinical attention. Risk factors for chronic grief are loss of a child (Raphael 1983), a dependent or clinging relationship with the deceased (Parkes 1983), or an unnatural death (Rynearson 1987b). Treatment often is protracted and difficult.

High-Risk Medical and Psychiatric Complications

Medical morbidity and mortality. Whether and to what extent medical health is compromised after the death of a loved one is somewhat controversial. Some investigators have found bereavement poses minimal risk to the health of survivors (Clayton 1979; Murrell et al. 1988; Norris and Murrell 1990), particularly in individuals not already ill before the death.

Other investigators have presented evidence that bereavement is associated with declining health status in a larger than expected number of bereaved persons. For example, elderly widows and widowers have been found to increase use of medical health care compared to married men and women (McHorney and Mor 1988; Mor et al. 1986; Parkes 1964; Shuchter and Zisook 1993; Weiner et al. 1975). Complaints of somatic symptoms and poor health are more numerous in elderly persons who have lost a spouse than in married individuals (Maddison and Viola 1968; Parkes 1972; Raphael 1983; Thompson et al. 1984). Evidence regarding an increased incidence of specific medical disorders after loss is meager (Jacobs and Douglas 1979; Klerman and Izen 1977; Osterweis et al. 1984; Stroebe et al. 1981, 1982); cardiovascular disease is the most frequently mentioned disorder that may be linked to bereavement (Chambers and Reiser 1953; Engle 1961; Parkes 1972; Weiner et al. 1975).

Even though the most frequently given risk factor for declining health after bereavement is preexisting health problems, Thompson et al. (1984) reported that elderly bereaved spouses (especially widows) were at risk for worsening of old illnesses and for development of new ones in the months immediately following the death. However, this vulnerability to poor health was not found at 30 months follow-up (Gallagher-Thompson et al. 1983). Perhaps the increased health risk in widows immediately after the death is related to the increased caretaking burden assumed by wives (Hutchin 1993; Moss et al. 1993) and the likelihood that these women have neglected their own health while focusing on the needs of their dying husbands. Shuchter and Zisook (1993) suggested that a reasonable preventive health intervention would be to ensure that caregivers and recently bereaved spouses receive the necessary medical attention during these high-risk periods.

Most studies on medical morbidity are limited by flaws in design and small sample sizes (Osterweis et al. 1984), but several large-scale studies have demonstrated higher mortality rates for widows/widowers compared to their married counterparts (Cox and Ford 1964; Helsing and Szklo 1981; Kaprio et al. 1987; Kraus and Lilienfeld 1959; Levav et al. 1988; Rees and Lutkins 1967). In a comprehensive review of the mortality of bereavement, Stroebe and Stroebe (1993a) concluded that the vast majority of studies support an excess mortality rate in bereaved versus nonbereaved individuals. Death rates appear lowest for married individuals, followed (in order) by single, widowed, and divorced persons.

Elderly persons are afflicted with more chronic illnesses than younger people, but the group at greatest risk of dying (relative to their peers) following the death of a loved one are younger widows (Helsing and Szklo

1981; Jones 1987; Kaprio et al. 1987; Mellstrom et al. 1982). One study, however, found that the oldest old persons may be at relatively higher risk compared to controls (Bowling and Charlton 1987). The highest period of risk for widowers appears to be during the first 6 months after the loss (Helsing and Szklo 1981; Rees and Lutkins 1967; Young et al. 1963); this period of risk for widows may be delayed 1 or 2 years (Cox and Ford 1964; Helsing and Szklo 1981). Other risk factors include moving into a chronic care facility (Helsing and Szklo 1981), social isolation and lack of social support (Bowling and Charlton 1987; Gallagher-Thompson et al. 1993; Helsing and Szklo 1981), living alone or not remarrying (for widowers) (Helsing and Szklo 1981), sudden deaths for widowers or widows under 50, and death from a chronic illness for widowers between 50 and 64 years (Stroebe and Stroebe 1993a). One well-known study of survivors of Israeli soldiers killed in war did not reveal an overall increase in mortality, but found that widowed or divorced parents who lost a son had an increased mortality rate that was statistically significant in the mothers (Levav et al. 1988).

No consistent pattern emerges for the causes of excess mortality during bereavement (Stroebe and Stroebe 1993a). The most compelling data implicate death from suicide (Kaprio et al. 1987; MacMahon and Pugh 1965), accidents (Helsing and Szklo 1981; Jones 1987; Mellstrom et al. 1982), and heart disease (Jones et al. 1984; Kaprio et al. 1987; Mellstrom et al. 1982; Parkes et al. 1969); but cancer, liver cirrhosis, diabetes, and infectious diseases also are mentioned (Klerman and Izen 1977; Osterweis et al. 1984; Stroebe and Stroebe 1993a).

Psychiatric morbidity.   The loss of a spouse is a severe life stress event that has been linked to the onset, exacerbation, or maintenance of a variety of psychiatric disorders.

Substance use.   Widows and widowers have been found to be at high risk for increased use of alcohol, tobacco, and other substances (Blankfield 1983; Klerman and Izen 1977; Osterweis et al. 1984). For example, Maddison and Viola (1968) found that middle-aged widows were more likely than married women to report increased cigarette smoking and use of alcohol and drugs (primarily sedatives and hypnotics). Clayton (1979) found a higher incidence of alcohol use in a sample of older widows and widowers compared to married controls. These increases occurred for the most part in people who had preexisting alcohol problems. Similarly, Valanis et al. (1987) found more widows and widowers than controls use alcohol, but no new cases of heavy or problem drinking were found. Furthermore, Valanis reported that most bereaved persons did not change patterns of drinking; 16% of widows and widowers increased their drinking after the death of the spouse, 11% decreased their drinking, and 57% did not change the quantity of alcohol they consumed. Those most vulnerable to increasing alcohol consumption tended to be women who were depressed and who had fewer economic resources. Measuring changes in alcohol use in a sample of middle-aged and elderly widows and widowers (mean age = 61 years), Zisook et al. (1990a) found approximately equal numbers of those who increased (30%) versus those who decreased (26%) the number of days per month they drank. However, when changes in alcohol use was measured by the quantity of alcohol consumed per drinking day, Zisook reported that more widows and widowers increased (34%) than decreased (10%) their quantity of alcohol consumption. Risk factors for increased drinking included the quantity of drinking before the death, being male, a past history of major depression, dissatisfaction with social and emotional supports, and experiencing a depressive episode soon after the death.

Anxiety symptoms and syndromes.   Although bereavement may be a better paradigm for separation anxiety (Clayton 1990; Parkes 1972) than for depression, anxiety symptoms and syndromes have received little emphasis in the literature. Anxiety is not listed as one of the "morbid" complications of bereavement, but Lindemann's (1944) description of "normal" grief highlights symptoms of somatic anxiety (tightness in throat, choking sensation, sighing) and intense subjective anxiety (tension, mental pain, restlessness, feelings of unreality, and depersonalization). The "waves of grief" Lindemann describes resemble the "pangs of pining and yearning" that Bowlby (1969) ascribed to separation anxiety and that he conceptualized as the characteristic features of grief. Lending some biological support to the close relationship of separation anxiety to bereavement, Shuchter et al. (1986) reported that dexamethasone nonsuppression was related more to anxiety levels than to depressive symptoms or syndromes in a group of recently bereaved widows.

Parkes (1964) found that grief can precipitate a variety of anxiety symptoms and states. He noted that 1) restlessness, tension, insomnia, headaches, and irritability are common during the first year of spousal bereavement and 2) panic attacks were common in the first several months. Clayton (1968, 1974) found that some anxiety symptoms were more prevalent in widows than in married controls. Widows reported an increased frequency of anxiety attacks, insomnia, weight loss, fatigue, decreased concentration, poor memory, shortness of breath, palpitations, and blurred vision. Maddison and Viola (1968) found increased nervousness, panic feelings, fears, insomnia, and trembling in widows 1 year after the deaths of their husbands. Zisook et al. (1990b, 1993) reported high risk rates of several anxiety symptoms during the first 7 months of spousal bereavement, elevated scores on Hopkins Symptom Checklist scales of anxiety, somatization, interpersonal sensitivity, and obsessions in older widows and widowers compared to community norms. There was an increased use of prescribed antianxiety medications, hypnotics, and over-the-counter "nerve pills." Factors predicting continued high anxiety 7 months after the death of a loved one included female gender, increased depression and anxiety symptom intensity soon after the loss, nonresolution of grief, lower income, younger age, and less environmental support.

While most of the bereavement studies noted above emphasized the symptoms of anxiety rather than syndromes or disorders, Jacobs et al. (1990) used the modified Structured Clinical Interview for DSM-III to determine the prevalence of anxiety disorders during the first year of spousal bereavement (mean age = 55 years). He found more than 40% of bereaved spouses reported at least one type of anxiety disorder. There were higher than expected rates for panic and for generalized anxiety disorders during the entire first year, for agoraphobia in the first 6 months, and for social phobia in the latter 6 months. The risks for panic and generalized anxiety disorders were highest among those who had a past personal history of anxiety disorders.

Posttraumatic stress. The DSM-III-R specifically uses bereavement as an example of an event that does not fulfill the "stressor" criteria for the diagnosis of posttraumatic stress disorder (PTSD); that is, bereavement is not an unnatural event in an ordinary life. Some investigators consider bereavement to be an appropriate example of a posttraumatic stress syndrome (Horowitz 1986), and others limit the association of bereavement and PTSD to instances where the death occurred in association with traumatic circumstances (Raphael and Maddison 1976). Sudden, unexpected, violent, and untimely deaths may increase the risk of a number of unfavorable outcomes (Raphael 1977, 1983) including unresolved grief and poor health (Lundin 1984), anxiety symptoms (Lehman et al. 1987), and poor overall functioning (Parkes 1975). Rynearson (1981, 1984, 1987a, 1987b, 1990) and Parkes (1993) have compared the reactions to severely traumatic losses (such as suicide, homicide, or other forms of unnatural dying) to PTSD. Rynearson pointed out that people bereaved by a homicide event experience intrusive, vivid, and repetitive images of the death; impaired cognitive processes; nightmares; heightened arousal; hypervigilance; and avoidance.

Schut et al. (1991) reported that the duration of a deceased spouse's terminal illness does not correlate with high rates of developing PTSD in widows and widowers, but the bereaved spouses' perceptions that the death was unanticipated or that there had not been a satisfactory opportunity to make farewells correlated with development of PTSD. According to Middleton et al. (1993), bereavement complicated by PTSD can be differentiated from other bereavement reactions by the intrusive phenomena that often reflect the scene of the death or other traumatic images, anxiety, hyperarousal, nightmares, and other ongoing reexperiencing or avoidant phenomena. Some investigators have not found the suddenness or unexpectedness of the death of a loved one to be related to poor outcome in elderly individuals (Breckenridge et al. 1986); there is not much data on when or whether losses are likely to lead to PTSD in elderly persons. PTSD, as defined by DSM-III-R, is not a widely studied phenomenon in elderly persons under any circumstances. More work is warranted in this area.

Depression.   A large and growing body of literature documents the importance of grief and bereavement to the pathogenesis of depression. After the death of a spouse, most widows and widowers will experience intermittent symptoms of depression as part of their grief (Clayton 1990; Gallagher-Thompson et al. 1983; Nuss and Zubenko 1992). Symptoms frequently may be persistent and pervasive enough to meet criteria for a major depressive syndrome. Prevailing clinical wisdom suggests these depressive syndromes are not major depression but are aspects of uncomplicated bereavement. According to the DSM-III-R, if a major depressive syndrome occurs within "a few months" of the death of a loved one, the depression generally should not be considered major depression but should be considered uncomplicated bereavement (APA 1987). Such episodes are common, occurring in between 29% and 58% of widows and widowers 1 month after their spouse's death (Clayton et al. 1972; Gilewski et al. 1991; Harlow et al. 1991), 24% and 30% 2 months after the death (Futterman et al. 1990; Zisook and Shuchter 1991a), and approximately 25% 4 months after the death (Clayton et al. 1972; McHorney and Mor 1988). It is not at all clear, however, that such early depressive syndromes are as self-limiting or benign as the name "uncomplicated bereavement" might imply. For example, Zisook and Shuchter (1991a) and Gilewski et al. (1991) independently found that these early depressive syndromes were potent predictors of continued depression over longer follow-up. Zisook and Shuchter (1993a) found "uncomplicated bereavement" to be associated with frequent physician visits and self-perceived poor medical health; increased use of alcohol, other nonprescribed substances, and psychotropic medications; disrupted work performance and social adjustment; and poor overall adaptation to bereavement.

Although many studies on widowhood contain large percentages of elderly subjects, few bereavement studies have focused on elderly persons until recently. In the late 1970s, the National Institute on Aging established bereavement and aging as research funding priorities and funded three controlled, prospective, longitudinal studies that looked at depression and its risk factors after late-life bereavement (Lund et al. 1993). The first of these studies took place in California (Breckenridge et al. 1986; Gallagher-Thompson et al. 1982, 1983; Gilewski et al. 1991; Futterman et al. 1990; Thompson et al. 1984), the second in Utah (Caserta and Lund 1992; Caserta et al. 1989; Dimond et al. 1987; Lund 1989; Lund et al. 1985, 1986a, 1986b, 1990, 1993), and the third in Florida (Faletti et al. 1989). They were followed by a number of other investigations that examined depressive reactions in late-life bereavement (Bruce et al. 1990; Goldberg et al. 1988; Harlow et al. 1991; McHorney and Mor 1988; Norris and Murrell 1990; Zisook and Shuchter 1991b).

In general, these studies reveal that there are more similarities than differences between the depressive reactions experienced by older versus younger individuals. As in younger individuals, the risk for depressive symptoms and syndromes in late life is substantial (Breckenridge et al. 1986; Bruce et al. 1990; Gallagher-Thompson et al. 1983; Harlow et al. 1991) and remains greater than the risk for married controls for at least 2 years beyond the death of a loved one (Harlow et al. 1991; Zisook and Shuchter 1993b). On the other hand, several investigators have found that the frequency and intensity of depressive symptoms and syndromes after late life bereavement may be less than in younger individuals (Faletti et al. 1989; McHorney and Mor 1988; VanZandt et al. 1989). Zisook and Shuchter (1993b) found that risks for major depressive syndrome in older widows and widowers is less than in their younger counterparts only for the first year; by the end of the second year of bereavement the frequency of major depressive syndrome in widows and widowers older than 65 years is identical to the frequency in those under 65 years. Therefore, it may not be that older widows and widowers are less distressed or depressed than younger ones, but rather that it takes somewhat longer for the full impact of bereavement to be experienced.

There are more similarities than differences in the nature of the major depressive syndrome associated with bereavement in late life compared with non-bereavement-related major depression. Gallagher-Thompson et al. (1982) and Breckenridge et al. (1986) emphasized that the depressions experienced by late-life widows and widowers tend to be milder than other major depressive syndrome and that self-depreciation rarely is observed in bereavement reactions. Similarly, Bruce et al. (1990) found bereavement increased the risk for dysphoria and major depressive syndrome and that the major depressive syndrome experienced by widows and widowers was symptomatically similar to other major depressive syndrome except for fewer reports of guilt or worthlessness. One sleep study found abnormal sleep architecture in depressed elderly widows; this finding supports the similarity of bereavement-related major depressive syndrome to other forms of major depression (Reynolds et al. 1992). More studies using structured diagnostic interviews and carefully selected ambulatory depressed controls are needed to confirm or expand these observations.

Increased attention has been given in recent years to subsyndromal depressions (painful symptoms of depression that do not quite meet full criteria for major depression) (Judd et al. 1994). These subsyndromal depressions may be quite frequent in elderly persons and may be associated with substantial suffering and morbidity (Blazer 1994; Blazer and George 1987; Broadhead et al. 1990). A large number of elderly, bereaved individuals may experience subsyndromal depressions, although most of these depressions go unrecognized (Pasternak et al. 1994; Zisook et al. 1994). It is possible that subsyndromal depressions may represent early preclinical major depression, may be the aftermath of partially remitted major depression, or may be a form of attenuated major depression important in its own right. Much more investigation is needed on the frequency, course burden, and treatment of subsyndromal depressions.

The course of depressive symptoms and syndromes associated with bereavement may be very variable. Most investigators have found a decreasing frequency of depressive symptoms and major depressive syndrome during the first year of widowhood (Bornstein et al. 1973; Futterman et al. 1990; Gilewski et al. 1991; Harlow et al. 1991; Zisook and Shuchter 1991a). However, two studies that continued to track depressive syndromes during the second year of bereavement found little evidence of further decrease in their frequency. In one of the studies, the frequency of depressive syndromes was 16% compared with 10% in married control subjects at the end of 2 years of bereavement (Harlow et al. 1991); in the other study the frequency was 14% versus 4% (Zisook and Shuchter 1993b). Murrell et al. (1988) initially reported that the depressive symptoms in elderly bereaved individuals were intense but temporary; however, the same group later reported that conjugal bereavement (but not loss of a parent or child) in elderly persons is associated with an increased risk for depression that is not transient (it lasts at least 9 months) (Norris and Murrell 1990). The course of major depressive syndrome for many widows and widowers may be much more episodic than previously thought (Zisook and Shuchter 1993a).

Not all bereaved individuals experience major depressive syndrome after their loss. The adaptive capacities of individuals undergoing severe life stressors are impressive (Pollock 1987; Shuchter and Zisook 1993; Silverman 1972), but, because risk for developing a major depressive syndrome after bereavement is substantial and the morbidity of untreated depression so great, it is important to identify risk factors. In general, there are no consistent findings on risk factors that relate to gender. Some studies found that older widows are at higher risk (Bruce et al. 1990; Gallagher-Thompson et al. 1983) and other studies reported that older widowers are most vulnerable (Richards and McCallum 1979), but most studies have not found substantial differences between bereaved men and women (Clayton 1990; Feinson 1986; Zisook and Shuchter 1991a). Loss of a spouse may be a greater risk than most other types of losses (Norris and Murrell 1990). Poor prior physical and mental health (McHorney and Mor 1988; Nuss and Zubenko 1992) and prebereavement depression (Norris and Murrell 1990) or dysphoria (Bruce et al. 1990) are additional risk factors. A particularly traumatic loss, such as a suicide, may be especially likely to result in persistent depressive syndromes (Gilewski et al. 1991). Several investigators have emphasized the protective role of social supports in attenuating the risks for depression associated with late-life bereavement (Dimond et al. 1987; Goldberg et al. 1988; Norris and Murrell 1990; Nuss and Zubenko 1992). Others have identified early intense reactions soon after the loss (Farberow et al. 1987; Lund et al. 1985; Parkes and Weiss 1983; Zisook and Shuchter 1991a) and early depressive reactions (Dimond et al. 1987; Gilewski et al. 1991; Zisook and Shuchter 1991a) as powerful predictors of later depression. Additional risk factors include financial problems and global stress (Norris and Murrell 1990), recent disability (Goldberg et al. 1988), and subsequent losses in widowers (Siegel and Kuykendall 1990). Using a stepwise logistic regression procedure, Zisook and Shuchter (1993b) were able to identify a six-variable model that explained 27% of the variance and correctly classified 91% of widows and widowers in terms of major depressive syndrome 2 years after loss. The six variables are 1) presence of a major depressive syndrome soon after the loss, 2) intense symptoms of depression soon after the death, 3) family history of major depression, 4) increased alcohol consumption soon after the loss, 5) poor physical health around the time of the death, and 6) a sudden and unexpected death.

Treatment

Most bereaved individuals grieve, adapt to their loss, and get on with their lives (Pollock 1987; Shuchter and Zisook 1993) without requiring any professional intervention. Time is the great healer for the majority of persons who are not at high risk for complications. People do not necessarily "get over it," but they do "get used to it" and " get on with it" over time (Goin et al. 1979). Healthy and secure persons whose life experiences have led to a reasonable trust in themselves and others can be expected to cope effectively and to adjust to the death of a loved one. Multiple or unexpected and untimely deaths of people on whom the bereaved person depends or who depended on the bereaved person can overwhelm even the most secure person. Lack of security and support can undermine a person's capacity to cope with all types of bereavement (Parkes 1990), and poor physical or psychological health can render an otherwise secure and well supported individual vulnerable. In such circumstances, preventive interventions may help ward off the development of full-blown complications. Once complications develop, prompt and focused treatment may help reverse symptoms and/or may minimize long-term disability.

Prebereavement Counseling

The first level of primary prevention may occur before the death occurs. Most late-life bereavement occurs in the context of chronic illness and provides the possibility of "anticipatory" mourning (Schoenberg et al. 1974). Although data concerning the benefits of "anticipatory grief" are sparse, there is some support for the value of counseling families and loved ones before the death of a terminally ill family member occurs (Cameron and Parkes 1983). It is important that this counseling does not encourage a sense of helplessness in the bereaved person. Counseling should not encourage premature withdrawal from the dying person; the bereaved person should not act as though the dying person were already dead. Honest and open communication builds trust and allows the family to address unresolved conflicts, repair miscommunications, and begin to prepare for inevitable changes. Information is given in a straightforward way that can be heard but that does not constitute an overwhelmingly traumatic confrontation with the impending loss (Parkes and Weiss 1983).

Before the death of a loved one, especially if survivors are involved in a substantial caregiving role, it is likely that bereaved persons may neglect their own medical needs. Such neglect may add to the already heightened risks of medical and psychiatric complications after the death of the loved one. Sound preventive principles ensure that caregivers take care of their medical needs, eat and sleep well, and visit their physician for routine care. If they have a past history of major depression or anxiety disorders, their families and health providers should be alert to the heightened risk for exacerbation of their primary condition.

Hospice.   Hospice offers comprehensive care to dying patients and their families during the terminal stage of illness and is committed to continued bereavement care for the bereaved person. In one small study of a hospice treatment program in Britain, Parkes (1981) randomly assigned high risk survivors to no special treatment or to a brief supportive intervention 10 to 14 days after the death. After a 20-month follow-up, the supported group had better health scores and less use of drugs, alcohol, and tobacco. Hospice programs offer great opportunities for prebereavement and postbereavement intervention studies; few such studies have been completed.

Mutual support.   Since the development of Phyllis Silverman's Widows-to-Widows Program (1972, 1986), self-help interventions have played an important role in bereavement outcome (Liebermann 1993). Barrett (1978) was unable to demonstrate benefits for self-help groups, but several studies have suggested their effectiveness, especially for high-risk individuals. For example, in a controlled study of relatively young widows (mean age = 52), Vachon and colleagues (1980) found that the emotional support and practical assistance from a "widow contact" accelerated the rate of achieving landmark stages, especially for widows who were most distressed initially. Constantino (1988) reported lower depression scores and better social adjustment in widows treated with self-help groups than in a nontreatment control group; Liebermann and Videka-Sherman (1986) found that self-help groups significantly decrease depression scores and psychotropic medication use compared to no such treatment. Marmar et al (1988) found self-help groups are approximately as effective as brief, dynamic psychotherapy in bereaved women who were depressed and experiencing adjustment disorder, posttraumatic stress disorder, or major depression. Referral to self-help groups may provide needed support and "protection" for elderly bereaved individuals, especially for those with high-risk indicators or whose support system is weak.

Group psychotherapy.   Yalom and Vinogradov (1982) argued that bereavement groups constitute a particularly efficient preventive intervention for a large at-risk population and represent excellent preventive mental health practice. In a controlled study of brief group therapy for widows and widowers, Lieberman and Yalom (1992) found that group participants showed modest improvement on role functioning and positive psychological states compared with untreated controls. Both groups, however, showed improvement during the year; overall, the two groups' adjustment to their loss were more alike than different. Group therapy clearly is a form of treatment that requires further study.

Individual psychotherapy.   Surprisingly few controlled studies have evaluated the efficacy of individual psychotherapy for preventing or lessening the impact of bereavement complications. Two studies were unable to provide strong support for the efficacy of brief therapy for preventing long-term complications. In the first of these studies, Polak et al. (1975) found no differences between bereaved individuals who received immediate crisis intervention after the sudden death of a family member and those who did not receive treatment. In the second study, Gerber et al. (1975) found no differences in outcome between elderly widows and widowers assigned either to brief supportive psychotherapy or to no active treatment. In contrast to these two negative studies, Raphael (1977, 1978) found that high-risk widows benefited from early supportive psychotherapy. In widows who were at risk because of perceived nonsupportiveness of their social networks, such psychotherapy led to a reduction in health care use; those at risk because of ambivalent relationships with their husbands benefited from an attenuation of the severity of depressive symptoms. Raphael's study did not include elderly widows; therefore, it is important to replicate these important findings in older widows and widowers.

There are several published treatment studies, in addition to the preventive studies reviewed above, that support the usefulness of prompt treatment once complications arise. For example, Horowitz et al. (1984) found dynamic psychotherapy to be an effective treatment for adults with postbereavement adjustment disorders following the death of a parent or spouse. Interpersonal therapy using grief as its primary paradigm may be suited for dealing with chronic grief, depression, or anxiety disorders associated with bereavement (Klerman 1989). A small case report series suggests the potential effectiveness of interpersonal psychotherapy for bereavement-related depression following loss of a spouse in late life (Miller et al. 1994). Other forms of psychotherapy that have been described include "guided mourning" (Mawson et al. 1981), "re-grief work" (Volkan 1971), "grief resolution therapy" (Melges and De Maso 1980), and conjoint family therapy (Paul and Grosser 1965). Lazare (1979) advocates an individualized approach for treating unresolved grief; Worden (1991) and Shuchter and Zisook (1987) describe individualized, task-specific forms of treatment that may involve multiple modalities of care. These modes of treatment have not yet been systematically compared to each other in bereaved individuals; therefore, it is difficult for clinicians to know when one form of treatment may be preferable to others. These psychotherapies may have more in common than they have differences. Most of these therapies include some degree of education, support, attention to the relationship with the deceased as it developed before the death and as it has changed since, provocative techniques for those whose expression of grief is blocked, and assurances of "normality" for bereaved individuals who need to be reminded that their wide-ranging feelings and experiences are not deviant, abnormal, or fixed (Raphael et al. 1993).

Medications. Although many clinicians have strong opinions about the use of medication in grief reactions, there are no controlled studies on any medications for prevention or treatment of grief complications. Sleep is a frequent and persistent bereavement-related problem (Clayton 1979, 1990); therefore, hypnotics may be helpful on an as-needed basis. Persistent lack of sleep does not help anyone's health or well-being. There are few data on pharmacological approaches to anxiety disorders associated with bereavement, but there is no reason to think that treatment should not be similar to that given to nonbereaved individuals with anxiety syndromes. Depression is perhaps the best documented complication of bereavement. There are no current data on whether medication treatment of symptoms of depression or subsyndromal depressions does more good than harm, but data on the negative consequences of these "mild" depressive reactions are being collected (Broadhead et al. 1990; Judd et al. 1994; Pasternak et al. 1994). Two open studies with tricyclic antidepressants support the safety and efficacy of these medications for bereavement-related major depressive syndromes (Jacobs et al. 1987; Pasternak et al. 1991), but controlled trials are needed. It is possible that treatment of the early depressive syndromes often seen within months of the death of a loved one may help prevent some of the prolonged suffering, morbidity, and even mortality associated with bereavement. Longitudinal controlled trials are lacking, however.

Special Concerns

Most information on late-life bereavement comes from studies on widows and widowers. More information is needed on the natural history and epidemiology of other losses—such as loss of children, siblings, friends, and nondeath losses—faced in late life. Little is known of how different cultures and subcultures deviate from the white, middle class norms described in this chapter. The oldest old persons have not been well described in the bereavement literature, and the particular characteristics or needs of bereaved persons with cognitive difficulties are unknown. There are few treatment studies specifically of late life bereavement. Should subsyndromal depressions be treated? If so, how? How soon after the death should a major depressive syndrome be considered pathological and be treated? Under what circumstances are particular psychotherapeutic approaches, or antidepressant medications, or combinations indicated? How long should treatment continue? There are many unanswered questions that require further inquiry.

References

American Psychiatric Association: Diagnostic and Statistical Manual of Mental Disorders, 3rd Edition, Revised. Washington, DC, American Psychiatric Association, 1987

Barrett CJ: Effectiveness of widows' groups in facilitating change. J Consult Clin Psychol 46:20, 1978

Blankfield A: Grief and alcohol. Am J Drug Alcohol Abuse 9:435–446, 1983

Blazer DG: Epidemiology of depressive disorders in late life, in Diagnosis and Treatment of Depression in Late Life: Results of the NIMH Consensus and Development Conference. Edited by Schneider LS, Reynolds CF, Leibowitz BD, et al. Washington, DC, American Psychiatric Press, 1994, pp 9–20

Blazer DG, George LK: The epidemiology of depression in an elderly community population. Gerontologist 27:281–287, 1987

Bornstein PE, Clayton PJ, Halikas JA, et al: The depression of widowhood after thirteen months. Br J Psychiatry 122:561–566, 1973

Bowlby J: Processes of mourning. Int J Psychoanal 42:317–340, 1961

Bowlby J: Attachment and Loss: Attachment, Vol 1. New York, Basic Books, 1969

Bowlby J: Attachment and Loss. Separation: Anxiety and Anger, Vol 2. New York, Basic Books, 1973

Bowlby J: Attachment and Loss. Loss: Sadness and Depression, Vol 3. New York, Basic Books, 1980/1981

Bowling A, Charlton J: Risk factors for mortality after bereavement: a logistic regression analysis. J R Coll Gen Pract 37:551–554, 1987

Breckenridge JN, Gallagher D, Thompson LW, et al: Characteristic depressive symptoms of bereaved elders. J Gerontol 41:163–168, 1986

Broadhead WE, Blazer DG, George LK, et al: Depression, disability days, and days lost from work in a prospective epidemiologic survey. JAMA 264:2524–2528, 1990

Bruce M, Kim K, Leaf P, et al: Depressive episodes and dysphoria resulting from conjugal bereavement in a prospective community sample. Am J Psychiatry 147:608–611, 1990

Cameron J, Parkes CM: Terminal care: evaluation of effects on surviving family of care before and after bereavement. Postgrad Med J 59:73–78, 1983

Caserta MS, Lund DA: Bereaved older adults who seek early professional help. Death Studies 16:17–30, 1992

Caserta MS, Van Pelt J, Lund DA: Advice on the adjustment to loss from bereaved older adults: an examination of resources and outcomes, in Older Bereaved Spouses: Research With Practical Applications. Edited by Lund DA. New York, Taylor & Francis/Hemisphere, 1989, pp 123–133

Caserta MS, Lund DA, Dimond MF: Understanding the context of perceived health ratings: the case of spousal bereavement in later life. Journal of Aging Studies 4:231–243, 1990

Chambers WN, Reiser MF: Emotional stress in the precipitation of congestive heart failure. Psychosom Med 15:38–60, 1953

Clayton PJ: Mortality and morbidity in the first year of bereavement. Arch Gen Psychiatry 30:747–750, 1974

Clayton PJ: The sequelae and nonsequelae of conjugal bereavement. Am J Psychiatry 136:1530–1534, 1979

Clayton PJ: Bereavement and depression. J Clin Psychiatry 51:34–40, 1990

Clayton PJ, Desmarais L, Winokur G: A study of normal bereavement. Am J Psychiatry 125:168–178, 1968

Clayton PJ, Halikas JA, Maurice WL: The depression of widowhood. Br J Psychiatry 120:71–76, 1972

Cleiren MPHD: Adaptation After Bereavement. Leiden University, Leiden, DSWO Press, 1991

Constantino RE: Comparison of two group interventions for the bereaved. Image 20:83–87, 1988

Cox PR, Ford JR: The mortality of widows shortly after widowhood. Lancet 1:163–164, 1964

Cumming E, Henry WR: Growing Old. New York, Basic Books, 1961

Deutsch H: Absence of grief. Psychoanal Q 6:12–22, 1937

DeVaul RA, Zisook S, Faschingbauer TR: Clinical aspects of grief and bereavement. Prim Care 6:391–402, 1979

Dimond MF, Lund DA, Caserta MS: The role of social support in the first two years of bereavement in an elderly sample. Gerontologist 27:599–604, 1987

Engel GL: Is grief a disease? Psychosom Med 23:18–22, 1961

Faletti MV, Gibbs JM, Clark C, et al: Longitudinal course of bereavement in older adults, in Older Bereaved Spouses: Research With Practical Applications. Edited by Lund DA. New York, Taylor & Francis/Hemisphere, 1989, pp 37–51

Farberow NL, Gallagher DE, Gilewski MJ, et al: An examination of the early impact of bereavement on psychological distress in survivors of suicide. Gerontologist 27:592–598, 1987

Feinson MC: Aging widows and widowers: are there mental health differences? Int J Aging Hum Dev 23:241–255, 1986

Freud S: Mourning and melancholia (1917), in The Standard Edition of the Complete Psychological Works of Sigmund Freud. Translated and edited by Strachey J. London, Hogarth Press, 1957, p 217

Futterman A, Gallagher D, Thompson LW, et al: Retrospective assessment of marital adjustment and depression during the first two years of spousal bereavement. Psychol Aging 5:277–283, 1990

Gallagher DE, Thompson LW, Peterson JA: Psychosocial factors affecting adaptation to bereavement in the elderly. Int J Aging Hum Dev 14:79–95, 1981

Gallagher-Thompson DE, Breckenridge JN, Thompson LW: Similarities and differences between normal grief and depression in older adults. Essence 5:127–140, 1982

Gallagher-Thompson DE, Breckenridge J, Thompson LW, et al: Effects of bereavement on indicators of mental health in elderly widows and widowers. J Gerontol 38: 565–571, 1983

Gallagher-Thompson D, Futterman A, Farberow N, et al: The impact of spousal bereavement on older widows and widowers, in Handbook of Bereavement: Theory, Research and Intervention. Edited by Stroebe MS, Stroebe W, Hansson RO. Cambridge, Cambridge University Press, 1993, pp 227–239

Gerber I, Weiner A, Battin D, et al: Brief therapy to the aged bereaved, in Bereavement: Its Psychosocial Aspects. Edited by Schoenberg B, Gerber I. New York, Columbia University Press, 1975, pp 310–313

Gilewski MJ, Farberow NL, Gallagher DE, et al: Interaction of depression and bereavement on mental health in the elderly. Psychol Aging 6:67–75, 1991

Glick IO, Weiss RS, Parkes CM: The First Year of Bereavement. New York, Wiley, 1974

Goin MK, Burgoyne RW, Goin JM: Timeless attachment to a dead relative. Am J Psychiatry 136:988–989, 1979

Goldberg EL, Comstock GW, Harlow SD: Emotional problems and widowhood. J Gerontol 3:5206–5208, 1988

Hansson RO, Carpenter BN, Fairchild SK: Measurement issues in bereavement, in Handbook of Bereavement. Edited by Stroebe MS, Stroebe W, Hansson RO. Cambridge, England, Cambridge University Press, 1993, pp 62–74

Harlow SD, Goldberg EL, Comstock GW: A longitudinal study of the prevalence of depressive symptomatology in elderly widowed and married women. Arch Gen Psychiatry 48:1065–1068, 1991

Helsing KJ, Szklo M: Mortality after bereavement. Am J Epidemiol 114:41–52, 1981

Holmes T, Rahe R: The social readjustment rating scale. J Psychosom Res 11:213–218, 1967

Horowitz MJ: Stress Response Syndromes. Northvale, NJ, Aronson, 1986

Horowitz MJ, Marmar C, Weiss DS, et al: Brief psychotherapy of bereavement reactions. Arch Gen Psychiatry 41:438–448, 1984

Hutchin S: The distress of care giving. Presented at the 146th annual meeting of the American Psychiatric Association, San Francisco, CA, May 22–27, 1993

Information Please Almanac (46th Edition). Boston, MA, Houghton-Mifflin, 1993

Jacobs S: Pathologic Grief. Washington, DC, American Psychiatric Press, 1993

Jacobs SC, Douglas L: Grief: a mediating process between a loss and illness. Compr Psychiatry 20:165–175, 1979

Jacobs SC, Nelson JC, Zisook S: Treating depression of bereavement with antidepressants: a pilot study. Psychiatr Clin North Am 10:501–510, 1987

Jacobs SC, Hansen F, Kasl S, et al: Anxiety disorders in acute bereavement: risk and risk factors. J Clin Psychiatry 51:267–274, 1990

Jones DR: Heart disease mortality following widowhood: some results from the OPCS longitudinal study. J Psychosom Res 31:325–333, 1987

Jones DR, Goldblatt PO, Leon DA: Bereavement and cancer: some results using data on deaths of spouses from the Longitudinal Study of the Office of Population Censuses and Surveys. Br Med J 298:461–464, 1984

Judd LL: Subsyndromal depression. Presented at the 146th annual meeting of the American Psychiatric Association, San Francisco, CA, May 22–27, 1993

Kaprio J, Koskenvuo M, Rita H: Mortality after bereavement: a prospective study of 95,647 widowed persons. Am J Public Health 77:283–287, 1987

Klerman GL: Depressive disorders: further evidence for increased medical morbidity and impairment of social functioning. Arch Gen Psychiatry 46:856–858, 1989

Klerman GL, Izen J: The effects of bereavement and grief on physical health and general well being. Adv Psychosom Med 9:63–104, 1977

Kraus AS, Lilienfeld AM: Some epidemiological aspects of the high mortality rate in the young widowed group. J Chronic Dis 10:207–217, 1959

Lazare A: Unresolved grief, in Outpatient Psychiatry. Edited by Lazare A. Baltimore, MD, Williams & Wilkins, 1979, pp 498–512

Lehman DR, Wortman CB, Williams AF: Long-term effects of losing a spouse or child in a motor vehicle crash. J Pers Soc Pathol 52:218–231, 1987

Levav I, Friedlander Y, Kark J, et al: An epidemiologic study of mortality among bereaved parents. N Engl J Med 319:457–461, 1988

Lieberman MA: Bereavement self-help groups: a review of conceptual and methodological issues, in Handbook of Bereavement: Theory, Research and Intervention. Edited by Stroebe MS, Stroebe W, Hansson RO. Cambridge, England, Cambridge University Press, 1993, pp 411–426

Lieberman MA, Videka-Sherman L: The impact of self-help groups on the mental health of widows and widowers. Am J Orthopsychiatry 56:435–449, 1986

Lieberman MA, Yalom I: Brief group psychotherapy for the spousally bereaved: a controlled study. Int J Group Psychother 42:117–132, 1992

Lindemann E: Symptomatology and management of acute grief. Am J Psychiatry 101:141–148, 1944

Lund DA: Older Bereaved Spouses: Research With Practical Applications. New York, Taylor & Francis/Hemisphere, 1989

Lund DA, Dimond MF, Caserta MS, et al: Identifying elderly with coping difficulties after two years of bereavement. Omega 16:213–223, 1985

Lund DA, Caserta MS, Dimond MF: Gender differences through two years of bereavement among the elderly. Gerontologist 26:314–320, 1986a

Lund DA, Caserta MS, Dimond MF, et al: Impact of bereavement on self-conceptions of older surviving spouses. Symbolic Interaction 9:235–244, 1986b

Lund DA, Caserta MS, Van Pelt J, et al: Stability of social support networks after late life spousal bereavement. Death Studies 14:53–73, 1990

Lund DA, Caserta MS, Dimond MF: The course of spousal bereavement in later life, in Handbook of Bereavement: Theory, Research and Intervention. Edited by Stroebe MS, Stroebe W, Hansson RO. Cambridge, Cambridge University Press, 1993, pp 240–254

Lundin T: Morbidity following sudden and unexpected bereavement. Br J Psychiatry 144:84–88, 1984

MacMahon B, Pugh TF: Suicide in the widowed. Am J Epidemiol 81:23–31, 1965

Maddison D, Viola A: The health of widows in the year following bereavement. J Psychosom Res 12:297–306, 1968

Marmar CR, Horowitz MJ, Weiss DS, et al: A controlled trial of brief psychotherapy and mutual-help group treatment of conjugal bereavement. Am J Psychiatry 145:203–212, 1988

Mawson D, Marks IM, Ramm L, et al: Guided mourning for morbid grief: a controlled study. Br J Psychiatry 138:185–193, 1981

McHorney CA, Mor V: Predictors of bereavement depression and its health services consequences. Med Care 26:882–893, 1988

Melges FT, DeMaso DR: Grief resolution therapy: reliving, revising and revisiting. Am J Psychother 34:51–61, 1980

Mellstrom D, Nilsson A, Oden A, et al: Mortality among the widowed in Sweden. Scand J Soc Med 10:33–41, 1982

Middleton W, Raphael B, Martinek N, et al: Pathological grief reactions, in Handbook of Bereavement: Theory, Research and Intervention. Edited by Stroebe MS, Stroebe W, Hansson RO. Cambridge, Cambridge University Press, 1993, pp 44–61

Miller MD, Frank E, Cornes C, et al: Applying interpersonal psychotherapy to bereavement-related depression following loss of a spouse in late-life. Journal of Psychotherapy Practice and Research 3:149–162, 1994

Mor V, McHorney C, Sherwood S: Secondary morbidity among the recently bereaved. Am J Psychiatry 143:158–163, 1986

Moss MS, Moss SZ, Rubinstein R, et al: Impact of elderly mother's death on middle age daughters. Int J Aging Hum Dev 37:1–22, 1993

Murrell SA, Himmelfarb S, Phifer JF: Effects of bereavement/loss and pre-event status on subsequent physical health in older adults. Int J Aging Hum Dev 27:87–107, 1988

Norris FH, Murrell SA: Social support, life events, and stress as modifiers of adjustment to bereavement by older adults. Psychol Aging 5:429–436, 1990

Nuss WS, Zubenko GS: Correlates of persistent depressive symptoms in widows. Am J Psychiatry 149:346–351, 1992

Osterweis M, Solomon F, Green M (eds): Bereavement: Reactions, Consequences, and Care. Washington, DC, National Academy Press, 1984

Parkes CM: The effects of bereavement on physical and mental health: a study of the medical records of widows. BMJ 2:274–279, 1964

Parkes CM: Bereavement and mental illness. Br J Med Psychol 38:388–397, 1965

Parkes CM: Psycho-social transitions: a field for study. Soc Sci Med 5:101–115, 1971

Parkes CM: Bereavement: Studies of Grief in Adult Life, 2nd Edition. New York, International Universities Press, 1972

Parkes CM: Determinants of outcome following bereavement. Omega 6:303–323, 1975

Parkes CM: Evaluation of a bereavement service. Journal of Preventive Psychiatry 1:179–188, 1981

Parkes CM: Risk factors in bereavement: implications for the prevention and treatment of pathologic grief. Psychiatric Annals 20:308–313, 1990

Parkes CM: Psychiatric problems following bereavement by murder or manslaughter. Br J Psychiatry 162:49–54, 1993

Parkes CM, Weiss RS: Recovery From Bereavement. New York, Basic Books, 1983

Parkes CM, Benjamin B, Fitzgerald RG: Broken heart: a statistical study of increased mortality among widowers. Br Med J 1:740–743, 1969

Pasternak RE, Reynolds CF III, Schlernitzauer M, et al: Acute open-trial nortriptyline therapy of bereavement-related depression in late life. J Clin Psychiatry 52:307–310, 1991

Pasternak RE, Reynolds CF, Miller MD, et al: The symptom profile and two-year course of subsyndromal depression in spousally bereaved elders. American Journal of Geriatric Psychiatry 2:210–219, 1994

Paul N, Grosser G: Operational mourning and its role in conjoint family therapy. Community Ment Health J 1:339–345, 1965

Polak PR, Egan D, Vandenburgh R, et al: Prevention in mental health: a controlled study. Am J Psychiatry 132:146–149, 1975

Pollock GH: The mourning-liberation process in health and disease. Psychiatr Clin North Am 10:345–354, 1987

Raphael B: Preventive intervention with the recently bereaved. Arch Gen Psychiatry 34:1450–1454, 1977

Raphael B: Mourning and the prevention of melancholia. Br J Med Psychol 41:303–310, 1978

Raphael B: The Anatomy of Bereavement. New York, Basic Books, 1983

Raphael B, Maddison D: The care of bereaved adults, in Modern Trends in Psychosomatic Medicine. Edited by Hill OW. London, Butterworth, 1976

Raphael B, Middleton W, Martinek N, et al: Counseling and therapy of the bereaved, in Handbook of Bereavement: Theory, Research and Intervention. Edited by Stroebe MS, Stroebe W, Hansson RO. Cambridge, England, Cambridge University Press, 1993, pp 427–453

Rees W, Lutkins S: Mortality of bereavement. BMJ 4:13–16, 1967

Reynolds C, Hoch CC, Buysse DJ, et al: Electroencephalographic sleep in spousal bereavement and bereavement-related depression of late life. Biol Psychiatry 31:69–82, 1992

Richards JG, McCallum J: Bereavement in the elderly. N Z Med J 89:201–204, 1979

Rubin S: Treating the bereaved spouse: a focus on the loss process, the self and the other. Psychotherapy Patient 6:189–205, 1990

Rynearson EK: Suicide internalized: existential sequestrum. Am J Psychiatry 138:84–87, 1981

Rynearson EK: Bereavement after homicide: a descriptive study. Am J Psychiatry 141:1452–1454, 1984

Rynearson EK: Psychotherapy of pathologic grief: revisions and limitations. Psychiatr Clin North Am 10:487–500, 1987a

Rynearson EK: Psychological adjustment to unnatural dying, in Biopsychosocial Aspects of Bereavement. Edited by Zisook S. Washington, DC, American Psychiatric Association, 1987b

Rynearson EK: Pathologic grief: the queen's croquet ground. Psychiatric Annals 20:295–303, 1990

Rynearson EK, McCreery JM: Bereavement after homicide: a synergism of trauma and loss. Am J Psychiatry 150:250–261, 1993

Sanders CM: A comparison of adult bereavement in the death of a spouse, child and parent. Omega 10:303–322, 1980

Sanders CM: Comparison of younger and older spouses in bereavement outcome. Omega 11:217–232, 1981

Sanders CM: Risk factors in bereavement outcome, in Handbook of Bereavement: Theory, Research and Intervention. Edited by Stroebe MS, Stroebe W, Hansson RO. Cambridge, Cambridge University Press, 1993, pp 255–267

Schoenberg B, Carr AC, Kutscher AH, et al (eds): Anticipatory Grief. New York, Columbia University Press, 1974

Schut HAW, de Keijser J, van den Bout J, et al: Incidence and prevalence of post traumatic stress symptomatology in the conjugally bereaved. Paper presented to the Third International Conference on Grief and Bereavement in Contemporary Society, Sydney, Australia, 1991, June/July 1991

Shuchter SR: Dimensions of Grief: Adjusting to the Death of a Spouse. San Francisco, CA, Jossey-Bass, 1986

Shuchter SR, Zisook S: Multidimensional approach to widowhood. Psychiatric Annals 16:295–308, 1986

Shuchter SR, Zisook S: A multidimensional model of spousal bereavement, in Biopsychosocial Aspects of Bereavement. Edited by Zisook S. Washington, DC, American Psychiatric Association, 1987, pp 35–47

Shuchter SR, Zisook S: The course of normal grief, in Handbook of Bereavement: Theory, Research and Intervention. Edited by Stroebe MS, Stroebe W, Hansson RO. Cambridge, Cambridge University Press, 1993, pp 23–43

Shuchter SR, Zisook S, Kirkorowicz C, et al: The dexamethasone test in acute grief. Am J Psychiatry 143:879–881, 1986

Siegel JM, Kuykendall DH: Loss, widowhood, and psychological distress among the elderly. J Consult Clin Psychol 58:519–524, 1990

Silver RL, Wortman CB: Coping with undesirable life events, in Human Helplessness: Theory and Applications. Edited by Gabor J, Seligman MEP. New York, Academic Press, 1980, pp 279–340

Silverman PR: Widowhood and prevention intervention. Family Coordinator 21:95–102, 1972

Silverman PR: Widow-to-Widow. New York, Springer Press, 1986

Stern K, Williams GM, Prados M: Grief reactions in later life. Am J Psychiatry 108:289–294, 1951

Stroebe MS, Stroebe W: The mortality of bereavement: a review, in Handbook of Bereavement: Theory, Research and Intervention. Edited by Stroebe MS, Stroebe W, Hansson RO. Cambridge, England, Cambridge University Press, 1993a, pp 175–195

Stroebe W, Stroebe MS: Determinants of adjustment to bereavement in younger widows and widowers, in Handbook of Bereavement: Theory, Research and Intervention. Edited by Stroebe MS, Stroebe W, Hansson RO. Cambridge, England, Cambridge University Press, 1993b, pp 208–226

Stroebe MS, Stroebe W, Gergen KJ, et al: The broken heart: reality or myth? Omega 12:87–105, 1981

Stroebe W, Stroebe MS, Gergen K, et al: The effects of bereavement on mortality: a social psychological analysis, in Social Psychology and Behavioral Medicine. Edited by Eiser JR. Chichester, England, Wiley, 1982, pp 527–560

Thompson LW, Breckenridge JN, Gallagher D, et al: Effects of bereavement on self-perception of physical health in elderly widows and widowers. J Gerontol 39:309–314, 1984

U.S. Bureau of the Census: Current Population Reports: Demographic and Socioeconomic Aspects of Aging in the United States (Series P-23, No 138). Washington, DC, U.S. Government Printing Office, 1984

Vachon MLS: Predictors and correlates of adaptation in conjugal bereavement. Am J Psychiatry 139:998–1002, 1982

Vachon MLS, Sheldon AR, Lancee WJ, et al: A controlled study of self-help intervention for widows. Am J Psychiatry 137:1380–1384, 1980

Valanis B, Yeaworth RC, Mullis MR: Alcohol use among bereaved and nonbereaved older persons. J Gerontol Nurs 13:26–32, 1987

VanZandt S, Mou R, Abbott R: Mental and physical health of rural bereaved and nonbereaved elders: a longitudinal study, in Older Bereaved Spouses: Research With Practical Applications. Edited by Lund DA. New York, Hemisphere, 1989, pp 25–35

Volkan VD: "Regrief" therapy, in Bereavement: Its Psychosocial Aspects. Edited by Schoenberg G, Gerber IE, Wiener A, et al. New York, Columbia University Press, 1971, pp 334–350

Weiner A, Gerber IE, Battin D, et al: The process and phenomenology of bereavement, in Bereavement: Its Psychosocial Aspects. Edited by Schoenberg B, Berger I, Weiner A, et al. New York, Columbia University Press, 1975

Worden JW: Grief Counseling and Grief Therapy: A Handbook for the Mental Health Practitioner. New York, Springer, 1991

Wortman CB, Silver RC: The myths of coping with loss. J Consult Clin
    Psychol 57:349–357, 1989

Yalom ID, Vinogradov S: Bereavement groups: techniques and themes.
    Int J Group Psychother 34:419–430, 1982

Young M, Benjamin B, Wallis C: Mortality of widowers. Lancet 2:254–
    256, 1963

Zisook S: Unresolved grief, in Biopsychosocial Aspects of Bereavement.
    Edited by Zisook S. Washington, DC, American Psychiatric Associa-
    tion, 1987, pp 23–34

Zisook S, Shuchter SR: Depression through the first year after the death of
    a spouse. Am J Psychiatry 148:1346–1352, 1991a

Zisook S, Shuchter SR: Early psychological reaction to the stress of wid-
    owhood. Psychiatry 54:320–333, 1991b

Zisook S, Shuchter SR: Uncomplicated bereavement. J Clin Psychiatry
    54:365–372, 1993a

Zisook S, Shuchter S: Major depression associated with widowhood. Am J
    Geriatr Psychiatry 1:316–326, 1993b

Zisook S, Shuchter SR, Mulvihill M: Alcohol, cigarette and medication
    use during the first year of widowhood. Psychiatric Annals 20:318–
    326, 1990a

Zisook S, Mulvihill M, Shuchter SR: Widowhood and anxiety. Psychiatr
    Med 8:99–116, 1990b

Zisook S, Shuchter SR, Sledge P, et al: Aging and bereavement. J Geriatr
    Psychiatry Neurol 6:137–143, 1993

Zisook S, Shuchter SR, Sledge P: Diagnostic and treatment considerations
    in depression associated with late-life bereavement, in Diagnosis and
    Treatment of Depression in Late Life: Results of the NIMH Consen-
    sus and Development Conference. Edited by Schneider LS, Reynolds
    CF, Leibowitz BD, et al. Washington, DC, American Psychiatric Press,
    1994, pp 419–435

George S. Alexopoulos, M.D.

Affective Disorders

A ffective disorders in elderly individuals are a major clinical and public health problem with far-reaching medical, social, and economic consequences. In addition to the enormous suffering by the patient, geriatric depression exacerbates medical morbidity and disability and leads to family disruption. Since the mid-1980s there has been significant progress in the diagnosis and treatment of depression in elderly individuals, as well as in the understanding of potential risk factors. On the other hand, the field of geriatric mania is relatively nascent. The Consensus Development Conference on the Diagnosis and Treatment of Depression in Late Life (NIMH Panel 1992) recognized this progress by collecting and reviewing the opinions of experts and establishing what currently constitutes reliable knowledge in this area. This chapter is not an exhaustive review of geriatric affective disorders; instead, selected accomplishments in the field that form the basis of our current understanding and may become the fulcrum for research over the next decade will be highlighted.

Epidemiology of Depression

The National Institute of Mental Health Epidemiologic Catchment Area Survey observed that major depression is less frequent in elderly than in younger adults. The overall prevalence of major depression among persons ages 65 years or older was estimated to be 1.4% in women and 0.4% in men, with an overall prevalence of 1% (Weissman et al. 1988). This prevalence rate is approximately one-fourth of that of adults ages 18 to 44 years. These findings were confirmed by other investigators (Feldman et al. 1987; Hagnell et al. 1982; Klerman 1988; Koenig and Blazer 1992). Approximately 2% of the elderly population have dysthymic disorder, and 4% have an adjustment disorder with depressed mood (Blazer et al. 1987). A rather large percentage of elderly persons, approximately 15%, have depressive symptomatology that does not meet criteria for a specific depressive syndrome (Koenig and Blazer 1992). Nonetheless, nonsyndromic depression does not appear to increase with age (Koenig and Blazer 1992).

The relatively low prevalence of depressive syndromes identified in elderly populations may be due in part to methodological problems, including the tendency of elderly persons to express psychiatric symptoms in somatic terms, reluctance to recall and report psychiatric symptoms, and use of diagnostic categories that are unsuitable for elderly individuals (Koenig and Blazer 1992). In addition to methodological problems, a cohort effect has been suggested as a reason for the low prevalence of depression in this generation of elderly persons. The cohort effect is also supported by suicide studies showing that white men born in 1922 had lower suicide rates than cohorts born earlier (Blazer et al. 1986). Depression appears to have an increasingly earlier onset in cohorts born in more recent years, and there is a narrowing in the differential risk for depression between genders. However, the Stirling County Study failed to demonstrate a cohort effect (Murphy et al. 1984). Finally, depression appeared to be more frequent between 1960 and 1975 than in earlier years. This increase in the rates of major depression over time has been confirmed in large cross-national samples (Klerman et al. 1985).

Depression occurs at relatively high rates in special geriatric populations. In elderly medical outpatients, the prevalence of depression ranges from 7% to 36%, an average of 5% higher than that of community samples (Koenig and Blazer 1992). Medically hospitalized elderly patients have an even higher prevalence of depression, with a rate of 40% for combined major and minor depression (Koenig et al. 1991). In nursing home residents, major depression occurs at a rate of 12%–16%, and other depressive disorders were observed in 30%–35% of the institutionalized population (Parmelee et al. 1989; Rovner et al. 1986; Weissman et al. 1991).

Geriatric depression is associated with female gender, divorced or separated marital status, low socioeconomic level, poor social support, and recent adverse and unexpected life events. Severe impairment in medical health resulting in disability constitutes an important risk factor. Neurological and endocrinological disorders, as well as chronic obstructive pulmonary disease, myocardial infarction, and malignancies are associated with increased incidence of depression.

In conclusion, depressive syndromes occur in the older geriatric population at a rate lower than that of younger adults. However, very high rates of depression occur in socioeconomically deprived, medically ill, disabled, and institutionalized elderly persons; this depression must be recognized and treated. With the increase in the elderly population and the aging of birth cohorts who appear to be particularly prone to depression, an unprecedented number of elderly patients are expected to be in need of antidepressant treatment.

Underuse of mental health services has been noted in all age groups but is particularly common in the population over 65 (Blazer et al. 1987). The frequency of depression and the underutilization of mental health services in elderly individuals can only contribute to the disturbing rate of suicide in this age group. Until relatively recently, the lack of recognition of depression in elderly individuals was at least partly related to a health care provider bias that depression is a normal consequence of aging. Hopefully, this collusion of hopelessness between caregiver and patient will be dissipated through education about the normal consequences of aging and the realization that advances in therapeutics offer much hope for relief in frail elderly persons who have depression.

Diagnosis

In elderly individuals, depressive syndromes often occur in the context of medical and neurological disorders. Sometimes these conditions appear to predispose or trigger depression, for example, depression occurring in the context of hypothyroidism or after a myocardial infarction. In other cases, the relationship of medical or neurological illness to depression is less clear. However, overall medical severity and disability appear to be important risk factors for depression. For these reasons, geriatric depression is viewed as a heterogeneous entity. The hypothesis has been advanced that depression with onset in late life occurs in a heterogeneous group that includes a large subgroup of patients with neurological brain disorders that may or may not be evident when the depression first appears (Alexopoulos 1990). This assertion is supported by differences observed between late- and early-onset geriatric depression. Compared with patients with early-onset depression, patients with late-onset depression appear to have less frequent family history of mood disorders (Mendlewicz and Baron 1991), higher prevalence of dementing disorders (Alexopoulos et al. 1993b), more impairment in neuropsychological tests (Alexopoulos et al. 1993b), higher rate of dementia development on follow-up (Alexopoulos et al. 1993b), greater enlargement in lateral brain ventricles (Alexopoulos et al. 1992a), and more white-matter hyperintensities (Coffey et al. 1988, 1990). The heterogeneity of late-life depression imposes methodological limitations on studies of illness onset. Further research is needed to identify specific clinical and biological parameters that can further characterize subgroups of patients with late-onset depression and clarify their pathogenesis.

Dementia patients develop depression at a rate higher than that of the general population. Depressive manifestations of varying intensity occur in approximately 50% of dementia patients (Alexopoulos and Abrams 1991). Reports of the rate of major depression in Alzheimer's patients have been highly discrepant, ranging from 0% to 87% (Cummings et al. 1987; Knesvich et al. 1983; Merriam et al. 1988), with most studies showing a range of 17% to 31% (Wragg and Jeste 1989). Dementia patients being treated at psychiatric centers (Lazarus et al. 1987), as well as patients with mild to moderate dementia syndromes, are more likely to report depression (N. E. Miller 1980). Depressive symptomatology appears to be elicited more often when reports of relatives are used than when evaluation relies exclusively on the interviewer's impressions (Alexopoulos and Abrams 1991; Burns et al. 1990; Merriam et al. 1988). There is some evidence that a family history of mood disorder predisposes Alzheimer's patients to develop depression (Lawlor et al. 1989; Pearlson et al. 1990). However, further studies are needed to confirm this observation.

A review of nine studies revealed that depression occurs in approximately 24% of patients with cerebrovascular disease (Kramer and Reifler 1992). Cortical and lacunar infarct had the highest comorbidity with depression, and Binswanger's disease had the lowest. Left hemisphere lesions, especially those close to the frontal pole, are most frequently associated with post-stroke depression, and subcortical atrophy appears to be a predisposing factor (Starkstein et al. 1988a). It should be pointed out, however, that epidemiological studies failed to confirm the high incidence of post-stroke depression (House et al. 1991).

In addition to patients with Alzheimer's disease or cerebrovascular syndromes, Parkinson's disease patients appear to develop depression at a rate of up to 50% (Sano et al. 1989). The severity of depression does not appear to be related to the severity of motor disability.

The similarity of depressive manifestations to symptoms and signs of dementing disorders often poses diagnostic problems. Vegetative features seem to overlap with symptoms and signs of dementia (N. E. Miller 1980), whereas early-stage Alzheimer's patients show loss of interest, decreased energy, difficulty in concentration, agitation, or retardation (Alexopoulos and Abrams 1992). Apathy, a characteristic of frontal lobe syndrome, may be misidentified as retarded depression. Sad, downcast mood (N. E. Miller 1980) and psychic rather than vegetative features (Lazarus et al. 1987) have been found useful in distinguishing depression-dementia patients from patients with dementia alone. It remains unclear whether depression is associated with the degree of cognitive impairment in dementia patients. Dementia patients may be unable to identify and express dysphoric feelings. For this reason, examination should rely on caregiver reports, as well as examination of the patient (Alexopoulos et al. 1988). Identification of depression in dementia patients, Parkinson's disease patients, and patients with cerebrovascular disease is important, because they may respond to drug therapy or electroconvulsive therapy (ECT).

Some elderly depressed patients develop a dementia syndrome that improves or is completely abated after remission of depression. This syndrome has been termed *pseudodementia, dementia of depression,* or *depression with reversible dementia* and has attracted considerable clinical and heuristic interest. Depressed elderly patients who remain with considerable cognitive impairment even after improvement of depression usually have an early-stage dementing disorder whose cognitive manifestations are exacerbated when the depressive syndrome is superimposed. Although some disagreement exists (Rabins et al. 1984; Sachdev et al. 1990) it appears that even patients with more or less complete cognitive recovery develop high rates of irreversible dementia (about 20% per year) on follow-up (Alexopoulos et al. 1993c; Copeland et al. 1992; Kral and Emery 1989; Reding et al. 1985). Many of these patients may even remain cognitively unimpaired for 1–2 years before the development of irreversible dementia. The heterogeneity of the course of depression with reversible dementia suggests that these patients can be ordered along a continuum. At the one end of the continuum lie cases in which the cognitive disturbance results predominantly from the depressive syndrome itself. At the other end are cases in which the intellectual impairment originates from a progressive subclinical dementing disorder with some contribution by the depressive syndrome. Therefore, identification of a reversible dementia syndrome in elderly depression patients constitutes an indication for thorough diagnostic workup and frequent follow-up aimed at the identification of treatable neurological disorders.

Psychotic depression occurs in 20%–45% of hospitalized elderly depression patients (Meyers 1992) and in 3.6% of elderly depression patients living in the community (Kivela et al. 1988). Patients with psychotic depression as a rule have delusions, and hallucinations are less frequent. The usual themes of depressive delusions are guilt, hypochondriasis, nihilism, persecution, and sometimes jealousy. Depressive delusions can be distinguished from delusions of dementia patients in that the latter are less systematized and less congruent to the affective disturbance (Greenwald et al. 1989). Sometimes it is difficult to distinguish depressive delusions from overvalued ideas of worthlessness and hopelessness. Nondelusional depression patients as a rule are able to recognize the exaggerated nature of overvalued ideas, although they are unable to free themselves from their excessive concerns. The clinical value of identifying depressive delusions lies in the fact that psychotic depression requires treatment with combinations of tricyclic and neuroleptic agents or ECT, as it rarely responds to antidepressants alone.

Atypical depression, anxious depression, dysthymia, adjustment disorder with depressed mood, as well as depressive syndromes of institutionalized populations and of old-old individuals, have obvious clinical interest. However, the limited empirical knowledge base prevents a conclusive discussion.

Course and Outcome

Despite progress in antidepressant treatments, longitudinal studies of 1–6 years' duration suggest a chronicity rate of 7%–30% of geriatric patients with major depression (Alexopoulos and Chester 1992; Baldwin and Jolley 1986; Burvill et al. 1991; Murphy 1983). If partially remitted subjects are considered chronic, the rate of chronicity reaches 40% (Alexopoulos and Chester 1992). Chronicity of depression may be predicted by a history of a long current episode (Alexopoulos et al. 1992b; Murphy 1983) or long previous episodes (Keller et al. 1986) of coexisting medical illness (Baldwin and Jolley 1986; Murphy 1983), high severity of depression (Baldwin and Jolley 1986; Georgotas et al. 1989), non-melancholic presentation (Murphy 1983), and delusions (Murphy 1983).

Naturalistic treatment studies of geriatric populations observed a 13%–19% rate of relapse/recurrence at 1 year (Baldwin and Jolley 1986; Burvill et al. 1991; Murphy 1983). This percentage is lower than the relapse/recurrence rate (34%) reported in younger adults. However, if the follow-up of elderly depression patients is extended to 3–6 years, the recurrence rate increases to 38% (Baldwin and Jolley 1986; Cole 1990). A 20-year follow-up study of mixed-age depressive patients showed that 95% of patients had a recurrence (Lee and Murray 1988). Relapse/recurrence appear to have different predictors than recovery of depression (Keller et al. 1984). The likelihood of relapse/recurrence may be high in patients with a history of frequent episodes (Georgotas and McCue 1989a; Keller et al. 1983), late age at illness onset (Angst and Weiss 1967; Keller et al. 1983), a history of dysthymia (Keller et al. 1984), concurrent medical illness (Baldwin and Jolley 1986; Murphy 1983; Kukull et al. 1986), and possibly high severity and chronicity of the index depressive episode (Georgotas and McCue 1989a; Georgotas et al. 1988). However, some disagreement exists (Baldwin and Jolley 1986).

A large proportion of geriatric depressive patients have cognitive dysfunction or dementia. Approximately 40% of geriatric major depression patients consecutively hospitalized in a tertiary care academic psychiatric center also met criteria for dementia (Alexopoulos and Chester 1992). The large percentage of elderly depression patients with evidence of brain disease suggests that it is clinically meaningful to examine predictors of dementia in these populations. With some exceptions (Rabins et al. 1984; Sachdev et al. 1990), follow-up data show that elderly depression patients who initially had reversible dementia develop permanent dementia at a rate of 9%–25% per year (Alexopoulos et al. 1993c; Copeland et al. 1992; Kral and Emery 1989; Reding et al. 1985). The presence of an initially reversible dementia leads to a yearly rate of irreversible dementia 2.5 to 6 times higher than that in the general geriatric population.

Knowledge of risk factors and periods of high risk for particular adverse outcomes enable the clinician to use appropriate diagnostic methods and offer preventive treatments with favorable benefit-risk ratios. Outcome studies using naturalistic and controlled treatment designs are needed to further investigate the treatment needs of specific populations of geriatric depression patients, including patients with cognitive impairment, very advanced age, medical illnesses, and disabilities.

Biological Dysfunction in Geriatric Depression

Although the etiology of geriatric depression remains unclear, some differences have been noted in measures of brain structure and function, as well as in neurochemical and neuroendocrine measures in the periphery.

Studies of monoamine metabolites in peripheral fluids yielded relatively inconsistent findings. In mixed-age depression patients, a significant correlation was noted between age at onset and plasma methoxyhydroxyphenylglycol (MHPG) (Karege et al. 1989). Studies using agonists of the platelet α_2-adrenoreceptor have shown increased binding in mixed-age and elderly depressed patients (Kafka and Paul 1986). Increased α_2-receptor binding was associated with early-onset depression (Sacchetti et al. 1985). A weak correlation was also noted between age at onset and urinary MHPG. Geriatrics studies are needed to replicate these findings and examine whether low urine and plasma MHPG and high α_2-adrenoreceptor binding can differentiate early-onset, perhaps familial, depression from late-onset depression, an entity associated with medical or neurological disorders.

Platelet monoamine oxidase (MAO) activity has been thought to be a marker of vulnerability for bipolar disorder (Leckman et al. 1977), alcoholism, and perhaps other disorders (Alexopoulos et al. 1983). Platelet MAO activity appears to be elevated in Alzheimer's disease patients with (Alexopoulos et al. 1987) and without depression (Alexopoulos et al. 1984d). Hospitalized women with late-onset depression were found to have higher platelet MAO activity than elderly women with early-onset depression (Alexopoulos et al. 1984c). Studies are needed to examine whether high platelet MAO activity can identify subgroups of late-onset depression patients with high medical morbidity or subclinical Alzheimer's disease. Elevated platelet MAO activity was reported in elderly depression patients with reversible dementia compared with nondementia depression patients (Alexopoulos et al. 1987). Future research may examine whether high platelet MAO activity can identify depression patients with reversible dementia who develop permanent dementia on follow-up.

Platelet imipramine binding is thought to reflect the function of a modulating system of serotonin uptake. Low platelet imipramine binding has been found in geriatric depression patients compared with controls (Nemeroff et al. 1988; Schneider et al. 1988a). Platelet imipramine binding is lower in primary depression than in depression occurring in the context of medical illness (Schneider et al. 1988a). Furthermore, reduced platelet imipramine binding is associated with poor response to antidepressant treatment

(Schneider et al. 1986). Because platelet imipramine binding is within normal range in Alzheimer's disease patients (Nemeroff et al. 1988), it is important to study whether this test can identify depression patients with clinical or subclinical states of dementia.

Plasma cortisol escape from dexamethasone suppression (an abnormal dexamethasone suppression test [DST]) is more frequent in geriatric than in younger depression patients (Alexopoulos et al. 1984a). Therefore, the DST is more sensitive in geriatric than in younger depression patients. However, abnormal DST results occur in one-third of dementia patients (Skare et al. 1990), thus suggesting a low specificity for geriatric depression. Although inadequate geriatric data exist, studies of younger adults suggest that lack of normalization of DST after adequate clinical response is associated with early relapse of depression.

Blunted thyroid-stimulating hormone (TSH) response to thyrotropin-releasing hormone (TRH) has been observed in 25% of depression patients; this abnormality may be trait related in at least some patients. Blunted TSH response has been reported in geriatric depression patients and also in Alzheimer's patients (Sunderland et al. 1985). Therefore, blunted TSH response to TRH is not specific for geriatric depression.

The development of brain imaging techniques has allowed studies of brain structure and function. Brain computed tomography (CT) studies demonstrated enlargement of lateral brain ventricles in geriatric depression. Ventricular enlargement is more pronounced in late-onset depression patients than in similarly aged early-onset depression patients (Jacoby and Levy 1980); the ventricles of late-onset depression patients appear to be comparable to those of Alzheimer's disease patients (Alexopoulos et al. 1992a). The biological meaning of ventricular enlargement is unclear, but it appears to be associated with poor response to antidepressant treatment (Young et al. 1988), as well as with functional abnormalities of depression, including hypercorticolemia (Kellner et al. 1983), hypothyroidism (Johnstone et al. 1986), decreased dopamine β-hydroxylase (Meltzer et al. 1984), and increased cerebral spinal fluid (CSF) 5-hydroxyindoleacetic acid (5-HIAA) (Standish-Barry et al. 1986).

Brain magnetic resonance imaging (MRI) studies showed white-matter hyperintensity in young and middle-aged bipolar patients (Dupont et al. 1990) and in elderly depression patients (Coffey et al. 1988). This finding was more frequent and more pronounced in late-onset than in early-onset depression (Coffey et al. 1988) and was associated with poor response to drug treatment. However, replication of these studies is needed in samples controlled for cerebrovascular risk factors.

Treatment

Psychotherapy, family therapy, drug therapy, and ECT are effective in the treatment of geriatric mood disorders. Psychotherapies, including cognitive behavior therapy, interpersonal therapy and perhaps psychodynamic psychotherapies have been found effective in mild geriatric depression (Reynolds et al. 1992). Monthly interpersonal psychotherapy sessions have been observed to reduce the recurrence rate in younger adults who recovered from major depression (Frank et al. 1991). The efficacy of psychotherapy in preventing recurrences of geriatric depression is currently under investigation. Despite its efficacy and the lack of side effects, psychotherapy remains underutilized in geriatric depression. Family approaches are important in geriatric mood disorders, as most patients depend on family members not only for emotional support, but also for their day-to-day functioning.

Drug Therapy

Nortriptyline and desipramine are the most frequently used tricyclic antidepressants in geriatric depression. Their advantages over tertiary amines include their low anticholinergic and sedative effects. Elderly patients have decreased tolerance for anticholinergic and hypotensive side effects. Nortriptyline, in particular, appears to have a lower potential for orthostatic hypotension than do other tricyclic agents. Plasma levels of amitriptyline and imipramine tend to be higher in elderly individuals than in younger adults (Abernethy et al. 1985; Burch 1988) and do not appear to correlate with antidepressant response. A similar lack of relationship between plasma levels and response has been observed for doxepin and trazodone (Spar 1987). Elderly patients require plasma levels of antidepressants similar to those required by young adults. However, some elderly patients may develop therapeutic blood levels while receiving subtherapeutic dosages of tricyclic antidepressants (Dawling et al. 1981; Katz et al. 1989). Elderly patients appear to have higher plasma levels of hydroxylated metabolites of nortriptyline and desipramine than do young patients, even when plasma levels of the parent compounds are similar (Nelson et al. 1988; Young 1987). The difference may be due in part to reduced renal clearance resulting from the aging process or disease. Elevated hydroxylated metabolites of nortriptyline may contribute to cardiac conduction problems in elderly patients (Schneider et al. 1986; Young et al. 1985). It has been suggested that the onset of antidepressant response occurs later in elderly adults than in young adults (Georgotas et al. 1989). Therefore, an antidepressant drug trial may not be complete until after 6–9 weeks have elapsed. During antidepressant treatment, higher intellectual functions, orthostatic blood pressure, the electrocardiogram (ECG), and the ability to urinate should be monitored frequently. Pretreatment systolic orthostatic hypotension has been found to correlate with antidepressant response to nortriptyline in some elderly patients (Schneider et al. 1986). However, the clinical usefulness of this finding has not been adequately tested.

If a depressed patient fails to respond to tricyclic agents, MAO inhibitors, selective serotonin reuptake inhibitors (SSRIs), or bupropion may be considered. MAO inhibitors appear to be well tolerated and effective in geriatric major depression patients, but they have not been systematically studied in the very old. The dosages of MAO inhibitors required in elderly individuals are considerably lower than those required in younger depression patients (Georgotas et al. 1986). The most frequent side effect of MAO inhibitors is orthostatic hypotension, leading to a high risk of falls and fractures. Other important limitations of the drugs are the diet restrictions and the potential for multiple adverse drug interactions. Inhibition of platelet MAO activity by 80% has been found to predict antidepressant response in younger depression patients (Georgotas et al. 1986), but the clinical usefulness of monitoring platelet MAO activity in elderly patients remains uncertain.

SSRIs appear to be well tolerated and effective in geriatric depression, although placebo-controlled studies are still lacking (Cohn et al. 1990; Dunner et al. 1992; Falk et al. 1989). SSRIs appear to have fewer overall side effects than tricyclic antidepressants and trazodone. Studies of elderly outpatients observed that SSRIs are equally effective with tricyclics in the acute treatment of depression. It is unknown, however, whether SSRIs can be helpful in severe major geriatric depression. There is some evidence that fluoxetine may prevent relapse or recurrence in elderly patients who recovered from depression. Bupropion has not been extensively investigated in elderly individuals (Kane et al. 1983). However, it appears to be tolerated by mixed-age cardiac patients; therefore, it should be considered in patients with heart disease (Roose et al. 1991). Exacerbation of preexisting hypertension has been observed in patients treated with bupropion.

Psychostimulants such as dextroamphetamine and methylphenidate have been used in geriatric patients. Their efficacy in treatment of geriatric major depression has not been established. However, psychostimulants appear to improve apathy and anergy in medical patients (Kaplitz 1975; Katon and Raskind 1980). In these populations, psychostimulants have rapid onset of action, minimal side effects, little tolerance development, and minimal risk for addiction. Nonetheless, placebo-controlled studies are needed to identify the magnitude of improvement induced by psychostimulants and the exact type of symptoms that respond to these agents.

It has been suggested that lithium may augment tricyclic antidepressant response in elderly patients (Katona and Finch 1991; Zimmer et al. 1991). The dose of lithium required by elderly depression patients receiving tricyclic agents may be one-third to one-half that of younger adults.

In younger depression patients, combinations of tricyclic agents with SSRIs have led to an antidepressant response sooner than tricyclic agents alone (Nelson et al. 1991). Systematic studies of such combinations in elderly individuals are lacking.

Electroconvulsive Therapy

ECT is an important treatment modality for geriatric depression patients because of its safety and rapid onset of action. Approximately 80% of the population in the seventh or eighth decade of life have one or more medical illnesses. Medical illness and depression tend to occur in the same persons (Kukull et al. 1986). Therefore, the percentage of medical illness in elderly depression patients is even higher than that in the general population. Cardiac conduction defects, prostatic hypertrophy, glaucoma, and other conditions increase the risk of drug therapy. Moreover, even when antidepressants are tolerated, the need for gradual introduction of antidepressants and the slow onset of antidepressant action in elderly individuals prolong the time during which patients remain depressed and increase the risk for suicide, debilitation, dehydration, and electrolyte disturbances, all further reasons ECT often is an important therapeutic option in elderly individuals.

Controlled studies have demonstrated that ECT is an established acute antidepressant treatment (Greenberg and Fink 1992). Administration of three ECTs weekly appears to produce a more rapid recovery than ECT given once a week (Kellner et al. 1992). Less frequent ECT is associated with less cognitive impairment, but no differences in cognitive function were found 1 month after ECT completion between a group that had undergone ECT three times and one that had undergone ECT twice weekly (Kellner et al. 1992). It appears that electrode placement and electrical dose influence both efficacy and memory side effects of ECT (Weiner 1984). Low electrical dose (just above seizure threshold) unilateral ECT was found to be less effective than high-dose (2.5 times the threshold) unilateral ECT (Sackeim et al. 1993). However, disagreement exists (American Psychiatric Association 1990). Use of a high- or low-dose electrical stimulus does not appear to influence the efficacy of bilateral ECT. Regardless of electrode placement, high dosage increases the speed of improvement. These data challenge earlier findings suggesting that long duration of seizures is associated with high treatment efficacy. High-dose unilateral ECT is associated with prolonged time to recover orientation after seizure induction (Sackeim et al. 1993). Bilateral ECT results in longer recovery time than high-dose unilateral ECT (Sackeim et al. 1993). Compared with unilateral ECT, bilateral ECT leads to greater retrograde amnesia within a short period after completion of ECT, but there may not be significant memory differences after 2 months (Sackeim et al. 1993). Most of these observations used mixed-age samples. Geriatric studies are needed to compare the benefit-risk ratio of high-dose unilateral with that of bilateral ECT especially in dementia or cognitively impaired depression patients or patients at high risk for future development of dementia (e.g., depression patients with a history of reversible dementia).

Anecdotal literature suggests that ECT is an effective continuation of maintenance antidepressant treatment (Decina et al. 1987). Controlled studies of continuation and maintenance ECT are needed, as there is evidence of a high relapse/recurrence rate in ECT responders who previously had a medication-resistant depressive disorder.

ECT is a safe treatment, with a mortality rate of .01% (Kramer 1985). The majority of deaths (67%) related to ECT are due to cardiac complications and occur immediately after or within a few hours of ECT. Compared with younger adults, elderly patients and patients with preexisting cardiac disease are more prone to cardiovascular events occurring in the context of ECT, including ischemic syndromes, arrhythmias, decompensation of heart failure, and transient severe rise in blood pressure (Alexopoulos et al. 1984b; Burke et al. 1987). However, with adequate medical evaluation, monitoring during and after ECT, and appropriate intervention, most cardiovascular events related to ECT have a benign outcome.

ECT leads to cerebrovascular contraction, heightened blood-brain barrier permeability, and increased brain oxygen consumption (Alexopoulos et al. 1989b). Nonetheless, ECT appears to be reasonably safe 1 month after a cerebrovascular accident (Hsiao et al. 1987). ECT is generally contraindicated in patients with intracranial tumors, because it may lead to delirium, major neurological events, or death (Maltbie et al. 1980). However, anecdotal evidence (Alexopoulos et al. 1989b) suggests that patients with small asymptomatic tumors without surrounding edema or obstruction of CSF flow may tolerate ECT.

Elderly patients have a longer recovery than younger adults, especially after bilateral ECT (Frazer and Glass 1978). Moreover, geriatric patients sometimes develop prolonged confusion after ECT (Alexopoulos et al. 1984b; Burke et al. 1987), and falls occur in up to 15% of patients (Burke et al. 1987). However, controlled studies are needed to examine whether and to what extent ECT-related confusion is responsible for these falls. The practice of favoring ECT over antidepressants in medically ill depression patients may have led to inflated reports of ECT-related morbidity (Alexopoulos et al. 1989b). Anecdotal literature suggest that ECT was used uneventfully in patients more than 100 years old (Bracken et al. 1987; O'Shea et al. 1987) and in elderly patients with aortic aneurisms (Karliner 1978a); cardiac pacemakers (Abiuso et al. 1975; Alexopoulos and Frances 1980); a history of myocardial infarction (Karliner 1978a), stroke (Hsiao et al. 1984; Karliner 1978b), transient ischemic attacks, severe hypertension, or arrhythmias (Regestein and Lind 1980); or in patients in need of anticoagulants (Alexopoulos et al. 1982).

Long-Term Treatment

Once an affective episode is terminated, continuation antidepressant treatment should be administered for the purpose of preventing the reemergence (relapse) of the previously treated episode. Continuation treatment generally consists of 6-month therapy with the same drug and the same dosage used for treatment of the acute episode. Maintenance therapy consists of use of antidepressant treatments beyond the first 6 months after recovery and by convention is intended for presentation of new depressive episodes. In mixed-age bipolar disorder patients, lithium maintenance reduces the occurrence of manic-depressive episodes by 50%. However, there is disagreement as to whether low lithium plasma levels (0.4 to 0.6 mEq/L) or levels similar to those used for acute treatment (0.8 to 1.2 mEq/L) are required for maintenance therapy. Lithium and tricyclic agents both are effective maintenance therapies in preventing recurrences of major depression. The efficacy and the side effects of maintenance antidepressant therapies in elderly depression patients require further investigation. At present, elderly patients with a history of multiple episodes or with a late age at illness onset are at particularly high risk for recurrence and should be considered for maintenance therapies.

Bipolar Disorder

Mania or hypomania constitutes 5%–10% of the diagnoses of elderly patients (Roth 1955; Yassa et al. 1988; Young and Klerman 1992). However, limited information is available concerning the prevalence of bipolar disorders in the elderly community. In a sample of 923 elderly persons studied in the Epidemiologic Catchment Area Study, no manic cases were identified (Kramer et al. 1985).

Most patients with manic syndromes have bipolar mood disorder. Some cases of mania may be etiologically related to medical diseases and drugs (Krauthammer and Klerman 1978). Manic symptoms and signs may be part of schizoaffective disorder, a condition related to bipolar disorder (Klerman 1987). Schizoaffective disorder is infrequently diagnosed in geriatric patients.

Klerman (1987) subcategorized bipolar disorder on the basis of course and family history. Type I consists of patients who are hospitalized at least once for a manic episode and also have a history of major depressive episodes. Type II includes patients with mild manic (hypomania) and depressive episodes. Type III patients have cyclothymic mood fluctuations without major depression or mania. Type IV patients have manic states resulting from medical illness or drugs; manic emerging during antidepressant treatment is not considered organic mood disorder. Type V patients have histories of major depression only with a family history of bipolar disorder.

Mania first occurring in late life is a heterogeneous condition (Young and Klerman 1992). A substantial subgroup of late-onset mania patients consists of patients with unipolar major depression who changed polarity in late life. Some of these patients have had a family history of bipolar disorder and were classified as Type V before they changed polarity. Bipolar disorders associated with medical illnesses or drugs (Type IV) may be particularly prevalent among late-onset cases.

The incidence of late-onset mania is unknown. Studies of first hospital admissions suggest that the risk for mania declines with aging (Shulman and Post 1980). However, there is some evidence that first admissions for mania increase after 60 years of age, especially in men (Eagles and Whalley 1985; Spicer et al. 1973). Late-onset bipolar disorder patients have a lower rate of affective disorders among relatives compared with early-onset mania patients (Rice et al. 1987). It has been suggested that mania associated with medical disorders or drug treatment as a rule has onset after 40 years of age (Krauthammer and Klerman 1978). Mania with onset during senescence is associated with coarse brain disease. Cerebrovascular disease, especially right-sided lesions, has been implicated in late-onset mania (Starkstein et al. 1988b).

The course and outcome of manic states in geriatric patients are unclear. As manic states in this age group probably represent various disorders with multiple biological determinants, no single characterization of "mania" can be considered to be prototypic (Young and Klerman 1992). Disorientation, delirium, and reversible cognitive dysfunction have been described in mania patients. It is unclear whether reversible cognitive dysfunction in mania leads to persistent cognitive dysfunction and dementia at follow-up, as it does in depression. Older age appears to be associated with chronic mania (Wertham 1929), and there is a suggestion of an association between later age at onset and greater duration of episode, as well as shorter intervals between episodes (MacDonald 1918). However, further studies are needed to establish these relationships. There is no clear difference in relapse rate between early- and late-onset geriatric mania patients, but prospective studies are needed (Young and Klerman 1992). The mortality rate for elderly bipolar disorder patients seems to be greater than the community base rate for this age group (Dhingra and Rabins 1991) and also appears to exceed that of geriatric depression patients (Shulman et al. 1992). It remains to be determined whether late-onset mania patients are at greater risk for the development of dementia than early-onset elderly patients.

Treatment of Geriatric Mania

Lithium is an effective treatment for elderly mania patients. However, lithium may be less effective in mania complicated by neurological and medical disorders than in uncomplicated mania. Elderly patients tend to show high lithium plasma levels at relatively low dosages because of an age-associated reduction in renal clearance. About one-half to two-thirds of the dosage required for young adults is usually sufficient for elderly individuals. The half-life of lithium is about 24 hours in the seventh decade of life. Therefore, steady-state pharmacokinetics are anticipated 5 or more days after the stabilization of the daily dosage. Elderly persons have a high increase of pharmacodynamic sensitivity to lithium and tend to have a fine tremor and even myoclonus at plasma levels considered to be therapeutic for young adults. It has been suggested that lithium plasma levels of 0.3 to 0.6 mEq/L are clinically effective in elderly individuals. However, controlled studies are lacking. The onset of action of lithium is slow and may require several days or weeks. Lorazepam or low dosages of high-potency antipsychotics may be used in the early treatment of acutely agitated elderly mania patients. A large number of elderly patients develop side effects when treated with lithium. Elderly patients develop lithium-induced tremor more frequently than younger patients (Murray et al. 1983). Lithium may induce or worsen cognitive impairment, and this side effect is more prominent in dementia patients (Kelwala et al. 1984). In elderly mania patients, delirium can develop at lithium levels at or even below the therapeutic lithium plasma level range. Patients with Parkinson's disease (Schaffer and Garvey 1984) and patients receiving neuroleptics (F. Miller and Menninger 1987) are prone to lithium-induced delirium. Delirium and cerebellar dysfunction may last for weeks after lithium discontinuation (Schou 1984). Lithium can worsen rigidity and tremor in patients with Parkinson's disease or produce parkinsonism in neurologically intact patients (Jefferson et al. 1981). Sinoatrial block can be caused by lithium (Roose et al. 1979). Cardiac drugs, including digitalis and β-blockers, increase the risk for sinoatrial block. Salt depletion caused by vomiting or diarrhea, thiazide diuretics, nonsteroidal anti-inflammatory drugs, and angiotensin-converting enzyme inhibitors may raise lithium plasma levels and lead to toxicity.

Anticonvulsant drugs such as carbamazepine and sodium valproate appear to have antimanic action in younger adults (Bowden et al. 1994). Anecdotal evidence suggests that carbamazepine (Kellner and Neher 1991) and sodium valproate are effective in elderly mania patients (Gnam and Flint 1993; McFarland et al. 1990; Yassa and Cvejic 1994). History of poor response to lithium does not preclude response to anticonvulsants (Bowden et al. 1994). Some evidence exists that carbamazepine and valproate are more effective than lithium in rapidly cycling patients with dysphoric mania (Bowden et al. 1994). Patients with neurological brain diseases may be responsive to sodium valproate (Stoll et al. 1994). Complete blood count and liver function tests should be obtained before treatment with carbamazepine and valproate. Elderly mania patients tend to develop a higher valproate plasma free fraction of valproate than younger patients, but the clinical significance of a high valproate free fraction in unclear (Rimmer and Richens 1985). Carbamazepine may cause sedation, confusion, and ataxia in a dose-dependent fashion (Schneier and Khan 1990). Carbamazepine-treated patients should have frequent complete blood counts because carbamazepine can cause leukopenia (white blood cells below 4,000/mm^3) in approximately 2% of cases (Tohen et al. 1995). Approximately one-half of the patients who develop carbamazepine-induced leukopenia have a drop in white count within the first 16 days of treatment. Valproate causes leukopenia in 0.4% of patients, a percentage comparable to that of tricyclic antidepressants.

ECT is highly effective in mania. Approximately 80% of ECT-treated mania patients achieve remission or marked clinical improvement (Mukherjee et al. 1994). ECT is effective even in mania patients who are resistant to drug therapy. Clinical improvement after ECT is a primary therapeutic effect rather than a result of an ECT-induced organic brain syndrome. Mania patients require a comparable number of ECT treatments to depressed patients. Mania patients often have a lower seizure threshold than depressed patients (Mukherjee et al. 1994). Because it is well-tolerated by most geriatric patients, ECT is the treatment of choice for elderly mania patients who are unable to tolerate drug therapy or have a severe behavioral disturbance that necessitates rapid response.

Suicide

Suicide is more frequent in elderly individuals than any other population. In 1989, the suicide rate in the United States was 12.2/100,000 population (McIntosh et al. 1994; National Center for Health Statistics, 1992). Americans older than 65 years of age had a suicide rate of 20.1/100,000, almost twice that of the general population. Suicide rates consistently increase in males and reach their highest level in the oldest age group. In contrast, female suicide rates increase slightly with age, peak in middle adulthood, and decline in late life. In 1989, the suicide rate for men older than 65 years was 40.7/100,000, while the suicide rate for women of similar age was 5.9/100,000. White men older than 65 years had the highest suicide rate (43.5/100,000), followed by nonwhite men (15.7/100,000), white women (6.3/100,000), and nonwhite women (2.8/100,000) (McIntosh et al. 1994; National Center for Health Statistics 1992). Although suicide is more frequent in elderly patients than in younger patients, the rate of suicide for elderly individuals steadily decreased from the 1930s to 1980. However, the suicide rate began to rise again in the 1980s (Allen and Blazer 1991). Demographic differences between persons who contemplate or attempt suicide and those who commit suicide suggest that these populations are dissimilar. About 60% of suicide victims are men, but 75% of those who attempt suicide are women. Suicide victims as a rule use guns or hang themselves, whereas 70% of suicide attempters take a drug overdose, and 22% cut or slash themselves. Difficulties in extrapolating conclusions from suicide attempters led to the development of "psychological autopsy" as the main technique for studying suicide. Psychological autopsy seeks to reconstruct the medical, psychiatric, and social profiles of suicide victims through postmortem review of medical records and systematic interviews of persons closely associated with the suicide victims. Psychological autopsy studies observed that almost all elderly suicide victims have had a psychiatric disorder, most commonly late-onset depression (Conwell et al. 1991). However, psychiatric disorders in suicide victims often do not receive medical or psychiatric attention. When compared with younger adults, more elderly suicide victims are widowed and fewer are single, separated, or divorced. Violent methods of suicide are more prevalent, and alcohol use and psychiatric histories appear to be less common with aging (Conwell et al. 1990). Physical illness and loss seem to be the most common suicide precipitants in late life, whereas employment, financial, and family relationship problems are the most frequent precipitants in younger adults (Conwell et al. 1990).

Most elderly persons who commit suicide communicate their suicidal thoughts to family or friends prior to the act of suicide. Education of physicians, other health and social agents, and the public on the role of depression, substance abuse, and suicide warnings may effectively reduce the incidence of suicide.

References

Abernethy DR, Greenblatt DJ, Shader RI: Imipramine and desipramine disposition in the elderly. J Pharmacolol Exp Ther 232:183–188, 1985

Abiuso P, Dunkelman R, Proper M: Electroconvulsive therapy in patients with pacemakers. JAMA 240:2459–2460, 1975

Alexopoulos GS: Clinical and biological findings in late-onset depression, in American Psychiatric Press Review of Psychiatry, Vol 9. Edited by Tasman A, Goldfinger SM, Kaufmann CA. Washington, DC, American Psychiatric Press, 1990, pp 249–262

Alexopoulos GS, Abrams RC: Depression in Alzheimer's disease. Psychiatr Clin North Am 14:327–340, 1991

Alexopoulos GS, Chester JG: Outcomes of geriatric depression. Clin Geriatr Med 8:363–373, 1992

Alexopoulos GS, Frances RJ: ECT and cardiac patients with pacemakers. Am J Psychiatry 137:1111–1112, 1980

Alexopoulos GS, Nasr H, Young RC: Electroconvulsive therapy in patients on anticoagulants. Can J Psychiatry 27:46–47, 1982

Alexopoulos GS, Lieberman KW, Frances R: Platelet MAO activity in alcoholic patients and their first degree relatives. Am J Psychiatry 140:1501–1504, 1983

Alexopoulos GS, Young RC, Kocsis JH, et al: Dexamethasone suppression test in geriatric depression. Biol Psychiatry 19:1567–1571, 1984a

Alexopoulos GS, Shamoian CA, Lucas J, et al: Medical problems of geriatric patients and younger controls during electroconvulsive therapy. J Am Geriatric Soc 32:651–654, 1984b

Alexopoulos GS, Lieberman KW, Young RC: Platelet MAO activity and age at onset of depression in elderly depressed women. Am J Psychiatry 141:1276–1278, 1984c

Alexopoulos GS, Lieberman KW, Young RC: Platelet MAO activity in primary degenerative dementia. Am J Psychiatry 14:97–99, 1984d

Alexopoulos GS, Lieberman KW, Young RC, et al: Platelet MAO activity in geriatric patients with depression and dementia. Am J Psychiatry 144:1480–1483, 1987

Alexopoulos GS, Abrams RC, Young RC, et al: Cornell scale for depression in dementia. Biol Psychiatry 23:271–284, 1988

Alexopoulos GS, Young RC, Abrams RC, et al: Chronicity and relapse in geriatric depression. Biol Psychiatry 26:551–564, 1989a

Alexopoulos GS, Young RC, Abrams RC: ECT in the high-risk geriatric patient. Convuls Ther 5:75–87, 1989b

Alexopoulos GS, Young RC, Shindledecker RD: Brain computed tomography findings in geriatric depression and primary degenerative dementia. Biol Psychiatry 31:591–599, 1992a

Alexopoulos GS, Meyers BS, Young RC, et al: Chronicity in geriatric depression. New research presented at the annual meeting of the American Psychiatric Association, 1992b

Alexopoulos GS, Meyers BS, Mattis S, et al: Cognitive dysfunction in late-onset depression. New research presented at the annual meeting of the American Psychiatric Association, San Francisco, CA, May 22–27, 1993a

Alexopoulos GS, Young RC, Meyers BS: Geriatric depression: age of onset and dementia. Biol Psychiatry 34:141–145, 1993b

Alexopoulos GS, Meyers BS, Young RC, et al: The course of geriatric depression with "reversible dementia": a controlled study. Am J Psychiatry 150:1693–1699, 1993c

Allen A, Blazer DG: Mood disorders, in Comprehensive Review of Geriatric

Psychiatry. Edited by Sadavoy J, Lazarus LW, Jarvik LF. Washington, DC, American Psychiatric Press, 1991, pp 337–351

American Psychiatric Association, Task Force on Electroconvulsive Therapy: The Practice of Electroconvulsive Therapy: Recommendations for Treatment, Training, and Privileging. Washington, DC, American Psychiatric Association, 1990

Angst J, Weiss P: Periodicity of depressed psychoses, in Proceedings of the Fifth International Medical Foundation (International Congress Series 129). Edited by Brill H, Cole JO, Deniker, P, et al. Amsterdam, The Netherlands, Excerpta Medica, 1967, pp 703–710

Baldwin RC, Jolley DJ: The prognosis of depression in old age. Br J Psychiatry 149:574–583, 1986

Blazer DG, Bachar JR, Manton KG: Suicide in late life: review and commentary. J Am Geriatr Soc 34:519–525, 1986

Blazer DG, Hughes DC, George LK: The epidemiology depression in an elderly community population. Gerontologist 27:281–287, 1987

Bowden CL, Brugger AM, Swann AC, et al: Efficacy of divalproex vs. lithium and placebo in the treatment of mania: The Depakote Mania Study Group. JAMA 271:918–924, 1994

Bracken P, Ryan M, Dunne D: Electroconvulsive therapy in the elderly (letter). Br J Psychiatry 150:713, 1987

Burch JE: Antidepressive effect of amitriptyline treatment with plasma drug levels controlled within three different ranges. Psychopharmacology 94:197–205, 1988

Burke WJ, Rubin EH, Zorumski CE, et al: The safety of ECT in geriatric psychiatry. J Am Geriatr Soc 35:516–521, 1987

Burns A, Jacoby R, Levy R: Psychiatric phenomena in Alzheimer's disease, III: disorders of mood. Br J Psychiatry 157:81–86, 1990

Burvill PN, Hall WD, Stampfer HG, et al: The prognosis of depression in old age. Br J Psychiatry 158:64–71, 1991

Clark DC: Suicide risk assessment and prediction in the 1990s. Crisis 11:104–112, 1990

Coffey CE, Figiel GS, Djang WT, et al: Leukencephalopathy in elderly depressed patients. Biol Psychiatry 24:143–161, 1988

Coffey CE, Figiel GS, Djang WT, et al: Subcortical hyperintensity on magnetic resonance imaging: a comparison of normal and depressed elderly subjects. Am J Psychiatry 147:187–189, 1990

Cohn CK, Shrivastava R, Mendels J, et al: Double-blind, multicenter comparison of sertraline and amitriptyline in elderly depressed patients. J Clin Psychiatry 51:12 (suppl B)28–33, 1990

Cole MG: The prognosis of depression in the elderly. Can Med Assoc J 142:633–639, 1990

Conwell Y, Rotenberg M, Caine ED: Completed suicide at age 50 and over. J Am Geriatr Soc 38:640–644, 1990

Conwell Y, Olsen K, Caine ED, et al: Suicide in later life: psychological autopsy findings. Int Psychogeriatr 3:59–66, 1991

Copeland JRM, Davidson IA, Dewey ME, et al: Alzheimer's disease, other dementias, depression and pseudodementia: prevalence, incidence and three-year outcome in Liverpool. Br J Psychiatry 161:230–239, 1992

Cummings JL, Miller B, Hill MA, et al: Neuropsychiatric aspects of multi-infarct dementia and dementia of the Alzheimer type. Arch Neurol 44:389–393, 1987

Dawling S, Crome P, Heyer EJ: Nortriptyline therapy in elderly patients: dosage prediction from plasma concentration at 24 hours after a single 50 mg dose. Br J Psychiatry 139:413–416, 1981

Decina P, Guthrie EB, Sackheim HA, et al: Continuation ECT in the management of relapses of major affective episodes. Acta Psychiatr Scand 75:559–562, 1987

Dhingra U, Rabins PV: Mania in the elderly: a five- to seven-year follow-up. J Am Geriatr Soc 39:581–583, 1991

Dunner DL, Cohn JB, Walshe T, et al: Two combined, multicenter double-blind studies of paroxetine and doxepine in geriatric patients with major depression. J Clin Psychiatry 53:2 (suppl)57–60, 1992

Dupont RM, Jernigan TL, Butter N, et al: Subcortical abnormalities detected in bipolar affective disorder using magnetic resonance imaging. Arch Gen Psychiatry 144:488–492, 1990

Eagles JM, Whalley LJ: Ageing and affective disorders: the age at first onset of affective disorders in Scotland 1966–1978. Br J Psychiatry 147:180–187, 1985

Falk WE, Rosenbaum JE, Otto MW, et al: Fluoxetine versus trazodone in depressed geriatric patients. J Geriatr Psychiatry Neurol 2:208–214, 1989

Feighner JP, Cohn JB: Double-blind comparative trials of fluoxetine and doxepin in geriatric patients with major depressive disorder. J Clin Psychiatry 46:20–25, 1985

Feldman E, Mayo R, Hawton K, et al: Psychiatric disorder in medical in-patients. Q J Med 63:405–412, 1987

Frank E, Kupfer DJ, Wagner EF, et al: Efficacy of interpersonal psychotherapy as a maintenance treatment of recurrent depression: contributing factors. Arch Gen Psychiatry 48:1053–1059, 1991

Frazer RM, Glass IB: Recovery from ECT in elderly patients. Br J Psychiatry 133:524–528, 1978

Georgotas A, McCue RE: Relapse of depressed patients after effective continuation therapy. J Affect Disord 17:159–164, 1989a

Georgotas A, McCue RE: The additional benefit of extending an antidepressant trial past seven weeks in the depressed elderly. Int J Geriatr Psychiatry 4:191–195, 1989b

Georgotas A, McCue RE, Hapworth W, et al: Comparative efficacy and safety of MAOIs vs TCAs in treating depression in the elderly. Biol Psychiatry 21:1155–1166, 1986

Georgotas A, McCue RE, Cooper TB, et al: How effective and safe is continuation therapy of elderly depressed patients? Arch Gen Psychiatry 45:929–932, 1988

Georgotas A, McCue RE, Cooper TB, et al: Factors affecting the delay of antidepressant effect in responders to nortriptyline and phenelzine. Psychiatry Res 28:1–9, 1989

Gnam W, Flint AJ: New onset rapid cycling bipolar disorder in an 87 year old woman. Can J Psychiatry 38:324–326, 1993

Gosselin C, Ancill RJ: Comparative plasma levels of doxepin and despiramine in the elderly. Can J Psychiatry 34:921–924, 1989

Greenberg L, Fink M: The use of electroconvulsive therapy in geriatric patients. Clin Geriatr Med 8:349–354, 1992

Greenwald BS, Kramer-Ginsber E, Marin DB, et al: Dementia with coexistent major depression. Am J Psychiatry 146:1472–1478, 1989

Hagnell O, Lanke J, Rorsman B, et al: Are we entering an age of melancholy? Psychol Med 12:279–289, 1982

House A, Dennis M, Mogridge L, et al: Mood disorders in the year after first stroke. Br J Psychiatry 158:83–92, 1991

Hsiao JK, Evans DL: ECT in a depressed patient after craniotomy. Am J Psychiatry 141:442–444, 1984

Hsiao JK, Messenheimer JA, Evans DL: ECT and neurological disorders. Convuls Ther 3:121–136, 1987

Jacoby RJ, Levy R: Computer tomography in the elderly, 3: affective disorder. Br J Psychiatry 136:270–275, 1980

Jefferson JW, Griest JH, Baudhuin M: Lithium: interactions with other drugs. J Clin Psychopharmacol 1:124–131, 1981

Johnstone EC, Owens DG, Crow TJ, et al: Hypothyroidism as a correlate of lateral ventricular enlargement in manic depressive and neurotic illness. Br J Psychiatry 148:317–321, 1986

Kafka MS, Paul SM: Platelet alpha$_2$ adrenergic receptors in depression.

Arch Gen Psychiatry 43:91–95, 1986

Kane JM, Cole K, Sarantakos S, et al: Safety and efficacy of bupropion in elderly patients: preliminary observations. J Clin Psychiatry 44:134–136, 1983

Kaplitz SE: Withdrawn, apethetic geriatric patients responsive to methylphenidate. J Am Geriatr Soc 13:271–276, 1975

Karege F, Bovier P, Gaillard JM, et al: Plasma MHPG and age of onset in depressed patients. Psychiatry Res 30:103–105, 1989

Karliner W: Cardiovascular disease and ECT. Psychosomatics 19:238–241, 1978a

Karliner W: ECT for patients with CNS disease. Psychosomatics 19:781–783, 1978b

Katon W, Raskind M: Treatment of depression in the medically ill elderly with methylphenidate. Am J Psychiatry 137:963–965, 1980

Katona CLE, Finch EJL: Lithium augmentation for refractory depression in old age. Advances in Neuropsychiatry and Psychopharmacology 2:177–184, 1991

Katz IR, Simpson GM, Jethanandani V, et al: Steady state pharmacokinetics of nortriptyline in the frail elderly. Neuropsychopharmacology 2:229–236, 1989

Keller MB, Lavori PW: Double depression, major depression and dysthymia: distinct entity or different phases of a single disorder? Psychopharmacol Bull 20:399–402, 1984

Keller MB, Lavori PW, Lewis CE, et al: Predictors of relapse in major depressive disorder. JAMA 250:3299–3304, 1983

Keller MB, Klerman GL, Lavori PW: Long-term outcome of episodes of major depression. JAMA 252:788–792, 1984

Keller MB, Lavori PW, Rice J, et al: The persistent risk of chronicity in recurrent episodes of nonbipolar major depressive disorder: a prospective follow-up study. Am J Psychiatry 143:24–28, 1986

Kellner CH, Rubinow DR, Gold PW, et al: Relationship of cortisol hypersecretion to brain CT scan alterations in depressed patients. Psychiatry Res 8:191–197, 1983

Kelwala S, Pomara N, Stanley M, et al: Lithium-induced accentuation of extrapyramidal symptoms in individuals with Alzheimer's disease. J Clin Psychiatry 45:342–344, 1984

Kellner CH, Monroe RR, Pritchett J, et al: Weekly ECT in geriatric depression. Convuls Ther 8:245–252, 1992

Kellner MB, Neher F: A first episode of mania after age 80: a case report. Can J Psychiatry 36:607–608, 1991

Kivela SL, Pahkala K, Laippala P: Prevalence of depression in an elderly Finnish population. Acta Psychiatr Scand 78:401–413, 1988

Klerman GL: The classification of bipolar disorders. Psychiatr Ann 17:13–17, 1987

Klerman GL: The current age of youthful melancholia: evidence for increase in depression among adolescents and young adults. Br J Psychiatry 152:4–14, 1988

Klerman GL, Lavori PW, Rice J, et al: Birth cohort trends in rates of major depressive disorder among relatives of patients with affective disorders. Arch Gen Psychiatry 42:689–693, 1985

Knesvich J, Martin R, Berg L, et al: Preliminary report on affective symptoms in the early stages of senile dementia of the Alzheimer's type. Am J Psychiatry 140:233–235, 1983

Koenig HG, Blazer DG: Epidemiology of geriatric affective disorders. Clin Geriatr Med 8:235–251, 1992

Koenig HG, Meador KG, Shelp F, et al: Depressive disorders in hospitalized medically ill patients: a comparison of young and elderly men. J Am Geriatr Soc 39:881–890, 1991

Kral VA, Emery OB: Long-term follow-up of depressive pseudodementia of the aged. Can J Psychiatry 34:445–446, 1989

Kramer BA: Use of ECT in California, 1977–1983. Am J Psychiatry 142:1190–1192, 1985

Kramer M, German PS, Anthony JC: Patterns of mental disorders among the elderly residents of eastern Baltimore. J Am Geriatr Soc 33:236–245, 1985

Kramer SI, Reifler BV: Depression, dementia and reversible dementia. Archives in Geriatric Medicine 8:289–297, 1992

Krauthammer C, Klerman GL: Secondary mania. Arch Gen Psychiatry 35:1333–1339, 1978

Kukull WA, Koepsell TD, Inui TS, et al: Depression and physical illness among elderly general medical clinic patients. J Affect Dis 10:153–162, 1986

Lawlor BA, Sunderland T, Mellow AM, et al: Family history of depression and alcoholism in Alzheimer's patients and age-matched controls. Int J Geriatr Psychiatry 4:327–331, 1989

Lazarus L, Newton N, Cohler B, et al: Frequency in presentation of depressive symptoms in patients with primary degenerative dementia. Am J Psychiatry 144:41–45, 1987

Leckman JF, Gerson ES, Murphy DL: Reduced MAO activity in first degree relatives of individuals with bipolar affective disorders: a preliminary report. Arch Gen Psychiatry 34:601–606, 1977

Lee AS, Murray RM: The long-term outcome of Maudsley depressives. Br J Psychiatry 153:741–751, 1988

MacDonald JB: Prognosis in manic-depressive insanity. J Nerv Ment Dis 47:20–30, 1918

Maltbie AA, Wingfield MS, Volow MR, et al: Electroconvulsive therapy in the presence of brain tumor. J Nerv Ment Dis 106:400–405, 1980

McFarland BH, Miller MR, Straumfjord AA: Valproate use in the older manic patient. J Clin Psychiatry 51:479–481, 1990

McIntosh JL, Santos JF, Hubbard RW, et al: Epidemiology, in Elder Suicide Research Theory and Treatment. Washington, DC, American Psychological Association, 1994, pp 7–61

Meltzer HY, Tong C, Luchins DJ: Serum dopamine beta-hydroxylase activity and lateral ventricular size in affective disorders and schizophrenia. Biol Psychiatry 19:1395–1402, 1984

Mendlewicz J, Baron M: Morbidity risks in subtypes of unipolar depressive illness: differences between early- and late-onset forms. Br J Psychiatry 134:463–466, 1991

Merriam A, Aronson N, Gaston P, et al: The psychiatric symptoms of Alzheimer's disease. Am Geriatr Soc 36:7–12, 1988

Meyers BS: Geriatric delusional depression. Clin Geriatr Med 8:299–308, 1992

Miller F, Menninger J: Lithium-neuroleptic neurotoxicity is dose dependent. J Clin Psychopharmacol 7:89–91, 1987

Miller NE: The measurement of mood in senile brain disease: examiner ratings and self-reports, in Psychopathology of the Aged. Edited by Cole JO, Barrett JE. New York, Raven Press, 1980

Mukhergee S, Sackeim HA, Schnur DB: Electroconvulsive therapy of acute manic episodes; a review of 50 years' experience. Am J Psychiatry 151:169–176, 1994

Murphy E: The prognosis of depression in old age. Br J Psychiatry 142:111–119, 1983

Murphy JL, Sobol AM, Neff RK, et al: Stability of prevalence: depression and anxiety disorders. Arch Gen Psychiatry 41:990, 1984

Murray N, Hopwood S, Balfour DJK, et al: Influence of age on lithium efficacy and side effects in outpatients. Psychol Med 13:53–60, 1983

National Center for Health Statistics: Advance report of final mortality statistics, 1989. NCHS Monthly Vital Statistics Report 40 (8, suppl 2), 1992

National Institutes of Health Consensus Development Panel on Depression in Late Life: Diagnosis and treatment of depression in late life. JAMA 268:1018–1024, 1992

Nelson JC, Atillasoy E, Mazure C, et al: Hydroxydesipramine in the elderly. J Clin Psychopharmacol 428–433, 1988

Nelson JC, Mazure CM, Bowers MB Jr, et al: A preliminary open study of the combination of fluoxetine and desipramine for rapid treatment of major depression. Arch Gen Psychiatry 48:303–307, 1991

Nemeroff CB, Knight DL, Krishnan KRR, et al: Marked reduction in the number of platelelt ^{3}H-imipramine binding sites in geriatric depression. Arch Gen Psychiatry 45:914–923, 1988

O'Shea B, Lynch T, Falvey J, et al: Electroconvulsive therapy and cognitive improvement in a very elderly depressed patient. Br J Psychiatry 150:255–257, 1987

Parmelee PA, Katz IR, Lawton MP: Depression among institutionalized aged: assessment and prevalence estimation. J Gerontol 44:M22–M29, 1989

Pearlson GD, Ross CA, Lohr WD, et al: Family history of affective disorder is associated with depressive syndrome of Alzheimer's disease. Am J Psychiatry 147:452–456, 1990

Rabins P, Merchant A, Nestadt G: Criteria for diagnosing reversible dementia caused by depression: validation by 2-year follow-up. Br J Psychiatry 144:488–492, 1984

Reding M, Haycox J, Blass J: Depression in patients referred to a dementia clinic. Arch Neurol 42:894–896, 1985

Regestein QR, Lind LJ: Management of electroconvulsive treatment in an elderly woman with severe hypertension and cardiac arrhythmias. Compr Psychiatry 21:288–291, 1980

Reynolds CE, Frank E, Perel JM, et al: Combined pharmacotherapy and psychotherapy in the acute and continuation treatment of elderly patients with recurrent major depression: a preliminary report. Am J Psychiatry 149:1687–1692, 1992

Reynolds CF III, Kupfer DJ, Hock CC, et al: Two-year follow-up of elderly patients with mixed depression and dementia: clinical and electroencephalographic sleep findings. J Am Geriatr Soc 34:793–799, 1986

Rice J, Reich T, Andreasen NC, et al: The familial transmission of bipolar illness. Arch Gen Psychiatry 44:441–447, 1987

Rimmer EM, Richens A: An update on sodium valproate. Pharmacotherapy 5:171–184, 1985

Roose SP, Bone S, Haidofer C, et al: Lithium treatment in older patients. Am J Psychiatry 136:843–844, 1979

Roose SP, Dalack GW, Glassman AH, et al: Cardiovascular effects of buproprion in depressed patients with heart disease. Am J Psychiatry 148:512, 1991

Roth M: The natural history of mental disorder in old age. Journal of Mental Science 101:281–301, 1955

Rovner BW, Kafonek S, Filipp L, et al: Prevalence of mental illness in a community nursing home. Am J Psychiatry 143:1446–1449, 1986

Sacchetti E, Conte G, Pennatti A, et al: Platelet alpha$_2$ adrenoreceptors in major depression: relationship to urinary 4-hydroxy-3-methoxyphenylglycol and age of onset. J Psychiatr Res 19:579–586, 1985

Sachdev PS, Smith JS, Angus-Lepan H, et al: Pseudo-dementia twelve years on. J Neurol Neurosurg Psychiatry 53:254–159, 1990

Sackeim HA, Prudic J, Devanand DP, et al: Effects of stimulus intensity and electrode placement on the efficacy and cognitive effects of electroconvulsive therapy. N Engl J Med 328:882–883, 1993

Sano M, Stern Y, Williams J, et al: Coexisting dementia and depression in Parkinson's disease. Arch Neurol 46:1284–1286, 1989

Schaffer CB, Garvey MJ: Use of lithium in acutely manic elderly patients. Clin Gerontol 3:58, 1984

Schneider LS, Frederickson E, Severson J, et al: ^{3}H-imipramine binding in depressed elderly: relationship to family history and clinical response. Psychiatry Res 19:257–266, 1986

Schneider LS, Severson JA, Sloane RB, et al: Decreased platelet ^{3}H-imipramine binding in elderly outpatients with primary depression compared to secondary depression. J Affect Disord 15:195–200, 1988a

Schneider LS, Cooper TB, Severson JA: Electrocardiographic changes with nortriptyline and 10-hydroxynortriptyline in elderly depressed outpatients. J Clin Psychopharmacol 8:402–408, 1988b

Schneier HA, Khan D: Selective response to carbamazepine in a case of organic mood disorder. J Clin Psychiatry 51:485, 1990

Schou M: Long-lasting neurological sequelae after lithium intoxication. Acta Psychiatr Scand 10:594–602, 1984

Shulman K, Post F: Bipolar affective disorder in the old age. Br J Psychiatry 136:26–32, 1980

Shulman KI, Tohen M, Satlin A, et al: Mania compared with unipolar depression in old age. Am J Psychiatry 149:341–345, 1992

Skare S, Pew B, Dysken M: The dexamethasone suppression test in dementia: a review of the literature. J Geriatr Psychiatry Neurol 3:124–138, 1990

Spar JE: Plasma trazodone concentrations in elderly depressed inpatients:

cardiac effects and short-term efficacy. J Clin Psychopharm 7:406–409, 1987

Spicer CC, Hare EH, Slater E: Neurotic and psychotic forms of depressive illness: evidence from age incidence in a national sample. Br J Psychiatry 123:35–39, 1973

Standish-Barry HMAS, Bouras N, Hale AS, et al: Ventricular size and CSF transmitter metabolite concentrations in severe endogenous depression. Br J Psychiatry 148:386–392, 1986

Starkstein SE, Boston JD, Robinson RG: Mechanism of mania after brain injury. J Nerv Ment Dis 176:87–100, 1988a

Starkstein SE, Robinson RG, Price TR: Comparison of patients with and without post-stroke major depression matched for size and location of lesion. Arch Gen Psychiatry 45:247–252, 1988b

Stoll AL, Banov M, Kolbrener M, et al: Neurologic factors predict a favorable valproate response in bipolar and schizoaffective disorders. J Clin Psychopharmacol 14:311–313, 1994

Sunderland T, Tariot PN, Mueller EA: TRH stimulation test in dementia of the Alzheimer's type and elderly controls. Psychiatry Res 16:269–275, 1985

Tohen M, Castillo J, Baldessarini RJ, et al: Blood dyscrasias with carbamazepine and valproate: a pharmacoepidemiological study of 2,228 patients at risk. Am J Psychiatry 152:413–418, 1995

Weiner RD: Does electroconvulsive therapy cause brain damage? The Behavioral and Brain Sciences 7:1–53, 1984

Weissman MM, Leaf PJ, Tischler GL, et al: Affective disorders in five United States communities. Psychol Med 18:141–153, 1988

Weissman MM, Bruce ML, Leaf PJ, et al: Affective disorders, in Psychiatric Disorders in America: The Epidemiologic Catchment Area Study. Edited by Robins LN, Regier DA. New York, Free Press, 1991, pp 53–80

Wertham FI: A group of benign chronic psychoses: prolonged manic excitements with a statistical study of age, duration, and frequency in 2,000 manic attacks. Am J Psychiatry 86:17–78, 1929

Wragg RE, Jeste DV: Overview of depression and psychosis in Alzheimer's disease. Am J Psychiatry 146:577–589, 1989

Yassa R, Cvejic J: Valproate in the treatment of posttraumatic bipolar disorder in a psychogeriatric patient. J Geriatr Psychiatry Neurol 7:55–57, 1994

Yassa R, Nair V, Nastase C, et al: Prevalence of bipolar disorder in a psychogeriatric population. J Affect Disord 14:197–201, 1988

Young RC: Plasma 10-hydroxynortriptyline and ECG changes in elderly depressed patients. Am J Psychiatry 142:866–868, 1985

Young RC, Klerman GL: Mania in late life: focus on age of onset. Am J
    Psychiatry 149:867– 876, 1992

Young RC, Alexopaulos GS, Shamoian GA, et al: Plasma 10-hydroxy-
    nortriptyline and renal function in elderly depressives. Biol Psychia-
    try 22:1283–1287, 1987

Young RC, Nambudiri D, Alexopoulos GS, et al: VBR and response to
    nortriptyline in geriatric depression (abstract). Presented at the an-
    nual meeting of the Society of Biological Psychiatry, 1988

Zimmer B, Rosen J, Thorton JE, et al: Adjunctive lithium carbonate in
    nortriptyline-resistant elderly depressed patients. J Clin Psycho-
    pharmacol 11:254–256, 1991

Dilip V. Jeste, M.D.
M. Jackuelyn Harris, M.D.
Jane S. Paulsen, Ph.D.

Psychoses

Psychoses are among the most severe psychiatric disorders in persons in any age group, including elderly individuals. These disorders are characterized by delusions, hallucinations, thought disorder, bizarre behavior, or other evidence of loss of touch with reality. Almost any type of psychosis that occurs in younger persons can be seen in older patients. There are, however, some important epidemiological and clinical differences between early-onset and late-onset psychoses. Discussed in this chapter are the more common psychoses such as schizophrenia, delusional disorder, and psychotic features complicating dementia. Psychotic symptoms secondary to other organic mental syndromes and mood disorders with psychotic features are considered elsewhere in this book.

Late-Onset Schizophrenia

Historical Background

Nearly 100 years ago Kraepelin used the term *dementia praecox* to refer to a disorder currently known as schizophrenia. Dementia praecox suggested

This work was supported in part by National Institute of Mental Health Grants 5R37-MH43693, MH45131, and P30MH49671 and by the Department of Veterans Affairs.

an onset in youth and a deterioration of function in the "emotional and volitional spheres of mental life" (Kraepelin 1899). Kraepelin (1919/1971) himself later came to doubt the appropriateness of his terminology because the "dementia" of dementia praecox was not always accompanied by permanent deterioration; remissions did occur in some cases. In addition, not all of the patients first presented in youth. There was a subset of patients with onset of symptoms well into the 5th, 6th, or 7th decade of life. Kraepelin applied the diagnosis paraphrenia to those patients with relatively late onset of delusions and hallucinations, characterized by a predominance of paranoid symptoms. Although Kraepelin stressed the disintegration of personality in dementia praecox as opposed to paraphrenia, he described some paraphrenia patients with a predominantly downhill course, whereas a subset of patients with dementia praecox did not have a marked deterioration in social and personal functioning. Indeed, follow-up studies of Kraepelin's paraphrenia patients by other investigators indicated that some of the patients diagnosed as having paraphrenia had symptoms similar to those of patients with dementia praecox (Mayer 1921).

The earlier versions of the DSM of the American Psychiatric Association did not have an upper age limit for the diagnosis of schizophrenia. It was not until DSM-III (American Psychiatric Association 1980) that it was first stipulated that onset of symptoms for schizophrenia must begin before age 45. DSM-III-R (American Psychiatric Association 1987), on the other hand, allowed an onset of schizophrenic symptoms after age 45, applying the term *late-onset schizophrenia* to these individuals. DSM-III-R did not include paraphrenia as a diagnostic entity. DSM-IV (American Psychiatric Association 1994) does not specify an upper age limit for the diagnosis of schizophrenia nor is the term *late-onset* specified.

Epidemiology

Although there is a body of literature on late-onset schizophrenia dating back to 1913, there are several important problems with its interpretation. First, there has been no general agreement on the definition of late onset. Some studies chose 40 years of age, but others examined patients with onset after ages 45, 60, or 65 years (Harris and Jeste 1988). Second, the criteria used to establish the diagnosis of schizophrenia were not always mentioned in these studies. Third, it is often difficult to objectify the assessment of age at onset of schizophrenia. Elderly patients may not remember, and significant others may have passed away, making corroboration of the patient's history difficult. Finally, the presence of premorbid paranoid or schizoid personality traits may make the evaluation of premorbid functioning difficult, and older patients with schizophrenic symptoms may be thought to have organic mental syndromes, mood disorders, or simple sensory deficits.

Harris and Jeste (1988), on analyzing data from the psychiatric literature, estimated that 13% of all hospitalized schizophrenic patients were reported to have onset of psychosis in their 40s, 7% had onset in their 50s, and only 3% first presented after age 60. Most studies of late-onset schizophrenia show a 2–10 times higher proportion of women than men (Bland 1977; Blessed and Wilson 1982; Bleuler 1943; Kay and Roth 1961). Several factors, such as greater longevity of women, psychosocial stressors, and neuroendocrine changes, have been suggested as possible explanations for the higher prevalence of late-onset schizophrenia in women. The precise contribution of these and other factors to the onset of schizophrenia in women in later life is unclear.

Diagnosis

The patient should meet DSM-IV (American Psychiatric Association 1984) criteria for schizophrenia (including duration of at least 6 months), with the additional requirement that onset of symptoms—including the prodrome—must be at or after age 45. Documentation of a decrease in functioning markedly below the highest level achieved may be difficult in older patients, who may be retired, widowed, or relatively socially inactive. The typical clinical picture is that of an older woman who exhibits persecutory delusions; frequently has auditory hallucinations, a chronic course, premorbid schizoid and paranoid traits; and shows improvement in positive symptoms with low-dose neuroleptic therapy.

Symptomatology

Late-onset schizophrenia is often characterized by bizarre delusions, which have a predominantly persecutory characteristic. Auditory hallucinations are the second most prominent psychotic symptom. Schneiderian first-rank symptoms, such as thought broadcasting or two voices arguing with each other, may be present. Symptoms of depression are reported by a number of these patients. Systematized delusions of physical or mental influence are seen in a considerable proportion of patients. Grandiose, erotic, or somatic delusions may occur in some cases. Looseness of association and inappropriateness of affect are less common than in younger schizophrenic patients (Jeste et al. 1988). There is an insidious deterioration of personal and social adjustment. To exclude the diagnosis of early-onset schizophrenia, it is important to make certain that there were no prodromal symptoms of schizophrenia (e.g., marked social isolation, blunted or inappropriate affect, marked impairment in personal hygiene) before age 45.

Pathogenesis and Etiology

The etiology and pathophysiology of late-onset schizophrenia are not well understood. Several variables have been explored in some detail, including genetics, premorbid personality, neuropsychology and brain imaging, and sensory deficits.

Genetics. Studies that have examined the prevalence of schizophrenia in families of late-onset schizophrenic patients have had methodological problems (Harris and Jeste 1988). For example, not all family members have been followed into old age to ensure that every case of late-onset schizophrenia in other family members is detected. Physical illness and geographic relocation of relatives also make it difficult to conduct such studies. The published studies suggest that the prevalence of schizophrenia is approximately 7% in siblings and 3% in parents of all probands with late-onset schizophrenia (Bleuler 1943; Herbert and Jacobson 1967; Kay and Roth 1961; Larson and Nyman 1970; Rokhlina 1975). The overall prevalence of schizophrenia in first-degree relatives of late-onset schizophrenic patients (Rokhlina 1975) has been reported to be slightly lower than that in families of early-onset schizophrenic patients but greater than that in families of normal probands.

Premorbid personality. Some studies (Herbert and Jacobson 1967; Kay and Roth 1961) noted that a sizable proportion of late-onset schizophrenic patients had abnormal premorbid personality traits of a paranoid or schizoid nature. Many patients had never been married and were considered by neighbors to be eccentric. Nevertheless, when compared with earlier onset schizophrenia patients, patients with late-onset schizophrenia are more likely to have been married, held a job or been a homemaker, and had children (Jeste et al. 1988).

Neuropsychology and brain imaging. Despite a considerable amount of published research on neuropsychological functioning in schizophrenia

(Braff 1993; Green and Walker 1985; Gur and Pearlson 1993; Levin et al. 1989; Saykin et al. 1991; Strauss 1993), little is known about the cognitive deficits associated with late-onset schizophrenia. Heaton et al. (1994) compared the neuropsychological performance of late-onset schizophrenia patients with that of two groups of early-onset schizophrenia patients (those younger than 45 years, and those older than 45 years), patients with Alzheimer's disease, and elderly control subjects. All the schizophrenia groups showed more impairment than the control group in all neuropsychological ability areas, except for memory; no schizophrenia group showed memory impairment. By contrast, the Alzheimer's disease group showed more impairment than the control group in memory as well as all other ability areas. The Alzheimer's disease group demonstrated greater learning and memory impairments than the schizophrenia groups; the three schizophrenia groups did not differ from one another. Although the patient groups (those with schizophrenia and Alzheimer's disease) all showed verbal, complex perceptual-motor, abstraction, attention, sensory, and motor impairments relative to the control subjects, the three schizophrenic groups were strikingly similar but were different from the Alzhemier's disease group. Discriminant function analyses were able to correctly classify 70.3% of the schizophrenia group, 88.2% of the Alzheimer's disease group, and 89.7% of the control group. The results further indicated that the neuropsychological discriminant functions rarely misclassified a schizophrenia subject as having Alzheimer's disease, or vice versa; moreover, there was no tendency for this type of error to be made more often with late-onset schizophrenia patients than with early-onset schizophrenia patients. In general, these findings suggest that late-onset and early-onset schizophrenia patients share a common cognitive profile that is distinctly different from that of dementia patients.

One structural brain finding in late-onset schizophrenia that has been reported by several groups of investigators is an increased ventricle-to-brain ratio as seen on magnetic resonance imaging (MRI) or computed tomography (CT) scans (Krull et al. 1991; Naguib and Levy 1987; Rabins 1989). In addition to the quantification of ventricular and sulcal size, several reports have documented large areas of subcortical white-matter hyperintensities (in the periventricular regions as well as elsewhere) in patients with late-onset schizophrenia and related psychoses when compared with age-matched control subjects (Breitner et al. 1990; Coffey et al. 1990; Lesser et al. 1991, 1992; Miller and Lesser 1988; Miller et al. 1991). In addition, some reports have noted an increased number of vascular lesions in patients with late-life psychoses of different types (Breitner et al. 1990; Flint et al. 1991).

In the few studies of functional brain imaging conducted in late-onset schizophrenia patients, single photon emission computed tomography (SPECT) findings have revealed lower global cortical uptake (particularly in the left posterior frontal region and bilateral inferior temporal regions) in late-life schizophrenia patients than in control subjects (Dupont et al. 1994; Lesser et al. 1993). The uptake did not correlate with age at onset, duration of illness, current daily neuroleptic dose, severity of psychopathology, or global cognitive impairment. In the only available published study of positron-emission tomography (PET) in late-onset schizophrenia, Pearlson et al. (1993) reported elevated B_{max} (receptor density) values for dopamine D_2 receptors in 13 late-onset schizophrenia patients never treated with neuroleptics when compared with age- and gender-matched control subjects; this indicated that the higher dopamine D_2 values in the patients were not secondary to neuroleptic effects. Unfortunately, none of these functional imaging results in late-onset schizophrenia patients have been compared with those in age-matched early-onset schizophrenia patients. An important question arises as to whether brain abnormalities associated with late-onset schizophrenia have pathogenetic significance.

Sensory deficits.   Several studies have reported an association between sensory impairment and late-onset schizophrenia. Cooper and Porter (1976) noted an increased incidence of cataracts in a population of patients with "paranoid psychosis" compared with patients with affective psychosis, whereas Cooper and Curry (1976) demonstrated an association between bilateral conductive hearing loss and paranoid psychosis. A review found that more than 85% of published studies (i.e., 23 of 27) suggested a positive association between sensory impairment (visual or hearing) and a somewhat heterogeneous group of late-life psychoses with paranoid symptoms (Prager and Jeste 1993). However, because of methodological limitations in much of the available literature (e.g., variable and poorly defined diagnostic terminology for psychosis and a lack of objective, quantified techniques for measuring sensory impairment), the relative contribution of sensory deficits to late-onset schizophrenia remains unclear. Prager and Jeste (1993) evaluated visual and hearing impairments in 87 middle-age and elderly subjects (16 with late-onset schizophrenia, 25 with early-onset schizophrenia, 20 with mood disorder, and 26 control subjects). Although psychiatric patients had greater impairments on measures of corrected (with eyeglasses) visual acuity and in self-reported hearing deficit, impairment levels on uncorrected (constitutional) visual acuity or on pure-tone audiometry were similar to those in the control group. These findings suggest that the observed relationship between sensory deficits and late-life psychosis may be due, at least in part, to inadequate correction of sensory deficits (e.g., not getting the appropriate eyeglasses) in older psychiatric patients. Although a causal relationship between sensory impairment and late-life psychosis remains to be illuminated, interventions targeted toward increased correction of sensory impairment in elderly individuals could be potentially effective in decreasing the morbidity of late-life psychotic disorders.

Differential Diagnosis

Whenever an elderly patient presents with psychotic symptoms, organic abnormality must first be ruled out in the differential diagnosis. This is especially important because a number of potentially reversible medical illnesses—for example, certain endocrinopathies—can have clinical presentations similar to that of schizophrenia (Table 20–1). A careful neurological examination accompanied by complete blood chemistry tests, including tests of thyroid function and vitamin deficiencies (e.g., B_{12} and folic acid), as well as serological tests for syphilis, are usually part of the assessment. Other appropriate laboratory tests may be needed in individual patients. Modern imaging methods (e.g., MRI or CT scan) may identify cases in which structural abnormalities coexist with late-onset psychosis. Because structural abnormalities may not always produce neurological deficits, at least in the early stages, it is useful to have at least a CT scan of the brain in a newly diagnosed elderly patient with a late-onset psychotic disorder of uncertain etiology.

Another important differential diagnosis is early-onset schizophrenia. Caution is required in using the diagnosis of late-onset schizophrenia strictly on the basis of a first psychiatric hospitalization for psychosis after age 45. It is prudent to obtain a detailed history of the disorder from both the patient and his or her family or friends, because some patients may have had prodromal or even overt psychotic symptoms for some time prior to the first hospitalization. The prodrome differs from premorbid personality traits in that it requires a clear deterioration from a previous level of functioning. Also, some patients with an apparent late-onset psychosis may have had a more benign psychotic illness that did not require hospitalization until age 45.

Mood disorders with psychotic features may present for the first time after age 45 and can be confused with late-onset schizophrenia. The

Table 20–1.   Disorders associated with secondary psychosis in the elderly

Endocrinopathies	Viral encephalitis
Hyperthyroidism	Spinocerebellar degeneration
Hypothyroidism	Neurosyphilis
Addison's disease	
Cushing's disease	**Vitamin deficiencies**
Hyperparathyroidism	Thiamine
Hypoparathyroidism	Niacin
Hypoglycemia	B_{12}
	Folate
Neurological disorders	
Parkinson's disease	**Other conditions**
Alzheimer's disease	Iatrogenic (secondary to drugs
Pick's disease	such as L-dopa) and other drugs
Multi-infarct dementia	potentially toxic to the central
Seizure disorders	nervous system
Hydrocephalus	Systemic lupus erythematosus
Demyelinating diseases (e.g.,	Temporal arteritis
multiple sclerosis)	Hyponatremia
Neoplasms	Delirium (e.g., as a result of hypoxia)
Encephalopathies (posttraumatic,	
hepatic, postanoxic, toxic)	

predominance of affective symptoms and periodicity of the illness should make the clinician consider a mood disorder.

Delusional disorder may mimic late-onset schizophrenia, but the latter diagnosis is more likely in the presence of bizarre delusions or prominent auditory hallucinations, Schneiderian first-rank symptoms, deteriorated functioning, and flattening of affect. (See "Late-Life Delusional Disorder" below for further discussion of this differential diagnosis.)

Treatment

In patients with late-onset schizophrenia, as well as in those with early-onset schizophrenia, neuroleptic drugs are the mainstay of therapy. Available studies suggest that a large majority of late-onset schizophrenia patients improve symptomatically with neuroleptic treatment (Jeste et al. 1993). An important consideration is the higher incidence of side effects seen in elderly individuals, as compared to younger patients, with administration of a given amount of neuroleptic. Some studies have shown positive correlations between age and serum level of neuroleptic when equivalent doses of neuroleptic are administered (Tran-Johnson et al. 1992; Yesavage et al. 1982). Usually, small doses of neuroleptics (e.g., 0.5–2.5 mg of haloperidol per day) are sufficient to produce improvement in older patients.

The clinician should advise the patient and family of the possibility of adverse effects, including sedation, anticholinergic effects, parkinsonian reactions, postural hypotension, neuroleptic malignant syndrome, and tardive dyskinesia (the incidence of which is higher in patients who begin neuroleptic treatment in later life) (Jeste and Caligiuri 1993; Saltz et al. 1991). Frequent monitoring is necessary to detect these side effects. Periodic assessment (at least once in several months) for the emergence of involuntary movements is also recommended. At present, there is no satisfactory evidence to indicate superiority of one or more specific neuroleptic drugs in the treatment of late-onset schizophrenia. In individual patients, specific drugs may be preferred on the basis of their side effect profiles. For example, low-potency neuroleptics with marked anticholinergic activity (e.g., thioridazine) should be avoided in men with prostatic hypertrophy and urinary retention. Similarly, high-potency neuroleptics with an increased risk of parkinsonian reactions (e.g., haloperidol) may not be the drugs of choice for patients with preexisting rigidity or tremor.

Course and Prognosis

Studies of the course of late-onset schizophrenia have generally found it to be chronic (Herbert and Jacobson 1967; Kay and Roth 1961). Spontaneous remissions seem to be uncommon, and discontinuation of neuroleptics (frequently because of noncompliance) tends to exacerbate psychosis. Good compliance and supportive psychosocial therapies can improve the outlook for the patient.

Aging of Early-Onset Schizophrenia Patients

Many early-onset schizophrenia patients survive into old age, yet comparatively little is known about the long-term course of schizophrenia. A review of the literature on the course of schizophrenia suggests that approximately one-third of patients either undergo remission or are left with mild symptoms over the long term (McGlashan 1988). The more positive, dramatic symptoms of schizophrenia seem to lessen in severity with the passage of time, whereas negative symptoms persist. The deterioration in schizophrenia usually occurs shortly after the onset of the disorder and is often limited to the first 5 or 10 years after illness. A review of neuropsychological deficits in chronic schizophrenia suggested that cognitive dysfunction typically remains stable following the initial deterioration (Heaton and Drexler 1987). Partial or complete remission, ranging in incidence from 6% to greater than 50%, has been reported in individual studies (Belitsky and McGlashan 1993; Harding et al. 1987; McGlashan 1988). However, heterogeneity of outcome is a constant finding in these studies. Many attempts have been made to uncover associations between specific factors and outcome in schizophrenia. A number of patient-related factors (e.g., better prognosis in women, those ever married, and those with normal neurological evaluations) and illness-related factors (e.g., better prognosis with acute-onset, short-duration illness with affective symptoms) have been associated with outcome in the literature, but most of these are of little value for predicting the course in a particular patient (Prudo and Blum 1987; Ram et al. 1992). Differences in the methods by which information was obtained, lack of adequate control groups, and inattention to such details as drug history or specific subtype of schizophrenia make conclusions difficult to draw.

Research is needed to examine the impact of changes in social structure and other age-related changes on the course and outcome of schizophrenia. Retirement, for example, may markedly alter the pattern of psychosocial stressors and may have a favorable impact (owing to removal of work-related stresses) or an unfavorable effect (secondary to a reduction in income as well as a decrease in employment-associated self-esteem) on the outcome of schizophrenia. Biological factors (e.g., hormonal changes during menopause) also may be important. Any related differences in pharmacokinetics and pharmacodynamics of neuroleptics and other psychotropic medications and a tendency for milder positive symptoms in elderly schizophrenia patients may result in the need for lower doses of these drugs.

Late-Life Delusional Disorder

Persecutory delusions in the elderly patient usually occur in the context of another, underlying neuropsychiatric disorder (e.g., schizophrenia, mood disorder, or dementia). Occasionally, however, primary delusional disorder is implicated. Conceptualization and study of this disorder have been hampered by inconsistencies in nomenclature and diagnostic criteria.

Kraepelin (1919/1971) defined paranoia as an often incurable disorder characterized by the development of a chronic, well-systematized, delusional state of nonbizarre quality with little or no impairment of orientation, memory, or intellect and an absence of hallucinations, thought disorder, disturbed volition, or personality deterioration. Kraepelin's paraphrenia, on the other hand, included both paranoid delusions and systematized hallucinations and typically had its onset in later life.

DSM-III (American Psychiatric Association 1980) described *paranoid disorder* as consisting of the occurrence of at least 1 week of persistent delusions of persecution or jealousy with emotion appropriate to the content of the delusions, without evidence of schizophrenia or affective disorder and without prominent hallucinations or evidence of organic dysfunction. *Paranoia* was described as a chronic and stable persecutory delusional system of greater than 6 months' duration. In DSM-III-R (American Psychiatric Association 1987), the term *paranoid disorder* was replaced by *delusional disorder*, and the criteria for the delusional content were broadened to include erotomanic, grandiose, jealous, persecutory, somatic, and unspecified types; also, the minimum required duration of symptoms was increased to 1 month. DSM-IV criteria (American Psychiatric Association 1994) for delusional disorders do not differ significantly from DSM-III-R criteria, except for the addition of a "mixed" type that has delusions characteristic of more than one of the above types but without any one theme predominating.

Prevalence

Studies suggest that between 2% and 8% of the psychiatric population has some type of paranoid symptoms (Leuchter and Spar 1985). In DSM-IV (American Psychiatric Association 1994), the population prevalence of delusional disorder was estimated at 0.03%, with a lifetime risk of 0.05% to 0.1%. A study of the incidence of paranoid or delusional disorder by Heston (1987) indicated that although only about 2% of patients satisfied DSM-III (American Psychiatric Association 1980) criteria for paranoid disorder, another 13% had paranoid ideation.

Delusional disorder can occur in young people but usually presents first in mid- to late adulthood. The average age at onset is somewhat earlier for men (40–49 years) than for women (60–69 years).

Diagnosis and Symptomatology

The patient should meet DSM-IV (American Psychiatric Association 1994) criteria for delusional disorder. The occurrence of nonbizarre delusions (defined by DSM-IV as delusions involving situations that may occur in real life—for example, being followed, having a disease, being deceived by one's spouse or lover) is fundamental to this illness. Auditory or visual hallucinations, if present, are not prominent, and affective symptoms, if any, are of brief duration and do not antedate the delusional syndrome. The predominant theme or themes of the delusion may be erotomanic, grandiose, jealous, persecutory, somatic, or of unspecified or mixed types.

Pathogenesis and Etiology

Four factors have been postulated to contribute to the development of delusional disorder, although the available evidence in favor of each of these requires verification.

1. *Genetics:* Some studies have found an increased incidence of schizophrenia in families of patients with paranoid or delusional disorder (Kendler and Davis 1981; Winokur 1977).
2. *Premorbid personality:* Persons with premorbid avoidant, paranoid, or schizoid personality disorders may be more likely to develop delusional disorder (American Psychiatric Association 1987).
3. *Sensory deficits:* Some studies have demonstrated an association between hearing loss and paranoia in elderly individuals (Cooper and Curry 1976), whereas other systematic studies have failed to confirm this relationship (Moore 1981).
4. *Socioeconomic status:* There is some evidence that immigration or low socioeconomic status can predispose to delusional disorder (American Psychiatric Association 1987; Gurian et al. 1992).

Differential Diagnosis

To make the diagnosis of late-life delusional disorder, organic causes must first be investigated and excluded. Delusional syndromes associated with early dementia can resemble delusional disorder (American Psychiatric Association 1994). The relative absence of cognitive impairment in delusional disorder should help to rule out dementia. Differentiation from late-onset schizophrenia has been discussed previously.

Delusions can accompany mood disorders. Therefore, for a diagnosis of delusional disorder to be made, the clinician must establish that the delusions preceded the onset of mood disorder. Depressive symptoms frequently occur in delusional disorder but usually begin subsequent to the development of delusions.

DSM-IV (American Psychiatric Association 1994) requires symptoms to have been present for at least 1 month. Otherwise, a diagnosis of psychotic disorder, not otherwise specified, may be considered.

Treatment

Antipsychotic drugs are often efficacious, especially in agitated delusional patients, but they must be administered cautiously in the elderly patient. Some patients may be refractory to neuroleptic therapy. One common problem in the treatment of patients with delusional disorder is noncompliance. Raskind et al. (1979) have suggested that parenteral depot neuroleptics may be preferable to oral daily medication because of problems with compliance. From the viewpoint of therapeutic efficacy, however, there is little evidence that any one type of neuroleptic is superior to others. Supportive psychotherapy is an important modality of treatment. For some delusional patients, especially those who are paranoid, a somewhat distant medical approach is more acceptable and less threatening. Antidepressant drugs, electroconvulsive therapy, and psychotherapeutic approaches have all been tried, with variable success.

Course and Prognosis

The data on prognosis are limited, making it difficult to draw conclusions. The course may be chronic, especially in those with persecutory delusions, whereas others may have remissions and relapses. The diagnostic consistency of the disorder has been questioned. Kraepelin (1909) noticed that diagnostic inconsistency was extremely high, with 80% of the patients later meeting his criteria for dementia praecox or paraphrenia. In other, more recent studies, diagnostic consistency ranged from 3% to 56% (Koehler and Hornstein 1986; Winokur 1977). This wide range is probably due, at least in part, to differences in length of follow-up.

Psychotic Disorders Not Elsewhere Classified

DSM-IV (American Psychiatric Association 1994) describes several other less well defined psychotic disorders. There is a relative paucity of literature on the characterization of these disorders in elderly individuals. The conditions in this category include the following:

1. *Brief psychotic disorder:* This is characterized by sudden onset of psychotic symptoms of less than 1 month's duration, precipitated by a stressful situation, with eventual complete return to premorbid level of functioning.
2. *Schizophreniform disorder:* This disorder is similar to schizophrenia except that the duration of symptoms (including the prodromal and residual phases) is less than 6 months.
3. *Schizoaffective disorder:* This diagnosis is applied when patients do not meet criteria for schizophrenia but have schizophrenic symptoms (criterion A) and a history of a mood disturbance at some time, along with psychotic features in the absence of prominent mood symptoms for at least 2 weeks.
4. *Shared psychotic disorder:* This diagnosis is used when a close relationship with a person (or persons) with an already present delusion results in the new development of a similar delusion in the second person. McNiel et al. (1972) described shared psychotic disorder (also called folie à deux) in two elderly persons with shared persecutory delusions. The authors noted that the disorder in their patients was similar to that in younger persons, except for an unusually strong interdependence in the elderly couple.

Psychotic Disorder Not Otherwise Specified (Atypical Psychosis)

DSM-IV (American Psychiatric Association 1994) describes psychotic disorder, not otherwise specified (NOS) as a disorder with clearly psychotic symptoms that do not meet the criteria for any other "nonorganic" psychotic disorder. In essence, this is a residual category to be used in those situations in which either the patient's history and symptoms do not fit into any other category, or not enough information is available to make a diagnosis. The diagnosis of atypical psychosis, the DSM-III (American Psychiatric Association 1980) equivalent of psychotic disorder NOS, was often made for patients with onset of a schizophrenia-like illness in later life, as DSM-III did not recognize late-onset schizophrenia. With removal of the restriction on age at onset of schizophrenia in DSM-III-R and DSM-IV (American Psychiatric Association 1987, 1994), it is expected that the number of patients with the diagnosis of psychotic disorder NOS will decrease. In a study of 16 middle-age and older patients diagnosed with psychotic disorder NOS, 7 had pure hallucinatory states (primarily auditory), and 9 did not meet criteria for schizophrenia because of a lack of deterioration in functioning markedly below the highest level achieved before the disturbance (Lesser et al. 1992).

The prevalence of visual hallucinosis in patients with eye abnormality ranges from 18% to 57%, and many of these patients were not aware that what they were seeing was not real. Therefore, such physical disorders must be carefully ruled out as factors causing and maintaining the disturbance before considering the diagnosis of psychosis NOS (Beck and Harris 1994).

Psychosis in Patients With Dementia

Alzheimer's disease is the most common type of dementia in elderly individuals. Psychotic symptoms and disruptive behaviors are present in a sizable proportion of Alzheimer's patients and can cause considerable stress to family members. Patients with both Alzheimer's disease and delusions have been found to have significantly more wandering, agitation, and family and marital problems and significantly less self-care in comparison with patients with Alzheimer's disease without delusions (Rockwell et al. 1994). This may be one possible explanation for the high rate of institutionalization among patients with Alzheimer's disease with delusions (Steele et al. 1990). DSM-III-R (American Psychiatric Association 1987) listed only one psychotic symptom among behavioral complications of Alzheimer's disease—that is, delusions. DSM-IV (American Psychiatric Association 1994) has expanded this list to include other behavioral disturbances.

Prevalence

In a review of psychiatric features occurring in patients with Alzheimer's disease, Wragg and Jeste (1989) noted that about 30% of patients (range, 10%–73%) exhibit delusions, often of a persecutory nature. The delusions are usually concrete and interpersonal and may be stimulated by environmental stress. The more common types of delusions refer to specific persons (e.g., daughter-in-law or neighbor) stealing things or spying on the patient or someone impersonating the spouse or a significant other. Complex or elaborate, systematized delusions that characterize schizophrenia or delusional disorder are rarely seen in Alzheimer's disease patients. Hallucinations are reported to occur in about 21%–49% of patients, with a tendency toward a higher incidence in hospitalized and nursing home populations. Visual hallucinations are slightly more frequent than auditory hallucinations.

Diagnosis and Symptomatology

Psychotic symptoms in the patient with dementia may present as disordered perception and thought content. Because of cognitive impairment, patients may be unable to verbalize their thoughts or perceptions properly. In such cases, the occurrence of delusions or hallucinations can only be inferred from patients' behavior (e.g., responding to a visual or auditory hallucination). Isolated psychotic symptoms such as persecutory delusions are more frequent than diagnosable psychotic or mood disorders in patients with Alzheimer's disease (Teri et al. 1988; Wragg and Jeste 1989).

Pathogenesis/Etiology

Association of psychotic symptoms with specific neuropsychiatric features has been attempted. For example, Mayeux et al. (1985) noted an increased incidence of psychotic symptoms in Alzheimer's disease patients with coexistent extrapyramidal disorder. Both visual and auditory deficits have been positively associated with psychotic symptoms in dementia patients. There is no consistent association of psychosis with stage of Alzheimer's disease. Nevertheless, there has been some suggestion of increased frontal temporal dysfunction on neuropsychological testing (Jeste et al. 1992) and increased densities of senile plaques and neurofibrillary tangles in specific cortical areas, especially the middle frontal cortex and the presubiculum (Zubenko et al. 1991) in patients with Alzheimer's disease and psychosis. A past history of psychiatric disorder may be positively associated with psychotic symptoms in patients with Alzheimer's disease (Berrios and Brook 1985).

Differential Diagnosis

Delirium may occur as a result of medications or medical disorders in the context of dementia and is an important consideration in the differential diagnosis of psychotic symptoms in patients with Alzheimer's disease. The onset of dementia of the Alzheimer's type or other dementing illness prior to the development of psychotic symptoms should help differentiate these patients from elderly schizophrenia or delusional disorder patients who have subsequently developed some cognitive impairment.

Treatment

Few well-controlled, systematic studies have examined the effects of the treatment of psychotic symptoms in patients with Alzheimer's disease or other dementing illnesses. The available data suggest that treatment with neuroleptic medications results in improvement (Lohr et al. 1992). The various neuroleptic drugs seem to be equally effective in these patients, but as stated previously, caution is advised when administering these medications. Sometimes a particular neuroleptic that is least likely to aggravate existing medical problems is selected. For example, particular care is taken to exclude delirium before commencing neuroleptic therapy with drugs possessing substantial anticholinergic effects, as these may worsen cognitive impairment. Alternative treatment options for the management of the dementia patient should be considered (Wragg and Jeste 1989). These include benzodiazepines, which may be of benefit in reducing anxiety and agitation but not specific psychotic symptoms. Trazodone, because of its sedative effects, may also have efficacy in this regard. Supportive psychotherapy may be beneficial for patients in the earlier stages of dementia, and behavioral modification may also be valuable in various stages of the illness. Families can benefit considerably from education and support with appropriate ways of coping with the afflicted family member.

Course and Prognosis

Although there have been few systematic studies of the course of psychosis in Alzheimer's disease, Cummings et al. (1987) have suggested that as the severity of the dementia increases, the psychotic symptoms tend to decrease (i.e., some level of cognitive integrity is necessary for the expression of psychotic symptoms).

Summary

Psychotic symptoms can develop in elderly individuals in a variety of different conditions. As a result of increased research in this area, the terminology and classification have improved, although much remains to be learned about the etiopathology of these disorders. Late-onset schizophrenia (i.e., schizophrenia with onset at or after age 45) is usually characterized by bizarre, persecutory delusions; auditory hallucinations; chronic course; and a variable degree of symptomatic improvement with low-dose neuroleptics. Delusional disorder presents with nonbizarre delusions (as defined previously) without prominent hallucinations. It is of utmost importance to exclude neurological, endocrine, and other medical conditions when evaluating an older patient with new onset of psychosis in the absence of a past history of a psychotic disorder. Patients diagnosed as having Alzheimer's disease or other dementias may also develop psychotic symptoms. Other conditions associated with late-life psychosis include mood disorders with psychotic features, recurrence of earlier onset schizophrenia, and psychoses not otherwise specified. A detailed medical, psychosocial, and laboratory workup and a comprehensive biopsychosocial approach to management, with an emphasis on using relatively low doses of medications, are highly recommended.

References

American Psychiatric Association: Diagnostic and Statistical Manual of Mental Disorders, 3rd Edition. Washington, DC, American Psychiatric Association, 1980

American Psychiatric Association: Diagnostic and Statistical Manual of Mental Disorders, 3rd Edition, Revised. Washington, DC, American Psychiatric Association, 1987

American Psychiatric Association: Diagnostic and Statistical Manual of Mental Disorders, 4th Edition. Washington, DC, American Psychiatric Association, 1994

Beck J, Harris MJ: Visual hallucinosis in non-psychotic elderly. International Journal of Geriatric Psychiatry 9:531–536, 1994

Belitsky R, McGlashan TH: At issue: the manifestations of schizophrenia in late life, a dearth of data. Schizophr Bull 19:683–685, 1993

Berrios GE, Brook P: Delusions and the psychopathology of the elderly with dementia. Acta Psychiatr Scand 72:296–301, 1985

Bland RC: Demographic aspects of functional psychoses in Canada. Acta Psychiatr Scand 55:369–380, 1977

Blessed G, Wilson ID: The contemporary natural history of mental disorder in old age. Br J Psychiatry 141:59–67, 1982

Bleuler M: Late schizophrenic clinical pictures. Fortschr Neurol Psychiatr 15:259–290, 1943

Braff DL: Information processing and attention dysfunctions in schizophrenia. Schizophr Bull 19:233–259, 1993

Breitner J, Husain M, Figiel G, et al: Cerebral white matter disease in late-onset psychosis. Biol Psychiatry 28:266–274, 1990

Coffey CE, Figiel GS, Djang WT, et al: Subcortical hyperintensity on magnetic resonance imaging: a comparison of normal and depressed elderly subjects. Am J Psychiatry 47:187–189, 1990

Cooper AF, Curry AR: The pathology of deafness in the paranoid and affective psychoses of later life. J Psychosom Res 20:97–105, 1976

Cooper AF, Porter R: Visual acuity and ocular pathology in the paranoid and affective psychoses of later life. J Psychosom Res 20:107–114, 1976

Cummings JL, Miller B, Hill MA, et al: Neuropsychiatric aspects of multi-infarct dementia and dementia of the Alzheimer type. Arch Neurol 44:389–393, 1987

Dupont RM, Lehr P, Lamoureaux G, et al: Preliminary report: cerebral blood flow abnormalities in older schizophrenic patients. Psychiatry Research Neuroimaging 51:121–130, 1994

Flint AJ, Rifat SI, Eastwood MR: Late-onset paranoia: distinct from paraphrenia? International Journal of Geriatric Psychiatry 6:103–109, 1991

Green M, Walker E: Neuropsychological performance and positive and negative symptoms in schizophrenia. J Abnorm Psychol 94:460–469, 1985

Gur RE, Pearlson GD: Neuroimaging in schizophrenia research. Schizophr Bull 19:337–353, 1993

Gurian BS, Wexler D, Baker EH: Late-life paranoia: possible association with early trauma and infertility. International Journal of Geriatric Psychiatry 7:277–284, 1992

Harding CM, Brooks GW, Ashikaga T, et al: The Vermont longitudinal study, II: long-term outcome of subjects who once met the criteria for DSM-III schizophrenia. Am J Psychiatry 144:727–735, 1987

Harris MJ, Jeste DV: Late-onset schizophrenia: an overview. Schizophr Bull 14:39–55, 1988

Heaton R, Paulsen J, McAdams LA, et al: Neuropsychological deficits in schizophrenics: relationship to age, chronicity and dementia. Arch Gen Psychiatry 51:469–476, 1994

Heaton RK, Drexler M: Clinical neuropsychological findings in schizophrenia and aging, in Schizophrenia and Aging. Edited by Miller NE, Cohen GD. New York, Guilford Press, 1987, pp 145–161

Herbert ME, Jacobson S: Late paraphrenia. Br J Psychiatry 113:461–469, 1967

Heston LL: The paranoid syndrome after mid life, in Schizophrenia and Aging. Edited by Miller NE, Cohen GD. New York, Guilford Press,

1987, pp 249–257

Jeste DV, Caligiuri MP: Tardive dyskinesia. Schizophr Bull 19:303–315, 1993

Jeste DV, Harris MJ, Pearlson GD, et al: Late-onset schizophrenia: studying clinical validity. Psychiatr Clin North Am 11:1–14, 1988

Jeste DV, Wragg RE, Salmon DP, et al: Cognitive deficits of patients with Alzheimer's disease with and without delusions. Am J Psychiatry 149:184–189, 1992

Jeste DV, Lacro JP, Gilbert PL, et al: Treatment of late-life schizophrenia with neuroleptics. Schizophr Bull 19:817–830, 1993

Kay DWK, Roth M: Environmental and hereditary factors in the schizophrenias of old age ("late paraphrenia") and their bearing on the general problem of causation in schizophrenia. Journal of Mental Science 107:649–686, 1961

Kendler S, Davis KL: The genetics and biochemistry of paranoid schizophrenia and other paranoid psychoses. Schizophr Bull 7:689–709, 1981

Koehler K, Hornstein C: 100 years of DSM-III paranoia—how stable a diagnosis over time? Eur Arch Psychiatry Neurol Sci 235:255–258, 1986

Kraepelin E: Psychiatrie, Ein Lehrbuch fur Studierende und Artzte, 6th Edition. Leipzig, Barth, 1899

Kraepelin E: Psychiatrie ein Lehrbuch fur Studierende und Aertzte, 8th Edition. Leipzig, Barth, 1909

Kraepelin E: Dementia Praecox and Paraphrenia (1919). Translated by Barclay RM. Huntington, NY, Krieger, 1971

Krull AJ, Press G, Dupont R, et al: Brain imaging in late-onset schizophrenia and related psychoses. International Journal of Geriatric Psychiatry 6:651–658, 1991

Larson CA, Nyman GE: Age of onset in schizophrenia. Hum Hered 20:241–247, 1970

Lesser IM, Miller BL, Boone KB, et al: I. Brain injury and cognitive function in late-onset psychotic depression. J Neuropsychiatry Clin Neurosci 3:33–40, 1991

Lesser IM, Jeste DV, Boone KB, et al: Late-onset psychotic disorder, not otherwise specified: clinical and neuroimaging findings. Biol Psychiatry 31:419–423, 1992

Lesser IM, Miller BL, Swartz JR, et al: Brain imaging in late-life schizophrenia and related psychosis. Schizophr Bull 19:773–782, 1993

Leuchter AF, Spar JE: The late-onset psychoses. J Nerv Ment Dis 173:488–494, 1985

Levin S, Yurgelun-Todd D, Craft S: Contributions of clinical neuropsychology to the study of schizophrenia. J Abnorm Psychol 98:341–356, 1989

Lohr JB, Jeste DV, Harris MJ, et al: Treatment of disordered behavior, in Clinical Geriatric Psychopharmacology, 2nd Edition. Edited by Salzman C. Baltimore, MD, Williams & Wilkins, 1992, pp 79–113

Mayer W: On paraphrenic psychoses (in German). Zeitschrift fur die Gesamte Neurologie und Psychiatrie 71:187–206, 1921

Mayeux R, Stern Y, Spanton S: Heterogeneity in dementia of the Alzheimer type: evidence of subgroups. Neurology 35:453–461, 1985

McGlashan TH: A selective review of recent North American long-term follow-up studies of schizophrenia. Schizophr Bull 14:515–542, 1988

McNiel JN, Verwoerdt A, Peak D: Folie à deux in the aged: review and case report of role reversal. J Am Geriatr Soc 20:316–323, 1972

Miller BL, Lesser IM: Late-life psychosis and modern neuroimaging. Psychiatr Clin North Am 11:33–46, 1988

Miller BL, Lesser IM, Boone KB, et al: Brain lesions and cognitive function in late-life psychosis. Br J Psychiatry 158:76–82, 1991

Moore NC: Is paranoid illness associated with sensory defects in the elderly? J Psychosom Res 25:69–74, 1981

Naguib M, Levy R: Late paraphrenia: neuropsychological impairment and structural brain abnormalities on computed tomography. International Journal of Geriatric Psychiatry 2:83–90, 1987

Pearlson GD, Tune LE, Wong DF, et al: Quantitative D_2 dopamine receptor PET and structural MRI changes in late onset schizophrenia. Schizophr Bull 19:783–795, 1993

Prager S, Jeste DV: Sensory impairment in late-life schizophrenia. Schizophr Bull 19:755–772, 1993

Prudo R, Blum HM: Five-year outcome and prognosis in schizophrenia: a report from the London Field Research Centre of the International Pilot Study of Schizophrenia. Br J Psychiatry 150:345–354, 1987

Rabins P: Coexisting depression and dementia. J Geriatr Psychiatry 22:17–24, 1989

Ram R, Bromet EJ, Eaton WW, et al: The natural course of schizophrenia: a review of first-admission studies. Schizophr Bull 18:185–207, 1992

Raskind M, Alvarez C, Herlin S: Fluphenazine enanthate in the outpatient treatment of late paraphrenia. J Am Geriatr Soc 27:459–463, 1979

Rockwell E, Jackson E, Vilke G, et al: A study of delusions in a large cohort of Alzheimer disease patients. Am J Geriatr Psychiatry 2:157–164, 1994

Rokhlina ML: A comparative clinico-genetic study of attack-like schizophrenia with late and early manifestations with regard to age (in

Russian). Zh Nevropatol Psiikhiatr Im S S Korsakova 75:417–424, 1975

Saltz BL, Woerner MG, Kane JM, et al: Prospective study of tardive dyskinesia incidence in the elderly. JAMA 266:2402–2406, 1991

Saykin AJ, Gur RC, Gur RE, et al: Neuropsychological function in schizophrenia: selective impairment in memory and learning. Arch Gen Psychiatry 48:618–624, 1991

Steele C, Rovner B, Chase GA, et al: Psychiatric symptoms and nursing home placement of patients with Alzheimer's disease. Am J Psychiatry 147:1049–1051, 1990

Strauss ME: Relations of symptoms to cognitive deficits in schizophrenia. Schizophr Bull 19:215, 1993

Teri L, Larson EB, Reifler BV: Behavioral disturbance in dementia of the Alzheimer's type. J Am Geriatr Soc 36:1–6, 1988

Tran-Johnson TK, Krull AJ, Jeste DV: Late life schizophrenia and its treatment: the pharmacologic issues in older schizophrenic patients. Clin Geriatr Med 8:401–410, 1992

Winokur G: Delusional disorder (paranoia). Comp Psychiatry 18:511–521, 1977

Wragg R, Jeste DV: Overview of depression and psychosis in Alzheimer's disease. Am J Psychiatry 146:577–587, 1989

Yesavage JA, Becker J, Werner PD, et al: Serum level monitoring of thiothixene in schizophrenia: acute single-dose levels at fixed doses. Am J Psychiatry 139:174–178, 1982

Zubenko GS, Moossy J, Martinez AJ, et al: Neuropathologic and neurochemical correlates of psychosis in primary dementia. Arch Neurol 48:619–624, 1991

Javaid I. Sheikh, M.D.

Anxiety Disorders

A nxiety is a normal emotion with adaptive value in that it acts as a warning system alerting a person of noxious events or impending danger. This warning system can be considered maladaptive, however, when it becomes unjustifiably excessive and thus morbid. This morbid anxiety usually manifests itself in the form of a multitude of cognitive (e.g., worry, fearfulness), behavioral (e.g., hyperkinesis, phobias), and physiological (e.g., palpitations, hyperventilation) symptoms. The severity of such anxiety may range from excessive worrying about everyday concerns regarding job and relationships to episodes of intense anxiety and fear (panic attacks). Anxiety disorders are diagnostic entities comprising various combinations of signs and symptoms of morbid anxiety with criteria regarding their intensity and duration, as described in DSM-IV (American Psychiatric Association 1994). Typically, patients or their families or both seek medical attention when symptoms of anxiety disorders interfere with functioning at work, family, and social settings. Although anxiety disorders in elderly people are among the most frequent psychiatric conditions, they remain among the least studied (Sheikh 1992). This chapter describes the symptomatology and diagnostic classification of anxiety disorders based on DSM-IV, summarizes findings from epidemiological data in the literature, discusses pathogenesis, presents a systematic way of completing diagnostic work-up, and describes treatment methods for anxiety in elderly people.

Diagnostic Classification and Symptomatology

DSM-IV describes operationally defined, phenomenologically oriented diagnostic criteria for various anxiety disorders. A list of various anxiety disorders based on DSM-IV classification appears in Table 21–1. Brief descriptions of the symptomatology associated with various anxiety disorders along with additional features specific to the elderly population follow.

Panic Disorder

Panic disorder is manifested by recurrent episodes of severe anxiety or fear (panic attacks) that are accompanied by multiple somatic and cognitive symptoms. For example, during a panic attack one may experience palpitations, shortness of breath, chest pain or discomfort, sweating, hot and cold flashes, tingling in hands or feet, fear of dying, fear of losing control, and so forth. The panic attacks can occur either unexpectedly (uncued) or can be situationally bound (cued), that is, occurring in specific feared situations. Many patients with recurrent panic attacks develop fear of being in places from which escape might be difficult in case of incapacitating panic attacks. Such a fear of panic may lead over time to multiple avoidance responses (agoraphobia). Thus panic disorder can be present with or without agoraphobia. Panic disorder is typically chronic

Table 21–1.   DSM-IV anxiety disorders

Panic disorder
with agoraphobia
without agoraphobia
Agoraphobia without history of panic disorder
Social phobia
Specific phobia
Generalized anxiety disorder
Obsessive-compulsive disorder
Acute stress disorder
Posttraumatic stress disorder
Anxiety disorder due to a general medical condition and substance-induced anxiety disorder
Anxiety disorder not otherwise specified (NOS)

in its course with frequent recurrences and remissions. Preliminary investigations suggest that many older patients with onset of panic attacks in early life seem to continue with their symptomatology in later life, while receiving inadequate or no treatment over the years (Sheikh et al. 1991). It also appears that, although it may not be very common for panic disorder to appear de novo in old age, it does occur (Luchins and Rose 1989; Sheikh et al. 1988). Data from ongoing studies in our program suggest that late-onset panic disorder may be characterized by fewer panic symptoms, less avoidance, and lower scores on somatization measures compared to the early-onset panic disorder in older populations (Sheikh 1991, 1993).

Agoraphobia Without History of Panic Disorder

The central feature of this rare disorder is a fear of being in public places or situations from which escape might be difficult, in the absence of a history of panic attacks. It is not clear whether some of these patients are presenting with a variant of panic disorder. This disorder has not been studied in older adults.

Social Phobia

Social phobia is diagnosed in the presence of a persistent fear of one or more social situations. Common examples include fear of public speaking or inability to eat food or write in the presence of others. Attempts to enter the phobic situation are typically accompanied by marked anticipatory anxiety. Epidemiological evidence (Blazer et al. 1991) suggests that this disorder is chronic and persists in old age. Though systematic studies of this disorder in elderly people are lacking, our clinical experience suggests that eating or writing in public may be more bothersome to older people than public speaking as a result of the presence of dentures and tremors, respectively.

Specific Phobia

The diagnostic characteristic here is a marked and excessive or unreasonable and persistent fear of an object or situation. Examples include fear of flying, animals, receiving an injection, and seeing blood. The diagnosis is made only if avoidance or anxious anticipation causes significant distress or dysfunction. Systematic studies of specific phobias in elderly people are lacking, in general. However, it does appear that in urban settings, fear of crime is particularly prevalent in the elderly population (Clarke and Lewis 1982) leading to nocturnal neurosis in some cases (Cohen 1976).

Generalized Anxiety Disorder

This disorder is manifested by excessive anxiety or worry (apprehensive expectations) on most days for 6 months or longer. The worry is pervasive in that it focuses on many life circumstances, and the person finds it difficult to control the worry and to focus attention on tasks at hand. The worry is associated with six of the following symptoms of motor tension, autonomic hyperactivity, or hyperarousal:

1. *Motor tension:* trembling, muscle tension, restlessness, fatigability;
2. *Autonomic hyperactivity:* shortness of breath, rapid heart rate, sweating or cold clammy hands, dry mouth, dizziness, digestive disturbances, hot flashes or chills, frequent urination, and trouble swallowing or "lump in throat"; and
3. *Hyperarousal:* feeling on edge, exaggerated startle response, difficulty concentrating, insomnia, and irritability.

Many elderly patients with this syndrome may also present with features of depression, thus making the diagnosis and therapeutic decisions difficult at times.

Acute Stress Disorder

This new category in DSM-IV describes acute reactions manifesting anxiety as a response to extreme stress that last no more than 1 month. Little information is available about this disorder at this time, though it may be a harbinger of the development of posttraumatic stress disorder in some cases.

Posttraumatic Stress Disorder

The central criterion for this disorder is the development of characteristic symptoms after a person has experienced, witnessed, or been confronted with an event or events that involve actual or threatened death or serious injury, or a threat to the physical integrity of oneself or others. The person's response to the stressor must involve intense fear, helplessness, or horror. The symptoms experienced are usually a combination of three categories: 1) reexperiencing the traumatic event (in the form of images, thoughts, perceptions, dreams, illusions, hallucinations, or flashbacks);

2) avoidance of stimuli associated with the trauma or numbing of general responsiveness (depressionlike symptoms); and 3) symptoms of increased arousal (anxietylike symptoms). The symptoms usually begin soon after the trauma but can be delayed for a number of months or years. The disorder itself can be acute or chronic if the duration is less or more than three months, respectively. Clinical experience with elderly patients suggests presentations similar to those of younger people, though systematic studies of this syndrome in elderly people are lacking.

Obsessive-Compulsive Disorder

This disorder is characterized by recurrent obsessions or compulsions that are sufficiently severe to cause marked distress or dysfunction in occupational or personal matters. Obsessions are thoughts, impulses, or images that are experienced as intrusive and ego-dystonic and that cause marked anxiety or distress. Obsessions are not simply worries about real-life problems; common examples include repetitive thoughts of violence toward a loved one, contamination by germs or dirt, and doubts about injuring or offending someone. Compulsions are ritualistic behaviors (e.g., handwashing, ordering, checking) or mental acts (e.g., praying, counting, repeating words silently) that are performed in response to an obsession or according to certain rigid rules. Usually the compulsive behavior or mental act is designed to prevent discomfort or some dreaded situation and is often recognized by the individual as being either excessive or unrealistic. Attempting to resist a compulsion produces tension that can be relieved by yielding to the compulsion. Epidemiological data for this disorder suggest a 6-month prevalence of about 1.5% in elderly populations (Blazer et al. 1991), although little is known about any special manifestations in older adults.

Anxiety Disorder as a Result of a General Medical Condition and Substance-Induced Anxiety Disorder

These two anxiety disorders are new categories in DSM-IV. They are defined by etiology.

Anxiety Disorder Not Otherwise Specified

This category includes disorders with prominent anxiety symptoms that are not classifiable as specific anxiety disorders. Examples include clinically significant symptoms of anxiety and depression where criteria are not met for either a specific mood or anxiety disorder, or situations in which a clinician is unable to determine whether an anxiety disorder is primary, secondary, or substance-induced.

Epidemiology

There have been few epidemiological studies of anxiety disorders in elderly people. Studies belonging to the era before the introduction of the DSM-III (American Psychiatric Association 1980) have tended to categorize anxiety and depression into a mixed, anxious-depressive neurosis following the tradition at that time (Bergman 1971; Post 1972). It is thus difficult to discern the prevalence of different anxiety disorders based on those studies.

More recently, in a comparison of the epidemiological catchment area data of age groups 45–64 years (middle-aged) and 65-plus years (older-aged), Blazer et al. (1991) document the 6-month and lifetime prevalence in the Duke Community Sample for all anxiety disorders excluding posttraumatic stress disorder. Their analysis shows that both 6-month and lifetime prevalence of all anxiety disorders declines somewhat from the middle-age to the older-age group, though in the older adults it still stands at a formidable combined (all anxiety disorders) prevalence of 19.7% for the 6-month period and 34.05% for the lifetime (see Table 21–2). These data indicate that anxiety disorders as a group are the most common psychiatric conditions in elderly people, as they are in younger populations. There also is the suggestion that anxiety disorders may result in higher medical and psychiatric comorbidity. For example, in a study from Great Britain, Lindesay (1991) indicates that in elderly people phobic disorders are associated with considerably higher psychiatric and medical morbidity when elderly individuals with phobic disorders are matched for age and sex to case control subjects without history of phobic disorders. It also appears that despite higher rates of contact with general practitioners among phobic elderly patients compared with control subjects, only one phobic elderly person in this study was receiving psychiatric help. It appears that anxiety disorders are among the most common psychiatric ailments experienced by older adults and among the least studied in that age group.

Pathogenesis and Etiology

Several theories of the pathogenesis of various anxiety disorders in the general population have been in vogue at different times during the last

Table 21–2. Six-month and lifetime prevalence of anxiety disorders by age for the Duke ECA community sample

| | Age groups (years) | | | |
| | 6 month | | Lifetime | |
Diagnosis	45–64	65+	45–64	65+
Simple phobia	13.29	9.63	18.11	16.10
Social phobia	2.04	1.37	3.18	2.64
Agoraphobia	7.30	5.22	9.40	8.44
Panic disorder	1.10	0.04	2.04	0.29
Obsessive-compulsive disorder	2.01	1.54	3.33	1.98
Generalized anxiety disorder	3.10	1.90	6.70	4.60

Source. Reprinted from Blazer D, George LK, Hughes D: "The Epidemiology of Anxiety Disorders: An Age Comparison," in *Anxiety in the Elderly*. Edited by Saltzman C, Lebowitz BD. New York, Springer, 1991, pp. 17–30. Used with permission.

few decades. They can best be divided among psychological and biological models of anxiety.

The psychological models have ranged from postulating anxiety as signaling danger from unconscious conflictual impulses, to anxiety expressed as phobias being caused by traumatic conditioning. More recently, cognitive-behavioral paradigms have become more popular. These assume that individuals prone to anxiety states, particularly panic attacks, misinterpret normal body sensations and create "catastrophic" cognitions about such sensations that may spiral into full-blown panic attacks (Barlow 1988). Unlike studies of depression in old age, which seem to show a strong association of depression with chronic physical illness, financial problems, and assumption of the care-giving role (George et al. 1989; Schulz et al. 1990), studies of the psychological factors contributing to anxiety in old age are lacking. Thus the role of the well-known stressors of old age (including decline in physical functioning, illness, retirement, economic deprivation, loss of a spouse, social isolation) as potential contributors to the development of anxiety states in old age, remains unknown.

The biological models have been influenced by Klein's (1981) postulation that bodily dysfunction may underlie panic attacks, and thus researchers have mostly focused on panic disorder as their field of study. Over the years, panic induction using lactate infusions (Liebowitz et al. 1984), various assertions of involvement of central noradrenergic activation in anxiety and fear states (Charney et al. 1982; Redmond and Huang 1979), and findings of Reiman et al. (1984) documenting increased parahippocampal activity during panic attacks provoked by lactic acid have stimulated excitement and discussion in the field regarding biological factors underlying anxiety. Finally, some family and genetic studies seem to suggest familial transmission of panic disorder. For example, Cloninger et al. (1981) found that the lifetime risk for panic disorder in the first-degree relatives of panic disorder patients was 20.5% and as much as 50% in a small sample of female relatives. These figures contrast sharply with the approximately 2%–5% lifetime risk in the general population. Similar results have also been reported by Crowe et al. (1983) and Harris et al. (1983). In a study of 29 adult twins of the same sex, the concordance rate for monozygotic twins for panic disorder with or without agoraphobia was 31% compared with no concordance in dizygotic twins (Torgersen 1983). Note that panic disorder is the only anxiety syndrome for which such specificity of genetic transmission has been noted.

A review of the normal age-related changes in different neurotransmitter systems suggests that there is a decline in central noradrenergic functioning in old age, including a decrease in the number of locus coeruleus neurons, a decreased norepinephrine content in many brain areas, and an increase in monoamine oxidase (type B) levels (Sunderland et al. 1991). These findings explain and support the phenomenological research documenting a milder symptomatology in late-onset panic disorder (Sheikh et al. 1991). Studies of serotonin function (Gottfries et al. 1979; Meek et al. 1977) and the GABAergic system (Allen et al. 1983; Bareggi et al. 1985) in normal aging have demonstrated either normal or decreased levels, and any role of serotonin function in the anxiety states of old age remains unknown.

Diagnostic Workup and Differential Diagnosis

Several factors can confound proper assessment of anxiety in elderly populations. To begin with, many medical conditions can masquerade as somatic manifestations of anxiety. These may include cardiovascular problems (e.g., angina pectoris, cardiac arrhythmias), endocrine disorders (e.g., hyperthyroidism, hypoglycemia), pulmonary disorders (e.g., pulmonary embolism, chronic obstructive pulmonary disease), and neurological illnesses (e.g., temporal-lobe epilepsy, movement disorders). Second, any major medical illness can produce anxiety as an expected response to a physical stressor. Third, many medications can produce symptoms of anxiety. Examples of such medications include sympathomimetic compounds such as pseudoephedrine hydrochloride in over-the-counter drugs, thyroid replacement therapies, neuroleptics, antidepressants, and steroids, among others. In addition, withdrawal from sedatives, hypnotics, or alcohol needs to be considered in the differential diagnosis. Finally, depression can be the possible principle disorder with concomitant anxiety as a comorbid condition. With these caveats in mind, evaluation of geriatric anxiety is usually accomplished in three major ways: clinical evaluation, assessment by rating scales, and laboratory investigations.

Clinical Evaluation

The clinical evaluation includes a history of present and past illness (e.g., panic disorder usually has remissions and relapses), medication usage (e.g., cold medications, anticholinergic medications), drug (e.g., over-the-counter hypnotic or stimulant) and alcohol use, and a family history (e.g., panic disorder). A mental status examination may reveal some of the cognitive and behavioral signs and symptoms of anxiety including apprehension, distractibility, hyperkinesis, and startled response. Physiological signs and symptoms detected during the physical examination including increased heart rate, rapid breathing, sweating, and trembling can provide additional clues.

Psychometric Assessment

Clinical evaluation of anxiety in elderly people can be aided by using anxiety rating scales. These also can serve as instruments to document effectiveness of various psychological and pharmacological therapeutic interventions. These scales are primarily of two kinds: observer-rated and self-rated. The most commonly used observer-rated scale is the Hamilton Anxiety Rating Scale (Hamilton 1959). It has 14 items consisting of 89 symptoms measuring psychic and somatic components of anxiety, with each item rated on five levels of severity from "none" (0) to "very severe" (4). A rating of 18 or above is generally considered to be suggestive of clinically significant anxiety. The scale should however be used selectively, as it may be cumbersome for many elderly people to go through the list of 89 symptoms without getting very fatigued. Also, it is worth considering while interpreting the score that elderly people tend to overendorse the somatic items.

There are several self-rated anxiety scales including the State-Trait Anxiety Inventory (Spielberger et al. 1970), the Beck Anxiety Inventory (Beck et al. 1988), and the SCL-90-R (Derogatis 1975), which can be quite useful as adjuncts to clinical evaluation. A more detailed discussion of the advantages and disadvantages of various anxiety rating scales in elderly populations is available elsewhere (Sheikh 1991).

Laboratory Tests

Laboratory tests can aid in diagnosing anxiety disorders induced by underlying medical conditions and substance abuse. A complete blood count, electrocardiogram, vitamin B_{12} and folate levels, thyroid-function tests, blood-glucose levels, and a drug/alcohol screening can be helpful when used appropriately to rule out medical causes of anxiety.

Treatment

Safe and effective management of anxiety in elderly patients can be accomplished by using pharmacological treatments, psychological treatments, or both. A variety of compounds, including benzodiazepines, buspirone, antidepressants, and β-blockers, seem to show effectiveness for various anxiety disorders.

Pharmacological Treatments

While prescribing any medications to elderly patients, one needs to consider age-related physiological changes in absorption, distribution, protein binding, metabolism, and excretion of drugs. In addition to significantly altering plasma levels of drugs, these changes can lead to excessive accumulation of medications in various body tissues and make elderly patients particularly prone to experiencing toxic side effects even at dose ranges average for the general population. Numerous compounds belonging to several different classes have been used as anxiolytics over the past few decades. These include alcohol, barbiturates, antihistamines, antidepressants, neuroleptics, β-blockers, benzodiazepines, and azapirones. A brief description of different classes of compounds commonly used at present as anxiolytics follows.

Benzodiazepines.   These medications have been the most frequently prescribed anxiolytics for both young and older patients in the last three decades. Several researchers have demonstrated the efficacy of benzodiazepines in generalized anxiety disorder (Hoehn-Saric et al. 1988; Rickels

1978), panic disorder (Ballenger et al. 1988; Tesar et al. 1987), and obsessive-compulsive disorder (Bacher 1990; Hewlett et al. 1990). Systematic investigations of these medications in anxiety disorders of elderly adults are lacking in general, though these medications are used routinely in clinical practice in this population. In elderly patients, short half-life benzodiazepines such as lorazepam, oxazepam, and temazepam may be preferable in that they are inactivated by direct conjugation in the liver, a mechanism that does not seem to be affected by aging (Moran et al. 1988). Most other benzodiazepines such as diazepam, chlordiazepoxide, chlorazepate, and flurazepam tend to be metabolized via oxidative pathways into active metabolites, which tend to linger in elderly people for long periods of time. Several studies have documented undesirable side effects in elderly patients of long-acting benzodiazepines (e.g., diazepam, chlorazepate, chlordiazepoxide), including drowsiness, fatigue, psychomotor impairment, and cognitive impairment (Boston Collaborative Drug Surveillance Program 1973; Curran et al. 1987; Larson et al. 1987; Pomara et al. 1984; Pomara et al. 1991). It also appears that long-acting benzodiazepines can have prolonged half-lives in elderly people. For example, Rosenbaum (1979) documented that the half-life of diazepam's metabolites increased from 20 hours in a 20-year-old to 90 hours in an 80-year-old individual. Alprazolam, a commonly used, intermediate half-life, antipanic medication, also was shown to have a half-life of more than 21 hours in elderly people compared to 11 hours in young people (Kroboth et al. 1990). In a preliminary analysis of an 8-week-long study of older panic disorder patients (ages 55 and older) in our program, we found alprazolam to be more effective in blocking panic attacks compared to a placebo. Data on long-term effectiveness or safety of this medication in older patients with panic disorder are, however, lacking. Given the probability that, if taken for long periods of time, even short-acting benzodiazepines will tend to accumulate in older people, any use of benzodiazepines in this population should be for specific indications and time-limited, preferably to less than 6 months.

Buspirone. This anxiolytic medication with serotonin-1A agonist properties has demonstrated efficacy in younger patients with generalized anxiety disorder (Rickels et al. 1982; Rickels and Schweizer 1987). Studies of buspirone in geriatric populations have shown the following: the pharmacokinetics are very similar in both elderly and younger people; buspirone is well-tolerated and does not cause sedation or cognitive or psychomotor impairment; it does not produce adverse interactions when coprescribed with a variety of other medications (including antihypertensives, cardiac glycosides, and bronchodilators); and it is effective for remediation of chronic anxiety symptoms (Gammans et al. 1989; Napoliello 1986; Robinson et al. 1988). It also appeared to be effective in mixed anxiety-depression syndromes (Robinson et al. 1990). Finally, there was some evidence that buspirone may be effective in treating agitated patients with dementia (Colenda 1988). It must be mentioned, however, that in contrast to research data, clinical experience with this medication suggests that a therapeutic response is somewhat inconsistent.

Antidepressants.   Several reports over the last three decades have documented the effectiveness of various antidepressants in younger patients with anxiety disorders. For example, the tricyclic imipramine and the monoamine oxidase inhibitor phenelzine have proven effective in panic disorder and agoraphobia (Mavissakalian and Michaelson 1986; Sheehan et al. 1980; Zitrin et al. 1983). More recently, several researchers have demonstrated efficacy of the serotonin reuptake inhibitors (SRIs) such as fluoxetine, paroxetine, and sertraline in panic disorder (Ohrstrom et al. 1992; Schneier et al. 1990). In the same vein, the tricyclic antidepressant clomipramine (Insel et al. 1983; Thoren et al. 1980; Volavka et al. 1985), and the SRIs fluoxetine and sertraline (Chouinard et al. 1990; Greist et al. 1992) have shown efficacy for alleviating symptoms of obsessive-compulsive disorder. Because controlled studies in various anxiety disorders are lacking, evidence is at best inconclusive for the efficacy of secondary amine tricyclics (like desipramine or nortriptyline) or of atypical antidepressants (like bupropion or trazodone), which may otherwise be preferable in elderly patients because they are less anticholinergic than imipramine or clomipramine (Ballenger 1994). Our practice is thus to use one of the SRIs as the first line of treatment in older patients with panic disorder or obsessive-compulsive disorder as they seem to be much better tolerated by elderly people compared to imipramine or clomipramine.

β-Blockers, antihistamines, and neuroleptics.   Although β-blockers have been used for the treatment of various anxiety disorders for about three decades now, their effectiveness remains controversial. One area where they appear to be consistently useful is to manage somatic anxiety by blocking autonomic reactions commonly associated with anxiety conditions (Lader 1976; Noyes 1985; Tyrer and Lader 1974). Some reports suggest that β-blockers such as propranolol and oxprenolol may be quite suitable for some geriatric patients with anxiety and agitation (Petrie 1983;

Petrie and Ban 1981). Greendyke et al. (1986) suggested their use in extremely agitated individuals with dementia in very high doses of up to 520 mg/day. A 10-mg dose of propranolol twice a day, to be gradually increased to 20 to 30 mg twice a day if no response occurs, may be sufficient in some of these cases. Caution should be exercised, however, in using nonselective β-blockers (β_1 and β_2 blockade) such as propranolol or pindolol in medically ill elderly patients. These are generally contraindicated in patients with chronic obstructive pulmonary disease, diabetes mellitus, and congestive cardiac failure. Cardioselective β_1 agents such as atenolol and metoprolol may be used with caution in some of these patients. Antihistamines such as hydroxyzine and diphenhydramine are also used sometimes in the short term with monitoring for anticholinergic side effects to manage mild anxiety, with varying degrees of success. Finally, our clinical experience suggests that low-dose, high-potency neuroleptics such as haloperidol and fluphenazine (e.g., 0.25 mg–0.5 mg twice a day of haloperidol) can be quite effective in severe anxiety and agitation associated with organic brain syndromes.

Psychological Treatments

Psychological treatments can be quite useful for management of anxiety disorders in elderly patients, either in combination with pharmacological treatments or as alternatives to them. Studies in younger populations suggested that dynamic psychotherapy is of limited therapeutic usefulness as a primary treatment for various anxiety disorders (Sheehan et al. 1980; Weiss 1964; Zitrin et al. 1978). No such studies of dynamic psychotherapy in elderly people exist. Many psychiatrists believe, however, that a psychodynamically oriented supportive therapy can be a valuable adjunct to medication treatment by enabling the patient to view the therapist as understanding and empathic, thus improving patient compliance with the prescribed medication.

Numerous reports describing the efficacy of cognitive-behavior therapy in anxiety disorders of younger patients have been published over the years. For example, a number of cognitive and behavioral interventions are efficacious for the treatment of generalized anxiety (Barlow 1988; Beck 1988), panic disorder (Barlow and Cerny 1988; Clark 1989; Clark et al. 1985), phobias (Marks 1981, 1987), and obsessive-compulsive disorder (Marks 1981; Rachman and Hodgson 1980) in the general population. In general, systematic studies of the effectiveness of cognitive-behavior therapy in anxious elderly people are lacking. One has to settle for inference based on studies in younger patients and to hope that the methods in these studies will be similarly effective in the geriatric population. Preliminary data from our ongoing studies indicate that cognitive-behavior therapy can be quite effective in older patients with panic disorder (Swales et al., in press). Cognitive-behavior treatment should thus be considered as an alternative to pharmacological treatment where the possibility of side effects and drug interactions is high because of intercurrent medical problems and polypharmacy, or where compliance with a medication regimen is an issue. It can also be considered as a valuable adjunct to pharmacological treatments in cases where patients have behavioral symptoms that can be targeted (e.g., moderate to severe degree of agoraphobia in panic disorder patients). Table 21–3 summarizes strategies for effective management of anxiety disorders in elderly patients.

Table 21–3. Strategies for effective management of anxiety disorders in the elderly

Disorder	Treatment of choice	Alternative treatments
Panic disorder with or without agoraphobia	Serotonin reuptake inhibitors (e.g., fluoxetine, paroxetine, sertraline)	Alprazolam, imipramine, phenelzine; cognitive-behavior therapy
Generalized anxiety disorder	Benzodiazepines or buspirone	Cognitive-behavior therapy
Obsessive-compulsive disorder	Serotonin reuptake inhibitors	Clomipramine; cognitive-behavior therapy
Social phobia— generalized	Phenelzine + cognitive-behavior therapy	Benzodiazepines
Social phobia— specific	β-Blockers + cognitive-behavior therapy	Buspirone
Specific phobia	Cognitive-behavior therapy or benzodiazepines	β-Blockers
Acute and posttraumatic stress disorders	As indicated	—

Source. Adapted from Sheikh JI: "Anxiety Disorders," in *Textbook of Geriatric Neuropsychiatry.* Edited by Coffey CE, Cummings JL. Washington, DC, American Psychiatric Press, 1994, pp. 279–296. Used with permission.

Complications

Alcohol abuse seems to be a common complication of anxiety disorders in younger populations. For example, Boyd et al. (1984) estimated that the risk of alcohol problems in phobic patients is about two-and-a-half times that of the general population, and the risk in patients with panic disorder is more than four times. A review of the literature (Kushner et al. 1990) suggested that in many cases of agoraphobia and social phobia, alcohol problems may be related to attempts at self-medication. Though these studies have focused on younger patients, a similar comorbidity with alcoholism may also exist in the older population.

Anxiety disorders can create problems in initiating and maintaining sleep as well as significantly affect the quality of sleep. In a study assessing vegetative signs and symptoms of anxiety, Mathew et al. (1982) found that restless sleep was the only vegetative symptom consistently related to anxiety. On the other hand, anxiety appears to be a common finding in patients with chronic insomnia. Inquiry into the duration and quality of sleep should be an integral component of any management plans for anxiety in elderly patients. Since sleep disturbances are frequently reported by both anxious and nonanxious elderly patients, such inquiry should take into account the common clinical observation that older people tend to go to bed early and may nap during the day. Thus a seemingly early wake-up time may not be so in reality, and the total amount of sleep, including nap time, may be sufficient for many.

Increased mortality of cardiovascular origin may be another potential complication of panic disorder. In a series of long-term studies, Coryell et al. (1982, 1986) have documented increased mortality as a result of cardiovascular disease among male, but not female, patients with panic disorder. Specifically, it appears in these studies that males with a panic disorder diagnosis were twice as likely to die compared with age- and sex-matched control subjects. After a review of causes of death in his sample of men, Coryell (1988) attributes the excess mortality to chronic hyperarousal and exercise intolerance in panic disorder patients, and possibly to the additional deleterious effects of associated smoking or alcohol abuse. These findings are controversial, however, because of the small number of patients involved and other methodological problems of this series of studies, and they should thus be considered inconclusive.

Prognosis and Outcome

Anxiety disorders tend to be chronic, interspersed with remissions and relapses of varying degrees. Proper education of the patient, leading to better compliance with the treatment regimen, and recent advances in treatment will almost certainly improve in the future the outlook for these patients for better functioning and a more optimistic prognosis.

Summary

Despite increasing research interest in the area of anxiety in younger age groups, few systematic studies of the phenomenology and treatment of anxiety disorders in elderly people have been performed. Data from epidemiologic catchment area studies suggest that anxiety disorders remain among the most prevalent of all psychiatric disorders in this age group. Several reports suggest that panic disorder can have its onset in late-life and that it may be a distinct subtype with differences in vulnerability factors, phenomenology, treatment, course, and prognosis (Luchins and Rose 1989; Sheikh 1993; Sheikh et al. 1988, 1991). Any evaluation of anxiety in elderly adults should take into account multiple medical illnesses and medications that can produce a similar symptom picture. Use of effective and safe treatments presently available for anxiety disorders should minimize complications and improve prognosis.

References

Allen SJ, Benton JS, Goodhardt MJ, et al: Biochemical evidence of selective nerve cell changes in the normal aging human and rat brain. J Neurochem 41:256–265, 1983

American Psychiatric Association: Diagnostic and Statistical Manual of Mental Disorders, 3rd Edition. Washington, DC, American Psychiatric Association, 1980

American Psychiatric Association: Diagnostic and Statistical Manual of Mental Disorders, 4th Edition. Washington, DC, American Psychiatric Association, 1994

Bacher NM: Clonazepam treatment of obsessive compulsive disorder (letter). J Clin Psychiatry 51:168–169, 1990

Ballenger JC: Pharmacological treatment of panic disorder, in Handbook of Depression and Anxiety: A Biological Approach. Edited by den Boer

JA, Ad Sitsen JM. New York, Marcel Dekker, 1994, pp 275–289

Ballenger JC, Burrows GD, DuPont RL, et al: Alprazolam in panic disorder and agoraphobia: results from a multicenter trial, I: efficacy in short-term treatment. Arch Gen Psychiatry 45:413–422, 1988

Bareggi SR, Franceschi M, Smirne S: Neurochemical findings in cerebrospinal fluid in Alzheimer's disease, in Normal Aging, Alzheimer's Disease, and Senile Dementia: Aspects on Etiology, Pathogenesis, Diagnosis, and Treatment, Proceedings of Two Symposia held at the Collegium Internationale Neuropsychopharmacogicum 14th Congress, June 22 and 23, 1984, Florence, Italy. Edited by Gottfries CG. Brussels, Editions de l'Universite de Bruxelles, 1985, pp 203–212

Barlow DH: Anxiety and Its Disorders: The Nature and Treatment of Anxiety and Panic. New York, Guilford Press, 1988

Barlow DH, Cerny JA: Psychological Treatment of Panic (Treatment Manuals for Practitioners Series). New York, Guilford Press, 1988

Beck AT: Cognitive approaches to panic disorder: theory and therapy, in Panic: Psychological Perspectives. Edited by Rachman S, Maser JD. Hillsdale, NJ, Lawrence Erlbaum, 1988, pp 91–110

Beck AT, Epstein N, Brown G, et al: An inventory for measuring clinical anxiety: psychometric properties. J Consult Clin Psychol 56:893–897, 1988

Bergman K: The neuroses of old age, in Recent Developments in Psychogeriatrics: A Symposium (Br J Psychiatry Special Publication No 6). Edited by Kay DWK, Walk A. Ashford, UK, Headley Brothers, 1971, pp 39–50

Blazer D, George LK, Hughes D: The epidemiology of anxiety disorders: an age comparison, in Anxiety in the Elderly. Edited by Salzman C, Lebowitz BD. New York, Springer, 1991, pp 17–30

Boston Collaborative Drug Surveillance Program: Clinical depression of the central nervous system due to diazepam and chlordiazepoxide in relation to cigarette smoking and age. N Engl J Med 288:277–280, 1973

Boyd JH, Burke JD, Greenberg E, et al: Exclusion criteria of DSM-III: a study of co-occurrence of hierarchy-free syndromes. Arch Gen Psychiatry 41:983–989, 1984

Charney DS, Heninger GR, Sternberg DE: Assessment of α-2-adrenergic autoreceptor function in humans: effects of oral yohimbine. Life Sci 30:2033–2041, 1982

Chouinard G, Goodman W, Greist J, et al: Results of a double-blind placebo controlled trial of a new serotonin uptake inhibitor, sertraline, in the treatment of obsessive-compulsive disorder. Psychopharmacol

Bull 26:279–284, 1990

Clark DM: Anxiety states: panic and generalized anxiety, in Cognitive Behaviour Therapy for Psychiatric Problems: A Practical Guide. Edited by Hawton K, Salkovskis PM, Kirk J, et al. New York, Oxford University Press, 1989, pp 52–96

Clark DM, Salkovskis PM, Chalkley AJ: Respiratory control as a treatment for panic attacks. J Behav Ther Exp Psychiatry 16:23–30, 1985

Clarke AH, Lewis MJ: Fear of crime among the elderly. British Journal of Criminology 232:49, 1982

Cloninger CR, Martin RI, Clayton P, et al: A blind follow-up and family study of anxiety neurosis: preliminary analysis of the St. Louis 500, in Anxiety: New Research and Changing Concepts. Edited by Klein DF, Rabkin JG. New York, Raven, 1981, pp 137–154

Cohen CI: Nocturnal neurosis of the elderly: failure of agencies to cope with the problem. J Am Geriatr Soc 24:86–88, 1976

Colenda CC: Buspirone in treatment of agitated demented patient (letter). Lancet 1:1169, 1988

Coryell W: Mortality of anxiety disorders, in Handbook of Anxiety, Vol 2: Classification, Etiological Factors and Associated Disturbances. Edited by Noyes JR, Roth M, Burrows GD. Amsterdam, The Netherlands, Elsevier, 1988, pp 311–320

Coryell W, Noyes R, Clancy J: Excess mortality in panic disorder: a comparison with primary unipolar depression. Arch Gen Psychiatry 39:701–703, 1982

Coryell W, Noyes R, Hause JD: Mortality among outpatients with anxiety disorders. Am J Psychiatry 143:508–510, 1986

Crowe RR, Noyes R, Pauls DL, et al: A family study of panic disorder. Arch Gen Psychiatry 40:1065–1069, 1983

Curran HV, Allen D, Lader M: The effects of single doses of alprazolam and lorazepam on memory and psychomotor performance in normal humans. Journal of Psychopharmacology 2:81–89, 1987

Derogatis LR: The SCL-90-R. Baltimore, MD, Clinical Psychometric Research, 1975

Gammans RE, Westrick ML, Shea JP, et al: Pharmacokinetics of buspirone in elderly subjects. J Clin Pharmacol 29:72–78, 1989

George LK, Landerman R, Blazer D, et al: Concurrent morbidity between physical and mental illness: an epidemiological examination, in Mechanisms of Psychological Influence on Physical Health, With Special Attention to the Elderly. Edited by Carstensen LL, Neale J. New York, Plenum, 1989, pp 9–22

Gottfries CG, Adolfsson R, Oreland L, et al: Monoamines and their metabolites and monoamine oxidase activity related to age and to some dementia disorders, in Drugs and the Elderly: Perspectives in Geriatric Clinical Pharmacology. Edited by Crooks J, Stevenson IH. Baltimore, MD, University Park Press, 1979, pp 189–197

Greendyke RM, Kanter DR, Schuster DB, et al: Propranolol treatment of assaultive patients with organic brain disease: a double-blind crossover, placebo-controlled study. J Nerv Ment Disord 174:290–294, 1986

Greist J, Chouinard G, DuBoff E, et al: Double-blind comparison of three doses of sertraline and placebo in the treatment of outpatients with obsessive-compulsive disorder. Poster presented at the Collegium Internationale Neuropsychopharmacologicum 18th Congress, Nice, France, June 1992

Hamilton M: The assessment of anxiety states by rating. Br J Med Psychol 32:50–55, 1959

Harris EL, Noyes R, Crowe RR, et al: Family study of agoraphobia: report of a pilot study. Arch Gen Psychiatry 40:1061–1064, 1983

Hewlett WA, Vinogradov S, Agras WS: Clonazepam treatment of obsessions and compulsions. J Clin Psychiatry 51:158–161, 1990

Hoehn-Saric R, McLeod DR, Zimmerli WD: Differential effects of alprazolam and imipramine in generalized anxiety disorder: somatic vs. psychic symptoms. J Clin Psychiatry 49:293–301, 1988

Insel TR, Murphy DL, Cohen RM, et al: Obsessive-compulsive disorder: a double-blind trial of clomipramine and clorgyline. Arch Gen Psychiatry 40:605–612, 1983

Klein DF: Anxiety reconceptualized, in Anxiety: New Research and Changing Concepts. Edited by Klein DF, Rabkin JG. New York, Raven Press, 1981, pp 235–263

Kroboth PD, McAuley JW, Smith RB: Alprazolam in the elderly: pharmacokinetics and pharmacodynamics during multiple dosing. Psychopharmacology 100:477–484, 1990

Kushner MG, Sher KJ, Beitman BD: The relation between alcohol problems and the anxiety disorders. Am J Psychiatry 147:685–696, 1990

Lader M: Somatic and psychiatric symptoms in anxiety, in Neuropsychiatric Effects of Adrenergic Beta-Receptor Blocking Agents. Edited by Carlsson C, Engel J, Hansson L. London, ICI Pharmaceuticals, 1976, pp 21–28

Larson EB, Kukull WA, Buchner D, et al: Adverse drug reactions associated with global cognitive impairment in elderly persons. Ann Intern Med 107:169–173, 1987

Liebowitz MR, Fryer AJ, Gorman JM, et al: Lactate provocation of panic attacks, I: clinical and behavioral findings. Arch Gen Psychiatry 41:

764–770, 1984

Lindesay J: Phobic disorders in the elderly. Br J Psychiatry 159:531–541, 1991

Luchins DJ, Rose RP: Late-life onset of panic disorder with agoraphobia in three patients. Am J Psychiatry 146:920–921, 1989

Marks IM: Cure and Care of Neuroses: Theory and Practice of Behavioral Psychotherapy. New York, Wiley, 1981

Marks IM: Fears, Phobias, and Rituals: Panic, Anxiety, and Their Disorders. New York, Oxford University Press, 1987

Mathew RJ, Swilhart AA, Weinman ML: Vegetative symptoms in anxiety and depression. Br J Psychiatry 141:162–165, 1982

Mavissakalian M, Michaelson L: Agoraphobia: relative and combined effectiveness of therapist-assisted in vivo exposure and imipramine. J Clin Psychiatry 47:117–122, 1986

Meek JL, Bertilsson L, Cheney DL, et al: Aging-induced changes in acetylcholine and serotonin content of discrete brain nuclei. J Gerontol 32:129–131, 1977

Moran MG, Thompson TL II, Nies AS: Sleep disorders in the elderly. Am J Psychiatry 145:1369–1378, 1988

Napoliello MJ: An interim multicentre report on 677 anxious geriatric outpatients treated with buspirone. Br J Clin Pract 40:71–73, 1986

Noyes R: Beta-adrenergic blocking drugs in anxiety and stress. Psychiatr Clin North Am 8:119–132, 1985

Ohrstrom JK, Judge R, Manniche PM, et al: Paroxetine in the treatment of panic disorder. Proceedings of the Annual Scientific Meeting of the American College of Neuropsychopharmacology, San Juan, Puerto Rico, December 1992

Petrie WM: Drug treatment of anxiety and agitation in the aged. Psychopharmacol Bull 19:238–246, 1983

Petrie WM, Ban TA: Propranolol in organic agitation. Lancet 1:324, 1981

Pomara N, Stanley B, Block R, et al: Diazepam impairs performance in normal elderly subjects. Psychopharmacol Bull 20:137–139, 1984

Pomara N, Deptula D, Singh R, et al: Cognitive toxicity of benzodiazepines in the elderly, in Anxiety in the Elderly. Edited by Salzman CL, Lebowitz BD. New York, Springer, 1991, pp 175–196

Post F: The management and nature of depressive illnesses in late life: a follow-through study. Br J Psychiatry 121:393–404, 1972

Rachman SJ, Hodgson RJ: Obsessions and Compulsions. Englewood Cliffs, NJ, Prentice-Hall, 1980

Redmond DE, Huang YH: Current concepts, II: new evidence for a locus coeruleus–norepinephrine connection with anxiety. Life Sci 25:2149–

2162, 1979

Reiman EM, Raichle ME, Butler FK, et al: A focal brain abnormality in panic disorder, a severe form of anxiety. Nature 310:683–685, 1984

Rickels K: Use of antianxiety agents in anxious outpatients. Psychopharmacology 58:1–17, 1978

Rickels K, Schweizer EE: Current pharmacotherapy of anxiety and panic, in Psychopharmacology: The Third Generation of Progress. Edited by Meltzer HY. New York, Raven, 1978, pp 1193–1203

Rickels K, Weisman K, Norstad N, et al: Buspirone and diazepam in anxiety: a controlled study. J Clin Psychiatry 43:81–86, 1982

Robinson DS, Napoliello MJ, Schenk J: The safety and usefulness of buspirone as an anxiolytic drug in elderly versus young patients. Clin Ther 10:740–746, 1988

Robinson DS, Rickels K, Feighner J, et al: Clinical effects of the 5HT$_{1A}$ partial agonists in depression: a composite analysis of buspirone in the treatment of depression. J Clin Psychopharmacol 10:67S–76S, 1990

Rosenbaum JK: Anxiety, in Outpatient Psychiatry: Diagnosis and Treatment. Edited by Lazare A. Baltimore, MD, Williams & Wilkins, 1979, pp 252–256

Schneier FR, Liebowitz MR, Davies SO, et al: Fluoxetine in panic disorder. J Clin Psychopharmacol 10:119–121, 1990

Schulz R, Visintainer P, Williamson GM: Psychiatric and physical morbidity effects of caregiving. Journal of Gerontology: Psychological Sciences 45:P181–P191, 1990

Sheehan DV, Ballenger J, Jacobsen G: Treatment of endogenous anxiety with phobic, hysterical, and hypochondriacal symptoms. Arch Gen Psychiatry 37:51–59, 1980

Sheikh JI: Anxiety rating scales for the elderly, in Anxiety in the Elderly. Edited by Salzman C, Lebowitz BD. New York, Springer, 1991, pp 251–265

Sheikh JI: Anxiety disorders and their treatment, in Clinics in Geriatric Medicine: Psychiatric Disorders in Late Life, Vol 8. Edited by Alexopoulos GS. Philadelphia, PA, WB Saunders, 1992, pp 411–426

Sheikh JI: Is late-onset panic disorder a distinct syndrome? Proceedings of the 146th Annual Scientific Meeting of the American Psychiatric Association, San Francisco, CA, May 1993

Sheikh JI: Anxiety disorders, in Textbook of Geriatric Neuropsychiatry. Edited by Coffey CE, Cummings JL. Washington, DC, American Psychiatric Press, 1994, pp 279–296

Sheikh JI, Taylor CB, King RJ, et al: Panic attacks and avoidance behavior in the elderly. Proceedings of the 141st Annual Scientific Meeting of the American Psychiatric Association, Montreal, Canada, May 1988

Sheikh JI, King RJ, Taylor CB: Comparative phenomenology of early-onset versus late-onset panic attacks: a pilot survey. Am J Psychiatry 148:1231–1233, 1991

Spielberger C, Gorsuch R, Lushene R: STAI Manual for the State-Trait Anxiety Inventory. Palo Alto, CA, Consulting Psychologists Press, 1970

Sunderland T, Lawlor BA, Martinez RA, et al: Anxiety in the elderly: neurobiological and clinical interface, in Anxiety in the Elderly. Edited by Salzman C, Lebowitz BD. New York, Springer, 1991, pp 105–129

Swales PJ, Sheikh JI: Clinical and research perspectives on anxiety in the elderly. Proceedings of the 146th Annual Meeting of the American Psychiatric Association, San Francisco, CA, May 1993

Swales PJ, Solfrin JF, Sheikh JI: Cognitive-behavior therapy in older panic disorder patients. Am J Geriatric Psychiatry (in press)

Tesar GE, Rosenbaum JF, Pollack MH, et al: Clonazepam vs. alprazolam in the treatment of panic disorder: interim analysis of data from a prospective double-blind, placebo-controlled trial. J Clin Psychiatry 48:16–21, 1987

Thoren P, Asberg M, Cronholm B, et al: Clomipramine treatment of obsessive-compulsive disorder, I: a controlled clinical trial. Arch Gen Psychiatry 37:1281–1285, 1980

Torgersen S: Genetic factors in anxiety disorders. Arch Gen Psychiatry 40:1085–1089, 1983

Tyrer PJ, Lader MH: Response to propranolol and diazepam in somatic and psychiatric anxiety. Br Med J 2:14–16, 1974

Volavka J, Neziroglu F, Yaryura-Tobias JA: Clomipramine and imipramine in obsessive-compulsive disorder. Psychiatry Res 14:85–93, 1985

Weiss E: Agoraphobia in the Light of Ego Psychology. New York, Grune & Stratton, 1964

Zitrin CM, Klein DF, Woerner MG: Behavior therapy, supportive psychotherapy, imipramine, and phobias. Arch Gen Psychiatry 35:307–316, 1978

Zitrin CM, Klein DF, Woerner MG, et al: Treatment of phobias, I: comparison of imipramine hydrochloride and placebo. Arch Gen Psychiatry 40:125–138, 1983

C H A P T E R   2 2

Barry S. Fogel, M.D.
Joel Sadavoy, M.D., F.R.C.P.C.

Somatoform and Personality Disorders

Somatoform Disorders

Definitions

The essential features of somatoform disorders are physical symptoms with no demonstrable organic findings, together with presumptive evidence of underlying psychological precipitants. DSM-IV (American Psychiatric Association 1994) describes seven categories of somatoform disorders: body dysmorphic disorder; conversion disorder; hypochondriasis; somatization disorder; pain disorder; undifferentiated somatoform disorder; and somatoform disorder, not otherwise specified. DSM-IV confines reference to age-relevant facts to the observation that the onset of all of these disorders is generally prior to age 30, but hypochondriasis and somatoform pain may develop at any age.

The nature of the research on somatoform disorders is such that it is sometimes difficult to reliably know which of these disorders has been included in study samples. Often patients and subjects are grouped under broad terms such as *hypochondriasis, hysteria, somatization, somatic burden,* or *somatic complaints.* Consequently, these disorders are still most appropriately conceptualized as a single category when interpreting data, especially from older studies.

Epidemiology

Relatively little is known about the epidemiology of these disorders in elderly individuals, and the data on their incidence and prevalence in old age are somewhat conflicting. A number of studies support the commonly held view that somatoform symptoms are more common in elderly individuals (Brink et al. 1981; Busse 1976; Leon et al. 1979), whereas others contradict these findings (Costa et al. 1987; Levkoff et al. 1987). Estimates of the presence of hypochondriasis in general medical populations vary widely from 0.4% to 14% (Barsky et al. 1990; Beaber and Rodney 1984; Kellner 1986), with an even wider range in elderly individuals (3.9%–33%) (Palmore 1970; Stenback et al. 1978).

Data from the Epidemiologic Catchment Area Study revealed no significant differences in the lifetime prevalence of somatization disorder or the total number of symptoms between women younger than 45 and those older than 45. In those older than 65, the 6-month prevalence rate of somatization disorder was 0 (Wittchen 1992).

Barsky et al. (1991), in a carefully diagnosed general medical clinic population (60 hypochondriasis patients, 100 control patients), found that hypochondriasis was unrelated to age. Kramer-Ginsberg et al. (1989) found no association between age and hypochondriasis in a sample of elderly depressed patients. Lyness et al. (1993), in a similar sample of depressed patients, found no contribution of age to somatic concerns if the elderly group alone was examined. However, increased age was a predictor of somatic concern if the entire age spectrum of their sample was included (i.e., those ages 20 and older). In a study of very old individuals (>85 years) living at home, Bowling (1990) found that patients with high depression scores were most often worried about their health. Interestingly, the higher the degree of psychiatric morbidity, the less likely these very old individuals were to report psychological distress to their physicians. Musalek et al. (1989), in a retrospective study of age at onset of delusional themes in patients of a psychiatric clinic, found that two-thirds of cases of "hypochondriasis" arose prior to age 40. However, there was a second peak (23% of cases) after age 60.

In contrast, McDonald (1973), utilizing data from a sample of patients admitted to a psychiatric hospital, showed a decreased incidence of diagnosed anxiety in elderly patients at admission; however, hypochondrial reactions increased in those older than 65 years. In an earlier study, McDonald (1967) had found significantly more psychosomatic disorders in elderly neurotic patients living at home compared with those admitted to the hospital. Taking all these data into account, McDonald concluded that as age increases, neuroticism has a tendency to present with somatic symptoms.

Hale and Cochran (1992) used the Brief Symptom Inventory to study 841 college graduates in four cohorts ranging in age from 22 to over 86. In analyzing results, they removed the somatic- and memory-related items of the scale (which they presumed to be normatively related to aging). They found that the younger cohorts reported more psychological distress than the older cohorts, but the older cohorts showed greater distress on somatic and obsessive-compulsive scale items.

Still other studies have shown an age-related increase in the hypochondriasis scale score on the Minnesota Multiphasic Personality Inventory (MMPI) (Lawton et al. 1980). However, it is important to remember that these scales rely on questions that include somatic complaints. Because elderly individuals are generally less healthy, they will score higher on the hypochondriasis scale because of a larger number of actual disease-engendered complaints.

Costa and McCrae (1987) described an elegant analysis of data on the diagnosis and expression of hypochondriasis in aging. Citing Coates and Janoff-Bulman (1978), they suggested that physical illness alone does not have a lasting effect on personality, as most individuals adapt to even the most catastrophic medical conditions. Hence, they argued, the illnesses associated with old age are unlikely to be the cause of personality change. This observation becomes most relevant in relation to neuroticism, a broad dimension of normal personality that encompasses many traits, including self-consciousness; inability to inhibit cravings; vulnerability to stress; and the tendency to experience hostility, anxiety, and depression. In their analysis of data, Costa and McCrae concluded that neuroticism is a much stronger predictor of somatic complaints than age. Consequently, hypochondriacal behavior should not be considered a normal aspect of aging (i.e., secondary to physical decline), but instead should be considered the result of longstanding personality factors; a comorbid condition, usually depression; or some other form of poor psychological adjustment. This position is indirectly supported by studies of health care utilization. Older subjects are no different from younger subjects in seeking treatment for conditions deemed serious by physicians (Hoag 1981), and they do not make disproportionately large numbers of visits to physicians (Eckstein

1978). Eckstein suggested that, given the large burden of illness and disabilities, the complaints of elderly individuals are remarkably low-keyed and valid (Eckstein 1978). Ford (1983) offered further support in stating that hypochondriacal behavior should not therefore be considered a normal aspect of aging, but a symptom of another underlying problem, usually depression or some other form of poor psychological adjustment. Affleck et al. (1992) supported the relationship between neuroticism and pain expression. They found that in a group of 54 subjects with rheumatoid arthritis, individuals with higher neuroticism scores showed more chronic distress, mediated by a tendency to catastrophize their pain.

In summary, despite sometimes conflicting data, the bulk of the evidence indicates that although somatoform disorders are present in old age, elderly individuals are no more likely than younger individuals to present a somatoform picture. Moreover, it is probable that age and associated physical illnesses per se are not sufficient etiological explanations of somatoform disorders. Rather, these disorders are more reliably explained by longstanding personality traits and vulnerabilities or the presence of a comorbid disturbance such as depression.

Etiology

The early determinants of late-life psychological disturbance are difficult to establish, but the etiology of somatoform disorders is probably multifactorial. As indicated earlier, personality and developmental factors likely are central causative factors, and several aspects of development have been implicated as precursors to later somatoform symptoms. Whitehead et al. (1981) suggested that children who learn to adopt the "sick role," reinforced by attention and "treats" from parents, are more likely to assume a sick role as adults.

Gender, education, ethnicity, and social class also seem to affect the expression of somatoform symptoms (Jacob and Turner 1991). For example, Maddocks (1964) reported that hypochondriasis in elderly individuals is found more often in women and lower socioeconomic class groups. Patterson et al. (1992) found that "greater childhood social deprivation and misfortune" was associated with "relatively more psychological disturbance" in the elderly men in their sample, but not in the women.

Lowenthal (1971) proposed that overall physical health status may be either a stressor or the result of a stressor. The effect of events and whether they are experienced as stressors varies depending on whether the events are the result of voluntary action (e.g., a move to a retirement or nursing home) and on the coping styles and life context of the individual (Busse 1976).

Busse (1976) asserted that hypochondriacal patients use their symptoms as a means of adapting to the psychosocial changes of aging through escape to the sick role. In his view the major precipitants for hypochondriacal expression are exposure to prolonged criticism without the option of escape, partial isolation secondary to socioeconomic restrictions, and deteriorated marital relations secondary to the prolonged infirmity of one of the partners. Symptomatic behavior is reinforced further by the availability and acceptability of medical care.

Busse (1976) went on to hypothesize three psychodynamic etiological elements of hypochondriasis: 1) withdrawal of psychic interest in others and centering of it on one's self-body and its functioning (hence these patients appear self-centered, uncaring, and manipulative); 2) shift of anxiety from a threatening psychic source to the less threatening focus of the body (e.g., intolerable guilt over the earlier death of a child is converted to anxious worry about health status); and 3) use of physical symptoms as a means of self-punishment and atonement for unacceptable hostile feelings toward ambivalently loved objects.

Bianchi (1973) examined the variables associated with hypochondriasis (which included disease phobia, disease conviction, somatic preoccupation, and psychogenic pain) in 118 patients. Five chief components were found to be related to hypochondriasis:

1. An inhibition of anger/maternal oversolicitude component (programmed augmentation leading to disease phobia)
2. An anxiety component (current augmentation leading to disease phobia)
3. A psychogenic pain/somatic preoccupation component
4. A somatic preoccupation/hypochondriacal personality component
5. A disease conviction/disordered cognition component

Disease phobia (as opposed to the conviction of having a disease) was the hypochondriacal symptom most often preceded by early life events. A pervasive inability to express negative emotion, especially anger, as a causal explanation for chronic pain symptoms was supported by Kerns et al. (1994), who used multiple regression analysis to study 142 patients with chronic pain. Inhibition of expressed anger was the strongest predictor of reports of pain intensity and pain behavior.

Bianchi's (1971) multifactorial etiological model of disease phobia hypothesizes that the behavior is promoted by early experiences with illness in self and family, reinforced by maternal oversolicitude. Hypochondriasis arises in the vulnerable individual when anxieties emerge (perhaps secondary to stressors that further reduce an already diminished sensation and pain threshold), thereby releasing hypochondriacal symptoms.

Barsky et al. (1991) also suggest that hypochondriasis may serve a coping function, fostering adoption of the sick role. Such behavior may be seen as a vehicle for enhancing social contact and support and forcing caregiving responses. In addition, it reflects loss of self-esteem and may be a means of communicating psychological distress.

From a psychodynamic perspective, somatic expressions of distress in elderly individuals reflect underlying age-associated conflicts. Busse (1976) summarized these as fear of irrelevance and abandonment; sexual decline; a regressed expression of rage, jealousy, or helplessness; and a symbolic reaction to a sense of being assaulted by negative internalized objects. This latter formulation is illustrated by the case of an elderly woman admitted to a psychogeriatric unit because of increasing anxiety, dangerous behaviors (e.g., smoking in bed, burning holes in her carpet), and bizarre preoccupations with her health. She was transferred to the unit from her home in an apartment building for elderly individuals, where she had managed independently. Her past history included a stormy, conflicted relationship with her two daughters, who withdrew from her once she was safely institutionalized. The withdrawal of her family was the apparent immediate precipitant for her decompensation, although she had had a lifelong history of Cluster B personality disorder with highly self-centered narcissistic and acting-out characteristics. Her cognitive state was unimpaired, and her general health was good except for a colostomy performed for inflammatory bowel disease some years previously, which was the main center of her somatic preoccupation.

In the hospital the patient was incessantly preoccupied with her stoma, excoriating it by scratching and inserting foreign objects such as paper and pins to "clean it." She was convinced it was dirty, dreaded its normal action, and thought about it constantly. However, she was not delusional, nor did she fulfill criteria for any other Axis I disorder. This self-mutilating attack on herself became understandable during psychotherapy as the therapist became aware of the unconscious association between the stoma and her mother. The patient described her mother as rigid, perfectionistic, and punitive, especially with regard to the patient's self-control and cleanliness. As the patient experienced the rejection of her daughters (similar to the rejection of her mother), she regressed to a phase of fear and conflict with her rejecting, punitive mother. In this process the stoma came to symbolize her uncontrollable, dirty, and unacceptable self, which she turned against with all the loathing and viciousness she had internalized from her mother.

Stoudemire (1991) examined the communication value of somatoform symptoms from various points of view, focusing on alexithymia. This is a psychodynamically based concept that describes an individual's diminished capacity for symbolization of feeling through language. Such individuals have difficulty identifying and communicating feeling states, together with a relative incapacity to distinguish between feelings and bodily sensations. Stoudemire suggested that such individuals communicate through somatic language that can be understood if attended to. He termed this form of somatic communication *somatothymia*. He also agreed with others (Bianchi 1971; Busse 1976) that the origins of somatic expression may derive from learned behaviors (i.e., adoption of the sick role in childhood), which predisposes patients to reliance on somatic communication, especially when under stress.

Clinical Picture

The presentation of somatoform disorders in old age has not been well described, although in general older individuals probably have a presentation similar to that of younger populations. Most studies confirm the important comorbid relationship between somatoform disorders and depression and anxiety (DeAlarcon 1964; Gurland 1976; Post 1963). Kramer-Ginsberg et al. (1989), in a sample of 70 elderly patients (mean age 75) with unipolar major depressive episodes and no acute medical illness, found that 60% had a concurrent diagnosis of hypochondriasis on admission; 40% retained this diagnosis after treatment of depression. There was no relationship between hypochondriasis and age, age at onset of depression, severity of depression, short-term outcome, or suicidality. However, there was a significant correlation between hypochondriasis and psychic and somatic anxiety. These and other results (Kay and Bergmann 1966) support the contention that new-onset hypochondriasis is a marker for depression in elderly individuals that may be "masked" by the somatoform component. Lipowski (1990) pointed out that somatization linked to depression is highly associated with suicide and that 90% of female patients with a primary diagnosis of somatization disorder have a major depression. He suggested three reasons for the close relationship between depression and somatic complaints: 1) depression promotes recall of past illness-related memories, 2) depression may lower the threshold for perception of pain and other somatic symptoms, and 3) pain may exacerbate depression in a vicious cycle.

Pasnau and Bystritsky (1990) have highlighted the connection between anxiety and somatization, listing headache, tachycardia, abdominal distress, insomnia, flatulence, and exhaustion as prominent somatic anxiety symptoms. Other symptoms cited as common are pain, dizziness, dyspnea, paresthesias, and tinnitus.

Management of Somatoform Disorders

Empirical data on treatment approaches and efficacy are lacking, although clearly an integrated approach (Sadavoy 1994) to treatment is most likely indicated based on the complex interplay of early life problems, personality features, alexithymia, depressive and anxiety disorders, and comorbid physical conditions.

Because of the strong association between comorbid psychiatric factors (especially depression, anxiety, and suicidality) and somatoform disorders, management begins with a diligent examination of the patient for these factors, together with ensuring an appropriate full medical workup. (For example, Katon et al. [1993], in a 12-week placebo-controlled double-blind trial using nortriptyline, found a significant correlation between improved depression scores and decreases in measures of functional disability in elderly individuals with chronic tinnitus.) Similarly, the clinician must maintain an initial high index of suspicion of a comorbid Axis II diagnosis, which should be the object of specific inquiry, and must differentiate carefully between depression and somatoform disorder with or without comorbid personality disorder. Even simple, detailed history taking, however, may be difficult, as many of these patients resist a search for psychological factors, insisting that their symptoms are only physical and fearing being told "once again" that nothing is wrong. Despite resistance, clinicians are most effective if they pursue data collection from both the patient and collateral informants.

Treatment choice is determined by the capacity of the patient to engage in the process and willingness to accept the diagnosis. Because of the frequent interplay of various immediate life stressors, personality factors, and interpersonal issues, the psychotherapies are an important component of management. This conclusion is reinforced by the finding of Kramer-Ginsberg et al. (1989) that 40% of patients with comorbid depression and hypochondriasis, retained the diagnosis of hypochondriasis after successful treatment of their depression.

Any form of psychotherapeutic intervention is complicated by the difficulty that this patient group demonstrates in forming an alliance with treatment. Gurian (1991), for example, asserted that cure is impossible and implied that the physician must make special efforts to understand that the patient has a pathological abnormality and is not merely nasty. This therapeutic perspective may be difficult to maintain in light of the personality features, which often include help-rejecting complaintiveness, physician "shopping," time-engulfing demandingness, and refractoriness to treatment. These factors all conspire to make these patients easy targets for systematic rejection by the therapeutic community as the record of failed therapeutic relationships mounts.

Management has several components that incorporate two basic principles: 1) containment of the patient's anxiety-based somatoform symptoms, not unlike management of Cluster B personality disorders; and 2) active, vigorous treatment for identified depressive or dysthymic disorder. The frequent interplay of social and interpersonal factors in the precipitation and perpetuation of some somatoform disorders requires the clinician to be prepared to intervene in an active, supportive manner with regard to these issues. However, caution is in order to avoid becoming enmeshed in the frequently demanding and overly dependent stance that often characterizes these patients. Any referrals to social support agencies should be carefully coordinated by the therapist with an eye toward avoiding duplication and splitting of services.

The core of long-term management, both psychotherapeutic and pharmacological, resides in the therapeutic relationship. This is best maintained by adoption of a clear, structured relationship with openly identified, nonpunitive limits on frequency of contact, use of emergency services and other physicians, telephone contact, use of medications, and duration of sessions.

Because long-term cure is unlikely, pharmacological management of anxiety should be cautious, although because this patient group is prone to heightened expressions of anxiety, anxiolytic or hypnotic agents may be used judiciously and intermittently. Pasnau and Bystritsky (1990) advocated educating the anxious elderly patient about the interplay between symptoms and stress and using cognitive therapy and relaxation training to improve the patient's sense of control and self-esteem.

Because of the important role of interpersonal factors, family therapy may be a useful mode of intervention. Goldstein and Birnbom's (1976) case review, although anecdotal, supported the utility of this approach.

Personality Disorders

Although personality traits increasingly are recognized as an important modifier of illness behavior and disease outcomes, the study of personality disorders has remained limited by conceptual and methodological difficulties. Unlike personality traits, which can be measured reliably and validly, personality disorders are defined by clinically derived clusters of behavioral manifestations that usually can be determined only by history. Collateral informants often are needed for diagnostic accuracy, and retrospective diagnoses are plagued by the imperfect recall of individuals and the changing trend of material recorded in or withheld from medical records. The overlap and interaction of personality traits is expected; the overlap of personality disorder diagnoses is problematic, because it suggests significant heterogeneity within personality disorder categories. The nosological problems associated with personality disorder diagnoses are worse when older people are studied, because recall may be worse, informants less available, and diagnostic behavioral criteria less typical of the manifestations of personality disorder seen in later life.

Notwithstanding the nosological issues, clinicians continue to find utility in diagnostic categories (e.g., antisocial, borderline, narcissistic, histrionic, or schizoid personality) that communicate in a few words clinical descriptions and management advice and increasingly are seen as powerful incremental predictors of course and outcome in Axis I disorders. The personality disorders most discussed by general psychiatrists are not necessarily those with the most robust diagnostic criteria, but those that orient clinicians toward an approach to management and clinician-patient interaction.

Classification of Personality Disorders

The diagnostic criteria for personality disorders can be found in DSM-IV (American Psychiatric Association 1994). The personality disorders are often grouped into the following clusters that share a common behavioral theme:

- Cluster A, which consists of odd or eccentric personalities; these include the paranoid, schizoid, and schizotypal personality disorders
- Cluster B, which consists of dramatic, emotional, and erratic personalities; these include the antisocial, borderline, narcissistic, and histrionic personality disorders

- Cluster C, which consists of the anxious and fearful personalities; these include the avoidant, dependent, and obsessive-compulsive personality disorders

Patients with personality traits that cause sufficient distress or functional impairment to merit designation as mental disorders are said to have *trait disturbances,* or *subsyndromal personality disorders.* Those with personality traits of several personality disorders who do not meet full criteria for any of them, yet are seen as sufficiently impaired to warrant a personality disorder diagnosis, receive a diagnosis of *personality disorder, not otherwise specified.* This creates a potential diagnostic ambiguity: When does a patient with multiple (subsyndromal) trait disturbances warrant a diagnosis of personality disorder, not otherwise specified? The ambiguity has not been officially resolved.

Stability of Personality Traits With Aging

It is in accord with everyday experience that personality traits such as extroversion and neuroticism are reasonably stable over the life course. In the absence of such major confounders as manic illness, introverts do not become gregarious at age 70, nor do fearful individuals develop nerves of steel at the end of life. Costa and his colleagues, developers of the NEO Personality Inventory and champions of the five-factor theory of personality, have shown that when personality traits are measured with standard questionnaires and tested again several years later, the results are highly correlated (Costa and McCrae 1980). These correlations remain high even when major life events have intervened (Costa et al. 1987; McCrae and Costa 1988). However, such studies do not rule out aging-related changes in entire cohorts in ways that leave the relative ranking of individuals unchanged. Cross-sectional comparisons of populations of different ages do suggest differences, but it is not possible to determine whether the differences are due to age, period, or cohort effects. For example, Johnson et al. (1985) found that older Hawaiians were more orderly, stable, and conscientious and less active than younger Hawaiians. Eysenck et al. (1985) found that impulsiveness and venturesomeness were lower in subjects older than 60. Costa et al. (1986) showed that extroversion, neuroticism, and openness to experience decreased slightly but significantly with age in a cross-sectional analysis of 10,063 subjects examined by questionnaire in a national epidemiological survey.

A decrease in extroversion and other "active" traits with age may be the most replicated difference between younger and older subjects in trait studies (Gutman 1966; Heron and Chown 1967; Sealey and Cattell 1965). In the only major longitudinal study of the question, Spiro (1990), examining 13-year longitudinal data from the Veterans Administration Longitudinal Study, showed that aggregate mean levels of extroversion declined with aging.

Despite the relative lack of generic age-related personality changes, the experience of "personality change" is commonly described by patients and by caregivers in connection with mood disorders and brain diseases, especially traumatic brain injury and dementia.

Personality Change in Later Life

Personality change in later life can be viewed as comprising five different clinical situations:

1. A personality trait changes qualitatively because of a major change in brain function, whether owing to a mood disorder, a toxic-metabolic insult, or gross brain disease. Examples include loss of extroversion in major depression and loss of conscientiousness as a result of frontal lobe degeneration.

2. A personality trait changes quantitatively because of a change in brain function. Examples include aggravation of passive-dependent traits by Parkinson's disease, aggravation of impulsiveness by frontal lobe disease, or aggravation of hostility by chronic pain.

3. A personality trait changes qualitatively because of a change in the physical or social environment or because of a major life event. Examples include new development of paranoid traits in a person who has recently been assaulted and whose neighborhood has become unsafe and development of extroversion in a previously withdrawn person after the death of a controlling, domineering spouse.

4. A personality trait changes quantitatively because of a change in physical or social environment or because of a major life event. Examples include an increased emotional display when a person with a borderline personality disorder is placed in a nursing home with a roommate he or she does not like, and social withdrawal in a man with lifelong poor social skills following the loss of a wife who orchestrated relationships with children and with other couples.

5. A personality trait changes qualitatively or quantitatively as a result of intrapsychic change induced by experience and reflection. Examples include increased assertiveness as self-consciousness and the importance of the opinions of others diminish, or softening and enhanced capacity for intimacy as past personal deficiencies are acknowledged in late life.

The 10th revision of the *International Classification of Diseases* (World Health Organization 1991) distinguishes personality change from personality disorder and requires that personality change be linked to an identifiable environmental stressor or brain disease. However, the difficulty of distinguishing personality change from the increased symptomatic expression of a preexisting personality disorder or trait disturbance is acknowledged. The classification offered above aims to make this fine distinction explicit in theory, although it is sometimes difficult in practice.

DSM-IV (American Psychiatric Association 1994) classifies situations 1 and 2 as personality change resulting from a general medical disorder but excludes dementia and delirium from its list of causes.

Age-Related Changes in Symptoms of Patients With Personality Disorders

Empirical studies of personality disorder symptoms in relation to age have tended to focus on the progression of symptoms between young adulthood and middle age, with few or no elderly subjects included. The general thrust of these studies is that middle-age persons with borderline personality or antisocial personality show less overt, high-energy acting out than younger ones (Arboleda-Florez 1991; Maddocks 1970; McGlashan 1986; Snyder et al. 1985; Tyrer and Seivewright 1988). Notwithstanding, some individuals with antisocial personalities remain actively criminal into old age (Arboleda-Florez 1991). By contrast, individuals with eccentric, odd, or suspicious Cluster A personalities do not become less symptomatic during progression from youth to midlife (Reich et al. 1988; Tyrer and Seivewright 1988).

Personality change with early dementia has received attention in several systematic studies. Not only are personality changes common in early dementia, but those who know the patient well tend to agree on what the changes are (Strauss et al. 1993). Petry et al. (1989) identified the development of apathy and/or self-centered behavior as the most common manifestations of early Alzheimer's disease. Personality disturbance characteristically is the first manifestation of the frontal lobe dementias, including Pick's disease, pure frontal lobe degeneration, and other related neuropathological entities. Either apathy and withdrawal or an uncharacteristic impulsiveness and disinhibition may be the presenting signs (Miller et al. 1994). The different presentations may depend partly on premorbid personality traits and partly on the part of the frontal system that is first affected by the degenerative disease. The relative weights of disease-specific and patient-specific determinants of personality change remain to be determined by further study.

Epidemiology of Personality Disorder in Old Age

Empirically established estimates of the prevalence of personality disorder in old age are few, and estimates based on recorded clinical diagnoses are notoriously inaccurate. The problem of chart-based diagnoses may be especially great in elderly individuals, because the presence of an "organic" diagnosis greatly reduces the chance that a personality disorder diagnosis will be recorded on Axis II.

A fairly solid estimate of the prevalence of antisocial personality disorder in the community comes from the Epidemiologic Catchment Area Study, which found a prevalence of 0.8% in persons older than 65 (Robins et al. 1984). No other personality disorders were systematically sought in the Diagnostic Interview Schedule that formed the basis of the Epidemiologic Catchment Area Study, nor has any large population-based study provided the basis for an estimate of personality disorder prevalence in the general elderly population.

The prevalence of personality disorder in psychiatric hospital inpatients has been studied more extensively. Kastrup (1985), studying a sample of more than 2,000 patients older than 65 admitted for the first time to a psychiatric facility, found that 0.7% of men and 2.8% of women had a diagnosis of personality disorder. Diagnostic criteria were not specified, and the estimate is surely low, because diagnosis of comorbid personality disorder in persons with a primary diagnosis of another psychiatric disorder was not counted. Fogel and Westlake (1990) studied recorded personality disorder diagnoses in a sample of 2,322 adults admitted to a private psychiatric hospital with major depression. The rate of personality disorder comorbidity was 15.8% in the entire sample, whereas only 12% of the patients older than 65 had a comorbid personality disorder diagnosis. Obsessive-compulsive personality was diagnosed in 46% of elderly depression patients with Axis II comorbidity; borderline and histrionic personality disorders were practically never diagnosed in elderly patients. Kunik et al. (1994) found that of 547 older psychiatric inpatients (ages 51–96) with various Axis I diagnoses, 13% received a personality disorder diagnosis on Axis II. The rate of comorbid personality disorder ranged from 6% in patients with an organic mental disorder on Axis I to 24% in patients with major depression on Axis I. Within the age range of these patients, and after controlling for diagnosis, there was no correlation between age and the rate of personality disorder diagnoses.

Although the true prevalence of personality disorder in elderly individuals is essentially unknown, there is reasonable support for a minimum estimate of between 10% and 20% for personality disorder as a comorbid condition in older psychiatric inpatients. This prevalence warrants systematic efforts to determine the presence of personality disorder in an older psychiatric inpatient, in view of the potential relevance of personality disorder diagnoses to treatment strategy and prognosis.

Relevance of Personality Disorder as a Comorbidity

Studies of personality disorder as a comorbidity in older psychiatric patients have focused on patients with major depression and patients with psychosis. Brodaty et al. (1993) studied the prognosis of unipolar major depression treated in a mood disorders specialty unit in Australia. Of the 61 patients older than 60 in their total sample of 242 consecutive patients, 41% had a durable remission at follow-up nearly 4 years later. Premorbid personality disturbance was a negative prognostic factor. Thompson et al. (1988) studied the efficacy of 16–20 sessions of psychotherapy in a sample of 79 depression patients with a mean age of 66 years. Subjects with a personality disorder were less likely to show a reduction in depressive symptoms with short-term psychotherapy. Abrams et al. (1994) focused attention on the different rates for comorbid personality disorder in early-onset and late-onset elderly depression patients. In a study of 30 volunteers older than 60 who had fully recovered from an episode of major depression, the 16 with early-onset depression had significantly more avoidant and dependent traits than the 14 with first-onset depression after age 60. However, the small sample and retrospective design limit the interpretability and generalizability of the finding.

A similar theme of less personality abnormality in late-onset mental illness was suggested by the observations of Yassa and Suranyi-Cadotte (1993) in a study of 40 elderly patients with psychosis (20 with late-onset schizophrenia, 13 with paraphrenia, and 7 with pure delusional disorder).

The patients with pure delusional disorder (paranoia) had the latest onset of symptoms and the least premorbid personality disturbance; the schizophrenia and paraphrenia patients tended to have paranoid or schizoid premorbid personality.

Symptomatic Expression of Personality Disorder in Old Age

The symptomatic expression of personality disorder in elderly individuals may differ from that in younger individuals for several reasons, including 1) different normative life stressors tasks, events, and living arrangements; 2) diminished energy, drive, impulsiveness, and/or extroversion (see earlier discussion); 3) learning from accumulated life experience; and 4) effects of gross brain disease or indirect effects of systemic illness. These factors can aggravate, attenuate, or alter the focus of personality disorder–related behavior. Alternatively, if these age-associated factors block the use of long-established and rigid patterns of adaptation, the patient may develop depression (Akiskal 1983), somatic preoccupation (Verwoerdt 1987), or overwhelming anxiety, or may commit suicide. Clinical wisdom holds that isolated drug treatment of anxiety or depression under these circumstances without addressing the underlying personality disorder by psychotherapeutic, environmental, or social interventions is likely to have a disappointing outcome. This wisdom has not been empirically tested.

Reports concerning life events and personality disorder expressions have focused mainly on Cluster B personalities and on the negative life events of institutionalization, forced intimacy, and bereavement; the narcissistic wounds of ill health; and the burdens of caring for a cognitively impaired spouse. These will be discussed further later. Regarding patients with Cluster A personalities, particularly those with paranoid and schizoid personalities, it has been observed that the social isolation typical of these patients becomes highly problematic if they develop functional impairments or medical conditions necessitating personal care, whether institutional or community based. In either case they find themselves with the unpleasant choice of accepting social contacts that have always caused anxiety or suffering adverse medical consequences if they do not. If an institution forces them to be intimate (e.g., sharing a room in a nursing home), they can become agitated, anxious, or delusional (Sadavoy and Fogel 1992). Efforts by community-based care agencies to provide services to such patients in their homes are often thwarted by these patients' dislike of social contact or their mistrust and apparent rejection of service providers.

For patients with Cluster B personality disorders, close relationships have always been both necessary and problematic. Their core psychodynamic problems, which include impaired affect tolerance (Krystal 1987), real or fantasized narcissistic injury (Lazarus 1980), and fear or experience of abandonment, make them especially vulnerable to the normative life events of bereavement, separation from friends or family members, loss of occupational status through retirement, and financial problems. Acting out, however, takes forms typical of the patient's age and social situation. Rather than splitting lovers or parents, an elderly patient with borderline disorder may split physicians or family caregivers. Impulsiveness may be manifested by self-administration of prescription drugs rather than abuse of street drugs. The dynamics of patient-staff interaction in institutional care settings, however, resemble those encountered when borderline disorder patients are treated in psychiatric hospitals (Sadavoy and Dorian 1983), with scapegoating, chaotic care, and a threatened breakdown of the treatment plan.

Treatment Considerations

When treating the older patient with personality disorder, the central task is to establish a stable clinician-patient relationship that regulates interpersonal distance and affective expression in a way that holds and comforts the patient and provides stability. With Cluster A patients, the relationship usually is cool and professional but evidently caring; with Cluster B patients, there is an inevitable ebb and flow of transference and countertransference, but the therapist recurrently restores a stable framework and supplies an observing ego. In institutions, the clinician should endeavor to educate staff regarding the patient's dynamics and help to formulate a written treatment plan to be followed consistently by all caregivers. Elderly patients with borderline disorder, like younger ones, do not easily tolerate inconsistency and ambivalence in their caregivers.

The use of drug therapy in elderly outpatients with personality disorder is always constrained by the risks of drug misuse. Notwithstanding, patients with major depression should receive drug treatment, with the usual precautions. Elderly patients with borderline, schizotypal, or paranoid disorders and with fleeting delusions, paranoia, or micropsychotic episodes should be treated with a relatively low dose of an antipsychotic drug with some anxiolytic effect (e.g., thioridazine, perphenazine, or risperidone). Haloperidol is often poorly tolerated by these patients, who experience its near-universal extrapyramidal side effects as a narcissistic injury as well as a discomfort.

References

Abrams R, Rosendahl E, Card C, et al: Personality disorder correlates of late and early onset depression. J Am Geriatr Soc 42:727–731, 1994

Affleck G, Tennen H, Urrows S, et al: Neuroticism and the pain-mood relation in rheumatoid arthritis: insights from a prospective daily study. J Consult Clin Psychol 60:119–126, 1992

Akiskal HS: Dysthymic disorder: psychopathology of proposed chronic depressive subtypes. Am J Psychiatry 140:11–20, 1983

American Psychiatric Association: Diagnostic and Statistical Manual of Mental Disorders, 4th Edition. Washington, DC, American Psychiatric Association, 1994

Arboleda-Florez J: Antisocial burnout: an exploratory study. Bull Am Acad Psychiatry Law 19:173–183, 1991

Barsky A, Wyshak G, Klerman G: The prevalence of hypochondriasis among medical outpatients. Soc Psychiatry Psychiatr Epidemiol 24:89–94, 1990

Barsky AJ, Frank C, Cleary P, et al: The relation between hypochondriasis and age. Am J Psychiatry 148(7):923–928, 1991

Beaber R, Rodney W: Under diagnosis of hypochondriasis in family practice. Psychosomatics 25:39–45, 1984

Bianchi GN: The origins of disease phobia. Aust N Z J Psychiatry 5:241–257, 1971

Bianchi GN: Patterns of hypochondriasis: a principal components analysis. Br J Psychiatry 122:541–548, 1973

Bowling A: The prevalence of psychiatric morbidity among people aged 85 and over living at home. Soc Psychiatry Psychiatr Epidemiol 25:132–140, 1990

Brink T, Janakes C, Martinez N: Geriatric hypochondriasis: situational factors. J Am Geriatr Soc 29:37–39, 1981

Brodaty H, Harris L, Peters K, et al: Prognosis of depression in the elderly: a comparison with younger patients. Br J Psychiatry 163:589–596, 1993

Busse EW: Hypochondriasis in the elderly: a reaction to stress. J Am Geriatr Soc 24:145–149, 1976

Coates D, Janoff-Bulman R: Lottery winners and accident victims: is happiness relative? J Pers Soc Psychol 36:917–927, 1978

Costa P, McCrae R: Somatic complaints in males as a function of age and neuroticism: a longitudinal analysis. J Behav Med 3:245–257, 1980

Costa PT, McCrae R, Zonderman A, et al: Cross-sectional studies of personality in a national sample, II: stability in neuroticism, extroversion and openness. Psychol Aging 1:144–149, 1986

Costa PT, McCrae RR, Zonderman A: Environmental and dispositional influences on well-being: longitudinal follow-up of an American national sample. Br J Psychol 78:299–306, 1987

DeAlarcon R: Hypochondriasis and depression in the aged. Gerontol Clin 6:266–267, 1964

Eckstein D: Common complaints of the elderly, in The Geriatric Patient. Edited by Reichel W. New York, HP Publishing, 1978

Eysenck SBG, Pearson PR, Easting G, et al: Age norms for impulsiveness, venturesomeness, and empathy in adults. Personality and Individual Differences 6:613–619, 1985

Fogel BS, Westlake R: Personality disorder diagnosis and age in inpatients with major depression. J Clin Psychiatry 51:232–235, 1990

Ford CV: The Somatizing Disorders: Illness as a Way of Life. New York, Elsevier, 1983, pp 89–90

Goldstein SE, Birnbom F: Hypochondriasis and the elderly. J Am Geriatr Soc 24:150–154, 1976

Gurian B: Coping with hypochondriasis in older patients. Geriatrics 46:71–77, 1991

Gurland B: The comparative frequency of depression in various adult age groups. J Gerontol 31:283–292, 1976

Gutman GM: A note on the MMPI: age and sex differences in extroversion and neuroticism in a Canadian sample. Br J Soc Clin Psychol 5:128–129, 1966

Hale WD, Cochran CD: Age differences in self-reported symptoms of psychological distress. J Clin Psychol 48:633–637, 1992

Heron A, Chown SM: Age and Function. London, England, Churchill Livingstone, 1967

Hoag MR: Age and medical care utilization patterns. J Gerontol 36:103–111, 1981

Jacob R, Turner S: Somatoform disorders, in Adult Psychopathology and Diagnosis. Edited by Jacob R, Turner S. New York, Wiley, 1991

Johnson RC, Ahern FM, Nagoshi CT, et al: Age- and group-specific cohort effects on personality test scores: a study of three Hawaiian populations. Journal of Cross-Cultural Psychology 16:467–481, 1985

Kastrup M: Characteristics of a nationwide cohort of psychiatric patients—

with special reference to the elderly and the chronically admitted. Acta Psychiatr Scand 71:107–115, 1985

Katon W, Sullivan M, Russo J, et al: Depressive symptoms and measures of disability: a prospective study. J Affect Disord 27:245–254, 1993

Kay PWK, Bergmann K: Physical disability and mental health in old age. J Psychosom Res 10:3–12, 1966

Kellner R: Somatization and Hypochondriasis. New York, Praeger, 1986

Kerns RD, Rosenberg R, Jacob M: Anger expression and chronic pain. J Behav Med 17:57–67, 1994

Kramer-Ginsberg E, Greenwald B, Aisen P, et al: Hypochondriasis in the elderly depressed. J Am Geriatr Soc 35:507–510, 1989

Krystal H: The impact of massive psychic trauma and the capacity to grieve effectively: later life sequelae, in Treating the Elderly With Psychotherapy. Edited by Sadavoy J, Leszcz M. Madison, CT, International Universities Press, 1987, pp 95–155

Kunik ME, Mulsant B, Rifai H, et al: Diagnostic rate of comorbid personality disorder in elderly psychiatric inpatients. Am J Psychiatry 151:603–605, 1994

Lawton MP, Whilihan W, Belsky J: Personality tests and their use with older adults, in Handbook of Mental Health and Aging. Edited by Birsen J, Slane RB. Englewood Cliffs, NJ, Prentice-Hall, 1980, pp 537–553

Lazarus LW: Self psychology and psychotherapy with the elderly: theory and practice. J Geriatr Psychiatry 13:69–88, 1980

Leon G, Gillum B, Gillum R, et al: Personality stability and change over a 30 year period—middle age to old age. J Consult Clin Psychol 47:517–524, 1979

Levkoff SE, Cleary P, Wetle T: Differences in the appraisal of health between aged and middle-aged adults. J Gerontol 42:114–120, 1987

Lipowski ZJ: Somatization and depression. Psychosomatics 31:13–21, 1990

Lowenthal ML: Social stress and adaptation toward a developmental perspective. Paper presented at the Task Force on Aging Panel, Developmental Aspects of Aging, American Psychological Association, Washington, DC, September 1971

Lyness JM, King D, Conwell Y, et al: Somatic worry and medical illness in depressed inpatients. Am J Geriatr Psychiatry 1:288–295, 1993

Maddox GL: Self assessment of health status: a longitudinal study of selected elderly subjects. J Chronic Dis 17:449–460, 1964

Maddox PD: A five-year followup of untreated psychopaths. Br J Psychiatry 116:511–575, 1970

McCrae R, Costa P: Psychological resilience among widowed men and women: a 10-year follow-up of a national sample. Journal of Social Issues 44:129–142, 1988

McDonald C: The pattern of neurotic illness in the elderly. Aust N Z J Psychiatry 1:203–210, 1967

McDonald C: An age-specific analysis of the neuroses. Br J Psychiatry 122:477–480, 1973

McGlashan TH: The Chestnut Lodge followup study, III: long-term outcome of borderline personalities. Arch Gen Psychiatry 43:20–30, 1986

Miller BL, Chang L, Oropilla G, et al: Alzheimer's disease and frontal lobe dementias, in Textbook of Geriatric Neuropsychiatry. Edited by Coffey CE, Cummings JL. Washington, DC, American Psychiatric Press, 1994, pp 389–404

Musalek M, Berner P, et al: Delusional theme, sex and age. Psychopathology 22:260–267, 1989

Palmore E (ed): Normal Aging. Durham, NC, Duke University Press, 1970

Pasnau R, Bystritsky A: Importance of treating anxiety in the elderly ill patient. Psychiatr Med 8(3):163–173, 1990

Patterson TL, Smith L, Smith T, et al: Symptoms of illness in late adulthood are related to childhood social deprivation and misfortune in men but not in women. J Behav Med 15:113–125, 1992

Petry S, Cummings JL, Hill MA, et al: Personality alterations in dementia of the Alzheimer type: a three-year followup study. J Geriatr Psychiatry Neurol 2:203–207, 1989

Post F: Depressive reactions in the elderly: a reappraisal. Gerontologist 3:156–159, 1963

Reich J, Ndvaguba M, Yates W: Age and sex distribution of DSM-III personality cluster traits in a community population. Compr Psychiatry 29:298–303, 1988

Robins LN, Helzer SC, Weissman MM, et al: Lifetime prevalence of specific psychiatric disorders in three sites. Arch Gen Psychiatry 41:949–958, 1984

Sadavoy J: Integrated psychotherapy for the elderly. Can J Psychiatry 39:S19–S26, 1994

Sadavoy J, Dorian B: Management of the characterologically difficult patient in the chronic care setting. J Geriatr Psychiatry 16:233–240, 1983

Sadavoy J, Fogel B: Personality disorders in the elderly, in Handbook of Mental Health and Aging. Edited by Birren J, Sloan, Cohen G. Academic Press, 1992, pp 433–462

Sealey AP, Cattell RB: Standard trends in personality development in men and women of 16 to 70 years, determined by 16 PF measurements. Paper presented at the British Psychological Society Conference, April 1965

Snyder S, Goodpaster WA, Pitts WM, et al: Demography of psychiatric patients with borderline traits. Psychopathology 18:38–49, 1985

Spiro A: Change and stability in personality. Abstract submitted to the Gerontological Society of America Annual Meeting, Boston, MA, November 16, 1990

Stenback A, Kumpulainen M, Vaukhenen M: Illness and health in septuagenarians. J Gerontol 33:57–61, 1978

Stoudemire A: Somatothymia parts I and II. Psychosomatics 32(4):365–381, 1991

Strauss ME, Pasupathi M, Chatterjec A: Concordance between observers in descriptions of personality change in Alzheimer's disease. Psychol Aging 8:475–480, 1993

Thompson LW, Gallagher D, Czirr R: Personality disorder and outcome in the treatment of late-life depression. J Geriatr Psychiatry 21:133–146, 1988

Tyrer P, Seivewright H: Studies of outcome, in Personality Disorders: Diagnosis, Management and Course. Edited by Tyrer P. London, Wright, 1988, pp 119–136

Verwoerdt A: Psychodynamics of paranoid phenomenon in the aged, in Treating Elderly With Psychotherapy. Edited by Sadavoy J, Leszcz M. Madison, CT, International Universities Press, 1987, pp 67–93

Whitehead WE, Winget C, Fedoravicius A, et al: Learned illness behavior in patients with irritable bowel syndrome and peptic ulcer. Dig Dis Sci 27:202–208, 1981

World Health Organization: International Classification of Diseases, 10th Revision. Geneva, World Health Organization, 1991

Yassa R, Suranyi-Cadotte B: Clinical characteristics of late-onset schizophrenia and delusional disorder. Schizophr Bull 19:201–207, 1993

Linda Ganzini, M.D.
Roland M. Atkinson, M.D.

Substance Abuse

Substance abuse constitutes a leading public health problem, yet there has been little attention paid to alcohol and drug addiction among elderly persons. Recent studies, however, indicate that substance abuse, particularly alcohol abuse, is a substantial source of psychiatric and physical morbidity in elderly individuals.

Elderly individuals are a highly heterogeneous population with substantial variability in physical and functional status. As such, the presentations, complications, and consequences of substance abuse are wide ranging. In this chapter we review the recent literature on the use of alcohol, prescription drugs (especially benzodiazepines), and nonprescription drugs by elderly persons. For further information and a general overview of the field of substance abuse, standard texts are referenced (Lowinson et al. 1992; Schuckit 1989). Standard pharmacology texts offer further information on drug classes discussed (Gilman et al. 1990).

Alcohol Use Disorders and Problem Drinking

Introduction and Definitions

Interest in geriatric alcoholism has developed only in the past few years, and for that reason current understanding of the phenomenology and treatment of older alcoholic patients is still fragmentary and often based on unreplicated studies. Definitions of alcohol use disorders (alcohol dependence and alcohol abuse) and the more inclusive term *alcoholism* are given in Table 23–1. Problem drinking includes more circumscribed adverse medical or social consequences of alcohol use in cases that may not meet criteria for an alcohol use disorder or alcoholism. Heavy drinking is even more inclusive and more variably defined, although most authorities agree that regular consumption of alcoholic beverages in excess of two standard drinks per day, or occasional consumption of five or more drinks, constitutes heavy drinking. (A standard drink contains about 10 g of absolute alcohol and is equivalent to 12 oz domestic beer, 4 oz table wine, or a cocktail containing 1–1.25 oz hard liquor.) For narrative ease, we use *alcoholism* and *alcoholic patient* as general terms in this chapter.

Epidemiology

Prevalence. A majority of persons older than 60 continue to drink beverage alcohol (Atkinson 1990). Community surveys suggest that the prevalence of alcoholism declines with age and that older men are far more likely to be diagnosed than women. These trends in general apply to blacks and Hispanics as well as whites (Helzer et al. 1991). The Epidemiologic Catchment Area (ECA) study, using DSM-III criteria, determined that the 1-year prevalence of alcohol use disorders in persons ages 65 and older was 3.10% in men and 0.46% in women (compared with 7.85% and 1.04%, respectively, in those ages 45 to 64 years old) (Helzer et al. 1991). The prevalence of alcoholism is higher in clinical than in community settings. For example, current or recent alcoholism was identified in 11% of Veterans Administration nursing home admissions (Joseph et al. 1992), 14% of elderly emergency department patients (Adams et al. 1992), and 23% of geriatric psychiatry inpatients (Speer and Bates 1992). A study of Medicare claims for 1989 reported a prevalence of alcohol-related hospitalizations in persons ages 65 and older of 54.7 per 10,000 population for men and 14.8 per 10,000 for women, rates that were similar to those for myocardial infarction (Adams et al. 1993).

Table 23–1. Definitions: alcohol dependence, alcohol abuse, and alcoholism

1a. **DSM-IV alcohol dependence criteria** (American Psychiatric Association 1994, p. 181)
A maladaptive pattern of alcohol use, leading to clinically significant impairment or distress, as manifested by three (or more) of the following, occurring at any time in the same 12-month period:
1. Tolerance, as defined by either of the following:
    a. Need for markedly increased amounts of alcohol to achieve intoxication or desired effect
    b. Markedly diminished effect with continued use of the same amount of alcohol
2. Withdrawal, as manifested by either of the following:
    a. Alcohol withdrawal syndrome
    b. Alcohol taken to relieve or avoid withdrawal symptoms
3. Alcohol is often taken in larger amounts or over a longer period than was intended
4. There is a persistent desire or unsuccessful efforts to cut down or control use of alcohol
5. A great deal of time is spent in activities necessary to obtain, use, or recover from the effects of alcohol
6. Important social, occupational, or recreational activities are given up or reduced because of use
7. Continued use despite knowledge of having a persistent or recurrent physical or psychological problem that was likely to have been caused or exacerbated by alcohol consumption

1b. **DSM-IV alcohol abuse criteria** (American Psychiatric Association 1994, pp. 182–183)
A maladaptive pattern of alcohol use leading to clinically significant impairment or distress, as manifested by one (or more) of the following, occurring within a 12-month period:
1. Recurrent use resulting in a failure to fulfill major role obligations at work, school, or home
2. Recurrent use in situations in which it is physically hazardous (e.g., driving an automobile while impaired by alcohol)
3. Recurrent alcohol-related legal problems
4. Continued alcohol use despite having persistent or recurrent social or interpersonal problems caused or exacerbated by the effects of alcohol

and

Has never met the criteria for alcohol dependence.

1c. **National Council on Alcoholism and Drug Dependence and the American Society of Addiction Medicine definition of alcoholism** (Morse and Flavin 1992)
Alcoholism is a primary, chronic disease with genetic, psychosocial, and environmental factors influencing its development and manifestations. The disease is often progressive and fatal. It is characterized by impaired control over drinking; preoccupation with the drug alcohol; use of alcohol despite adverse consequences; and distortions in thinking, most notably denial. Each of these symptoms may be continuous or periodic.

Source. Adapted from DSM–IV. Used with permission.

Factors contributing to age-associated decline in reported prevalence of alcoholism. Many chronic alcoholism patients die prematurely (Moos et al. 1994), whereas others become securely abstinent before old age or gradually moderate their alcohol intake (Atkinson et al. 1992; Liberto et al. 1992). Some social drinkers also moderate their drinking (Adams et al. 1990), but in others lifelong consumption patterns persist into old age (Liberto et al. 1992). Drinkers may underreport their consumption of alcohol because of impaired recall and shame about excessive drinking. Elderly individuals are less likely to encounter the proxy sources who often first report alcoholism in younger persons (e.g., employer, family, court). Clinicians, trained to the view made popular in the 1960s that alcoholism is not a significant problem in old age, may not recognize or report drinking problems (Atkinson et al. 1992). In one revealing study, physicians were more likely to miss the diagnosis of alcoholism in older patients than in younger ones, and when they did make the diagnosis, they were less likely to refer elderly patients for alcohol treatment (Curtis et al. 1989).

Cohort effects are also important. Lifelong substance use habits and attitudes typically are established by early adulthood and depend on prevailing but ever changing social norms (Atkinson et al. 1992). Recent prevalence data reviewed in Atkinson 1990, illustrates how the older cohorts were influenced by negative values about alcohol use in the Prohibition Era (1920–1933). Higher levels of alcohol consumption and problems in old age might be expected in birth cohorts entering their 60s in the 1990s and beyond, and narrowing of the "gender gap" is likely (Atkinson et al. 1992).

Incidence of late-onset alcoholism. According to DSM-III-R, onset of an alcohol use disorder after the age of 45 in men is rare (American Psychiatric Association 1987). In contrast, the ECA incidence study (using repeated interviews of the same households) indicated that in men the annual incidence of alcohol use disorders (as defined by DSM-III [American Psychiatric Association 1980]) per 100 person-years of risk was 5.78 for those ages 18–29, 4.00 for those ages 30–44, 1.68 for those ages 45–64, and 1.20 for those ages 65 and older (Eaton et al. 1989). Respective rates for women were 1.11, 0.50, 0.31, and 0.27. The findings portray a reduced but continued risk for development of these disorders beyond age 45. Consistent with these data, onset of initial drinking problems at age 60 or older was reported by 29%–68% of elderly alcoholic patients in treatment (Atkinson et al. 1990).

Risk factors.   A family history of alcoholism or a personal history of previous heavy alcohol consumption or alcohol dependence increases the risk of a new episode of problem drinking, although late-onset cases frequently have no family history of alcoholism (Atkinson et al. 1990). It has been hypothesized that life stress may precipitate late-onset or relapse of alcohol problems, but in systematic studies support for this hypothesis has not been consistently demonstrated. The complexity of stress (Finney and Moos 1984) and the difficulty of determining whether stressors are caused by or are a cause of drinking are issues that plague research on this theme. In many cases discretionary time and money increase opportunities to drink, and when there is a history of earlier heavy drinking, or when drinking partners are at hand, the line that separates social from problem drinking may be easily crossed.

Age-associated biological and medical factors can influence the effects and abuse potential of alcohol. Because of age-related changes in the volume of distribution (reduced body water and lean body mass), a standard alcohol load produces a peak blood level that averages about 20% higher in a 65-year-old man than in a 30-year-old man (Vestal et al. 1977). Even when peak blood alcohol level is controlled, older persons show greater central nervous system sensitivity to alcohol, as measured by tests of cognition and motor coordination (Vogel-Sprott and Barrett 1984). Thus an alcohol consumption level that did not produce problems years earlier might, if unmoderated, lead to hazards or dependence at a later age. The presence of chronic medical disorders that produce pain or insomnia may also foster habitual self-medication with alcohol, with development of tolerance and dependence. Secondary alcohol use disorders may be precipitated in patients with other psychiatric disorders such as major depression.

Diagnosis and Symptomatology

Clinical presentations.   An alcohol use disorder in an elderly individual may not be suspected because the presenting picture often does not correspond with stereotypes based on younger patients. Severe primary alcoholism, with major social consequences, is certainly seen in elderly individuals, but antisocial behavior and lower socioeconomic status are less common, and clinical manifestations are more variable. The following four presentations are common in older alcoholic individuals and may make diagnosis difficult:

1. *Circumscribed or focal problems.* Frequent alcohol use can cause, aggravate, or complicate the management of medical problems as diverse as hypertension, diabetes mellitus, osteoporosis, gastritis and peptic ulcer disease, macrocytic anemias, hypercholesterolemia, parkinsonism, and gout. Alcohol-drug interactions can confound medical prescribing: acute alcohol intake reduces the metabolism of many drugs, whereas, conversely, chronic alcohol use may increase drug metabolism by inducing microsomal enzyme activity. Alcohol may also be a factor in psychosocial problems, (e.g., simple depressed mood or demoralization, insomnia, anxiety, persistent family discord, or arrests for driving while intoxicated). Alcohol may impair memory function in an elderly patient without dementia (Atkinson and Ganzini 1994). The findings and pattern may or may not meet DSM-IV criteria (American Psychiatric Association 1994) for an alcohol use disorder.

2. *Uncomplicated mild dependence.* The patient who is mildly dependent on alcohol may not have any specific complaint or finding, but may simply report consumption levels that are high. Tolerance may accompany this pattern. Because the risk of later medical or psychiatric complications may be increased by sustained heavy drinking, intervention is justified.

3. *Medically complex dependence.* The medically complex patient typically presents in the emergency department or on the medical ward because of severe illness. The symptoms, although obvious, may be nonspecific and thus are easily attributed to a cause other than alcohol abuse (Gambert 1992). Presenting features include delirium, dementia, lack of self-care, dehydration, malnutrition, bladder and/or bowel incontinence, muscle weakness or frank myopathy, gait disorder, recurring falls, burns, head trauma, or accidental hypothermia. Hypoglycemia, congestive heart failure, and aspiration pneumonia can also be caused or aggravated by alcohol dependence.

4. *Psychiatrically complex dependence.* These patients have an alcohol use disorder that is associated with another psychiatric disorder ("dual diagnoses"). Most commonly in an older alcoholic, the coexisting problem is an affective or organic mental disorder (Atkinson 1994; Finlayson et al. 1988), although anxiety disorders and schizophrenia also commonly coexist with alcoholism in older patients treated in general psychiatric clinic settings (Blow et al. 1992). Accurate differential diagnosis often requires repeated assessment over time (see section, "Differential Diagnosis").

Course.   Very little is known about the subsequent course of alcoholism after diagnosis in older adults. Persistent drinking in the presence of dementia or alcohol-related liver disease carries high short-term mortality rates (Atkinson et al. 1992).

Approaches to diagnosis.   Diagnosis of alcohol use disorders and problem drinking requires openness to the possibility of the problem; skillful interviewing, sometimes aided by screening tests and home visits; physical and neurological examination; and appropriate laboratory tests.

Interview.   Information elicited from interviews provides the foundation for accurate diagnosis of alcohol use disorders. The task of acquiring information is by no means easy and may be especially daunting in elderly individuals. Sensitive inquiry about drinking practices is sometimes necessary to elicit this information and should be a routine part of the geriatric psychiatric workup. Denial of alcohol problems and defensiveness when asked about alcohol use are common in alcoholic patients. Reasons include alcohol-induced amnesia for many intoxication episodes, shame about reliance on alcohol, pessimism about recovery, and the desire to continue drinking. For these reasons, careful rapport building through repeated contacts; thorough inquiry with relatives, caregivers, and others in the social network; reviews of medical records; and home visitation are especially useful assessment methods. The DSM-IV alcohol use disorder criteria (see Table 23–1) offer a reasonable framework for acquiring information to establish a diagnosis (American Psychiatric Association 1994).

Screening instruments.   The CAGE test (CAGE = Cut + Annoyed + Guilty + Eye-opener) and the geriatric version of the Michigan Alcoholism Screening Test (MAST-G) (Table 23–2) have both shown promise as preliminary screens for alcohol problems in older clinical populations (F. C. Blow, unpublished data, 1992; Buchsbaum et al. 1992; Joseph et al. 1992). Although a positive result on either test does not make the diagnosis of a currently active problem drinking, these questionnaires can help identify patients who need a more detailed clinical assessment.

Physical and laboratory findings.   Physical stigmata of alcoholic liver disease, peripheral polyneuropathy, and cerebellar ataxia are among physical findings that may help confirm a diagnosis, but these are often absent. Laboratory data may be helpful, especially in mild dependence or in differential diagnosis of complex cases. Findings from one large

Table 23–2. Screening measures for alcohol problems

2a. **Ewing's CAGE Screening Measure** (Ewing 1984)
   1. Have you ever felt you ought to Cut down your drinking?
   2. Have people Annoyed you by criticizing your drinking?
   3. Have you ever felt bad or Guilty about your drinking?
   4. Have you ever had a drink first thing in the morning to steady your nerves or get rid of a hangover ("Eye-opener")?

(Positive answers to two or more questions suggest an alcohol problem at some time, although the problem may not currently be active.)

2b. **Michigan Alcoholism Screening Test—Geriatric Version** (MAST-G) (F. C. Blow, unpublished manuscript, 1991)
   1. After drinking, have you ever noticed an increase in your heart rate or beating in your chest?
   2. When talking with others, do you ever underestimate how much you actually drink?
   3. Does alcohol make you sleepy so that you often fall asleep in your chair?
   4. After a few drinks, have you sometimes not eaten or been able to skip a meal because you didn't feel hungry?
   5. Does having a few drinks help decrease your shakiness or tremors?
   6. Does alcohol sometimes make it hard for you to remember parts of the day or night?
   7. Do you have rules for yourself that you won't drink before a certain time of the day?
   8. Have you lost interest in hobbies or activities you used to enjoy?
   9. When you wake up in the morning, do you ever have trouble remembering part of the night before?
   10. Does having a drink help you sleep?
   11. Do you hide your alcohol bottles from family members?
   12. After a social gathering, have you ever felt embarrassed because you drank too much?
   13. Have you ever been concerned that drinking might be harmful to your health?
   14. Do you like to end an evening with a "night cap"?
   15. Did you find your drinking increased after someone close to you died?
   16. In general, would you prefer to have a few drinks at home rather than go out to social events?
   17. Are you drinking more now than in the past?
   18. Do you usually take a drink to relax or calm your nerves?
   19. Do you drink to take your mind off your problems?
   20. Have you ever increased your drinking after experiencing a loss in your life?
   21. Do you sometimes drive when you have had too much to drink?
   22. Has a physician or nurse ever said he or she was worried or concerned about your drinking?
   23. Have you ever made rules to manage your drinking?
   24. When you feel lonely, does having a drink help?

(Positive answers to five or more questions suggest an alcohol problem at some time, although the problem may not currently be active.)

group of older alcoholic patients are compared with findings in younger alcoholic patients in Table 23–3 (Hurt et al. 1988). Macrocytic red blood cells, with or without anemia, and liver transferase enzyme elevations are the most typical findings. Toxicological examination of blood or breath samples for alcohol may help establish a diagnosis of severe alcohol intoxication in the moribund patient. In the ambulatory patient, a high blood alcohol level (>150 mg/100 ml) in the presence of a relatively normal mental and neurological examination is strong evidence for tolerance and physical dependence.

Complications. Alcohol withdrawal disorders include the tremulous syndrome, hallucinosis, seizures, and delirium tremens. Although there is no evidence that these disorders occur at different rates in elderly individuals, some data from animal studies have shown increasing alcohol dependence liability with age (Atkinson 1988; Atkinson and Ganzini 1994). In older persons, alcohol withdrawal disorders can be more intensely symptomatic and difficult to treat (Liskow et al. 1989) and may be associated with greater mortality. Other organic central nervous system complications include reversible cognitive impairment (Brandt et al. 1983; Grant et al. 1984); Wernicke-Korsakoff syndrome (Victor et al. 1989); dementia associated with alcoholism (Lishman 1987; Smith and Atkinson 1994); and deterioration of another form of dementia, such as Alzheimer's (King 1986), among others (see Atkinson and Ganzini [1994] for a more full review). Alcohol-associated insomnia resembles the age-associated pattern of sleep disorganization: both show frequent awakenings, especially from deep, slow-wave sleep, and reduced rapid eye movement (REM) sleep (Dustman 1984).

Psychosocial complications are diverse. Alcohol problems are found in 7%–30% of older suicides (Blazer 1982; Conwell et al. 1990; Martin and Streissguth 1982). The association of alcoholism with suicide may be stronger in late middle-aged men than in elderly men or women of any age (Conwell et al. 1990). Case material has demonstrated that alcohol intoxication may be a factor in geriatric pedophilia and other sexual misconduct and in violent events (e.g., abuse or attacks by and on elderly individuals).

Differential diagnosis. Two problems—depression and cognitive impairment—deserve special emphasis because they are commonly associated with aging and also can be sequelae of sustained heavy drinking in otherwise non–mentally ill persons.

Table 23–3. Frequency of laboratory abnormalities in alcoholic inpatients

| | Results[a] | | | |
| | Patients ≥ 65 years[b] | | Younger patients[b] | |
Blood tests	No.	%	No.	%
MCH increased	213	71	123	57[c]
AST increased	214	56	123	42[d]
GGT increased	123	55	101	48
MCV increased	213	44	124	17[c]
Glucose increased	206	32	124	36
Uric acid increased	201	21	123	<1[c]
Albumin decreased	186	17	115	3[c]
Alkaline phosphatase increased	213	11	123	15
Triglycerides increased	191	16	122	19
Phosphorus increased	198	9	124	11

Note. MCH = mean corpuscular hemoglobin; AST = aspartate aminotransferase; GGT = gamma-glutamyltransferase; MCV = mean corpuscular volume.
[a]No. = number of patients tested in each age group; % = percentage of patients tested in the age group who had an abnormal value.
[b]Older patients: $n = 216$; mean age, 69.6 years; age range, 65–83 years; younger patients: $n = 125$; mean age, 44.3 years; age range, 19–64 years.
[c]$P < .05$; for others $P > .3$.
[d]$P < .01$ using Wilcoxon two-sample rank sum test to compare age groups for proportion having an abnormal value.
Source. Adapted from Hurt et al. 1988.

Depression. As in younger patients, depressive symptoms are reported by a majority of older alcoholic patients entering treatment (Atkinson 1990; Atkinson and Ganzini 1994). Such findings generally are interpreted as correlates or consequences of recent heavy drinking in alcoholic patients rather than as evidence of a primary affective disorder, because scores on depression self-report measures usually fall to normal levels without specific antidepressant treatment after 2 to 4 weeks of sobriety. Affective disorders are diagnosed much less often than simple depressed mood: 12% of elderly patients in one large group hospitalized for alcoholism treatment had concurrent affective disorders, usually major depression (Finlayson et al. 1988). Antidepressant treatment should be withheld for at least 2 weeks in the depression patient who has been drinking heavily up to the time of admission. If the depressed mood is a consequence of alcohol effects, at least partial "spontaneous" resolution of depression should be apparent after this time. A history of previous heavy alcohol use can be a risk factor for occurrence

(Saunders et al. 1991) and high severity (B. L. Cook et al. 1991) of subsequent depressive disorders in elderly individuals.

Cognitive impairment.   Defects in memory, visual-spatial skills, abstraction, and problem solving increase in frequency, severity, and duration with age in recovering alcoholic patients; the deficits may not fulfill criteria for dementia, yet may resolve over a course of months to years (Atkinson and Ganzini 1994; Brandt et al. 1983; Grant et al. 1984). In some cases residual deficits after a few weeks of sobriety can be sufficiently subtle that a coarse screen for dementia such as the Mini-Mental State Examination (MMSE) will not indicate them. Frank dementia is also commonly associated with alcohol excess. In the Liverpool community epidemiological survey, men with histories of heavy drinking were 4.6 times more likely to have dementia than other men (Saunders et al. 1991). In a large group of elderly alcoholic inpatients, 25% had a coexisting dementia (Finlayson et al. 1988). In dementia registries, more than 20% of patients may have a history of alcoholism or heavy drinking (King 1986; Smith and Atkinson 1994). Differential diagnosis between dementia associated with alcoholism and dementia of the Alzheimer type can be difficult, because the criteria for each require exclusion of the other, yet there are no clear-cut biological markers for either disease. Some findings that are potentially useful in differential diagnosis are offered in Table 23–4.

Treatment, Prognosis, and Outcome

General issues.   Treatment for alcohol problems has three aims: 1) reduce alcohol consumption, 2) treat medical and psychiatric comorbidities, and 3) engender psychosocial changes to reduce risk of relapse. In mild cases the clinician's advice to cut down or abstain may be effective. The person with more pervasive alcohol problems should receive outpatient psychosocial alcoholism treatment and/or attend Alcoholics Anonymous meetings. Ambulatory, gradual detoxification is often achieved without resorting to medications or hospital admission. Use of deterrent drugs such as disulfiram can be hazardous and is seldom necessary in elderly individuals.

In the most serious cases, including those involving patients who are not helped by outpatient treatment, patients should be referred to a specialized inpatient alcoholism treatment unit. If severe medical or psychiatric complications are present or major withdrawal is anticipated or already occurring, initial treatment should take place in an acute medical ward, geriatric evaluation and management unit, or psychiatric inpatient unit, followed by transfer to the alcoholism treatment unit after stabilization. Intractable heavy drinking in the presence of dementia or other co-existing major mental disorder may force placement of the patient in residential care where, unfortunately, alcoholic patients are not always welcomed. In a few locales, alcohol-free foster homes and other residential facilities have been established, staffed by personnel trained to care for recovering alcoholic patients in an accepting manner.

Interventions.   Medical advice is often a simple and effective way to influence patients to cut down on drinking (Edwards 1988). The efficacy of brief intervention (i.e., patient education and advice by primary medical care providers) for older heavy drinking patients is currently being investigated (W. L. Adams, personal communication, Medical College of Wisconsin, Milwaukee 1993). The term *intervention* is also used to refer to a form of "crisis management" in which a skilled professional arranges a firm, factual, but emotionally supportive confrontation between the alcoholic person and key figures in his or her social network, with the aim of overcoming the alcoholic person's denial sufficiently to prompt an agreement to enter treatment (Atkinson 1985). The efficacy of this strategy with older adults has not been studied systematically, but case experience cautions that the more typical approach used with younger adults requires

Table 23–4.   Features that may distinguish between alcohol-associated dementia and dementia of the Alzheimer type

Feature	Dementia associated with alcoholism[a]	Dementia of Alzheimer type[a]
Ataxia	Common	Uncommon
Peripheral polyneuropathy	Common	Uncommon
Naming deficit (anomia, dysnomia)	Uncommon	Common
Stable or improved cognitive function over many months with abstinence from alcohol	Common	Does not occur
Reduced cortical atrophy with abstinence from alcohol	Can occur	Does not occur

[a]Findings will be variable in mixed dementias (e.g., Alzheimer's complicated by alcoholism or heavy drinking).
Source.   Adapted from Smith and Atkinson (1994).

modification for many elderly patients: there should only be one or two participants (e.g., spouse or other primary caregiver and primary medical provider), young grandchildren usually should not participate, and emotional support is crucial to mitigate catastrophic shame and refusal to participate further.

Psychosocial treatments. Psychosocial approaches address the recovering alcoholic patient's needs with regard to socialization, housing and financial problems, existential issues, and ability to acknowledge alcohol problems and modify behavior to avoid circumstances that have been associated with drinking in the past (i.e., relapse prevention). Age-specific psychosocial approaches are indicated for most persons not handicapped by severe dementia, chronic psychosis, or severe personality disorder (Atkinson 1994; Kofoed et al. 1984). In age-heterogeneous group meetings, whether Alcoholics Anonymous or clinical treatment, elderly persons may be offended by profanity and disclosure of antisocial behavior by younger members. Elderly persons are more apt to engage successfully if the group is composed of age peers and led in a low-key, slow-paced, emotionally supportive manner (Kofoed et al. 1987). Frank discussion of problems often follows months of more superficial discourse. Peer bonding and shared reminiscing in such groups are probably important factors in retention, as are family and court involvement in treatment (Atkinson et al. 1993; Dunlop et al. 1982). Inclusion of cognitive-behavioral training that addresses such themes as self-efficacy, self-esteem, and relapse prevention may also aid recovery (Dupree et al. 1984; Rice et al. 1993; Schonfeld and Dupree 1991).

Drinking relapses during treatment. Surreptitious drinking is common during alcoholism treatment. When abstinence is the goal of treatment, it is desirable to monitor substance use in recovering elderly problem drinkers by means of randomly conducted, unannounced breath and urine examinations. Such monitoring is conducted in the spirit of assisting rather than intruding. Patients, relatives, and fellow group members (who may establish social ties outside the meetings) are also encouraged to offer information on drinking, a form of support for the relapsed patient's recovery. Patients who resume drinking may fail to keep scheduled appointments. In this circumstance, an unannounced home visit by a staff member may clarify whether a drinking relapse has occurred. Patients are maintained in the program unless they persist in recurrent bouts of heavy drinking.

Treatment setting and outcome.   In general, older alcoholic patients seem to respond to treatment as well as or better than younger alcoholic patients (Atkinson 1994). The age-specific social treatments described previously have been conducted principally with outpatients treated over 6 to 12 months, either in an elder-specific outpatient program within a general substance abuse treatment program, or within a geriatrics mental health center. Some variables affecting outpatient treatment retention have been studied, but no outcome studies have been reported. Older patients are more likely to remain in outpatient treatment than younger patients (Atkinson et al. 1993; Kofoed et al. 1987). Court-supervised older drinking drivers and married elderly patients whose spouses participate in treatment are more likely to stay in treatment than their age peers who lack such third-party involvement (Atkinson et al. 1993). In a single study comparing 1-year drinking outcomes of older alcoholic patients randomly assigned either to an age-specific inpatient alcoholism treatment unit or to an age-heterogeneous alcoholism treatment unit in the same facility, patients treated in the age-specific program were more likely to be abstinent 1 year later (Kashner et al. 1992).

Alcohol and Health Maintenance

Does moderate drinking help to maintain good health?   The use of small amounts of beverage alcohol has been advocated as a safe social adjuvant in elder residential care facilities, but more comprehensive management of the facility milieu may better ensure optimal socialization (Atkinson and Kofoed 1984). Alcohol has also long been touted as an appetite stimulant. In healthy elderly persons, caloric intake and blood levels of some micronutrients may increase with alcohol intake, although other micronutrient levels decrease (Jacques et al. 1989). Use of alcohol to aid sleep is problematic, because regular alcohol late in the evening is apt to disorganize sleep (Dustman 1984). A report from France demonstrated that elderly individuals who consumed moderate amounts of wine scored higher on the MMSE than individuals who abstained from alcohol (Letenneur et al. 1993), but abstaining individuals may be predisposed to cognitive dysfunction. If moderate drinking is advised, several cautions apply. The list of potentially hazardous interactions among alcohol, chronic medical disorders, and medications is lengthy (Gambert 1992). Clinicians who advise outpatients to use alcohol should recall that in residential studies in the literature, quantity was carefully regulated, and use within a social context was ensured (Atkinson and Kofoed 1984).

Does moderate alcohol use prevent coronary artery disease? An intriguing aspect of the alcohol and health maintenance debate is the well-validated association in men of regular but moderate alcohol use (up to two drinks per day) with lower morbidity and mortality from coronary artery disease, when compared with heavy alcohol users and abstainers. Why should abstainers have higher morbidity and mortality than moderate drinkers? Alcohol elevates plasma levels of high-density lipoprotein (HDL) cholesterol, including a subfraction (HDL_3) with antiatherogenic activity, but apparently it does not elevate the most antiatherogenic subfraction (HDL_2) (Davidson 1989). Alcohol also reduces blood platelet aggregation and has other anticoagulant effects that could explain the epidemiological finding, although under some circumstances alcohol also increases selected hemostatic processes. Another interpretation is that the heterogeneous abstaining group includes subgroups at high risk for coronary disease (e.g., ex-heavy drinkers and others who stopped using alcohol for health reasons) (Atkinson and Ganzini 1994). Unfortunately, most reported studies were not designed to account for this possibility. Studies that have closely examined abstainers report conflicting findings (i.e., that abstainers either were or were not more predisposed to coronary disease than moderate drinkers). The hypothetical alcohol-protective effect in coronary artery disease needs further study before acceptance.

Benzodiazepine Dependence

Elderly individuals rarely abuse or illicitly use benzodiazepines (Busto et al. 1986; Pinsker and Suljaga-Petchel 1984). Physicians, however, frequently prescribe benzodiazepines for extended periods of time in elderly individuals, a practice that presents several hazards (American Psychiatric Association 1990). Adverse effects of benzodiazepines increase with age and may deleteriously affect functioning. When patients use these drugs over the long term (defined in most studies as daily use for more than 1 year), they are likely to develop a dependence disorder and have characteristic, unpleasant symptoms when the drug is discontinued.

Benzodiazepines, which are among the most widely prescribed drugs in the United States, are indicated in the treatment of insomnia or anxiety (American Psychiatric Association 1990). Use of these agents as short-term treatments has been emphasized. Complaints of insomnia increase with age, yet benzodiazepine hypnotics offer an imperfect solution, because their efficacy diminishes after several weeks of treatment (American

Psychiatric Association 1990). Rebound insomnia can be especially severe after discontinuation of short half-life agents such as triazolam (Kales et al. 1979). Benzodiazepines are efficacious in the long-term treatment of some anxiety disorders such as panic disorder; however, this is a relatively rare diagnosis in older persons (Eaton et al. 1989). The role of these agents in the long-term treatment of other anxiety disorders such as generalized anxiety disorder is not well defined. Most studies have examined the relative risks of extended use of benzodiazepines; empirical assessment of long-term benefit is lacking (Rickels and Schweizer 1990).

Epidemiology and Characteristics of Long-Term Benzodiazepine Users

Prolonged daily use of benzodiazepines is a pattern all too common in elderly individuals. One national study of more than 3,000 community-dwelling persons reported that 1.6% had taken benzodiazepines daily for more than 1 year (Mellinger et al. 1984). Older persons were overrepresented among these long-term users: 71% were older than 50 years, and one-third were older than 65 years. Studies in both the United States and other countries confirm that whether these agents are used to treat anxiety or insomnia, young and middle-age persons are prescribed benzodiazepines for briefer periods than are elderly persons (Dunbar et al. 1989; Isacson et al. 1992; Mant et al. 1988; Smart and Adlaf 1988).

Long-term users of benzodiazepines are likely to have poor physical health (Mellinger et al. 1984; Rodrigo et al. 1988). Unlike younger benzodiazepine abusers who take these drugs outside of medical supervision, elderly long-term users obtain these agents from primary care physicians and see these physicians at reasonably frequent intervals. Despite treatment with these psychotropic agents, however, elderly patients continue to have chronic anxiety and depression, yet only a minority seek assistance from mental health professionals (Mellinger et al. 1984; Rodrigo et al. 1988). Caregivers of patients with dementia have a substantially higher prevalence of use of sedative or hypnotic agents than comparable populations (Clipp and George 1990). Older persons rarely ingest these agents for their euphoric effects.

Young adults who abuse benzodiazepines often abuse other substances, especially alcohol, stimulants, and heroin (Busto et al. 1986). They escalate the dosage of the drug over time, culminating in high-dose dependence. Both polysubstance abuse and dosage escalation are rare in older persons (Busto et al. 1986; Salzman 1991). In one study of 93 elderly users of benzodiazepines, few took more than the equivalent of 4 mg diazepam per day. Although half of the continuous users had received their first prescription 5 years or more before, only 1.8% were using higher daily doses than originally prescribed (Pinsker and Suljaga-Petchel 1984).

The prescription of benzodiazepines for elderly patients in long-term care settings has been a source of concern. Studies indicate that approximately one-fourth of elderly patients in these settings receive sedative or hypnotic agents, frequently long half-life agents such as diazepam and flurazepam, which are more likely to cause toxicity (Beardsley et al. 1989; Beers et al. 1988; Buck 1988). Inadvisable prescribing practices, such as benzodiazepine use in the absence of documentation of a mental disorder, and standing orders for hypnotics as opposed to as-needed prescribing, are common in nursing homes (Beardsley et al. 1989; Beers et al. 1988).

Adverse Effects of Benzodiazepines

When physicians prescribe benzodiazepines to elderly persons, they expose these patients to several hazards. Benzodiazepines cause both acute and chronic toxicity syndromes, characterized by cognitive impairment and balance problems. When patients who have taken benzodiazepines over an extended period stop the drug, unpleasant discontinuance symptoms develop as a result of dependence. Each of these hazards will be discussed below.

Toxic effects. Elderly patients are more troubled by adverse effects of benzodiazepines than younger patients. When compared with younger persons, elderly individuals clear these drugs more slowly, and repeated doses produce higher steady-state serum concentrations (Greenblatt and Shader 1991; Greenblatt et al. 1991). Yet even at similar serum or plasma drug concentrations, elderly individuals, when compared with younger persons, develop more sedation and psychomotor impairment (Castleden et al. 1977; Greenblatt and Shader 1991). Adverse effects may occur with both brief and extended treatment and are more prominent in patients treated with high dosages of long half-life agents (Greenblatt and Shader 1991), but also occur with short half-life agents such as triazolam (Greenblatt et al. 1991).

Benzodiazepines impair attention, memory, arousal, and psychomotor ability (Pomara et al. 1991). Although this effect is dose related, single doses of diazepam as low a 2.5 mg may cause measurable impairment in memory and psychomotor performance in elderly persons (Pomara et al.

1985). Although some tolerance develops to the adverse effects on cognition (Pomara et al. 1991), continual use of benzodiazepines may result in a dementia-like syndrome (Golombok et al. 1988; Higgitt 1988). Larson et al. (1987), in a study of 300 patients at a dementia evaluation clinic, found that 12% had had an adverse drug reaction causing cognitive impairment and that long-acting benzodiazepines were the most common offending agents. Memory impairment may persist for at least several weeks after drug withdrawal (Rummans et al. 1993).

Elderly individuals may have substantial daytime balance impairments following nightly hypnotic treatment (Bonnet and Kramer 1981), and results from epidemiological studies suggest that benzodiazepine-treated elderly individuals are at increased risk of both falls and hip fractures (Granek et al. 1987; Ray et al. 1987, 1989; Tinetti et al. 1988). It is likely that benzodiazepines impair the driving skills of elderly persons (American Psychiatric Association 1990; Salzman 1991).

Dependence.   Long-term therapeutic prescribing of benzodiazepines leads to dependence in the majority of patients, and sudden discontinuation of these drugs will lead to unpleasant symptoms and signs. Discontinuation symptoms are substantially more likely following 8–12 months of daily benzodiazepine use (Rickels et al. 1983). Three forms of discontinuance phenomena are recognized: 1) recurrence symptoms, which include the gradual reemergence and persistence of former anxiety symptoms for which the drug was originally prescribed; 2) rebound symptoms—that is, former symptoms that, following drug cessation, are transiently more intense than before treatment; and 3) a true withdrawal syndrome—that is, novel signs and symptoms unlike those for which the drug was originally prescribed (American Psychiatric Association 1990).

Some studies report that 90%–100% of mixed-age patients who discontinue long-term benzodiazepine treatment have at least mild recurrence and rebound symptoms (Rickels et al. 1990b; Schweizer et al. 1990). Commonly occurring symptoms include anxiety, insomnia, fatigue, tremulousness, concentration difficulties, irritability, muscle tension, restlessness, and diaphoresis (American Psychiatric Association 1990; Rickels et al. 1990b; Roy-Byrne and Hommer 1988; Schweizer et al. 1990). True withdrawal symptoms, which include tinnitus; ataxia; nausea; and perceptual distortions such as hyperacusis, derealization, and depersonalization, develop in 20%–50% of patients and persist for 2–4 weeks (American Psychiatric Association 1990; Atkinson and Ganzini 1994; Roy-Byrne and Hommer 1988). Severe withdrawal can include convulsions, delirium, and psychosis but occurs very infrequently, usually following abrupt discontinuation of high dosages (American Psychiatric Association 1990; Noyes et al. 1988). Whether withdrawal symptoms can persist beyond a few weeks is controversial (Higgitt 1990).

Among mixed-age patients, severity of benzodiazepine discontinuance symptoms is increased by abrupt withdrawal, dependence on high dosages or short half-life agents, comorbid or current alcohol problems, personality abnormality, and presence of panic disorder (American Psychiatric Association 1990; Atkinson and Ganzini 1994). Although studies that specifically examined the effect of age on discontinuance phenomena are few, they suggest that advanced age does not necessarily confer an increased risk of symptoms. In one study of gradual benzodiazepine withdrawal, elderly subjects were compared with young subjects matched for benzodiazepine dosage and duration of use. Elderly patients reported significantly less severe withdrawal symptoms and were as likely as young subjects to complete the study and remain benzodiazepine free for 4 weeks (Schweizer et al. 1989). Whether old age alters the risk of severe withdrawal phenomena such as seizures or delirium is unknown (Atkinson and Ganzini 1994). Clinically, however, benzodiazepine withdrawal is frequently overlooked in elderly individuals, and the symptoms are instead attributed to other medical illnesses (Whitcup and Miller 1987).

Treatment and Outcome

Between 50% and 70% of persons who are able to withdraw from benzodiazepines remain abstinent (Ashton 1987; Golombok et al. 1987; Rickels et al. 1991). Despite the fact that age does not appear to increase liability for discontinuance phenomena, elderly persons who can be withdrawn from benzodiazepine treatment have more difficulty remaining abstinent and are likely to relapse (Ashton 1987; Golombok et al. 1987; Holton et al. 1992).

Several guidelines are proposed to lessen the severity of benzodiazepine withdrawal and improve long-term outcome. A gradual taper of the benzodiazepine over a minimum of 1 month, but in some cases up to several months, is recommended. Dosage decrements must be especially small during the second half of the taper (Higgitt et al. 1985; Noyes et al. 1988; Schweizer et al. 1990). Patients who are dependent on short half-life agents may be able to more comfortably withdraw by switching to a long half-life agent (Rickels et al. 1990a). Adjuvant pharmacological treatment with carbamazepine may improve outcome but has not been studied in elderly patients (Schweizer et al. 1991). Treatment of comorbid depressive disorders is recommended (American Psychiatric Association 1990; Rickels et al. 1990a). Alternative anxiety reduction techniques are no more likely to improve outcome than a physician's advice to reduce consumption (Fraser et al. 1990; Hopkins et al. 1982; Onyett and Turpin 1988).

Prescription Narcotic Analgesic Abuse

Very few studies have been published on the prevalence and characteristics of elderly abusers of prescription narcotic analgesics. In one community survey, the 2-week prevalence of prescribed narcotic use was 2.1% for elderly women and 2.3% for elderly men (Chrischilles et al. 1990). Case series of hospitalized elderly patients indicate that dependence on prescribed narcotics was less common than dependence on anxiolytic or sedative-hypnotic agents (Finlayson 1984; Jinks and Raschko 1990; Whitcup and Miller 1987). Abuse of narcotics by elderly patients is rare unless the patient was a narcotic abuser when young (Jinks and Raschko 1990). However, narcotics are prescribed for a variety of painful, nonmalignant, but chronic conditions such as arthritides and neuropathies, and tolerance and dependence can occur even in the absence of abuse (Portenoy and Payne 1992).

Illegal Drug Use

Prevalence

The ECA studies reported that 1.6% of persons older than 65 years had a lifetime prevalence of illegal drug use; however, current use of illegal drugs (i.e., for the preceding 6 months) was virtually nonexistent (Anthony and Helzer 1991). Surveys of homeless individuals, reports of adverse drug reactions, and drug arrests also indicate that the current cohorts of elderly persons have very low rates of illegal drug abuse (Atkinson et al. 1992). The majority of older persons who have a diagnosis of illegal drug dependence also have a history of alcohol dependence (N. S. Miller et al. 1991).

Opiate Abuse

Opiate abusers are the most well studied of the illegal drug abusers, but elderly individuals constitute a very small portion of heroin addicts. For example, in 1985 only 2% of all methadone maintenance clients in New

York City were older than 60 years (Pascarelli 1985). Data from the Drug Abuse Warning Network in 1991 indicated that 1.8% of all reports of heroin/morphine abuse in United States urban emergency departments are in persons older than 55 (National Institute on Drug Abuse 1992a). Development of addiction after young adulthood is rare, and mortality over the course of addiction is high (Atkinson et al. 1992). One United States study, which followed heroin addicts for 24 years, reported that 27.7% died during this period (Hser et al. 1993). Medical examiner data from the Drug Abuse Warning Network in 1991 showed that 5.6% of deaths from heroin or morphine were in persons older than 55 years (National Institute on Drug Abuse 1992b). Older addicts often have comorbid addictions, especially to tobacco and alcohol, contributing to disability and early mortality.

One theory to account for the decrease in elderly addicts was that over time they "matured out"—that is, gradually became abstinent (Winick 1962). More recent studies do not support this theory that increasing proportions of addicts become abstinent over time, especially once addiction exceeds 5–10 years (Haastrup and Jepsen 1988; Hser et al. 1993). Studies from the 1970s paint a picture of elderly addicts who are isolative and secretive about their drug use, who are not otherwise criminally involved, and who often support their drug habit with licit employment (Atkinson et al. 1992). A more recent study of elderly addicts followed for more than two decades and approaching 50 years of age showed that many remain highly involved in criminal activities (Hser et al. 1993).

Other Illegal Drugs

Little information is available regarding the use of other illegal drugs by elderly individuals. The 1-year prevalence of marijuana use in persons older than 50 years was 1% in 1982, and there are rare case reports of cocaine abuse in older persons (Atkinson et al. 1992). Little is known about age-related changes in the pattern of drug-induced psychiatric syndromes or altered treatment needs of elderly substance abusers.

Nonprescription Drugs

Epidemiology

Currently there are more than 300,000 nonprescription preparations in the United States containing more than 700 active ingredients (Gilbertson

1986). In recent years, the Food and Drug Administration has removed many drugs with low therapeutic indices but has made other former prescription drugs such as diphenhydramine and ibuprofen available in nonprescription form (Lamy 1989). The most common nonprescription drugs used by elderly individuals are vitamins, analgesics, laxatives, antacids, and cold remedies (Conn 1992; Delafuente et al. 1992; Helling et al. 1987; Mant et al. 1992).

Misuse of nonprescription drugs. For the most part, elderly persons turn to nonprescription drugs as an initial treatment for mild illnesses (Stoller 1988). Expectations about these drugs are modest, and users rarely describe these drugs as necessary for functioning (Guttman 1978; Parry et al. 1973). Concerns, however, have been raised about misuse of these medications by all individuals of all ages, especially elderly individuals. One study of hospital admissions found that 19% of elderly patients had at least one adverse drug reaction, and the likelihood of an adverse drug reaction was associated with increases in the number of diseases and number of drugs used (Grymonpre et al. 1988; Ives et al. 1987). Adverse effects of nonprescription and prescription drugs are additive, making elderly individuals—the largest consumers of prescribed drugs—especially vulnerable to the effects of nonprescription drugs (Mant et al. 1992; Lamy 1989). One study indicated that as few as one in six consumers of nonprescription drugs report use to a physician (Guttman 1978). Many consumers are unaware of possible adverse effects and fail to read directions and warnings (Conn 1992).

Characteristics of users. Although some writers have suggested that nonprescription drug use may result from poverty, lack of access to medical care, or resistance to medical treatment, several studies show that nonprescription drug use is associated with increasing educational level and higher income but not with fewer physician visits (Conn 1991; Johnson and Pope 1983; Stoller 1988). A correlation among nonprescription drug use, depressive symptomatology, and poor mental health was found in several studies (Chrischilles et al. 1992; Johnson and Pope 1983; Simons et al. 1992; Svarstad 1983; Verbrugge 1985). Data suggest that this is not just because depression is more likely with worsening medical illnesses. One possible explanation is that an increased focus on somatic sensations often found in depression may lead to more self-medication with nonprescription drugs (Jacobsen and Hansen 1989).

Psychoactive Nonprescription Drugs

Consumption of psychoactive nonprescription drugs, primarily hypnotics and stimulants, declines with age (Parry et al. 1973). Nonprescription hypnotics are predominantly agents with antihistamine/anticholinergic properties, such as diphenhydramine and doxylamine succinate. Use of these agents in community-living elderly individuals ranges from 0.1% to 4%, and nonprescription hypnotics are taken less frequently than prescribed hypnotics (Chrischilles et al. 1992; Svarstad 1983). The infrequency of use among elderly individuals is surprising considering age-related increases in complaints of insomnia. Use of drugs with anticholinergic properties may be the most common drug-induced cause of delirium in elderly individuals (Gustafson et al. 1988), and even mild concentration and memory problems produced by these agents may result in functional decline, especially in frail or cognitively impaired elderly persons (P. S. Miller et al. 1988; Peters 1989; Rovner et al. 1988; Tune and Bylsma 1991). Anticholinergic agents are common in prescribed medications, and these effects may be additive with nonprescription anticholinergics (Tune et al. 1992). Anticholinergics may also cause or exacerbate other common age-related illnesses, such as urinary retention, constipation, and impaired visual acuity (Peters 1989).

Caffeine is the active ingredient in nonprescription stimulants. Use of nonbeverage caffeine by older persons is very rare, with one study showing less than 1% use (Svarstad 1983). Nonprescription cold remedies often contain sympathomimetics (e.g., phenylpropanolamine), which have prominent stimulant effects and may produce psychiatric syndromes with both manic and psychotic features (Lake et al. 1985). Sympathomimetics are often combined with antihistamines in nonprescription cold remedies, which may increase the risk of toxicity (Pentel 1984).

Other Nonprescription Drugs

Laxatives and antacids. Most studies indicate an age-related increase in self-medication with both laxatives and antacids; in fact, misuse of laxatives may be the most common nonprescription misuse by elderly individuals (Conn 1992). Compulsive laxative consumption may assume addictive proportions.

Vitamins and minerals.   Although vitamin and mineral supplementation is not currently recommended for healthy elderly individuals, studies indicate that between 25% and 69% of elderly persons take some supplements (Gray et al. 1986; Koplan et al. 1986; Schneider and Nordlund 1983; Sobal et al. 1986). Although some studies show an age-related increase in vitamin use, others show no increase or a decrease (Schneider and Nordlund 1983; Sobal et al. 1986; Yearick et al. 1980). Use of some vitamin products among elderly individuals, such as vitamin E and vitamin C, has increased substantially since the 1970s (Stewart 1989). In general, white elderly persons with greater affluence and higher education are more likely to take vitamins (Koplan et al. 1986). The majority of users spend no more than $1 per week on vitamins (Sobal et al. 1986). One study of elderly individuals living in a retirement community found that a small number consumed very high, potentially harmful doses of vitamins. In this study 3.2% took potentially toxic doses of vitamin A, 23% consumed 10 times the recommended dietary allowance (RDA) of vitamin C, and 28% took 10 times the RDA for vitamin E (Gray et al. 1986). Some reasons endorsed for taking these vitamins include tiredness, need for more energy, and coping with stress (Sobal et al. 1986).

Nonprescription analgesics.   Between one-third and one-half of all elderly individuals use nonprescription analgesics, predominantly salicylates, acetaminophen, and ibuprofen (Chrischilles et al. 1992; Conn 1992; Delafuente et al. 1992). The risk of salicylate toxicity increases with age, in part because age-related changes in renal function result in higher blood levels (Grigor et al. 1987). Salicylate toxicity presents with a dementia-like picture associated with tinnitus and irritability. In one series of patients with chronic salicylate toxicity, the median age was 77 years. Eighty percent showed abnormal mental status, and 85% had some functional dependence when first evaluated (Bailey and Jones 1989). Analgesic preparations may contain alcohol or caffeine, and dependence and abuse of the psychoactive ingredient may result in toxicity from the analgesic (Murray 1980). Use of multiple analgesics, a practice that has no clear benefits but likely increases the risk of adverse drug reactions, is found in 10%–15% of elderly users of analgesics (Chrischilles et al. 1990).

References

Adams WL, Garry PJ, Rhyne R, et al: Alcohol intake in the healthy elderly: changes with age in a cross-sectional and longitudinal study. J Am

Geriatr Soc 38:211–216, 1990

Adams WL, Magruder K, Trued S, et al: Alcohol abuse in elderly emergency department patients. J Am Geriatr Soc 40:1236–1240, 1992

Adams WL, Yuan Z, Barboriak JJ, et al: Alcohol-related hospitalizations of elderly people: prevalence and geographic variation in the United States. JAMA 270:1222–1225, 1993

American Psychiatric Association: Diagnostic and Statistical Manual of Mental Disorders, 3rd Edition. Washington, DC, American Psychiatric Association, 1980

American Psychiatric Association: Diagnostic and Statistical Manual of Mental Disorders, 3rd Edition, Revised. Washington, DC, American Psychiatric Association, 1987

American Psychiatric Association: Benzodiazepine Dependence, Toxicity, and Abuse. Washington, DC, American Psychiatric Association, 1990

American Psychiatric Association: Diagnostic and Statistical Manual of Mental Disorders, 4th Edition. Washington, DC, American Psychiatric Association, 1994

Anthony JC, Helzer JE: Syndromes of drug abuse and dependence, in Psychiatric Disorders in America: The Epidemiologic Catchment Area Study. Edited by Robins LN, Regier DA. New York, Free Press, 1991, pp 116–154

Ashton H: Benzodiazepine withdrawal: outcome in 50 patients. Br J Addict 82:665–671, 1987

Atkinson RM: Persuading alcoholic patients to seek treatment. Compr Ther 11:16–24, 1985

Atkinson RM: Alcoholism in the elderly population. Mayo Clin Proc 63:825–829, 1988

Atkinson RM: Aging and alcohol use disorders: diagnostic issues in the elderly. Int Psychogeriatr 2:55–72, 1990

Atkinson RM: Treatment programs for aging alcoholics, in Alcohol and Aging. Edited by Beresford TP, Gomberg ESL. New York, Oxford University Press, 1994, pp 297–321

Atkinson RM, Kofoed LL: Alcohol and drug abuse, in Geriatric Medicine. Vol 2. Edited by Cassell CK, Walsh JR. New York, Springer-Verlag, 1984, pp 219–235

Atkinson RM, Ganzini L: Substance abuse, in American Psychiatric Press Textbook of Geriatric Neuropsychiatry. Edited by Coffey CE, Cummings JL. Washington, DC, American Psychiatric Press, 1994, pp 297–321

Atkinson RM, Tolson RL, Turner JA: Late versus early onset problem drinking in older men. Alcoholism 14:574–579, 1990

Atkinson RM, Ganzini L, Bernstein MJ: Alcohol and substance-use disorders in the elderly, in Handbook of Mental Health and Aging, 2nd Edition. Edited by Birren JE, Sloane RB, Cohen GD. New York, Academic Press, 1992, pp 515–555

Atkinson RM, Tolson RL, Turner JA: Factors affecting outpatient treatment compliance of older male problem drinkers. J Stud Alcohol 54:102–106, 1993

Bailey RB, Jones SR: Chronic salicylate intoxication: a common cause of morbidity in the elderly. J Am Geriatr Soc 37:556–561, 1989

Beardsley RS, Larson DB, Burns BJ, et al: Prescribing of psychotropics in elderly nursing home patients. J Am Geriatr Soc 37:327–330, 1989

Beers M, Avorn J, Soumerai SB, et al: Psychoactive medication use in intermediate-care facility residents. JAMA 260:3016–3020, 1988

Blazer DG: Depression in Late Life. St. Louis, MO, CV Mosby, 1982

Blow FC, Cook CAL, Booth BM, et al: Age-related psychiatric comorbidities and level of functioning in alcoholic veterans seeking outpatient treatment. Hosp Community Psychiatry 43:990–995, 1992

Bonnet MH, Kramer M: The interaction of age, performance and hypnotics in the sleep of insomniacs. J Am Geriatr Soc 29:508–512, 1981

Brandt J, Butters N, Ryan C, et al: Cognitive loss and recovery in long-term alcohol abusers. Arch Gen Psychiatry 40:435–442, 1983

Buchsbaum DG, Buchanan RG, Welsh J, et al: Screening for drinking disorders in the elderly using the CAGE questionnaire. J Am Geriatr Soc 40:662–665, 1992

Buck JA: Psychotropic drug practice in nursing homes. J Am Geriatr Soc 36:409–418, 1988

Busto U, Sellers EM, Naranjo CA, et al: Patterns of benzodiazepine abuse and dependence. Br J Addict 81:87–94, 1986

Castleden CM, George CF, Marcer D, et al: Increased sensitivity to nitrazepam in old age. Br Med J 1(6052):10–12, 1977

Chrischilles EA, Lemke JH, Wallace RB, et al: Prevalence and characteristics of multiple analgesic drug use in an elderly study group. J Am Geriatr Soc 38:979–984, 1990

Chrischilles EA, Foley DJ, Wallace RB, et al: Use of medications by persons 65 and over: data from the established populations for epidemiologic studies of the elderly. Journal of Gerontolology: Medical Sciences 47:M137–M144, 1992

Clipp EC, George LK: Psychotropic drug use among caregivers of patients with dementia. J Am Geriatr Soc 38:227–235, 1990

Conn VS: Older adults: factors that predict the use of over-the-counter medication. J Adv Nurs 16:1190–1196, 1991

Conn VS: Self-management of over-the-counter medications by older adults. Public Health Nurs 9:29–36, 1992

Conwell Y, Rotenberg M, Caine ED: Completed suicide at age 50 and over. J Am Geriatr Soc 38:640–644, 1990

Cook BL, Winokur G, Garvey MJ, et al: Depression and previous alcoholism in the elderly. Br J Psychiatry 158:72–75, 1991

Curtis JR, Geller G, Stokes EJ, et al: Characteristics, diagnosis, and treatment of alcoholism in elderly patients. J Am Geriatr Soc 37:310–316, 1989

Davidson DM: Cardiovascular effects of alcohol. West J Med 151:430–439, 1989

Delafuente JC, Meuleman JR, Conlin M, et al: Drug use among functionally active, aged, ambulatory people. Ann Pharmacother 26:179–183, 1992

Dunbar GC, Perera MH, Jenner FA: Patterns of benzodiazepine use in Great Britain as measured by a general population survey. Br J Psychiatry 155:836–841, 1989

Dunlop J, Skorney B, Hamilton J: Group treatment for elderly alcoholics and their families. Social Work Groups 5:87–92, 1982

Dupree LW, Broskowski H, Schonfeld L: The Gerontology Alcohol Project: a behavioral treatment program for elderly alcohol abusers. Gerontologist 24:510–516, 1984

Dustman RE: Alcoholism and aging: electrophysiological parallels, in Alcoholism in the Elderly: Social and Biomedical Issues. Edited by Hartford JT, Samorajski T. New York, Raven, 1984, pp 201–225

Eaton WW, Kramer M, Anthony JC, et al: The incidence of specific DIS/DSM-III mental disorders: data from the NIMH Epidemiologic Catchment Area program. Acta Psychiatrica Scand 79:163–178, 1989

Edwards G: Which treatments work for drinking problems? Br Med J 296:4–5, 1988

Ewing JA: Detecting alcoholism: the CAGE questionnaire. JAMA 252:1905–1907, 1984

Finlayson RE: Prescription drug abuse in older persons, in Alcohol and Drug Abuse in Old Age. Edited by Atkinson RM. Washington, DC, American Psychiatric Press, 1984, pp 61–70

Finlayson RE, Hurt RD, Davis LJ, et al: Alcoholism in elderly persons: a study of the psychiatric and psychosocial features of 216 inpatients. Mayo Clin Proc 63:761–768, 1988

Finney JW, Moos RH: Life stressors and problem drinking among older persons, in Recent Developments in Alcoholism, Vol 2. Edited by Galanter M. New York, Plenum, 1984, pp 267–288

Fraser D, Peterkin GSD, Gamsu CV, et al: Benzodiazepine withdrawal: a pilot comparison of three methods. Br J Clin Psychol 29:231–233, 1990

Gambert SR: Substance abuse in the elderly, in Substance Abuse: A Comprehensive Textbook, 2nd Edition. Edited by Lowinson JH, Ruiz P, Millman RB, et al. Baltimore, MD, Williams & Wilkins, 1992, pp 843–851

Gilbertson WE: The FDA's OTC drug review, in American Pharmacy Association Handbook of Non-Prescription Drugs, 8th Edition. Washington, DC, American Pharmacy Association, 1986, pp 1–8

Gilman AG, Rall TW, Nies AS, et al (eds): Goodman and Gilman's The Pharmacological Basis of Therapeutics, 8th Edition. New York, Pergamon, 1990

Golombok S, Higgitt A, Fonagy P, et al: A follow-up study of patients treated for benzodiazepine dependence. Br J Med Psychol 60:141–149, 1987

Golombok S, Moodley P, Lader M: Cognitive impairment in long-term benzodiazepine users. Psychol Med 18:365–374, 1988

Granek E, Baker SP, Abbey H, et al: Medications and diagnoses in relation to falls in a long-term care facility. J Am Geriatr Soc 35:503–511, 1987

Grant I, Adams KM, Reed R: Aging, abstinence, and medical risk factors in the prediction of neuropsychologic deficit among long-term alcoholics. Arch Gen Psychiatry 41:710–718, 1984

Gray GE, Paganini-Hill A, Ross RK, et al: Vitamin supplement use in a southern California retirement community. J Am Diet Assoc 86:800–802, 1986

Greenblatt DJ, Shader RI: Benzodiazepines in the elderly: pharmacokinetics and drug sensitivity, in Anxiety in the Elderly: Treatment and Research. Edited by Salzman C, Lebowitz BD. New York, Springer, 1991, pp 131–145

Greenblatt DJ, Harmatz JS, Shapiro L, et al: Sensitivity to triazolam in the elderly. N Engl J Med 324:1691–1698, 1991

Grigor RR, Spitz PW, Furst DE: Salicylate toxicity in elderly patients with rheumatoid arthritis. J Rheumatol 14:60–66, 1987

Grymonpre RE, Mitenko PA, Sitar DS, et al: Drug-associated hospital admissions in older medical patients. J Am Geriatr Soc 36:1092–1098, 1988

Gustafson Y, Berggren D, Brannstrom B, et al: Acute confusional states in elderly patients treated for femoral neck fracture. J Am Geriatr Soc 36:525–530, 1988

Guttman D: Patterns of legal drug use by older Americans. Addict Dis

3:337–356, 1978

Haastrup S, Jepsen PW: Eleven year follow-up of 300 young opioid addicts. Acta Psychiatr Scand 77:22–26, 1988

Helling DK, Lemke JH, Semla TP, et al: Medication use characteristics in the elderly: the Iowa 65+ rural health study. J Am Geriatr Soc 35:4–12, 1987

Helzer JE, Burnam A, McEvoy LT: Alcohol abuse and dependence, in Psychiatric Disorders in America: The Epidemiologic Catchment Area Study. Edited by Robins LN, Regier DA. New York, Free Press, 1991, pp 81–115

Higgitt A: Indications for benzodiazepine prescriptions in the elderly (editorial). International Journal of Geriatric Psychiatry 3:239–243, 1988

Higgitt AC, Lader MH, Fonagy P: Clinical management of benzodiazepine dependence. Br Med J 291:688–690, 1985

Holton A, Riley P, Tyrer P: Factors predicting long-term outcome after chronic benzodiazepine therapy. J Affect Disord 24:245–252, 1992

Hopkins DR, Sethi KBS, Mucklaw JC: Benzodiazepine withdrawal in general practice. J R Coll Gen Pract 32:758–762, 1982

Hser Y-I, Anglin D, Powers K: A 24-year follow-up of California narcotics addicts. Arch Gen Psychiatry 50:577–584, 1993

Hurt RD, Finlayson RE, Morse RM, et al: Alcoholism in elderly persons: medical aspects and prognosis of 216 inpatients. Mayo Clin Proc 63:753–760, 1988

Isacson D, Carsjo K, Bergman U, et al: Long-term use of benzodiazepines in a Swedish community: an eight-year follow-up. J Clin Epidemiol 45:429–436, 1992

Ives TJ, Bentz EJ, Gwyther RE: Drug-related admissions to a family medicine inpatient service. Arch Intern Med 147:1117–1120, 1987

Jacobsen BK, Hansen V: Mental problems and frequent use of analgesics. Lancet 1:273, 1989

Jacques PF, Sulsky S, Hartz SC, et al: Moderate alcohol intake and nutritional status in nonalcoholic elderly subjects. Am J Clin Nutr 50:875–883, 1989

Jinks MJ, Raschko RR: A profile of alcohol and prescription drug abuse in a high-risk community-based elderly population. Ann Pharmacother 24:971–975, 1990

Johnson RE, Pope CR: Health status and social factors in nonprescribed drug use. Med Care 21:225–233, 1983

Joseph C, Atkinson R, Ganzini L, et al: Screening for alcohol problems in the nursing home. Poster presented at the annual meeting of the American

Geriatrics Society, Washington, DC, November 1992

Kales A, Scharf MB, Kales JD, et al: Rebound insomnia: a potential hazard following withdrawal of certain benzodiazepines. JAMA 241:1692–1695, 1979

Kashner TM, Rodell DE, Ogden SR, et al: Outcomes and costs of two VA inpatient treatment programs for older alcoholic patients. Hosp Community Psychiatry 43:985–989, 1992

King MB: Alcohol abuse and dementia. International Journal of Geriatric Psychiatry 1:31–36, 1986

Kofoed LL, Tolson RL, Atkinson RM, et al: Elderly groups in an alcoholism clinic, in Alcohol and Drug Abuse in Old Age. Edited by Atkinson RM. Washington, DC, American Psychiatric Press, 1984, pp 35–48

Kofoed LL, Tolson RL, Atkinson RM, et al: Treatment compliance of older alcoholics: an elder-specific approach is superior to "mainstreaming." J Stud Alcohol 48:47–51; correction 48:183, 1987

Koplan JP, Annest JL, Layde PM, et al: Nutrient intake and supplementation in the United States (NHANES II). Am J Public Health 76:287–289, 1986

Lake RC, Alagna SW, Quirk RS, et al: Does phenylpropanolamine cause psychiatric disorders? in Phenylpropanolamine: Risks, Benefits and Controversies. Edited by Morgan JP, Kagan DV, Brody JS. New York, Praeger, 1985, pp 285–314

Lamy PP: Nonprescription drugs and the elderly. Am Fam Physician 39:175–179, 1989

Larson EB, Kukull WA, Buchner D, et al: Adverse drug reaction associated with global cognitive impairment in elderly persons. Ann Intern Med 107:169–173, 1987

Letenneur L, Dartigues JF, Orgogozo JM: Wine consumption in the elderly. Ann Intern Med 118:317–318, 1993

Liberto JG, Oslin DW, Ruskin PE: Alcoholism in older persons: a review of the literature. Hosp Community Psychiatry 43:975–984, 1992

Lishman WA: Organic Psychiatry, 2nd Edition. Oxford, England, Blackwell, 1987, pp 517–521

Liskow Bl, Rinck C, Campbell J, et al: Alcohol withdrawal in the elderly. J Stud Alcohol 50:414–421, 1989

Lowinson JH, Ruiz P, Millman RB, et al (eds): Comprehensive Textbook of Substance Abuse, 2nd Edition. Baltimore, MD, Williams & Wilkins, 1992

Mant A, Duncan-Jones P, Saltman D, et al: Development of long term use of psychotropic drugs by general practice patients. Br Med J (Clin Res Ed) 296:251–254, 1988

Mant A, Whicker S, Kwok YS: Over-the-counter self-medication: the issues. Drugs Aging 2:257–261, 1992

Martin JC, Streissguth AP: Alcoholism and the elderly: an overview, in Treatment of Psychopathology in the Aging. Edited by Eisdorfer C, Fann WE. New York, Springer, 1982, pp 242–280

Mellinger GD, Balter MB, Uhlenhuth EH: Prevalence and correlates of the long-term regular use of anxiolytics. JAMA 251:375–379, 1984

Miller NS, Belkin BM, Gold MS: Alcohol and drug dependence among the elderly: epidemiology, diagnosis, and treatment. Compr Psychiatry 32:153–165, 1991

Miller PS, Richardson JS, Jyu CA, et al: Association of low serum anticholinergic levels and cognitive impairment in elderly presurgical patients. Am J Psychiatry 145:342–345, 1988

Moos RH, Brennan PL, Mertens JR: Mortality rates and predictors of mortality among late-middle-aged and older substance abuse patients. Alcoholism 18:187–195, 1994

Morse RM, Flavin DK: The definition of alcoholism. JAMA 268:1012–1014, 1992

Murray RM: Minor analgesic abuse: the slow recognition of a public health problem. Br J Addict 75:9–17, 1980

National Institute on Drug Abuse: Annual Emergency Room Data 1991: Data From the Drug Abuse Warning Network (DAWN), Series 1, No 11-A, DHHS Publication No (ADM) 92-1955, 1992a

National Institute on Drug Abuse: Annual Medical Examiner Data 1991: Data From the Drug Abuse Warning Network (DAWN), Series 1, No 11-B, DHHS Publication No (ADM) 92-1956, 1992b

Noyes R Jr, Garvey MJ, Cook BL, et al: Benzodiazepine withdrawal: a review of the evidence. J Clin Psychiatry 49:382–389, 1988

Onyett SR, Turpin G: Benzodiazepine withdrawal in primary care: a comparison of behavioural group training and individual sessions. Behavioral Psychotherapy 16:297–312, 1988

Parry HJ, Balter MB, Mellinger GD, et al: National patterns of psychotropic drug use. Arch Gen Psychiatry 28:769–783, 1973

Pascarelli EF: The elderly in methadone maintenance, in The Combined Problems of Alcoholism, Drug Addiction and Aging. Edited by Gottheil E, Druley KA, Skoloda TE, et al. Springfield, IL, Charles C Thomas, 1985, pp 210–214

Pentel P: Toxicity of over-the-counter stimulants. JAMA 252:1898–1903, 1984

Peters NL: Snipping the thread of life: antimuscarinic side effects of medications in the elderly. Arch Intern Med 149:2414–2420, 1989

Pinsker H, Suljaga-Petchel K: Use of benzodiazepines in primary care geriatric patients. J Am Geriatr Soc 32:595–597, 1984

Pomara N, Stanley B, Block R, et al: Increased sensitivity of the elderly to the central depressant effects of diazepam. J Clin Psychiatry 46:185–187, 1985

Pomara N, Deptula D, Singh R, et al: Cognitive toxicity of benzodiazepines in the elderly, in Anxiety in the Elderly: Treatment and Research. Edited by Salzman C, Lebowitz BD. New York, Springer, 1991, pp 175–196

Portenoy RK, Payne R: Acute and chronic pain, in Substance Abuse: A Comprehensive Textbook, 2nd Edition. Edited by Lowinson JH, Ruiz P, Millman RB, et al. Baltimore, MD, Williams & Wilkins, 1992, pp 691–721

Ray WA, Griffin MR, Schaffner W, et al: Psychotropic drug use and the risk of hip fracture. N Engl J Med 316:363–369, 1987

Ray WA, Griffin MR, Downey W: Benzodiazepines of long and short elimination half-life and the risk of hip fracture. JAMA 262:3303–3307, 1989

Rice C, Longabaugh R, Beattie M, et al: Age group differences in response to treatment for problematic alcohol use. Addiction 88:1369–1375, 1993

Rickels K, Schweizer E: The clinical course and long-term management of generalized anxiety disorder. J Clin Psychopharmacol 10:101S–110S, 1990

Rickels K, Case WG, Downing RW, et al: Long-term diazepam therapy and clinical outcome. JAMA 250:767–771, 1983

Rickels K, Case WG, Schweizer E, et al: Benzodiazepine dependence: management of discontinuation. Psychopharmacol Bull 26:63–68, 1990a

Rickels K, Schweizer E, Case WG, et al: Long-term therapeutic use of benzodiazepines, I: effects of abrupt discontinuation. Arch Gen Psychiatry 47:899–907, 1990b

Rickels K, Case WG, Schweizer E, et al: Long-term benzodiazepine users 3 years after participation in a discontinuation program. Am J Psychiatry 148:757–761, 1991

Rodrigo EK, King MB, Williams P: Health of long term benzodiazepine users. Br Med J 296:603–606, 1988

Rovner BW, David A, Lucas-Blaustein MJ, et al: Self-care capacity and anticholinergic drug levels in nursing home patients. Am J Psychiatry 145:107–109, 1988

Roy-Byrne PP, Hommer D: Benzodiazepine withdrawal: overview and implications for treatment of anxiety. Am J Med 84:1041–1052, 1988

Rummans TA, Davis LJ, Morse RM, et al: Learning and memory impairment in older, detoxified, benzodiazepine-dependent patients. Mayo Clin Proc 68:731–737, 1993

Salzman C: Pharmacologic treatment of the anxious elderly patient, in Anxiety in the Elderly: Treatment and Research. Edited by Salzman C, Lebowitz BD. New York, Springer, 1991, pp 149–173

Saunders PA, Copeland JRM, Dewey ME, et al: Heavy drinking as a risk factor for depression and dementia in elderly men. Br J Psychiatry 159:213–216, 1991

Schneider CL, Nordlund DJ: Prevalence of vitamin and mineral supplementation in the elderly. J Fam Pract 17:243–247, 1983

Schonfeld L, Dupree LW: Antecedents of drinking for early and late-onset elderly alcohol abusers. J Stud Alcohol 52:587–592, 1991

Schuckit MA: Drug and Alcohol Abuse, 3rd Edition. New York, Plenum, 1989

Schweizer E, Case WG, Rickels K: Benzodiazepine dependence and withdrawal in elderly patients. Am J Psychiatry 146:529–531, 1989

Schweizer E, Rickels K, Case WG, et al: Long-term therapeutic use of benzodiazepines, II: effects of gradual taper. Arch Gen Psychiatry 47:908–915, 1990

Schweizer E, Rickels K, Case WG, et al: Carbamazepine treatment in patients discontinuing long-term benzodiazepine therapy: effects on withdrawal severity and outcome. Arch Gen Psychiatry 48:448–452, 1991

Simons LA, Tett S, Simons J, et al: Multiple medication use in the elderly: use of prescription and non-prescription drugs in an Australian community setting. Med J Aust 157:242–246, 1992

Smart RG, Adlaf EM: Alcohol and drug use among the elderly: trends in use and characteristics of users. Can J Public Health 79:236–242, 1988

Smith DM, Atkinson RM: Substance abuse in the elderly, in Textbook of Geriatric Neuropsychiatry. Edited by Coffey CE, Cummings JL. Washington, DC, American Psychiatric Press, 1994, pp 306–307

Sobal J, Muncie HL, Baker AS: Use of nutritional supplements in a retirement community. Gerontologist 26:187–191, 1986

Speer DC, Bates K: Comorbid mental and substance disorders among older psychiatric patients. J Am Geriatr Soc 40:886–890, 1992

Stewart RB: Nutritional supplements in the ambulatory elderly population: patterns of use and requirements. DICP 23:490–495, 1989

Stoller EP: Prescribed and over-the-counter medicine use by ambulatory elderly. Med Care 26:1149–1157, 1988

Svarstad BL: Stress and the use of nonprescription drugs: an epidemiological study. Research in Community and Mental Health 3:233–254, 1983

Tinetti ME, Speechley M, Ginter SF: Risk factors for falls among elderly persons living in the community. N Engl J Med 319:1701–1707, 1988

Tune L, Carr S, Hoag E, et al: Anticholinergic effects of drugs commonly prescribed for the elderly: potential means for assessing risk of delirium. Am J Psychiatry 149:1393–1394, 1992

Tune LE, Bylsma FW: Benzodiazepine-induced and anticholinergic-induced delirium in the elderly. Int Psychogeriatr 3:397–408, 1991

Verbrugge L: Triggers of symptoms and health care. Soc Sci Med 20:855–876, 1985

Vestal RE, McGuire EA, Tobin JD, et al: Aging and ethanol metabolism in man. Clin Pharmacol Ther 21:343–354, 1977

Victor M, Adams RD, Collins GH: The Wernicke-Korsakoff Syndrome and Related Neurologic Disorders Due to Alcoholism and Malnutrition (Contemporary Neurology Series, Vol 3). Philadelphia, PA, FA Davis, 1989

Vogel-Sprott M, Barrett P: Age, drinking habits and the effects of alcohol. J Stud Alcohol 45:517–521, 1984

Whitcup SM, Miller F: Unrecognized drug dependence in psychiatrically hospitalized elderly patients. J Am Geriatr Soc 35:297–301, 1987

Winick C: Maturing out of narcotic addiction. United Nations Bulletin on Narcotics 14:1–7, 1962

Yearick ES, Wang ML, Pisias SJ: Nutritional status of the elderly: dietary and biochemical findings. J Gerontol 35:663–671, 1980

Charles F. Reynolds III, M.D.

Sleep Disorders

C omplaints of disturbed nocturnal sleep and daytime sleepiness are
common among older Americans in general and are very important
symptoms in late-life psychiatric disorders, particularly mood and
dementing disorders. Furthermore, the prevalence of sleep medication use
increases steadily with advancing age, as does the prevalence of many types
of sleep-related behavioral disturbances. These disturbances, including
nocturnal wandering, confusion, and agitated behavior, are not well tolerated by caregivers (Sanford 1975) and may thus trigger a family's decision to institutionalize an older, often demented relative (Pollak and Perlick
1987). It is not surprising that prescription of sedating medication is highly
prevalent among institutionalized elderly individuals (James 1985; U.S.
Public Health Service 1976). Finally, as epidemiological work has indicated, complaints of disturbed sleep are frequent among community-
residing elderly individuals, particularly those who live alone, are unemployed, or are depressed or bereaved (Clayton et al. 1972; Ford and
Kamerow 1989; Rodin et al. 1988).

Supported in part by National Institute of Mental Health Grants MH00295, MH37869,
MH52247, and MH30915.

Clinical Epidemiology of Late-Life Sleep Disorders

Earlier epidemiological surveys reported that as many as 30% of the older population (i.e., persons ages 60 and older) suffer from and complain of poor sleep quality on a chronic basis (Bliwise 1993; Miles and Dement 1980). The National Institute of Mental Health (NIMH) and the National Institute on Aging Epidemiologic Catchment Area (ECA) study of 7,954 respondents (who were questioned between 1981 and 1985, at baseline and 1 year later) found that 10.2% reported persistent insomnia and 3.2% reported persistent hypersomnia at the first interview (Ford and Kamerow 1989). Rates of prevalent and incident insomnia complaints were highest among the 1,801 respondents ages 65 and older (12.0% and 7.3%, respectively). By contrast, rates of prevalent and incident hypersomnia complaints in elderly individuals were lower than rates of complaints of insomnia. Thus, 1.6% of those ages 65 and older had complaints of persistent hypersomnia at the initial interview ("prevalent" hypersomnia). Importantly, the risk of developing new major depression was much higher in those respondents (of any age) who had insomnia at both interviews versus those without insomnia (odds ratio: 39.8) and those whose insomnia had resolved by the second visit (odds ratio: 1.6). This finding led Ford and Kamerow (1989) to raise the intriguing suggestion that early recognition and treatment of sleep disturbances may prevent future psychiatric disorders. The authors found that "those with sleep complaints were more likely to have received services from both the general medical and specialty mental health sectors" (Ford and Kamerow 1989, p. 1479). Other surveys of nighttime sedation in community-resident elderly individuals have shown that 20%–25% regularly use sleeping pills (1983 NIH Concensus Conference on Drugs and Insomnia 1984). Older patients frequently complain that their sleep is nonrestorative and that they have difficulty maintaining sleep, whereas younger subjects are more likely to complain of difficulty initiating sleep. Trouble maintaining alertness during the day is also a frequent complaint in elderly individuals, and, consistent with this complaint, sleep laboratory studies have demonstrated an increase in sleepiness during the day in late life. Most sleep researchers believe that this increase reflects unmet sleep need, a reflection of nocturnal sleep fragmentation (Carskadon et al. 1982).

Sleep-related behavioral disturbances (including nocturnal agitation, night wandering, shouting, and incontinence) are particularly important among institutionalized elderly individuals with dementing disorders. It is likely that the widespread use of tranquilizing medication in nursing home residents reflects in part the clinical importance of "sundowning" (agitated verbal or physical behavior at the time of sunset) and related nocturnal agitation, wandering, and screaming. An earlier survey of physicians' prescribing practices in nursing homes and other institutional settings suggested that as many as 90% of patients in nursing homes may receive medication for sleep on a regular basis (U.S. Public Health Service 1976). A more recent report by James (1985) estimated that 35% of such patients receive tranquilizing medication.

Finally, sleep disturbance is a major and debilitating symptom of bereavement, particularly following the death of a spouse. For example, Clayton et al. (1972) found that complaints of sleep disturbance were about as prevalent at 13 months (48%) as at 1 month following the loss of a spouse. The frequency of spousal death has been estimated at 1.6% and 3.0% yearly for older men and women, respectively (Murrell et al. 1984). Given the large number of spousally bereaved elderly persons, the strong likelihood of concurrent sleep disturbance, and the risk for developing major depression posed by persistent sleep disturbance (Ford and Kamerow 1989), the public health importance of sleep disturbance in late-life bereavement is clear. It also seems plausible to suggest that persistent sleep loss in bereavement may lead not only to bereavement-related depression, but also to self-medication with alcohol and sleeping medication.

Our ongoing studies of physiological sleep changes associated with spousal bereavement in late life have shown that sleep in bereavement-related depression is very similar to sleep in endogenous recurrent major depression (with shortened rapid eye movement [REM] sleep latency and other REM and slow-wave sleep changes described later) (Reynolds et al. 1992). By contrast, among spousally bereaved individuals who do not become depressed, sleep as measured by electroencephalogram (EEG) remains essentially normal over the first 2 years of bereavement, with the exception of elevated REM generation during REM sleep (Reynolds et al. 1993). (The last finding could correlate with the increased burden of affective information processing that occurs during bereavement.)

Rodin and associates (1988) examined the relationship among aging, sleep, and depression by focusing on how the frequency of depressed affect over time related to poor sleep in community-residing elderly individuals (ages 62 or older; $N = 264$). The frequency of depressed affect over a 3-year period was "related positively to sleep disturbance, even when subjects' age, gender, and health status were considered simultaneously." Furthermore, the authors noted that "early morning awakening was the sleep symptom most consistently related to depressed mood over the course of study. Poor health and female gender showed positive but less consistent relationships to the sleep complaints than depressed affect." Sleep laboratory studies of elderly depressed patients have confirmed the correlation between severity of depression and early morning awakening (Reynolds et al. 1985), as well as the predictive validity of early morning awakening in distinguishing depression from dementia (Reynolds et al. 1989).

The observation that longitudinal fluctuation in sleep complaints (particularly of sleep continuity disturbance and early morning awakening) covaries strongly with intensity of depressive symptoms was confirmed and extended by Kennedy et al. (1991). These investigators studied the persistence or remission of depressive symptoms in late life in a sample of 1,885 adults ages 65 or older from the ECA study. Changes in health and sleep disturbance and added formal support services were distinguishing characteristics of elderly patients with persistent or remitted depression.

The weight of epidemiological evidence reviewed here and elsewhere (Reynolds et al. 1995) suggests that sleep disturbance is a consequence of depressive symptoms, a significant correlate of help-seeking behavior, and a major risk factor for the subsequent development of syndromal major depression. Other studies have shown that sleep-related behaviors often precipitate the decision of families to institutionalize an elderly demented relative (Pollak et al. 1990). Thus, any understanding of how to attenuate the sleep changes and disturbances of usual and pathological aging in a way that would reduce psychiatric morbidity, burden to families, and the rate of institutionalization would be of enormous public health significance. Hence, I believe that a basic challenge confronting those who care for elderly patients with sleep disturbances is how to preserve the successful functioning of the aging circadian time-keeping system in the face of multiple medical and psychosocial challenges.

Diagnosis

Consistent with the sleep disorders section of DSM-IV (American Psychiatric Association 1994), two major categories of dyssomnia (sleep disorder) will be reviewed: insomnias (disorders of initiating and maintaining sleep) and hypersomnias (disorders of excessive daytime sleepiness). The importance of these categories to psychiatry is underscored by the ECA data cited previously (Ford and Kamerow 1989). Specifically, 40% of respondents with persistent insomnia and 46.5% of those with hypersomnia had a psychiatric disorder, as determined by the

Diagnostic Interview Schedule (Robins et al. 1981). Thus, psychopathological disorders are of major importance in the differential diagnosis of the dyssomnias. However, they do not exhaust the differential diagnostic possibilities.

In the following discussion the terms *nonrapid eye movement (NREM)* and *REM* sleep are used. These terms denote two very different operating states of the central nervous system during sleep: REM sleep represents an activated brain, and NREM sleep, a quiescent brain. Also, during REM sleep, heart rate, respiratory rate, and blood pressure all tend to increase relative to NREM sleep, and ventilatory response to increased concentrations of inhaled carbon dioxide is decreased compared with that in NREM sleep. Furthermore, the onset of REM sleep is mediated by the firing of cholinergic cells in the pontine tegmentum, whereas NREM sleep depends on the basal forebrain area and the midbrain raphe. In addition, REM sleep represents the circadian component of sleep-wake regulation, occurring near the low point of the circadian temperature rhythm. NREM sleep (and particularly the slow-wave sleep component) represents the homeostatic component of sleep-wake regulation. It is particularly slow-wave sleep that is diminished with age. For further discussion of the physiological correlates of sleep and sleep regulation, see Kryger et al. (1989).

The key symptoms in the diagnosis of late-life sleep disorders are complaints of insomnia; nonrestorative sleep; excessive daytime sleepiness; a shift in the timing of the major sleep period; frequent periods of sleep and wakefulness during the 24-hour day (rather than consolidation of major sleep and wake periods); and decrease in mood, performance, and alertness related to the foregoing symptoms.

The initial aim of clinical assessment is to determine the duration of the patient's complaint and likely contributing factors. Transient disturbances (i.e., lasting less than 2 to 3 weeks) are usually situationally determined; more persistent disturbances (i.e., lasting longer than a month) often indicate more serious underlying medical or psychiatric problems and thus may require more detailed medical, physiological, and psychiatric evaluation (1983 NIH Consensus Conference on Drugs and Insomnia 1984; Consensus Development Conference 1990). Sources of diagnostic information should include interviews with both the patient and a bed partner, as well as a sleep-wake log kept daily over a 2-week period to determine the distribution and quality of the patient's sleep during the 24-hour day. The usefulness of such a log is enhanced if daily data concerning scheduling of sleep and naps as well as social activities are obtained, together with information about the timing of meals, medications, exercise, and other indicators of social rhythms. Further assessment should attend to physician- and self-prescribed drug use.

Sleep disturbances in late life reflect the following factors:

- Age-dependent decreases in the ability to sleep
- An increased prevalence of sleep-disordered breathing (sleep apnea) and nocturnal periodic limb movements
- Sleep-phase alterations, particularly advancement of the major sleep period to an earlier time of day
- Psychiatric disorders, such as depression, dementia, anxiety, and paranoid disorders
- Medical disorders, particularly those involving nocturia, pain, and limitation of mobility
- Poor sleep habits, particularly the tendency to spend excessive amounts of time in bed
- Iatrogenic factors, particularly the use of sedating medications during the daytime
- Adverse environmental factors, such as inadequate lighting that may encourage sleeping at the "wrong" time of the 24-hour day, or excessive heat or noise
- Psychosocial factors, such as loneliness, inactivity, and boredom

Bearing these factors in mind, the clinician should evaluate the patient for the following possibilities:

- Irregular sleep-wake scheduling, including spending excessive amounts of time in bed (more than 7 or 8 hours per 24 hours)
- Evening self-medication, especially with nicotine, alcohol, or caffeinated beverages
- Obsessive worry about sleep and the use of the bed for activities not conducive to sleep
- Dependence on sleeping pills
- Temporal displacement of the major sleep period to an earlier time in the 24-hour day
- Heavy snoring or obstructive breathing during sleep, which may indicate the presence of sleep apnea
- Feelings of restlessness in the legs at sleep onset, which may indicate nocturnal myoclonus
- The presence of an affective, psychotic, anxiety, or dementing disorder

- Medical disorders known to be specifically exacerbated by sleep (parasomnias), such as nocturnal angina, congestive heart failure, and esophageal reflux
- The use, timing, and dosage of other medications known to have psychotropic effects, such as antihypertensive medications, antihistamines, and antiparkinsonian drugs (for example, propranolol may lead to insomnia, L-methyldopa to daytime sedation, and L-dopa to insomnia or nightmares)

Sleep laboratory evaluation (polysomnography) can be helpful to the elderly person with a sleep disorder and is indicated if the physician suspects sleep apnea (suggested particularly by the presence of heavy snoring and excessive daytime sleepiness) or nocturnal myoclonus (suggested by complaint of restless legs or akathisia-like sensations in the legs interfering with sleep onset). Sleep laboratory evaluation should also be considered if routine treatment measures have not resolved the problem. In this context, "routine" treatment should include the following:

1. Consistent attention to the sleep-wake schedule and a comfortable sleep environment, limiting time in bed to approximately 7 hours nightly (temporal control)
2. Reduction in or elimination of self-medication with nicotine, alcohol, or excessive liquid ingestion
3. Use of the bedroom for sleep and intimacy only, with avoidance of activities that are not conducive to sleep (stimulus control)
4. Careful attention to the timing of physical activity, meals, medication, and sleep periods (including naps)
5. Detoxification from depressant or stimulant drugs
6. Appropriate behavioral treatment for insomnia

Etiology and Pathogenesis of Late-Life Sleep Disorders

As has been suggested elsewhere (Reynolds et al. 1994), successful adaptation in late life depends on preservation of nocturnal sleep quality, ability to maintain daytime alertness, and physiological integrity of nocturnal EEG sleep. Neither poor sleep nor excessive daytime sleepiness is an inevitable accompaniment of growing old. Rather, the preservation of vigorous health, vitality, and engagement in life ("successful aging," in the words of Rowe and Kahn [1987]) appears to be correlated with three behavioral strategies on the part of "successfully aging" elderly individuals to circumvent the effects of the age-related loss in the ability to sleep:

1. The adoption of extremely stable sleep-wake schedules, within the context of a life-style characterized by high stability of social rhythms generally
2. Limitation of time in bed to approximately 7 hours out of 24
3. Choosing a schedule of activities that generally reflects morning-type or "lark" circadian orientation (Monk et al. 1991; Reynolds et al. 1991a, 1991b, 1993b)

Nonetheless, there is an age-dependent decrease in the ability to sleep that reflects both the aging process per se and the impact of concurrent physical and psychiatric disorders. The most important age-dependent decrements in the ability to sleep include the following:

*   Decreased continuity of sleep, manifested particularly by an increase in the number of microarousals (3–15 seconds in duration)
*   Decreased slow-wave sleep (the deepest level of NREM sleep and perhaps the most restorative sleep)
*   A tendency for the major sleep period to occur earlier in the night (phase advancement)
*   A tendency for REM sleep to occur earlier in the night
*   Increased napping during the day
*   A general tendency to spend more time in bed, which may be a response to poor sleep but tends only to perpetuate the problem and make sleep quality worse

Other age-associated changes in sleep include a decrement in growth hormone secretion (which typically is maximal during the first 2 hours of sleep, in association with NREM sleep stages 3 and 4), decreases in sleep-associated prolactin and testosterone release, increases in plasma norepinephrine levels, and increases in cortisol secretion (particularly in elderly depression patients). A general reference on age-dependent changes in sleep, biological rhythms, and sleep-related neuroendocrine activity is the work by Roth and Roehrs (1989).

Sleep researchers generally agree that it is the ability to sleep, rather than the need for sleep, that diminishes with age. The belief that many older people have unmet sleep need is substantiated by findings of increased daytime sleepiness among elderly individuals. Unmet sleep need in late life probably results from sleep fragmentation, loss of sleep depth, and the redistribution of sleep in the 24-hour period. In essence, the nocturnal sleep of many older people who demonstrate more "usual" rather than "successful" aging is brittle and shallow and is characterized by numerous transient arousals and by a decrease in or total loss of the deepest levels of NREM (slow-wave) sleep.

Previous reports of sleep in healthy elderly individuals have also noted gender-related differences in sleep continuity and slow-wave sleep, with elderly men having more impaired sleep maintenance and less slow-wave sleep than elderly women. Paradoxically, however, older women are more likely than men to complain of sleep disturbance and to receive sleeping pills. It is possible that older women may be more sensitive to sleep quality and sleep losses, and particularly to the mood-disrupting effects of sleep loss, than older men (Reynolds et al. 1986, 1991b).

With respect to observable behaviors during sleep in late life, snoring has received considerable attention. Koskenvuo et al. (1985, 1987) found habitual, severe snoring in 9% of men ($n = 3,847$) and 3.6% of women ($n = 3,664$) ages 40 to 67. Snoring was more prevalent in men and women with hypertension (relative risks of 1.91 and 3.19, respectively) and in men with ischemic heart disease or stroke ($n = 4,388$; relative risk, 1.91 and 2.38, respectively). Clinically it is believed that severe snoring is likely to reflect frank or complete occlusion of the airway during sleep, leading to sleep apnea.

Numerous studies have shown that sleep-disordered breathing increases with advancing age, more so in men than in women. The best epidemiological work in this area has been done by Ancoli-Israel (1989) and Ancoli-Israel et al. (1985), who showed an overall prevalence for sleep disordered breathing of about 25% among a large sample of community-residing elderly individuals in San Diego.

From a sleep physiological perspective, both major depression and dementia of the Alzheimer's type are associated with characteristic changes in the physiological organization and intensity of sleep (Reynolds et al. 1988, 1993b). The sleep physiological correlates of late-life depression include

- Short REM sleep latencies (i.e., diminished time between sleep onset and REM sleep onset)
- Prolonged first REM sleep periods with enhanced density of rapid eye movements

- Shifting of electroencephalogram slow-wave activity from the first to the second NREM sleep period
- Early morning awakening

By contrast, sleep in Alzheimer's dementia deteriorates as the dementia progresses, with the development of an arrhythmic, polyphasic sleep-wake pattern, gradual loss of all phasic activity (i.e., decreased spindles and K complexes in stage 2, decreased rapid eye movements in stage REM), normal or prolonged REM sleep latency, and increased prevalence of sleep apnea (Prinz et al. 1982). Sleep physiological alterations in depressive pseudodementia are similar to those of endogenous depression, including a transient antidepressant response to all-night sleep deprivation and a robust REM sleep rebound during recovery sleep after acute sleep deprivation (Buysse et al. 1988). Patients afflicted with primary degenerative dementia and secondary depression do not show an antidepressant response to acute total sleep deprivation or an REM sleep rebound during the recovery sleep that follows sleep deprivation. As reviewed by Wu and Bunney (1990), more than half of patients with depression experience transient improvement in symptoms of depression after a night of sleep deprivation. The authors also reported that more than 80% of these patients, if unmedicated with thymoleptic agents, would relapse after one night of sleep.

EEG sleep measures in elderly patients with mixed depression and cognitive impairment appear to correlate with 2-year survival status. Such "mixed-symptom" patients lacking a short REM latency but showing evidence of sleep-disordered breathing have a significantly elevated risk of mortality by the time of 2-year follow-up (Hoch et al. 1989), as well as diminished capacity for REM sleep rebound following all-night sleep deprivation. I have interpreted the finding of diminished REM sleep generation and sleep-disordered breathing as correlates of brain failure that predict early mortality.

Generalized anxiety disorder and panic disorder are characterized by sleep continuity disturbances, such as sleep onset and sleep maintenance difficulties, but generally lack the REM sleep stigmata of major or endogenous depression. Sleep in mania and psychotic depression are characterized by extreme sleep fragmentation and early-onset REM sleep. (For further review, see Vogel et al. 1989.)

The occurrence of "sundowning" was empirically studied by Evans (1987) and found to be associated with a diagnosis of dementia and/or fluid or electrolyte abnormalities; it occurred more frequently in patients who had recently been admitted to a nursing facility, in patients whose rooms had been changed in the preceding month, and in patients who participated in fewer daytime activities. Sundowning has been linked to sensory deprivation, loneliness, diminished social and physical time cues (e.g., visits, lighting), partial arousal from REM sleep (Feinberg et al. 1967), and sleep apnea (Hoch et al. 1989). Thus, it appears that sundowning may be the final common expression of numerous different underlying mechanisms, some related to changes in sleep-wake rhythmicity and some to the physical and psychosocial time cues that impinge on "internal clocks." Bliwise (1993) has published a landmark review of sleep in dementia.

In the context of internal clocks, the circadian temperature rhythm exerts powerful effects on the regulation of sleep. Conversely, sleep disturbances such as insomnia are associated with diminished amplitude in the body temperature rhythm. The body temperature cycle is the generally accepted "marker" or output of the circadian clock, which drives the daily cycle (Weitzman et al. 1982). REM sleep is most likely near the low point of the daily temperature rhythm under free-running conditions (internal desynchronization). It is generally accepted that human temperature rhythms tend to flatten and shorten with "usual" aging. This reduction in amplitude appears to result from an increase in low point of daily temperatures. There may also be a change with age in circadian "type." Thus, older people tend to prefer earlier bedtimes and wake-up times than their younger counterparts and tend to be rated as "larks" (morning types) rather than as "owls" (evening types). This shift in circadian type from owl to lark may be related to an age-dependent shortening in the duration or period of the circadian temperature rhythm.

It is likely that life-style changes play an important contributory role in late-life sleep disorders. For example, the fact that many older people spend increased time in bed may reflect a feeling that they have little reason to get up, including few opportunities for social and physical activity as well as loss of important social time cues that may attend retirement. Among institutionalized elderly individuals, environmental factors such as temperature, noise, and lighting undoubtedly provide important and perhaps deleterious changes in time cues for the circadian regulation of sleep and wakefulness.

Treatment of Late-Life Sleep Disorders

Elderly persons and their families may need to be told that some sleep disturbance, particularly insomnia, may be an unavoidable consequence of aging—not that less sleep is needed, but rather that ability to sleep may diminish with age. Reinforcement of a regular sleep-wake schedule, together with limiting time in bed to no more than 7 or 8 hours nightly, may be effective countermeasures to the age-related tendency to lose the consolidation of sleep and develop a polyphasic sleep-wake cycle. In practical terms, the elderly person with a complaint of insomnia should be encouraged to go to bed only when sleepy, get up at the same time each morning, reduce naps to no more than 30 to 45 minutes daily, and limit nightly time in bed to 7 hours (all examples of temporal control). The older patient with the complaint of sleep disturbance, particularly insomnia, should also be instructed to maintain "stimulus control" by using the bedroom only for activities conducive to sleep. Stimulus control serves to keep the bed as a powerful stimulus to sleep. In practice, strengthening temporal and stimulus control, together with education and reassurance, help the older person achieve a sense of increased control and diminished need for medication.

Although controlled studies are lacking, there is reason to believe that regular exercise, particularly if it leads to improved aerobic fitness, may enhance the quality and depth of sleep in late life. There is also reason to believe that the use of a behavioral technique known as *sleep restriction therapy* may be particularly useful among elderly individuals with insomnia. As developed by Spielman and colleagues (1987), sleep restriction therapy teaches the patient to spend less time in bed at night in order to create a modest sleep debt, which then overrides sleep fragmentation.

With respect to the use of sleeping pills in late life, diagnosis is the most salient of all clinical considerations. Most sleep disorder experts agree that sedative-hypnotic agents have a place in 1) the management of transient or situational insomnia, 2) persistent sleep loss that is associated with bad habits and does not respond to behavioral interventions, and 3) persistent insomnia associated with nonpsychotic psychiatric disorders. Additional clinical considerations include

- A review of the relative indications and contraindications for using low-dose sedating antidepressants, benzodiazepines, or antipsychotic compounds
- Age-dependent changes in the rate of metabolism
- Effects on daytime alertness and performance
- Concurrent medications that might potentiate the effects of sedative-hypnotic agents
- The potentially exacerbating effect on borderline and full-blown sleep apnea syndrome

There are few controlled trials of sedative-hypnotic agents in well-diagnosed samples of geriatric patients. In one review, only six controlled studies of the use of sedating medication in elderly patients with dementia or organic brain syndromes had been published during the preceding 15 years (Reynolds et al. 1989). These studies involved a total of 134 inpatients, some with mild to moderate dementia and others with "organic brain syndrome" with agitation. None of the studies employed sleep laboratory or objective methods to assess drug effects, but all used a placebo control and were double blinded; nursing observations of sleep onset time, sleep duration, and duration of arousals were the main outcome measures. In general, the studies reported that compared with placebo, the use of active compounds was associated with nurses' observations of increased sleep time (less time to sleep onset and fewer intermittent wakenings). The drugs investigated included butabarbital, nitrazepam, flurazepam, chloral hydrate, lorazepam, temazepam, hydroxyzine, and thioridazine. With the exception of thioridazine, all compounds were associated with significant negative side effects, such as increased daytime sleepiness, drug withdrawal insomnia, and diminished capability for performing activities of daily living (Linnoila and Viukari 1976).

These findings strongly suggest that benzodiazepines do not offer a viable long-term strategy for successful management of sleep disturbance in dementia. Furthermore, given the finding that sleep apnea appears to occur significantly more often in dementia patients than in the general elderly population (Hoch et al. 1989), the use of sleeping pills might exacerbate sleep apnea and thereby increase the burden of cognitive deterioration in dementia. Accordingly, it may be preferable to use an antipsychotic compound, such as perphenazine (4–8 mg), thioridazine (25–50 mg), thiothixene (2–4 mg), risperidone (2–4 mg), or haloperidol (0.5–1 mg), for patients with marked behavioral disturbances at night who have dementia associated with psychosis and/or nocturnal wandering or agitated behavior. The use of such medications in elderly individuals necessitates monitoring for orthostatic blood pressure changes, extrapyramidal symptoms, and tardive dyskinesia.

In other older patients with chronic insomnia who cannot function without maintenance sleep-promoting medication, the use of a low-dose sedating antidepressant (e.g., 25–50 mg of trazodone or trimipramine; or 50–100 mg of nefazodone) may be preferable to using a benzodiazepine on a long-term basis. Antidepressants may retain their sedating effects longer than benzodiazepines, without the development of tolerance, daytime sequelae, or withdrawal symptoms. However, orthostatic blood pressure changes during therapy must be monitored. Moreover, such patients often have diagnosable affective disorders, and they frequently have low-grade sleep apnea that might be diminished by a tricyclic antidepressant but exacerbated by a benzodiazepine. When prescribed to patients with major depression, tricyclic antidepressants usually prolong REM sleep latency and suppress REM sleep to between 8% and 10% of time spent asleep. More sedating antidepressants such as amitriptyline also shorten sleep latency and decrease intermittent wakefulness and early morning awakening. (The atropinic side effects of amitriptyline may make it unsuitable for use in most geriatric patients.) Maintenance benzodiazepine therapy should be considered in chronic insomnia associated with a diagnosable anxiety disorder, if there is no sleep apnea.

When using benzodiazepines in elderly individuals, the physician should recall that compounds with longer onset of action may not help sleep-onset insomnia, that short duration of action may not sustain sleep that is less likely to cause daytime sedation, and that active metabolites may prolong duration of action. Probably the key pharmacokinetic issue is the elimination half-life of the compound (Carskadon et al. 1983). Long-acting benzodiazepines (e.g., flurazepam) are likely to produce daytime sedation of "hangovers." Benzodiazepines with shorter elimination half-lives (e.g., temazepam 15 mg, lorazepam 0.5–2 mg, and triazolam 0.125 mg, or zolpidem 5 mg) tend to be better tolerated by elderly individuals. (*Note:* Triazolam, however, has been associated with anterograde amnesia, which could lead to confusional syndromes in elderly individuals.) A physician who determines that a benzodiazepine is indicated for an elderly patient should establish the smallest effective dose, often one-third to one-half that prescribed for middle-age patients. The patient should take the medication about 30 minutes before bedtime. Daytime consequences should be monitored, particularly daytime sleepiness and amnesic episodes. The patient should be followed regularly, with an effort to limit the use of the benzodiazepine to less than 20 doses per month over a period of not more than 3 months. At the same time, the clinician should teach the patient to use nonpharmacological approaches to sleep disturbance to avoid the long-term use of these compounds. The recently approved agent zolpidem may also prove to be useful for the treatment of transient insomnia in elderly individuals.

Diphenhydramine (25–50 mg) has long been used to promote sleep in elderly people. Its effectiveness as a sedative-hypnotic agent is not as great as that of benzodiazepines, and its usefulness in cholinergically brittle older patients may be limited. Similarly, although L-tryptophan (500–2,000 mg) may induce sleep, there is no evidence that it maintains sleep, the major problem for elderly insomniacs. In January 1990, the Food and Drug Administration recalled L-tryptophan for clarification of safety issues.

If it is determined that the period of leg jerks during sleep (nocturnal myoclonus) is a major factor in the patient's complaint of insomnia (a judgment that depends on the results of sleep laboratory evaluation), then the use of a benzodiazepine may be helpful. The cause of nocturnal myoclonus is unknown; although benzodiazepine therapy does not suppress myoclonus, it overrides the arousal effect of periodic leg jerks, allowing the maintenance of sleep continuity. In an elderly sleeper, the use of benzodiazepines with shorter elimination half-lives is generally preferable (see Table 24–1).

The judgment that sleep disturbance is related to sleep apnea also depends on the findings of sleep laboratory evaluation. The causes of sleep apnea are multiple, complex, and imperfectly understood; hypotonus of upper airway muscles leading to airway occlusion is probably an important element in the pathogenesis. The decision of whether to treat and, if so, how to intervene is also complex and depends on the severity and type of apnea, together with its physiological and behavioral sequelae. Interventions range from the behavioral (e.g., weight loss, training the patient to sleep on his or her side) and the prosthetic (e.g., continuous positive airway pressure) to the pharmacological (e.g., acetazolamide) and surgical (e.g., uvulopalatopharyngoplasty or tracheotomy). For detailed reviews of therapy for nocturnal myoclonus and sleep apnea, the reader is referred to Kryger et al. (1989).

Table 24–1. Elimination half-lives of various benzodiazepines and zolpidem

Drug	Usual range of elimination half-life (hours)
Diazepam	10–70
Alprazolam	8–15
Lorazepam	10–20
Oxazepam	5–15
Flurazepam	36–120
Temazepam	8–20
Triazolam	1.5–5
Clonazepam	30–60
Zolpidem	2.5–2.9
Estazolam	12–15
Quazepam	40+

There is a great need for intervention research to establish chronic efficacy for treatments of recurring or persistent insomnia in late life (and at other times in the life cycle). Because primary insomnia (as defined in DSM-IV) tends to be chronic and recurring, interventions must be efficacious over long periods of time. Based on the work of Spielman et al. (1987) and Friedman et al. (1991), therapy utilizing sleep restriction techniques holds particular promise for short- and long-term efficacy in the management of primary (i.e., idiopathic) sleep maintenance insomnia, particularly in late life. Another promising lead, although less well researched to date, is the use of bright-light exposure in the evening (Campbell and Dawson 1991). Properly timed bright-light exposure may help reduce sleep maintenance difficulties and improve daytime alertness via internal phase realignments of circadian temperature and sleep-wake rhythms. Finally, enhancing aerobic fitness may lead to improved sleep quality in elderly individuals (Vitiello et al. 1990).

Prognosis and Outcome

Most clinicians believe that late-life sleep disturbance tends to be a chronic, intermittent problem. However, there are relatively few studies of the natural history of sleep disorders in late life. It is reasonable to assume that the prognosis for sleep disturbance is related to the prognosis for any associated medical and psychiatric conditions.

A major aspect of the clinical and epidemiological importance of sleep duration in late life is its well-established relationship to mortality. In analyzing data on more than 1 million adults interviewed by the American Cancer Society in 1959–1960, Kripke et al. (1979) observed that "men who reported usually sleeping less than four hours were 2.80 times as likely to have died within six years as men who reported 7.0 to 7.9 hours of sleep" (p. 103). Ancoli-Israel's (1989) reexamination of the Kripke data indicated that 86% of the deaths associated with reported short (less than 7 hours) or long (more than 8 hours) sleep periods occurred among respondents more than 60 years old.

In reviewing the data available from epidemiological surveys of sleep complaints in later life, Webb (1989) issued an important caveat:

> Sleep disorders, in the sense of pathologic conditions which interfere with vital and life style functioning in the aged will be present in the midst of "sleep difficulties" which are associated with aging. It is important that the latter not be elevated to the status of "disorders" or be

permitted to distract from the detection and treatment of a more profound and threatening sleep problem (p. 285).

References

American Psychiatric Association: Diagnostic and Statistical Manual of Mental Disorders, 4th Edition. Washington, DC, American Psychiatric Association, 1994

Ancoli-Israel S: Epidemiology of sleep disorders. Clin Geriatr Med 5:347–362, 1989

Ancoli-Israel S, Kripke DF, Mason W, et al: Sleep apnea and periodic movements in an aging sample. J Gerontol 40:419–425, 1985

Bliwise DL: Sleep in normal aging and dementia. Sleep 16:40–81, 1993

Buysse DJ, Reynolds CF, Kupfer DJ, et al: EEG sleep in depressive pseudodementia. Arch Gen Psychiatry 45:568–576, 1988

Campbell SS, Dawson D: Bright light treatment of sleep disturbance in older subjects. Sleep Research 20:448, 1991

Carskadon MA, Brown ED, Dement WC: Sleep fragmentation in the elderly: relationship to daytime sleep tendency. Neurobiol Aging 3:321–327, 1982

Carskadon MA, Seidel WF, Greenblatt DJ, et al: Daytime carryover of triazolam and flurazepam in elderly insomniacs. Sleep 5:361–371, 1983

Clayton PJ, Halikas JA, Mauria WL: The depression of widowhood. Br J Psychiatry 120:71–78, 1972

Consensus Development Conference: Diagnosis and Treatment of Sleep Disorders in Late Life. Bethesda, MD, National Institute of Health, 1990

Evans LK: Sundown syndrome in institutionalized elderly. J Am Geriatr Soc 35:101–108, 1987

Feinberg I, Koresko RL, Heller N: EEG sleep patterns as a function of normal and pathological aging in men. J Psychiatr Res 5:107–144, 1967

Ford DE, Kamerow DB: Epidemiological studies of sleep disturbances and psychiatric disorders: an opportunity for prevention? JAMA 262:1479–1484, 1989

Friedman L, Bliwise DL, Yesavage JA, et al: A preliminary study comparing sleep restriction and relaxation treatments of insomnia in older adults. J Gerontol Psychol Sci 46:1–8, 1991

Hoch CC, Reynolds CF, Nebes RD, et al: Clinical significance of sleep-disordered breathing in Alzheimer's disease: preliminary data. J Am

Geriatr Soc 37:138–144, 1989

James DS: Survey of hypnotic drug use in nursing homes. J Am Geriatr Soc 33:436–439, 1985

Kennedy GJ, Kelman HR, Thomas C: Persistence and remission of depressive symptoms in late life. Am J Psychiatry 148:174–178, 1991

Koskenvuo M, Kaprio J, Partinen M, et al: Snoring as a risk factor for hypertension and angina pectoris. Lancet 1:893–896, 1985

Koskenvuo M, Kaprio J, Telaviki T, et al: Snoring as a risk factor for ischemic heart disease and stroke in men. Br Med J 294:16–19, 1987

Kripke DF, Simons RN, Garfinkel L, et al: Short and long sleep and sleeping pills: is increased mortality associated? Arch Gen Psychiatry 36:103–116, 1979

Kryger MH, Roth T, Dement WC (eds): Principles and Practice of Sleep Medicine. Philadelphia, PA, WB Saunders, 1989, pp 413–430

Linnoila M, Viukari M: Efficacy and side effects of nitrazepam and thioridazine as sleeping aides in psychogeriatric inpatients. Br J Psychiatry 128:566–569, 1976

Miles LE, Dement WC: Sleep and aging. Sleep 3:119–220, 1980

Monk TH, Reynolds CF, Buysse DJ, et al: Circadian characteristics of healthy 80-year-olds and their relationship to objectively recorded sleep. J Gerontol 46:M171–M175, 1991

Murrell SA, Norris F, Hutchins G: Distribution and desirability of life events in older adults: population and policy implications. J Community Psychol 12:301–311, 1984

1983 NIH Consensus Conference on Drugs and Insomnia. Drugs and insomnia: the use of medications to promote sleep. JAMA 251:2410–2414, 1984

Pollak CP, Perlick D: Sleep problems and institutionalization of the elderly. Sleep Research 16:407, 1987

Pollak CP, Perlick D, Linsner JP, et al: Sleep problems in the community elderly are predictors of death and nursing home placement. J Community Health 15:123–135, 1990

Prinz P, Peskind ER, Vitaliano PP, et al: Changes in the sleep and waking EEGs of nondemented and demented elderly subjects. J Am Geriatr Soc 30:86–93, 1982

Reynolds CF, Hoch CC, Monk TH: Sleep and chronobiologic disturbances in late life, in Geriatric Psychiatry. Edited by Busse EW, Blazer DG. Washington, DC, American Psychiatric Press, 1985, pp 475–488

Reynolds CF, Kupfer DJ, Hoch CC, et al: Sleep deprivation in healthy elderly men and women: effects on mood and on sleep during recovery.

Sleep 9:492–501, 1986

Reynolds CF, Kupfer DJ, Taska LS, et al: EEG sleep in healthy elderly depressed and demented subjects. Biol Psychiatry 20:431–442, 1988

Reynolds CF, Jennings JR, Hoch CC, et al: Daytime sleepiness in the healthy "old old": a comparison with young adults. J Am Geriatr Soc 39:957–962, 1991a

Reynolds CF, Monk TH, Hoch CC, et al: EEG sleep in the healthy "old old": a comparison with the "young old" in visually scored and automated measures. J Gerontol 46:M39–M46, 1991b

Reynolds CF, Hoch CC, Buysse DJ, et al: EEG sleep in spousal bereavement and bereavement-related depression of late life. Biol Psychiatry 31:69–82, 1992

Reynolds CF, Hoch CC, Buysse DJ, et al: Sleep after spousal bereavement: a study of recovery from stress. Biol Psychiatry 34:791–797, 1993a

Reynolds CF, Hoch CC, Buysse DJ, et al: REM sleep in successful, usual and pathological aging: the Pittsburgh experience 1980–1993. J Sleep Res 2:203–210, 1993b

Reynolds CF, Dew MA, Monk TH, et al: Sleep disorders in late life: a biopsychosocial model for understanding pathogenesis and intervention, in Textbook of Geriatric Neuropsychiatry. Edited by Cummings J, Coffey CE. Washington, DC, American Psychiatric Press, 1994, pp 323–331

Reynolds CF, Buysse DJ, Kupfer DJ: Disordered sleep: developmental and biopsychosocial perspectives on the diagnosis and treatment of insomnia, in Psychopharmacology: The Fourth Generation of Progress. Edited by Bloom F, Kupfer DJ. New York, Raven Press, 1995, pp 1617–1629

Robins LN, Helzer JE, Croughan J, et al: National Institute of Mental Health Diagnostic Interview Schedule: its history, characteristics and validity. Arch Gen Psychiatry 38:381–389, 1981

Rodin J, McAvay G, Timko C: Depressed mood and sleep disturbances in the elderly: a longitudinal study. J Gerontol 43:45–52, 1988

Roth T, Roehrs TA: Drug sleep disorders and aging (review). Clin Geriatr Med 5(2):395–404, 1989

Rowe JW, Kahn RL: Human aging: usual and successful. Science 237:143–149, 1987

Sanford JRA: Tolerance of debility in elderly dependents by supporters at home: its significance for hospital practice. Br Med J 3:471–473, 1975

Spielman A, Saskin P, Thorpy MJ: Treatment of chronic insomnia by restriction of time in bed. Sleep 10:45–56, 1987

U.S. Public Health Service: Physician's drug prescribing patterns in skilled nursing facilities (PHS Publ No 76-50050). Bethesda, MD, U.S. Department of Health, Education and Welfare, 1976

Vitiello MV, Schwartz RS, Bradbury RL, et al: Improved subjective sleep quality following fitness training in healthy elderly males. Sleep Research 19:154, 1990

Vogel GW, Reynolds CF, Akiskal HS, et al: Psychiatric disorders, in Principles and Practice of Sleep Medicine. Edited by Kryger MH, Roth T, Dement WC. Philadelphia, PA, WB Saunders, 1989, pp 413–430

Webb WB: Age-related changes in sleep. Clin Geriatr Med 5:275–287, 1989

Weitzman ED, Moline ML, Czeisler CA, et al: Chronobiology of aging: temperature, sleep/wake rhythms, and entertainment. Neurobiol Aging 3:299–309, 1982

Wu JC, Bunney WE: The biological basis of an antidepressant response to sleep deprivation and relapse: review and hypothesis. Am J Psychiatry 147:14–21, 1990

Domeena C. Renshaw, M.D.

Sexuality and Aging

C ondescending humor, silence, disbelief, and benign neglect have pervaded the topic of geriatric sexual expression throughout the centuries. Fertility and virility were so inextricably linked in ancient times that, when King David (Book of Kings) was unable to provide an heir with a maiden brought to him for that purpose, he abdicated in favor of young Adonijah. Nothing is mentioned about David's aging queen, perhaps because childbearing and sexuality were considered synonymous at that time. Sexual disenfranchisement of the aged has continued since ancient times despite laboratory studies (Masters and Johnson 1966) and numerous substantiating reports that sexual interest, activity, fantasy, arousal, and activity may continue into old age for both sexes (Brecher 1983; Butler and Lewis 1977; Kinsey et al. 1948; Marsiglia and Donnelly 1991). One physician's oldest sexually active patient is 96.

Current technology can document a man's sexual responses and test for anatomical, vascular, hormonal, and tissue changes. Silicone penile implants were being used by the mid-1950s, and a new bionic era dawned in the 1970s with the dramatic development of the first inflatable penile prosthesis (Krauss 1987). Since then, despite litigation risks, the United States has witnessed a thriving industry that includes chemical injections into the penis to aid men with erectile problems (Virag 1982). There are hundreds of impotence clinics in large and small hospitals across the country; "potency fairs" display treatment options; Impotence Anonymous, US TOO, and similar self-help or support groups advertise and attract elderly men and their partners. These developments defied predictions that privacy concerns and social shame would deter seniors from seeking assistance for sexual dysfunction.

Sexual Dysfunctions After Age 50

During one 10-year period, only 3% of the patients at the Johns Hopkins Sex Clinic were older than 60, and none were older than 70 (Wise 1983). Erectile disorder was the predominant presenting complaint in 70% of patients. Approximately 28% (460 of 1,658) of couples seen during a 23-year study at Loyola Sex Therapy Clinic were older than 50; 258 were older than 65; and several were in their 80s (Annual Report of L.U.S.D.C. June 1995 [unpublished]; Renshaw 1988a). In 51%, erectile complaints presented (see Table 25–2).

Concurrent physical problems in the Loyola group included hypertension, diabetes, arthritis, chronic renal disease, cerebrovascular disease, postprostatectomy, and postcoronary bypass. Most patients were educated, middle class, and white; 6% were black; religious preferences included 32% Catholic, 30% Protestant, 25% Jewish, and a few Muslim or Hindu or nonreligious.

Kinsey et al. (1948) reported that 125 of 5,000 men were older than 60; erection problems were reported in 2% of 40-year-olds, 7% of 50-year-olds, 18% of 60-year-olds; 27% of 70-year-olds, and 75% of 80-year-olds. In the mailed response to the Consumer's Union study (Brecher 1983), 44% of those older than 50 reported less firm erections than in their younger days, and 32% reported frequent lost erections during sexual activity. Neither study was conducted in a treatment setting.

The Loyola clinic study is a structured 7-week sex therapy training clinic with married couples. Solo patients with sexual problems are seen in 6-week all-male or all-female special sexual therapy groups or in open-ended sex therapy.

Of the 1,658 couples, 9 men (0.4%) older than 50 admitted to bisexual orientation and activity. One woman said she was bisexual. Eight of the male patients presented with secondary impotence; the other male patient, age 64 years who had undergone prostatectomy, presented with secondary impotence and retrograde ejaculation. The bisexual woman was

53 years old, had 3 children, a (secret) lesbian lover, and selective hypoactive sexual desire (Gibson 1992; Weisbord 1991).

Brief Sex Therapy

Brief therapy for any sexual dysfunction is individualized; several general therapeutic steps usually are prescribed for practice at home.

Once an individual or a couple determines that there is a problem, the first step is to seek help from a physician who has special training in sexual medicine. Sexual partners should go to the evaluation together.

The physician takes an explicit history of the sexual complaints of both partners and the partners' reactions to these complaints; this is followed by a routine medical, personal, family, and marital history. Some patients can express their feelings in writing to the partner with less embarrassment. Asking each partner to review past accomplishments in the relationship by writing a letter to the other partner can be supportive personally and can enhance bonding. The therapist selects, facilitates, interprets, and shares the letters to enhance closeness, encourage honesty, and thereby improve communication.

Psychological evaluation begins with an in-depth interview about the present problem; early and current family life history; illness; and both partners' dating, love, and sexual relationships. Sexual questionnaires are administered as part of sex therapy so that 1) each partner will know himself or herself better; 2) partners will know each other better; 3) how each partner regards the relationship can be determined; and 4) organicity, (particularly head injury), mental, or psychiatric disorders can be excluded. There is no standard blood test battery performed as part of the sexual evaluation, but tests such as testosterone, prolactin, or thyroid levels are ordered when clinically indicated.

Much sexual distress relates to sexual uncertainties and needless guilt about sexual expression or fantasy, all of which can cause anxiety. A sensitive, explicit sexual history can, therefore, be therapeutic and educational. For example, the clinician may say that "masturbation has been studied and found to be natural, not at all abnormal, and practiced privately by nearly everyone. However, people worry about it. How often per month do you masturbate? Do you have any questions about it?" Sex education can provide profound relief to the patient; this is illustrated in a letter from a 62-year-old woman 2 years after evaluation who said: "You will never know what it meant for me to hear that the clitoris was solely a pleasure organ. For over 50 years I secretly worried that I was weird." Sex education provides powerful sex therapy by cognitive correction of restrictive misinformation. This process of sex education may be further reinforced by suggesting relevant readings (Brecher 1983; Butler and Lewis 1977; Masters et al. 1986; Renshaw 1995; Zilbergeld 1992).

A thorough physical and genital examination of both partners is needed to carefully exclude, or take into account, overt physical problems. Visible or palpable genital abnormalities, the strength of male peripheral pulses, and local causes for vaginal or pelvic pain (atrophic vaginitis) may be diagnosed during such examinations. Additional tests may be needed if the problem is not discovered during this evaluation. (Table 25–1 outlines common causes of impotence, 60% of which arise from organic causes.) If there are no gross abnormalities, the next step may be a diagnostic trial of brief sex therapy that includes sex education, relationship therapy, and direction for sexual activities at home. This therapy may proceed while additional investigation is progressing.

Table 25–2 gives a sample of sexual symptoms seen at Loyola Clinic, and the 1994 diagnostic codes are outlined in Table 25–3.

At home the couple is instructed in the use of sensate focus technique (nongenital foreplay), which allows them to learn to relax, discover how highly erotic the skin is, and enjoy loving foreplay while delaying intercourse (Masters et al. 1986). Both partners are encouraged to be open and

Table 25–1.   Common etiology of erectile disorders

Organic
   Vascular: arteriosclerosis, pelvic trauma or surgery
   Postsurgical: prostatectomy, cystectomy; penectomy; priapism;
      abdominoperineal resection of rectum
   Neurological: diabetes mellitus; cord trauma; demyelinating lesions; pituitary
      adenoma
   Chemical: alcohol; tranquilizers; antihypertensives; diuretics; β-blockers;
      antidepressants
   Hormonal: hyperprolactinemia; low testosterone; high estrogen, low thyroid
   Carcinoma: prostatic; related radiotherapy and chemotherapy
Somatopsychic
   Mild organic changes with heavy psychogenic overlay
Psychological
   Anxiety; anger; conflict; sexual trauma; depression; separation, divorce;
      inhibitions; job, financial, or personal (spouse, close family member, or
      friend) loss; deliberate control; gender conflict; situational symptom

Table 25–2.   Sexual disorders in aging patients

Disorder	*n*	%
Symptomatic males (*n* = 1,272/1,658)		
Erectile disorder	637	51
No sexual symptom (came with symptomatic spouse)	495	30
Hypoactive sexual desire	451	35
Premature ejaculation	238	19
Hypoactive sexual desire + other symptom	124	10
Erectile disorder + premature ejaculation	91	7
Inhibited orgasm (delayed/retrograde ejaculation)	47	3
Dyspareunia	5	0.004
Symptomatic females (*n* = 1,159/1,658)		
Inhibited orgasm	542	46
No sexual symptom (came with symptomatic spouse)	618	37
Hypoactive sexual desire	499	43
Dyspareunia	95	8
Vaginismus	62	5
Inhibited orgasm + dyspareunia + vaginismus	89	8
Unconsummated marriages	124	10

Note.   Loyola Sex Therapy Clinic Study of 1,658 couples evaluated 1/1/72 to 6/30/95.
Source.   Annual report, Renshaw 1995.

honest and to use private sexual fantasy to stimulate erections and vaginal lubrication. Women often are helped greatly by such foreplay because the average female arousal response is four times longer than a man's (the man's arousal response becomes longer after age 50, however, and the time difference is shortened). This foreplay-only approach may relieve some men of anxiety associated with performance and penetration.

Cooperative patients may risk change and take the time at home for playful touching, kissing, sexual surprises, laughter, showering together, and enjoying their own and each other's total bodies rather than focusing only on the genitals and genital arousal. Positive, even surprising, sexual responses may occur, often recapitulating the affection these partners shared during courtship. Such a bonding, therapeutic approach is a modified Masters-Johnson technique that may bring about considerable symptomatic improvement in relatively few visits (Masters et al. 1986). In the Loyola study, symptom reversal to coitus occurred in 72% of patients after 7 weeks of therapy (Renshaw 1988a; Renshaw 1995).

Table 25–3.   DSM-IV diagnostic categories of sexual dysfunction

Specify: Psychogenic only or psychogenic and biogenic
 (Note: If biogenic only, code on Axis III)
Specify: Lifelong or acquired
Specify: Generalized or situational

Sexual desire disorders
  302.71   Hypoactive sexual desire disorder
  302.79   Sexual aversion disorder
Sexual arousal disorders
  302.72   Female sexual arousal disorder
  302.72   Male erectile disorder
Orgasmic disorders
  302.73   Female orgasmic disorder
  302.74   Male orgasmic disorder
  302.75   Premature ejaculation
Sexual pain disorders
  302.76   Dyspareunia
  306.51   Vaginismus
  302.70   Sexual dysfunctions not otherwise specified

Source.   Reprinted from DSM-IV. Used with permission.

Brief sex therapy by itself may be totally effective; additional expensive laboratory studies may be unnecessary. If brief sex therapy (7 weeks) does not solve the problem, additional diagnostic assessment may be indicated to discover physical or psychological problems.

Impotence or Erectile Disorder

Impotence, or erectile disorder, is the persistent inability to obtain or maintain a penile erection suitable for sexual intercourse. It is estimated that more than 10 million men in the United States are chronically impotent.

Every man older than 50 needs to know that partial erections are normal, natural, and predictable because of general and peripheral arteriosclerotic vascular changes and diminished connective tissue elasticity. The amount of semen and the intensity of orgasm decrease with increasing age; the postejaculatory, refractory phase increases (Masters and Johnson 1966). This is not impotence. Erection improves with longer, stronger, foreplay directly on the penis so that penetration and climax can follow.

The sophisticated diagnostic procedures for evaluating erectile disorders that have evolved since 1980 are not entirely conclusive. To exclude endocrine causes of impotence, a medical workup should include fasting blood sugar and levels of testosterone, luteinizing hormone, prolactin, estradiol, thyroid-stimulating hormone, and thyroxine (T_4). Pancreatic, thyroid, and pituitary disorders must be excluded. Because reduced blood flow may be a factor, special, noninvasive tests of the penis that include measurement of nonerect penile blood pressure (normally 80% of brachial pressure) should be performed. Penile pulse is measured by a Doppler amplification device. Penile width during sleep erections may be measured in a nocturnal penile tumescence study; this test must include an 8-hour electroencephalogram to identify the sleep stages. This study is expensive and may not be conclusive. Vascular problems may be identified with arteriography studies. Injection of dye into the vas deferens, followed by masturbation and radiography of the penis, can exclude rare, but surgically correctable, congenital crural leakage points (Wagner and Green 1981). Evaluation of afferent and efferent innervation of the penis may be tested with sacral evoked potential studies. Intrapenile injections are used for diagnosis and for treatment (Wagner and Kaplan 1993). Alcohol and necessary prescription medications can contribute to or cause impotence (Buffum et al. 1981).

There are specific "high risk for impotence" situations that may be superimposed on mild or moderate organic change. For example, divorce or death of a spouse may lead to loss of potency. Erections commonly are vulnerable to emotional problems, pain, and losses such as personal or financial loss. Marital conflict, marriage breakdown, and bereavement may lead to secondary impotence; resolution of the sexual disorder may be delayed because of unresolved emotional and interpersonal conflict (Zilbergeld 1992). The possibility of a physical cause or contributing factor for impotence should not be ignored even in very stressful divorce or grief situations. It is a great injustice to suggest a psychological etiology when, for example, reduced penile blood flow is responsible for the impotence. Physical and psychological causes are not mutually exclusive and usually coexist.

The more extensive, time-consuming, and costly tests for impotence may be appropriate in cases when the patient 1) reports he has never been functional in intercourse (male virgin), 2) was formerly functional but now reports recurrent or frequent erectile failure with intercourse, 3) has "soft tip" erections (i.e., rigidity is insufficient for penetration of the vagina), or 4) a course of brief sex therapy fails despite the cooperation of both partners.

Treatment

Chemical Treatment

Aphrodisiacs have been sought since the days of alchemy, but there has been no scientific validation of any substances purported to have aphrodisiac effects. The latest "aphrodisiac"—injections of papaverine and combinations of vasodilators into the penile corpora—became widely used in the United States by 1987 and went beyond diagnostic use to treatment at home after clinical effectiveness had been demonstrated and the dose established (Virag 1982; Wagner and Kaplan 1993; Zorgniotti and Lafleur 1985). The injections were popular for home use because they caused an instant, chemically induced erection (especially in men who were not cooperative in "talking therapy") (Hartmann and Langer 1993; Virag 1982; Virag et al. 1991; Wagner and Kaplan 1993). Abuse resulted in "group papaverine parties." Complications include discontinuance because of aversion to injections, one unexpected death, nonresponsiveness, local infections, crural scarring, and priapism that may require an emergency room chemical intrapenile injection or, rarely, surgical reduction. Various patches or creams rubbed onto the penis are under investigation, but the partner is at risk for absorption of these products during coitus unless a condom is used (Cavallini 1991; Heaton et al. 1990; Laaban et al. 1985; Owen et al. 1989).

Surgical Treatment

Surgical treatment for impotence resulting from physical causes is widely available and includes several types of inflatable or semirigid, surgically implanted penile prostheses (Krauss 1987; Scott et al. 1973). These devices have made headlines in the past decade, heralding an era of "bionic sex." Such an implant may not ensure satisfactory intercourse if the relationship with the partner is conflicted or if the partner is not interested. Penile devices are not free of complications such as mechanical failure, local infection, and tissue erosion of the device. Both partners must consider such surgery carefully. The implant may afford great sexual pleasure and closeness if a man's partner is receptive. The implant does not, however, give the man a climax or an ejaculation. It provides an erectile splint and assurance that penetration is possible.

Mechanical Devices

Vacuum erection devices are noninvasive and are useful to many impotent men including elderly men who may not be interested in surgery or injections (Nadig and Cookson 1993; Nadig et al. 1986). A pump builds a vacuum in a long plastic cylinder that covers the penis to the perineum. Blood is drawn into the penis and a wide rubber band is slipped onto the penile root (this band should be removed not more than 30 minutes later). The 1995 cost with a safety valve for rapid deflation and a motor was a minimum of $450. Vacuum erection devices can be highly effective even after prostate cancer. A willing partner, a sense of humor, practice, and patience improve its value. New models are "senior friendly" with battery or electrical inflation and a light touch release lever. Some men may become impatient, may not practice, or may not use their vacuum erection devices, whereas other men request a prescription for a "spare."

Premature Ejaculation

Premature ejaculation rarely is the sole symptom in elderly men, but occurs with or prior to secondary impotence or inhibited sexual desire. Very few cases of premature ejaculation have biological or chemical causes. A major medical workup rarely is indicated. Premature ejaculation self-corrects in some men when practice and confidence reduce sexual anxiety. Sexual self-esteem and confidence may decline unless premature ejaculation is corrected, and secondary impotence often follows because of the pervasive fear of recurrence of instant ejaculation. In a young man, a thorough, explicit sexual history may reveal that rapid (less than 1 minute) erection and ejaculation is a new or transient symptom. If the physical-genital examination is normal, then the physician can inquire about possible recent causes of premature ejaculation (e.g., a long time interval between the intercourse contact; a new, awkward, or unfamiliar setting; a fear of being seen; a return to sex after a long abstinence; or infrequent coitus). Such psychosocial causes of occasional premature ejaculation respond well to reassurance and directives from the physician to make love in a relaxed atmosphere. For men older than 60, these same questions can establish whether there was earlier premature ejaculation underlying the erectile disorder or hypoactive sexual desire. Premature ejaculation usually responds readily to sex education, reassurance, and sex therapy techniques practiced at home alone or with a cooperative partner (Renshaw 1995).

Masturbation does not cause premature ejaculation. Instead, masturbating to ejaculation before intercourse might assist in early correction of the problem because the second erection will last longer. Patients of any age should be informed of this. The squeeze technique is a frequently prescribed sex therapy exercise. The partner squeezes the penis at the coronal ridge for 15 seconds during foreplay when told ejaculation is imminent. The erection then is allowed to subside. After waiting 50 seconds, the couple plays again, squeezes again for 15 seconds, and repeats this sequence several times to gain confidence in controlling the man's orgasm before intercourse. This procedure usually occurs with the man supine (relaxed with no pressure to penetrate) and the woman on top (Masters et al. 1986), but there are variations such as the man sitting on a low armless chair with the woman on his lap. The success rate for this technique is high—up to 90% (Masters et al. 1986).

Inhibited Male Orgasm
(Delayed or Absent Ejaculation)

A medical workup for this problem begins with a careful history of general health, medication use, or use of other exogenous substances (e.g., drugs or alcohol or both). Physical and genital examinations are accompanied by explicit questions about whether the symptom is situational or selective (only with intercourse, after alcohol indulgence, or after ingestion of medications) or global/generalized (with intercourse and with masturbation and apparently unrelated to chemical ingestion).

Mechanical factors that could obstruct the flow of semen must be sought if the ejaculation delay is generalized. These factors include congenital absence of seminal vesicles, an inflammation obstructing the urethra, neurological problems affecting the neck of the bladder, or problems after prostate surgery that may lead to retrograde ejaculation into the bladder. The latter may be quite compatible with good erections, intercourse, and climax. If the patient becomes aware of, and understands, his internal ejaculation, he may be able to enjoy it rather than become anxious when he does not feel the warmth of an external ejaculate. Because approximately 30% of men older than 60 have a prostatectomy, this diagnostic question is important (Wennenberg et al. 1988). Neurological lesions and some endocrine lesions may affect ejaculation; therefore, a neurological exam and blood hormone tests (as for impotence) may be indicated because early diabetic neuropathy, for example, may cause retrograde ejaculation. Vasectomy, which causes a barely notice-able reduction in volume of ejaculate, is not the cause of delayed or ab-sent ejaculation.

Female Sexual Dysfunction

Inhibited orgasm may be primary (never attained a climax by hand, mouth, vibrator, coitus, or in any other way), secondary, or situational. Sexual pain disorders include dyspareunia and vaginismus. Dyspareunia is pain on intercourse. Vaginismus is spasm of the vaginal pubococcygeus muscles.

For any female sexual problem, a full physical and genital-pelvic ex-amination should follow an explicit history. The examination should be educational, with instruction from the physician about the position of the clitoris, its attachments, and the circular pubococcygeus muscle of the lower vagina that a woman can contract voluntarily (as if to stop urination) and relax (by open-mouth exhalation). During the examination, the patient may be given a hand mirror for viewing her genitals and may be offered accurate education about her genital anatomy so that she can explore at home on her own or with her partner.

The sexological examination is standard practice in sex therapy. It is done with the partner present, so both may learn from the sex education (Masters et al. 1986). A nurse chaperon, whose name and presence during the examination is substantiated on the chart, always is present because of physician concern about litigation.

Standard sex therapy home exercises for anorgasmia include self-stimulation to orgasm. A woman finds where her pleasure areas are and can direct her partner (if she has one) or can find release and normal relaxation on her own at any time. Brief sex therapy with home massage and foreplay is helpful regardless of age. Anorgasmic women in their 50s to late 70s have had the satisfaction of finally experiencing a first orgasm.

At menopause, or after an early total hysterectomy, the vaginal wall may be thin or dry and less elastic (atrophic) because of reduced estrogen. Orgasm may be less intense (Masters and Johnson 1966). Hormonal re-placement treatment may be indicated (unless contraindicated because of risk of cancer), because many older women remain interested in sexual activity. The older woman responds rapidly and well to estrogen alone or combined with progesterone but needs regular gynecology follow-up every 6 months. A culture is done and specific medications prescribed if there is a vaginal infection. Localized or focal vaginal pain may be caused by a minute vestibular area that is infected and may require excision under a local anesthetic if it has not responded to antibiotics.

Hypoactive Sexual Desire

Explicit sex history questions determine whether the hypoactive sexual desire is situational (relating to sex with a specific partner or to sex under particular conflictual circumstances) or generalized (at all times). If it is generalized, then hormonal blood tests may be indicated because thyroid, pituitary, secondary prolactinemia, or other disorders may be causative. Neurological problems such as intracranial lesions are investigated in some uncommon cases, underscoring the need for thorough medical evaluation as an integral part of the overall treatment of sexual problems at any age. Fear of coitus following cardiac bypass surgery routinely is addressed (Renshaw 1987).

The most common (but not age specific) underlying causes of selective hypoactive sexual desire are related to fatigue; career, financial, or time pressures; major depression; medications; alcohol abuse; and conflict between partners. If both partners are motivated to change, sex therapy (often combined with other approaches such as marital therapy, individual therapy, or pharmacotherapy) can be effective. Relaxed, early morning love play after a restful night's sleep often is best for highly stressed, fatigued, older, or disabled persons. Pleasurable closeness can encourage open, honest communication, avoidance of blame, and respect for normal libido differences. Patients are advised to take turns giving and receiving affection with sustained touch, so that both may be emotionally nurtured and pleasurable sexual exchange may be restored. Outcome data of controlled studies of the efficacy of these treatment approaches in persons older than 65 are not available. In clinical treatment the success in those older than 50 has been the same as for those younger than 50.

Libido Differences

Libido differences are so common in marriages and in relationships that they are not considered to be a diagnostic category. They are individual differences that are neither good nor bad; they are simply differences. When a couple is unable to negotiate a compromise regarding the frequency of sexual encounters, the issue may reach crisis proportions. Negotiation may be open and constructive or there may be veiled threats ("I'm going to look for it elsewhere") or taunts ("It's fine with me, go find someone else").

Distress about sexual desire discrepancies is coded diagnostically as an adjustment disorder when a couple with libido differences seeks help. The wife may be upset enough to arrange an appointment, but with older couples, it is more common for a husband to initiate sexual counseling.

For example, a 64-year-old man on the verge of retirement said, "I want more than golf; it's time she stops being so frigid." The pejorative term was upsetting to his coitally compliant wife. His wife, 63, was a "good wife" who waited for his initiation, felt "good" about intercourse, could "take it or leave it, but looked forward to being held." She was nonorgasmic, yet she blossomed when sex therapy encouraged massage, cuddling, bathing together, and permission to use sexual fantasy. She said, "The bedroom has gone from mechanical to marvelous." Despite her newfound pleasure, she still could not be a sexual initiator. "I still can't do that," she said. "What if he doesn't want to? It's a man's role. I'll be 64 years old next month."

Special Circumstances

Several single, elderly homosexuals presented with impotence resulting from recurrent depression, demoralization, active grieving over the loss of a valued partner, loss of attractiveness to young urban gays, hurt, and feelings of being exploited and rejected. One 63-year-old man came because of anxiety about how to cope when his 40-year-old partner developed AIDS. The unaffected partner said: "He didn't get it from me. He swore he was faithful these 10 years. I tried to be, but when I failed I always use rubbers. It's that I'm chicken about hospitals. I can't stand blood but I get an HIV test every 60 days. I'd rather die first than watch him deteriorate. Besides, I need sex and I'm also chicken to ask him to leave my house; he doesn't have a job." Altruism was not an attribute of this wealthy art dealer. He stayed in treatment only for four sessions, which were centered on obtaining residential care, counseling sessions, and health insurance for his former lover. He canceled his fifth appointment by explaining: "I'm off to Cairo for some [rest and recreation]." He did not call back.

Personal styles of being gay and individual adjustment to aging will determine relationships and sexual expressions. Some gay persons are content and satisfied with their looks, finances, career achievement, friendships, and family—all of which are major factors. Others worry about poverty, illness, loneliness, increased vulnerability to random matings, alcohol, drug use, and sexually transmitted diseases such as AIDS. Black gay individuals and "gray gays" view themselves as minorities within a minority with added stresses resulting from illness and finances. Senior gay individuals who are in nursing homes or who are solitary and live alone (at home) face risks similar to all senior heterosexuals (e.g., physical or sexual elder abuse by family or caretakers). Older gay people are not immune to sexually transmitted diseases (Ramsey 1991; Rogstad and Bignell 1991). Medical and sex education must be part of their total health care. Literature from self-help groups can be recommended for senior or black gays to gain perspective and integration (Berger 1982; Poor 1982; Vacha 1985).

A small group of cognitively impaired persons came to clinical attention in one study (Boller and Frank 1982) because of inappropriate sexual behaviors. Although some of these were young (with developmental disabilities or head injuries), there were some older men and women with chronic neurological or psychiatric illness who required assistance at home, in day hospitals, or in long-term settings. Family, neighbors, and staff may become upset, rejecting, or severely punitive when sexual behavior caused by organicity occurs in public or intrudes on weaker, younger, or unwilling partners. However, clinical experience suggests that behavior modification therapy is possible and effective through sex education and directive techniques (sometimes with small doses of antipsychotic medication) that help implement external controls, allaying observer anxiety and improving the care of the afflicted men and women (Renshaw 1988b).

If a minor is molested by an older person, evaluation includes search for a previous history of such behavior because young pedophiles, exhibitionists, and voyeurs become old ones (Macnamara and Sagarin 1977). However, organic mental disorders also can lead to sexually deviant behavior.

Even if cognitive impairment is documented by the physician, a report to child protective authorities is mandatory by law. When an organic mental disorder is advanced, the patient's family may ask the court to consider them as personal guardians of the older family member. Family, neighbors, and children require education about the sexual disinhibition sometimes associated with cognitive impairment so that the patient can be told to stop, even by a 5-year-old.

When an institutionalized, cognitively impaired, elderly patient displays inappropriate or disinhibited sexual behavior in public, caregivers may feel needless concern about the potential for rape, even though coercive sexual behavior is rare in cognitively impaired older adults. Elderly persons usually are too frail and impaired to carry out rape or other inappropriate sexual behaviors. More common are verbal obscenities or clumsy sexual overtures to staff or to other impaired patients. Although the risk of such dangerous behavior is minimal, staff may be alarmed and fearful.

Management consists of performing a careful mental status examination, noting the sexual behaviors, having open staff discussion about the meaning and management of such behaviors, and introducing such behavioral techniques as extinction (nonattention if possible), firm limit setting, privilege reduction, and/or positive reinforcement for appropriate behavior.

Caregivers are instructed in specific approaches to deal with inappropriate sexual behavior. These approaches include anticipating repetition of the behavior, clearly defining staff members' roles, telling the patient to stop the sexual behavior while it is occurring, and using external controls if the initial verbal call proves ineffectual. Adjunctive use of small daily doses of psychotropic medication (haloperidol concentrate 0.5 to 1.5 mg b.i.d.) may enhance management of a particularly difficult to treat elderly patient.

Conclusion

There are occasional special situations that draw senior patients to clinicians for sexual help and guidance. The majority of seniors will seek sex counseling from their physicians about sexual questions and problems related to normal changes of aging in sickness and in health. Much can be done in these situations to provide a careful physical check, health care where needed, and reassurance when indicated. Brief sex therapy can be tried with a few 20-minute visits, or home reading can be suggested. Referral to a sexual dysfunction clinic may be necessary to provide further assistance if brief sex therapy and home reading fail.

References

American Psychiatric Association: Diagnostic and Statistical Manual of Mental Disorders, 4th Edition. Washington, DC, American Psychiatric Association, 1994

Annual Report, Loyola University Sexual Dysfunction Clinic, June 1995

Berger RN: Gay and Gray. Urbana, University of Illinois Press, 1982

Boller F, Frank E: Sexual dysfunction, in Neurological Disorders: Diagnosis, Management, and Rehabilitation. New York, Raven, 1982

Brecher, EM (ed): Consumer Reports Books: Love, Sex, and Aging.

Boston, MA, Little, Brown, 1983

Buffum J, Smith DE, Moser C, et al: Drugs and sexual function, in Sexual Problems in Medical Practice. Edited by Lief H. Monroe, WI, American Medical Association, 1981, pp 211–242

Butler R, Lewis M: Sex After Sixty. New York, Harper & Row, 1977

Cavallini G: Minoxidil versus NTG: a prospective double-blind controlled trial in transcutaneous erection facilitation for organic impotence. J Urol 146:50–53, 1991

Gibson, HB: Emotional and Sexual Lives of Older People: A Manual for Professionals. New York, Chapman & Hall, 1992

Hartmann U, Langer D: Combination of psychosexual therapy and intrapenile injections in the treatment of erectile dysfunctions: rationale and predictors of outcome. Journal of Sex Education and Therapy 19:1–12, 1993

Heaton JPW, Morales A, Owen J, et al: Topical glyceryltrinitrate causes measurable penile arterial dilatation in impotent men. J Urol 143:729–730, 1990

Kinsey AC, Pomeroy WB, Martin CE: Sexual Behavior in the Human Male. Philadelphia, PA, WB Saunders, 1948

Krauss DJ: Management of impotence, II: selected surgical procedures: penile prostheses. Clin Ther 9:149–156, 1987

Laaban JP, Bodenan P, Rochemaure J: Transdermal nitrate, penile erection, and spousal headache. Ann Intern Med 103:804, 1985

Macnamara DE, Sagarin E: Sex, Crime and the Law. New York, Free Press, 1977

Marsiglia W, Donnelly D: Sexual relations in later life: a national study of married persons. J Gerontol 46(6): S338–S344, 1991

Masters WH, Johnson VE: Human Sexual Response. Boston, MA, Little, Brown, 1966

Masters WH, Johnson VE, Kolodny RC: Sex and Human Loving. Boston, MA, Little, Brown, 1986

Nadig PW, Cookson MS: Long-term results with vacuum constriction device. J Urol 149:290–294, 1993

Nadig PW, Ware JC, Blumoff R: Noninvasive device to produce and maintain an erection-like state. Urology 2:126–131, 1986

Owen JA, Saunders F, Harris C, et al: Topical nitroglycerin: a potential treatment for impotence. J Urol 141:546, 1989

Poor M: The older lesbian, in Lesbian Studies. Edited by Crickshank M. Old Westbury, NY, Feminist Press, 1982

Ramsey KH: Elder sexual abuse: preliminary findings. Journal of Elder

Abuse and Neglect 3:78–90, 1991

Renshaw DC: Wives of impotent men. Consultant 19:41–48, 1979

Renshaw DC: Sex after coronary bypass surgery. Cardiology 4:46–48, 1987

Renshaw DC: Profile on 2,376 patients treated at Loyola Sex Clinic between 1972 and 1987. Sexual and Marital Therapy 3:111–117, 1988a

Renshaw DC: Sex and cognitively impaired patients. Consultant 28:133–137, 1988b

Renshaw DC: Seven Weeks to Better Sex. New York, Random House, 1995

Rogstad KE, Bignell CJ: Age is no bar to sexually acquired infection. Age Aging 20:377–378, 1991

Scott FB, Bradley WE, Timm GW: Management of erectile impotence: use of implantable inflatable prosthesis. Urology 2:80–82, 1973

Vacha K: Quiet Fire: Memoirs of Older Gay Men. New York, Crossing Press, 1985

Virag R: Intracavernous injection of papaverine for erectile failure (letter). Lancet 2(8304):938, 1982

Virag R, Shoukry K, Floresko J, et al: Intracavernous self-injection of vasoactive drugs in the treatment of impotence: 8-years experience with 615 cases. J Urol 145:287–293, 1991

Wagner G, Green R: Differential diagnosis of erectile failure, in Impotence, Physiological, Psychological, Surgical Diagnosis and Treatment. New York, Plenum, 1981, pp 114–118, 123–127, 151

Wagner G, Kaplan HS: The New Injection Treatment for Impotence. New York, Brunner/Mazel, 1993

Weisbord M: Our Future Selves: Love, Life, Sex and Aging. Toronto, Canada, Random House of Canada, 1991, p 202

Wennenberg JE, Mulley AG, Hanley D, et al: An evaluation of prostatectomy for benign urinary tract obstruction: geographic variations and the assessment of medical care outcomes. JAMA 259:3027–3030, 1988

Wise TN: Sexual disorders in medical and surgical conditions, in Clinical Management of Sexual Disorders. Edited by Meyer JK, Schmidt CW, Wise TN. Baltimore, MD, Williams & Wilkins, 1983, pp 317–332

Zilbergeld B: The New Male Sexuality. New York, Bantam, 1992

Zorgniotti AW, Lafleur RS: Auto-injection of the corpus cavernosum with a vasoactive drug combination for vasculogenic impotence. J Urol 133:39–41, 1985

SECTION IV

Treatment

Donald P. Hay, M.D.
Linda K. Hay, Ph.D.

Electroconvulsive Therapy

With more than one-half century of electroconvulsive therapy (ECT) use worldwide, and with many clinical and research studies completed, it is evident that ECT is a remarkably safe and effective treatment for several psychiatric illnesses, especially depressive disorders (Abrams and Essman 1982; American Psychiatric Association 1978, 1990; Fink 1979; Greenberg and Fink 1992; NIMH Consensus Conference 1985; Palmer 1981). Lack of familiarity with information on ECT has allowed fear and apprehension about this treatment to continue. However, progress is being made in educating the public and professionals about this often poorly understood procedure (Endler and Persad 1988; Hay and Hay 1990).

The frequency with which depression is encountered by psychiatrists, the increased vulnerability of older patients to side effects from pharmacotherapeutic agents, and the demonstrated safety and efficacy of ECT make this treatment especially suitable for use in elderly patients (Alexopoulos et al. 1984, 1989; Ancil and Holliday 1990; Atkinson et al. 1991; Avery and Winokur 1976; Benbow 1987; Bidder 1981; Burke et al. 1985; Cattan et al. 1990; Fogel 1988; Fraser 1981; Fraser and Glass 1980; Gaspar and Samarasinghe 1982; Godber et al. 1987; Hay 1989; Karlinsky and Shulman 1983; Meyers and Mei-tal 1985; Mielke et al. 1984; Raskind 1983; Regestein and Reich 1985; Rosenvinge 1991; Rubin et al. 1991; Salzman 1982; Weiner 1982, 1983).

The low risk of complications from ECT must be considered with the findings suggesting that depression itself can increase the mortality rate in elderly medical inpatients with severe physical illness (Koenig et al. 1989). Several reports indicate that elderly patients with major depressive illness respond to ECT as well as or better than younger individuals (Benbow 1987; Heshe et al. 1978; Stromgren 1973).

The efficacy of ECT in elderly patients is well established; the primary concern remains evaluation of the relative safety of ECT in older adults. The increased number of medical problems and the pharmacotherapy for these coexistent illnesses place older individuals at higher risk for side effects or complications from ECT. However, ECT frequently is considered the safest procedure for this population, especially when careful attention is given to the patient's medical state (Alexopoulos et al. 1984, 1989; Bidder 1981; Hay 1989; Huang et al. 1989; Regestein and Reich 1985; Weiner and Coffey 1988).

Indications

The indications for ECT in elderly patients generally are the same as those for younger patients. The American Psychiatric Association Task Force on electroconvulsive therapy listed affective disorders and certain forms of schizophrenia (e.g., schizoaffective and catatonic schizophrenia) as two of the primary indications for ECT (American Psychiatric Association 1978). Other indications for use of ECT, in addition to major depression and mania, include severe organic affective psychoses. These indications are defined by the 1990 Task Force, which reports that the efficacy of ECT does not diminish with advancing age and that ECT generally may be less risky than pharmacotherapy in this group. Major depressive disorder by far is the illness most frequently treated with ECT in the elderly population.

ECT's efficacy in treating major depressive disorder has been studied extensively: there have been comparison trials of ECT versus tricyclics, versus monoamine oxidase inhibitors (MAOIs), versus sham ECT, and in patients in whom antidepressant medications were ineffective (Kumar et al. 1991). The American Psychiatric Association Task Force on Treatments in Psychiatry summarized the literature and found that ECT is as effective for depression as, if not more effective than, all other treatment modalities (Welch 1989).

The syndrome of "depressive pseudodementia" with symptoms of disorientation and impaired cognition often is misdiagnosed as "profound dementia." Such individuals may respond well to a course of ECT and frequently tolerate this treatment better than antidepressant medication (Abrams 1992; Bright-Long and Fink 1993).

The clinical features that predict good outcome for ECT in the depressed elderly include mood disorder, guilt, psychomotor retardation, and coexistent symptoms of agitation and anxiety (Fraser 1981; Fraser and Glass 1980). Other indications for ECT in the depressed elderly include nonresponsiveness to psychotropic medication, serious suicidal risk, refusal to eat or drink resulting in malnutrition or dehydration, insomnia, history of better response to ECT than to other treatment, and the presence of delusions. A long duration of depressive illness correlates with a poorer outcome of ECT and of pharmacotherapy (Gaspar and Samarasinghe 1982; Karlinsky and Shulman 1983; Salzman 1982; Zorumski et al. 1988). A less favorable response has been noted in depressed individuals with other coexisting psychiatric syndromes, especially dementia or somatization disorder (Zorumski et al. 1988).

The issue of whether ECT would be safer or more effective as the first choice of treatment for depression has been reviewed but not answered. For patients with delusional depression, tricyclics alone have been found to be effective less than half the time, and although tricyclic-neuroleptic combinations can approach the efficacy of ECT in young adults (Spiker et al. 1986), these combinations are riskier and less well tolerated by elderly patients because of their greater vulnerability to orthostatic hypotension, tardive dyskinesia, drug-induced parkinsonism, and other side effects. Therefore, ECT can be considered a first choice for the delusionally depressed older patient (Fogel 1988; Meyers 1992; Welch 1989).

Similarly, nondelusional depression with somatic preoccupation and profound agitation may respond better and more rapidly to ECT than to antidepressants. Depression with vegetative signs but without the cognitive verbal expressions of dysphoria, such as may occur in Alzheimer's disease or poststroke disorders (Fogel 1988), is another psychiatric disorder in elderly patients that may benefit from ECT. Agitated depressed patients with moderate to severe dementia and patients with parkinsonism accompanied by psychosis and paraphrenia are other clusters of symptoms for which ECT may be effective (Fogel 1988). A retrospective study of elderly patients with dementia and major depression who were treated with ECT showed that they responded well to treatment (Nelson and Rosenberg 1991). Many published reports of the use of ECT show improvement of depression when present as a comorbity with dementia (Ancil and Holliday 1990; Bright-Long and Fink 1993;

Frances et al. 1989; Greenwald et al. 1989; Liang et al. 1988; Meyers and
Mei-tal 1985–1986; Nelson and Rosenberg 1991; Price and McAllister
1989; Reynolds et al. 1987; Snow and Wells 1981).

Risks

As with younger adult populations, there are no absolute contraindications
to ECT and the decision whether to proceed with this treatment requires an
assessment of the risk-benefit ratio of ECT with the risk-benefit ratio of not
using ECT (including the effects of continuing depression and the alternative treatments). Specific conditions that traditionally have been of concern
for the psychiatrist considering ECT include depression with coexisting cardiac illness (especially recent myocardial infarction), congestive heart failure, conduction abnormalities, hypertension, and impaired pulmonary
function. These illnesses may require specific medical measures prior to ECT
to lessen the risk of complications. One study of elderly patients identified
major risk factors to be cardiac failure, myocardial infarction in the previous
year, angina, stroke in the preceding 2 years, chronic renal failure, and significant arrhythmias or conduction disturbances (Gaspar and Samarasinghe
1982). Subsequent studies, however, have shown that most contraindications
to ECT are relative rather than absolute; ECT has been given successfully to
elderly poststroke patients within 1 month of the stroke (Murray et al. 1986).
Several additional reports have been documented of a variety of poststroke
patients receiving ECT successfully and without adverse reactions
(Alexopolous et al. 1984; Allman and Hawton 1987; Kwentus et al. 1984).
Note that ECT is effective and sometimes essential in poststroke patients
with depression. Although increasing age does not predispose to increased
complications from ECT, the comorbid conditions listed above occur with
greater frequency in elderly patients.

Increased intracranial pressure, such as that caused by brain tumor,
has been considered an absolute contraindication to ECT (Chen et al. 1989;
Welch 1989). Although use of ECT has been associated with untoward
consequences in the presence of a variety of cerebral diseases, knowledge
is limited based on the tendency to report adverse outcomes. There is not
a large body of systematic data on risks versus benefits in at-risk populations; but the successful use of ECT to treat carefully selected patients with
brain tumors in the absence of significantly increased intracranial pressure has been reported in a review by Alexopoulos et al. (1989).

Adverse Effects

The mortality risk of ECT has been estimated at approximately 3 to 4 per 100,000 treatments or per 10,000 patients treated (Abrams 1992; Fink 1979), and it may be even lower (Kramer 1985). The death rate from ECT is similar to that of anesthetic induction alone (Abrams 1992; Fink 1979). The leading cause of death associated with ECT is cardiovascular complication (reference). This risk of death from ECT with anesthesia is less than the risk of death from anesthesia with childbirth.

An ECT treatment rarely results in the treated individual experiencing prolonged seizure activity, status epilepticus, or other unusual behavioral manifestations. Although such consequences are unusual, a pretreatment electroencephalogram (EEG) may be useful for later comparison for patients with histories of seizures or who had prior atypical neurological responses to ECT.

Confusion after ECT treatments differs from patient to patient; the extent of any confusion depends on the variables of electrode placement, type of stimulus, length of seizure activity, number of previous treatments, and spacing between treatments. Less postictal confusion is reported after unilateral than bilateral electrode placement; it has been reported that reorientation usually occurs earlier after brief-pulse stimulation than after sine-wave stimulation (Abrams 1992).

Memory problems have been difficult to assess in depressed patients receiving ECT because of the effect of the depression itself on memory. This is a sensitive area in elderly patients because they are vulnerable to memory deficits caused by multiple system problems. It is important to be aware that treating depression often results in improved memory; therefore, preexisting memory impairment need not be considered a contraindication to ECT in elderly patients (Salzman 1982; Stoudemire et al. 1991). Numerous reports have concluded that bilateral ECT results in a greater degree of memory loss than unilateral ECT, and that brief-pulse right unilateral ECT appears to produce the least impairment of memory (Abrams 1992).

There have been many reports in the literature of individuals with preexisting cognitive deficits undergoing ECT without any worsening of confusion or memory difficulties (Demuth and Rand 1980; McAllister and Price 1982; Perry 1983; Snow and Wells 1981). Memory frequently may improve with ECT, notably as a result of the reduction of cognitive impairment associated with depression (Dubovsky et al. 1985). Another report described no differences between memory scores of patients under 45 from those 45 to 64 who had undergone ECT (Aronson et al. 1990). Other reports illustrate an age dependent effect of ECT on memory: they show more of an effect of ECT on memory in older patients, but this effect is mitigated by differences in older and younger populations and is less of an effect of age 6 months after ECT (Giordanni et al. 1992; Zervas et al. 1993).

Procedures

Consent

Patients with moderate-to-severe cognitive impairment will not be able to give informed consent. Most states require a court order before ECT can proceed, even though these patients may appear to acquiesce to treatment. In most states a court order is necessary even when there is a guardian or durable power of attorney.

Obtaining informed consent from an elderly patient may be complicated, especially if the patient is exhibiting symptoms of cognitive impairment. Major depression may limit competency to request or refuse treatment (Sullivan and Ward 1992). Treatment cannot begin if the patient does not consent to ECT. Legal assistance is required when patients are considered incompetent to give informed consent and refuse to do so, especially when delaying treatment is life threatening. A court order may be required as a lifesaving intervention. More frequently, however, the patient does not refuse ECT but is perceived as not having full cognition and appreciation of the procedure. In this situation, further in-depth discussions with the patient and the family may be essential to ensure adequate understanding by all. This discussion procedure may include a high degree of family involvement in decision making and extensive use of outside consultants to document decision incapacity and the need for treatment (Levine et al. 1991). Risks, benefits, and treatment alternatives are explained and the discussions are recorded in the patient's chart. Use of written, descriptive information about ECT, use of informed consent videotapes, and a second or third opinion from a psychiatrist who is not involved in the patient's care may be helpful. When the patient exhibits "mild" cognitive dysfunction and is agreeing to treatment, it is helpful to keep the patient and the family well informed and to request informed consent from all of them.

Pretreatment Assessment

Pretreatment assessment should include the same laboratory evaluation routinely done for younger adults. This assessment includes a chemistry screening panel, thyroid function tests (especially tests for thyroid-stimulating hormone), a urinalysis, an electrocardiogram, chest radiographs, and a physical and neurological (optional) examination; the primary care physician's opinion regarding medical stability for ECT should be recorded in the patient's chart. Specific evaluations may include complete spinal radiographs to apprise the psychiatrist of fractures, osteoporosis, or significant spinal degeneration requiring closer attention or precautionary measures (e.g., increased amounts of succinylcholine or increased support of the head and neck). Such radiographs document preexisting lesions; occasionally, calcified abdominal aortic aneurysms have been noted on radiographs of the spine, allowing the clinician to determine whether further evaluation or intervention is required (however, reports have noted no untoward effects in patients receiving ECT with either treated or untreated aneurysms [Abrams 1992]). In the presence of neurological findings, a computed tomography brain scan or magnetic resonance imaging scan alerts the practitioner to recent or old infarctions or other central nervous system lesions that may be contributing to the depression or cognitive dysfunction.

Obtaining an EEG prior to ECT is not recommended routinely but can be part of the diagnostic work-up of patients with evidence of intracranial disease. Once the ECT series is initiated, the changes brought about by the treatment (generalized slowing with increased amplitude) do not allow a reference baseline EEG until 30 days after the end of the series (Abrams 1992).

Careful evaluation of the dentition of the elderly patient prior to ECT is essential because many patients have dentures (partial or full) or loose or missing teeth. If there are no loose teeth and only a few teeth are missing, then it is safe to use a rubber semicircular bite block that helps to distribute the pressure of contraction of the masseter (the strongest muscle in the body). A semicircular rubber bite block should be used rather than a padded or rubberized tongue blade because direct stimulation of the temporalis muscles may not be blocked by succinylcholine, and in the elderly patient there is a greater risk of further loosening of teeth if the jaw pressure is focused at only one point (Abrams 1992).

Full or partial denture plates should be removed prior to ECT to prevent damage. However, there can be instances in which a partial plate surrounds and supports only a few or even just one tooth and its removal might result in damage to the unsupported teeth during the ECT. In situations such as these, a consultation with the patient's dentist (or hospital dentist) can determine the best way to proceed. It usually is preferable during the procedure to support the existing permanent teeth with the dentures if they are found to be strong enough to withstand the pressure. It is important that the anesthesiologist hold the jaw up against the bite block at the time of administering the stimulus; this measure prevents a sudden slapping of the jaw against the maxilla and prevents dental damage or biting of the lip.

If there is any question of the patient's physical status prior to ECT, a consultation should be obtained from the appropriate specialist. Consultation with a cardiologist, neurologist, anesthesiologist, orthopedist, rheumatologist, or other specialist may be indicated depending on the patient's physical state. If there is any question about appropriateness for ECT, another psychiatrist skilled in use of ECT can be consulted.

Electrical Stimulus

Stimulus dosing, alternative use of fixed dose versus titration methods, has been discussed in the recent literature. Sackeim et al. (1993) found that increasing the electrical dosage increases the efficacy of right unilateral ECT although not to the level of bilateral treatments. They also found that high electrical dosage is associated with a more rapid response (Sackeim et al. 1987a, 1987b, 1991, 1993). Other reports indicate that for most patients, especially elderly ones, higher energy levels than the seizure threshold are necessary (Fink 1989). Pettinati et al. (1990) found more improvement in patients with a fixed-high-dose ECT at a duration of between 2 and 3 seconds. Sackeim et al. (1992) reported that high levels of electrical stimulus may not be effective if the stimulus time is too short. Abrams et al. found a 68% reduction in Hamilton depression scores with 3-second stimulus compared with the 51% reduction in scores found with 1-second stimulus used by Sackeim. Abrams recommends a fixed-high-dose stimulus delivered over several seconds; Sackeim recommends the titration method.

Most studies indicate that the brief-pulse, square-wave stimulus is preferable to the sine-wave stimulus because the latter is thought to contribute to confusion and memory loss but not to the therapeutic effect (Abrams 1992). Research on wave form and stimulus intensity in ECT for elderly patients has been recommended; older patients have a higher seizure threshold and may have different patterns of physiological response to particular stimulus parameters (Fogel 1988).

Laterality of Stimulus

Although bilateral ECT is viewed by many to be the most effective form of treatment (Abrams et al. 1983), unilateral treatments are reported to be just as effective but without the side effects of memory loss and confusion (Fraser and Glass 1980; Kroessler 1985; Salzman 1982; Welch 1982). Many studies have reported equivalent efficacy of unilateral and bilateral ECT (Fogel 1988). No significant differences were noted in 29 depressed elderly patients receiving randomly assigned unilateral or bilateral ECT (Fraser and Glass 1980). Another study of elderly patients showed equivalent improvement but found the rate of recovery of respiration, consciousness, and orientation to be prolonged with bilateral treatments (Fraser 1981). One study of 122 elderly patients who received bilateral ECT with few problems argued that those who do not respond to unilateral treatments should be given bilateral ECT (Benbow 1987). Other studies indicate a greater number of missed seizures or a higher relapse rate associated with unilateral ECT (Pettinati and Nilsen 1985); some experts have recommended bilateral ECT as the treatment of choice for severely agitated, psychotic, and suicidal patients (Fogel 1988). Several reports have indicated increased efficacy of right unilateral ECT if it is administered with a supra-threshold stimulus greater than 75% of maximum device output (Abrams 1992). Unilateral ECT can be initiated in nonemergency cases and can be changed to bilateral treatment if improvement does not begin rapidly; unilateral placement is used also for patients who exhibit cognitive worsening during the course of treatment (Fink 1989).

Stimulus Dosage

Seizure threshold increases with age (Sackeim et al. 1987a); conversely, seizure duration decreases with age and number of treatments in the series (Sackeim et al. 1987a), and the stimulus dosage needs to be increased accordingly as seizure duration can be increased by increasing the energy of the ECT stimulus (Weiner 1979).

Treatment frequency varies; most practitioners in the United States and Canada provide three treatments per week on alternate days; in Great Britain treatments traditionally have been given twice per week (Fogel 1988). A double-blind study comparing the two methods reported the actual number of treatments required to reach improvement to be the same, with improvement occurring more rapidly in the three times per week group (Shapira et al. 1989). Some studies have reported that multiple treatments of ECT during one treatment session (multiple monitored ECT [MMECT]) may achieve the same degree of clinical improvement with the advantages of shorter treatment duration, fewer sessions of general anesthesia, fewer intravenous administrations, lower dosages of anesthetic agents, and a reduction in the time the patient is at risk for suicide (Berens et al. 1982). Other studies have reported that MMECT does not show increased efficacy over singly monitored ECT (Salzman 1982). However, a study of 44 elderly patients with severe depression found MMECT to be as safe and efficacious for elderly patients as for younger patients and that elderly patients tolerate multiple seizures as well as nonelderly patients; this finding suggests that MMECT may be used safely with elderly patients (Mielke et al. 1984). The question of whether this approach is more effective or, conversely, might be more toxic on a cardiovascular or neurological basis requires additional study. MMECT, given with unilateral high dosage brief-pulse stimuli (instead of the way it was initially studied), may prove to be extremely helpful for rapid treatment even if it is not found to increase cognitive impairment. Rapid treatment methods fit in well with managed care and medicare health care reforms and requirements.

The total number of ECT treatments required in a series for elderly patients usually is 6 to 9, although 12 or more treatments may be needed for complete remission (Fogel 1988). The potential for greater improvement must be weighed against the risk of anesthetic complications when deciding to continue any ECT series (Fogel 1988). Typically, treatment continues until the patient is symptom free unless side effects of confusion or significant memory loss become apparent.

Medications and Anesthesia

Premedication with an anticholinergic agent, such as atropine or glycopyrrolate, generally is recommended to diminish or block the direct vagal effects on the heart during and immediately after the electrical stimulus (Abrams 1992). The advantages of glycopyrrolate (a synthetic agent that does not enter the central nervous system) are the low likelihood of inducing postictal confusion (Abrams 1992; Kramer et al. 1986) and the reduced frequency of cardiac arrhythmias (Swartz and Saheba 1989). Regarding the necessity of atropinic premedication (Wyant and MacDonald 1980), a case report (Decina et al. 1984) of cardiac arrest in an elderly patient who received a β-blocker without pretreatment with an atropinic agent suggests that an atropinic drug should be used if a β-blocker may be administered during ECT.

The most commonly used anesthetic agent is methohexital. It reportedly induces fewer cardiac arrhythmias than thiopental (Abrams 1992; Pitts et al. 1965). Methohexital induces a shorter sleep time and less postanesthetic confusion (Egbert and Wolfe 1960; Osborne et al. 1963; Woodruff et al. 1968).

Adequate muscle relaxation during ECT is necessary to prevent strain on the cardiovascular system, prevent fractures in osteoporotic patients, and limit increases in blood pressure and heart rate (Salzman 1982). The muscle relaxant of choice is succinylcholine. It is given intravenously by rapid bolus push after the anesthetic at a dosage of 0.5 mg to 1.0 mg per kilogram of body weight (Abrams 1992). Higher doses of succinylcholine may be required for the elderly patient with a greater potential for fractures; the benefit needs to be weighed against potential complications for prolonged respiratory paralysis.

After administering the succinylcholine, the treatment team observes the patient for muscle fasciculations that begin in the neck region and travel to the legs and feet. Fasciculations in the gastrocnemius muscles and in the toes must be observed carefully; otherwise, those unaware that circulation in elderly patients often is slow may proceed to give ECT to patients who are not sufficiently paralyzed, placing them at greater risk of fracture. It is important, therefore, to establish the absence of the patellar deep tendon reflex and facial or radial nerve reflex (by means of a hand-held nerve stimulator), to observe the course and cessation of fasciculations, and to watch for abdominal relaxation (Baker 1986; Hay 1989).

Because elderly patients are more likely to exhibit an elevated seizure threshold, which often increases as the treatment series continues (Sackeim et al. 1987a), it is critical to determine that a seizure has indeed been induced; if not, it is necessary to re-treat with different settings or electrode placement while the anesthetic and muscle relaxant are still exerting their full effect. Failure to check for this may result in missed seizures, which may lead to the erroneous conclusion that the ECT treatment (or series) was ineffective.

The cuffing-off of an extremity prior to administration of succinylcholine to observe the presence of the seizure in the cuffed-off limb is extremely important, even if the ECT apparatus has a built-in EEG recording device. It may be difficult to tell from the EEG recording alone if a seizure has occurred, and the peripheral seizure has a different duration (usually shorter) than the centrally recorded one.

Oxygenation with 100% oxygen is essential since cerebral oxygen requirements are increased during a seizure (Abrams 1992; Abrams and Essman 1982). Pretreatment oxygenation may minimize side effects of memory loss and cardiac arrhythmias (Holmberg 1953; Posner et al. 1969; Salzman 1982). Elderly patients requiring ECT may have a higher frequency of respiratory difficulties (such as chronic obstructive pulmonary disease, emphysema, or asthma [Fawver and Milstein 1985]) that suggest evaluation of respiratory function and, when indicated, consultation with the anesthesiologist prior to initiation of the ECT series. The use of a pulse oximeter is required for all ECT treatments in the same way it is required for all anesthetic procedures. Theophylline has been reported to lower the seizure threshold; a case of status epilepticus as a complication of concurrent ECT and theophylline therapy has been reported (Peters et al. 1984). It is preferable, therefore, not to have theophylline as a medication during ECT and to use inhalers instead of theophylline when possible during the ECT series. The use of caffeine, however, as a seizure threshold lowering technique has been found to be effective and safe in elderly patients.

The cardiovascular system receives the most significant physiological stress from ECT. Tachycardia and hypertension develop in many elderly patients, and cardiac work increases significantly during the seizure. There can be an abrupt shift to bradycardia at the end of the seizure, and occasional potentially dangerous bradyarrhythmias can develop (Welch 1989). Various strategies of premedication have been proposed to prevent development of hypertension, tachycardia, rebound hypotension, bradycardia, and bradyarrhythmias. These premedications include nitroprusside, propranolol, and diazoxide (Fogel 1988; Regestein and Reich 1985; Weiner 1983). The most frequently recommended pre-ECT antihypertensives, labetalol and esmolol, are advantageous because of their short duration of action (Hay 1989).

Some elderly patients referred for ECT exhibit cardiac arrhythmias. Pretreating the patient with lidocaine may cause an elevation of the seizure threshold and prevent the induction of or shorten the duration of a seizure (Abrams 1992). Most arrhythmias noted before the ECT series begins are relatively benign premature ventricular contractions and need not be treated. Premature ventricular contractions sometimes are anxiety induced and tend to disappear after ECT. If they persist or worsen after the treatment, lidocaine or another antiarrhythmic such as verapamil can be administered. If the arrhythmia is of concern, and treatment of the arrhythmia appears to be indicated before ECT is initiated, cardiac consultation may be requested (Hay 1989).

It is the responsibility of the psychiatrist who administers the ECT to alert the anesthesiologist and the rest of the treatment team (recovery room nurses, psychiatric nurses for the patient's unit, nurse anesthetists) to the special needs of the elderly patient and to encourage the use of techniques conducive to a good and safe outcome: adequate preoxygenation, a rubber bite block instead of a padded tongue blade, adequate amounts of succinylcholine, observations for fasciculations and the absence of patellar and other reflexes, and the cuffing-off of the distal portion of an extremity before administering succinylcholine (Hay 1989).

Management of Concurrent Medication

Elderly patients referred for ECT may be receiving anticoagulation therapy; this raises the question of whether to continue warfarin during the ECT treatment. Studies suggest that it is preferable to continue warfarin anticoagulation throughout the ECT series rather than to switch to intermittent bolus heparin before and after, but not during, ECT (Hay 1987, 1989; Tancer and Evans 1989). Concurrent administration of ECT and various medications may pose problems. Lithium coincident with ECT may prolong the muscular blockade of succinylcholine; this has been implicated as causing acute confusional states (Abrams 1992).

Despite a report that concurrent treatment with tricyclics and ECT may improve the response of some elderly patients, most authors suggest that concurrent antidepressant treatment does not increase ECT response or may be associated with diminished affective improvement (Abrams 1975; Price et al. 1978; Siris et al. 1982). One report suggests that outcome may be improved for those patients who receive tricyclic antidepressant drugs concurrent with ECT (Nelson and Benjamin 1989).

Benzodiazepines increase the seizure threshold (Abrams 1992) and, therefore, should be tapered and discontinued, if possible, prior to ECT.

The use of monoamine oxidase inhibitors (MAOIs) during ECT has been avoided in the past because of the concern for the adverse interaction of the MAOI with anesthesia. Some authors suggest this precaution may be unnecessary (Abrams 1992), but they add that no therapeutic advantage has been noted from combining ECT and MAOIs.

Many older patients referred for ECT exhibit coexistent movement disorders of idiopathic Parkinson's disease, neuroleptic-induced parkinsonism, dystonia, akathisia, and tardive dyskinesia. Various studies have reported improvement in the movement disorder and in the affective illness being treated by ECT (Fink 1988; Hay et al. 1990).

Continuation or Maintenance ECT

Relapse after completion of a series of ECT treatments may approach 50% (even in patients receiving post-ECT maintenance medication) (Sackeim 1990). A customary approach is to place patients on an antidepressant drug or lithium after the ECT series. Continuation ECT, provided as an outpatient procedure at the conclusion of the ECT series, has been recommended for patients who have shown adequate improvement with a prior course of ECT and who have relapsed before within 6 months despite adequate maintenance antidepressant therapy (Abrams 1992). Continuation ECT may be recommended for patients with a poor pretreatment response to medication (Sackeim et al. 1990). Continuation ECT is begun approximately 1 week after the initial series is completed; thereafter, the interval is increased and the frequency of treatment decreased. The first continuation ECT treatment is given approximately 1 week after the last of the series; the second treatment is given 2 weeks later; the third, 3 or 4 weeks later; and so on. The interval is steadily increased so that the patient usually receives approximately 4 to 6 treatments over the 6-month period after the series.

Maintenance ECT is a similar series of decreasing frequency ECT treatments given on an outpatient basis after the initial treatment series. The maintenance series is initiated after a period when treatments are withheld until the patient becomes symptomatic. This is the usual course of treatment for the patient undergoing a first series because of the probability that the patient may not relapse if placed on prophylactic antidepressant medication. After a patient has received an initial series of ECT, been put on prophylactic antidepressant medication, and has relapsed, it is advisable to initiate continuation ECT after any future ECT series and not to wait for the patient to relapse.

Summary

Fifty-six years of experience with ECT have shown this treatment to be effective, safe, and—at times—a lifesaving procedure. The treating psychiatrist must identify those individuals whose symptoms are appropriate indicators for ECT and must administer ECT in a manner that minimizes side effects. The clinician needs to continue to be familiar with modern techniques of administering ECT including delivery of the stimulus, anesthesia, muscular relaxation, and ways of minimizing stress to the cardiovascular system.

ECT can be especially valuable for geriatric patients who have failed to respond to pharmacotherapy, those intolerant of the side effects of antidepressant drugs, the delusionally depressed, and patients (such as suicidal and/or malnourished persons) who need immediate relief from a life-threatening psychiatric illness.

References

Abrams R: Drugs in combination with ECT, in Drugs in Combination With Other Therapies. Edited by Greenblatt M. New York, Grune & Stratton, 1975, pp 157–164

Abrams R: Electroconvulsive Therapy, 2nd Edition. New York, Oxford University Press, 1992

Abrams R, Essman W: Electroconvulsive Therapy: Biological Foundations and Clinical Applications. New York, Spectrum Publications, 1982

Abrams R, Taylor MA, Faber R, et al: Bilateral versus unilateral electroconvulsive therapy: efficacy in melancholia. Am J Psychiatry 140:463–465, 1983

Alexopoulos G, Shamoian C, Lucas J, et al: Medical problems of geriatric psychiatric patients and younger controls during electroconvulsive therapy. J Am Geriatr Soc 32:651–654, 1984

Alexopoulos G, Young R, Abrams RC: ECT in the high risk geriatric patient. Convulsive Therapy 5:75–87, 1989

Allman P, Hawton K: ECT for post-stroke depression: beta blockade to modify rise in blood pressure. Convulsive Therapy 3:218–221, 1987

American Psychiatric Association Task Force Report on Electroconvulsive Therapy: Task Force Report No 14. Washington, DC, American Psychiatric Association, 1978

American Psychiatric Association Task Force Report on Electroconvulsive Therapy: The Practice of ECT: Recommendations for Treatment, Training, and Privileging. Washington, DC, American Psychiatric Association, 1990

Ancil RJ, Holliday SG: Treatment of depression in the elderly: a Canadian view. Prog Neuropsychopharmacol Biol Psychiatry 14:655–661, 1990

Aronson SM, et al: Short term memory effects of ECT in elderly versus young depressed inpatients. American Psychiatric Association Annual Conference Proceedings: Abstract #61. New York, 69, May 1990

Atkinson SD, Smith C, Smith EM, et al: Electroconvulsive therapy revisited. J Okla State Med Assoc 84:219–221, 1991

Avery D, Winokur G: Mortality in depressed patients treated with electroconvulsive therapy and antidepressants. Arch Gen Psychiatry 33:1029–1037, 1976

Baker NJ: Electroconvulsive therapy and severe osteoporosis: use of a nerve stimulator to assess paralysis. Convulsive Therapy 2:285–288, 1986

Benbow S: The use of electroconvulsive therapy in old age psychiatry. International Journal of Geriatric Psychiatry 2:25–30, 1987

Berens ES, Yesavage JA, Leirer VO: A comparison of multiple and single electroconvulsive therapy. J Clin Psychiatry 43:126–128, 1982

Bidder T: Electroconvulsive therapy in the medically ill patient. Psychiatr Clin North Am 4:391–405, 1981

Bright-Long LE, Fink M: Reversible dementia and affective disorder: the Rip Van Winkle syndrome. Convulsive Therapy 9:209–216, 1993

Burke W, Rutherford J, Zormuski C, et al: Electroconvulsive therapy and the elderly. Compr Psychiatry 26:480, 1985

Burke W, Rubin E, Zormuski C, et al: The safety of ECT in geriatric psychiatry. J Am Geriatr Soc 35:516–521, 1987

Cattan RA, Barry PP, Mead G, et al: Electroconvulsive therapy in octogenarians. J Am Geriatr Soc 38:753–758, 1990

Chen LS, McNamara JO, Maltby DA, et al: Effect of intranigral application of clinically affective anticonvulsants on electroshock induced seizure. Neuropharmacology 28:781–786, 1989

Decina P, Malitz S, Sackeim HA, et al: Cardiac arrest during ECT modified by beta-adrenergic blockade. Am J Psychiatry 141:298–300, 1984

Demuth GW, Rand BS: Atypical major depression in a patient with severe primary degenerative dementia. Am J Psychiatry 137:1609–1610, 1980

Dubovsky SL, Gay M, Franks RD, et al: ECT in the presence of increased intracranial pressure and respiratory failure: case report. J Clin Psychiatry 46:489–491, 1985

Egbert LD, Wolfe SW: Evaluation of methohexital for premedication in electroshock therapy. Anesth Analg 39:416–419, 1960

Endler NS, Persad E: Electroconvulsive Therapy: The Myths and the Realities. Toronto, Canada, Hans Huber Publishers, 1988

Fawver J, Milstein V: Asthma/emphysema complication of electroconvulsive therapy: a case report. Convulsive Therapy 1:61–64, 1985

Fink M: Convulsive Therapy: Theory and Practice. New York, Raven, 1979

Fink M: ECT for Parkinson's disease? Convulsive Therapy 4:189–191, 1988

Fink M: ECT: an adequate treatment? Convulsive Therapy 5:311–313, 1989

Fogel B: Electroconvulsive therapy in the elderly: a clinical research agenda. International Journal of Geriatric Psychiatry 3:181–190, 1988

Frances A, Weiner RD, Coffey CE: ECT for an elderly man with psychotic depression and concurrent dementia. Hosp Community Psychiatry 40(3):237–238, 242, 1989

Fraser R: ECT and the elderly, in Electroconvulsive Therapy: An Appraisal. Edited by Palmer R. New York, Oxford University Press, 1981

Fraser RM, Glass IB: Unilateral and bilateral ECT in elderly patients. Acta Psychiatr Scand 62:13–31, 1980

Gaspar D, Samarasinghe A: ECT in psychogeriatric practice: a study of risk factors, indications, and outcome. Compr Psychiatry 23:170–175, 1982

Giordanni B, Grunhaus LJ, Metler LE: Cognitive/behavioral effects of ECT in the elderly. APA 145th Annual Conference Proceedings Abstract:238–239. Washington, DC, May 1992

Godber C, Rosenvinge H, Wilkinson D, et al: Depression in old age: prognosis after ECT. International Journal of Geriatric Psychiatry 2:19–24, 1987

Greenberg L, Fink M: The use of electroconvulsive therapy in geriatric patients. Clinics in Geriatric Medicine 8:349–354, 1992

Greenwald BS, Kramer-Ginsberg E, Marin DB, et al: Dementia with coexistent major depression. Am J Psychiatry 146(11):1472–1478, 1989

Hay DP: Anticoagulants and ECT. Convulsive Therapy 3:236–237, 1987

Hay DP: Electroconvulsive therapy in the medically ill elderly. Convulsive Therapy 5:8–16, 1989

Hay DP, Hay LK: The role of ECT in the treatment of depression, in Depression: New Directions in Research, Theory, and Practice. Edited by McCann CD, Endler NS. Toronto, Canada, Wall & Emerson, 1990, pp 255–272

Hay DP, Hay LK, Blackwell B, et al: ECT and tardive dyskinesia. J Geriatr Psychiatry Neurol 3:106–109, 1990

Heshe J, Roeder E, Theilgaard A: Unilateral and bilateral ECT: a psychiatric and psychological study of therapeutic effect and side effects. Acta Psychiatr Scand Suppl 275:1–180, 1978

Holmberg G: The influence of oxygen administration on electrically induced convulsions in man. Acta Psychiatr Neurol Scand 28:365–386, 1953

Huang KC, Lucas LF, Tsueda K, et al: Age related changes in cardiovascular function associated with electroconvulsive therapy. Convulsive

Therapy 5:17–25, 1989

Karlinsky H, Shulman K: The clinical use of electroconvulsive therapy in old age. J Am Geriatr Soc 32:183–186, 1983

Koenig H, Shelp F, Goli V, et al: Survival and health care utilization in the elderly medical inpatients with major depression. J Am Geriatr Soc 37:599–606, 1989

Kramer BA: Use of ECT in California. Am J Psychiatry 142:1190–1192, 1985

Kramer BA, Allen RE, Friedman B: Atropine and glycopyrrolate as ECT preanesthesia. J Clin Psychiatry 47:199–200, 1986

Kroessler D: Relative efficacy rates for therapies of delusional depression. Convulsive Therapy 1:173–182, 1985

Kumar A, Mozley D, Dunham C, et al: Semiquantitative I-123 IMP SPECT studies in late onset depression before and after treatment. International Journal of Geriatric Psychiatry 6:775–777, 1991

Kwentus JA, Schultz SC, Hart RP: Tardive dystonia, catatonia, and electroconvulsive therapy. J Nerv Ment Disord 172:171–173, 1984

Levine SB, Blank K, Schwartz HI: Informed consent in the electroconvulsive treatment of geriatric patients. Bull Am Acad Psychiatry Law 19:395–403, 1991

Liang RA, Lam RW, Aniell RJ: ECT in the treatment of mixed depression and dementia. Br J Psychiatry 152:281–284, 1988

McAllister TW, Price TR: Severe depressive pseudodementia with and without dementia. Am J Psychiatry 139:626–629, 1982

Meyers B: Geriatric delusional depression. Clin Geriatr Med 8:299–308, 1992

Meyers B, Mei-tal V: Empirical study on an inpatient psychogeriatric unit: biological treatment in patients with depressive illness. Int J Psychiatry Med 15:111–124, 1985–1986

Mielke D, Winstead D, Goethe J, et al: Multiple-monitored electroconvulsive therapy: safety and efficacy in elderly depressed patients. J Am Geriatr Soc 32:180–182, 1984

Murray GB, Shea V, Conn DK: Electroconvulsive therapy for post-stroke depression. J Clin Psychiatry 47:258–260, 1986

Nelson JP, Benjamin L: Efficacy and safety of combined ECT and tricyclic antidepressant drugs in the treatment of depressed geriatric patients. Convulsive Therapy 5:321–329, 1989

Nelson JP, Rosenberg DR: ECT treatment of demented elderly patients with major depression: a retrospective study of efficacy and safety. Convulsive Therapy 7:157–165, 1991

NIMH Consensus Conference: Electroconvulsive therapy. JAMA 254:2103–2108, 1985

Osborne RG, Tunakan B, Barmore J: Anaesthetic agent in electroconvulsive therapy: a controlled comparison. J Nerv Ment Disord 137:297–300, 1963

Palmer R: Electroconvulsive Therapy: An Appraisal. New York, Oxford University Press, 1981

Perry GR: ECT for dementia and catatonia (letter). J Clin Psychiatry 44:117, 1983

Peters SG, Wochos DN, Patterson GC: Status epilepticus as a complication of concurrent electroconvulsive and theophylline therapy. Mayo Clin Proc 59:568–570, 1984

Pettinati HM, Nilsen S: Missed and brief seizures during ECT: differential response between unilateral and bilateral electrode placement. Biol Psychiatry 20:506–514, 1985

Pitts FN, Desmaris GM, Stewart W, et al: Induction of anesthesia with methohexital and thiopental in electroconvulsive therapy. N Engl J Med 273:353–360, 1965

Posner JB, Plum F, Van Poznak A: Cerebral metabolism during electrically induced seizures in man. Arch Neurol 20:388–395, 1969

Price TR, McAllister TW: Safety and efficacy of ECT in depressed patients with dementia: a review of clinical experience. Convulsive Therapy 5:1–74, 1989

Price TR, Mackenzie TB, Tucker GJ, et al: The dose response ratio in electroconvulsive therapy: a preliminary study. Arch Gen Psychiatry 35:1131–1136, 1978

Raskind M: Electroconvulsive therapy in the elderly. J Am Geriatr Soc 32:177–178, 1983

Regestein OR, Reich P: Electroconvulsive therapy in patients at high risk for physical complications. Convulsive Therapy 1:101–114, 1985

Reynolds CF, Pered JM, Kuper DJ, et al: Open-trial response to antidepressant treatment in elderly patients with mixed depression and cognitive impairment. Psychiatry Res 21(2):111–122, 1987

Rosenvinge H: The real value of electroconvulsive therapy in the elderly. Dementia 2:225–228, 1991

Rubin EH, Kinscherf DA, Wehrman SA: Response to treatment of depression in the old and very old. Journal of Geriatric Psychiatry and Neurology 4:65–70, 1991

Sackeim HA, Decina P, Prohovnik I, et al: Seizure threshold in electroconvulsive therapy: effects of sex, age, electrode placement, and number of treatments. Arch Gen Psychiatry 44:355–360, 1987a

Sackeim HA, Decina P, Portnoy S, et al: Studies of dosage, seizure threshold, and seizure duration in ECT. Biol Psychiatry 22:249–268, 1987b

Sackeim HA, Prudic J, Devanand DP, et al: The impact of medication resistance and continuation pharmacotherapy on relapse following response to electroconvulsive therapy in major depression. J Clin Psychopharmacol 10:96–104, 1990

Sackeim HA, Devanand DP, Prudic J: Stimulus intensity, seizure threshold, and seizure duration: impact on the efficacy and safety of electroconvulsive therapy. Psychiatr Clin North Am 14:803–843, 1991

Sackeim HA, Prudic J, Devanand DP, et al: Stimulus dosing strategies and the efficacy of unilateral ECT. Convulsive Therapy 8:46–52, 1992

Sackeim HA, Prudic J, Devanand DP, et al: Effects of stimulus intensity and electrode placement on the efficacy and cognitive effects of electroconvulsive therapy. N Engl J Med 328:839–846, 1993

Salzman C: Electroconvulsive therapy in the elderly patient. Psychiatr Clin North Am 5:191–197, 1982

Shapira B, Kindler S, Lere B: Treatment schedule and rate of response to ECT. Biol Psychiatry 25:106A–107A, 1989

Siris SG, Glassman AH, Stetner F: ECT and psychotropic medication in the treatment of depression and schizophrenia, in Electroconvulsive Therapy: Biological Foundation and Clinical Applications. Edited by Abrams R, Essman WB. New York, Spectrum, 1982, pp 91–112

Snow SS, Wells CE: Case studies in neuropsychiatry: diagnosis and treatment of coexistent dementia and depression. J Clin Psychiatry 42:439–441, 1981

Spiker DG, Dealy RS, Hanin I, et al: Treating delusional depression with amitriptyline. J Clin Psychiatry 47:243–245, 1986

Stoudemire A, Hill CD, Morris R, et al: Cognitive outcome following tricyclic and electroconvulsive treatment of major depression in the elderly. Am J Psychiatry 148:1336–1340, 1991

Stromgren LS: Unilateral versus bilateral electrotherapy: investigations into therapeutic effect in endogenous depression. Acta Psychiatr Scand 240:8–65, 1973

Sullivan MD, Ward NG: The woman who wanted electroconvulsive therapy and do-not-resuscitate status: questions of competence on a medical–psychiatry unit. Gen Hosp Psychiatry 14:204–209, 1992

Swartz CM, Saheba NC: Comparison of atropine with glycopyrrolate for use in ECT. Convulsive Therapy 5:56–61, 1989

Tancer M, Evans D: Electroconvulsive therapy in geriatric patients undergoing anticoagulation therapy. Convulsive Therapy 5:102–109, 1989

Weiner RD: The psychiatric use of electrically induced seizures. Am J Psychiatry 136:1507–1517, 1979

Weiner RD: The role of electroconvulsive therapy in the treatment of depression in the elderly. J Am Geriatr Soc 30:710–712, 1982

Weiner RD: ECT in the physically ill. Journal of Psychiatric Treatment and Evaluation 5:457–462, 1983

Weiner RD, Coffey CE: Indication for use of electroconvulsive therapy, in American Psychiatric Press Review of Psychiatry, Vol 7. Edited by Frances AJ, Hales RE. Washington, DC, American Psychiatric Press, 1988, pp 458–481

Welch CA: The relative efficacy of unilateral nondominant and bilateral stimulation. Psychopharmacol Bull 18:68–70, 1982

Welch CA: Electroconvulsive therapy, in Treatments of Psychiatric Disorders: A Task Force Report of the American Psychiatric Association. Edited by Karasu TB. Washington, DC, American Psychiatric Association, 1989, pp 1803–1813

Woodruff RA, Pitts FN Jr, McClure JN: The drug modification of ECT. Arch Gen Psychiatry 18:605–611, 1968

Wyant GM, MacDonald WB: The role of atropine in electroconvulsive therapy. Anaesthesia and Intensive Care 8:445–450, 1980

Zervas IM, Calev A, Jandorf L, et al: Age-dependent effects of electroconvulsive therapy on memory. Convulsive Therapy 9:39–42, 1993

Zorumski C, Rubin E, Burke W: Electroconvulsive therapy for the elderly: a review. Hosp Commun Psychiatry 39:643–647, 1988

Robert C. Young, M.D.
Barnett S. Meyers, M.D.

Psychopharmacology

G eriatric psychopharmacology is a broad field. It is a relatively new discipline, however, and the amount of available, clinically relevant empirical information is limited. Some texts (Jenike 1985a; Salzman 1992) and review articles (Meyers and Kalayam 1989; Rockwell et al. 1988; Shamoian 1988; Wragg and Jeste 1988) are helpful and so are discussions focusing on psychopharmacological issues from the perspectives of age and age-related disease effects on particular organ systems (Jarvik 1989; Jefferson and Greist 1979; Roose et al. 1987). Some discussions of general psychopharmacology include mention of geriatric issues (Janicak et al. 1993; Schatzberg and Cole 1986).

This chapter is organized around classes of treatments, rather than disorders, because specific agents are prescribed for many different disorders. The chapter emphasizes certain themes: 1) a thorough understanding of the geriatric patient is necessary for safe and effective pharmacotherapy, an accurate psychiatric diagnosis is necessary but not sufficient, and the clinician must obtain a thorough knowledge of the patient's physical health including the functioning of various physiological systems; 2) treatment is based on the specific situation, which includes the effects of age- and aging-related disease on a particular patient and on the medication being considered; and 3) the injunction to "start low and go slow" is neither sufficiently precise nor informed.

Particular attention is paid to the psychiatric implications of organic brain diseases. Psychopharmacology in these clinical situations is an important and evolving dimension of this field; the limited knowledge base is reviewed according to class of drug. Information in this chapter follows the suggestion of Leibovici and Tariot (1988) that the selection of drug class for syndromes in the context of organic brain disease follows the same strategy as for the analogous idiopathic syndromes.

A chapter on geriatric psychopharmacology must consider the 5% of elderly individuals who reside in long-term care facilities. The Nursing Home Reform Amendments to the Omnibus Budget Reconciliation Acts of 1987 (OBRA 1987) provided the Health Care Financing Administration with the mandate to regulate use of psychopharmacological agents in facilities accredited by Medicare. The initial focus on neuroleptic medications, designed to prevent the unnecessary use of medications for purposes of chemical restraint or the convenience of staff, was based on literature indicating misuse of antipsychotic medications in nursing homes at which a small number of physicians treat large numbers of patients (Ray et al. 1980). Subsequent data (Ray et al. 1987) demonstrated that older nursing home residents have a dose-related increase in risk of hip fractures in association with exposure to a number of categories of pharmacotherapeutic drugs, and these data contributed to the development of these regulations.

OBRA regulations, which are somewhat class specific, require that a physician review the indications for continued use of each psychopharmacological agent at specific intervals (every 3 months in the case of short-acting benzodiazepines and every 6 months for neuroleptics and antidepressants). The physician is expected to taper the medication or to document the rationale for maintaining the treatment. Side effects should be noted. Because compliance with OBRA regulations is reviewed annually by state surveyors, many nursing homes currently retain pharmacy consultants to ensure that compliance is maintained and that stiff penalties are avoided. Professional organizations have taken a leading role in conceptualizing and defining the appropriate use of pharmacotherapeutic medications (Board of Directors of the American Association for Geriatric Psychiatry, Clinical Practice Committee of the American Geriatrics Society, Committee on Long-Term Care and Treatment for the Elderly of the American Psychiatric Association 1992). This response occurred in part because of the pejorative wording and restrictive approach used in the Health Care Financing Administration's publication of guidelines (Health Care Financing Administration 1991).

General Considerations

Selecting a class of medication, choosing specific agents within classes, and determining dosages for elderly patients require very careful risk-benefit analyses.

Accurate diagnosis merits special attention because of the increased prevalence of physical diseases in elderly patients and because of the overlap between the signs and symptoms of physical diseases and those of primary psychiatric illness (Kathol and Perry 1981). Therefore, a thorough assessment of physical health status is essential. On the other hand, the presence of physical illness should not dissuade clinicians from treating psychopathology adequately.

As with young adults, pharmacological treatments have a role in acute symptom reduction, reversal of episodes of illness, and prevention of relapse and recurrence. Weighing the risks against the benefits of long-term pharmacotherapy is very important in geriatric patients; the increased vulnerability of these patients to medication side effects must be balanced against the morbidity of prolonged psychiatric illnesses. Late-life paranoid disorders, for example, are chronic illnesses (Kay 1962; Post 1966); chronicity and frequent relapses are common outcomes of geriatric depression (Alexopoulos et al. 1989; Baldwin and Holley 1986; Post 1972). Furthermore, chronicity and relapse have been associated with increased morbidity and mortality (Murphy 1983).

Compliance can be a special problem in elderly patients. Among ambulatory outpatients living independently, compliance can be compromised by lack of information, cognitive dysfunction, physical disability, and dissatisfaction with side effects and with complex drug regimens. Compliance with long-term drug therapy may be more problematic because the costs (financial and in terms of side effects) may be greater than the perceived benefits. More than 50% of geriatric patients fail to take medications as prescribed within 10 days of hospital discharge (Parkin et al. 1976), and compliance decreases further in subsequent weeks (Kruse et al. 1992). In outpatients, compliance decreases over time after a clinical visit (Cramer et al. 1990). Approximately 70% of patients on tricyclics miss 25%–50% of their daily dose (Kessler 1978). Lamy et al. (1992) provided commonsense guidelines for improving compliance in psychogeriatric patients by maximizing patient motivation through direct and open communication. Simple dosing strategies (once or twice daily) are preferable; dosage timing should minimize the experience of, and dysfunction from, side effects. Perel (1988) suggested using large deviations from previously established dose-to-plasma ratios to identify compliance, but this technique is most suitable for research use and is limited to medications for which blood level determinations are readily available. Finally, the psychiatrist should be aware of each medication's side effects and how these may change as a function of age. For example, older patients are less likely to develop acute dystonias from neuroleptic medications but are more vulnerable to bradykinesia and tremor (Salzman et al. 1970). Similarly, anticholinergic activity of low-potency neuroleptic drugs and tricyclic antidepressants (TCAs) can lead to severe constipation, fecal impaction, and, more rarely, paralytic ileus in older patients who have less physical activity and decreased bowel motility.

Principles of Clinical Pharmacology in Elderly Patients

Clinical thinking about drugs in elderly patients can be clarified by considering two distinct general conceptual issues: pharmacokinetics and pharmacodynamics. Pharmacokinetics can be described as the "effect of a patient on a drug"; pharmacodynamics as the "effect of a drug on a patient."

Pharmacokinetics and Aging

Pharmacokinetic factors determine concentrations of a drug in tissue compartments over time. Consideration of pharmacokinetic issues precedes consideration of pharmacodynamic differences, because much of the interindividual differences in response to drugs in mixed-age populations is accounted for by pharmacokinetic differences. Pharmacokinetics includes the component processes of absorption, distribution, and elimination; elimination involves both metabolism and excretion.

Absorption. Psychotropic drugs are well absorbed from the gastrointestinal tract by diffusion. Some physiological changes that occur with aging theoretically decrease drug absorption (see Table 27–1), and the rate of absorption of lipid soluble drugs may decrease with age. There is no evidence, however, that a clinically significant decrease in total absorption of psychotropic drugs occurs with normal aging in the absence of gastrointestinal disease (Israili and Wenger 1981).

Table 27–1. Effects of age on pharmacokinetics

Component	Age effect	Consequence
Absorption	Decreased gastric pH, motility; decreased intestinal surface area and blood flow	Decreased rate of absorption, but no apparent effect on total bioavailability
Metabolism	Decreased hepatic blood flow	Decreased metabolism
	Decreased activity of some catabolic enzymes	Increased plasma levels of medications requiring demethylation (e.g., tertiary amine TCAs, diazepam)
Distribution	Increase in fat/lean body ratio	Increased volume of distribution and prolonged half-lives of lipid-soluble drugs
	Decrease in albumin	Increased free fraction of benzodiazepines
	Increase in α-acid glycoprotein	Possible decreased free fraction of polycyclic antidepressants
Excretion	Decrease in renal glomerular filtration	Decreased clearance of lithium and hydroxy metabolites of antidepressants

Metabolism. The liver is the principal site for metabolic transformation of lipid-soluble psychotropic drugs. Metabolites can be pharmacologically active or inactive. Phase I metabolic pathways include demethylation, ring hydroxylation, and sulfoxidation. Conjugation of parent compound or metabolites (Phase II) produces generally inactive, water-soluble forms (e.g., glucuronides) that are cleared renally. The activity of the hepatic cytochrome P450 enzymes that moderate Phase I processes varies widely among individuals and has important genetic determinants. Some drugs are metabolized largely on the initial transit through the hepatic circulation (the "first-pass effect").

Age-associated effects on hepatic metabolism are outlined in Table 27–2. Some metabolic pathways (e.g., demethylation) may be influenced particularly by age (Abernathy et al. 1985), and these effects may contribute to increased plasma concentrations of particular drugs in elderly patients (e.g., tertiary amine TCAs [Nies et al. 1977] and benzodiazepines with active metabolites [Greenblatt and Shader 1981]). Other pathways,

Table 27–2. Effects of age-related diseases on pharmacokinetics

Component	Type of medical condition	Consequence
Absorption	Gastric or small bowel resection; heart failure; use of antacids	Possible decreased absorption
Metabolism	Severe liver disease; heart failure	Decreased metabolism
Distribution	Inflammatory states	Increased α-acid glycoprotein causing increased plasma total antidepressant levels
	Malnutrition; chronic illness; liver disease	Decreased binding proteins (albumin and α-acid glycoprotein)
Excretion	Renal failure; heart failure	Decreased clearance of lithium and hydrophilic metabolites

such as hydroxylation, may be less affected by age (Abernathy et al. 1985; Pollock et al. 1992). However, it is difficult to separate the effects of altered metabolism on drug plasma concentrations and half-lives from effects of changes in distribution and excretion.

Distribution. Drugs are distributed throughout the body in three compartments: fat tissue, body water, and binding to plasma proteins. The "volume of distribution" indicates how widely a particular drug is distributed in the body.

The distribution of particular drugs is determined in part by their lipid solubility. Most psychotropic drugs are highly lipid soluble; the notable exception is lithium, which is a hydrophilic ion. The increase in proportion of body fat to water with increasing age (Hollister 1981) increases the volume of distribution for lipid soluble psychotropic agents in elderly patients.

Psychotropic drugs, with the exception of lithium, are extensively bound to plasma proteins. Polycyclic antidepressants are bound extensively to α-acid glycoprotein, whereas benzodiazepines are bound predominantly to albumin (Curry 1981). Aging or age-associated factors can change intravascular protein concentrations; these changes may alter drug distribution (see Table 27–1).

Excretion. Psychotropic drugs are eliminated mainly by the kidneys. Renal excretion of lipid-soluble drugs occurs mainly as hydrophilic forms that are either glucuronide conjugated or unconjugated. For TCAs, hepatic hydroxylation followed by renal excretion is the major elimination pathway. The decrease in glomerular filtration that is associated with aging (Rowe 1980) accounts for part of the increased accumulation of hydrophilic metabolites in some elderly patients (Kitanaka et al. 1981; Nelson et al. 1988a; Young et al. 1984). This age-related decrease also leads to decreased clearance of lithium in elderly patients (Chapron et al. 1982; Hardy et al. 1987).

Related terms. *Clearance* refers to the volume of blood from which all drug is removed per unit of time. The *half-life* of a drug is the time required for half of the amount of drug to be eliminated; this is directly proportional to the volume of distribution and is inversely proportional to clearance.

Steady-state concentrations are obtained when the amount of a drug entering plasma on repeat administration balances its clearance. Such concentrations are directly proportional to dose, at a given dosing interval, and are inversely proportional to clearance. Steady-state concentrations are achieved after five or six half-lives of repeated administration. Age-related prolongation of the half-life of certain drugs increases the time required to achieve steady state concentrations.

Physical illness effects on pharmacokinetics. Elderly psychiatric patients frequently have one or more nonpsychiatric illnesses. These potentially can modify pharmacokinetics by decreasing absorption, altering the concentration of plasma proteins, slowing hepatic metabolism, or diminishing renal clearance (see Table 27–2). Drugs and restricted diets used for managing physical disorders also may interact with psychotropic medications. Such interactions can occur at a pharmacokinetic level; the concentration of either the psychotropic or nonpsychotropic drug, or of both drugs, can be affected. Such influences on psychotropic drugs may or may not be clinically significant. These influences include decreases or delays in absorption, displacement from binding proteins, increases or decreases in hepatic metabolism, and decreases in renal excretion. Salzman's text (1992) lists possible interactions. Important examples are given in Table 27–3 and are described below in the sections that discuss specific drugs.

Pharmacodynamics and Aging

In addition to having different pharmacokinetic characteristics, individuals may differ in tissue response to a given concentration of drug, or pharmacodynamics. Age-associated changes occur in peripheral and

Table 27–3.   Examples of pharmacokinetic drug interactions

Drug interaction	Consequence
Phenothiazines, tricyclics, or benzodiazepine with antacids	Decreased absorption
Tricyclics with methylphenidate	Inhibition of tricyclic metabolism
Tricyclics or benzodiazepines with cimetidine	Decreased tricyclic or benzodiazepine metabolism
Tricyclics with barbiturates, carbamazepine, and hydantoin	Induced tricyclic metabolism
Lithium carbonate with thiazide diuretics or nonsteroidal anti-inflammatory agents	Decreased lithium excretion

central neurotransmitters and organ systems. These changes may alter therapeutic and toxic effects of drugs at a given concentration.

Age effects have been reported on responses to acute administration of pharmacological agonists and some psychotropic agents. These effects include blunted prolactin response to neuroleptic medications (presumably related to altered dopaminergic neurotransmission) (Rolandi et al. 1982), decreased response of peripheral β-adrenergic receptors to agonist drugs (Vestal et al. 1979), and decreased noradrenergic response to desipramine administration (Bickford-Wimer et al. 1987).

There is little empirically derived information concerning age-related differences in behavioral response to pharmacological challenge. Increased sensitivity of elderly patients to cognitive effects of diazepam has been reported (Pomara et al. 1984; Reidenberg et al. 1978).

Considerations of pharmacodynamics are complex for several reasons. Most psychotropic drugs interact with many neurotransmitter systems, these neurotransmitter systems themselves interact, and biological consequences of drug action change as a function of time during chronic administration.

The concept that older persons have increased sensitivity to toxic effects of psychotropic drugs administered at conventional doses and concentrations comes from case reports of adverse reactions; systematic studies of this question are lacking. It is possible, but also remains to be demonstrated, that geriatric patients have a narrower margin between therapeutic and toxic doses or concentrations. Similarly, clinical lore that therapeutic effects of psychotropic drugs generally occur at lower doses or concentrations in elderly patients have not been supported by empirical studies. It is not known whether elderly patients treated with a broad range of plasma concentrations of TCAs or lithium have the same concentration-response relationship as younger adults. Studies assessing whether elderly patients respond to concentrations comparable to those effective in young adults will be discussed in sections related to the specific agents.

The increased risk of falls in older patients receiving pharmacotherapeutic agents results from the pharmacodynamic properties of their medications interacting with physiological changes related to aging. Falls can be mediated through the adverse reactions of orthostatic hypotension, extrapyramidal side effects, ataxia, and impaired cognition. The public health importance of falls in older patients is supported by data demonstrating that approximately 5% of falls in older individuals result in fractures (Tinetti 1987). Falls are the most frequent cause of death by injury in late life (Baker and Harvey 1985); they contribute to more than one-third of admissions to nursing homes (Wild et al. 1980). An increased incidence of falls has been associated with use of a number of pharmacotherapeutic agents (including antidepressants, antipsychotics, and benzodiazepines) in studies of older outpatients (Tinetti 1987) and residents of nursing homes (Tinetti et al. 1988). Ray et al. (1987) used epidemiological data to demonstrate a dose-response relationship between the incidence of hip fractures and use of psychotropics in residents of long-term care facilities. Thus, aging-related pharmacodynamic effects that predispose to falls may lead to secondary morbidities and mortalities.

Physical-neurological illness effects on pharmacodynamics. Certain brain disorders in elderly patients are associated with additional neuronal changes and may thereby influence drug effects. Such illnesses include Parkinson's disease, cerebrovascular disease, and primary degenerative dementia. Evidence for central disruption of biogenic amine and acetylcholine neurotransmitter systems by these disorders has been summarized (Addonizio 1987; Meyers and Young 1989). Clinically relevant manifestations include increased sensitivity of patients with Parkinson's disease to neuroleptic-induced exacerbation of motor dysfunction and to anticholinergic delirium (Figiel et al. 1989), and sensitivity of dementia patients to the sedative side effects of these agents (Sunderland and Silver 1988). The psychiatrist who prescribes a neuroleptic drug to treat agitation or psychosis in a patient with Parkinson's disease must recognize that this treatment can aggravate dopaminergic dysfunction and can increase neuromuscular symptoms. Alternative approaches of lowering the dosage of an antiparkinsonian medication (e.g., L-dopa) that could be causing the psychiatric signs and symptoms, or using new generation antipsychotics, should be considered.

Drug-drug interaction at the pharmacodynamic level. Drugs for medical or neurological disorders can interact with psychotropic agents at the pharmacodynamic level. Examples of such interactions, provided in Table 27–4, include instances in which drug interactions are additive (e.g., anticholinergic effects from low-potency neuroleptic medications add to those of antiparkinsonian drugs) and those in which there is inhibition of the effect of one class of agents by those of another (e.g., guanethidine and phenothiazines or TCAs).

Types of Antidepressant Drugs

Among antidepressant agents, the TCAs have been first-line agents for pharmacotherapy of depressive syndromes in older and younger patients (see Table 27–5 for antidepressant drugs marketed in the United States). Other polycyclic agents, and other drugs, have been introduced in the United States market in recent years. Monoamine oxidase inhibitors (MAOIs) have received renewed attention as clinically useful alternatives. Stimulant drugs are occasionally used in depressed patients, but systematic studies of their efficacy for major depression are unavailable.

Tricyclic Antidepressants

Indications

These drugs are of central importance in treating acute unipolar and bipolar major depressive disorders. TCAs also are indicated for continuation and maintenance treatment in major depression.

Efficacy

Rockwell et al. (1988) reviewed 17 controlled acute treatment studies of polycyclic antidepressants in patients older than 60 years. Twelve involved TCAs; six of these (Branconnier et al. 1982; Cohn et al. 1984; Georgotas et al. 1989; Gerner et al. 1980; Meredith et al. 1984; Wakelin 1986) used placebo control and demonstrated therapeutic superiority to placebo. The six TCA studies that did not use placebo control involved comparisons with "second generation" antidepressants. All of these TCA studies except that of Georgotas et al. (1986) dealt with tertiary amines.

Table 27–4. Examples of pharmacodynamic drug interactions

Drug interaction	Consequence
Tricyclics, neuroleptic medications, or benzodiazepines with other sedative drugs	Increased sedative effect
Tricyclics or low-potency neuroleptic medications with antihypertensives	Increased vulnerability to orthostatic hypotension
Tricyclics and phenothiazine with guanethidine	Blockage of neuronal uptake prevents activity of either agent
Tricyclics with clonidine	Competition at α_2 receptor may interfere with activity of either agent
Lithium with neuroleptic medications	Increased extrapyramidal side effects
Tricyclics with quinidine	Increased quinidine-like effects; decreased cardiac conduction

The secondary amine TCAs nortriptyline and desipramine are especially useful in elderly depressed persons because of the side effect profile of these drugs (see below). Georgotas et al. (1986) demonstrated superiority of nortriptyline to placebo in ambulatory geriatric depressed patients. Nelson et al. (1985) reported that elderly patients with melancholic depression require and respond to plasma desipramine levels comparable to those effective in younger adults.

Salzman et al. (1993) reviewed efficacy data from studies that included and identified patients 75 years and older. Their findings, based on a review of the 171 patients identified, suggest that some (but not all) of the oldest old patients demonstrate only a modest therapeutic benefit from standard antidepressant treatment; the authors call for additional studies of this age group. Continuation treatment is designed to prevent relapse of the index episode during the first 6 months of therapy. Georgotas et al. (1989) prospectively treated recovered elderly patients with major depression for 4 to 8 months with nortriptyline at an average dose of 80 mg per day. Only 17% of the patients completing nortriptyline treatment continuation experienced relapses. Similarly, Reynolds et al. (1992) reported that 24% of patients continued on nortriptyline for 16 weeks after recovering from an episode of major depression experienced a recurrence during a 4-week to 6-week period of discontinuation; in comparison, none of the 24 patients who continued on nortriptyline during this period experienced another depressive episode.

Table 27–5. Antidepressant drugs marketed in the United States

Classes	Examples
Cyclic antidepressants	
Tertiary amine tricyclic	Amitriptyline, imipramine, doxepin
Secondary amine tricyclic	Nortriptyline, desipramine, protriptyline
Heterocyclic antidepressants	Maprotiline
Monocyclic antidepressants	Bupropion
Selective serotonin reuptake inhibitors	Fluoxetine, sertraline, paroxetine
Noradrenaline-serotonin reuptake inhibitor	Venlafaxine
Others	Trazodone, amoxapine, nefazodone
Monoamine oxidase inhibitors	Phenelzine, tranylcypromine, selegiline
Stimulants	Dextroamphetamine, methylphenidate

Maintenance treatment is defined as the use of medication beyond the continuation interval to prevent the occurrence of new episodes. Georgotas et al. (1989) found the recurrence rate over 1 year was 13.3% for phenelzine and more than 50% for nortriptyline; the latter did not differ from placebo. Of note, interim analyses of additional data from this research group indicated prophylactic efficacy in individuals maintained on nortriptyline (A. Georgotas, personal communication). Similarly, an open study by Reynolds et al. (1989) reported a low rate of recurrence (14.7%) over a 3-year period in older patients experiencing major depression who were maintained on higher plasma levels of nortriptyline following successful hospital treatment for major depression.

Practical Guidelines

Pretreatment assessment. Treatment history concerning previous successful or unsuccessful drug trials guides selection of particular agents. Adequacy of prior treatment efforts needs to be assessed by noting drug dose, duration of administration, and drug blood levels. Therapeutic response needs to be judged, and any treatment-limiting side effects need to be noted. Clinicians can make use of psychopathology rating scales to help monitor change during treatment. For example, the Hamilton Depression Rating Scale (HDRS) (Hamilton 1960) is applicable for rating depressive signs and symptoms in cognitively intact patients. The Cornell Scale (Alexopoulos et al. 1988) is useful for elderly patients with cognitive impairment. The 30-item Geriatric Depression Rating Scale is a self-report instrument with established reliability and validity for identifying geriatric depression (Yesavage et al. 1983).

Cognitive function should be evaluated before and during treatment. The Mini-Mental State Exam (Folstein et al. 1975) is a convenient and widely used instrument for screening although it has limited sensitivity. Instruments that are more sensitive and more detailed can be used (e.g., the Dementia Rating Scale [Mattis 1988]).

The importance of an initial complete "review of systems" derives in part from the fact that side effects can be related to psychopathological or pathophysiological state. It is critical to compare physical complaints evaluated during treatment with complaints before treatment to judge whether these complaints represent drug toxicity.

Blood pressure assessment before and during treatment should include determination of orthostatic change. Baseline measurement of orthostatic blood pressure change is especially important because pretreatment orthostatic changes predict changes that occur during TCA treatment (Glassman et al. 1979).

Laboratory assessment includes an electrocardiogram. Ischemia, dysrhythmia, and conduction abnormalities need to be assessed in planning antidepressant pharmacotherapy.

Pretreatment assessment guides evaluation of antidepressants and selection of the proper medication. Secondary amine TCAs, specifically nortriptyline and desipramine, have advantages over tertiary amine TCAs for use in elderly patients. They have less anticholinergic and sedative potency, which may be related to diminished affinities for muscarinic, histaminic, and adrenergic receptors (Richelson 1982). Nortriptyline has a relatively low potential for inducing orthostatic hypotension (Roose et al. 1981). The use of protriptyline is complicated by its long half-life.

Dosing

Treatment is initiated at a low dose that is increased gradually. The target dose can be achieved in 1 to 2 weeks in most cases, but each patient's tolerance of side effects must be considered. Gradual increments allow patients to become accustomed to side effects and may increase compliance. There is no systematic evidence that divided dose administration is more effective or produces less toxicity than a single dose. A single nighttime dose usually is well tolerated and improves sleep.

Duration of treatment required for adequate response in elderly patients experiencing major depression may be somewhat longer than in younger adults (Georgotas et al. 1986), although early reduction in symptoms may predict good outcome (Jarvik and Mintz 1987). Some patients may require at least 9 weeks for symptoms to resolve (Georgotas et al. 1989). Duration of treatment to achieve optimal acute response in elderly patients has not been studied sufficiently, and some investigators recommend extending medication trials to 8 weeks in this age group.

The optimal target dose for elderly patients is not well delineated for any agent. Clinical studies show that older patients respond to doses and steady-state plasma levels of nortriptyline and desipramine that are comparable to those effective in younger adults (i.e., 50 to 150 ng/ml of nortriptyline and more than 125 ng/ml of desipramine (Georgotas et al. 1986; Nelson et al. 1985). Low steady-state plasma levels should not be treated, however, in patients who respond well.

Increased plasma 10-hydroxynortriptyline-to-nortriptyline ratios (Young et al. 1984) and plasma 2-hydroxy-desipramine-to-desipramine ratios (Kitanaka et al. 1981; Nelson et al. 1988a) have been reported in elderly patients. These compounds have pharmacodynamic activity that may influence efficacy (Nelson et al. 1988b; Young et al. 1987; Young 1991).

An early study using imipramine in outpatients experiencing major depression suggested response at low dosage of imipramine (Gerner et al. 1980), but this investigation was hampered by lack of imipramine plasma levels. Tertiary amine TCA concentrations often are increased per milligram dose in elderly patients. In contrast, plasma concentrations of secondary amine TCAs per milligram dose often overlap those in younger patients.

Although patients occasionally fail to respond to an antidepressant that was effective previously, there is no body of evidence that tolerance to therapeutic effects develops after prolonged use. Most patients fail to respond because they have not been treated adequately (Lydiard 1985). The possibility that an undiagnosed medical condition is presenting as a clinical depression must be reconsidered in nonresponders. Treatment resistance has been defined as lack of response to adequate blood levels for at least 4 weeks in young adults; longer duration may be appropriate for such a definition in elderly patients. Reviews of approaches used to overcome this clinical impasse in young adults (Extein 1989) and elderly patients with depression (Goff and Jenike 1986) are available.

Switching between agents with different types of neurotransmitter activity (e.g., from desipramine, which is noradrenergic, to fluoxetine, which is serotonergic) has theoretical appeal but is not supported by clinical trials. Switching to another class of agents (e.g., from a TCA to an MAOI) can be effective, but the conservative approach of waiting 2 weeks between discontinuing the TCA and starting the MAOI is recommended; a longer hiatus might be considered in the oldest old patients or if the TCA is a tertiary amine. The use of lithium augmentation before making this change ensures that there is an active mood stabilizer at work during the pharmacological waiting period.

Joffe et al. (1993) reported efficacy of lithium augmentation in mixed-age adults in a placebo controlled study, but there are limited data concerning the risk-benefit ratio of lithium augmentation in geriatric major depression. van Marwijk et al. (1990) reported therapeutic benefit in 33 of 51 geriatric patients, although serious side effects occurred in 20%. Zimmer et al. (1991) found equivocal benefit and noted side effects; however, the study design may not have been optimal for detecting benefit.

Potentiation of response to TCA by adding triiodothyronine (T_3) has been demonstrated in mixed-age adults (Joffe et al. 1993). The appropriateness of this strategy for treatment-resistant geriatric depression remains to be determined. The older patient's cardiac status is of special concern when using thyroid augmentation because increasing heart rate and cardiac work can lead to coronary insufficiency in patients with marginal cardiac status; consultation with the patient's cardiologist prior to instituting thyroid augmentation is recommended. The possible presence of subclinical hypothyroidism (elevated thyroid-stimulating hormone with normal T_3 and thyroxine T_4 values) should be considered in cases of treatment resistance or incomplete response. Intervention with supplemental thyroid medication involves consultation with the patient's primary care physician.

Combination of selective serotonin reuptake inhibitors (SSRIs) with standard TCAs may augment efficacy (Nelson et al. 1991; Weilburg et al. 1989). This strategy has been reported to be effective in a series of elderly patients with depression (McCue and Aronowitz 1994). Combination treatment with either fluoxetine or paroxetine can increase TCA blood levels markedly through inhibiting hepatic metabolism (Crewe et al. 1992). Sertraline has been found to have a similar inhibitory effect in vitro (Crewe et al. 1992), but an in vivo study demonstrated approximately 30% increases in plasma desipramine levels in association with sertraline compared with fourfold increases with fluoxetine (Preskorn et al. 1992).

Dosing in continuation and maintenance treatment requires study in geriatric patients. Data from the young adult literature indicates that higher plasma levels are associated with lower rates of recurrence (Frank et al. 1990). Furthermore, reduction to half the acute dosage markedly increases the likelihood of a new episode (Frank et al. 1990). Reynolds et al. (1992) reported much lower rates of recurrence in elderly patients with depression during high dose nortriptyline maintenance (levels = 116 ± 17 ng/ml) than Georgotas et al. (1989) had found at lower levels (90 ± 1 ng/ml).

Toxicity

Elderly patients with osteoporosis and coronary artery disease have a high risk of orthostatic hypotension. Orthostatic hypotension is not correlated with age (Glassman et al. 1979), but it can be more severe and have serious consequences in patients with decreased cardiac output and/or those treated with diuretics or β-blockers (Glassman et al. 1983). Orthostatic hypotensive effects can occur early in treatment at low doses and low plasma concentrations of tertiary and secondary amine TCAs.

TCAs may increase heart rate. The magnitude of the increase is dependent on baseline rate and usually is small. Such increases typically are associated only weakly with plasma TCA concentration (Glassman and Bigger 1981). Ischemia can be exacerbated, however, by tachycardia. Faced with significant tachycardia, clinicians may add selective β-blockers or may change antidepressant treatment.

Quinidine-like Type I antiarrhythmic effects of TCAs delay conduction through the His-Purkinje system and can produce heart block in patients with underlying conduction abnormalities (Roose et al. 1987). The limited data available for TCAs indicate prolongation of conduction peaks after 3 or 4 weeks of treatment (Glassman and Bigger 1981); this suggests that patients with borderline conduction defects before treatment should have weekly ECGs for the first 4 weeks on TCAs; then routine monitoring can be resumed. Conduction effects of TCAs are dependent on plasma drug concentrations in elderly and young adult patients (Glassman and Bigger 1981). Increased plasma concentrations of hydroxylated metabolites can contribute to such effects when they occur in elderly patients (Kutcher et al. 1986; Schneider et al. 1988; Young et al. 1985).

Glassman et al. (1993) called for studies of the risk-benefit ratio of TCAs and other antidepressants in elderly patients with ischemic heart disease. Recent studies of nonpsychiatric patients treated with specific Class I antiarrhythmic drugs after experiencing postmyocardial infarction ventricular arrhythmias have demonstrated increased rather than decreased cardiac mortality associated with continued prophylactic treatment, presumably in association with new ischemic events (Echt et al. 1991). The implications for use of maintenance TCA treatment of elderly depressed patients, a population at risk for myocardial infarctions, have yet to be determined.

Adverse effects on cognitive performance have been reported at high plasma TCA concentrations in mixed-age adults (Preskorn and Simpson 1982) and are concentration dependent in elderly patients with depression treated with nortriptyline (Young et al. 1991). However, TCA-induced delirium occurs far less frequently in elderly patients than previously thought and usually is associated with extremely high blood levels (Meyers 1991). A discontinuation study demonstrated that subjectively impaired memory functioning at therapeutic nortriptyline levels disappeared on placebo; memory complaints on nortriptyline occurred in association with delayed storage of novel information (Meyers 1991).

Additional Clinical Situations

Delusional symptoms are relatively common among elderly patients with major depression. The pharmacological treatment approach to the delusionally depressed elderly patient is not well studied. Mixed-age, delusionally depressed adults treated with TCAs alone respond less well than do nondelusional patients (Glassman et al. 1975). Combination of neuroleptic and antidepressant drugs is necessary for optimal response in many of these patients, and response rates to combined treatment can approach those in patients treated with electroconvulsive therapy (ECT) (Nelson and Bowers 1978; Perry et al. 1982; Spiker et al. 1985). Elderly patients may not tolerate aggressive combination treatment, however, particularly with the high neuroleptic doses associated with effectiveness (Nelson et al. 1986; Spiker et al. 1985), and use of ECT as an initial treatment may be preferable.

Depression Associated With Brain Disease

A recent study showing that imipramine treatment of Alzheimer's patients was associated with improved Mini-Mental State Exam (MMSE) scores in depressed patients, with no decrease in MMSE scores in patients without depression, and with no cases of delirium (Reifler et al. 1989) disputes the clinical lore that the central cholinergic deficits associated with Alzheimer's disease precludes use of TCAs in this population; however, depressed and nondepressed imipramine-treated patients in this study demonstrated significant decreases on the Mattis Dementia Rating Scale (Mattis 1988), a more sensitive measure of cognitive functioning. Consistent with these data, Reynolds et al. (1987) reported that geriatric depression associated with cognitive impairment improves in response to nortriptyline treatment and to ECT; improvement in dementia scores correlated with decreases in severity of depression. Whether optimal antidepressant doses or concentrations are the same in cognitively impaired patients and patients with dementia as in intact patients remains to be determined (Young et al. 1991).

Patients with poststroke depression tolerate and respond to nortriptyline (Lipsey et al. 1984). The doses used were comparable to those used to treat young adults with depression.

Monoamine Oxidase Inhibitors

Indications

Monoamine oxidase inhibitors (MAOIs) are indicated for acute treatment of unipolar and bipolar major depressive episodes. They can be used in continuation and maintenance pharmacotherapy. Although the fact that platelet and brain monoamine oxidase activity can increase with increasing age (Robinson 1981) is consistent with the use of MAOIs in geriatric patients, the clinical significance of such changes is unknown.

Recent trends include developing MAOIs that are more pharmacologically selective against MAO-A or MAO-B and, therefore, produce differential augmentation of concentrations of the neurotransmitters metabolized by these enzymes. MAOIs that are cleared more rapidly, called reversible MAOIs or RIMAs, are becoming available. Differences in indications for these compared with nonselective MAOIs await definition.

Efficacy

Experience with MAOIs in elderly patients has been reviewed by Rockwell et al. (1988). The acute efficacy of phenelzine in ambulatory elderly patients with an "endogenous" symptom profile experiencing major depression was found superior to placebo and comparable to nortriptyline (Georgotas et al. 1986).

Other MAOIs have received limited study in acute treatment of geriatric major depression. Harris and Hoelscher (1961) reported a placebo-controlled trial of tranylcypromine in which efficacy was demonstrated in a clinically heterogeneous patient group. Harris and Hoelscher (1961) reported superior response to isocarboxazid compared to placebo in a nursing home sample of depressed patients.

Moclobemide, an RIMA in widespread use outside the United States, has specificity for MAO-A (Freeman 1993); it primarily alters noradrenaline and serotonin oxidative metabolism and, to a lesser extent, tyramine and dopamine oxidative metabolism. Moclobemide has been reported equally effective in the acute treatment of geriatric depressed patients when compared to maprotiline (De Vanna et al. 1990) and mianserin (De Vanna et al. 1990; Tiller et al. 1990). In one study, moclobemide treatment was associated with a better outcome than fluvoxamine (Bocksberger et al. 1993).

Selegiline (L-deprenyl) in low dosage is associated with selective inhibition of MAO-B activity. Oxidative metabolism of benzylamine and phenylethylamine and to a lesser extent dopamine and tyramine is inhibited; oxidative metabolism of noradrenaline and serotonin is not inhibited. Antidepressant effects of selegiline occur primarily at nonselective dosages in young adults with major depression, antidepressant effects may occur at selective doses in patient subgroups (Mann et al. 1989). Sunderland et al. (1994) demonstrated statistically significant improvement during treatment with selegiline at doses that would inhibit MAO-A and MAO-B in geriatric patients with depression who had previously failed at least two trials of adequate pharmacotherapy. These data do not address whether such high-dose selegiline treatment is more effective than standard MAOIs.

Georgotas et al. (1989), reporting on the use of phenelzine in continuation treatment of ambulatory geriatric major depression, found a relapse rate of 24% in patients treated for 4 to 8 months with an average of 54 mg of phenelzine.

The efficacy of phenelzine in maintenance treatment of geriatric major depression was compared with placebo and nortriptyline by Georgotas et al. (1989), who studied a subgroup of patients who had completed continuation treatment studies. Initial data indicate that phenelzine had a strong prophylactic effect compared with placebo and nortriptyline over 1 year.

Practical Guidelines

Therapeutic response to phenelzine in elderly patients with depression can occur at doses comparable to those used with younger depressed patients (Georgotas et al. 1986). Systematic data on dose-response relationships in elderly patients are unavailable. Plasma levels of phenelzine may be higher in elderly patients versus younger patients receiving equivalent doses (Robinson 1981); the clinical significance of this is not known.

In geriatric patients with depression, Maguire et al. (1991) reported similar single-dose pharmacokinetics of moclobemide compared with younger patients, suggesting that clinicians can expect to use similar doses across the age spectrum.

Special concerns with nonselective MAOIs such as phenelzine and tranylcypromine include the need for dietary restriction of foods rich in tyramine and avoidance of drug-drug interactions, particularly with sympathomimetic agents and meperidine. In elderly patients, compliance may be reduced by cognitive and physical deficits. Analysis of the tyramine content of commonly prohibited foods suggests the lists usually given to patients are overrestrictive (McCabe and Tsuang 1982; Shulman et al. 1989; Sullivan and Shulman 1984). The availability of clear, easy-to-follow guidelines is especially relevant to treatment of elderly patients with depression who frequently must depend on others for shopping or food preparation. The rare spontaneous hypertensive crises that have been reported may have greater potential morbidity in elderly patients, but whether advanced age increases vulnerability to such reactions is uncertain.

More evidence is needed to determine whether a potential advantage of selective MAO inhibitors and RIMAs, when used in selective doses, is reduced risk of tyramine pressor response and, therefore, less need for dietary restriction. There appears to be a lower rate of drug-drug interactions associated with the use of selective MAOIs (Freeman 1993).

Toxicity

Standard MAOIs have weak anticholinergic activity and do not have quinidine-like effects. Their principal side effect, orthostatic hypotension, emerges more slowly than with TCAs but is more profound (Kronig et al. 1983). Pedal edema, presumably related to the vasodilating property of these agents, can complicate treatment; whether this adverse reaction is more common in elderly patients than in young adults is not clear.

Toxicity associated with selective MAO inhibition is relatively low in elderly patients. Neither acute nor subchronic moclobemide administration produced detectable effects on cognitive function or psychomotor performance in normal elderly volunteers (Kerr et al. 1992a). Moclobemide side effects include nausea and sleep disturbance (Freeman 1993; Tiller et al. 1990). The reversible characteristics of moclobemide's pharmacological activity has potential advantage on discontinuation in event of toxicity. Selegiline has been described as well tolerated in studies in geriatric patients when used as monotherapy (Agnoli et al. 1992; Magnani et al. 1991). Tariot et al. (1988) reported that tranylcypromine produced orthostatic hypotension in geriatric patients who had tolerated selegiline well.

Additional Clinical Situations

The use of MAOIs in depressive syndromes in patients with dementia has not received systematic study. The increase in MAO activity in brain and platelets in patients with senile dementia of Alzheimer type suggests a particular rationale for use of MAOIs in this context. Case reports have demonstrated that MAOIs can be used safely and effectively in Alzheimer patients (Jenike 1985b).

Use of selegiline in patients with Alzheimer's disease has been associated with improvement in behavioral disturbance (Agnoli et al. 1992; Mangoni et al. 1991; Tariot et al. 1987). It may potentiate effects of cholinomimetic treatment (Schneider et al. 1993).

In Parkinson's disease, selegiline at selective doses has been reported to improve motor and cognitive performance and delay need for L-dopa when used alone (Allain et al. 1993; Myllyla et al. 1993); it may also potentiate the therapeutic and toxic effects of L-dopa or L-dopa/carbidopa. Allain et al. (1993) reported that depressed mood was alleviated by selegiline.

Other Antidepressants

Maprotiline, a tetracyclic drug, is more selective for noradrenaline reuptake than are TCAs but does not have special clinical advantages in elderly patients because it shares the TCA side effect profile and carries some increased seizure risk. Amoxapine has a neuroleptic-related structure and can produce extrapyramidal side effects that can be especially problematic in elderly patients.

Other polycyclic antidepressants that have been developed and marketed more recently are potentially useful alternatives to TCAs or MAOIs for treating geriatric depressive disorders. Trazodone, nefazadone, bupropion, and the selective serotonin reuptake inhibitors (SSRIs) fluoxetine, sertraline, and paroxetine are FDA-approved antidepressants that have a narrower spectrum of pharmacological effects than TCAs. Venlafaxine combines selective reuptake inhibition of noradrenaline and serotonin (NSRI).

Indications

Despite the well-documented efficacy of intensive treatment using standard antidepressants in approximately 70% of cases (Klein et al. 1980), newer polycyclic antidepressants may have special uses in treating geriatric major depression. Because some older patients have difficulty tolerating anticholinergic and other side effects at therapeutic TCA doses, newer polycyclic antidepressants can be used to increase patient comfort and likelihood of compliance. Additional rationales include failing a course of adequate treatment with a standard TCA and a contraindication to TCAs (e.g., significant intraventricular conduction delay or pretreatment orthostatic hypotension).

Effects of some newer antidepressant medications may prove useful for patients with particular depressive symptom profiles. Sedative effects of trazodone can relieve insomnia; however, trazodone may promote sleep at doses inadequate to bring about remission of a depressive episode. As reviewed by Boyer et al. (1991), SSRI treatment has been associated with improvement in mixed-aged samples of patients with panic (Gorman et al. 1987) and obsessive-compulsive disorders (Goodman et al. 1989). If efficacy of SSRIs in specific anxiety disorders is demonstrated, these agents may have a special role in major depression associated with panic attacks or ruminative preoccupations; this awaits evaluation.

Efficacy

Randomized placebo-controlled treatment trials of patients with severe depression became unethical after the demonstration of safety and efficacy of intensive treatment with standard TCAs; furthermore, hospitals cannot justify reimbursement for controlled studies that use a placebo cell. For these reasons, knowledge of the efficacy of non-TCA polycyclic antidepressants and SSRIs has been gained largely through studies of outpatients with mild to moderately severe major depression. Controlled studies of at-risk populations (such as the most severely depressed, who generally require hospital treatment, and the physically frail elderly) are lacking. Clinicians should be aware that treatment of these populations with newer antidepressants assumes that findings from younger, less severely depressed and physically healthier patients can be generalized to more vulnerable and complicated patients. Because of the limited knowledge about concentration-response relationships for newer agents, little is known about optimizing dosage.

Phase III placebo-controlled treatment trials using non-TCA polycyclic compounds and SSRIs have included elderly patients with depression. Although exceptions do exist (Branconnier et al. 1983; Gerner et al. 1980; Tollefson et al. 1993), geriatric patients have not been the focus of most of these studies. Controlled studies in geriatric samples have, generally, compared the new agent with a tertiary amine TCA. Comparisons using target plasma levels of secondary amine TCAs are unavailable.

Trazodone, a triazolopyridine with minimal anticholinergic activity, was thought to be especially promising for geriatric depression. A placebo-controlled trial in older depressed outpatients (mean age 68.4 yrs) demonstrated a robust response, in study completers, to an average of either 305 mg/day of trazodone or 145 mg/day of imipramine; responses to the antidepressants were comparable and significantly better than to placebo (Gerner et al. 1980). However, the study demonstrated poor tolerance of the doses that produced drug-placebo differences; less than 60% of patients completed the study, with high dropout rates in all three groups (60% for imipramine and 30% each for trazodone and placebo). Although overall response rates were not provided, trazodone was effective in completers who tolerated aggressive pharmacotherapy. It is not known whether older patients with depression would tolerate or respond to lower doses of trazodone, and it is not known how trazodone response rates would compare with plasma level controlled treatment with a secondary amine TCA.

Three SSRIs (fluoxetine, sertraline, and paroxetine in order of pharmacological specificity) have been approved as antidepressants in the United States. Clinical trials have indicated antidepressent activity for two other SSRIs: citalopram and fluvoxamine. Most controlled studies using SSRIs to treat geriatric depression have used mixed-age patients experiencing major depression and compared the SSRIs with tertiary amine TCAs (e.g., Feighner and Cohn 1985). A 6-week placebo-controlled study of 771 older patients with major depression demonstrated a significantly greater response to a target dose of 20 mg/day of fluoxetine, measured by 50% improvement in HDRS scores and endpoint scores equal to or greater than 8 (Tollefson et al. 1995). Fewer than 50% of fluoxetine patients met the response criterion, however, and endpoint HDRS scores for fluoxetine and placebo-treated subjects were comparable. These results must be considered in light of data demonstrating that longer treatment periods can be associated with increased rates of response (Georgotas and McCue 1989; Schweizer et al. 1990).

The most promising fluoxetine data come from a controlled comparison of fluoxetine to desipramine in young adults with major depression, more than 40% of whom were hospitalized (Bowden et al. 1993). Efficacy was comparable at 6 weeks, and fluoxetine was associated with significantly fewer side effects.

Studies comparing sertraline and paroxetine with tertiary amine TCAs have produced similar results. Using endpoint analyses, treatment of geriatric patients with major depression who received an average of 116 mg/day of sertraline for more than 6 weeks was associated with 69.5% response rate compared with 62.5% for a comparable period of treatment with an average of 88 mg of amitriptyline (Cohn et al. 1990). Combined data from two studies comparing paroxetine (23.4 mg/day) with doxepin (105.2 mg/day) demonstrated comparable levels of improvement; HDRS scores decreased from an average of 25 at the point of assignment to an average of between 10 and 15 at week 5 (Dunner et al. 1992).

The safety and efficacy of SSRIs in acutely psychiatrically hospitalized geriatric patients (a population that experiences severe forms of depression) has not been established; neither have benefits and risks in patients with severe physical illness.

Bupropion has been assessed in controlled studies of older patients with depression. Two studies of outpatients older than 55 found that low (150 mg/day) and high (450 mg/day) doses of bupropion were equivalent in antidepressant efficacy to 150 mg/day of imipramine (Branconnier et al. 1983; Kane et al. 1983). Data indicating that a dose of 300 mg/day or greater was associated with earlier onset of action and greater anxiolytic activity than lower dosages in these older subjects (Branconnier et al. 1983) will require replication in a controlled study.

Nefazodone, which both blocks serotonin reuptake and acts as a 5-HT$_2$ receptor antagonist, has demonstrated antidepressant efficacy comparable with that of imipramine (Fontaine et al. 1994; Rickels et al. 1994). Nefazodone produces weaker α_1-adrenergic receptor blockade than trazodone, to which it is structurally related (Eison et al. 1990); this may explain the low frequency of both orthostatic hypotension and sedation in treatment studies. Venlafaxine, a recently approved antidepressant that inhibits neuronal uptake of both norepinephrine and serotonin, has demonstrated efficacy comparable with that of imipramine as well (Cunningham et al. 1994). Published data on the efficacy, safety, and dose-response relationships of these agents in elderly depressive patients are not available. Importantly, dose-response relationships in mixed-age depressive patients have been demonstrated for both nefazodone (Fontaine et al. 1994) and venlafaxine (Mendels et al. 1993), highlighting the need to study the ability of older patients to tolerate dose ranges associated with greatest antidepressant efficacy.

Practical Guidelines

Additional studies are needed to determine the optimal dosage and duration of treatment of these new agents in geriatric patients and in younger adult patients. This will augment their clinical utility and provide guidelines for mixed-age patients. Use of drug plasma concentrations as guidelines to geriatric or mixed-age management has not been established, but studies designed to establish concentration-effect relationships have been initiated for some of these agents.

Trazodone clearance is decreased in elderly patients (Greenblatt et al. 1982). One fixed-dose study suggested better response at steady-state trazodone concentration above 650 ng/ml (Monteleone and Gnocchi 1990). Trazodone's one active metabolite, *m*-chlorophenylpiperazine, is a serotonin receptor agonist.

Fluoxetine has a longer half-life than that of sertraline or paroxetine (van Harten 1993). Norfluoxetine, the major active metabolite of fluoxetine, has a half-life several times longer than that of fluoxetine. Limited published data show that metabolism of fluoxetine appears to be unaffected by aging (Bergstrom et al. 1988; Lemberger et al. 1985).

Sertraline has a longer half-life than paroxetine. It has a demethylated metabolite that is a less potent serotonin reuptake inhibitor than sertraline and has a half-life that is several times longer than that of sertraline. Increased plasma steady-state sertraline concentration/dose ratios in elderly patients have been reported (Warrington 1991).

No major metabolites of paroxetine have been identified. Steady-state plasma paroxetine concentrations have been reported as higher in elderly patients compared with young adults at doses of 30–40 mg/day but not at doses of 20 mg per day (Hebenstreit et al. 1989).

Bupropion has several active metabolites, including a hydroxylated form, that are present in plasma in higher concentrations than the parent compound. These metabolites are implicated in clinical effects (Golden et al. 1988). Pollock et al. (1993) noted higher plasma concentrations of bupropion metabolite in geriatric patients with depression who did not respond to bupropion compared with those who responded.

Venlafaxine is metabolized to one major active metabolite: o-desmethylated venlafaxine. Data concerning age effects and both nefazodone and venlafaxine pharmacokinetics are needed.

Toxicity

Early recommendations for use of trazodone in geriatric patients were based on the finding of fewer anticholinergic and overall side effects with trazodone than with imipramine (Gerner et al. 1980). Clinically significant ECG effects were not identified in healthy older outpatients (Hayes et al. 1983). Trazodone treatment has been associated with ventricular ectopy (Janowsky et al. 1983), excessive sedation, and orthostatic hypotension with syncope (Nambudiri et al. 1989; Spivak et al. 1989), presumably mediated through competitive blockade at the α-adrenergic receptor. Clinicians must, therefore, consider the patient's baseline cardiovascular status and risks versus benefits of sedative side effects prior to prescribing this antidepressant.

Fluoxetine, sertraline, and paroxetine have low propensity for cardiovascular and anticholinergic side effects. Kerr et al. (1992b) reported that paroxetine did not produce detectable adverse cognitive effects in geriatric patients with depression. Paroxetine can, however, increase anxiety, motor restlessness, and insomnia.

A number of cases of drug-induced parkinsonism have been reported in middle-aged adults in association with SSRI treatment (Bouchard et al. 1989; Broud 1989). Data on the incidence and severity of EPS development in elderly patients treated with SSRIs from systematic prospective studies are not available. However, reports from younger patients, and the reported association between sertraline treatment and postural imbalance in older patients with depression (Laghrassi-Thode et al. 1995), are consistent with the need for clinicians to monitor older patients with depression for the development of EPS during SSRI therapy.

Hyponatremia can occur during SSRI treatment. Case report literature suggests that elderly patients may be particularly vulnerable to this effect, which is believed to be mediated by inappropriate antidiuretic hormone secretion (Pillans and Coulter 1994).

Drug-drug interactions are an important issue with SSRIs. SSRIs are metabolized primarily by the hepatic P450-2 D6 system and most SSRIs are potent inhibitors of these enzymes. As reviewed by van Harten (1993), use of SSRIs (particularly fluoxetine and paroxetine) is associated with increased plasma TCA levels and other drugs used to treat medical disorders that are metabolized by the same system. There is a potentially lethal interaction between SSRIs and MAOIs.

Despite the association of seizures with doses of bupropion exceeding 450 mg/day, bupropion has a side effect profile especially suitable for geriatric patients. Anticholinergic, antihistaminic, and cardiovascular side effects are minimal; hypertension may be exacerbated, however. History of prior seizure, but not age, appears to increase the occurrence of seizures in patients treated with bupropion (Davidson 1989).

Because nefazodone inhibits the P450 3A4 isoenzyme, combined use with either of the antihistamines terfenadine or astemizole is contraindicated to prevent potential cardiotoxicity. Inhibition of the 3A4 isoenzyme increases levels of alprazolam and triazolam, requiring 50%–75% reductions in doses of these medications when prescribed with nefazodone.

The side effect profiles of venlafaxine and nefazodone are similar to that of SSRIs and, therefore, may be generally advantageous in elderly individuals. Dose-dependent hypertension can occur with venlafaxine, however, and this needs careful consideration in elderly patients with cardiovascular comorbidity.

Stimulants

Indications

The absence of controlled studies makes it difficult to assess benefits, risks, or appropriate indications for psychostimulant use in geriatric patients with symptoms of depression.

Efficacy

Stimulants, which include dextroamphetamine, methylphenidate, and pemoline, can reduce apathy and psychomotor retardation in some patients with depression. Reports that low doses of methylphenidate improve depressive symptoms in patients ages 80 to 105 who do not meet diagnostic criteria for a depressive disorder (Gurian and Rosowsky 1993) and that 10 mg of methylphenidate reverses anorexia occurring in association with apathy in patients with severe dementia (Maletta and Winegarden 1993) are consistent with a tradition of psychostimulant literature on the treatment of frail, cognitively impaired, and physically ill elderly patients. Despite the numerous reports that stimulants can reverse symptoms of depression or anergic symptoms (particularly those occurring in association with dementia or debilitating physical illness [Chiarello and Cole 1987]), controlled studies demonstrating efficacy in systematically diagnosed patients with major depression are not available. A recent review (Satel and Nelson 1989) concluded that most controlled studies in patients with primary depression have not demonstrated greater efficacy with stimulants than with placebo.

Methylphenidate was found in a retrospective study by Lingam et al. (1988) to be effective for elderly patients with poststroke depression.

Toxicity

The increased energy and improved behavior reported in patients with dementia or physical illness must be balanced against stimulant-induced emergence of agitation or cognitive deterioration in patients with organic brain disease and against potential cardiovascular toxicity in patients with severe physical illness (Satel and Nelson 1989).

Antimanic Drugs

Types

Lithium salts are first-line antimanic agents in patients of all ages. Other antimanic compounds such as anticonvulsants that have been used to treat mania may be appropriate as well for elderly patients (see Table 27–6 for antimanic drugs marketed in the United States).

Lithium Salts

Indications

The primary indications for lithium salts in elderly patients are acute mania or hypomania (Mirchandani and Young 1993). Additional indications are bipolar depression and potentiation of antidepressants in unipolar major depression. Lithium salts can be used in continuation and maintenance treatment for bipolar and unipolar patients.

Table 27–6. Antimanic drugs marketed in the United States

Classes	Examples
Lithium salts	Lithium carbonate
Anticonvulsants	Carbamazepine, valproate
Neuroleptic medications	Haloperidol
Benzodiazepines	Lorazepam, clonazepam
Other	Verapamil

Efficacy

Response to lithium in acute mania has not been compared with placebo in geriatric patients, partly because of ethical concerns. Response to lithium in elderly patients has not been compared with other drugs such as neuroleptic medications. The same limitations in the literature regarding lithium in geriatric manic patients also pertain to the other indications noted.

Shulman and Post's study (1980) of elderly patients with mania showed that more than 40% had late-onset bipolar illness, and many of these cases had coarse brain pathology. Of the late-onset cases, 24% had overt brain disease. Lithium was tolerated well and was effective, but doses and levels were not reported. Other open studies have suggested satisfactory response to lithium salts in geriatric populations (Glasser and Rabins 1984; Stone 1989).

Predictors of poor response by young adult manic patients to lithium have not been evaluated in geriatric patients. These predictors are greater severity, dysphoric mood, negative family history, frequent episodes, and psychiatric comorbidity. While some older patients have attenuated treatment response (Young and Falk 1989), age does not seem to be a strong predictor of poor response based on limited geriatric data (Young et al. 1992).

Adequacy of treatment with lithium or other mood stabilizers in geriatric bipolar patients presenting with depressive syndrome needs to be documented with plasma levels and dose adjusted if necessary. If symptoms persist, the usual clinical approach is continuation of the mood-stabilizing drug and addition of an antidepressant.

Practical Guidelines

Pretreatment assessment. A baseline ECG to assess sinus functioning is indicated prior to use of lithium salts because of the risk of sick sinus syndrome (Roose et al. 1979b). This complication may be encountered in older patients with coronary artery disease that has compromised the sinus node.

Baseline evaluation includes thyroid and renal function tests. Serum creatinine is not a sensitive index of renal function; patients with renal insufficiency who require careful monitoring and for whom collection of 24-hour urine output is not feasible can have creatinine clearance approximated from age, body weight, and serum creatinine (Friedman et al. 1989). Assessment of thyroid status, including thyroid-stimulating hormone, is especially important in elderly patients. Lithium's antagonism of thyroid gland function, in combination with the diminished thyroid reserve that accompanies aging (Sawin et al. 1985), makes an elderly population vulnerable to developing hypothyroidism during lithium treatment.

Dosing

The lithium dose necessary to achieve a targeted blood level usually is one-half to two-thirds of that required in younger adults (Hardy et al. 1987). This is consistent with beginning at low doses in the range of 150 mg to 300 mg per day and increasing slowly with small increments while monitoring plasma levels. The half-life for lithium approximates 24 hours in patients older than 70 without renal disease (Chapron et al. 1982; Hardy et al. 1987). The plasma level obtained 5 days after a patient has started a specific dose of lithium does not change significantly unless medical illness or use of medications that influence lithium excretion supervene (see Tables 27–2 and 27–3).

Foster et al. (1990) and others have suggested that erythrocyte-to-plasma lithium ratio may be a better predictor of lithium toxicity than plasma concentrations alone. This suggestion requires systematic study, however.

Salt depletion, which may be caused by vomiting and diarrhea or by a low-sodium diet, can increase renal reabsorption of lithium and can raise plasma levels (Jefferson and Greist 1979). The presence of renal disease does not preclude use of lithium. Despite persistent controversy, there is no clear evidence that lithium causes or accelerates the course of renal failure in the vast majority of patients (Meyers and Kalayam 1989); however, a small number of patients treated with lithium have been identified who developed impaired renal concentrating ability (DePaulo et al. 1986) and/or diminished glomerular function that may progress to insufficiency (Gitlin 1993).

The potential for causing lithium toxicity by concurrent administration of agents that diminish lithium clearance is of special concern in geriatric patients. Jefferson and Greist (1979) reviewed the effects of diuretics on lithium clearance. Thiazide diuretics block reabsorption of sodium in the distal tubule, leading to increased proximal reabsorption of sodium and lithium and an increase in lithium plasma levels of 33% or more. Potassium-sparing diuretics may have a similar, although less profound, effect. Furosemide, a loop diuretic, is not associated with significant increase in lithium level (Crabtree et al. 1991).

Nonsteroidal anti-inflammatory medications are used commonly by elderly patients. Some of these agents diminish renal clearance of lithium by nearly 50% (Jefferson et al. 1981). Availability of over-the-counter forms of these agents (e.g., ibuprofen) makes it necessary for the psychiatrist to instruct elderly patients not to begin a new medication without discussion.

A few cases of elevated lithium levels in association with use of angiotensin-converting enzyme inhibitors have been reported. A study of lithium combined with enalapril in 10 healthy young volunteers failed to find an effect of the angiotensin-converting enzyme inhibitor, although one subject did have a 31% increase in lithium level (Das Gupta et al. 1992). Additional information on this possible pharmacokinetic interaction is needed; clinicians are advised to monitor lithium levels carefully when an angiotensin-converting enzyme inhibitor is added to a patient's lithium regimen.

Lithium pharmacodynamics (i.e., the relationship between specific plasma concentrations and therapeutic or toxic responses) in elderly patients is not well understood despite clinical lore suggesting increased sensitivity. Case reports dealing with acute efficacy (Schaffer and Garvey 1984) have suggested response in geriatric patients with mania at lower levels (e.g., 0.4 to 0.8 mEq/L) than are optimal in mixed-age adults. One naturalistic study suggested better response to higher lithium levels in younger patients and in geriatric patients (Young et al. 1992).

The efficacy of lithium for prophylaxis has received little study in elderly bipolar patients. Abou-Saleh and Coppen (1983) noted no difference in affective morbidity over an average of 5 years in elderly patients versus younger patients maintained on comparable lithium levels. In a prospective study, Murray and associates (1983) reported greater manic psychopathology, although no more frequent hospitalizations, among older patients from a mixed-age sample. Both studies used maintenance levels between 0.6 and 1.0 mEq/L. These results are consistent with the conclusions that bipolar illness does not "burn out" and that lithium prophylaxis continues to play a crucial role as patients with bipolar illness age.

Toxicity

Acute lithium toxicity includes tremor, ataxia, gastrointestinal distress, cognitive impairment, and severe polyuria. Roose and associates (1979a) reported more instances of toxicity in elderly bipolar outpatients compared with younger patients in a maintenance treatment program.

Little suitable data exist for assessing whether lithium toxicity routinely occurs at lower levels in geriatric adults compared with younger adults. Although elderly patients may be more likely to present fine tremor at therapeutic lithium levels compared with younger patients at equivalent levels, the occurrence of polyuria and polydipsia apparently does not increase with age (Murray et al. 1983).

Concern about long-term adverse reactions to lithium involves impact on renal and thyroid function. Despite some persistence of controversy, damage to glomerular function from prolonged lithium use has not been established after more than 40 years of use, more than 18 of which were in the United States (Meyers and Kalayam 1989). Conservative management includes twice-yearly monitoring of renal function. Diminished renal function does not preclude use of lithium, but careful consideration must be given to the benefit of continued use versus the possibility that lithium has contributed to renal pathology. Thyroid function should be assessed twice yearly, especially if there is a change in the course of affective illness or physical health. Thyroid-stimulating hormone increases can be managed with thyroid hormone.

Additional Clinical Situations

Himmelhoch et al. (1980) found that neurological status (including extrapyramidal syndromes and dementia but not age) was associated with delayed and/or poor treatment response, including lithium-induced neurotoxicity; lithium levels were not specified. Black et al. (1988) reported that "complicated" manias (i.e., those with coexisting nonaffective psychiatric illness or with serious medical illness) had poorer immediate response to lithium treatment. Shukla et al. (1987) reported that mixed-age patients with secondary manias had a poor acute response.

Anticonvulsants

Carbamazepine, valproic acid, and clonazepam have been used for years in treating elevated mood states in mixed-age adults. The use of valproate in mania has been approved by the Food and Drug Administration (FDA) in the face of accumulating experimental evidence of efficacy (Bowden et al. 1994).

Indications

Anticonvulsants can be used as alternatives to lithium in geriatric manic patients. Indications are poor tolerance of, or failure to respond to, lithium salts.

Efficacy

There are no placebo-controlled studies of the efficacy of anticonvulsants alone in geriatric patients with mania. A case report has indicated that therapeutic response to carbamazepine can occur in geriatric manic patients (Kellner and Neher 1991). Experience with a larger number of cases indicates that valproate also can be useful in geriatric manic patients (Gnam and Flint 1993; McFarland et al. 1990). There is a need for data on experience with clonazepam in the acute treatment of mania in elderly patients.

These agents can be used as adjuncts in patients partially responsive to lithium salts. Such use requires study in geriatric patients.

Practical Guidelines

Pretreatment assessment. Patients treated with carbamazepine or valproic acid should undergo hematological assessment and liver function tests before treatment. An electrocardiogram should be obtained for patients being considered for carbamazepine treatment.

Dosing. Optimal dosing with these agents has not been established in geriatric patients. Relationships between carbamazepine and valproate plasma concentrations and antimanic response are not well delineated in any age group. Active metabolites for all compounds are generated; data are lacking on advanced age and pharmacokinetics. Valproate has a shorter half-life than carbamazepine. Valproate and carbamazepine affect the P450 isoenzymes. Carbamazepine induces P450 activity, thereby decreasing concentrations of some other medications. Valproate, conversely a P450 inhibitor, can cause increased levels of concurrently used medications.

Toxicity. Carbamazepine can cause side effects including sedation, confusion, ataxia, and sialorrhea. Central nervous system side effects generally are dose-dependent and occur most frequently at the high end of the anticonvulsant concentration range (Schneider and Subin 1991). Carbamazepine has quinidine-like properties and can cause prolongation of cardiac conduction; therefore, an electrocardiogram should be repeated during treatment. Hepatic enzyme elevations, usually small and transient, can occur. Complete blood count should be monitored because of the possibility of agranulocytosis; a slight reduction in leukocyte count occurs frequently.

Valproate may have a lower side effect profile than carbamazepine, including less sedative and anticholinergic effects, although direct comparisons are needed in elderly patients. Absence of cognitive toxicity on neuropsychological testing was reported by Craig and Tallis (1994) in a series of geriatric patients with seizure disorder. Valproate is reported in the case literature to be well tolerated in intact elderly patients and in elderly patients with dementia. It can inhibit platelet production and function; it can produce usually mild hepatic enzyme elevations.

The toxicity profile of clonazepam is the same as that for benzodiazepines.

Additional Clinical Situations

Carbamazepine has been used successfully to control agitated, aggressive behaviors in patients with organic brain disease. The literature consists mainly of case reports; however, Gleason and Schneider (1990) reported that hostility and irritability were most improved in an open study of probable Alzheimer patients. Chambers et al. (1982), reporting on a placebo-controlled trial in 19 patients with dementia, noted toxicity but no benefit.

Mazure et al. (1992) reported that adjunctive use of valproate can be helpful in patients with organic mental syndrome and behavioral disorders. Mellow et al. (1993) noted that valproate produced sustained improvement in two of four patients with dementia who were agitated and aggressive.

Neuroleptic Drugs

Types

Various classes of antipsychotic drugs are available for use in elderly patients. These drugs can be organized by chemical structure or ranked according to clinical potency (see Table 27–7 for a list of neuroleptic drugs marketed in the United States).

Indications

Typical neuroleptic drugs are first-line agents for managing psychotic symptoms in elderly patients. These drugs have a limited role in managing behavioral disturbances accompanying organic mental syndromes, especially if psychotic symptoms are present (Schneider et al. 1990; Sunderland and Silver 1988). Neuroleptic medications may be viewed as a single group of drugs that differ primarily in their side effect profiles. Less information on dose-response relationships is available for neuroleptic drugs than for antidepressant and antimanic agents. Neuroleptic medications should be prescribed empirically, in the lowest effective dose, given the absence of systematic data on dosage and the increased sensitivity of the elderly population to specific adverse reactions. A recent study demonstrated the occurrence of a 26.7% decrease in antipsychotic drug use in association with implementation of OBRA-87 (Schorr et al. 1994).

Experience is limited in geriatric patients with atypical antipsychotic agents (clozapine and risperidone) that recently have become available. Each of these drugs has potential advantages; efficacy, dosing requirements, and risks in elderly patients need to be assessed.

Schizophrenias

Neuroleptic drugs are used to treat elderly schizophrenic patients (Tran-Johnson et al. 1992). Post (1966) and others have indicated the therapeutic utility of neuroleptic drugs in late-onset chronic psychosis.

Dementia

The occurrence of behavioral disturbance and psychotic symptoms in patients experiencing dementia is receiving increasing attention. Caregivers seeking professional assistance to cope with dementia patients residing in the community report that approximately 70% of these patients demonstrate disturbed behavior and approximately 50% have psychotic symptoms (Rabins et al. 1982). The severity of the dementia may correlate with the number and type of behavioral problems (Teri et al. 1988); 82% of mildly impaired Alzheimer's patients reported behavior problems compared with 96% of patients with severe cognitive dysfunction (MMSE

Table 27–7. Neuroleptic drugs marketed in the United States

Classes	Examples
Phenothiazines	
Aliphatic	Chlorpromazine
Piperidine	Thioridazine, mesoridazine
Piperazine	Fluphenazine, trifluoperazine
Butyrophenones	Haloperidol
Thioxanthenes	Thiothixene
Diphenylbutylpiperidine	Pimozide
Dibenzepins	Loxapine
Dihydromorphines	Molindone
Dibenzodiazepines	Clozapine
Benzisoxazoles	Risperidone

score less than 10); 38% of patients with severe dementia had agitation compared with 10% with mild impairment; the rates for the presence of hallucinations were 30% and 10%, respectively. This issue has special public health relevance because persistently unmanageable and disruptive behavior is the principal reason reported by caregivers for seeking institutionalization (Ferris et al. 1985). Cohen-Mansfield (1986) applied a 13-item agitated behavior scale to nursing home residents and found that 73% of individuals assessed demonstrated a minimum of one agitated behavior at a frequency of several times a day; 56% of these individuals were receiving neuroleptic medications.

Efficacy

Schizophrenias. Raskind et al. (1979) noted that depot fluphenazine was more effective than oral haloperidol in the ongoing outpatient management of elderly patients with schizophrenia; blood levels were not determined and noncompliance may have contributed to these results.

Neuroleptic treatment has proven more effective in late-life psychoses than placebo (Post 1962) and more effective than no treatment (Post 1966). In open trials Jeste et al. (1988) suggested that late-onset schizophrenic patients may respond to lower doses of neuroleptic medication than geriatric early-onset cases.

A number of series of case reports on atypical neuroleptic drugs indicate response to clozapine in some geriatric patients refractory to typical neuroleptic drugs (Bajulaiye and Addonizio 1992; Ball 1992; Frankenburg and Kalunian 1994; Oberholzer et al. 1992; Salzman et al. 1995). These reports involve a diverse group of patients including chronic schizophrenic patients. Studies of clinical experience with risperidone in geriatric patients are needed.

Dementia. Reviews of neuroleptic drug treatment for behavioral disturbances such as agitation, assaultive tendencies, and wandering and for psychotic symptoms in patients with dementia (Raskind et al. 1987; Schneider et al. 1990; Sunderland and Silver 1988; Wragg and Jeste 1988) point to the dearth of controlled studies.

Neuroleptic drugs are superior to placebo in controlling agitation and psychosis in patients with dementia but do not abolish behavioral disturbance. For example, Barnes et al. (1982) noted improved functioning in a mixed sample with Alzheimer's and multi-infarct dementias who received loxapine or thioridazine compared to placebo. Efficacy of neuroleptic drugs appears to be proportional to the degree of disturbance. There is no evidence for the superiority of one neuroleptic drug or class of agents over another (Tune et al. 1991). Neuroleptic drug treatment has an uncertain impact on cognitive functioning in patients with dementia; adverse effects appear to be dose specific and medication specific (Raskind et al. 1987). Haloperidol can decrease agitation associated with dementia, but the higher doses needed for effectiveness are associated with greater extrapyramidal side effects (Devanand et al. 1989). Tune et al. (1991) caution that neuroleptic drug side effects can emerge over several months of treatment.

Practical Guidelines

Pretreatment assessment. Administration of neuroleptic drugs should be preceded by assessment of neuromuscular function. This approach enables the clinician to identify neuroleptic drug-induced parkinsonism and tardive dyskinesia. Elderly patients have an increased vulnerability to both forms of adverse reactions (Ayd 1976; Jeste and Wyatt 1987). A simple screening instrument such as the Abnormal Involuntary Movement Scale (Whittier 1969) can characterize and quantify baseline functioning.

Baseline assessment should include complete blood count for patients for whom clozapine is being considered.

Dosing. Steady-state concentration-dose ratios that increase with age have been reported for chlorpromazine (Aoba et al. 1986; Rosenblatt et al. 1981) and thioridazine (Axelsson 1976). Such differences have not been found consistently for haloperidol (Weisbard et al. 1993). These differences have been studied in other neuroleptic drugs on a limited basis.

Preliminary studies only have been made of dose-response relationships in using neuroleptic drugs to treat uncontrolled behavior caused by dementia or chronic paranoid states. Devanand et al. (1989) studied different strengths of the neuroleptic drug haloperidol and found that higher doses (close to 5 mg) were associated with greater improvement in behavior and with worsened cognitive performance than doses in the 1-mg range.

Devanand et al. (1992) examined 19 subjects with probable Alzheimer's disease who manifested psychosis or behavioral disturbance. Compared with oral dose, blood levels of haloperidol showed a stronger positive association with symptomatic improvement and with severity of extrapyramidal features.

Dysken et al. (1990) studied haloperidol and reduced haloperidol concentrations in 18 patients with primary degenerative dementia. A "good response" was seen over a low plasma haloperidol concentration range of 0.3 to 2.5 ng/ml, a range of concentrations in which many commercial laboratories do not detect plasma haloperidol. There was no significant linear or curvilinear relationship between response and plasma levels of haloperidol and reduced haloperidol.

Mazure et al. (1992) studied 10 geriatric psychiatric patients without dementia who received fixed dose of perphenazine (0.15 mg/kg/day). Neither Brief Psychiatric Rating Scale total nor symptom change scores correlated with perphenazine levels.

Available reports describe clozapine treatment in geriatric psychiatric patients at doses ranging from 75 mg per day to 350 mg per day. Some reports have suggested increased plasma concentrations/dose ratios of clozapine in elderly patients compared with younger patients (Haring et al. 1990). Clozapine has a major demethylated metabolite, norclozapine, that can contribute to toxicity. Concentration-effect relationships have not been described in elderly patients.

Risperidone has a 9-hydroxylated metabolite that accumulates and is pharmacologically active. Age effects on risperidone pharmacokinetics have not been studied.

Toxicity

Neuroleptic drugs can be placed on a continuum ranging from low-potency drugs (e.g., thioridazine and chlorpromazine) to high-potency agents (e.g., fluphenazine and haloperidol). Low-potency agents have greater anticholinergic, α_1-receptor antagonist, and antihistaminic activities (Richelson 1982); these agents have a greater potential for causing sedation, confusion, and orthostatic hypotension. The high-potency agents are relatively pure dopamine-2 receptor blockers and produce extrapyramidal side effects; whether these drugs are associated with greater risk of tardive dyskinesia or neuroleptic malignant syndrome compared to low-potency agents remains to be studied.

Neuroleptic drug treatment can impair cognitive performance (Devanand et al. 1989; Perlick et al. 1986). The pharmacological mechanisms may involve anticholinergic effects, but catecholamine receptor blockade may be involved. The relative risk posed by various classes of neuroleptic drugs remains to be determined.

Elderly patients receiving neuroleptic medications are at increased risk for falls and their related morbidity (Ray et al. 1987). The extent to which low-potency agents contribute to falls by increasing confusion and cardiovascular instability versus high-potency agents causing falls through drug-induced parkinsonism remains unclear.

Use of anticholinergic agents can improve neuroleptic drug-induced rigidity but are largely ineffective for tremor and akathisia (Shader and DiMascio 1970). These agents can cause central anticholinergic toxicity and can increase the risk for tardive dyskinesia or worsen existing dyskinesia (Jeste and Wyatt 1987).

In patients receiving neuroleptic drugs, cross-sectional studies have demonstrated a strong association between age and prevalence of tardive dyskinesia (Jeste and Wyatt 1987). Prevalence estimates exceed 40% in patients older than 60, and late-life tardive dyskinesia is reported to be more severe and less likely to spontaneously remit (Smith and Baldessarini 1980). Although female gender (Woerner et al. 1991) and a diagnosis of affective disorder (Gardos and Casey 1984; Kane et al. 1983; Yassa et al. 1992) have been reported to increase the prevalence of tardive dyskinesia in neuroleptic drug-treated patients, controversy about these risk factors exists (Jeste and Wyatt 1987; Kane et al. 1983). A prospective study of patients older than age 55 treated with neuroleptic drugs for the first time (Saltz et al. 1991) demonstrated cumulative incidence of 31% after 43 weeks of treatment. Although rates of tardive dyskinesia depend on criterion cutoff scores, most authorities agree that elderly patients are especially vulnerable to developing this side effect with neuroleptic treatment.

Some studies that included elderly patients have noted associations between relatively high neuroleptic plasma or serum concentration-to-dose ratios and tardive dyskinesia (Jeste et al. 1982; Yesavage et al. 1987). Other studies have been negative (Jeste et al. 1981; McCreadie et al. 1992).

Akathisia occurs across a broad range of ages. The behavioral manifestations of this adverse reaction are thought to result from an internal sense of restlessness (Crane and Naranjo 1971). The diminished ability of dementia patients to vocalize their sensations could lead to underdiagnosis in this population (Wragg and Jeste 1988). An unfortunate cycle of motor restlessness that leads to increasing doses of neuroleptic medication that causes worsening of akathisia can ensue. Alternatively, considering "agitated behavior" as a possible expression of akathisia and attempting to decrease the dose of neuroleptic medication reverses this form of iatrogenic suffering in some patients.

The neuroleptic malignant syndrome, involving a toxic response of extrapyramidal symptoms, delirium, hyperpyrexia, and autonomic dysfunction, can occur in elderly patients. A literature search completed in 1987 identified 18 reported patients older than 65 (Addonizio 1987) associated with neuroleptic malignant syndrome. The relative vulnerability of elderly patients to this life-threatening reaction to neuroleptic medications is unknown; it is possible that age masks the phenomenology of the syndrome and that dementia confounds diagnosis (Wragg and Jeste 1988).

Although controversy persists (Moleman et al. 1986), the preponderance of evidence indicates that elderly patients, particularly those with dementia (Peabody et al. 1987), have an increased vulnerability to extrapyramidal reactions during neuroleptic drug treatment. More than 50% of geriatric patients who receive these agents have parkinsonian side effects (Ayd 1976; Salzman 1992). These side effects may be aggravated by the degeneration of nigrostriatal pathways associated with aging (Meyers and Kalayam 1989), higher plasma levels per dose of neuroleptic medications, or a longer duration of drug exposure (Wragg and Jeste 1988).

Clozapine has a low propensity for inducing extrapyramidal side effects in mixed-age patients. This is a potential advantage in elderly patients and may be attributed to its potent anticholinergic properties or its relatively weak antagonism of striatal dopamine receptors compared with typical neuroleptic drugs. The frequency of other side effects including lethargy and sedation, respiratory distress, and leukopenia (despite treatment at relatively low doses in some reports) points out the need for controlled studies in elderly patients (Ball 1992; Salzman 1994). The clinician should be alert to the risk of agranulocytosis, particularly because of the reported higher risk of this complication with increasing age (Alvir et al. 1993).

Risperidone treatment in mixed-age populations is associated with less extrapyramidal side effects than conventional neuroleptic drugs; this and possible lower anticholinergic effects may be advantages in elderly patients. More data are needed to reach conclusions on risperidone's side effects and benefits.

Additional Clinical Situations

Neuroleptic medications can be useful adjuncts in acute management of mania. When used in this context, neuroleptic medications should be used only when behavioral interventions have not succeeded, and they should be used in the lowest possible dose. Neuroleptic drugs should be tapered off prior to hospital discharge, if possible; behavior should be assessed on lithium alone.

Use of neuroleptic drugs can be problematic in patients with Parkinson's disease because of exacerbation of baseline motor abnormalities and peripheral autonomic dysregulation. The use of clozapine reportedly is well tolerated in such patients (Scholz and Dichgans 1985; Wolters et al. 1990). Controlled studies are needed, however.

Antianxiety Agents and Hypnotics

Types

The primary anxiolytic agents are the benzodiazepines (see Table 27–8 for a list of anxiolytic/hypnotic drugs marketed in the United States). This class also includes buspirone, antihistamines, antidepressants, and β-blockers.

The hypnotics include benzodiazepines, barbiturates, and related compounds. Barbiturates are not recommended because of their potential risk

Table 27–8. Anxiolytic/hypnotic drugs marketed in the United States

Classes	Examples
Anxiolytics	
Benzodiazepines	Lorazepam
Azaspirodecanedione	Buspirone
β-Blockers	Propranolol
Hypnotics	
Benzodiazepines	Lorazepam
Barbiturates	Seconal
Barbiturate-like compounds	Chloral hydrate

of respiratory suppression in high dosage and their high potential for dependency and for drug-drug interactions. Others such as glutethimide, methaqualone, and ethyl chlorvinyl should also be avoided. Meprobamate can be problematic because it greatly induces the metabolism of other medications, has a narrow margin between toxic and therapeutic doses, and is associated with dependence and life-threatening withdrawal reactions. Unfortunately, some states now require special prescriptions for benzodiazepines, and this may lead to an increased use of agents that carry greater risk but are less restricted.

There are apparent pharmacodynamic differences among benzodiazepines. For example, the short half-life of triazolam must be weighed against the drug's propensity for causing anterograde amnesia (Scharf et al. 1988); this effect could lead to confusional syndromes in elderly patients.

Buspirone is structurally and pharmacologically distinct from benzodiazepines. It interacts with serotonin and dopamine receptors (Zimmer and Gershon 1991).

Indications

A comprehensive text on anxiety and anxiolytics in elderly patients has recently appeared (Salzman and Lebowitz 1991). The indications for anxiolytic use appear to be narrow and, in cognitively intact elderly patients, they are analogous to those in younger adults without dementia. Indications for anxiolytic use include generalized anxiety, panic disorder, and short-term use in the treatment of disturbed sleep. Anxiolytics also have a limited place in management of patients with dementia.

Efficacy

Anxiolytic and hypnotic effects. Clinical studies reported for patients older than 65 generally are based on small samples; consequently, the clinician needs to maintain a healthy skepticism toward the literature on treatment outcome (efficacy, side effects, and toxicity) for any specific drug.

The acute efficacy of anxiolytic agents has received limited investigation in elderly patients. Greater efficacy compared with placebo in reducing anxiety and insomnia has been reported for oxazepam (Koepke et al. 1982) and alprazolam (Cohn 1984). The association of anxiety with depression after middle age deserves special attention. Nearly one-third of older depressed patients continue to have morning anxiety more than 1 year after discharge from hospital treatment; two-thirds of these have symptoms of anxiety at other times (Blazer et al. 1989). Many of these patients may use anxiolytic agents despite absence of long-term efficacy data and the potential risk of dependence.

Buspirone in open treatment studies has been reported to reduce Hamilton Anxiety Rating Scale scores in elderly patients (Levine et al. 1989; Napoliello 1986; Robinson and Napoliello 1988; Singh and Beer 1988). The samples studied were clinically heterogeneous.

Agitation in dementia. In patients with dementia, diazepam has been found more calming than thioridazine, but thioridazine was associated with greater improvement of behavioral disturbance (Kirven and Montero 1973). Lorazepam has been found effective in reducing agitation, wandering, and restlessness in patients with dementia (Sizaret et al. 1974). Such studies have not distinguished sedation from an anxiolytic action. Although anxiety can be a concomitant of dementia, patients with dementia may be agitated without appearing to be anxious. It is not surprising, therefore, that a randomized comparison of the benzodiazepine oxazepam with haloperidol and diphenhydramine found all three agents to be effective, and comparably so, in reducing dementia-related agitation (Coccaro et al. 1990). Furthermore, benzodiazepines can increase agitation in some patients by worsening cognitive impairment. Discontinuation of benzodiazepines has been found to improve cognitive performance in nursing home patients with dementia (Salzman 1992).

An open trial of buspirone for dementia-related agitation reported 22% improvement on an operationalized agitation scale at an average dose of 35 mg/day (Sakauye et al. 1993). Placebo-controlled efficacy data are not available.

Practical Guidelines

Pretreatment assessment. In considering treatment with benzodiazepines and related drugs, history taking identifies and characterizes prior treatment including abuse and dependence.

Dosing. Pharmacokinetic and pharmacodynamic concomitants of aging make older patients especially vulnerable to toxic effects of benzodiazepines. The twofold to threefold increase in half-life of long-acting agents with active metabolites (diazepam, chlordiazepoxide, flurazepam) over short-acting compounds (lorazepam, oxazepam, temazepam, triazolam) in elderly patients versus young adults (Greenblatt et al. 1982; Salzman et al. 1983) argues for use of the latter group of medications in elderly patients to avoid drug accumulation.

Buspirone is not known to have pharmacologically active metabolites. It does not interact pharmacodynamically with alcohol, but does interact with haloperidol.

Toxicity. Toxic doses of anxiolytics can produce sedation, ataxia, and impaired cognitive performance. Even "therapeutic" doses of benzodiazepines can decrease memory consolidation in this population (Jenike 1985a; Pomara et al. 1984; Rickels et al. 1987).

A pharmacodynamic component to increased sensitivity to benzodiazepines in elderly patients has been demonstrated. Increased sensitivity to given concentrations of benzodiazepines in elderly adults compared with young adults was described by Reidenberg et al. (1978) and in the studies by Pomara et al. (1984).

"Paradoxical" reactions to benzodiazepines may occur (Pomara et al. 1984). These involve increased irritability, agitation, and loss of behavioral control. The triazolobenzodiazepines may have greater potential for producing this disinhibition, which generally occurs during the first week of treatment. Whether age influences the vulnerability to such reactions is not known.

Tolerance to the effects of benzodiazepines can occur. Dependence can become a problem with long-term use. Dependence and toxicity are of sufficient concern that therapeutic trials with careful monitoring and on a time-limited basis should be undertaken.

The side effect profile of buspirone differs from that of benzodiazepines in that it may be associated with less sedative and cognitive toxicity (Hart et al. 1991; Lawlor et al. 1992). It produces less euphoria than benzodiazepines and may have less potential for dependence and abuse. It can produce dizziness, headache, sleep disturbances, and gastrointestinal complaints in elderly patients, however. Tardive dyskinesia has been reported (Strauss 1988).

Additional Clinical Situations

The triazolobenzodiazepine anxiolytic alprazolam is thought to have antidepressant properties, although panic disorder is the primary indication for using this medication. Weissman and colleagues (1992) completed a study comparing alprazolam, imipramine, and placebo in outpatients older than 60 with major depression. All subjects received weekly sessions of concurrent interpersonal psychotherapy. Alprazolam was associated with significantly greater decreases in depression and anxiety ratings at 2 weeks, but the differences between treatment groups disappeared by week 6. This may be because of benefits resulting from the psychotherapy administered to all treatment groups. These data indicate that alprazolam may cause rapid improvement in some of the symptoms associated with geriatric depression; however, the antidepressant efficacy of this agent when used alone remains to be demonstrated.

Benzodiazepines have been used early in the management of major depression in conjunction with antidepressant medication with the intention of reducing anxiety symptoms prior to the onset of effects of the antidepressant. Studies evaluating the risks and benefits of this strategy are not available.

Benzodiazepines have been used in mixed-age populations to ameliorate neuroleptic drug side effects including akathisia and tardive dyskinesia. Potential increased risks in elderly patients need to be weighed and alternative strategies need to be considered thoroughly.

Benzodiazepines may serve as useful alternatives to neuroleptic drugs as adjuncts in management of acute mania in elderly patients (Mirchandani and Young 1993). Data concerning their risks and benefits in this context are needed.

References

Abernathy DR, Greenblatt DJ, Shader RI: Imipramine and desipramine disposition in the elderly. J Pharmacol Exp Ther 232:183–188, 1985

Abou-Saleh MT, Coppen A: The prognosis of depression in old age: the case for lithium therapy. Br J Psychiatry 143:527–528, 1983

Addonizio G: Neuroleptic malignant syndrome in elderly patients. J Am Geriatr Soc 35:1011–1012, 1987

Agnoli A, Fabbrini G, Fioravanti M, et al: CBF and cognitive evaluation of Alzheimer type patients before and after IMAO-B treatment: a pilot study. Eur Neuropsychopharmacol 2:31–35, 1992

Alexopoulos GS, Abrams RC, Young RC, et al: Cornell scale for depression in dementia. Biol Psychiatry 23:271–284, 1988

Alexopoulos GS, Young RC, Abrams RC, et al: Chronicity and relapse in geriatric depression. Biol Psychiatry 26:551–564, 1989

Allain H, Pollak P, Neukirch HC: Symptomatic effect of selegiline in de novo Parkinsonian patients: the French selegiline multicenter trial.

Mov Disord 8 (suppl 1):S36–S40, 1993

Alvir JY, Ma J, Lieberman JA, et al: Clozapine-induced agranulocytosis. N Engl J Med 329:162–167, 1993

Aoba A, Yamaguchi N, Shedo M: Plasma neuroleptic levels in aged patients on various neuroleptic, in Liver and Aging. Edited by Kitani K. New York, Elsevier, 1986, pp 115–126

Axelsson R: On the pharmacokinetics of thioridazine in psychiatric patients, in Antipsychotic Drugs: Pharmacodynamics and Pharmacokinetics. New York, Pergamon Press, 1976, pp 353–358

Ayd FJ: A survey of drug-induced extrapyramidal reactions. JAMA 175:1045–1060, 1976

Bajulaiye R, Addonizio G: Clozapine in the treatment of psychosis in an 82-year-old woman with tardive dyskinesia. J Clin Psychopharmacol 12:364–365, 1992

Baker SP, Harvey AH: Fall injuries in the elderly. Clin Geriatr Med 1:501–512, 1985

Baldwin RC, Holley DJ: The prognosis of depression in old age. Br J Psychiatry 149:574–583, 1986

Ball CJ: The use of clozapine in older people. International Journal of Geriatric Psychiatry 7:689–692, 1992

Barnes R, Veith R, Okimoto J, et al: Efficacy of antipsychotic medications in behaviorally disturbed dementia patients. Am J Psychiatry 139:1170–1174, 1982

Bergstrom RF, Lemberger L, Farid NA, et al: Clinical pharmacology and pharmacokinetics of fluoxetine: a review. Br J Psychiatry 153 (suppl 3):47–50, 1988

Bickford-Wimer PC, Parfitt K, Hoffer BJ, et al: Desipramine and noradrenergic neurotransmission in aging: failure to respond in aged laboratory animals. Neuropsychopharmacology 26:597–605, 1987

Black SW, Winokur D, Nasrallah A, et al: Complicated mania: comorbidity and immediate outcome in the treatment of mania. Arch Gen Psychiatry 45:232–236, 1988

Blazer D, Hughes DC, Fowler N: Anxiety as an outcome symptom of depression in elderly and middle-aged adults. International Journal of Geriatric Psychiatry 4:273–278, 1989

Board of Directors of the American Association for Geriatric Psychiatry, Clinical Practice Committee of the American Geriatrics Society, Committee on Long-Term-Care and Treatment for the Elderly of the American Psychiatric Association: psychotherapeutic medications in the nursing home. J Am Geriatr Soc 40:946–949, 1992

Bocksberger JP, Gachoud JP, Richard J, et al: Comparison of the efficacy of moclobemide and fluvoxamine in elderly patients with a severe depressive episode. Eur Psychiatry 8:319–324, 1993

Bouchard RH, Pourcher E, Vincent P: Fluoxetine and extrapyramidal side effects (letter). Am J Psychiatry 146:1352–1353, 1989

Bowden CL, Schatzberg AF, Rosenbaum A, et al: Fluoxetine and desipramine in major depressive disorder. J Clin Psychopharmacol 13:305–311, 1993

Bowden CL, Brugger AM, Swann AC, et al: Efficacy of divalproex vs lithium and placebo in the treatment of mania. JAMA 271(12):918–923, 1994

Boyer WF, McFadden GA, Feighner JP: The efficacy of selective serotonin reuptake inhibitors in anxiety and obsessive-compulsive disorder, in Perspectives in Psychiatry, Vol 1. Selective Serotonin Reuptake Inhibitors. Edited by Feighner JP, Boyer WF. New York, Wiley, 1991, pp 109–117

Branconnier RJ, Cole JO, Ghazvinian S, et al: Treating the depressed elderly patient: the comparative behavioral pharmacology of mianserin and amitriptyline, in Typical and Atypical Antidepressants: Clinical Practice. Edited by Costa E, Racagni G. New York, Raven, 1982

Branconnier RJ, Cole JO, Ghazvinian S, et al: Clinical pharmacology of bupropion and imipramine in elderly depressives. J Clin Psychiatry 44(2):130–133, 1983

Broud TM: Fluoxetine and extrapyramidal side effects (letter). Am J Psychiatry 146:1353, 1989

Chambers CA, Bain J, Rosbottom R, et al: Carbamazepine in senile dementia and overactivity: a placebo controlled double blind trial. IRCS J Med Sci 10:505–506, 1982

Chapron DJ, Cameron IR, White LB, et al: Observations on lithium disposition in the elderly. J Am Geriatr Soc 30:651–655, 1982

Chiarello RJ, Cole JO: The use of psychostimulants in general psychiatry. Arch Gen Psychiatry 44:286–295, 1987

Coccaro EF, Kramer E, Zemishlany Z, et al: Pharmacologic treatment of noncognitive behavioral disturbances in elderly demented patients. Am J Psychiatry 147:1640–1645, 1990

Cohen-Mansfield J: Agitated behaviors in the elderly, II: preliminary results in the cognitively deteriorated. J Am Geriatr Soc 34:722–727, 1986

Cohn CK, Shrivastava R, Mendels J, et al: Double-blind, multicenter comparison of sertraline and amitriptyline in elderly depressed patients. J Clin Psychiatry 51(12, suppl B):28–33, 1990

Cohn JB: Double-blind safety and efficacy comparison of alprazolam and placebo in the treatment of anxiety in geriatric patients. Curr Ther Res 35:100–112, 1984

Cohn JB, Varga L, Lyford A: A two-center double-blind study of nomifensine, imipramine, and placebo in depressed geriatric outpatients. J Clin Psychiatry 45:68–72, 1984

Crabtree BL, Mack JE, Johnson CD, et al: Comparison of hydrochlorothiazide and furosemide on lithium disposition. Am J Psychiatry 148:1060–1063, 1991

Craig I, Tallis R: Impact of valproate and phenytoin on cognitive function in elderly patients: results of a single-blind randomized comparative study. Epilepsia 35:381–390, 1994

Cramer JA, Scheyer RD, Mattson RH: Compliance declines between clinical visits. Arch Intern Med 150:1509–1510, 1990

Crane GE, Naranjo ER: Motor disturbances induced by neuroleptics. Arch Gen Psychiatry 24:179–184, 1971

Crewe HK, Lennard MS, Tucker GT, et al: The effect of selective serotonin re-uptake inhibitors on cytochrome P450-6 (CYP-6) activity in human liver microsomes. Br J Clin Pharmacol 34:262–265, 1992

Cunningham LA, Borison RL, Carman JS, et al: A comparison of venlafaxine, traxodone and placebo in major depression. J Clin Psychopharmacol 14:99–106, 1994

Curry SH: Binding of psychotropic drugs to plasma protein and its influence on drug disposition, in Clinical Pharmacology in Psychiatry. Edited by Usdin E. New York, Elsevier, 1981, pp 213–223

Das Gupta K, Jefferson JW, Kobak KA, et al: The effect of enalapril on serum lithium levels in healthy men. J Clin Psychiatry 53:398–400, 1992

Davidson J: Seizures and bupropion: a review. J Clin Psychiatry 50:256–261, 1989

DePaulo J Jr, Correa EI, Sapir DG: Renal function and lithium: a longitudinal study. Am J Psychiatry 143:892–895, 1986

Devanand D, Sackeim H, Brown R, et al: A pilot study of haloperidol treatment of psychosis and behavioral disturbance in Alzheimer's disease. Arch Neurol 46:854–857, 1989

De Vanna M, Kummer J, Agnoli A, et al: Moclobemide compared with second-generation antidepressants in elderly people. Acta Psychiatr Scand Suppl 360:64–66, 1990

Dunner DL, Cohn JB, Walshe T, et al: Two combined, multicenter double-blind studies of paroxetine and doxepin in geriatric patients with major depression. J Clin Psychiatry 53 (2 suppl):57–60, 1992

Dysken MW, Johnson SB, Holden L, et al: Haloperidol concentrations in patients with Alzheimer's dementia. Clin Pharmacol Ther 47:162, 1990

Echt DS, Liebson PR, Mitchell LB, et al: Mortality and morbidity in patients receiving encainaide, flecainide or placebo. N Engl J Med 324: 781–788, 1991

Eison AS, Eison MS, Torrente JR, et al: Nefazodone: preclinical pharmacolgy of a new antidepressant. Psychopharm Bull 26:311–315, 1990

Extein I: Treatment of Tricyclic-Resistant Depression. Washington DC, American Psychiatric Association, 1989, pp 51–79

Feighner JP, Cohn JB: Double-blind comparative trials of fluoxetine and doxepin in geriatric patients with major depressive disorder. J Clin Psychiatry 46:20–25, 1985

Ferris SH, Steinberg G, Shulman E, et al: Institutionalization of Alzheimer's patients: reducing precipitating factors through family counseling. Arch Found Thanatol 12:7, 1985

Figiel GS, Krishnan KRR, Breitner JC, et al: Radiologic correlates of antidepressant-induced delirium: the possible significance of basal-ganglia lesions. J Neuropsychiatry 1(2):188 –190, 1989

Folstein MF, Folstein SE, McHugh PR: Mini Mental State: a practical method for grading the cognitive state of patients for the clinician. J Psychiatr Res 12:189–198, 1975

Fontaine R, Ontiveros A, Elie R, et al: A double-blind comparison of nefazodone, imipramine and placebo in major depression. J Clin Psychiatry 55:234–241, 1994

Foster JR, Silver M, Boksay IJ: The potential use of adjunctive intra-erythrocyte (RBC) lithium levels in detecting serious impending neurotoxicity in the elderly: two case reports. International Journal of Geriatric Psychiatry 5(1):9–14, 1990

Frank E, Kupfer DJ, Perel TM, et al: Three-year outcomes for maintenance therapies in recurrent depression. Arch Gen Psychiatry 47:1093–1099, 1990

Frankenburg FR, Kalunian D: Clozapine in the elderly. J Geriatr Psychiatry Neurol 7:129–132, 1994

Freeman H: Moclobemide. Lancet 342:1528–1532, 1993

Friedman JR, Norman DC, Yoshikawa TT: Correlation of estimated renal function parameters versus 24-hour creatinine clearance in ambulatory elderly. J Am Geriatr Soc 37:145–149, 1989

Gardos G, Casey D (eds): Tardive Dyskinesia and Affective Disorders. Washington DC, American Psychiatric Association, 1984

Georgotas A, McCue RE: The additional benefit of extending an antidepressant trial past seven weeks in the depressed elderly. International Journal of Geriatric Psychiatry 4:191–195, 1989

Georgotas A, McCue RE, Hapworth W, et al: Comparative efficacy and safety of MAOIs versus TCAs in treating depression in the elderly. Biol Psychiatry 21:1155–1166, 1986

Georgotas A, McCue RE, Cooper TB: A placebo-controlled comparison of nortriptyline and phenelzine in maintenance therapy of elderly depressed patients. Arch Gen Psychiatry 46:783–786, 1989

Gerner R, Estabrook W, Steuer J, et al: Treatment of geriatric depression with trazodone, imipramine and placebo: a double-blind study. J Clin Psychiatry 41:216–220, 1980

Gitlin MJ: Lithium-induced renal insufficiency. J Clin Psychopharmacol 132:276–279, 1993

Glasser M, Rabins P: Mania in the elderly. Age Aging 13:210–213, 1984

Glassman AH, Bigger JT Jr: Cardiovascular effects of therapeutic doses of the tricyclic antidepressants: a review. Arch Gen Psychiatry 38:815–820, 1981

Glassman AH, Kantor SJ, Shostak M: Depression, delusions, and drug response. Am J Psychiatry 132:716–719, 1975

Glassman AH, Bigger JT Jr, Giardina EV, et al: Clinical characteristics of imipramine-induced orthostatic hypotension. Lancet 1:468–472, 1979

Glassman AH, Johnson GG, Giardina EV, et al: The use of imipramine in depressed patients with congestive heart failure. JAMA 280:1987–2001, 1983

Glassman AH, Roose SP, Bigger JT Jr: The safety of tricyclic antidepressants in cardiac patients: risk-benefit reconsidered (commentary). JAMA 269: 2673–2675, 1993

Gleason RP, Schneider LS: Carbamazepine treatment of agitation in Alzheimer's outpatients refractory to neuroleptic. J Clin Psychiatry 51(3):115–118, 1990

Gnam W, Flint AJ: New onset rapid cycling bipolar disorder in an 87 year old woman. Can J Psychiatry 38(5):324–326, 1993

Goff DC, Jenike MA: Treatment-resistant depression in the elderly. J Am Geriatr Soc 34:63–70, 1986

Golden RN, DeVane CL, Laizure SC, et al: Bupropion in depression, II: the role of metabolites in clinical outcome. Arch Gen Psychiatry 45:145–149, 1988

Goodman WK, Price LH, Rasmussen SA, et al: Efficacy of fluvoxamine in

OCD: a double-blind comparison with placebo. Arch Gen Psychiatry 46:36–44, 1989

Gorman JM, Liebowitz MR, Fyer AJ, et al: An open trial of fluoxetine in the treatment of panic attacks. J Clin Psychopharmacol 7:329–332, 1987

Greenblatt DJ, Shader RJ: Benzodiazepine kinetics in the elderly, in Clinical Pharmacology in Psychiatry. Edited by Usdin E. New York, Elsevier, 1981, pp 174–181

Greenblatt DJ, Sellers EM, Shader RI: Drug disposition in old age. N Engl J Med 306:1081–1088, 1982

Gurian B, Rosowsky E: Methylphenidate treatment of minor depression in very old patients. Am J Geriatric Psychiatry 1:171–174, 1993

Hamilton M: A rating scale for depression. J Neurol Neurosurg Psychiatry 23:56–62, 1960

Hardy BG, Shulman KI, Mackenzie SE, et al: Pharmacokinetics of lithium in the elderly. J Clin Psychopharmacol 7:153–158, 1987

Haring C, Meise U, Humpel C, et al: Influence of patient-related variables on clozapine plasma levels. Am J Psychiatry 147:1471–1475, 1990

Harris R, Hoelscher WE: Use of a new psychic energizer (Marplan) in an old age home double blind study. J Am Geriatr Soc 9:218–224, 1961

Hart RP, Colenda CC, Hamer RM: Effects of buspirone and alprazolam on the cognitive performance of normal elderly subjects. Am J Psychiatry 148:73–77, 1991

Hayes RL, Gerner RH, Fairbands L, et al: EKG findings in geriatric depressives given trazodone, placebo or imipramine. J Clin Psychiatry 44:180–183, 1983

Health Care Financing Administration, U.S. Department of Health and Human Services: Federal Register 56, 48:826–848, 879, 1991

Hebenstreit GF, Fellerer K, Zochling R, et al: A pharmacokinetic dose titration study in elderly depressed patients. Acta Psychiatr Scand 80 (suppl 350):81–84, 1989

Himmelhoch JM, Neil JF, May SJ, et al: Age, dementia, dyskinesias and lithium response. Am J Psychiatry 137:941–944, 1980

Hollister LE: General principles of treating the elderly with drugs, in Clinical Pharmacology and the Aged Patient. Aging. Edited by Jarvik L, et al. New York, Raven, 16:1–9, 1981

Israili ZH, Wenger J: Aging, gastrointestinal disease, and response to drugs, in Clinical Pharmacology and the Aged Patient. Aging. Edited by Jarvik L, et al. New York, Raven, 16:131–155, 1981

Janicak PG, Davis JM, Preskorn SH, et al (eds): Principles and Practice of

Psychopharmacotherapy. Baltimore, MD, Williams & Wilkins, 1993

Janowsky D, Curtis G, Zisook S, et al: Ventricular arrhythmias possibly aggravated by trazodone. Am J Psychiatry 140:796–797, 1983

Jarvik L: The patient with renal disease, in Treatments of Psychiatric Disorders: A Task Force Report of the American Psychiatric Association, Vol 2. Washington, DC, American Psychiatric Association, 1989, pp 915–930

Jarvik LF, Mintz J: Treatment of depression, in Old Age: What Works? Edited by Awad AG, Durost H, Mayer HMR, et al. New York, Pergamon, 1987, pp 51–57

Jefferson JW, Greist JH: Lithium and the kidney, in Psychopharmacology Update. Edited by David JM, Greenblatt D. New York, Grune & Stratton, 1979, pp 81–104

Jefferson JW, Greist JH, Baudhuin M: Lithium: interactions with other drugs. J Clin Psychopharmacol 1:124–131, 1981

Jenike MA: Handbook of Geriatric Psychopharmacology. Littleton, CO, PSG Publishing, 1985a

Jenike MA: Monoamine oxidase inhibitors as treatment for depressed patients with primary degenerative dementia (Alzheimer's disease). Am J Psychiatry 142:763–764, 1985b

Jeste DV, Wyatt RJ: Aging and tardive dyskinesia, in Schizophrenia and Aging. Edited by Miller NE, Cohen GD. New York, Guilford, 1987

Jeste DV, DeLisi LE, Zalcman S, et al: A biochemical study of tardive dyskinesia in young male patients. Psychiatry Res 4:327–331, 1981

Jeste DV, Linnoila M, Wagner RL, et al: Serum neuroleptic concentrations and tardive dyskinesia. Psychopharmacology 76:377–380, 1982

Jeste DV, Harris MJ, Pearlson GD, et al: Late-onset schizophrenia: studying clinical validity. Psychiatr Clin North Am 11:1–14, 1988

Joffe RT, Singer W, Levitt AJ, et al: A placebo-controlled comparison of lithium and triiodothyronine augmentation of tricyclic antidepressants in unipolar refractory depression. Arch Gen Psychiatry 50:387–393, 1993

Kane JM, Cole K, Sarantakos S, et al: Safety and efficacy of bupropion in elderly patients: preliminary observations. J Clin Psychiatry 44:134–136, 1983

Kathol RG, Perry F: Relationship of medical illness to depression: a central review. J Affect Disord 3:111–121, 1981

Kay DWK: Outcome and cause of death in mental disorders of old age: a long-term follow-up of functional and organic psychoses. Acta Psychiatr Scand 38:149–276, 1962

Kellner MB, Neher F: A first episode of mania after age 80: a case report. Can J Psychiatry 36:607–608, 1991

Kerr JS, Fairweather DB, Hindmarch I: The effects of acute and repeated doses of moclobemide on psychomotor performance and cognitive function in healthy elderly volunteers. Human Psychopharmacology 7:273–279, 1992a

Kerr JS, Fairweather DB, Mahendran R, et al: The effects of paroxetine, alone and in combination with alcohol on psychomotor performance and cognitive function in the elderly. Int Clin Psychopharmacol 7:101–108, 1992b

Kessler KA: Tricyclic antidepressants: mode of action and clinical use, in Psychopharmacology: A Generation of Progress. Edited by Lipton M, DiMascio A, Killam K, et al. New York, Raven, 1978, pp 1289–1302

Kirven LE, Montero EF: Comparison of thioridazine and diazepam in the control of nonpsychotic symptoms associated with senility: double-blind control study. J Am Geriatr Soc 21:545–551, 1973

Kitanaka I, Zavadil AP, Cutler NR, et al: Altered hydroxy-desipramine concentrations in the elderly. Clin Pharmacol Ther 29:258, 1981

Klein DF, Gittelman R, Quitkin FM, et al: Diagnosis and Drug Treatment of Psychiatric Disorders: Adults and Children. Baltimore, MD, Williams & Wilkins, 1980

Koepke HH, Gold RL, Linden ME, et al: Multicenter controlled study of oxazepam in anxious elderly patients. Psychosomatics 23:641–645, 1982

Kronig MH, Roose SP, Walsh BP, et al: Blood pressure effects of phenelzine. J Clin Psychopharmacol 3:307–310, 1983

Kruse W, Koch-Gwinner P, Nikolaus T, et al: Measurement of drug compliance by continuous electronic monitoring: a pilot study of elderly patients discharged from hospital. J Am Geriatr Soc 40:1151–1155, 1992

Kutcher SP, Reid K, Dubbin JD, et al: Electrocardiogram changes and therapeutic desipramine and 2-hydroxy-desipramine concentrations in elderly depressives. Br J Psychiatry 148:676–679, 1986

Lamy PP, Salzman C, Nevis-Olesen J: Drug prescribing patterns, risks and compliance guidelines, in Clinical Geriatric Psychopharmacology. Edited by Salzman C. Baltimore, MD, Williams & Wilkins, 1992, pp 15–37

Laghrassi-Thode F, Pollock BG, Miller M, et al: Comparative effects of sertraline and nortriptyline on body sway in older depressed patients. American Journal of Geriatric Psychiatry 3:217–228, 1995

Lawlor BA, Hill JL, Radcliffe JL: A single oral dose challenge of buspirone does not affect memory processes in older volunteers. Biol Psychiatry 32:101–103, 1992

Leibovici A, Tariot PN: Agitation associated with dementia: a systematic approach to treatment. Psychopharmacol Bull 24:49–53, 1988

Lemberger L, Bergstrom RF, Wolen RL, et al: Fluoxetine: clinical pharmacology and psychologic disposition. J Clin Psychiatry 46:14–19, 1985

Levine S, Napoliello MJ, Domantay AG: Open study of buspirone in octogenarians with anxiety. Human Psychopharmacology 4:51–53, 1989

Lingam VR, Lazarus LW, Groves L, et al: Methylphenidate in treating poststroke depression. J Clin Psychiatry 49:151–153, 1988

Lipsey JR, Robinson RG, Pearlson GD: Nortriptyline treatment of poststroke depression: a double-blind study. Lancet 1:297–300, 1984

Lydiard BR: Tricyclic-resistant depression: treatment resistance or inadequate treatment? J Clin Psychiatry 46:412–417, 1985

Maguire K, Pereira A, Tiller J: Moclobemide pharmacokinetics in depressed patients: lack of age effect. Human Psychopharmacology 6:249–252, 1991

Magnani A, Grassi MP, Frattola L, et al: Effects of MAO-B inhibitor in the treatment of Alzheimer's disease. Eur Neurol 31:100–107, 1991

Maletta GJ, Winegarden T: Reversal of anorexia by methylphenidate in apathetic, severely demented nursing home patients. Am J Psychiatry 1:234–243, 1993

Mann JJ, Aarons SF, Wilner PJ, et al: A controlled study of the antidepressant efficacy and side effects of deprenyl: a selective monoamine oxidase inhibitor. Arch Gen Psychiatry 46:45–50, 1989

Mattis S: Dementia Rating Scale. Odessa, FL, Psychological Assessment Resource, 1988

Mazure CM, Druss BG, Cellar JS: Valproate treatment of older psychotic patients with organic mental syndromes and behavioral dyscontrol. J Am Geriatr Soc 40:914–916, 1992

McCabe B, Tsuang MT: Dietary consideration in MAO inhibitor regimens. J Clin Psychiatry 43:178–181, 1982

McCreadie RG, Robertson LJ, Wiles D: The Nithsdale Schizophrenia Survey, IX: akathisia, parkinsonism and tardive dyskinesia and plasma neuroleptic levels. Br J Psychiatry 161:793–799, 1992

McCue RE, Aronowitz J: Accelerated antidepressent response in geriatric inpatients. American Journal of Geriatric Psychiatry 2:244–246, 1994

McFarland BH, Miller MR, Straumfjord AA: Valproate use in the older manic patients. J Clin Psychiatry 51:479–481, 1990

Mellow AM, Solano-Lopez C, Davis S: Sodium valproate in the treatment of behavioral disturbance in dementia. J Geriatr Psychiatry Neurol 6:205–209, 1993

Mendels J, Johnson R, Mattes J, et al: Efficacy of bid doses of venlafaxine in a dose-response study. Psychopharm Bull 29:169–174, 1993

Meredith CH, Feighner JP, Hendrickson G: A double-blind comparative evaluation of the efficacy and safety of nomifensine, imipramine, and placebo in depressed geriatric outpatients. J Clin Psychiatry 45:73–77, 1984

Meyers BS: Adverse cognitive effects of tricyclic antidepressants in the treatment of geriatric depression: fact or fiction, in Psychopharmacological Treatment Complications in the Elderly. Edited by Shamoian CA. Washington, DC, American Psychiatric Association, 1991, pp 1–16

Meyers B, Kalayam B: Update in geriatric psychopharmacology, in Advances in Psychosomatic Medicine, Vol 19. Basel, Switzerland, Karger, 1989, pp 114–137

Meyers B, Young RC: Dementia of the Alzheimer's type, in Treatments of Psychiatric Disorders: A Task Force Report of the American Psychiatric Association, Vol 2. Washington, DC, American Psychiatric Association, 1989, pp 975–989

Mirchandani I, Young RC: Management of mania in the elderly: an update. Ann Clin Psychiatry 5:67–77, 1993

Moleman P, Janzen G, von Bargen BA, et al: Relationship between age and incidence of parkinsonism in psychiatric patients treated with haloperidol. Am J Psychiatry 143:232–234, 1986

Monteleone P, Gnocchi G: Evidence for a linear relationship between plasma trazodone levels and clinical response in depression in the elderly. Clin Neuropharmacol 13:S84–S89, 1990

Murphy E: The prognosis of depression in old age. Br J Psychiatry 142:111–119, 1983

Murray N, Hopwood S, Balfour JK, et al: The influence of age on lithium efficacy and side-effects in out-patients. Psychol Med 13:53–60, 1983

Myllyla VV, Sotaniemi KA, Vuorinen JA, et al: Selegiline in de novo parkinsonian patients: the Finnish study. Mov Disord 8 (suppl 1):S41–44, 1993

Nambudiri DE, Mirchandani IC, Young RC: Two more cases of trazodone-related syncope in the elderly. J Geriatr Psychiatry Neurol 2:225, 1989

Napoliello MJ: An interim multicentre report on 677 anxious geriatric out-patients treated with buspirone. Br J Clin Practice, February, 1986, pp 71–73

Nelson JC, Bowers MB: Delusional unipolar depression: description and drug response. Arch Gen Psychiatry 35:1321–1328, 1978

Nelson JC, Jatlow P, Mazure C: Desipramine plasma levels and response in elderly melancholic patients. J Clin Psychopharmacol 5:217–220, 1985

Nelson JC, Price LH, Jatlow PI: Neuroleptic dose and desipramine concentrations during combined treatment of delusional depression. Am J Psychiatry 143:1151–1154, 1986

Nelson JC, Atillasoy E, Mazure C, et al: Hydroxydesipramine in the elderly. J Clin Psychopharmacol 8:428–433, 1988a

Nelson JC, Mazure C, Jatlow PI: Antidepressant activity of 2-hydroxy-desipramine. Clin Pharmacol Ther 44:283–288, 1988b

Nelson JC, Mazure CM, Bowers MB, et al: A preliminary open study of the combination of fluoxetine and desipramine for rapid treatment of major depression. Arch Gen Psychiatry 48:303–307, 1991

Nies A, Robinson DS, Friedman MJ, et al: Relationship between age and tricyclic antidepressant levels. Am J Psychiatry 134:790–793, 1977

Oberholzer AF, Hendricksen C, Monsch AU, et al: Safety and effectiveness of low-dose clozapine in psychogeriatric patients: a preliminary study. Int Psychogeriatr 4:187–195, 1992

Omnibus Reconciliation Act of 1987. P.L. 100-203, 101 Stat. 1330

Parkin DM, Heyyey CR, Quirk J, et al: Deviation from prescribed drug treatment after discharge from hospital. Br Med J 2:686–688, 1976

Peabody CA, Warner D, Whiteford HA, et al: Neuroleptics and the elderly. J Am Geriatr Soc 35:233–238, 1987

Perel JM: Compliance and optimal dosage during maintenance: pharmacokinetic and analytical issues. J Clin Chem 34:881–887, 1988

Perlick D, Stastny P, Katz I, et al: Memory deficits and anticholinergic levels in chronic schizophrenia. Am J Psychiatry 143:230–232, 1986

Perry PJ, Morgan DE, Smith RE, Tsuang MT: Treatment of unipolar depression accompanied by delusions: ECT versus tricyclic antidepressant-antipsychotic combinations. J Affect Disord 4:195–200, 1982

Pillans PI, Coulter DM: Fluoxetine and hyponatraemia: a potential hazard in the elderly. N Z Med J 107(973):85–86, 1994

Pollock BG, Perel JM, Altieri LP, et al: Debrisoquine hydroxylation phenotyping in geriatric psychopharmacology. Psychopharmacol Bull 28:163–168, 1992

Pollock BG, Perel JM, Wright B, et al: Bupropion: Need for hydroxy-metabolite monitoring in the elderly depressed (abstract 18). Ther Drug Mon 15:162, 1993

Pomara N, Stanley B, Block R, et al: Adverse effects of single therapeutic doses of diazepam on performance in normal geriatric subjects: relationship to plasma concentrations. Psychopharmacology 84:342–346, 1984

Post F: The impact of modern drug treatment on old age schizophrenia. Gerontol Clin 4:137–146, 1962

Post F: Persistent Persecutory States of the Elderly. Oxford, England, Pergamon, 1966

Preskorn SH, Simpson S: Tricyclic antidepressant induced delirium and plasma drug concentrations. Am J Psychiatry 139:822–823, 1982

Preskorn SH, Alderman J, Chung M, et al: Desipramine levels after sertraline or fluoxetine. New Research, Proceedings. Washington, DC, American Psychiatric Association, 1992

Rabins PV, Mace NL, Lucas MJ: The impact of dementia on the family. JAMA 248:333–335, 1982

Raskind MN, Alvarez C, Herlin S: Fluphenazine enanthate in the outpatient treatment of late paraphrenia. J Am Geriatr Soc 27:459–469, 1979

Raskind MA, Risse SC, Lampe TH: Dementia and antipsychotic drugs. J Clin Psychiatry 48:5 (suppl):16–18, 1987

Ray WA, Federspiel CF, Schaffner W: A study of antipsychotic drug use in nursing homes: epidemiologic evidence suggesting misuse. Am J Public Health 70:485–491, 1980

Ray WA, Griffin MR, Schaffner W, et al: Psychotropic drug use and the risk of hip fracture. N Engl J Med 316:363–369, 1987

Reidenberg MM, Levy M, Warner H, et al: Relationship between diazepam dose, plasma level, age, and central nervous system depression. Clin Pharm Ther 23:371–374, 1978

Reifler BV, Teri L, Raskind M, et al: Double-blind trial of imipramine in Alzheimer's disease in patients with and without depression. Am J Psychiatry 146:45–49, 1989

Reynolds CF III, Perel JM, Kupfer DJ, et al: Open-trial response to antidepressant treatment in elderly patients with mixed depression and cognitive impairment. Psychiatry Res 21:111–122, 1987

Reynolds CF III, Perel JM, Frank E, et al: Open-trial maintenance pharmacotherapy in late life depression: survival analysis. Psychiatry Res 27:225–231, 1989

Reynolds CF III, Frank E, Perel FM, et al: Combined pharmacotherapy and psychotherapy in the acute and continuation treatment of elderly patients with recurrent major depression: a preliminary report. Am J Psychiatry 149:1687–1692, 1992

Richelson E: Pharmacology of antidepressants in use in the United States. J Clin Psychiatry 43:4–13, 1982

Rickels K, Schweizer E, Lucki I: Benzodiazepine side effects, in American Psychiatric Association Annual Review, Vol 6. Washington, DC, American Psychiatric Association, 1987

Rickels K, Schwizer E, Clary C, et al: Nefazodone and imipramine in major depression: a placebo-controlled trial. Br J Psychiatry 164:802–895, 1994

Robinson D, Napoliello MJ: The safety and usefulness of buspirone as an anxiolytic in elderly versus young patients. Clin Ther 10:740–746, 1988

Robinson DS: Monoamine oxidase inhibitors and the elderly, in Age and the Pharmacology of Psychoactive Drugs. Edited by Raskin A, Robinson DS, Levine J. New York, Elsevier, 1981, pp 149–161

Rockwell E, Lam RW, Zisook S: Antidepressant drug studies in the elderly. Psychiatr Clin North Am 11:215–233, 1988

Rolandi E, Magnani G, Sannia A, et al: Evaluation of Prl secretion in elderly subjects. Acta Endocrinol 42:148–151, 1982

Roose SP, Bone S, Haidorfer C, et al: Lithium treatment in older patients. Am J Psychiatry 136:843–844, 1979a

Roose SP, Nurnberger J, Dunner D, et al: Cardiac sinus node dysfunction during lithium treatment. Am J Psychiatry 136:804–806, 1979b

Roose SP, Glassman AH, Siris SG, et al: Comparison of imipramine and nortriptyline-induced orthostatic hypotension: a meaningful difference. J Clin Psychopharmacol 1:316–319, 1981

Roose SP, Glassman AH, Giardina EGV, et al: Tricyclic antidepressants in patients with cardiac conduction disease. Arch Gen Psychiatry 44:273–275, 1987

Rosenblatt JE, Pary RJ, Bigelow LB, et al: Measurement of serum neuroleptic concentrations by radioreceptor assay: concurrent assessment of clinical response and toxicity, in Neuroreceptors—Basic and Clinical Aspects. Edited by Usdin E, Bunney WE, Davis JM. New York, Wiley, 1981, pp 165–188

Rowe JW: Aging and renal function. Annu Rev Gerontol Geriatr 1:161–179, 1980

Sakauye KM, Camp CJ, Ford PA: Effects of buspirone on agitation associated with dementia. American Journal of Geriatric Psychiatry 1:82–84, 1993

Saltz BL, Woerner MG, Kane JM, et al: Prospective study of tardive dyskinesia incidence in the elderly. JAMA 266:2402–2406, 1991

Salzman C: Clinical Geriatric Psychopharmacology, 2nd Edition. Baltimore, MD, Williams & Wilkins, 1992

Salzman C, Lebowitz B (eds): Anxiety in the Elderly: Treatment and Research. New York, Springer, 1991

Salzman C, Shader RI, Pearlman M: Psychopharmacology and the elderly, in Psychotropic Drug Side Effects. Edited by Shader RI, DiMascio A. Baltimore, MD, Williams & Wilkins, 1970

Salzman C, Shader RI, Greenblatt DJ, et al: Long versus half-life benzodiazepines in the elderly: kinetics and clinical effects of diazepam and oxazepam. Arch Gen Psychiatry 40:293–297, 1983

Salzman C, Fisher J, Nobel K, et al: Cognitive improvement following benzodiazepine discontinuation in elderly nursing home residents. International Journal of Geriatric Psychiatry 7:89–93, 1992

Salzman C, Schneider L, Lebowitz B: Antidepressant treatment of very old patients. American Journal of Geriatric Psychiatry 1:21–29, 1993

Salzman C, Vaccaro B, Lieff J, et al: Clozapine in older patients with psychosis and behavioral disruption. American Journal of Geriatric Psychiatry 3:26–33, 1995

Satel SL, Nelson JC: Stimulants in the treatment of depression: a critical overview. J Clin Psychiatry 50:241–249, 1989

Sawin CT, Castelli WP, Hershman JM, et al: The thyroid: thyroid deficiency in the Framingham study. Arch Intern Med 145:1386–1388, 1985

Schaffer CB, Garvey MJ: Use of lithium in acutely manic elderly patients. Clin Gerontol 3:58, 1984

Scharf MB, Fletcher K, Graham JP: Comparative amnestic effects of benzodiazepine hypnotic agents. J Clin Psychiatry 49:134–137, 1988

Schatzberg AF, Cole JO: Manual of Clinical Psychopharmacology. Washington, DC, American Psychiatric Press, 1986, pp 249–251

Schneider LS, Sobin PB: Non-neuroleptic medications in the management of agitation in Alzheimer's disease and other dementias. Int J Geriatr Psychiatry 6:691–708, 1991

Schneider LS, Cooper TB, Serverson JH, et al: Electrocardiographic changes with nortriptyline and 10-hydroxynortriptyline in elderly depressed outpatients. J Clin Psychopharmacol 8:402–408, 1988

Schneider LS, Pollock VE, Lyness SA: A metaanalysis of controlled trials of neuroleptic treatment in dementia. J Am Geriatr Soc 38:553–563, 1990

Schneider LS, Olin JT, Pawluczyk S: A double-blind crossover pilot study of l-deprenyl (selegiline) combined with cholinesterase inhibitor in Alzheimer's disease. Am J Psychiatry 150:321–323, 1993

Scholz E, Dichgans J: Treatment of drug-induced exogenous psychosis in parkinsonism with clozapine and fluperlapine. Eur Arch Psychiatry Clin Neurolsci 235:60–64, 1985

Schorr RI, Fought RL, Ray WA: Changes in antipsychotic drug use in nursing homes during implementation of OBRA-87 regulations. JAMA 271:358–362, 1994

Schweizer E, Rickels K, Amsterdam JD, et al: What constitutes an adequate antidepressant trial for fluoxetine? J Clin Psychiatry 51:8–11, 1990

Shader RI, DiMascio A: Clinical Handbook of Psychopharmacology. New York, Science House, 1970

Shamoian CA: Somatic therapies in geriatric psychiatry, in Essentials of Geriatric Psychiatry. Edited by Lazarus LW. New York, Springer, 1988, pp 173–188

Shukla S, Hoff A, Aaronson T, et al: Treatment outcome in organic mania. New Research Program, Annual Meeting. Washington, DC, American Psychiatric Association, 1987

Shulman K, Post F: Bipolar affective disorders in old age. Br J Psychiatry 136:26–32, 1980

Shulman KI, Walker SE, MacKenzie S, et al: Dietary restrictions, tyramine and the use of monoamine oxidase inhibitors. J Clin Psychopharmacol 9:397–402, 1989

Singh AN, Beer M: A dose range-finding study of buspirone in geriatric patients with symptoms of anxiety. J Clin Psychopharmacol 8:67–68, 1988

Sizaret P, Versavel MC, Engel G, et al: Clinical investigation of lorazepam. Psychol Med 6:591–598, 1974

Smith JM, Baldessarini RJ: Changes in prevalence, severity, and recovery in tardive dyskinesia with age. Arch Gen Psychiatry 37:1368–1375, 1980

Spiker DG, Stein J, Rich CL: Delusional depression and electroconvulsive therapy: one year later. Convulsive Therapy 1:167–182, 1985

Spivak B, Radvan M, Meltzer M: Side effects of trazodone in a geriatric population. J Clin Psychopharmacol 9:62–63, 1989

Stone K: Mania in the elderly. Br J Psychiatry 155:220–224, 1989

Strauss A: Oral dyskinesia associated with buspirone use in an elderly woman. J Clin Psychiatry 49:322–323, 1988

Sullivan EA, Shulman KI: Diet and monoamine oxidase inhibitors: a re-examination. Can J Psychiatry 29:707–711, 1984

Sunderland T, Silver MA: Neuroleptic in the treatment of dementia. International Journal of Geriatric Psychiatry 3:79–88, 1988

Sunderland T, Cohen RM, Molchan S, et al: High-dose selegiline in treatment-resistant older depressive patients. Arch Gen Psychiatry 51:607–615, 1994

Tariot PN, Cohen RM, Sunderland T, et al: L-Deprenyl in Alzheimer's disease: preliminary evidence for behavioral change with monoamine oxidase B inhibition. Arch Gen Psychiatry 44:427–433, 1987

Tariot PN, Sunderland T, Cohen RM, et al: Tranylcypromine compared with l-deprenyl in Alzheimer's disease. J Clin Psychopharmacol 8:23–27, 1988

Teri L, Larson EB, Reifler BV: Behavioral disturbances in dementia of the Alzheimer's type. J Am Geriatr Soc 36:1–6, 1988

Tiller J, Maguire K, Davies B: A sequential double-blind controlled study of moclobemide and mianserin in elderly depressed patients. International Journal of Geriatric Psychiatry 5:199–204, 1990

Tinetti ME: Factors associated with serious injury during falls by ambulatory nursing home residents. J Am Geriatr Soc 35:644–648, 1987

Tinetti ME, Speechley M, Ginter SF: Risk factors for falls among elderly persons living in the community. N Engl J Med 319:1701–1707, 1988

Tollefson GD, Bosonworth JC, Heiligenstein JH, et al: A double-blind, placebo-controlled trial of fluoxetine in geriatric depression. Int Psychogeriatr 7:89–109, 1995

Tran-Johnson TK, Krull AJ, Jeste DV: Late life schizophrenia and its treatment: pharmacologic issues in older schizophrenic patients. Clin Geriatr Med 8:401–410, 1992

Tune LE, Steele C, Cooper T: Neuroleptic drugs in the management of behavioral symptoms of Alzheimer's disease. Psychiatr Clin North Am 14(2):353–373, 1991

van Harten J: Clinical pharmacokinetics of selective serotonin reuptake inhibitors. Clin Pharmacokinetics 14:203–220, 1993

van Marwijk HW, Bekker FM, Molen WA, et al: Lithium augmentation in geriatric depression. J Affect Disord 20:217–223, 1990

Vestal RE, Wood AJ, Shand DG: Reduced beta adrenergic receptor sensitivity in the elderly. Clin Pharmacol Ther 26:181–186, 1979

Wakelin JS: Fluvoxamine in the treatment of the older depressed patient: double-blind, placebo-controlled data. Int Clin Psychopharmacol 1:221–230, 1986

Warrington SJ: Clinical implications of the pharmacology of sertraline. Int Clin Psychopharmacol 6 (suppl 2):11–21, 1991

Weilburg JB, Rosenbaum JF, Biederman J, et al: Fluoxetine added to non-MAOI antidepressants converts nonresponders to responders: a preliminary report. J Clin Psychiatry 50:447–449, 1989

Weisbard JJ, Young RC, Kalayam B, et al: Age and haloperidol (abstract). American Journal of Geriatric Psychiatry 1:267, 1993

Weissman MM, Prusoff B, Sholomskas AJ: A double-blind clinical trial of alprazolam, imipramine, or placebo in the depressed elderly. J Clin Psychopharmacol 12:175–182, 1992

Whittier JR: Psychotropic Drugs and Dysfunctions of the Basal Ganglia. Edited by Crane GE, Nardner RJ Jr. Washington, DC, United States Public Health, 1969

Wild D, Nayak USL, Isaacs B: Characteristics of old people who fall at home. J Clin Exp Gerontol 2:271–287, 1980

Woerner MG, Kane JM, Lieberman JA, et al: The prevalence of tardive dyskinesia. J Clin Psychopharmacol 11:34–42, 1991

Wolters EC, Hurwitz TA, Mak E, et al: Clozapine in the treatment of Parkinsonian patients with dopaminomimetic psychoses. Neurology 40:832–834, 1990

Wragg RE, Jeste DV: Neuroleptic and alternative treatments: management of behavioral symptoms and psychosis in Alzheimer's disease and related conditions. Psychiatr Clin North Am 11:195–213, 1988

Yassa R, Nastase C, Dupont D, et al: Tardive dyskinesia in elderly psychiatric patients: a 5-year study. Am J Psychiatry 149:1206–1211, 1992

Yesavage JA, Brink TL, Ross L, et al: The geriatric depression rating scale: comparison with other self report and psychiatric rating scales, in Assessment in Geriatric Psychopharmacology. Edited by Crook T, Ferris S, Bartus R. New Canaan, CT, Mark Pawley Associates, 1983

Yesavage JA, Tanke ED, Sheikh JI: Tardive dyskinesia and steady state serum levels of thiothixene. Arch Gen Psychiatry 44:913–915, 1987

Young RC: Hydroxylated metabolites of antidepressants. Psychopharmacol Bull 27:521–532, 1991

Young RC, Falk JR: Age, manic psychopathology and treatment response. International Journal of Geriatric Psychiatry 4:73–78, 1989

Young RC, Alexopoulos GS, Shamoian CA, et al: Plasma 10-hydroxy-nortriptyline in elderly depressed patients. Clin Pharmacol Ther 35:540–544, 1984

Young RC, Alexopoulos GS, Kent E, et al: Plasma 10-hydroxynortriptyline and ECG changes in elderly depressive patients. Am J Psychiatry 142:866–868, 1985

Young RC, Alexopoulos GS, Shamoian CA, et al: Hydroxylated metabolites of tricyclic antidepressants in the elderly. Br J Psychiatry 150:131–132, 1987

Young RC, Mattis S, Alexopoulos GS, et al: Verbal memory and plasma drug concentrations in elderly depressives treated with nortriptyline. Psychopharmacol Bull 27:291–294, 1991

Young RC, Kalayam B, Tsuboyama G, et al: Mania: response to lithium across the age spectrum. Abstracts, Annual Meeting. Society for Neuroscience, Vol 18, 669.4, 1992

Zajecka JM, Fawcett J, Guy C: Coexisting major depression and obsessive-compulsive disorder treated with venlafaxine. J Clin Psychopharmacol 10:152–153, 1990

Zimmer B, Gershon S: The ideal late life anxiolytic, in Anxiety in the Elderly: Treatment and Research. Edited by Salzman C, Lebowitz BD. New York, Springer, 1991, pp 277–303

Zimmer B, Rosen J, Thornton JE, et al: Adjunctive lithium carbonate in nortriptyline-resistant elderly depressed patients. J Clin Psychopharmacol 11:254–256, 1991

Lawrence W. Lazarus, M.D.
Joel Sadavoy, M.D., F.R.C.P.C.

Individual Psychotherapy

The data on geriatric psychotherapy are based largely on clinical consensus and single-case studies, with some empirical data available in specific areas such as cognitive-behavioral (Gallagher and Thompson 1982; Thompson et al. 1991); behavioral, group, and milieu (Sadavoy and Robinson 1989); institutional treatment (Goldfarb and Turner 1953); and brief psychotherapy (Lazarus et al. 1987; Silberschatz and Curtis 1991). Gallagher and Thompson (1983) compared cognitive-behavior and brief relational and insight therapies in 30 depression patients (15 endogenous and 15 nonendogenous). All three modalities produced positive results, comparable to studies of tricyclic antidepressants in similar populations.

Apparently contradictory opinions that arise in the literature about geriatric psychotherapy are generally the result of observations made in different age and health status cohorts. The contradictions frequently can be resolved if the therapist applies appropriate principles of psychotherapy to appropriate subgroups of elderly individuals, avoiding erroneous attempts to homogenize the elderly population. Age per se defines neither indications nor contraindications for specific therapies (Myers 1984; Nemiroff and Colarusso 1985; Rechtschaffen 1959; Sadavoy and Leszcz 1987; Steuer 1982; Yesavage and Karasu 1982). For example, some patients in their seventh or later decade may be candidates for psychodynamically oriented therapy.

Innovative psychiatric outpatient programs were developed in the late 1960s to encourage older patients in the community to avail themselves of treatment. The Langley Porter Neuropsychiatric Institute (Feigenbaum 1973) publicized its special outpatient program, and within 3 years the proportion of elderly patients doubled. Furthermore, it was the clinical impression of the therapists that the improvement of elderly patients was similar to that of younger patients. The San Francisco Geriatric Screening Project (Simon and Lowenthal 1970) demonstrated in an uncontrolled study that early detection, evaluation, and treatment of psychiatrically impaired elderly persons in the community reduced the admission rate of elderly patients to state mental hospitals.

Psychotherapeutic goals, indications, techniques, and process are best defined based on a functional, rather than chronological, perspective. Function in old age may be conceptualized as a continuum between two poles: normative aging at one extreme and physical and mental frailty at the other (Kahana 1979). Influencing the adjustment of elderly individuals to the aging process are a variety of life stressors, some presenting as crises and others as chronic strain (Figure 28–1).

Barriers to Psychotherapy

Elderly individuals, according to a study by Eisdorfer and Stotsky (1977), make up only about 2%–4% of patients seen in psychiatric outpatient clinics and even a smaller percentage of most private psychiatric practices. Reasons for this low use of outpatient services can be understood from the perspective of the patient, the family, the physician, and the health care system (Gaitz 1974).

Raised in an era when shame and embarrassment were associated with seeing a psychiatrist, older people may shun such intervention and become indignant when a family member or personal physician suggests it. Negative beliefs about psychiatry, common to their age-cohort; sociocultural stereotypes regarding psychiatry; and geographic inaccessibility reinforce this hesitation. Some aging individuals believe that depression and anxiety are to be expected with aging or attribute the symptoms to medical rather than psychiatric causes. Moreover, the psychiatric problems themselves (e.g., depression with its associated helplessness and apathy) are often deterrents to treatment.

Additional barriers include such practical problems as arranging transportation, and interruptions of therapy because of illness. Adult children of aging parents may harbor the same negative, stereotypical attitudes about

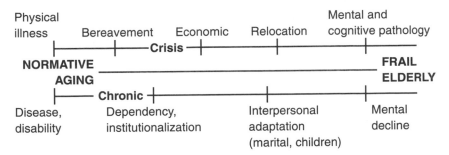

Figure 28–1. The continuum of functioning in old age.

psychiatry held by their parents, and they may minimize or deny their parents' psychiatric symptoms. The family may fear their parents' disapproval and anger if treatment were suggested. Conscious and unconscious resentment or ambivalence toward an aging parent or concerns about assuming financial responsibility may act as additional deterrents to adequate psychiatric care.

Primary care physicians may question the value of psychiatric intervention for frail, debilitated, elderly patients and may believe that their shortened life span renders them unsuitable for psychotherapy. Difficulty convincing elderly patients and their families of the usefulness of psychiatric treatment may be another deterrent.

General Principles of Individual Psychotherapy

The therapist of the elderly patient must individualize interventions in a flexible manner (Blau and Berezin 1975; Yesavage and Karasu 1982) and take into account the possible need to change to another therapeutic approach because of crises, health changes, family conflicts, and so on.

The therapist should use psychotherapy when appropriate, either as a primary or as an adjunctive treatment, in combination with medications, social and environmental manipulation, and patient advocacy. No single technique, principle, or rule of psychotherapy adequately addresses the heterogeneous geriatric population.

The complex interplay of medical, psychological, and sociocultural problems confronting frail elderly individuals requires flexibility and ingenuity on the part of the therapist. The therapist may be called on to function in different roles with the same patient; these may include family therapist, psychopharmacotherapist, primary care physician, and, at times, coordinator of the patient's treatment team. The psychiatrist is also concerned about previously undiagnosed medical problems and medication side effects that may be masquerading as, or aggravating, a psychiatric disorder. The initial office visit usually requires more than an hour to complete a comprehensive assessment of biopsychosocial factors and, when indicated, to obtain information from, and an assessment of, the patient's family. For a somatically oriented patient, beginning an initial interview in a medically oriented manner may provide the advantage of familiarity for the patient and place him or her at ease.

Therapists must be aware of concurrent physical problems that may accompany psychiatric symptoms and must ensure that psychotherapy or any other treatment has been preceded by a thorough medical workup. Families often may have to be involved for the clinician to obtain important collateral information not attainable from the patient and to gain their support and cooperation with the treatment plan, particularly when dealing with frail elderly individuals. However, the therapist should take care to respect the competent patient's wishes regarding confidentiality and other issues. Setting realistic psychotherapeutic goals helps both patient and therapist avoid mutual frustration and a sense of failure.

The identified elderly patient is usually first interviewed alone to convey respect for confidentiality and the patient's individuality and to elicit information that may not be obtainable in the family's presence. Some elderly patients are apprehensive about seeing a psychiatrist, so careful exploration of reactions and resistances to therapy should precede empathic explanations and realistic reassurances. When the patient and/or family is highly anxious, hopeless, or resistant to treatment, the therapist should adopt an active stance in working through patient and family resistances to therapy, demonstrate a willingness to help, and aid the patient and family to experience benefits from the very first interview; for example, explaining a treatment plan or confidently offering an expression of hope facilitates further therapy.

Goals of Psychotherapy

Normative Elderly Individuals

At the normative end of the continuum, structural change in psychoanalysis or psychoanalytic psychotherapy may be a realistic goal for some patients (M. Grotjahn 1955; Grunes 1987; Kahana 1987b; Myers 1984; Sadavoy and Leszcz 1987; Sandler 1982; Wheelright 1959; Zinberg 1963); as frailty increases, the goals of intensive psychotherapy become more modest. Goals for the healthier, more intact elderly patient include psychological mastery over past life stresses, leading to enhancement of current adaptation; formation and working through of conflicts in the therapeutic transference; resolution of childhood and adult sources of unconscious conflicts associated with shame, guilt, and humiliation; working through of unresolved grief reactions that were inhibited by earlier conflicts, thereby releasing restricted creativity and capacities for intimacy (e.g., in Pollock's [1987] terminology, "mourning-liberation"); resolution of current interpersonal conflict stemming from earlier, often unconscious, conflicts; working through loss and finding substitute sources of self-esteem; and coming to terms with failure to achieve one's ideal aspirations, as retirement and other forms of disengagement are imposed by life circumstances (Pollock 1987).

Crisis

When psychological defenses are overwhelmed by crisis, the first goal of therapy is aiding the patient to return to his or her best attainable level of function, rather than attempting structural or intrapsychic change. During and after the crisis, patients often require help to identify new, more realistic levels of function and to work toward them. Specific goals of psychotherapy during the crisis phases of old age, whether at the normative or frail end of the continuum, include mourning for lost capacities (if a patient retains enough ego strength to work through his or her losses); redirection of energy and creativity to realistic levels of functioning; redefinition of interpersonal relationships and acceptance of an appropriate level of dependency; acceptance and/or working through of separation and disengagement conflicts and fears; reengagement with new sources of gratification (e.g., new relationships with other patients and caregivers); control of regression and lessened need for using such primitive defenses as splitting, projection, primitive denial, and magical thinking (Sadavoy 1987); and reestablishment of healthy adaptive defenses to promote feelings of control and mastery (Goldfarb and Sheps 1954). Practical consequences of crisis therapy are improved adaptation to stress, including more appropriate use of the health care and social support systems.

Frail Elderly Individuals

The closer the patient's function to the more impaired end of the aging continuum, the more explicit, restricted, and focused become the goals of psychotherapy.

At the more debilitated, frail end of the continuum, therapeutic goals are often focused on narrowly defined behavioral change and problems in the "here and now." Psychodynamic formulations, however, remain useful and serve to humanize the patient and enhance the staff's understanding of him or her. The goal of therapy is to strengthen the roles of necessary caregivers and family and improve the environmental response so that it is in keeping with the patient's psychological and other needs (Cohen 1989).

The goals of therapy with frail elderly individuals include problem-oriented resolution of specific issues, such as the new role status imposed by sudden bereavement, physical illness, or relocation; acute psychosis; danger of suicide; psychiatric complications of dementia and confusional states; and terminal illness. The anxiety of family members over the deterioration of an elderly family member may focus therapy on the caregivers as well as, or instead of, the identified patient.

The goal of helping the elderly person work through anxieties and fears associated with death, although sometimes important (Segal 1958), is less clinically relevant than one might think. Elderly individuals, especially the very old, do not seem to express much death anxiety (Berezin 1972, 1987; Pollock 1987; Weisman and Hackett 1967). Indeed, death-related anxiety and conflict may be much more a phenomenon of earlier adult life (Jacques 1965; Yalom 1980). Elderly individuals who are confronting illness, decline, or death often tend to be more concerned with fears of pain, disability, abandonment, and dependency than with fear of death.

Indications for Individual Psychotherapy

Insight-oriented, intensive psychotherapy is indicated most frequently for the normative-aging cohort and is most productive if the patient is motivated; has a capacity for self-observation, insight, and mourning; is able to tolerate painful affects without excessive regression; and has demonstrated a capacity for productive work, intimacy, and pleasure (Pollock 1987).

Psychotherapy, and perhaps pharmacological intervention, may be necessary for bereaved patients who are identified as having a poor prognosis. Specific risk factors include an intense initial symptom response, absence of perceived or actual social support, a suddenness of the loss, and the presence of multiple concurrent stressful life events (Windholz et al. 1985).

Adaptation to the stresses and losses associated with aging can be accompanied by a variety of conflicts that may be indications for individual psychotherapy directed toward structural change. These issues include adaptation to loss; conflicts over feared or actual sexual decline; loss of identity and the accompanying narcissistic gratification as a productive worker; marital conflict; fears of dependency; failure to achieve goals that often arose from an idealized self-perception (classically termed *ego ideal* or, more recently, the self psychology term *grandiose self*); and coming to grips with one's mortality and the imminence of death (King 1980).

As aging progresses, crises often become the entrée to therapy, and crisis intervention techniques may be helpful. Supportive therapy is generally indicated until the patient's defenses and adaptive capacities can be reconstituted. Psychotherapy in these circumstances is often an adjunct to medical, pharmacological, and environmental support (Kahana 1987b). Although brief psychotherapy and cognitive therapy are particularly useful, long-term therapy may follow in selected cases. However, caution is necessary, because defenses should not be challenged by interpretative therapy unless the patient has the capacity to replace long-standing maladaptive defenses with new, adaptive, and fulfilling mechanisms for bolstering narcissistic supplies, protecting against damaged self-esteem, and replacing selfobject relationships (Yesavage and Karasu 1982).

Neugarten (1979) suggested that expectable and age-appropriate crises are handled more easily than crises that are temporally out of phase with an individual's life; for example, coming to terms with the death of a middle-age child may be exceedingly difficult because it is out of phase with the normal chronology of expectable life events. Psychotherapy is indicated when the individual is unable to master and adapt to the psychological impact of the crisis. Vulnerability is enhanced if there is a history of serious, early life deprivation; long-standing reliance on rigid and/or primitive defenses; over-reliance on the selfobject component of intimate relationships; previous unmourned losses; multiple or unbearably intense assaults on the individual's life circumstance, as may occur, for example, during war or severe deprivation; breakdown of ego capacities because of physical and/or emotional abnormality; and inability of caregivers, especially family, to tolerate the elderly family member's decline and disability.

Frailty usually interferes with the capacity to tolerate intensive psychotherapy and, in general, severely restricts or contraindicates its use. However, even in frail elderly individuals, focal therapy focused on specific, here-and-now issues can use techniques of insight and interpretation (Rosenthal 1985)—termed by Kahana (1987b)—in conjunction with cognitive, supportive, and educational techniques. Psychotherapy specifically adapted to the frail and institutionalized elderly person (Aronson 1958; Goldfarb 1956; Sadavoy and Dorian 1983; Sadavoy and Robinson

1989) has been used successfully. The more limited and frail the patient, the greater the indication for problem-oriented interventions such as behavioral therapies and environmental manipulation.

Often the frail patient welcomes a more familiar relationship with the therapist (e.g., sitting closer, physical contact, use of first names). However, this wish for closeness is not universal among geriatric patients and can be experienced as unprofessional or disturbing, especially by those in the normative-aging end of the spectrum. The therapist should be extremely careful to individualize his or her approach.

Themes and Issues Discussed in Psychotherapy

One of the most common issues discussed by elderly patients is that of loss. Many psychotherapists believe that a major developmental task for the aging individual is to find restitution for the myriad of biopsychosocial losses associated with this stage of the life cycle (Cath 1976; Meissner 1975). The significance of a particular loss is often associated with the amount of self-esteem that was invested in the lost function (e.g., the effect of arthritis on a concert pianist). What appears to be very devastating for some elderly persons is the rapidity and cumulative effect of repeated losses before sufficient time has passed to allow for mourning and resolution.

Erikson (1968) conceptualized the last phase of life as the struggle to attain and maintain ego integrity, with failure to do so leading to a state of despair and disgust. Cath (1976) characterized the middle and later years as a balance between factors that support a person's self-esteem, such as wisdom derived from life experience, attainment of a satisfying philosophical and religious world view, and past accomplishments, versus factors leading to emotional depletion, such as failing health and cognitive impairment. Cath asserts that, given adequate ego resources and a sustaining environment, most elderly people master the challenges of later life. Atchley (1982), a sociologist, stated that persons who lose self-esteem in late life do so because they have lost a feeling of control over their environment to such a degree that they feel defenseless, because self-esteem had previously been too dependent on work or social roles and/or because physical deterioration had become so extensive that the person must accept a less desirable self-image. Elderly individuals, according to Atchley, defend themselves against a negative self-image by choosing to interact with people who provide a positive egosyntonic experience, refusing to apply negative societal myths about aging to themselves, discounting messages that do not fit with their existing self-image, and focusing on past successes.

Transference

The literature on geriatric psychotherapy generally endorses the premise of the timelessness of the unconscious leading to the persistence of unconscious attitudes and fantasies from early life (Berezin 1972). These factors determine much of the content of the transference. There is little clinical evidence to strongly support the concept of a highly age-specific transference, although the stressors inherent in old age tend to mobilize certain reactions more often than others. Furthermore, developmental theory suggests that the transference not only derives from unconscious ties to significant childhood figures, but also contains elements of significant object relationships acquired (internalized) during adult life (e.g., spousal, child [or filial], and peer transferences) (Nemiroff and Colarusso 1985). Table 28–1 summarizes some of the age-related conflicts that tend to be associated with certain transferences that arise in therapy.

Frail elderly individuals, struggling with various fears and conflicts (including abandonment to institutions by their adult children and helpless reliance on caregivers), easily develop parental transferences with hopes for an idealized, magical protector and savior. The self in the transference constellation is experienced as weak and helpless, whereas the other (e.g., physician or nurse) is powerful and protective. At times the patient, especially when disappointed, may angrily reject the therapist and relate to the therapist as an abandoning parent, child, or spouse.

Narcissistic assaults inherent in lost beauty, power, and physical prowess often promote an idealizing and/or mirror transference to the therapist. To cope with narcissistic assaults on the self, the patient may experience himself or herself as a powerful, admired person, just as he or she perceives the therapist as powerful and admired. The patient unconsciously believes that the therapist is admiring and beneficent to him or her and basks in the fantasized approval of the therapist. Frail patients, who are often institutionalized and having to cope with pain, illness, and lost capacity, are prone to these idealizing transference constellations. This tendency for frail patients to develop an idealized type of transference can be useful therapeutically, as discussed in the section on psychotherapy with cognitively impaired individuals.

Bereavement and grief, especially for a lost spouse, may cause the patient to unconsciously turn to the therapist as a wished-for replacement, leading to spousal or "lover" transference that may be eroticized. The patient may identify with a much more youthful self-image and see himself or herself as sexually appropriate for the therapist (Crusey 1985). Similar eroticized transference may be mobilized as the patient becomes aware of

Table 28–1. Age-related conflicts associated with transference

Age-related conflicts	Developmental stage	Type of transference
Giving up of ideal goals (Kahana 1987a)	Normative	Sibling rivalry; envy; jealousy; peer; mirror transference
Sexual decline/unavailability	Normative	Erotic
Loss of roles	Normative	Sibling rivalry; idealized, filial, or peer
Conflict over death and mortality (Segal 1958)	Entire spectrum	Idealized protector, negative filial, or parental
Conflicts with adult children (Meerloo 1955; Myers 1984)	Entire spectrum	Filial
Bereavement (Levin 1965b)	Normative/crisis	Spousal, erotic, or peer
Narcissistic assaults (Grunes 1987; Lazarus 1980, 1988)	Normative/frail	Mirror, idealized, or peer; rivalry; envy
Dependency/abandonment (Levin 1965a)	Frail/crisis	Parental
Vulnerability/helplessness (Goldfarb 1956)	Frail/crisis	Idealized; magical savior
Pain, illness, lost capacity to adapt (Gitelson 1981)	Frail/crisis	Parental, idealized, or filial

his or her sexual decline and the unavailability of sexual objects. This normative stage of self-awareness may also lead to intense negative feelings toward the therapist, who may be perceived as unable or unwilling to restore to the patient his or her lost youth and sexuality. Beneath the anger lies depressive loss of self-esteem.

Classic oedipal conflicts also arise in the transference, leading the patient to experience libidinal, aggressive, and competitive feelings toward the therapist, associated with anxiety and neurotic behavior generated by the unconscious neurotic conflict.

The normative giving up of one's occupation through retirement can lead to loss of self-esteem and an angry or depressive sibling rivalry transference. The patient may begin to feel like the devalued, unloved child while perceiving the therapist as the successful, valued child. Conscious or unconscious conflicts over death and mortality may cause the patient to view the therapist as an idealized, magical protector with parental, filial, or spousal qualities, who will ward off the inevitability of death. The realistic inability of the therapist to provide the needed comfort and protection may then induce negative, angry feelings toward the perceived, disappointing parental, spousal, or filial transference figure.

Geriatric patients may develop "apparent" transference resistances to therapy in which they challenge the therapist, for example, as being too young and inexperienced and therefore incapable of understanding an elderly person. This defensive stance, however, often is the patient's initial defense against deeper fears of lost self-esteem. In this version of the so-called "reverse transference" (M. Grotjahn 1955; Levin 1965a; Myers 1984), the patient adopts the "old-experienced" self-perception, whereas the therapist is seen as young and therefore in need of help and education. Another version of the reverse transference may be evident when the patient adopts a kindly parental stance. However, beneath the surface interaction, whether positive or negative, often lurk feelings of helplessness and inferiority and fears of decline.

Countertransference

Therapists often do not advise or think of psychotherapy for elderly individuals (Ford and Sbordone 1980). Countertransference (unconscious reactions to the patient) and counterreactions (conscious reactions) may account for much of this apparent avoidance (Butler and Lewis 1977). Counterreactions include feeling that elderly individuals are unattractive, unproductive, close to death, chronic, unchangeable, and unrewarding. These ideas about therapy with elderly individuals are not supported by clinical experience.

Frail elderly individuals, especially those who are institutionalized, are more likely to mobilize the therapist's own unresolved conflicts about aging, including unconscious fears of illness, decline, and death (Nemiroff and Colarusso 1985; Yesavage and Karasu 1982). Therapists may become anxious about a patient's apparent helplessness and dependency; this anxiety in turn promotes fears of engulfment and can lead to withdrawal from or rejection of the patient. Conversely, in the face of the patient's decline, therapists may act on a grandiose need to conquer the forces of aging (Myers 1984). The therapist's narcissism is easily at risk in these circumstances, and he or she may experience depression or unreasonable anger when efforts to rescue the patient fail (Nemiroff and Colarusso 1985).

When the therapist overidentifies with the patient's problems, feelings of pity and sadness may arise (Hiatt 1971) that block accurate empathy and realistic exploration of the possibilities for change. Conversely, the therapist may unconsciously avoid the pain of accurately empathizing with the patient's loneliness and loss. If overwhelmed by the patient's problems, the therapist may avoid termination of therapy because of the conviction that he or she is keeping the patient alive, so that continuing therapy becomes a defense to ward off the patient's death (King 1980).

With geriatric patients, especially in the normative-aging group, therapists (particularly those who are younger and inexperienced) may be shocked and/or repelled by the patient's eroticized transference toward them and/or when they encounter erotic countertransference feelings in themselves. Belief in the asexuality of elderly individuals (Meerloo 1953) can act as a defense against unresolved conflicts over parental sexuality or oedipal conflicts (Myers 1984; Nemiroff and Colarusso 1985; Zinberg and Kaufman 1963).

Therapy with older patients may mobilize countertransference feelings associated with unresolved conflicts with parents more readily than occurs with younger patients (King 1980; Myers 1986). For example, unresolved hostility toward his or her parent may lead the therapist to a defensive idealization of the patient or inappropriate reliance on superficial, supportive modes of intervention—either way, avoidance of deeper areas of psychological conflict results (M. Grotjahn 1955; Lazarus and Weinberg 1980). Similar feelings may lead to an unconscious wish to dominate the patient (parent) and promote an overmedicalized or controlling stance.

To a greater or lesser extent, most therapists experience one or another of these transference-countertransference reactions. The therapist need not be dismayed when these reactions occur, but rather should recognize such reactions as universal and as a signal for self-reflection and possibly for discussion with a colleague.

Use of Defenses

In general, the dramatic defensive maneuvers of youth (e.g., promiscuity), self-destructive actions (e.g., self-mutilation), and antisocial behaviors seem to abate in old age (Sadavoy and Fogel 1992), although long-term follow-up and study of elderly individuals with regard to these behaviors has not yet been done. Frail elderly individuals are more likely to use defenses of withdrawal, infirmity, and physical preoccupation to deal with intrapsychic conflict and anxieties. Patients may use these defenses to avoid therapy, with claims of illness or immobility, or they may take refuge in past accomplishments, overusing reminiscence and avoiding the present, including the transference. The normative group demonstrates a fuller range of defenses, however, which take on an age-related coloration (e.g., denial of aging by attempts at youthful dress, seductiveness, or physical activity). In crises or periods of decline, regression may be intense.

Defenses and other unconscious material are expressed in a variety of forms, including dreams (Myers 1984) and acting out (Kahana 1987a, 1987b; Miller 1987; Nemiroff and Colarusso 1985; Sadavoy and Leszcz 1987). For example, a 65-year-old executive dealt with anxiety over illness, loss of physical energy, and sexual potency by canceling therapy sessions to take up white water rafting, despite his problems with chronic asthma and morbid obesity.

Termination

In general, clinical evidence suggests that open-ended therapeutic relationships are often necessary in psychotherapy of elderly individuals, especially frail elderly individuals, because of the frequency of recurrent crises in the life of the aging patient. Patients feel very reassured when the therapist expresses his or her concern and availability if problems occur in the future. The therapist can ease the appropriate return to therapy by anticipating with the patient the potential resistances that may inhibit reinstituting therapy, such as fear of dependency or admission of failure because of recurrent symptoms. The process of termination often mobilizes conflicts associated with issues such as the remaining life span and mortality, loneliness, abandonment, and dependency, as well as recurrence of the same issues and symptoms that led to the initiation of therapy. However, the older patient with good interpersonal supports and ego strengths often will be able to work through termination and other disengagement conflicts (Cath 1975).

Specialized Approaches to Psychotherapy With Elderly Individuals

Psychotherapy With Cognitively Impaired Individuals

Psychodynamic issues remain important in cognitively impaired individuals and influence interpersonal relationships, behavior expression, and response to treatment (Cohen 1989). Psychotherapeutic interventions with this group address the remaining reflective capacity of the individual patient and at the same time use psychodynamic understanding to intervene at the level of environmental manipulation and family and caregiver education and support. Often therapy is directed at minimizing excess disability (Brody et al. 1971; Kahn 1965). For example, correcting hearing and other sensory deficits, reducing isolation and withdrawal, maximizing independent function, treating concomitant depression, and improving medical status can significantly improve the patient's overall functioning.

A wide variety of psychotherapy techniques have been employed with these patients, most often in institutions. Cognitive-behavioral techniques often focus on changing specific target behaviors. Goals of therapy include increasing the patient's level of participation in activities of daily living; enhancing social interest and interaction; and improving skills in communication and such concrete tasks as toileting, bathing, ambulation, and feeding (Hussian 1984). Studies suggest that behavior therapies are most effective when integrated with milieu and other individual techniques (Sadavoy and Robinson 1989; Tobin 1989). Similar results have been shown for reality orientation techniques—that is, the more interactive and "person centered" the interventions, the greater the improvement (Hanley et al. 1981).

Individual psychotherapy may be useful for cognitively impaired individuals if employed judiciously and with well-defined goals (Cohen 1989; Sadavoy and Robinson 1989), although no controlled studies are yet available. The therapist should empathically communicate his or her understanding of the patient's distress over the loss of cognitive abilities, being sensitive to the patient's sense of a damaged self and propensity to shame. Because the patient's emotions, compared with his or her cognitive functioning, may remain relatively intact and can be understood by observing his or her posture and facial gestures, tuning in to the patient's emotional state may help to establish contact and to relieve loneliness and isolation. A touch on the patient's shoulder at the appropriate moment may augment verbal expressions of concern, particularly when an aphasia interferes with communication. The interviewer should refrain from asking stress-inducing questions, such as those that assess cognition, until rapport is established.

The dementia patient's tendency to reminisce about the past not only may represent a way to stave off depression and represent relatively unimpaired neurological functioning, but may also remind the patient of a time when he or she felt worthwhile, vital, and competent. In addition to encouraging constructive reminiscing, the therapist supports the patient's mastery of those current activities and interests from which he or she can still derive self-esteem and satisfaction. Occasional references to intensive psychotherapy are made in the literature (J. M. Grotjahn 1940; Hollos and

Ferenczi 1925; Sadavoy and Robinson 1989), but these efforts are best viewed as investigative rather than of general practical value.

Goldfarb and Turner (1953) pioneered a useful and practical psychotherapeutic intervention to bolster self-worth and a sense of mastery in institutionalized elderly persons. This method is based on the patient's need for sustaining selfobject relations and self-esteem enhancement (Lazarus 1980, 1988). During once-weekly, brief sessions, the therapist encourages an idealizing transference, enhancing the patient's sense of control and self-esteem by encouraging him or her to identify with and "borrow" the therapist's apparent power and prestige. The therapist tries to carry out a patient's request, thus fostering the patient's sense of mastery, control, and power over the therapist. Goldfarb's open, uncontrolled study showed this method to be effective if patients had neither psychosis nor major depression. Of 59 patients divided into three groups—psychosis without brain damage ($n = 5$), neurosis and personality disorder ($n = 13$), and chronic brain syndrome ($n = 41$)—28 improved and 18 stabilized (46 of the 59 patients) with the use of this method; only 15 of these patients were seen for more than 10 sessions.

Communication with the cognitively impaired patient begins with a basic understanding and knowledge of his or her behavior as well as its psychodynamic underpinnings. Behavior and verbal expression may be otherwise unintelligible to the uninformed caregiver (Cohen 1989; Sadavoy and Robinson 1989; Sadavoy 1991). Because the patient with moderate to severe dementia cannot convey his or her life story and achievements, uninformed staff in long-term care institutions have no way of understanding the patient's utterances and behavior. Cohen (1989) advocates that family members, health care professionals, and others knowledgeable about the patient convey the patient's personal history to the staff in various ways (e.g., conveying brief verbal histories or bringing memorabilia) to increase the staff's understanding, interest, and involvement. The more advanced the cognitive decline, the greater the patient's need to interact on a nonverbal level (for example, through activity, movement, or music).

Frequently, cognitive impairment is accompanied by delusions. Gentle redirection of the patient's attention to another focus, or simple distraction of the patient's attention, may be helpful (Cohen 1989), as is empathic reintroduction of reality and "jogging" the patient's memory, especially with the use of memory aids such as pictures and memorabilia. However, aggressive reality orientation can exacerbate psychosis or increase the patient's agitation. For example, confronting a patient who has the delusion that his or her long deceased parent has recently visited may precipitate agitation and depression. Instead, the therapist can refocus the patient's attention on real interactions with living family members. (For illuminating case reports of the effectiveness of this approach, the reader is directed to Cohen [1989]). For the most frail persons, individual therapy often is most effective and efficient when brief. Frequent contact is used (5 to 10 minutes several times a week), focused on day-to-day issues. Questions are brief, focused, and concrete rather than abstract. The flow of communication commonly is slow, with therapists giving the patient ample time to respond while avoiding being too reflective or unstructured.

The therapist is most helpful if he or she is able to tolerate the often ambiguous, impoverished, repetitive, and sometimes bizarre verbal interactions with these patients. Such patients frequently have a need to idealize the therapist, who must be able to tolerate the idealization despite his or her knowledge of therapeutic limitations.

Reminiscence or Life Review Therapy

Some authors have suggested that the realization of one's mortality leads the aging person to reflect on and reminisce about the past, a process that helps the person to conceptualize his or her life over time and to give it significance and meaning (Butler 1963). Reminiscence is characterized by the expression of memories of past experiences, especially those that were meaningful or conflictual.

To varying degrees, most patients in therapy, including elderly individuals, reminisce about the past, seek meaning for their life, and strive for some resolution of interpersonal and intrapsychic conflicts. The purpose of life review therapy is to enhance this process and make it more conscious and deliberate. Lewis and Butler (1974) reported that this technique helps to resolve old problems; increases tolerance of conflict; relieves guilt and fears; and enhances creativity, generosity, and acceptance of the present.

Life review therapy includes encouraging the patient to return to places of earlier experiences, write or tape his or her autobiography, reunite with family and old friends, review memorabilia, and attempt verbal or written summations of his or her life. However, despite its usefulness, this therapy may be contraindicated for patients who have realistic or overwhelming guilt about the past or who otherwise cannot cope with unmourned or unresolvable past disappointments and losses.

Brief Psychodynamic Psychotherapy

A brief psychodynamic therapy approach can be considered for elderly patients with clearly defined, circumscribed problems that can be expected to resolve within a limited amount of time. Examples of problems amenable to brief psychotherapy include adjustment disorder, grief reaction, and traumatic stress disorder that has not become chronic and entrenched. Setting a time limit on therapy reinforces the patient's confidence in his or her ability to resolve the problem, focuses and accelerates the therapeutic process, diminishes the patient's fear of protracted dependency on the therapist, and considers the patient's limited finances (Lazarus et al. 1987).

In one preliminary, uncontrolled study of the process and outcome of brief psychodynamic psychotherapy with eight elderly outpatients (four men and four women) ranging in age from 63 to 77, individually constructed outcome scales were used for each patient (Lazarus et al. 1987). Most outpatients met the DSM-III criteria (American Psychiatric Association 1980) for an adjustment disorder with depressed mood, and one patient had a panic disorder. Patients received 15 therapy sessions, and each session was videotaped for subsequent outcome ratings carried out by the researchers. Analysis of variance for measuring outcome on seven scales for each patient at the end of treatment and at 6 months follow-up demonstrated that seven of the eight patients showed significant lessening of their presenting symptoms ($P < .01$) and some resolution of their focal conflict. The four women showed greater improvement earlier and maintained the improvement longer than did the men.

Study of the process of therapy with these elderly outpatients revealed that patients often used the therapeutic relationship to reestablish a positive sense of self over time and/or to consolidate diverse and disparate aspects of the self into a more positive sense of self. The therapist was used by the patient for validation of competency and normalcy and for restoration of feelings of mastery and self-esteem. The generalizability of this preliminary study to other elderly outpatients is limited by the small sample size and reliance on unvalidated, individualized scales.

Silberschatz (1986) and Silberschatz and Curtis (1986, 1991) studied extensively the process and outcome of time-limited psychotherapy with older outpatients and found that patients entered treatment with specific conscious and unconscious goals that were essential for the therapist to understand. These goals sometimes included a wish for the therapist 1) to help the patient overcome his or her initial resistances to treatment (often based on ageist attitudes and myths) and guilt feelings over surviving or being successful while others (family and friends) have died or became disabled and 2) to provide support for overcoming negative attitudes and beliefs about the self. These investigators believed that what is most predictive of successful therapy is the ability of the therapist to ascertain and respond appropriately to the patient's goals for therapy and to help the patient disconfirm pathogenic beliefs about the self. It is likely that these researchers carefully selected patients who could articulately explore their presenting problems and were capable of an insight-oriented approach to therapy; therefore, the generalizability of their findings may be restricted to this patient cohort. Nevertheless, long-standing ageist biases that contend that most elderly patients require supportive rather than insight-oriented therapy may underestimate patients' abilities and provide a watered-down approach to therapy.

Cognitive-Behavior Psychotherapy

Cognitive psychotherapy (Beck et al. 1979) is a brief therapy approach that uses interpretations, explanations, and practical information to correct the depressed patient's stereotypical, self-defeating thoughts and dysfunctional attitudes. The goal is to promote integration of positive perceptions and thinking patterns and thereby diminish depression. Patients learn to reverse their negative cognitive sets by the following five processes: 1) learning to monitor negative thoughts, 2) recognizing connections between negative thoughts and feelings of depression, 3) examining the evidence for and against specific automatic thoughts, 4) learning to identify and alter dysfunctional beliefs that sustain these negative cognitions, and 5) developing more reality-oriented and adaptive strategies for coping with depression.

Modifications of cognitive therapy have been suggested to address the special problems of elderly depression patients (Gallagher and Thompson 1982). These modifications include the following:

- Acclimatizing patients for therapy (e.g., presenting therapy as a way to learn to adjust to the stress of life and encouraging active participation in the therapeutic process)
- Enhancing learning capabilities (e.g., by empathically understanding the patient's hesitation to try therapeutic suggestions)
- Terminating therapy gradually (e.g., anticipating future problems and leaving the door open for the patient to return)

- Extending treatment to 30 to 40 sessions, instead of the usual 15 to 20, for patients with chronic depression or a depressive episode superimposed on a dysthymic disorder

More modest goals are sometimes set for elderly individuals, and the general aim is for improved affective status rather than complete remission.

In the past few years, further modifications specific to elderly depression patients have been suggested (Thompson et al. 1991). These include greater flexibility and activity on the part of the therapist, keeping the patient focused on the "here and now," proceeding at a slower pace, and adopting the patient's own language when addressing certain issues. For patients with cognitive slowing or sensory deficits, it is helpful to present important information in several sensory modalities, such as repeating important themes or concepts, having the patient take notes, providing a tape recording of the interview for review between sessions, and giving specific work assignments between sessions. Several strategies may help reluctant patients overcome their resistance to therapy. If patients complain they are "too old to change," the therapist may respond, "Perhaps it is true that you cannot learn new ways of thinking about your problems, but how will you know this for certain unless you try?" If the patient complains that the therapist is "too young to help," the therapist can encourage temporary suspension of this belief so that a trial of therapy can proceed.

Clinical studies and experience to date indicate that cognitive therapy is especially efficacious for cognitively intact, motivated elderly patients with minor and major depressions. Greatest success, according to Thompson et al. (1991), comes in treating patients with reactive-type depressions for which a clear precipitant can be determined. A comparison of three brief therapy approaches—cognitive, behavioral, and psychodynamic—for elderly outpatients with major depression found that all three were equally efficacious at the completion of therapy; the overall positive response rate for the three therapies was 70%: 52% of patients had complete remission, and 18% showed significant symptomatic improvement. Improvement was defined as a change in the depression to a less severe level and improved self-reports on a measure such as the Beck Depression Inventory. There was a trend at follow-up for those treated with either cognitive or behavior therapy to maintain their improvement more than those treated psychodynamically (Thompson et al. 1987).

Age was not a predictor of outcome; very elderly patients responded as well as younger elderly patients to all three treatment modalities. Patients with major depression who tended to be less responsive to all three treatment modalities had many endogenous signs (a more biological type of depression), a concomitant personality disorder, and low expectations of improvement (Thompson et al. 1988). Only about half of these patients responded to cognitive-behavior therapy. Those with concomitant personality disorders or strong signs of endogenous-type depression often required a more protracted course of treatment (Thompson et al. 1991). (For more detailed information regarding the use of cognitive-behavior therapy with elderly individuals, the reader is referred to Gallagher and Thompson [1981], Hussian and Davis [1985], and Emery [1981].)

Pinkston and Linsk (1984) utilized behavioral therapy methods to teach 21 separate families at-home care for their impaired elderly relative. Although the elderly patients had a variety of psychiatric diagnoses, they all had severe mental and physical impairment. Also, their caregivers were willing to undergo rigorous study procedures involving assessment and training derived from operant and social learning theories of behavioral intervention. Impressive results were obtained. There was improvement in 73% of all behaviors (e.g., excessive negative verbalizations and self-care deficits) by the end of the study, and at 6 months follow-up, in 78% of previously targeted behaviors that had improved, the improvement was maintained. Also, at the end of the study most of the caregivers' own health status was self-rated as unchanged or improved. However, the high motivation of these caregivers (e.g., their resources, wherewithal, and willingness to engage in a comprehensive and time-consuming teaching program) limits the generalizability of these results.

Karasu (1986) reviewed therapeutic factors accounting for change in various psychotherapies. He believed that the positive aspects of cognitive therapy in adult patients (which probably have application to elderly individuals) include its structured procedures and time-limited nature, expectation of positive change, consideration of limited financial resources, support of higher-level defense mechanisms, encouragement of the patient's active participation, and potential for integration with other treatment modalities (e.g., behavioral or psychodynamic). Shortcomings include its restricted application to depression and less severely impaired patients and the potential (when used as the sole treatment modality) to produce overintellectualization and (if applied mechanically) to foster isolation of the patient's feelings.

Personality Disorders

Elderly patients with a Cluster B personality disorder (DSM-IV) (American Psychiatric Association 1994) tend to be excessively demanding, extremely sensitive, emotionally labile, and impulsive, and they may engage in destructive, acting-out behavior. They often have few or inadequate support systems because of their propensity for unstable relationships. Therapists may become frustrated because of the preponderance of demands and expectations.

The signs and symptoms that are present in the elderly personality disorder patient are similar to those that are present in the younger adult but with modifications brought on by age-relevant factors, such as confinement to a nursing home and physical infirmities. These elderly patients, because of impaired motoric behavior and generalized "slowing down," are less likely than their younger counterparts to flagrantly act out with criminal or promiscuous behavior. Passive-dependent behavior, social withdrawal, apathy, and vulnerability to depression may be prominent, and previous personality traits may become accentuated with cognitive and other health impairments. Whereas the elderly patient without significant character abnormality shows some resiliency and flexibility in dealing with change and trauma associated with aging, the personality disorder patient remains rigid, overwhelmed, and unable to adapt to age-related stresses.

Presentation

The elderly patient with a personality disorder in the dramatic, Cluster B spectrum carries with him or her psychopathology established in early stages of intrapsychic development. Sadavoy (1987) pointed to five unresolved intrapsychic maldevelopments that affect the elderly patient with a personality disorder: 1) fear of abandonment or loneliness; 2) real or fantasized narcissistic injury to self-esteem and failure of self and selfobject relationships; 3) impaired affect tolerance; 4) failure in the development of modulators of rage, which in turn leads to increased use of splitting; and 5) loss of self-cohesion induced by age-associated stressors, which may be so extreme as to cause brief psychotic episodes.

Dysfunction of intrapsychic structure can impair mourning and ability to cope with grief. This issue is a particularly familiar and difficult one to address in geriatric treatment, because elderly patients are routinely faced with the task of coping with losses.

Like similar patients at other ages, these geriatric patients express their personality disorders in many ways. Most frequent is their pathological way of relating to family and other caregivers. The patient may become increasingly helpless (Breslau 1987) and exhibit panicky behavior (e.g., calling family members for unreasonable reassurances). Patients may make incessant demands on caregivers that interfere with other obligations, expecting that others will change plans and cancel activities to respond to their requests. Such behavior eventually angers and frustrates family, caregivers, and/or staff. Treatment of concomitant anxiety can often lessen the patient's demands and acting out. Another common presentation consists of exaggerated somatic complaints that cannot be alleviated by reassurance.

A third presentation is depressive withdrawal. Some of these patients exhibit anhedonia, apathy, anorexia, and loss of the will to live. In these cases, life-threatening depressions may be superimposed on the personality disorder, requiring vigorous treatment. The therapist should be careful not to ascribe an Axis II personality disorder diagnosis without careful assessment for an Axis I diagnosis that may have a favorable prognosis. Treatable depressions and psychoses may be masked by readily apparent disruptive signs of a personality disorder.

Treatment

In developing a treatment plan, consideration is given to the patient's pathological behavior, to the stresses on the family and health care team, and to the patient's ability to engage in individual psychotherapy. Various treatment strategies have been suggested, although no formal studies of effectiveness have been undertaken to date. Sadavoy and Dorian (1983) described a psychodynamic approach that incorporates behavioral techniques for use in a long-term care setting. They enlist the help of the family and/or other caregivers in preparing a written statement of expected behavior from the patient. This approach takes into account the patient's underlying psychodynamics—as evident, for example, in his or her need for a sense of control—and recognizes the limitations of the staff's tolerance of the patient's unreasonable demands, acting out, and other disturbing behaviors. The staff sets nonpunitive limits on verbal and physical acting out, specific requirements for participation in prescribed activities, adherence to medication schedules, and conditions for privileges. With a clearly spelled out contract, a working alliance may be established that includes family and caregivers who work together to strive for mutually established goals.

In individual therapy with these patients, the therapist should adjust the frequency of sessions, titrating the intensity of therapy against the patient's sensitivity to rejection and forestalling the patient's feeling of being overwhelmed with rage and anxiety. Therapy focuses on helping the patient to connect feelings to causal events, thus promoting maintenance of self-esteem and self-cohesion. Developmental history is largely used for understanding the patient's needs and actions. Sadavoy and Dorian (1983) limit the emphasis on past unresolvable losses and mourning during the earlier phases of treatment, focusing instead on current here-and-now issues. This technique employs clarification and confrontation instead of deeper interpretations. In some cases, as a working alliance develops, a measure of working through of unresolved mourning may be attempted.

Gabbard (1989) addressed the issue of splitting, a common defense of the adult patient with a personality disorder that is also found in elderly patients. The reality of the caregiver's efforts is distorted by the disordered intrapsychic self of the patient. The caregiver is perceived as either good or bad, as defined by split-off, internal representations from the patient's past. For example, the patient may willingly accept medication from one caregiver but not from another. Thus, the same situation provokes either compliant or negativistic reaction, depending on the patient's intrapsychic assessment of a particular caregiver, despite the fact that each caregiver may behave toward the patient in a similar fashion. The psychotherapist deals with the internal world of the patient by using explanations, clarifications, and sometimes interpretations, with the goal of minimizing splitting of internal self and object representations. Staff intervention addresses the integration and moderation of the external world of the patient.

Use of Medication

Medication is often an important component of the comprehensive treatment plan. Patients' compliance with medication may be compromised because of distrust of the physician and staff; susceptibility to side effects; and negative beliefs and attitudes on the part of the patient, family, and other caregivers about these medications (Lazarus and Mershon 1987). Compliance is greatly enhanced by working through the patient's negative reactions and maintaining a very positive therapeutic relationship.

Reynolds et al. (1992) highlighted the importance of integrating pharmacotherapy with psychotherapy. In a sample of 61 elderly depression patients treated with a combination of nortriptyline and interpersonal psychotherapy, about 79% of treatment completers showed a full response to therapy based on their outcome criteria, compared with previous studies revealing treatment success rates of 50% to 70% using either treatment alone. The result of Reynolds et al.'s study might suggest some superiority for combined therapy during the acute and continuation phases of treatment of depression. The data, however, are preliminary and fail to include single-therapy control groups.

Integrating Psychotherapeutic Treatment Modalities

Three basic psychotherapy interventions, individual psychodynamic, cognitive-behavioral, and interpersonal, have been shown to be effective and may be productively combined (Sadavoy 1994). To utilize these therapies rationally, an organized assessment process is important and includes a tripartite evaluation at three levels: psychodynamic, interpersonal, and cognitive-behavior. The assessment attends not only to the analysis of the patient's current crisis, but also to the history of the patient's adult roles and relationships as well as his or her earlier developmental history. (It is important to note that the developmental history frequently is left out of geriatric assessments, perhaps because of the immediacy and importance of evaluating the more recent events in the patient's life.) The therapist determines the patient's strengths and weaknesses of function; the nature of his or her response to stresses throughout life, particularly during adult years; defense mechanisms and habitual modes of behavior; and earlier life trauma, whether in childhood or adulthood. This last issue is particularly relevant in ethnocultural communities of elderly persons, the histories of whom often include significant early trauma such as war experience, immigration, torture, assault, or accidents. Such events often lead to chronic symptoms of posttraumatic stress that may emerge with greater intensity in old age (Sadavoy 1987).

The assessment of interpersonal factors is of special relevance in old age, because this is a period of transition in several interpersonal areas and includes conflicts over increased dependency, loss, and bereavement. The vicissitudes of aging may lead to stressors that uncover preexisting and perhaps long-standing deficiencies in interpersonal relationships. For example, individuals who have relied on defensive personality styles requiring activity, intensity, and environmental control may have difficulty adapting to old age and its requirements for relinquishing appropriate control to others. Interpersonal conflicts or rebellious avoidance of using necessary support systems will sometimes emerge. Such individuals may experience strong longings for closeness while at the same time fearing rejection or engulfment. Intolerance of imposed intimate relationships may develop because of declining capacities and dependency on others.

As noted, cognitive-behavioral assessment is of relevance in elderly individuals, who are easily prone to cognitive distortions and vulnerable to developing inaccurate perceptions of their own roles and place in the world; their value to others; and fears of real or imagined assault from threatening forces and catastrophic images of decline, infirmity, pain, and abandonment. This element of inquiry focuses on the central themes of aging, particularly evaluating the patient's belief system, the presence of distortions, and concomitant affective responses.

In deciding on treatment interventions, the therapist of the geriatric patient is often placed in the position of having to make a triage decision—that is, evaluating the individual patient's capacity to utilize psychotherapy and, if so, at which level. Moreover, limited resources may force therapists into the position of deciding where to concentrate their efforts. It is important that this choice be made actively, based on the therapist's knowledge of a variety of therapeutic modalities. Unfortunately, all too often the therapist's preference for a particular therapy or his or her narrow range of expertise may determine the treatment choice. In making a triage decision, the therapist is faced with three decision points:

1. The accessibility of the patient to therapy (i.e., Is the patient able to attend? Does he or she have the mental and sensory capacity, or are there other barriers?)
2. Assessment of need (i.e., Does the patient require an active intervention, or does he or she have the psychological strength and supports, and will the natural course of the disorder lead to improvement over time without active psychotherapy?)
3. Which of the therapeutic modalities is most likely to be effective, and whether it is available. To make this decision, the therapist must be familiar with the indications for the three main therapeutic modalities. (Parenthetically, geriatric psychiatry training programs may not adequately address the need to train geriatric psychiatrists in the indications for and implementation of a range of psychotherapeutic modalities.)

Patients in institutions are highly vulnerable to triage decisions because they may be deemed inaccessible (i.e., too impaired in cognition and/or function to be reachable). More importantly, treatment, particularly psychotherapy treatment, is often unavailable.

Summary

Many clinical reports and a limited number of outcome studies support the contention that elderly patients are very responsive to various modalities of psychotherapy. Individual psychotherapy with elderly individuals is distinguished from that with younger adults by 1) attention to specific developmental tasks and challenges associated with aging; 2) the need for especially active therapeutic intervention to overcome patient, family, and health care system barriers to treatment; 3) the nature of the transference and countertransference reactions and resistances; and 4) the need to employ specialized psychotherapeutic approaches for frail, dementia, and personality disorder patients. The therapist of the elderly patient must maintain a flexible approach, because the patient's changing clinical status may require a shift from one treatment approach to another. For many elderly patients, insight-oriented psychotherapy provides an opportunity to resolve new and old conflicts while helping to give meaning to a lifetime of experience. For frail elderly individuals, supportive psychotherapy and environmental manipulation can shore up healthy defenses; provide for a caring, protective environment; help preserve self-respect and self-esteem; and provide understanding and guidance to an often bewildered family.

References

American Psychiatric Association: Diagnostic and Statistical Manual of Mental Disorders, 3rd Edition. Washington, DC, American Psychiatric Association, 1980

American Psychiatric Association: Diagnostic and Statistical Manual of Mental Disorders, 4th Edition. Washington, DC, American Psychiatric Association, 1994

Aronson MJ: Psychotherapy in a home for the aged. Arch Neurol Psychiatry 79:671–674, 1958

Atchley RC: The aging self. Psychotherapy: Theory, Research, and Practice 9:338–396, 1982

Beck A, Rush J, Shaw BF, et al: Cognitive Therapy of Depression. New York, Guilford, 1979

Berezin M: Psychodynamic considerations of aging and the aged: an overview. Am J Psychiatry 128:12, 33–41, 1972

Berezin M: Reflections on psychotherapy with the elderly, in Treating the Elderly With Psychotherapy: The Scope for Change in Later Life. Edited by Sadavoy J, Leszcz M. Madison, CT, International Universities Press, 1987, pp 45–63

Blau D, Berezin MA: Neurosis and character disorders, in Modern Perspectives in the Psychiatry of Old Age. Edited by Howells JG. New York, Brunner/Mazel, 1975, pp 201–233

Breslau L: Exaggerated helplessness syndrome, in Treating the Elderly With Psychotherapy: The Scope for Change in Later Life. Edited by Sadavoy J, Leszcz M. Madison, CT, International Universities Press, 1987

Brody E, Kleban MH, Lawton MP, et al: Excess disabilities of mentally impaired aged: impact of individualized treatment. Gerontologist 11(2):133, 1971

Butler RN: The life review: an interpretation of reminiscence in the aged. Psychiatry 26:65–70, 1963

Butler RN, Lewis MI: Aging and Mental Health: Positive Psychosocial Approaches. St. Louis, MO, CV Mosby, 1977

Cath SH: Some dynamics of middle and later years: a study in depletion and restitution, in Geriatric Psychiatry: Grief, Loss, and Emotional Disorders in the Aging Process. Edited by Berezin MA, Cath SH. New York, International Universities Press, 1975, pp 21–72

Cath SH: Functional disorders: an organismic view and attempt at reclassification, in Geriatric Psychiatry. Edited by Bellak L, Karasu TB. New York, Grune & Stratton, 1976

Cohen GD: Psychodynamic perspectives in the clinical approach to brain disease in the elderly, in Psychiatric Consequences of Brain Disease in the Elderly. Edited by Conn D, Grek A, Sadavoy J. New York, Plenum Press, 1989, pp 85–99

Crusey J: Short-term psychodynamic psychotherapy with a sixty-two-year-old man, in The Race Against Time. Edited by Nemiroff RA, Colarusso CA. New York, Plenum, 1985, pp 147–170

Eisdorfer C, Stotsky BA: Intervention, treatment and rehabilitation of psychiatric disorders, in The Handbook of the Psychology of Aging. Edited by Birren JE, Schaie KW. New York, Van Nostrand Reinhold, 1977, pp 724–748

Emery G: Cognitive therapy with the elderly, in New Directions in Cognitive Therapy. Edited by Emery G, Hollon SD, Bedrosian RC, et al. New York, Guilford, 1981, pp 84–98

Erikson EH: The human life cycle, in International Encyclopedia of the Social Sciences. Edited by Sills DL. New York, Macmillan, 1968, pp 286–292

Feigenbaum E: Ambulatory treatment of the elderly, in Mental Illness in Later Life. Edited by Busse EW, Pfeiffer E. Washington, DC, American Psychiatric Association, 1973, pp 153–166

Ford CV, Sbordone RT: Attitudes of psychiatrists toward elderly patients. Am J Psychiatry 137:571–575, 1980

Gabbard GO: Splitting in hospital treatment. Am J Psychiatry 146:

444–451, 1989

Gaitz GM: Barriers to the delivery of psychiatric services to the elderly. Gerontologist 14:210–214, 1974

Gallagher DE, Thompson LW: Depression in the Elderly: A Behavioral Treatment Manual. Los Angeles, University of Southern California Press, 1981

Gallagher DE, Thompson LW: Differential effectiveness of psychotherapies for the treatment of major depressive disorders in older adult patients. Psychotherapy: Theory, Research, and Practice 19:482–490, 1982

Gallagher DE, Thompson LW: Effectiveness of psychotherapy for both endogenous and non-endogenous depression in older adult outpatients. J Gerontol 38:707–712, 1983

Gitelson MA: The emotional problems of elderly persons, in Readings in Psychotherapy With Older People. Edited by Steury S, Blank ML. Washington, DC, National Institute of Mental Health, 1981, pp 8–17

Goldfarb AI: Psychotherapy of the aged: the use and value of an adaptational frame of reference. Psychoanal Rev 43:168–181, 1956

Goldfarb AI, Turner H: Psychotherapy of aged persons, II: utilization and effectiveness of "brief" therapy. Am J Psychiatry 109:916–921, 1953

Goldfarb AI, Sheps J: Psychotherapy of the aged. Psychosom Med 16:209–219, 1954

Grotjahn JM: Psychoanalytic investigation of a 71-year-old man with senile dementia. Psychoanal Q 9:80–97, 1940

Grotjahn M: Analytic psychotherapy with the elderly. Psychoanal Rev 42:419–427, 1955

Grunes JM: The aged in psychotherapy: psychodynamic contributions to the treatment process, in Treating the Elderly With Psychotherapy: The Scope for Change in Later Life. Edited by Sadavoy J, Leszcz M. Madison, CT, International Universities Press, 1987, pp 31–44

Hanley IG, McGuire RJ, Boyd WD: Reality orientation and dementia: a controlled trial of two approaches. Br J Psychiatry 138:10–14, 1981

Hiatt H: Dynamic psychotherapy with the aging patient. Am J Psychother 25:591–600, 1971

Hollos S, Ferenczi S: Psychoanalysis and the Psychic Disorder of General Paresis. New York, Nervous and Mental Disease, 1925

Hussian RA: Behavioral Geriatrics: Progress in Behavior Modification, Vol 16. New York, Academic Press, 1984, pp 159–183

Hussian RA, Davis RL: Responsive Care: Behavioral Interventions With Elderly Persons. Champaign, IL, Research Press, 1985

Jacques E: Death and the mid-life crisis. Int J Psychoanal 46:502–514, 1965

Kahana R: Strategies of dynamic psychotherapy with the wide range of older individuals. J Geriatr Psychiatry 12:71–100, 1979

Kahana R: Discussion: The Oedipus complex and rejuvenation fantasies in the analysis of a seventy-year-old woman. J Geriatr Psychiatry 20:53–60, 1987a

Kahana R: Geriatric psychotherapy: beyond crisis management, in Treating the Elderly With Psychotherapy: The Scope for Change in Later Life. Edited by Sadavoy J, Leszcz M. Madison, CT, International Universities Press, 1987b, pp 233–263

Kahn RS: Comments, in Proceedings of the York House Institute on the Mentally Impaired Aged. Philadelphia, PA, Philadelphia Geriatric Center, 1965

Karasu TB: The specificity versus nonspecificity dilemma: toward identifying therapeutic change agents. Am J Psychiatry 143:687–695, 1986

King PMH: The life cycle as indicated by the nature of the transference in the psychoanalysis of the middle-aged and elderly. Int J Psychoanal 61:153–159, 1980

Lazarus LW: Self-psychology and psychotherapy with the elderly: theory and practice. J Geriatr Psychiatry 13:69–88, 1980

Lazarus L: Self-psychology: its application to brief psychotherapy with the elderly. J Geriatr Psychiatry 21:109–125, 1988

Lazarus LW, Weinberg J: Treatment in the ambulatory-care setting, in Handbook of Geriatric Psychiatry. Edited by Busse EW, Blazer DG. New York, Van Nostrand Reinhold, 1980, pp 427–452

Lazarus LW, Mershon S: Psychiatric drugs and the elderly, in Handbook of Applied Gerontology. Edited by Lesnoff-Caravaglia G. New York, Human Sciences Press, 1987, pp 119–126

Lazarus LW, Groves L, Guttman D, et al: Brief psychotherapy with the elderly: a study of process and outcome, in Treating the Elderly With Psychotherapy: The Scope for Change in Later Life. Edited by Sadavoy J, Leszcz M. Madison, CT, International Universities Press, 1987, pp 265–293

Levin S: Depression in the aged, in Geriatric Psychiatry: Grief, Loss, and Emotional Disorders in the Aging Process. Edited by Berezin MA, Cath S. New York, International Universities Press, 1965a, pp 203–225

Levin S: Some comments on the distribution of narcissistic and object libido in the aged. Int J Psychoanal 46:200–208, 1965b

Lewis MI, Butler RN: Life-review therapy: putting memories to work in individual and group psychotherapy. Geriatrics 29:165–169, 172–173, 1974

Meerloo JAM: Contribution of psychoanalysis to the problem of the aged, in Psychoanalysis and Social Work. Edited by Hermann M. New York, International Universities Press, 1953, pp 321–337

Meerloo JAM: Transference and resistance in geriatric psychotherapy. Psychoanal Rev 42:72–82, 1955

Meissner WW: Normal psychology of the aging process revisited, I: discussion. Paper presented at the Annual Scientific Meeting of the Boston Society of Gerontologic Psychiatry, Boston, MA, 1975

Miller E: The Oedipus complex and rejuvenation fantasies in the analysis of a seventy-year-old woman. J Geriatr Psychiatry 20:29–51, 1987

Myers WA: Dynamic Therapy of the Older Patient. New York, Jason Aronson, 1984, p 6

Myers WA: Transference and countertransference issues in treatments involving older patients and younger therapists. J Geriatr Psychiatry 19:221–239, 1986

Nemiroff RA, Colarusso CA: The literature on psychotherapy and psychoanalysis in the second half of life, in The Race Against Time. Edited by Nemiroff RA, Colarusso CA. New York, Plenum, 1985, pp 25–43

Neugarten B: Time, age and the life-cycle. Am J Psychiatry 136:887–894, 1979

Pinkston EM, Linsk NL: Behavioral family intervention with the impaired elder. Gerontogist 26:576–583, 1984

Pollock GH: The mourning-liberation process: ideas on the inner life of the older adult, in Treating the Elderly With Psychotherapy: The Scope for Change in Later Life. Edited by Sadavoy J, Leszcz M. Madison, CT, International Universities Press, 1987, pp 3–29

Rechtschaffen A: Psychotherapy with geriatric patients: a review of the literature. J Gerontol 14:73–84, 1959

Reynolds CF, Frank E, Perel JM, et al: Combined pharmacotherapy and psychotherapy in the acute and continuation treatment of elderly patients with recurrent major depression: a preliminary report. Am J Psychiatry 149:1687–1692, 1992

Rosenthal HM: The use of psychoanalytic principles in the treatment of older people. Am J Psychoanal 45:119–134, 1985

Sadavoy J: Character disorders in the elderly: an overview, in Treating the Elderly With Psychotherapy: The Scope for Change in Later Life. Edited by Sadavoy J, Leszcz M. Madison, CT, International Universities Press, 1987, pp 175–229

Sadavoy J: Psychodynamic perspectives on dementia: Alzheimer's disease and the individual. American Journal of Alzheimer's Care and Research

6:12–20, 1991

Sadavoy J: Integrated psychotherapy for the elderly. Can J Psychiatry 39 (suppl 1):519–526, 1994

Sadavoy J, Dorian B: Treatment of the elderly characterologically disturbed patient in the chronic care institution. J Geriatr Psychiatry 16:223–240, 1983

Sadavoy J, Fogel B: Personality disorders in old age, in Handbook of Mental Health and Aging, 2nd Edition. Edited by Birren J, Slane RB, Cohen GD. San Diego, CA, Academic Press, 1992, pp 433–462

Sadavoy J, Leszcz M (eds): Treating the Elderly With Psychotherapy: The Scope for Change in Later Life. Madison, CT, International Universities Press, 1987

Sadavoy J, Robinson A: Psychotherapy and the cognitively impaired elderly, in Psychiatric Consequences of Brain Disease in the Elderly. Edited by Conn D, Grek A, Sadavoy J. New York, Plenum, 1989, pp 101–135

Sandler AM: A developmental crisis in an aging patient: comments on development and adaptation. J Geriatr Psychiatry 15:11–32, 1982

Segal H: Fear of death (notes on the analysis of an old man). Int J Psychoanal 39:178–181, 1958

Silberschatz G: Testing pathogenic beliefs, in The Psychoanalytic Process: Theory, Clinical Observation, and Empirical Research. Edited by Weiss J, Sampson H. New York, Guilford, 1986, pp 256–266

Silberschatz G, Curtis JT: Clinical implications on research on brief dynamic psychotherapy, II: how the therapist helps or hinders therapeutic progress. Psychoanal Psychol 3:27–37, 1986

Silberschatz G, Curtis JT: Time-limited psychodynamic therapy with older adults, in New Techniques in the Psychotherapy of Older Patients. Edited by Myers W, Washington, DC, American Psychiatric Press, 1991, pp 95–110

Simon A, Lowenthal MF: Crisis and Intervention: The Fate of the Elderly Mental Patient. San Francisco, CA, Jossey-Bass, 1970

Steuer J: Psychotherapy with the elderly. Psychiatr Clin North Am 5:199–213, 1982

Thompson LW, Gallagher D, Breckenridge JS: Comparative effectiveness of psychotherapies for depressed elders. J Consult Clin Psychol 55:385–390, 1987

Thompson LW, Gallagher D, Czirr R: Personality disorder and outcome in the treatment of late-life depression. J Geriatr Psychiatry 21:133–153, 1988

Thompson LW, Frank G, Florsheim M, et al: Cognitive-behavioral therapy for affective disorders, in New Techniques in the Psychotherapy of Older Patients. Edited by Myers WA. Washington, DC, American Psychiatric Press, 1991, pp 3–19

Tobin SS: Issues of care in long-term settings, in Psychiatric Consequences of Brain Disease in the Elderly. Edited by Conn D, Grek A, Sadavoy J. New York, Plenum, 1989, pp 163–187

Weisman AD, Hackett TP: Denial as a social act, in Psychodynamic Studies on Aging, Creativity, Reminiscing, and Dying. Edited by Levin S, Kahana RJ. New York, International Universities Press, 1967, pp 79–110

Wheelright JB: Some comments on the aging process. Psychiatry 22:407–411, 1959

Windholz MJ, Marmar CR, Horowitz MJ: A review of the research on conjugal bereavement: impact on health and efficacy of intervention. Compr Psychiatry 26:433–477, 1985

Yalom I: Existential Psychotherapy. New York, Basic Books, 1980

Yesavage JA, Karasu TB: Psychotherapy with elderly patients. Am J Psychother 36:41–55, 1982

Zinberg NE: The relation of regressive phenomena to the aging process, in Normal Psychology of the Aging Process. Edited by Zinberg NE, Kaufman I. New York, International Universities Press, 1963, pp 123–137

Zinberg NE, Kaufman I: Cultural and personality factors associated with aging: an introduction, in Normal Psychology of the Aging Process. Edited by Zinberg NE, Kaufman I. New York, International Universities Press, 1963, pp 17–71

Molyn Leszcz, M.D., F.R.C.P.C.

Group Therapy

T he appropriate application of group treatments to elderly individuals requires knowledge of the range of patients, settings, and techniques associated with this age group (Burnside 1978; MacLennan et al. 1988). Yalom (1995) notes the importance of the group leader's ability to identify the particular patient population as well as the patients' particular needs and concerns, to develop specific treatment objectives, and then to modify the structure of the group intervention to address these objectives. Homogenization may result in techniques and models that are appropriate for one patient population being misapplied to another. The designation *geriatric* fails to denote differences in age, ego function, education, sociocultural background, ethnic variables, and the capacity for introspection and self-reflection. Similarly, a broad range of group therapeutic approaches are applicable to elderly individuals. What links all effective group approaches is the creation of a context for interpersonal engagement between and among a number of patients and a therapist(s) that operates according to certain structures and group norms and aims to achieve a degree of group cohesiveness, reflected in feelings of mutual interest, attachment, and task effectiveness.

Table 29–1 lists the types of group therapy currently employed with geriatric patients. A large number of foci exist. These include the treatment

Table 29–1.   Group therapy approaches for the elderly

Verbal-centered groups for the cognitively intact
  Psychodynamic psychotherapy groups
  Reminiscence groups
  Cognitive-behavioral groups
  Homogeneous groups (e.g., widows, postretirement, and relocation groups)
  Burdened caregivers groups
Verbal-centered groups for the cognitively impaired
  Resocialization and remotivation groups
  Reality orientation groups
Creativity- and activity-centered groups
  Dance movement therapy groups
  Project groups
  Nutrition groups
  Drama, art, or poetry groups
Settings
  Outpatient groups
  Day hospital and partial hospitalization groups
  Acute hospital groups
  Institutional groups (i.e., chronic hospital groups, nursing home groups)

of specific functional disorders, most commonly, mood disorders; psychotherapeutic treatment of developmental and transitional phenomena and the impact of these life events on self-esteem, self-worth, and the individual's underlying personality; remediation of organic deficits in the cognitive and physical domains; addressing the desire for growth, creativity, and self-expression; and provision of support, education, and assistance in coping with caregiver burden.

A key concept in this chapter is the requirement that the therapist be flexible in conducting the group. Differences between supportive and insight-oriented groups, and between depth and nondepth groups, are frequently blurred. Many geriatric patients in fact are treated in some modified group that contains both insight-oriented and supportive approaches. In many instances, the therapist's awareness of both psychodynamic and process considerations, as well as structured techniques and content considerations, enhances therapeutic efficacy. Similarly, a realistic therapeutic perspective that recognizes the scope for growth for restoration of lost interpersonal, emotional, and cognitive capacities is essential.

In this chapter these considerations will be addressed by examining the indications for group therapy, the contemporary range of group therapy approaches, technical considerations for the therapist, and the effectiveness and outcome of these treatments.

Indications for Group Therapy

As with every treatment modality, a particular therapy for elderly individuals will not be equally effective with all individuals. In every instance, however, effective psychotherapy can proceed only with a clear anti-ageism bias: that the psychological difficulties of the elderly person are treatable and reversible until proven otherwise.

Social isolation, interpersonal alienation, maladaptive interpersonal skills, diminished self-worth, and depressive disengagement and withdrawal are common presenting features, and group therapy offers much opportunity for addressing these difficulties, promoting social engagement and the development of social networks (Wong 1991). Group therapy may be employed as the sole treatment or as adjunctive treatment to pharmacotherapy or individual therapy. When treatments are provided conjointly, they must be offered in an integrated and coherent fashion; the "therapeutic right hand" must know what the "therapeutic left hand" is doing. Because depression in elderly individuals is often a chronic, relapsing disorder even with initially effective pharmacological treatment (Murphy 1983), the importance of psychosocial therapies is underscored. Although it remains unclear whether social isolation and lack of social supports cause depression or whether depression-induced loss of social skills results in isolation, it is clear that elderly depressed patients are indeed more likely to have both diminished social supports and diminished social skills (Gallagher 1981; Grant et al. 1988). What is cause and what is effect is often unclear, but this self-perpetuating, reverberating cycle can be interrupted at either point. Group therapy may be more acceptable and less anxiety provoking than individual therapy owing to the sharing of concerns and mutual helpfulness. Regressive feelings related to dependency may also be diminished by participation in the group. In addition, the concrete opportunity for behavioral change and practice that occurs in most groups may hold special appeal for the older person, who may be less able to deal with abstract psychological issues.

In some instances, these objectives can be met entirely by the manifest content of the interaction around group activities. In other instances, these benefits can be accessed only by addressing the process of the group and effectively working through the patients' resistances to engagement.

The ideal treatment setting offers the broadest range of group modalities—a form of therapeutic "buffet." Resistance to engagement and the severity of presenting symptoms often determine the relative indications for verbal- or activity-centered groups. Depression is unlikely to be treated effectively by an activity- or creativity-centered group alone, and the resistive, devaluing patient is unlikely to connect effectively in such a setting. Activity-centered groups serve useful maintenance and prophylactic functions, and for the highly motivated individual, participation in such groups may be all that is required to maintain psychological integration. Referral to these groups should be linked to the special interests, talents, and concerns of the patient. The more depressed or functionally impaired patient may use activity-centered groups to good effect, in an ongoing fashion, following a period of more intensive treatment.

Group composition should be homogeneous for level of ego function, intellect, and degree of cognitive functioning. Age itself is generally not the main determining factor. In fact, active elderly individuals may be treated effectively in psychotherapy groups with younger patients. Such groups provide a rich opportunity to work through issues of feeling old and inadequate in a youthful society. On the other hand, even in homogeneous geriatric settings, mixing cognitively intact and cognitively impaired patients together can result in the former feeling an unwillingness to engage and the latter being unable to sustain engagement. The cognitively inaccessible patient may not benefit from the group and is likely to discourage participation by other members, who may see in the grossly impaired patient their worst fear of personal decline.

Homogeneous groups are more likely to become cohesive quickly and generally are more supportive (Salvendy 1993). Feelings of universality are enhanced, but there is a risk that excessive homogeneity will result in a lack of contrasting perspective that can diminish the range of problem solving. In general, the importance to group members of being able to identify positively with one another should be recognized in the selection and composition of groups. Individuals who are significantly deviant from the group norm are more likely to be early dropouts (Yalom 1995).

Group therapy is contraindicated for patients who are in acute crisis or who are suicidal; patients with drug or alcohol abuse; paranoid or violently aggressive patients; patients with persistent inability to attend to the process of the group because of severe cognitive impairment, sedation, irremediable hearing loss, or differences in language; and difficult, characterologically disturbed patients who persistently attack and devalue others in maladaptive efforts to bolster their own self-esteem. These contraindications are relative and are intended to serve as guidelines to maintain the viability and effectiveness of the group, as well as to avoid negative outcomes to any individual patient, such as group rejection or extrusion. A strong, well-established, and mature group is better able to contain a difficult patient than is a beginning, developmentally immature group. The group therapist must evaluate whether a particular group and a particular patient can benefit from one another at a particular point in time. Unlike the individual setting, in the group setting the therapist's selection of patients not only commits the therapist to the patient, but also commits each of the other group members to a relationship with that patient.

Preparation and training of patients prior to entry into group therapy has not been specifically researched with elderly individuals, but the evidence for its usefulness in other patient populations, as reviewed in detail by Yalom (1995), is quite substantial. Preparation and pretraining are incorporated in virtually all cognitive and behavioral group treatments (Thompson et al. 1991). Explaining the rationale of psychotherapy demystifies an otherwise anxiety-provoking situation; helps establish a therapeutic alliance; and sets group norms regarding regular attendance, confidentiality, and extra group socialization. Effective pretraining results in enhanced group tenure and task adherence, increased hopefulness, reduced anxiety, and increased interaction and self-disclosure, thereby increasing the chances for successful treatment (Yalom 1995). Dropout rates for group therapy with young patients range from 10% to 50% (Yalom 1995), and with elderly individuals the frequency rate is at least the same (Steuer et al. 1984). The likelihood of a premature dropout is increased with increased severity of depression; presence of severe physical illness; and a characterological style that devalues, externalizes, and blames.

Furthermore, in institutional settings group therapy is indicated to provide a forum to deal with the imposed accommodations to changes in life situation and reduced feelings of autonomy. The opportunity to work through and reconcile interpersonal difficulties in institutional relationships may enhance the quality of life available to residents in institutions. In addition, some settings have a heavy preponderance of female residents and staff, and group therapy may provide an opportunity for the relatively few men in the institution to meet together, stimulating models of identification with male figures in the matriarchal environment typical of many nursing homes (Leszcz et al. 1985).

Examination of the themes that emerge in group therapy (Table 29–2) illustrates that many of the psychological concerns of elderly individuals are generated by age-induced losses and changes and the patient's

Table 29–2. Themes in group therapy

Loss of significant relationships
Loss of physical and cognitive capacities
Loss of functions and tasks
Loss of self-worth and self-esteem
Loneliness and isolation
Depression and demoralization
Dependency-autonomy conflicts
Interpersonal conflict with spouse and family
Hopelessness, helplessness, and purposelessness
Wish for restoration of a sense of competence and mastery

difficulty in negotiating the late-life developmental challenge of maintaining a sense of self that is continuous in the present with the past (Leszcz 1987). These themes shape the overall objectives of group therapies with elderly individuals, as noted in Table 29–3.

Group Therapy Approaches

Psychodynamic Group Psychotherapy

Kohut's (1984) conceptualization of narcissism and self-psychology has greatly influenced the conduct of individual and group psychotherapy with elderly persons because of the understanding it provides of the internal and subjective experience of the elderly individual (Lazarus 1980). This conceptualization is particularly relevant to the individual faced with the challenge of maintaining a sense of self in the face of the narcissistic injuries of aging and the loss of central functions, capacities, and selfobject relationships. This conceptualization augments and facilitates the use of

Table 29–3. Objectives of treatment

Restoration of a sense of self-esteem and self-worth
Reduction of isolation and promotion of interpersonal engagement
Symptom reduction and mastery
Acquisition of coping skills and interpersonal skills
Grieving and adaptation to loss
Appropriate acceptance of dependency and rational utilization of available
    resources

the central dynamic and interactive group therapeutic mechanisms described by Yalom (1995).

Group therapy provides a self-esteem, self-sustaining treatment matrix in which the narcissistic injuries to the self may be addressed through the feeling of group cohesion and the providing of relationships that serve necessary selfobject functions, in addition to providing real objects for relatedness and support (Schwartzman 1984). The selfobject transference may be to the other individuals, the group as a whole, or the therapist, and it serves to restore a sense of self-stability and vitality by providing one or more central elements (Kohut 1984): 1) mirroring selfobjects that value, praise, and admire the individual; 2) idealized selfobjects in whose presence the individual feels safe, protected, and worthwhile; and 3) alter ego or twinning selfobjects with whom the individual can feel an essential alikeness and resonance through the process of pairing with another person (Lothstein and Zimet 1988). The emphasis on empathic recognition of the subjective experience of elderly individuals in the group deepens the therapist's understanding of the processes of relationships, interactions, and resistances in the group. With a self psychology perspective, it becomes more possible to understand empathically the interpersonal phenomena of defensive withdrawal, haughty devaluation, grandiose exhibitionism, monopolization, idealization, and the pursuit of special relatedness as attempts to protect or stabilize a vulnerable sense of self (Stone and Whitman 1977). Disruptive and alienating behavior that could threaten group cohesiveness can thereby be better contained, facilitating further opportunities for interpersonal engagement and interpersonal learning.

In addition to the considerations of the individual's sense of self, group therapy also is well suited to address other psychodynamic considerations, through the interpersonal articulation within the social microcosm of the group, of individual member's core concerns and conflicts. For some patients geriatric group therapy is a later installment in a sequence of psychotherapy that was first initiated in early or midlife, and echoes the earlier concerns.

Reminiscence Group Therapy

The process of reminiscing, or life review (Butler 1974; Poulton and Strassberg 1986) has been employed in a variety of ways in psychotherapy groups. Conceptualized as a developmentally appropriate and natural process of review through which elderly persons can organize and evaluate their lives, it has been used to promote reintegration of individuals' sense of who they are by having them reconnect to what they were. Although life review and reminiscence approaches are often used interchangeably, Burnside (1991) clarifies the distinction between the more comprehensive life review approaches that emphasize uncovering, exploration, and working through, and the more narrow, reminiscence approaches that emphasize ego support and aim to avoid generating anxiety. Reminiscence has been used to enhance the development of cohesion in beginning groups and groups experiencing demoralization in the face of group developmental difficulties (Leszcz et al. 1985). In addition, it has been used effectively as an organizing anchor in group psychotherapy for more impaired patients (Lesser et al. 1981), creating a clear and achievable self-esteem–enhancing focus. These processes may emerge spontaneously or follow a prescribed, chronological format (Goldwasser et al. 1982; Kavanagh and Burnside 1992). Only positive events may be addressed—a process known as *milestoning* (Lowenthal and Marrazzo 1990)—or the life review may be more complete to promote the individual's mourning and acceptance of his or her life as it indeed was.

In practice, the process of reminiscing may be used adaptively or maladaptively, according to the way it is experienced by the group members and managed by the group therapist. At its best, the reminiscing process fleshes out individuals within the group and makes them three-dimensional people rather than one-dimensional objects of projection for one another. It restores feelings of worth, stature, and competence through the articulation of past successes and the recollection of prior credentials and, through mutual reverberations and identifications, promotes feelings of affiliation and much needed social support (Wong 1991). What has been of greatest importance to any individual often cannot be assumed without confirmation, and subjective valuation may be very different from objective valuation. Reminiscing about previous challenges that have been mastered often helps to soothe the apprehension about facing the unknown future. Furthermore, appropriate grieving and conflict resolution may be facilitated, promoting better engagement in the current environment.

However, in patients who are profoundly depressed or withdrawn, reminiscing may result in a further preoccupation with the past; guilt over irreparable errors; and a heightened, morbid self-absorption that results in social alienation. In such instances group cohesion can be seriously undermined, and the therapist must determine whether reminiscing is serving the intended purpose of deepening the group members' understanding of one another, strengthening feelings of group cohesion and universality, and promoting both a sense of mastery and a willingness to engage. Benefits can be maximized and risks reduced if the therapist establishes a group norm that all reminiscing, and the experience of talking about, listening to, and sharing, be brought back centripetally into the "here and now" of the group and examined at the interpersonal level (Poulton and Strassberg 1986).

Cognitive-Behavior Group Therapy

Cognitive-behavior group therapy emphasizes conscious cognition and learning, adapting behavioral strategies and the cognitive therapy model to the group setting. It is well suited to addressing disturbances in mood and is the modality that has been best researched and evaluated in terms of effectiveness in the realm of geriatric group therapy (Thompson et al. 1991). Central elements include the identification of dysfunctional attitudes and cognitive distortions that engender depression. This process includes 1) helping patients identify and monitor their reactions in particular situations, 2) confronting and correcting distortions by realignment of the attributions of meaning made by the individual, 3) determining the basic assumptions and themes that shape these reactions, 4) practicing alternative cognitive and behavioral responses to anticipated stresses, by encouraging patients to tackle ever-increasing challenges, and 5) achieving mastery and maintenance of positive affects that breed alternative and more correct and objective assumptions (Rush 1983). Defocusing, depersonalizing, reducing dichotomous thinking, reframing, and focusing attention on partial positive outcomes as a way to counteract cognitive distortions of global negative outcome exemplify this approach (Thompson et al. 1991). In this model, the repetitive, maladaptive, depressogenic behaviors and cognitions are viewed as automatic. They reflect a form of learned behavior that is blind to other options. Psychodynamic considerations and questions of motivation are viewed as irrelevant.

Social isolation and the lack of alternative input exacerbate negative, self-devaluing, and self-blaming assumptions and make some elderly individuals particularly prone to distortions in the attribution of meaning to experience (Parham et al. 1982). The exchange and feedback that occur in a group are particularly well suited to confronting such assumptions and distortions. Treatment promotes the realignment and objectification of cognitive assumptions and the attribution of meaning to events and experiences.

More focused behavioral approaches (Gallagher 1981) employ modeling, role playing, didactic discussions, and feedback about each group member's efforts in using skills required to reengage with pleasurable experiences. The focus is on external and observable behavior only. The aim of treatment is to break the vicious cycle of depressed mood resulting in reduced interaction and reduced stimulation of positive interpersonal reinforcement, further social withdrawal, and the consequent erosion of social skills. The group serves as a supportive laboratory for prescribed behavioral practice, with homework assignments between sessions serving an additional important function. Relaxation techniques and problem-solving skills, as well as time management, self-assertion and self-expression, are taught. Psychoeducational approaches attempt to demystify depression, and there is a strong emphasis on the acquisition of behavioral skills. Patients are taught to log the relationship between their mood and either pleasurable or aversive behaviors and events to increase the frequency of pleasure-centered actions (Steinmetz-Breckenridge et al. 1985). Meditation, relaxation, and visual imagery techniques have also begun to be utilized with elderly individuals (Abraham et al. 1992).

Integrated Verbal-Centered Group Therapy

In clinical practice, the three models—psychodynamic, life review, and cognitive-behavior—may be effectively integrated into an approach that capitalizes on the strengths of each. This integrative approach requires empirical evaluation of its effectiveness, but it hinges on certain principles that emerge from clinical experience. Focusing on the elaboration of affect and self-disclosure is useful in gaining an understanding of the individual, and the life review further fleshes out this understanding. However, patients highly value skill acquisition (Gallagher and Thompson 1982). It aids in mastery, restoration of competence, and generalization of gains, and it amplifies the very important therapeutic factor of group cohesion by virtue of the feeling of shared achievement in the group. On the other hand, disregard for the group process or the subjective experience of the individual can result in a therapy group's assuming an unempathic, alienating, superficial, "pick yourself up by the bootstraps" orientation. Augmenting the documented effectiveness of "cold processing," role playing, simulations, and modeling to illuminate maladaptive interpersonal skills and interpersonal distortions, with the direct in vivo "hot processing" of a more interactive group that focuses on the actual interpersonal relationships created in the "here and now" of the group may generate additional benefit, particularly for patients with comorbid personality disturbance who are difficult to engage (Leszcz 1992; Safran and Segal 1990).

In an integrated model, individuals have the opportunity, for example, of examining their experience of isolation and loneliness in the group, exploring what they do that minimizes and maximizes their isolation and loneliness and practicing new skills and risk taking. A productive and logically consistent synthesis is formed of the patients' subjective experiences and the specific importance of their interpersonal relatedness, the historical context of the individuals and their relationships, their interpersonal contributions to their own current relational success and failure, along with the challenging of cognitive and interpersonal distortions and the direct behavioral practice of successful relating.

Issues of integration of psychotherapeutic and therapeutic approaches are being addressed broadly in the contemporary psychotherapy literature (Wachtel 1991), as practitioners recognize the reality that no one explanatory or therapeutic model can effectively address the vast scope of clinical and treatment needs. These modifications require ongoing construction and evaluation.

Schmid and Rouslin (1992) described another dimension to integrated group therapy: actively linking a predischarge hospitalized psychiatric patients' group with an aftercare group. This group includes significant family members along with the identified patients, facilitating both reentry to the community and continuity of care. Patient-caregiver issues can be addressed, and this approach also provides a forum for family members' clarification of active treatment issues.

Homogeneous Groups

A broad range of homogeneous groups generally meet over a short term of 8 to 20 sessions. Their composition is generally determined by a particular common problem, characteristic, or developmental issue. A relevant model is that of postretirement groups (Salvendy 1989), which may emphasize mutual support, countering the isolation and the loss of self-esteem induced by loss of the status of employment. Also prominent are groups for the recently bereaved (Lund and Caserta 1992). These may be led professionally or in a self-help model.

Groups for Burdened Caregivers

Caregiver groups have developed in response to the increasing number of frail individuals or individuals with cognitive impairment or dementia being cared for at home by their families (Kahan et al. 1985; Lazarus et al.

1981; Saul 1988). The rationale for these groups stems from the recognition that caregivers often are highly burdened, isolated, exhausted, and frequently depressed (Baldwin et al. 1989). The absence of social supports exacerbates the caregivers' strain (Zarit et al. 1980, 1982). Homogeneity of situation promotes rapidly cohesive groups with much self-disclosure and mutual support. Extra group contact is endorsed, and the self-help nature of the group is supported as well. A central psychological issue is the working through of the pain of providing care for a loved one who may have lost the capacity not only to express gratitude, but even to recognize the caregiver, or whose intermittent periods of recognition and lucidity may confuse and frustrate the caregiver. Hence providing personal validation within the group is highly valued by participants.

Objectives of these groups include the following:

- Education about the dementing or illness process and ways of interacting with the patient and providing care
- Working through loss and grief, promoting appropriate disengagement, and promoting realistic decisions about placement, if necessary
- Acquiring skills in problem solving and stress reduction
- Legitimizing the needs of the caregiver, thereby promoting self-care and regard to counter isolation and self-neglect
- Working through relationships with health care professionals
- Working through anger and guilt

The more affectively charged aspects of caregiving often are not readily accessed in a very highly focused and time-limited group treatment (Toseland et al. 1989).

Verbal-Centered Groups for Cognitively Impaired Individuals

Resocialization and Remotivation Groups

The objectives of verbal groups with the cognitively impaired stem from Linden's (1953) concept of "psychological senility." He first described this pattern of excess disability, beyond objective deficits, as a reversible picture of regressed dependency, morbid self-absorption, and disengagement arising from repeated losses and devaluation by society. Group therapy aims at stimulation, reengagement through leader- or patient-originated discussion and interaction, melded with the provision of as much sensory stimulation as possible. These groups focus on members' strengths and fundamental humanness and, although highly structured, do have a group process that must be attended to and understood by the therapist. These groups achieve interpersonal engagement more through the structure and content of the group than through the process. Patient engagement is both prompted and reinforced by the therapist repeatedly.

The array of content stimuli offered should be broad to maximize opportunities for effective activation and engagement. The leader may increase or decrease the amount of attention placed on process or activity according to patient needs. Cognitive exercises; activity and word games; life review; discussions; and participation in music, art, baking, and physical exercise are all components of these groups. The range is virtually limitless, but in each instance the emphasis should be on sensory stimulation, improved ego function, reality orientation, memory, judgment, problem solving, and interaction (Burnside 1978; Saul 1988).

Reality Orientation Groups

The objectives of reality orientation groups (Drummond et al. 1978) are the reversal of social and verbal disengagement and the diminished use of cognitive functions through continual stimulation and reorientation in an interactive environment. There is substantial overlap between reality orientation groups and resocialization and remotivation groups. Reality orientation occurs in two modes. The chief mode is a 24-hour milieu approach to provide consistent and persistent orientation of the individual, making the milieu as rational and knowable as possible. The second mode is classroom or group reality orientation. The reality orientation group room contains a full array of multisensory stimuli. Every opportunity is utilized to elucidate and remind individual patients of the who, where, what, and why of what is going on in a firm, friendly, nondemanding fashion, repeatedly bringing the patient back to the immediate present. Reinforcement for successful reorientation can be interpersonal or behavioral (Miller 1977) and can be linked to all activities of daily living. Reality orientation therapy may be utilized effectively to prepare for further resocialization therapy or reminiscence therapy. Prior reality orientation therapy has a significant, priming impact on the effective utilization of subsequent therapeutic interventions (Baines et al. 1987). Small group reality orientation enhances the 24-hour program but appears to be of minimal use in the absence of the more comprehensive milieu approach. Furthermore, without active therapeutic input and reinforcement, no generalization occurs, and learning is readily extinguished. The involvement of family members is essential to organize and coordinate the treatment program for their cognitively impaired relative (Teri and Gallagher-Thompson 1991).

Creativity- and Activity-Centered Groups

There is a broad range of creativity- and activity-centered groups, and there is substantial interplay among them (MacLennan et al. 1988). They provide opportunities for patients whose verbal skills may be diminished to express and rekindle a sense of self through the artistic or creative process, enhanced through working together with others. Both pleasure and mastery may be stimulated, challenging self-denigration and constricting distortions about the self. In many instances the nonverbal expression may be of even greater psychological depth than the verbal expression. The objective is not only to experience art, but to create it. These modalities are also important vehicles for retaining a sense of self in the midst of institutional life with its tendency toward homogenization and the blurring of individual differences. Creative expression is used as a form of engagement with one's world and with others, as well as an expression of self.

Dance movement therapy focuses on the integration of the self through reconnection of the individual with his or her own body (Samberg 1988). It is not task oriented like physical exercise, but instead is process oriented, promoting the opportunity to study the relationship between mood and movement and physical sensations. In a conceptual fashion analogous to the way that cognitive therapy challenges cognitive distortions and may treat depression by altering the way in which one thinks about oneself, dance movement therapy aims at ameliorating depression and demoralization by evoking positive and pleasurable bodily expressions. This therapy involves challenging negative or depressive assumptions of the physical self, its restrictions, and its limitations and increasing one's sense of physical mastery.

Technical Applications of Group Therapy

General Considerations

The objectives and indications of the various geriatric group therapies necessitate certain adaptations in therapist technique. Elderly individuals are often resistant to group psychotherapy and behave in ways that interfere with the development of group cohesion, especially when they are depressed. Withdrawal, devaluing self and others, hopelessness, and blaming generally are not conducive to group cohesion. It is striking that, regardless of the model of group therapy used, the recommended therapist posture and attitude are the same (Gallagher 1981). In their overview of the effectiveness of group therapy with elderly individuals, Tross and Blum (1988) concluded that the therapist's posture of respect, hopefulness, genuine warmth, and empathy appears to be as important as his or her theoretical rationale. In fact, Williams-Barnard and Lindell (1992) have confirmed this intuitive truth in a study that showed that patients' self-concept was significantly and powerfully affected by the degree to which rated group leaders demonstrated attitudes and behaviors toward group members that reflected the Rogerian concept of "prizing" (i.e., unconditional positive reward).

In general, the group leader carries a greater burden of responsibility to initiate and activate a group of geriatric individuals than is the case with groups of younger patients (Thompson et al. 1991). The group leader anchors the group, ensuring the psychological integrity of each individual and the logistical and functional integrity of the group as a whole. Determining a set and inviolate time for the group in a secure and comfortable location, free from time conflicts with other appointments, is essential. The format of the intervention should also reflect ethnic competence (Henderson et al. 1993), in that it is culturally attuned and respectful of cultural diversity and the unique beliefs, customs, and attitudes of the identified population. Active outreach by the group leaders to reduce fluctuations in composition of the group is a prerequisite for effective treatment. A cohesive group may not form spontaneously, and waiting for the group to activate itself is likely to result in a contagion of demoralization and group dropouts.

In view of the difficulty that some elderly persons have in getting started in the morning and the requirements of arranging transportation, it may be preferable to select a late morning or mid-afternoon time for the group. Normally such a time would foredoom a group of younger persons, but with elderly individuals it may be ideal, as it also promotes the opportunity for extra group contact around lunch and coffee. In younger persons' groups, extra group contact is generally prohibited because it often leads to subgrouping and, ultimately, to fragmentation in the group. In the geriatric population, however, extra group contact may be fostered, with the goal of providing opportunities for real relatedness, because elderly individuals do experience a realistic reduction in opportunities for such engagement. Furthermore, in institutional settings, extra group contacts are a fact of life. The key to successful management of this extra group contact or subgrouping is to diminish the boundary of secretiveness around the relationships and bring these interactions into the purview of the group, even if it is only to endorse and not to interpret them (Lothstein and Zimet 1988). Extra group contact can be a rich source of feedback about the individuals in the group, reducing treatment blind spots while providing an opportunity to practice interpersonal skills learned in the group proper.

While drawing attention to certain parameters that may be useful in conducting group therapy with elderly individuals, it is important also to recognize that excessive focus on patients' limits and vulnerabilities may emphasize deficits and underplay patients' strengths, and resources, and their capacity to tolerate the process of working through. The patient's readiness for change, growth, and resolution of long-standing concerns and psychological conflicts may be quite substantial. Pollock contended that elderly individuals are essentially dealing with forces and events that must be dealt with by all individuals across the entire life span. He described the process of mourning the loss of what was to facilitate the liberation of what will be as a lifelong process, often resulting in creativity and regeneration (Pollock 1987). Hence, the therapist must be alert to potential sources of ageism or countertransference that would tend to emphasize supportive interventions, when exploratory interventions would be better indicated (Leszcz 1987).

Verbal-Centered Groups

Verbal-centered groups function best with 6 to 10 patients and generally will meet weekly in ambulatory settings or as frequently as daily in partial hospitalization and day hospital institutional settings. Groups with larger membership appear to be less useful psychotherapeutically (Gorey and Cryns 1991). However, activity- and creativity-centered groups may function quite well with much larger numbers and may benefit from multiple leaders. The cognitively intact patients may participate in the group meeting for $1-1^1/_2$ hours, whereas cognitively impaired patients generally make better use of briefer time frames (i.e., 45 minutes) in light of their reduced attention and concentration.

The group therapist should ensure that the therapy is an esteem-enhancing and nonfailure experience for each member. A related task is that of protecting the group from fragmentation and rupture, a function more easily achieved when the therapist empathically recognizes the subjective experience of each group member. Awareness of what is subjectively important to each individual provides the therapist with a direction for the treatment and safeguards against the individual's loss of identity through group homogenization. Supporting even small gains and steps toward self-assertion and self-expression are essential.

Face-to-face interaction, direct contact, mutual support, and interaction in the "here and now" of the group will have to be reinforced repeatedly by the therapist, as should any pro-group cohesive interaction or feedback. Yalom and Terrazas (1967) advocated a model of "ego enhancement." They recommended that therapists always search for the central vulnerability, interpersonal core, or adaptive focus in every interchange. Externalization of blame for failures of the self and projection, devaluation, and denigration pose particular therapeutic challenges, as they are often quite ego syntonic and valued by the patient (Lazarus and Groves 1987). The therapist who focuses on inviting desired behavior rather than only rebuffing what is undesirable enhances group cohesion and the opportunities for the group to feel effective, without damaging members through hostile confrontation. For example, the therapist's efforts at accessing the loneliness that resides beneath manifest hostility may make an off-putting member of the group more approachable and comprehensible to his or her peers.

The relevance of each patient's comments and communications should be noted. The group language and metaphors should be familiar and resonant to the group members and voiced in a culturally acceptable form. At times the therapist has to reframe, integrate, translate, summarize, and underscore, ideally in a fashion that is not excessively gratifying of dependency needs but continues respectfully to insist on patients being accountable for themselves. In those instances when sensory impairment is prominent, the use of audio aids such as FM amplifying systems is an additional consideration, but this will be of little use if the hearing impairment is being used defensively by the patient to maintain his or her isolation and disengagement. When skill acquisition and homework assignments are a prominent aspect of the treatment, enlisting a reliable family member to prompt and support the patient between sessions can be invaluable.

Activity-Centered Groups

Activity-centered groups and verbal groups for cognitively impaired individuals also require substantial therapist activity. To safeguard against the group feeling patronized, structured exercises and activities cannot be prescribed without the therapist's own active and genuine participation. In resocialization and remotivation groups, patient initiative and responsibility enhance the group functions, and such groups are generally experienced as more cohesive than leader-dependent groups in which there is little patient initiation.

Special Problems

A broad range of countertransferential reactions may emerge in the treatment of elderly individuals. Along with the countertransferential issues faced by the individual therapist as a result of his or her exposure within the group, because of group pressures, the group therapist is more vulnerable to a complementary response to the group's depressive demoralization and feelings of futility. "What can a bunch of old, useless people do for one another?" is a common statement of patients in geriatric groups. If the therapist begins to identify with a position of hopelessness, therapeutic perspective is lost. Warning signs include the therapist's own boredom, lateness, or cancellation of meetings, with the rationalization that the group members will not notice the missed meeting (Leszcz 1987). In fact, the opposite appears true. Geriatric groups can be exquisitely sensitive to feeling devalued although their reaction and protest may be more silent and isolative than angry.

Conversely, the therapist may be an idealized object, the recipient of patients' projections of lost successes, health, and competence. The idealization is contained by the therapist more readily if he or she can recognize its transferential, selfobject roots and not feel personally overstimulated (Leszcz et al. 1985). Alternatively, if the idealization fails to strengthen and comfort group members and leaves them feeling bereft of any of their own power or efficacy, it must be actively confronted.

Resistances to intimacy and, frequently, inexperience in verbalization may slow the group work and make it more arduous than group work with younger patients. The therapist may feel devalued in identification with patients who devalue themselves. Consultation, supervision, and cotherapy serve to diminish these potential countertransferential difficulties by diluting their intensity and providing an opportunity for their recognition and exploration. The burden of activating the group and engaging resistant patients is decreased by sharing the responsibility between coleaders. Mixed-sex cotherapy teams may also evoke greater wishes for engagement among the group members (Linden 1953). In addition, cotherapy ensures that the group meets regularly, despite therapists' vacations or illness, and thereby reduces threats to the group's integrity.

In institutional settings it is useful if at least one of the coleaders is a regular team member of the ward or floor staff, to facilitate exchange of information and treatment planning. The group program should be experienced as an integrated and integral part of the overall treatment. Without administrative and institutional support, logistical obstacles to attendance emerge. Furthermore, both depth and nondepth approaches must be valued; otherwise, interdisciplinary rivalries produce subtle devaluation of various parts of the group treatment that can be detected by patients and lead to reluctance on their part to participate.

The general psychology of the milieu exerts significant influence on the actual group treatments (Astrachan et al. 1968). The therapy group may function as a psychological "biopsy" of the larger milieu, allowing exploration of the status of the larger milieu by exploring the smaller group process (Levine 1980). Group therapy both influences and is influenced by its setting, and generally staff morale is enhanced on wards where there is an opportunity for active psychological treatment (Reichenfeld et al. 1973).

An additional challenge in group therapy with elderly individuals is the presence of physical illness, notwithstanding the fact that real deficits may become the focus of specific skill acquisition, problem solving, and cognitive interventions. Physical impairment requires some adaptations of techniques in recognition of limitations placed on certain behavioral interventions by an individual's physical impairment (Gallagher 1981). Physical impairment interferes logistically with attendance and participation in the group and may result in group attrition. Steuer and Hammen (1983) similarly commented on the slower pace of cognitive approaches with elderly patients and their tendency to be more concrete and less abstract than younger patients.

The interplay among real and excess disability, true restriction, and treatment resistance is complex and requires diligence and patience in sorting out. The group is vulnerable to demoralization evoked by physical illness and impairment, but if contained effectively, the presence of real illness and real physical threats provides an opportunity for group members to address issues of quality of life and concerns about death.

Outcome of Group Therapy

Small sample size, brief time frames, study of nonpatient populations, lack of consensus on outcome measures, patients receiving more than one form of treatment at a time, and ethical difficulties in maintaining a nontreatment control group hamper evaluation of the outcome of group treatments

(Parham et al. 1982; Steuer et al. 1984). Many reports are anecdotal and clinical. Nonetheless, there is sufficient outcome research to point with optimism to a number of conclusions about the usefulness, efficacy, and practical considerations of group therapies with elderly individuals.

A meta-analysis of psychosocial interventions in geriatric depression concluded that treatment produces a significant effect size of 0.78 in contrast to a placebo or a no-treatment comparison (Scogin and McElreath, 1994). Group therapy and individual therapy are essentially equally effective, with no clearly demonstrable superiority of any particular modality or model. The overall effect size of 0.78 compares favorably with the often-cited effect size of 0.85 that is noted in the initial work of Smith et al. (1980) in their meta-analysis of 475 psychotherapy studies.

Cognitively Intact Patients

Although group psychotherapy is significantly superior to no treatment (Tross and Blum 1988), group therapy alone is probably less effective than psychopharmacotherapy in the treatment of depression (Gorey and Cryns 1991; Steuer and Hammen 1983). However, it can play a strong adjunctive role, and in some instances psychotherapy may be the only treatment patients can tolerate medically. The strongest and most methodologically sound efficacy data for group therapy of geriatric major depression are based on cognitive-behavioral approaches. However, there is also evidence that other coherent and rational models of group therapy, including the psychodynamic approaches, are significantly effective in reducing symptoms of depression, improving interpersonal and social functioning, and bolstering self-esteem (Beutler et al. 1987; Gallagher 1981; Steuer et al. 1984; Sweet et al. 1989; Thompson et al. 1991).

Structured reminiscing group therapy is significantly superior to unstructured group therapy in the treatment of elderly inpatients with depression, in terms of effectiveness, patient participation, and subjective valuation, and potential exists for patient deterioration in unstructured and undirected group treatments (Bachar et al. 1991). The effectiveness of reminiscence approaches, such as a structured autobiographical group, is reflected in significant improvements in measures of self-acceptance and feelings of validation of one's efforts in one's life (Botella and Feixas 1992–1993). In general, improvements in psychological well-being correlate significantly with both the amount of each individual's interpersonal engagement and interaction within the group (Rattenbury and Stones 1989), and the experience of interpersonal effectiveness and competence within the group (Moran and Gatz 1987). Group therapy decreases anxiety and enhances group members' ability to deal with emotions verbally and to use the present more than the past to sustain self-esteem (Lieberman and Gaurash 1979). There is evidence to suggest that specific behavioral and cognitive skill acquisition is directly linked to significantly improved outcome at follow-up 1 year after treatment cessation (Gallagher and Thompson 1982). Group cognitive therapy appears to be a modality that will draw much attention in the future because of its significant effectiveness and its manualization that lends itself to more widespread and reliable clinical application (Yost et al. 1986).

Some interesting questions regarding specific treatment benefits are also raised in the role of group therapy for the spousally bereaved. Participants are generally consistent in their report of high satisfaction and positive valuation of the group experience, both for peer- and leader-led groups, in particular regarding the provision of social and emotional support (Lieberman and Yalom 1992; Lund and Caserta 1992). However, Lieberman and Yalom (1992), in a methodologically sound study, concluded that in their sample of mid- and late-life bereaved spouses treated with brief group therapy, there were no significant treatment benefits at 1 year follow-up. Regardless of the degree of initial distress, all bereaved individuals improved, leaving open for further scrutiny the role of psychological interventions in spousal bereavement. Perhaps answers to this and related questions reside in the need to determine what is an effective dosage of psychotherapeutic intervention in terms of duration and intensity, along with improved assessment of who requires treatment and of treatment matching (Lund and Caserta 1992).

Tentative outcome research on groups for burdened caregivers indicates that participants in these groups value the groups highly, but the complexities of measurement of subjective and objective burden and the common situation of the progressive functional deterioration of the care receiver may translate into a lack of measurably significant intervention impact on measures of burden (Kosberg et al. 1990; Toseland et al. 1989). The burden of caregiving appears to be substantially greater in the care of cognitively impaired elderly family members, than in the care of cognitively intact, physically unwell elderly persons (Zarit and Toseland 1989). Much of the assistance offered to burdened caregivers is provided in time-limited groups meeting for 6 to 12 weekly sessions. However, longer term maintenance treatment—for example, once monthly for an additional 10 months—may sustain and broaden treatment effects, significantly reducing the subjective experience of burden and even improving the caregiver's evaluation of the ill relative's health status (Labrecque et al. 1992).

Significant and durable treatment benefits reported include improved feelings of mastery, self-directedness, and problem-solving ability; increased ability to consider appropriate alternatives to care for their family member; relationship improvement with the care receiver; increased capacity to grieve; and, quite importantly, an increased capacity to care for themselves (Kahan et al. 1985; Lazarus et al. 1981; Perkins and Poynton 1990; Toseland et al. 1989). Both professionally led and peer-led groups show significant effects, although the former emphasizes provision of information and problem solving, whereas the latter emphasizes peer support and social networking (Toseland et al. 1990). Although most participants value very highly the group and peer support, some severely distressed caregivers may require individual assistance (Toseland et al. 1989). Meta-analysis of controlled interventions for distressed caregivers documents that group interventions in general have only a small but positive effect on caregiver burden and dysphoria (Knight et al. 1993), notwithstanding the participants' subjectively high valuation of all groups.

Successful outcome in geriatric group therapy is linked to sufficient tenure in treatment; therefore, therapeutic strategies to facilitate treatment maintenance, as described earlier are essential. Although severe physical illness and chronicity of depression are negatively correlated with successful outcome (Gallagher 1981; Parham et al. 1982; Steuer et al. 1984), it is also evident that elderly persons with both depression and a disabling illness can in fact benefit significantly from active treatment, as reflected in improved mood scores and functional ability (Kemp et al. 1992). However, unlike physically well elderly depression patients, who may demonstrate even further gains in longer term follow-up, elderly physically disabled depression patients plateaued or failed to retain their gains. Further and ongoing physical difficulties likely are one mediator of this result, and ongoing or maintenance treatment appears to be indicated. In addition, physical disabilities, if not adequately encompassed psychotherapeutically, may interfere with or obstruct in-group participation and practice of between-meeting homework assignments (Brand and Clingempeel 1992).

Cognitively Impaired Patients

Evaluation of outcome effectiveness of group approaches with cognitively impaired elderly persons is hampered by a lack of consistency in measures utilized to determine improvements in cognition, behavior, and orientation.

In addition, in many instances the underlying dementing disorder is progressive. Hence evaluation of outcome must compare well-matched controlled and treated subjects over time. The literature demonstrates a broad range of creative approaches that blend elements of structured reality orientation, resocialization, and structured reminiscence therapy. Greater precision and description of the models employed will facilitate generalizability and better testing of the efficacy of particular models.

Early outcome studies (Linden 1953) based on populations of institutionalized, chronic, psychogeriatric patients treated in remotivation and resocialization groups documented improved discharge rates, hygiene and grooming, socialization, and participation in hospital activities. Reichenfeld et al. (1973) also documented statistically significant increases in hospital discharge rates and reductions in behavioral deterioration, although those who were physically more ill or more cognitively impaired at the outset improved less. Although improvements in verbal orientation and socially appropriate behavior may be produced by group interventions (Bower 1967), gains in orientation are rapidly extinguished without ongoing staff and family reinforcement (Gerber et al. 1991). It also appears that improvement is the result of behavioral reinforcement and not genuine changes in cognition (Gerber et al. 1991). However, some behavioral improvement may endure beyond the active treatment phase and may be readily reactivated by treatment resumption, as evidenced by one of the few controlled studies in this area (Baines et al. 1987). Prior reality orientation therapy has a significantly positive priming effect on subsequent utilization of reminiscence therapy (Baines et al. 1987). Structured reminiscence group therapy has produced significant, albeit short-lived, improvements in patient mood and depression scores (Goldwasser et al. 1982). Preliminary reports of significant improvement in cognitive functioning effected by focused visual imagery group therapy and cognitive therapy warrant further study and replication (Abraham et al. 1992).

It remains unclear how much of the improvements effected are linked not only to the specifics of reality orientation techniques, but also to the social engagement and behavioral reinforcement of more adaptive social functioning. Indeed, the active ingredients of treatment beyond social stimulation and interaction remain unclear (Baines et al. 1987). Exposure to reality orientation techniques is insufficient without actual interaction, encouragement, and consistent reinforcement by the staff. Staff's enthusiasm, realistic hopefulness, and behaviorally consistent responses are essential ingredients of effective treatment (Katz 1976). It is therefore particularly noteworthy that one less equivocal result in this area of study appears to be the fact that staff involved in these more active interventions appear to value highly the opportunity for more active treatment and the enhanced opportunity to know their patients in a more personal way. Staff's improved morale and involvement with their patients may be an important mediator of therapeutic impact (Baines et al. 1987).

References

Abraham IL, Neundorfer MM, Currie LJ: Effects of group interventions on cognition and depression in nursing home residents. Nursing Research 41:196–202, 1992

Astrachan BM, Harrow M, Flynn HR: Influence of the value system of a psychiatric setting on behavior in group therapy meetings. Soc Psychiatr 3:165–172, 1968

Bachar E, Kindler S, Schoflar G, et al: Reminiscing as a technique in the group psychotherapy of depression: a comparative study. Br J Clin Psychol 30:375–377, 1991

Baines S, Saxby P, Ehlert K: Reality orientation and reminiscence therapy. Br J Psychiatry 151:222–231, 1987

Baldwin BA, Kleeman KM, Stevens GL, et al: Family caregiver stress: clinical assessment and management. Int Psychogeriatr 1:185–193, 1989

Beutler L, Scogin F, Kirkish P, et al: Group cognitive therapy and alprazolam in the treatment of depression in older adults. J Consult Clin Psychol 55:550–556, 1987

Botella L, Feixas G: The autobiographical group: a tool for the reconstruction of past life experience with the aged. Int J Aging Hum Dev 36:303–319, 1992–1993

Brand E, Clingempeel WG: Group behavioral therapy with depressed geriatric inpatients: an assessment of incremental efficacy. Behav Ther 23:475–482, 1992

Bower HM: Sensory stimulation and the treatment of senile dementia. Med J Aust 22:1113–1119, 1967

Burnside IM: Working With the Elderly: Group Process and Techniques. North Scituate, MA, Duxbury Press, 1978

Burnside IM: Reminiscence: an independent nursing intervention for the elderly. Issues Ment Health Nurs 11:33–48, 1991

Butler R: Successful aging and the role of the life review. J Am Geriatr Soc 22:529–535, 1974

Drummond L, Kirschhoff L, Scarbrough DR: A practical guide to reality orientation: a treatment approach for confusion and disorientation. Gerontologist 18:568–573, 1978

Gallagher DE: Behavioral group therapy with elderly depressives: an experimental study, in Behavioral Group Therapy. Edited by Upper D, Ross SM. Champaign, IL, Research Press, 1981, pp 187–224

Gallagher DE, Thompson LW: Treatment of major depressive disorder in older adult outpatients with brief psychotherapies. Psychotherapy: Theory, Research, and Practice 19:482–490, 1982

Gerber GJ, Prince PN, Snider MC, et al: Group activity and cognitive improvement among patients with Alzheimer's disease. Hosp Community Psychiatry 42:843–845, 1991

Goldwasser AN, Averbach SM, Harkins SW: Cognitive, affective and behavioral effects of reminiscence group therapy on demented elderly. Int J Aging Hum Dev 25:209–222, 1982

Gorey KM, Cryns AG: Group work as interventive modality with the older depressed client: a meta-analytic review. Journal of Gerontological Social Work 16:137–157, 1991

Grant I, Patterson TL, Yager JC: Social supports in relation to physical health and symptoms of depression in the elderly. Am J Psychiatry 145:1254–1258, 1988

Henderson JN, Gutierrez-Mayka M, Garcia J, et al: A model for Alzheimer's disease support group development in African-American and Hispanic populations. Gerontologist 33:409–414, 1993

Kahan J, Kemp B, Staples RF, et al: Decreasing the burden in families caring for a relative with a dementing illness: a controlled study. J Am Geriatr Soc 33:664–670, 1985

Katz MM: Behavioral change in the chronicity pattern of dementia in the institutional geriatric resident. J Am Geriatr Soc 11:522–528, 1976

Kavanagh B, Burnside J: Reminiscing and life review: conducting the processes. J Gerontol Nurs 18:37–42, 1992

Kemp BJ, Corgiat M, Gill C: Effects of brief cognitive-behavioral group psychotherapy on older persons with or without disabling illness. Behavior, Health and Aging 2:21–28, 1991–1992

Knight BG, Lutzky SM, Macofsky-Urban F: A meta-analytic review of interventions for caregiven distress: recommendations for future research. Gerontologist 33:240–243, 1993

Kohut H: How Does Analysis Cure? Chicago, IL, University of Chicago Press, 1984

Kosberg JI, Cairl RE, Keller DM: Components of burden: intervention implications. Gerontologist 30:236–242, 1990

Labrecque MS, Peak T, Toseland RW: Long-term effectiveness of a group program for caregivers of frail elderly veterans. Am J Orthopsychiatry 62:575–588, 1992

Lazarus LW: Self-psychology and psychotherapy with the elderly: theory and practice. J Geriatr Psychiatry 13:69–88, 1980

Lazarus LW, Groves L: Brief psychotherapy with the elderly: a study of process and outcome, in Treating the Elderly With Psychotherapy: The Scope for Change in Later Life. Edited by Sadavoy J, Leszcz M. Madison, CT, International Universities Press, 1987, pp 265–294

Lazarus LW, Stafford B, Cooper K, et al: A pilot study of an Alzheimer patients' relatives discussion group. Gerontologist 21:353–358, 1981

Lesser J, Frankel R, Havasy S: Reminiscence group therapy with psychotic geriatric inpatients. Gerontologist 21:291–296, 1981

Leszcz M: Group psychotherapy with the elderly, in Treating the Elderly With Psychotherapy: The Scope for Change in Later Life. Edited by Sadavoy J, Leszcz M. Madison, CT, International Universities Press, 1987, pp 325–349

Leszcz M: The interpersonal approach to group psychotherapy. Int J Group Psychother 42:37–62, 1992

Leszcz M, Feigenbaum E, Sadavoy J, et al: A men's group: psychotherapy of elderly men. Int J Group Psychother 35:177–196, 1985

Levine HB: Milieu biopsy: the place of the therapy group on the inpatient ward. Int J Group Psychother 30:77–93, 1980

Lieberman MA, Gaurash N: Evaluating the effects of group changes on the elderly. Int J Group Psychother 29:283–304, 1979

Lieberman MA, Yalom ID: Brief group psychotherapy for the spousally bereaved: a controlled study. Int J Group Psychother 42:117–132, 1992

Linden M: Group psychotherapy with institutionalized senile women: study in gerontologic human relations. Int J Group Psychother 3:150–170, 1953

Lothstein LM, Zimet G: Twinship and alter ego selfobject transferences in group therapy with the elderly: a reanalysis of the pairing phenomenon. Int J Group Psychother 38:303–317, 1988

Lowenthal RI, Marrazzo RA: Milestoning, evoking memories for resocialization through group reminiscence. Gerontologist 30:269–272, 1990

Lund DA, Caserta MS: Older bereaved spouses' participation in self-help groups. Omega 25:47–61, 1992

MacLennan BW, Saul S, Bakur Weiner M: Group Psychotherapies for the Elderly (American Group Psychotherapy Association Monograph

No 5). Madison, CT, International Universities Press, 1988

Miller E: The management of dementia: a review of some possibilities. Br J Soc Clin Psychol 16:77–83, 1977

Moran JA, Gatz M: Group therapies for nursing home adults: an evaluation of two treatment approaches. Gerontologist 27:588–591, 1987

Murphy E: The prognosis of depression in old age. Br J Psychiatry 142:111–117, 1983

Parham JA, Priddy MJ, McGovern TU, et al: Group psychotherapy with the elderly: problems and prospects. Psychotherapy: Theory, Research, and Practice 19:437–447, 1982

Perkins RE, Poynton CF: Group counselling for relatives of hospitalized presenile dementia patients: a controlled study. Br J Clin Psychol 29:287–295, 1990

Pollock GH: The mourning-liberation process: ideas in the inner life of the older adult, in Treating the Elderly With Psychotherapy: The Scope for Change in Later Life. Edited by Sadavoy J, Leszcz M. Madison, CT, International Universities Press, 1987, pp 3–30

Poulton JL, Strassberg DS: The therapeutic use of reminiscence. Int J Group Psychother 36:381–398, 1986

Rattenbury C, Stones MJ: A controlled evaluation of reminiscence and current topics discussion groups in a nursing home context. Gerontologist 29:768–771, 1989

Reichenfeld HF, Csapo KG, Carriere L, et al: Evaluating the effect of activity programs on a geriatric ward. Gerontologist 13:305–310, 1973

Rush AJ: Cognitive therapy of depression. Psychiatr Clin North Am 6(1):105–127, 1983

Safran JO, Segal ZV: Interpersonal Processes in Cognitive Therapy. New York, Basic Books, 1990

Salvendy JT: Brief group psychotherapy at retirement. Group 13:43–52, 1989

Salvendy JT: Selection and preparations of patients and organizations of the group, in Comprehensive Group Therapy, 3rd Edition. Edited by Kaplan HI, Sadock BJ. Baltimore, MD, Williams & Wilkins, 1993, pp 72–84

Samberg S: Dance therapy groups for the elderly, in Group Psychotherapies for the Elderly (American Group Psychotherapy Association Monograph No 5). Edited by MacLennan BW, Saul S, Bakur Weiner M. Madison, CT, International Universities Press, 1988, pp 233–244

Saul SR: Group therapy with confused and disoriented people, in Group Psychotherapies for the Elderly (American Group Psychotherapy

Association Monograph No 5). Edited by MacLennan BW, Saul S, Bakur Weiner M. Madison, CT, International Universities Press, 1988, pp 199–208

Schmid AH, Rouslin M: Integrative outpatient group therapy for discharged elderly psychiatric inpatients. Gerontologist 32:558–560, 1992

Schwartzman G: The use of the group as selfobject. Int J Group Psychother 34:229–242, 1984

Scogin F, McElreath L: Efficacy of psychosocial treatments for geriatric depression: a quantitative review. J Consult Clin Psychol 62(1):69–74, 1994

Smith ML, Glass GV, Miller TI: Benefits of Psychotherapy. Baltimore, MD, Johns Hopkins University Press, 1980

Steinmetz-Breckenridge J, Thompson LW, Breckenridge JN, et al: Behavioral group therapy with the elderly, in Handbook of Behavioral Group Therapy. Edited by Upper D, Rose S. New York, Plenum, 1985, pp 275–302

Steuer JL, Hammen CL: Cognitive-behavioral group therapy for the depressed elderly: issues and adaptations. Cognitive Ther Res 7:285–296, 1983

Steuer JL, Mintz J, Hammen CL, et al: Cognitive-behavioral and psychodynamic group psychotherapy in treatment of geriatric depression. J Consult Clin Psychol 52:80–89, 1984

Stone WN, Whitman RM: Contributions of the psychology of self to group process and group therapy. Int J Group Psychother 27:343–359, 1977

Sweet M, Stoler N, Kelter R, et al: A community of builders: support groups for veterans forced into early retirement. Hosp Community Psychiatry 40:172–176, 1989

Teri L, Gallagher-Thompson D: Cognitive-behavioral interventions for treatment of depression in Alzheimer's patients. Gerontologist 31:413–416, 1991

Thompson LW, Gantz F, Florsheim M, et al: Cognitive-behavioral therapy in affective disorders in the elderly, in New Techniques in the Psychotherapy of Older Patients. Edited by Myers WA. Washington, DC, American Psychiatric Press, 1991, pp 3–19

Toseland RW, Rossiter CM, Labrecque M: The effectiveness of three group intervention strategies to support family caregivers. Am J Orthopsychiatry 59:420–429, 1989

Toseland RW, Rossiter CM, Peak T, et al: Therapeutic process in peer led and professionally led support groups for caregivers. Int J Group Psychotherapy 40(3):279–303, 1990

Tross S, Blum JE: A review of group therapy with the older adult: practice and research, in Group Psychotherapies for the Elderly (American Group Psychotherapy Association Monograph No 5). Edited by MacLennan BW, Saul S, Bakur Weiner M. Madison, CT, International Universities Press, 1988, pp 3–29

Wachtel PL: From eclecticism to synthesis: toward a more seamless psychotherapeutic integration. Journal of Psychotherapy Integration 1:43–54, 1991

Williams-Barnard CL, Lindell AR: Therapeutic use of "prizing" and its effect on self-concept of elderly clients in nursing homes and group homes. Issues Ment Health Nurs 13:1–17, 1992

Wong P: Social support functions of group reminiscence. Can J Commun Ment Health 10:151–161, 1991

Yalom ID: The Theory and Practice of Group Psychotherapy, 4th Edition. New York, Basic Books, 1995

Yalom ID, Terrazas F: Group therapy for psychotic elderly patients. Am J Nurs 68:1690–1694, 1967

Yost EB, Beutler LE, Corbishley MA, et al: Group Cognitive Therapy: A Treatment Approach for Depressed Older Adults. Oxford, England, Pergamon, 1986

Zarit SH, Reever KE, Bach-Peterson J: Relatives of the impaired elderly: correlates of feelings of burden. Gerontology 6:649–655, 1980

Zarit SH, Anthony CR, Boutselis M: Interventions with caregivers of dementia patients: comparison of two approaches. Psychol Aging 2:225–232, 1982

Zarit SM, Toseland RW: Current and future direction in family caregiving research. Gerontologist 29(4):481–483, 1989

Marion Zucker Goldstein, M.D.

Families of Older Adults

A s early as 1966, Brody suggested that the entire family, rather than the aged individual alone, should be considered the patient when an elderly person is brought for professional help (Brody 1966). In the practice of geriatric psychiatry, it has become quite apparent that above all else families would like to be better informed about the aging process, the psychopathology of late life, and the resources available to guide and help them in attending to the physical and mental health of themselves and their older relative. They would like access to comprehensive care by well-trained professionals who address the biopsychosocial vicissitudes of aging of body and mind within the family context. The desire of many families is to add years to life and quality of life to those years. Like parenting of children earlier in life, attentiveness to and knowledge of the issues of late life must be acquired and progressive learning through various stages and phases must take place. The one-on-one, dyadic model of assessment and intervention associated with a traditional medical model remains appropriate only in selected instances of professional care for the older adult and is rarely adequate as the only modality for the care of the frail elderly individual who can no longer function independently. The formal and informal networks of caregiving of older adults require an intensity of liaison work similar to that used between professional providers of care to improve effectiveness and compliance with the interventions recommended. Work with families can take place in the different settings where elderly individuals reside and require medical assessment and interventions. These settings include, for example, primary care practice, outpatient clinics, general hospital consultation-liaison services, psychiatric inpatient units, respite care, day hospitals, home health care, and long-term care facilities.

In this chapter, issues of family caregiving as well as those of elder abuse, neglect, and exploitation will be addressed. The incidence and prevalence of exploitation is rising, and physicians in general, and geriatric psychiatrists in particular, can be in the forefront of prevention, identification, intervention, and rehabilitation, as well as research and teaching.

In practice, psychoeducation of families of elderly individuals is carried out with greater frequency than family therapy based on prevailing theories of family systems, developmental theories, or intergenerational approaches to diminish stress and enhance coping styles. Various modalities of intervention will be addressed in this chapter, as will the benefits and limitations of family participation in mutual support groups.

A variety of professional efforts to involve the family of an elderly patient, be it to get collateral information; to educate the family about the patient's condition, prognosis, or interventions recommended; to assess the stresses experienced by various family members; or to involve the family in therapy are reimbursable by Medicare. Preservation of reimbursement of such professional services is vital to maintaining quality of care. Many current Medicare recipients are invited to sign up for managed care insurance. Before they agree to sign up, it is important that Medicare recipients and their families be well educated and informed of the conditions for their care.

Current Financial Realities of Practice: Families of Medicare Beneficiaries

A reimbursable code for seeing a patient's family with or without the patient is supplied by Medicare, although regional negotiations are needed at times to actually ensure that reimbursement is not denied, in spite of federal mandate. Medicare Current Procedural Terminology (CPT) code reimbursements are determined according to the Resource-Based Relative Value Scale by the Health Care Finance Administration and vary with the parameters listed in Table 30–1.

Although initial visits for patients can be billed for up to 70 minutes, follow-up time for charting, liaison activities, attention to physical comorbidities, and attention to legal issues is considerably more limited,

Table 30–1. Medicare CPT code reimbursement variables

Region
Site of service
Complexity
Length of time of service

although these issues add to the complexity and time required for service. These issues frequently involve active family participation and should be billed and reimbursed accordingly. A regional example of codes for services with families is presented in Table 30–2.

Administrators of a nursing home or rest home who are aware of the well-researched, high prevalence of psychiatric disorders in their residents and the severe stress most families experience when a relative resides in a nursing home, have several options for arranging for reimbursement for psychiatric consultation-liaison and family involvement. One option is a contractual arrangement with the consulting geriatric psychiatrist based on an hourly rate, with preplanned consultation and staff liaison time as well as availability to families. The billing office of the institution can assume responsibility for fee-for-service reimbursements to the institution. The liaison function with medical staff, nurses, social workers, and administration is essential for a consultation to be effective. With a contractual arrangement for a geriatric psychiatrist's time, consultation is not subject to the limitations of a coding system for the consultant. Managed care systems, which are entering the nursing home industry, are in need of professional ethical guidelines to keep economic motives from overriding the quality of services rendered, including the quality of liaison functions.

The family caregiver of elderly individuals who has become overstressed and depressed and seeks psychiatric help is beholden to his or her own insurance, be it a health maintenance organization (HMO) or other managed care insurance, to allow reimbursement of psychiatric intervention. Overstressed family members of elderly individuals who are insured

Table 30–2. Regional example of code and Medicare reimbursements for family participation

CPT E/M Code	Type of Rx	Reimbursement
90846	Family with patient	$86.61
90847	Family without patient	77.14
90887	Consultation with family	59.77

Source. New York State Psychiatric Association, Inc., Medicare Part B, 1992, for the WNY region.

by an HMO may require referral by primary care physicians who may not have been trained in assessing the need for a psychiatric referral of this nature. In such a situation, a self-referral for psychiatric care may lead to lack of insurance.

Developmentally and/or emotionally disabled children, including those engaged in substance abuse who have been taken care of by their parents throughout adulthood, become overstressed when their parents can no longer care for them and require care themselves. Abusive situations are not an infrequent occurrence when these adult children are unable to cope with role reversal. These situations require special expertise and awareness by formal providers of services. To date, DSM-IV codes are not yet available, nor have CPT Evaluation Management codes been developed for reimbursement of psychiatric diagnosis and interventions of elder abuse, neglect, or exploitation. These are very complex and professionally time-consuming situations that require extensive expertise and attention. So far, Medicare reimburses only 2.7 days of in-hospital care for *physical* harm done. This adult maltreatment syndrome has a diagnosis-related group (DRG) code and an *International Classification of Diseases* (World Health Organization 1991) code, but codes for the complexity and time needed to assess and treat abused individuals and perpetrators' mental conditions have yet to be developed.

Researchers have found that the family is the most important social group for older people, and in general, families do not abandon their elder members (Comptroller General of the United States 1977; Doty 1986; Horowitz 1985a; Shanas 1979a, 1979b; Stone et al. 1987). Family contacts remain especially frequent in the early and later parts of the life cycle. Powerful feelings and attitudes prevail, especially in times of crisis, and resurgence of past unresolved conflicts can occur. Unfinished developmental tasks from early life affect behaviors and family interactions in later life.

Family therapy can facilitate development to a level of filial maturity that will enhance appropriate role definition and more comfortable adaptation to midlife developmental stages as these relate to the care of aging parents (Fischer 1985; Goldstein 1989). A geriatric psychiatrist or general psychiatrist schooled in geriatric psychiatry can contribute substantially to increased motivation to attain filial maturity in those adult children who have not as yet reached this developmental phase. Participation and acceptance of the process of redefinition of roles in families with aging spouses, parents, grandparents, and/or great-grandparents can contribute to survival of the family unit, regardless of geographic proximity or distance. Identification of various levels of dependence and autonomy in elderly individuals, along with sharing of different family members' perceptions, can lead to emotional growth and conflict resolution when addressed alongside evaluation and assessment of the older adult.

To date, CPT codes and their reimbursement levels are inadequately connected with the mental health needs of elderly individuals and their families. In addition to the previously detailed inequities, psychiatric participation in court hearings 1) for judicial permission to treat a patient with neuroleptic medications over that patient's objection, 2) for competency, or 3) for guardianship, along with the concomitant added stress for patients and family members, the additional professional expertise required, and the time consumed, have not yet been addressed in reimbursement coding. A CPT E/M code for multifamily groups is currently being developed. Other efforts for changes are under way, especially an across-the-board 20% copayment for all medical services rendered regardless of site, the diagnosis of the patient, and the physician's specialty (or lack thereof). Such parity will no longer penalize the patient for having a psychiatric disorder or the psychiatrist for treating the patient and family. The current 50% copayment for psychiatric outpatient and most nursing home visits is a serious deterrent to access to mental health services. Managed care insurers have devised other limitations to the care of chronically mentally ill patients.

Family Demographics

Increased longevity has had major effects on family relationships. In addition to physical and mental health, age; gender; and sibling, marital, and parental status have considerable bearing on the role of the older adult in the family setting. Increased longevity with changing societal attitudes and family values have been the subject of research during recent decades (Brubaker 1990).

It is of importance to note that 73%–93% of persons ages 65 years or older have at least one living brother or sister (Brubaker 1983). Vaillant and Vaillant (1990) have shown the importance of sibling ties with advancing age. For the 4%–6% of elderly individuals who never married, it is often a niece or nephew who assists in dealing with the bureaucracy of support systems on behalf of a frail elderly relative (Brubaker 1983).

Marital status varies considerably by age and gender. Table 30–3 highlights the increasing percentage of widowed women with increasing longevity (U.S. Bureau of the Census 1992).

The number of unmarried (divorced, widowed, or never married) men ages 65 and older per 100 unmarried women ages 65 and older has ranged from 25 to 30 since the 1970s (U.S. Bureau of the Census 1992).

Table 30–3. Marital status of persons ages 65 years and older by age, sex, and race (in thousands, noninstitional population)

Age and	All races (N = 30,590)				White (n = 27,297)	
	Male		Female		Male	
marital status	No.	%	No.	%	No.	%
Ages 65–74						
Married, spouse present	6,372	77.1	5,234	51.4	5,808	79.3
Married, spouse absent	164	2.0	161	1.6	97	1.3
Widowed	841	10.2	3,648	35.9	680	9.3
Divorced	506	6.1	681	6.7	424	5.8
Never married	383	4.6	451	4.4	314	4.3
Ages 75–84						
Married, spouse present	2,683	71.6	1,693	28.6	2,494	73.2
Married, spouse absent	83	2.2	75	1.3	60	1.8
Widowed	747	19.9	3,576	60.5	634	18.6
Divorced	99	2.6	255	4.3	92	2.7
Never married	136	3.6	311	5.3	127	3.7
Ages 85 years and older						
Married, spouse present	393	50.1	162	9.5	362	51.6
Married, spouse absent	21	2.7	17	1.0	18	2.6
Widowed	329	41.9	1,377	80.8	282	40.2
Divorced	19	2.4	46	2.7	18	2.6
Never married	23	2.9	102	6.0	21	3.0

Note. — = zero or rounds to zero; (B) = the base for the derived figure is less than 75,000.
Source. Adapted from U.S. Bureau of Census (1992).

Whereas 19% of women ages 65 to 74 and about 33% of women ages 75 and older lived alone in 1992, only 6% of men between the ages of 65 and 74 and 8% of men ages 75 and older lived alone. Widowed women are the group of elderly who require the most care and have a great need for companionship, both of which are most frequently provided by daughters and daughters-in-law (Troll 1986). In the 1970s, one in five first marriages reached the 50th anniversary, with couples staying together regardless of the nature of the relationship (Ade-Ridder 1983; 1989). Since then, divorce and remarriage have increased considerably not only in younger couples, but among elderly individuals as well (Uhlenberg and Myers 1981). Divorce, remarriage, and the reconstituted family in one or more generations contribute to the complexities of the modern family (Cicirelli 1983a). The social, economic, and psychological experiences of aging are greatly influenced by divorce, especially for

Table 30–3. Marital status of persons ages 65 years and older by age, sex, and race (in thousands, noninstitional population) (*continued*)

| White (*n* = 27,297) | | Black (*n* = 2,607) | | | | Hispanic (*n* = 1,143) | | | |
| Female | | Male | | Female | | Male | | Female | |
No.	%	No.	%	No.	%	No.	%	No.	%
4,818	53.6	425	57.4	297	32.1	237	76.4	191	45.2
102	1.1	44	6.0	52	5.6	11	3.6	22	5.2
3,095	34.4	141	19.0	447	48.3	34	11.0	153	36.3
577	6.4	71	9.6	88	9.5	14	4.4	29	7.0
400	4.4	59	7.9	42	4.6	14	4.6	26	6.3
1,585	29.7	120	49.7	81	17.1	91	71.1	51	24.3
45	.9	15	6.3	29	6.1	7	5.2	6	2.7
3,214	60.2	91	37.6	306	64.4	21	16.6	125	59.2
214	4.0	7	2.9	32	6.8	6	4.7	11	5.1
280	5.3	9	3.6	27	5.7	3	2.3	18	8.7
153	9.9	27	35.1	7	4.4	14	(B)	1	(B)
14	.9	3	3.7	3	2.0	1	(B)	—	(B)
1,242	80.8	45	58.8	119	80.0	12	(B)	36	(B)
45	2.9	—	—	1	1.0	2	(B)	1	(B)
84	5.5	2	2.4	19	12.6	—	(B)	5	(B)

women, who live longer, remarry less frequently, and generally earn less than men (Uhlenberg et al. 1990).

Eighty percent of persons ages 65 and older have surviving children (Cicirelli 1983b). When the 76 million "baby boomers" born between 1946 and 1964 become "senior boomers" in 2010 to 2028, this scenario will have changed considerably. The number of children in a family is declining, and this trend is expected to continue. Whereas in the 1930s 50% of women had four or more children, in the 1980s only 25% of women had four or more children (Brubaker 1983). Twenty percent of babyboomers have no children, and 25% have only one child. The network of family caregivers will decline over the next decades, with decreases in numbers as well as availability.

Ten percent of persons ages 65 and older have living parents. With the high risk of disabilities and acute and chronic illness in both of these age groups, the need for extra familial supports is escalated when the old are helping the very old or, at times, visa versa.

Elderly individuals are generally members of multigenerational families. Seventy percent of persons ages 65 and older have grandchildren, and 40 percent have great-grandchildren (Hagsted 1985). Little is known about family solidarity, intimacy, and conflict in and among sets of related generations and distribution of responsibilities for frail and dependent elderly individuals in those families. Clinically, being or becoming a great-grandparent is generally perceived with great pride by elderly individuals who live long enough to experience this family role, which should be noted by the clinician. Considering the relatively high frequency of losses in the more advanced years of life, the gains and joys should not be overlooked, but given special recognition.

Living arrangements of elderly individuals influence their relationships with family markedly. Living arrangements for older adults vary with gender, race, and age, as shown in Table 30–4.

In the 65-and-older population, a far greater proportion of women live alone than men, and men are more likely to live with spouses. This phenomenon occurs in white, black, and Hispanic cultures. More women live with other relatives in the white and Hispanic populations, but in the black population, more men do so for those ages 65–74, and more women do so in the 75-and-older age group.

Data from the 1980s indicated that elderly men are more likely to live with their children than elderly women (40% versus 13.4%) (Brubaker 1983). However, more women than men live with a daughter or son prior to admission to a nursing home. These differences can be partly attributed to the fact that 1) women continue to do their own housekeeping as long as they are capable, and 2) women have greater relative longevity. Whereas 5% of elderly persons ages 65 and older live in institutional settings, 20% of elderly persons ages 80 and older reside in nursing homes or similar institutions. Type of living arrangement prior to admission to nursing home by gender and race is shown in Table 30–5 (National Center for Health Statistics 1985).

Primary care physicians and specialists are invariably involved in some way in these admissions, as many patients come from other health facilities, including general hospitals and other nursing homes, as indicated in Figure 30–1 (National Center for Health Statistics 1985).

Nursing home admissions are generally stressful for patient and family, especially when there is insufficient preplanning—a frequent occurrence when transitions are made from other health facilities. Timely, well-informed psychiatric consultation-liaison for both patient and family in the general hospital and in the nursing home has the potential to prevent harm and improve quality of life. For a poignant vignette by Kennedy that exemplifies this, the reader is referred to the work by the American Psychiatric Association Task Force on Models of Practice in Geriatric Psychiatry (1993). Under the current restrictive regulations that nursing homes must abide by, it is particularly difficult for families to place elderly relatives into a nursing home after a psychiatric hospitalization for reasons other than dementia. Of all admissions from health facilities to nursing homes, those from mental hospitals constitute only 5%, and those from another nursing home account for 61%, as reflected in Figure 30–2.

The determinants for transfers between nursing homes have not yet been researched. Clinical experiences verify the speculation that dissatisfaction of families with a nursing home and/or the inability of a nursing home to deal with resident and family are frequent motivating factors for such relocations. Case scenarios exemplifying stresses of relocation can be found in Goldstein (1995, in press).

Theoretical Models of Family Structure and Development

Because of the complexity of services needed for many elderly patients, optimal interventions are often multidisciplinary and practical in nature without much attention paid to theoretical models, although the latter may be inadvertently applied. When the sharing of power and responsibility among family members is considered at the center of family problems, interventions can bring about a more comfortable equilibrium (Committee on the Family 1970). For that matter, the sharing of power and responsibility between the professional and the family can also bring about a more comfortable equilibrium and greatly enhance the coordination and cooperation between the informal network of caregivers and formal providers of services.

Hesse-Bibers and Williamson (1984) emphasized the evolution of power in families over the course of the life cycle in terms of changing resources. Attention to shifts of resources between spouses and generations and the power shifts this can bring about can be used to improve adaptation and coping styles.

More complex theoretical models have evolved from studies of families with disturbed children, adolescents, or young adults and have been adapted for elderly individuals (Herr and Weakland 1979). Intergenerational conflicts were analyzed by Borszormenyi-Nagy and Spark (1973) in terms of loyalty, entitlement, ledger balance, justice, and legacy for posterity. An application of this model was described by Ginsberg-McEwan (1987).

Table 30–4. Living arrangements of elderly individuals by sex and race (in thousands, noninstitutional population)

Living arrangement and age	All races (N = 30,590)				White (n = 27,297)	
	Male		Female		Male	
	No.	%	No.	%	No.	%
Ages 65 years and older living:						
Alone	2,086	7	7,437	24	1,741	6
With spouse	9,448	31	7,089	23	8,664	32
With other relatives	897	3	2,917	10	723	3
With nonrelatives only	369	1	347	1	303	1
Ages 65–74 years living:	Total n = 18,440				Total n = 16,315	
Alone	1,100	6	3,461	19	867	5
With spouse	6,372	35	5,234	28	5,808	36
With other relatives	516	3	1,321	7	418	3
With nonrelatives only	278	2	158	1	230	1
Ages 75 years and older living:	Total n = 12,149				Total n = 10,983	
Alone	986	8	3,976	33	875	8
With spouse	3,076	25	1,855	15	2,856	26
With other relatives	380	3	1,596	13	305	3
With nonrelatives only	91	1	189	2	72	1

Source. Adapted from U.S. Bureau of Census (1992).

Bowen's well-known theory of re-relating with family members by redefining intergenerational roles has been applied to families with aging members by Quinn and Keller (1981). Bowen's family systems theory is grounded in analytical concepts and egopsychology with outcome goals of growth and development to reach conflict resolution. Hale and Mikita (1990) describe how Bowen's family systems approach can be applied in a consultation-liaison service in a teaching hospital with the availability of a family therapist. Solomon (1973) suggested five stages of family development and postulated that unless each stage is worked through in due time, the remaining stages are burdened by unresolved conflicts from the previous stage. The tasks of the fifth stage, or the stage that most older adults are in, are resolution of losses (economic, social, and physical) and dealing with possible dependence on children. This theoretical framework is useful in that it lends structure to traditional role definitions. However, Solomon's stages omit many complex vicissitudes of life, such as divorce, adult children who remain dependent, commitments to careers, sibling interactions, in-law relationships, grandparenting, family role variations among races, and alternative lifestyles (Brubaker 1985).

Table 30–4. Living arrangements of elderly individuals by sex and race (in thousands, noninstitutional population) (*continued*)

White (n = 27,297)		Black (n = 2,607)				Hispanic (n = 1,143)			
Female		Male		Female		Male		Female	
No.	%	No.	%	No.	%	No.	%	No.	%
6,722	25	312	9	626	19	50	4	169	15
6,556	24	572	29	384	17	342	30	243	21
2,275	8	124	19	514	4	63	6	246	22
313	1	50	2	25	1	11	1	19	2
		Total n = 1,665				Total n = 732			
3,051	19	210	13	357	21	29	4	92	13
4,818	30	425	26	297	18	237	32	191	26
987	6	68	4	251	15	35	5	127	17
136	1	36	2	21	1	9	1	12	2
		Total n = 941				Total n = 412			
3,671	33	102	11	269	29	21	5	77	19
1,738	16	147	16	88	9	105	25	52	13
1,289	12	54	6	256	27	29	7	118	29
177	2	15	2	10	1	2	0	8	2

Jarvik and Small (1988) suggested a six-step, self-observation, commonsense guide to improving relationships with elderly parents. These six steps are 1) monitoring mood, 2) reflecting on the intensity of reactions, 3) planning constructive strategies, 4) reassessing the situation, 5) listening and negotiating, and 6) planning compromise. The psychiatrist can be a facilitator of this process. Setting appropriate limits on a parent in the negotiation process requires a role reversal and level of filial maturity that is difficult to attain for many adult children.

In the absence of research validated outcome studies, one main advantage of the application of theoretical models is that such application involves family members above and beyond simply giving collateral information about the elderly family member. Another major advantage is in teaching programs, where their application can give the trainee a solid frame of reference for future practice, regardless of medical setting, and thus enhance professional development. An integrated focus on family issues, and how these can affect the course of illness of an elderly individual (and vice versa), has the potential to alleviate the frustrations for professionals and families that are often brought about by repetitive crisis interventions

Table 30–5.   Type of living arrangement prior to admission to nursing home by gender and race ($N = 1,306,800$)

Living arrangement	Male (%)	Female (%)	White (%)	Black/Other (%)
Alone	18.3	29.7	27.0	21.0
With spouse	17.0	7.9	10.8	6.1
Spouse and other relatives	3.6	1.1	1.7	
Son/daughter	6.9	16.2	13.7	13.0
Other relatives	9.4	8.1	7.8	15.8
Unrelated persons	2.9	3.2	2.9	6.0
Group quarters		5.0	6.1	5.9
Another health facility or unknown	36.9	27.7	30.2	31.0
Total	100.0	100.0	100.0	100.0

Source.   National Center for Health Statistics (1989).

for temporary symptomatic relief and behavioral manifestations of an elderly family member. The idea that repetitive crisis intervention, which is frequently mandated by reimbursement constraints, is more cost effective than an integrated focus on family issues may well prove to be an illusion, once business management and outcome studies are coordinated.

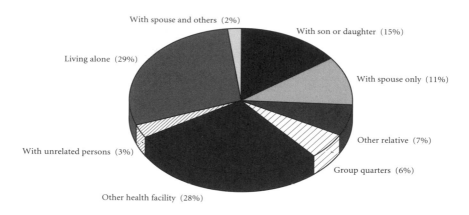

Figure 30–1.   Living arrangements prior to admission to nursing home of residents ages 65 and older living alone or with others ($N = 1,306,800$).
Source.   National Center for Health Statistics (1989).

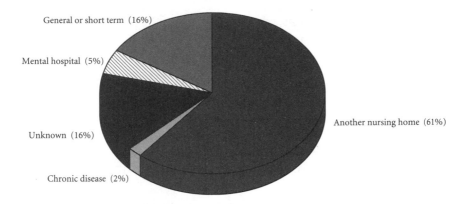

General or short term (16%)

Mental hospital (5%)

Unknown (16%)

Chronic disease (2%)

Another nursing home (61%)

Figure 30–2. Living arrangements prior to admission to nursing home for those living in other health facilities ($N = 358,700$).
Source. National Center for Health Statistics (1989).

A potential disadvantage of application of models of family theory to practice is that this practice can detract from problem assessment and resolution in a problem-focused, financially expedient, and practical manner in situations where positive short-term outcomes can be sustained over time.

Referral to mutual support groups can be very helpful to many families in alleviating the isolation that intense caregiving of a frail elderly relative frequently brings about. However, researchers have found that conflict-ridden topics, such as sexuality, money management, caregiver depletion, the right to die, and adaptation to life after an impaired elderly relative dies, are rarely raised or discussed in depth in mutual support groups (Hepburn and Wasow 1986). Mutual support groups rarely contribute to resolution of family or marital conflicts but can be a valuable adjunct to family and marital therapy (Goldstein 1990).

The frustrations experienced by families caring for an elderly relative with dementia require special attention. The symptoms and behaviors of dementia patients are particularly difficult to tolerate and cope with for most caregivers. Gradual and progressively more incapacitating loss of memory; repetitive verbal outbursts of uncontrolled, sometimes violent, behavior; accusations regarding the caregiver; wandering; incontinence; falling; and other manifestations take their toll on the caregiver. The continuous, unrelenting care and supervision required without sufficient respite leads to loss of other roles in life for the caregiver. Once the diagnosis of an irreversible progressive dementia has been made, the following interventions are recommended during the course of family therapy:

- Sharing of the diagnosis, with reassurance of the physician's commitment to the patient and family
- Systematic review of family myths about dementia, with substitution of a knowledge base about recognition of memory, concentration, attention loss, depression, anxiety, stressors, and expressions of frustration
- Acceptance of the need for repeated reminders and explanations within the context of the illness
- Alleviating guilt about delay of the diagnosis
- Recognition of family contributions to improving the patient's quality of life
- Reassurance of the availability of professional support and supervision of medications prescribed
- Routine inquiries about the caregiver's health, use of drugs and alcohol, or patient abuse
- Providing an opportunity for catharsis and ventilation in a secure, confidential, therapeutic environment
- Recommending formal care services when appropriate and working through resistances to acceptance
- Helping the entire family get together for care plans in which each family member can take a role within their resources and limitations
- Providing assistance through the terminal phases and thereafter (Gwyther and Blazer 1984)

Research has shown that brief family counseling without long-term commitment to either the elderly dementia patient or the family has limited benefit (Zarit et al. 1987). The family must be informed of the heightened vulnerability of elderly dementia patients to depression, delusions, and especially delirium during times of physical illness or medication toxicity.

Assessment of Family Members and Indications for Family Interventions

Indications for family participation in treatment occur often during life transitions, especially during times of mental and/or physical illness of one or more family members. One in every four of the 30 million Medicare beneficiaries enters a hospital at least once annually. With DRGs in all units except psychiatric and rehabilitation units serving as the standard for length of hospital stay, the geriatric patient is frequently sent home from the general hospital after only the acute condition that required the admission has been addressed.

Standards of care for elderly individuals with family must include early and immediate family assessment for need of further intervention and follow-up. Especially for elderly individuals with sensory, ambulatory, speech, or cognitive impairments or those who for other reasons are unable to articulate their needs at the time of relocation, family assessments should not be delayed. It is important that the assessment include the level of care the patient requires, as well as the level of care the family members need. Goals of assessment are many and include the prevention of fragmentation of mental and physical care needed by both patient and family and determining the nature and severity of stress and burden experienced by the caregiver. Although the impact of family dynamics among family members on symptom formation and outcome of illness is not usually considered part of the presenting complaint, results of family assessment should be integrated into an optimal treatment plan for the elderly patient. This approach can alleviate the anger engendered when family members are perceived as intruding in, interfering with, and disrupting the one-on-one, dyadic relationship between the formal provider of care and the elderly patient.

Life transitions that may be indications for family therapy include adult children leaving or not leaving home; excessive work demands or retirement; an ailing spouse or widowhood; relocations; grandparenthood or lack thereof (Kornhaber 1986); and loss of relationships through relocation, illness, disability, and death, with difficulties in finding a confidant and new relationships.

Although "on-time," so-called "normative" incidents are thought not to result in emotional crisis (Neugarten 1977), incidents perceived as normative by individuals, family units, or society vary with family value systems, generational differences, and current social and ethnic trends. Different perceptions and misinterpretations among family members about the level of health, strength, impairment, and weakness of elderly individuals and speculations about the etiology of the condition can contribute to conflict, lead to nonparticipation in care, and result in family criticism of one another and, at times, of the professionals involved. More than 80% of people ages 65 and older have at least one chronic medical problem, and multiple conditions are common (Tauber 1983). The presence of relative disability complicates adaptation to the normal aging processes by the elderly individual as well as by his or her family, although it is a "normative" event. When such issues are not addressed, they fester, become chronic, and hinder adequacy of care and equitable distribution of care among family members.

Research has shown that changes in the mental health status of an elderly family member tend to be more bewildering and anxiety provoking to others in the family than physical impairments that cause loss of independence and autonomy (Deimling and Bass 1986; Grad and Sainsbury 1966). Decline in the ability to perform physical activities of daily living (e.g., bathing, feeding, dressing, toileting) or instrumental activities of daily living (e.g., laundry and household chores, managing money, traveling, shopping) (Duke University 1978) requires not only modification of the lifestyle of other family members, but also access and acceptance of community resources.

Changes in the condition of an elderly family member that provoke symptomatic resentment, anger or violence, apprehension, fear, anxiety, distrust, worry, guilt, depression, ambivalence, or martyrdom in other family members is an indication for assessment for family therapy (M. D. Miller 1989).

Sibling rivalry (Ross and Milgram 1982) and unresolved resentments about past experiences can increase at the time when a parent can no longer live independently and the adult children, with or without consent of their parent, have to decide about a new living arrangement for the parent. The acquisition by all family members of a common knowledge base about the elderly person's condition is the first step in alleviating the discord that can ensue. Unrealistic insistence on independence on the part of the parent, as well as excessive clinging and overly dependent behaviors can be a source of great stress to family members of elderly individuals.

The clinician should be aware that one out of four elderly individuals has experienced the death of a parent before age 15. Loss of a parent at a young age and premature responsibility for others may contribute to current fears of abandonment, severe separation anxiety, recurrence of depression, and other unexpected behavior manifestations. Although results of Vaillant and Vaillant's (1990) study of normative aging did not find parent loss to be a predictor of late-life depression, clinical assessments of elderly depressed patients appear to reflect a high incidence of early parent loss. The variance in these observations may well have an as-yet-undetermined ecological basis. Experiences in the family of origin can adversely affect relationships with the family of procreation, especially when resultant behaviors are misperceived, taken personally, or taken out of context. Timely interventions by a clinician who is helping a family make quality of life decisions for a frail elderly relative who can no longer fully participate in decision making requires expertise and sensitivity to the patient's previous lifestyle.

Another recurring theme in the course of assessing indications for family interventions is the issue of appropriate money management by and for elderly individuals. Attitudes about finances must be put in an historical context to be effective in facilitating decision making. The effects of having lived through the Great Depression, World War I, and World War II and then of living on a fixed income with limited health care benefits must be taken into consideration. Families of elderly individuals must be knowledgeable about indications for power of attorney, health proxy, limited or general guardianship in case of cognitive decline, eligibility for Medicaid, estate planning, and how to communicate about preparation of a will and a living will in case of terminal illness. The family and the elderly relative must be informed about the limitations of premature acceptance of welfare and subsequent surrender of choices that only financial independence ensures. These choices can include choice of physician, choice of home health care, choice of long-term care facility, and choice of length of time for maintaining a long-term care bed during overnight visits with relatives or hospitalizations. Limitations in these potential choices under Medicaid vary from state to state. A well-meaning child's unwitting or intentional perpetuation of an elderly parent's maladaptive attitudes about spending money for personal care should be brought to the clinician's awareness at the time of consultation and motivations for alternative approaches assessed.

Epidemiology and Research About Caregivers of the Older Adult

In 1982, the U.S. Department of Health and Human Services reported that there were about 7.6 million informal caregivers providing unpaid assistance with activities of daily living for older adults. Selected caregiver characteristics according to the relationship of the caregiver to the disabled older person are reflected in Table 30–6.

The patient assessment process is not complete without taking the relationship and condition of the caregiver into account. The nature of some of these relationships is listed in Table 30–6. The condition of the caregiver is often manifested by symptoms of depression, anxiety, somatization, social isolation, and impaired personal growth and development. Informal caregivers were found to visit physicians more often on their own behalf and take more medications than matched control subjects who did not have caregiving responsibilities (Brody 1989). Caregivers experience more

Table 30–6. Selected caregiver characteristics by relationship of caregiver to disabled elderly person (United States 1982)

| | All caregivers | Relationship of caregiver to disabled elderly person | | | | | |
| | | Female | | | Male | | |
		Spouse	Child	Other[a]	Spouse	Child	Other[a]
Population (in thousands)	2,201	500	637	438	282	186	158
Percentage	100.0	22.7	28.9	19.9	12.8	8.5	7.2
Caregiver characteristics (%)							
Primary caregiver only	32.8	60.4	23.0	17.5	55.4	10.8	13.1
Lives with disabled person	73.9	99.3	60.6	54.0	98.6	60.6	73.3
Children less than 18 years old in home	21.1	5.8	24.2	36.8	5.2	24.5	37.9
Working	30.9	9.9	43.5	32.9	12.3	55.1	45.7
Quit work to become a caregiver	8.9	13.5	11.5	2.9	11.4	5.0	0.8
Not working for other reasons	59.7	76.2	44.7	64.2	76.3	39.9	53.5

[a]Includes sons- or daughters-in-law, siblings, grandchildren, other relatives, and nonrelatives. *Disabled* is defined as being limited in one or more activities of daily living (e.g., eating, bathing, getting in or out of bed or chair, and getting around indoors).

Source. 1982 National Long-Term Care Survey/Informal Caregivers Survey, U.S. Department of Health and Human Services.

psychiatric and health problems than those without caregiving responsibilities (Anthony et al. 1988; George and Gwyther 1986). Although a sizable research literature has accumulated about depressive symptoms in family caregivers (Deimling and Bass 1986; Fitting et al. 1986; Gallagher et al. 1989; George and Gwyther 1986; Pruchno and Resch 1989; Rosenthal 1993; Stommel et al. 1990; Zarit et al. 1986), ongoing therapeutic interventions are still the exception rather than the rule.

Caregiver gender, nature of relationship, stress, and coping styles have been the subjects of extensive scholarly attention. Studies show that caregiver stress is worsened by unsupportive attitudes and behaviors of family members (Brody 1966; Spark and Brody 1970). These research findings are guides for clinical assessment for stress etiology and interventions focused on stress alleviation. Studies of gender differences in caregiver burden have found that women caregivers experience more burden than men (Barusch and Spaid 1989; Borden and Berlin 1990; Coward and Dwyer 1990; Fitting et al. 1986; Parks and Pilisuk 1991). A recent meta-analysis of research in caregiver burden estimated that women caregivers are 20% more burdened than men caregivers (B. Miller and Cafasso 1992; B. Miller et al. 1991). The nature of stress experienced by both men and women depends greatly on type of relationship with the recipient of care, age, and cohort. Wives as caregivers have been reported to manifest higher rates of psychological distress and personal burden than husbands. Caregiving daughters experience more role strain and interpersonal burden (Boutselis 1985) than caregiving sons (Horowitz 1985b), and daughters are three times more likely to become caregivers (Coward and Dwyer 1990) than sons. Few communities provide adequate home health care, respite care, or institutional care to give caregivers a choice in the intensity of their caregiving commitments. Social policies reflect serious gender injustices in the imbalance between the availability of formal and informal caregiving. The majority of frail elderly individuals are women as are their unpaid family caregivers, the majority of whom are wives, daughters, and daughters-in-law.

In the course of assessment for family therapy with elderly individuals, evaluation of the individual patient precedes assessment of family members' perceptions of the elderly relative's condition. Psychiatric evaluation of the spouse, adult children, grandchildren, and other kin who contribute to or detract from the elderly patient's quality of life, or vice versa (i.e., the elderly patient detracts from their quality of life), focuses on conflicts and misperceptions that jeopardize the mental and physical health of each person involved. In the course of this assessment, family members

who have not yet assumed an active positive role can be invited to participate if desired by the patient.

Maltreatment of Elderly Individuals

Although most families put forth heroic efforts for the care of elderly individuals in their families, the House Select Committee on Aging (1990) concluded that 4% of elderly Americans might be victims of some sort of abuse.
This situation is now recognized as a serious public health problem. The prevalence of maltreatment of elderly individuals according to a random-sample
telephone survey of about 2,000 in the Boston, Massachusetts, metropolitan
area was 32 per 1,000 and in a Canadian study, 40 per 1,000 (Pillemer and
Finkelhor 1988; Podnieks 1992a, 1992b). In the Pillemer study, 60% of the
perpetrators were spouses, 20% were adult children, and 20% were other persons such as siblings, grandchildren, and boarders. Among the abusive adult
children, sons outnumbered daughters by a ratio of 2:1. The reported incidence rate in Massachusetts during that year was 1.8 per 1,000, indicating that
only 1 in 14 cases came to public attention.

Definitions and assessment criteria used by legislators, researchers,
and clinicians vary considerably and address a wide span of physical and
psychological abuse, neglect, and material exploitation (Hudson 1991;
Gebotys et al. 1992). Although all states currently have either mandatory
or voluntary reporting laws, they vary in terms of assessing, reporting,
investigating, monitoring, and issuing penalties. Mandatory reporting laws
regarding abuse of elderly individuals are based on a child abuse model
and are considered inappropriate by critics to ensure the safety of competent adult victims (Sellers et al. 1992).

Delays in addressing the problem since the 1960s are attributed to the
debate over how to best address the issues; lack of systematic, reliable research; delays in leadership by public officials in promoting the issues; philosophical differences about the role of government in family privacy; and
misconceptions that it was rare, did not appear in normal relationships,
and was a private matter. A major psychological barrier to recognition of
maltreatment of elderly individuals is the fact that abusers and many professional providers of care have common defenses—namely, denial, rationalization, and minimization. This has made the behavior of the abuser at
low risk for identification. Another factor to be considered that contributes
to low identification rates is the clinical observation that victimized
parents often fear 1) not being believed, 2) reprisal, 3) abandonment, and

4) institutionalization. They may be embarrassed about the situation and wish to protect their children, an attribute that the abusive adult child may not be able to identify with in relation to the now-dependent parent.

For competent adult victims of abuse, physicians must not disclose abuse to caregivers or any other third party without the consent of the patient. The patient should be educated regarding the resources available to him or her in order to arrive at a well-informed decision that will promote his or her best interests and safety.

Psychiatrists have the opportunity to discover abuse when a perpetrator discloses abusive behavior in the course of psychotherapy. Granting the psychiatrist the discretion to weigh, on a case-by-case basis, the threat to a victim of ongoing abuse versus the potential damage to the therapeutic relationship may well be a better approach to attain the eventual goal of ending the abuse than current reporting mandates.

In the course of research and the many clinical reports that have come to public attention about the nature of maltreatment of elderly individuals, profiles of victim and perpetrators have evolved. National statistics in 1988 revealed that the majority of victims are ages 75 and older, and 64.2% are women.

Categories of perpetrators of maltreatment of elderly individuals have evolved among those who find themselves intentionally or inadvertently in a family caregiving role. The family member involved in maltreatment of an elderly person may be 1) a criminal, 2) developmentally disabled, 3) mentally disabled, 4) a substance abuser, or 5) overstressed. A study by the National Aging Resource Center on Elder Abuse (NARCEA) revealed that 30% of domestic abuse of elderly persons involved adult children; 15%, spouses; and 17.8%, other relatives. According to the criteria used by NARCEA, 37% of abuse was identified as neglect, 26% as physical abuse, 20% as financial/material, and 17% as other. Case examples that have come to the attention of a protective service agency have been described (Goldstein 1995).

It is important for clinicians to be familiar with 1) definitions of maltreatment of elderly persons as accepted by their professional group (American Medical Association 1992); 2) assessment instruments that have validity, reliability, and specificity; 3) the adult protection laws of the state in which they practice; and 4) community resources provided by adult protective services and others. Intervention is optimal if it protects privacy, is carried out by a multidisciplinary team, and provides continuity of care and appropriate attention to each person involved in the situation identified as maltreatment of an elderly person.

Summary

The role of family members requires redefinition in later years, as does the role of the psychiatrist in the treatment of elderly individuals and their families. The modern family is complex and varied, and the role of elderly individuals is often poorly defined. The contemporary psychiatrist must be versed in clinical assessment and treatment from a biopsychosocial perspective that includes assessment and treatment of family members. Research findings by epidemiologists, gerontologists, nurses, sociologists, and psychologists must be integrated in the theoretical models of family dynamics and therapy.

Clinical attention to the rising incidence and prevalence of maltreatment of elderly individuals is needed in all settings where medical care is provided for the elderly population. Training, research, and advocacy require ongoing development if effective standards of clinical care are to be implemented. Reimbursement issues that enable implementation of quality care must be addressed by all concerned, including the families of elderly individuals.

References

Ade-Ridder L: Quality of long-term marriages, in Family Relationships in Later Life, Part I. Edited by Brubaker TA. Beverly Hills, CA, Sage, 1983, pp 21–30

Ade-Ridder L: Quality of marriage: a comparison between golden wedding couples and couples married less than 50 years, in Lifestyles of the Elderly: Diversity in Relationships, Health, and Caregiving. Edited by Ade-Ridder L, Hennon CB. New York, Human Sciences Press, 1989, pp 37–48

American Medical Association: Diagnostic and Treatment Guidelines on Elder Abuse and Neglect. Chicago, IL, American Medical Association 1992

Anthony CR, Zarit SH, Gatz M: Symptoms of psychological distress among caregivers of dementia patients. Psychol Aging 3:25–248, 1988

Barusch AS, Spaid WM: Gender differences in caregiving: why do wives report greater burden? Gerontologist 29:667–675, 1989

Borden W, Berlin S: Gender, coping and psychological well-being in spouses of older adults with chronic dementia. Am J Orthopsychiatry 60:603–610, 1990

Borszormenyi-Nagy IA, Spark GM: Invisible Loyalties: Reciprocity in Intergenerational Family Therapy. Hagerstown, MD, Harper & Row, 1973

Boutselis MA: The effects of gender and relationships on caregiver burden, distress and responsibility to interventions. PhD thesis, University of Southern California. Dissertation Abstracts, 1985

Brody EM: The aging family. Gerontologist 6:201–206, 1966

Brody EM: Family at risk, in Alzheimer's Disease: Treatment and Family Stress (DHHS Publ No (ADM) 89-1569). Edited by Light E, Lebowitz B. Rockville, MD, National Institute of Mental Health, 1989, pp 2–49

Brubaker TH: Family Relationships in Later Life. Beverly Hills, CA, Sage, 1983

Brubaker TH: Later Life Families. Family Studies Text Series I. Beverly Hills, CA, Sage, 1985

Brubaker TH: Family Relationships in Later Life, 2nd Edition. Newbury Park, CA, Sage, 1990

Cicirelli VG: A comparison of helping behavior to elderly parents of adult children with intact and disrupted marriages. Gerontologist 23:619–625, 1983a

Cicirelli VG: Adult children and their elderly parents, in Family Relationships in Later Life. Edited by Brubaker T. Beverly Hills, CA, Sage, 1983b, pp 31–46

Committee on the Family, Group for the Advancement of Psychiatry: The Field of Family Therapy, Vol VII, Report No 78. New York, Mental Health Materials Center, 1970

Comptroller General of the United States: Report to Congress on home health: the need for a national policy to better provide for the elderly (GAO Publ No HRD 78-19). Washington, DC, December 30, 1977

Coward RT, Dwyer JW: The association of gender, sibling network composition and patterns of parent care by adult children. Res Aging 12:158–181, 1990

Deimling GT, Bass DM: Symptoms of mental impairment among elderly adults and their effects on family caregivers. J Gerontol 41:778–784, 1986

Doty P: Family care of the elderly: the role of public policy. Milbank Q 64:34–75, 1986

Duke University: Multi-Dimensional Functional Assessment: The OARS Methodology; A Manual, 2nd Edition. Durham, NC, Center for the Study of Aging and Human Development, 1978

Fischer LR: Elderly parents and the caregiving role: an asymmetrical transition, in Social Bonds in Later Life: Aging and Interdependence. Edited by Peterson WA, Quadagno J. Beverly Hills, CA, Sage, 1985, pp 105–114

Fitting M, Rabins P, Lucas JL, et al: Caregivers for dementia patients: a comparison of husbands and wives. Gerontologist 26:248–252, 1986

Gallagher D, Rose J, Rivera P, et al: Prevalence of depression in family caregivers. Gerontologist 29:449–456, 1989

Gebotys RJ, O'Connor D, Mair KJ: Public perceptions of elder physical mistreatment. Journal of Elder Abuse and Neglect 4:151–171, 1992

George LK, Gwyther LP: Caregiver well-being: a multidimensional examination of family caregivers of demented adults. Gerontologist 26:253–259, 1986

Ginsberg-McEwan E: The whole grandfather: an intergenerational approach to family therapy, in Treating the Elderly With Psychotherapy: The Scope for Change in Later Life. Edited by Sadavoy J, Leszcz M. Madison, CT, International Universities Press, 1987, pp 295–324

Goldstein MZ: Parent care, in Family Involvement in the Treatment of the Frail Elderly. Edited by Goldstein MZ. Washington, DC, American Psychiatric Press, 1989, pp 1–22

Goldstein MZ: The role of mutual support groups and family therapy for caregivers of demented elderly. J Geriatr Psychiatry 23:117–128, 1990

Goldstein MZ: Elder abuse, in Comprehensive Textbook of Psychiatry/VI, 6th Edition. Edited by Kaplan I, Sadock BJ. Baltimore, MD, Williams & Wilkins, 1995, pp 2652–2656

Goldstein MZ: Working with families, in Psychiatric Care in the Nursing Home. Edited by Reichman W, Katz P. New York, Oxford University Press (in press)

Grad J, Sainsbury P: Problems of caring for the mentally ill at home. Proc R Soc Med, section on Psychiatry 59:20–23, 1966

Gwyther LP, Blazer DG: Family therapy and the dementia patient. Am Fam Physician 29:149–156,1984

Hagsted GO: Continuity and Connectedness in Grandparenthood. Edited by Bengston VL, Robertson J. Beverly Hills, CA, Sage, 1985, pp 31–48

Hale MS, Mikita MM: A family-systems model for consultation psychiatry. Adv Psychosom Med 20:17–32, 1990

Hepburn K, Wasow M: Support groups for family caregivers of dementia victims: questions, directions and future research, in The Elderly and Chronic Mental Illness (New Directions for Mental Health Services No 29). San Francisco, CA, Jossey-Bass, 1986, pp 83–92

Herr JJ, Weakland JH: Counseling Elders and Their Families: Practical Techniques for Applied Gerontology. New York, Springer, 1979

Hesse-Bibers S, Williamson J: Resource theory and power in families: life cycle considerations. Fam Process 23:261–278, 1984

Horowitz A: Family caregiving to the frail elderly, in Annual Review of Gerentology and Geriatrics, Vol 5. Edited by Eisdorfer C, Lawton MP,

Maddox GL. New York, Springer, 1985a, pp 194–246

Horowitz A: Sons and daughters as caregivers to older parents: differences in role performance and consequences. Gerontologist 25:612–617, 1985b

Hudson MF: Elder mistreatment: taxonomy with definitions by Delph. Journal of Elder Abuse and Neglect 3:1–20, 1991

Jarvik L, Small G: Parent Care. New York, Crown Publishers, 1988

Kornhaber A: Grandparenting: normal and pathological—a preliminary communication from the grandparent study. J Geriatr Psychiatry 19:19–37, 1986

Miller B, Cafasso L: Gender differences in caregiving: fact or artifact? Gerontologist 32:498–507, 1992

Miller B, McFall S, Montgomery A: The impact of elder health, caregiver involvement and global stress on two dimensions of caregiver burden. J Gerontol 46:S9–S19, 1991

Miller MD: Opportunities for psychotherapy in the management of dementia. J Geriatr Psychiatry Neurol 2:11–17, 1989

National Center for Health Statistics: The National Nursing Home Survey 1985 summary for the United States. Vital and Health Statistics, Series 12, No 97 (DHHS Publ No (PHS) 89-1758). Washington, DC, Public Health Service, US Government Printing Office, 1989

Neugarten BL: Adaptation and the life cycle, in Counseling Adults. Edited by Schlossberg NK, Entine AD. Monterey, CA, Brooks/Cole, 1977

Parks SH, Pilisuk M: Caregiver burden: gender and the psychological costs of caregiving. Am J Psychiatry 61:501–509, 1991

Pillemer K, Finkelhor D: The prevalence of elder abuse: a random sample survey. Gerontologist 28:51–57, 1988

Podnieks E: National survey of abuse of the elderly in Canada. Journal of Elder Abuse and Neglect 4:5–59, 1992a

Podnieks E: Emerging themes from a follow-up study of Canadian victims of elder abuse. Journal of Elder Abuse and Neglect 4:59–111, 1992b

Pruchno R, Resch N: Husbands and wives as caregivers: antecedents of depression and burden. Gerontologist 29:159–165, 1989

Quinn WH, Keller JF: A family therapy model for preserving independence. Am J Fam Ther 9:79–84, 1981

Rosenthal CJ, Sulman J, Marshall VW: Depressive symptoms in family caregivers of long-stay patients. Gerontologist 33(2):249–257, 1993

Ross HG, Milgram JJ: Important variables in adult sibling relationships, in Sibling Relationships: Their Nature and Significance. Edited by Lamb ME, Sutton ME. Hillsdale, NJ, Erlbaum, 1982

Select Committee on Aging, House of Representatives: A report by the chairman of the Subcommittee on Health and Long-Term Care. Elder abuse: a decade of shame and inaction (Committee Publ No 101-752). Washington, DC, US Government Printing Office, 1990

Sellers CS, Folts WE, Logan KM: Elder mistreatment: a multidimensional problem. Journal of Elder Abuse and Neglect 4:5–23, 1992

Shanas E: Social myth as hypothesis: the case of the family relations of old people. Gerontologist 19:3–9, 1979a

Shanas E: The family as a social system in old age. Gerontologist 19:169–174, 1979b

Solomon MA: A developmental conceptual premise for family therapy. Fam Process 12:179–188, 1973

Spark G, Brody EM: The aged are family members. Fam Process 9:195–210, 1970

Stommel M, Given C, Given B: Depression as an overriding variable explaining caregiver burdens. J Aging Health 2:81–102, 1990

Stone R, Cafferata GL, Sangi J: Caregivers of the frail elderly: a national profile. Gerontologist 27:616–626, 1987

Tauber CM: America in transition: an aging society. Current Population Reports, Series P-23, No 128, U.S. Bureau of the Census. Washington, DC, U.S. Government Printing Office, 1983

Troll LE: Family Issues in Current Gerontology. New York, Springer, 1986

Uhlenberg P, Myers MAP: Divorce and the elderly. Gerontologist 21:276–282, 1981

Uhlenberg P, Cooney T, Boyd R: Divorce for women after midlife. Journal of Gerontology: Social Sciences 45:S3–S11, 1990

US Bureau of the Census: Current Population Reports, Series P-20, No 468, Marital status and living arrangements. Washington, DC, US Government Printing Office, 1992

Vaillant GE, Vaillant CO: National history of male psychosocial health, XII: a 45 year study of predictors of successful aging at age 65. Am J Psychiatry 147:31–37, 1990

World Health Organization: International Classification of Diseases, 10th Revision. Geneva, World Health Organization, 1991

Zarit S, Todd P, Zarit J: Subjective burden of husbands and wives as caregivers: a longitudinal study. Gerontologist 26:260–266, 1986

Zarit SH, Anthony CR, Boutselis M: Interventions with care givers of dementia patients: comparison of two approaches. Psychol Aging 2:225–232, 1987

Joel E. Streim, M.D.
Barry W. Rovner, M.D.
Ira R. Katz, M.D., Ph.D.

Psychiatric Aspects of Nursing Home Care

Nursing homes provide care to injured, disabled, or sick patients who require medical, nursing, or rehabilitation services. They may provide convalescent care during recovery from acute illness or long-term care for chronic illness and disability. As documented in both the literature and several reviews (Beardsley et al. 1988; Larsen et al. 1989; Rabins et al. 1987; Rovner and Katz 1993), knowledge of the psychiatric aspects of nursing home care is growing rapidly. In parallel, the delivery of services is being shaped by federal legislation and evolving regulations. This chapter reviews the scientific and regulatory background of psychiatric care in the nursing home, presents current developments, and discusses the evolving roles of the psychiatrist in this setting. Psychiatric care in the nursing home is subject to change as a result of changes in federal regulations and industry practices as well as scientific advances; perhaps more than those describing other areas in geriatric psychiatry, this chapter must be considered a "snapshot" of the field.

Demographics

The 1985 National Nursing Home Survey (National Center for Health Statistics 1987) found that 5% of Americans age 65 or older (1.5 million people) resided in over 20,000 long-term care facilities and that 88% of all residents in nursing homes were 65 or older. One percent of the population ages 65–74, 3% of those 75–84, and 22% of those 85 or older live in these settings. These institutions care for a population that is both old and functionally impaired: 91% of residents required assistance in bathing; 78%, assistance in dressing; 63%, assistance in both toileting and transferring; and 40%, assistance in eating. Fifty-five percent were incontinent. Only 8% were independent in all activities of daily living. The average resident takes 3.2 medications daily. Eighty-four percent of residents were without spouses, and 57% had been transferred to the setting from another health-care facility, most commonly a hospital. The mean length of stay in a nursing home is 2.5 years; 67% of current residents have lived in a home for at least 1 year. One-half of elderly residents used their own or family finances to fund their first month in the nursing home. Most residents have exhausted their savings after only a few months (Benson and Gambert 1984; Campion et al. 1983; National Center for Health Statistics 1987). There are projections that 25% of Americans can now expect to spend part of their lives in nursing homes (Campion et al. 1983) and that the number of nursing home residents will more than triple by the year 2020 (McCarthy 1989).

Epidemiology and Clinical Characteristics of Psychiatric Disorders in the Nursing Home

The literature reports a high prevalence of psychiatric illness among nursing home residents. Recent studies that used rigorous methods report prevalence rates of 80%–90%. Rovner et al. (1990a) reported a prevalence of 80.2% among new admissions to a proprietary chain of nursing homes. Parmelee et al. (1989) surveyed the residents of a single large urban nursing home, confirmed diagnoses by clinical evaluation, and found psychiatric disorders, according to DSM-III-R (American Psychiatric Association 1987), in 91% of the residents. Other investigations, based on psychiatric interviews of randomly selected samples, found prevalence rates of disorders according to DSM-III (American Psychiatric Association 1980) or DSM-III-R as high as 94% (Chandler and Chandler 1988; Rovner et al. 1986; Tariot et al. 1993). Other studies have reported lower rates but appear to have used less rigorous methods or to have assessed only selected sub-populations of residents (Burns et al. 1988; Custer et al. 1984; German et al. 1986; National Center for Health Statistics 1987; Teeter et al. 1976).

Dementia

In all studies, the most common psychiatric disorder is dementia, with prevalence rates from one-half to three-quarters of residents (Chandler and Chandler 1988; Katz et al. 1989a; Parmelee et al. 1989; Rovner et al. 1986, 1990a; Tariot et al. 1993; Teeter et al. 1976). An Epidemiologic Catchment Area Study reported a lower prevalence of cognitive impairment, but the more severely impaired patients who could not complete testing procedures were excluded (German et al. 1986). Alzheimer's disease (primary degenerative dementia) accounts for 50%–60% of cases and multi-infarct dementia for 25%–30% (Barnes and Raskind 1980; Rovner et al. 1986, 1990a). Other causes of dementia are reported with lower prevalence and greater variability between sites.

Patients with dementia are at high risk for secondary complications, including delirium, psychosis, and depression that can increase cognitive and functional disability. Available studies report that 6%–7% of residents were delirious at the time of evaluation (Barnes and Raskind 1980; Rovner et al. 1986, 1990a). However, this probably underestimates the number of patients with reversible components to their cognitive impairment. One study found that nearly 25% of impaired residents have potentially reversible conditions (Sabin et al. 1982), and another, that 6%–12% of residential care patients with dementia improved in cognitive performance over the course of 1 year (Katz et al. 1991). In the nursing home and in other settings, the most common reversible cause of cognitive impairment may be cognitive toxicity from drugs used to treat medical or psychiatric disorders. Psychotic symptoms have been reported in 25%–50% of residents with a primary illness of dementia (Berrios and Brook 1985; Chandler and Chandler 1988; Rovner et al. 1986, 1990a; Teeter et al. 1976). Clinically significant depression is seen in about 25% of patients with dementia; one-third of these exhibit symptoms of a secondary major depression (Parmelee et al. 1989; Rovner et al. 1986, 1990a).

Behavioral Disturbances in the Nursing Home

Behavioral disturbances may be present in two-thirds to three-fourths of residents and multiple behavior problems in at least one-half (Chandler and Chandler 1988; Cohen-Mansfield 1986; National Center for Health Statistics 1979; Rovner et al. 1986, 1990a; Tariot et al. 1993; Zimmer et al. 1984). Disturbances of behavior, in addition to impaired ability to perform activities of daily living, have been identified as the most common reasons that patients with dementia are admitted to nursing homes (Steele et al. 1990), and disruptive behaviors frequently complicate care after admission (Cohen-Mansfield et al. 1989; Teeter et al. 1976; Zimmer et al. 1984). Most psychiatric consultations in long-term care settings are for the evaluation and treatment of behavioral disturbances, primarily in patients with dementia. Loebel et al. (1991) demonstrated that frequent, but not invariable, associations exist between the nature of behavioral problems that led to psychiatric consultation and the underlying diagnosis. The most common behavioral difficulties include pacing/wandering, verbal abusiveness, disruptive shouting, physical aggression, and resistance to necessary care. Risk factors for behavioral disturbances include both dementia and psychoses. Among patients with dementia, the association between psychosis and behavioral disturbance remains, even after controlling for the level of cognitive impairment (Rovner et al. 1990b). Other causes of agitation and hyperactivity may include agitated depression, delirium, sensory deprivation or overload, occult physical illness, pain, constipation, urinary retention, and adverse drug effects including akathisia caused by neuroleptics (Cohen-Mansfield and Billig 1986).

Cohen-Mansfield et al. (1989) have made major contributions to the characterization, description, and measurement of agitation and related behavioral disturbances as they occur among patients with dementia and have identified three distinct types of agitated behaviors: verbally agitated behavior, physically nonaggressive behavior, and aggressive behavior. The verbally agitated behaviors observed most frequently were constant requests for attention, negativism, repetitious sentences and questions, screaming, and complaining. The physically nonaggressive behaviors observed most frequently were pacing, inappropriate robing/disrobing, trying to get to a different place, handling things inappropriately, general restlessness, and inappropriate mannerisms. In contrast to agitation, apathy, abulia, inactivity, and withdrawal have received less attention in the literature. Marin (1990, 1991) has suggested guidelines for distinguishing the impaired motivation that is characteristic of depression from the apathy that is common in patients with dementia. A classic study by Kaplitz (1975) suggests that the apathy associated with dementia may be a treatable syndrome that is responsive to methylphenidate.

Depression

Depressive disorders are the second most common of the psychiatric diagnoses among nursing home residents. The epidemiology and clinical features of these disorders have recently been reviewed by Ames (1991) and by Katz and Parmelee (1993). Most studies report a prevalence of depression in 15%–50% of patients, according to the population studied and the instruments used, whether major depression or depressive symptoms are reported, and whether primary depression and depression occurring secondary to dementia are considered together or separately (Baker and Miller 1991; Chandler and Chandler 1988; Hyer and Blazer 1982; Katz et al. 1989a; Lesher 1986; Parmelee et al. 1989; Rovner et al. 1986, 1991; Tariot et al. 1993; Teeter et al. 1976). Studies from other countries have reported similar rates (Ames 1990; Ames et al. 1988; Harrison et al. 1990; Horiguchi and Inami 1991; Mann et al. 1984; Snowdon 1986; Snowdon and Donnelly 1986; Spagnoli et al. 1986; Trichard et al. 1982). The risk of depressive illnesses is significantly higher in nursing home residents than in the elderly individuals in the community (Blazer and Williams 1980; Kramer et al. 1985). Approximately 6%–10% of nursing home residents (or 20%–25% of those residents who are cognitively intact) meet DSM-III or DSM-III-R criteria for major depression; the prevalence of other, less severe, forms of depression is even higher. In contrast to prevalence data, little information is available on the incidence of depression in long-term care. One study reported that the 1-year incidence of major depression was 9.4% among those with minor or no depression at baseline, with a greater risk among those with minor depression; the incidence of minor depression among those euthymic at baseline was 7.4% (Parmelee et al. 1992a). Other, smaller scale studies reported comparable rates (Foster et al. 1991; Katz et al. 1989a).

Depression among nursing home residents tends to be persistent. Although Snowdon and Donnelly (1986) found a decrease in self-rated depression as a function of time after admission to the nursing home, Ames et al. (1988) found that only 17% of surviving patients with depression had recovered after an average 3.6 years of follow-up. Depression is associated with increased disability, but the directions of association remain to be established. Evidence for morbidity associated with depression comes from studies showing an increase in pain complaints among residents with depression (Parmelee et al. 1991), and an association between depression and biochemical markers of subnutrition (Katz et al. 1993). The association of depression with pain appeared to reflect an amplification of pain that could be attributed to physical illnesses confirmed by physicians rather than unfounded complaints. The relationship between depression and laboratory indicators of nutritional deficits suggests that these depressions are states of physiological as well as psychological significance; a significant component may be related to "failure to thrive" in the elderly as discussed by Braun et al. (1988). In addition to its association with morbidity, depression has been found to be associated with an increase in mortality in a number of studies, with effect sizes ranging from 1.6 to 3 (Ashby et al. 1991; Katz et al. 1989a; Parmelee et al. 1992b; Rovner et al. 1991). Controversy exists, however, about the mechanism involved. Although Rovner et al. (1991) report that the increased mortality remains even after controlling for the patients' medical diagnoses and level of disability, Parmelee et al. (1992a) found that the effect could be attributed to the interrelationships between depression, disability, and physical illness. Resolution of this issue will require additional study.

Major depression in long-term care patients is treatable. Katz et al. (1989b, 1990) conducted a double-blind, placebo-controlled study of the treatment of major depression in a study population (average age 84) from a nursing home and congregate apartment facility. Subjects were given either placebo or nortriptyline with doses adjusted to give plasma levels within the therapeutic range. Among study completers ($n = 23$), 58% of patients given active medication but only 9% of those given placebo were rated "much" or "very much" improved; 83% of those given drug, but only 22% of those given placebo exhibited improvement of any degree. Thus, even this small-scale study demonstrated a significant drug-placebo difference. The same study found that measures of self-care deficits and serum levels of albumin were highly intercorrelated and that both predicted a failure to respond to nortriptyline treatment. Thus, although the primary conclusion from this research must be that major depression remains a treatable disorder, even in long-term care patients with significant medical comorbidity, evidence also exists for a treatment-relevant subtype of depression, characterized by high levels of disability and low levels of serum albumin, that appears to emerge specifically in the long-term care setting. This latter disorder may be related to failure to thrive as discussed above. Additional studies are needed to replicate and validate these findings.

As many as two-thirds of nursing home residents with psychiatric disorders may be improperly diagnosed (German et al. 1986; Sabin et al. 1982). Lack of diagnosis and misdiagnosis is of grave concern when one considers the prevalence rates, the numbers of patients involved, the risks of excess disability, and the impact on quality of life. Standardized screening instruments administered on a regular basis by nursing home staff may be of use in identifying patients in need of psychiatric consultation. Both the Mini-Mental State Exam (Folstein et al. 1975) and the Blessed Memory-Information-Concentration Test (Blessed et al. 1968) have been used in screening for cognitive impairment. The Geriatric Depression Scale shows promise for use in identifying nursing home residents who need additional evaluation for depression (Brink et al. 1982). Although there is some controversy in this area (Burke et al. 1989), it remains reliable in screening for depression among those with a mild or moderate degree of dementia (Burke et al. 1992; Parmelee et al. 1989). However, structured instruments cannot replace evaluation by experienced clinicians. Nursing home residents with symptoms of major depression commonly have medical illnesses or medication effects that can confound the diagnosis of major depression. The model of Cohen-Cole and Stoudemire (1987) may be useful in considering how to approach the process of diagnosis: an etiological strategy that relies on clinical judgment regarding whether each symptom should be attributed to depression or other causes may be the most practical approach now; an inclusive strategy, in which all criterion symptoms are considered regardless of the possible contributions of medical causes, may optimize the sensitivity of diagnosis; and substitutive, or exclusive, strategies, in which ambiguous symptoms are either replaced or not considered at all may optimize specificity. For example, using an inclusive strategy, a severely anemic patient may be given a DSM-IV diagnosis of major depressive disorder based on the presence of persistent dysphoria, diminished appetite, sleep disturbance, impaired concentration, and fatigue, even if the fatigue could be partly or fully caused by the patient's anemia. By contrast, using an exclusive approach, fatigue attributable to anemia would not be considered among the symptoms used to meet the criteria for a diagnosis of major depression, and the patient would not be given a diagnosis of major depression unless another symptom, not ascribed to anemia, were present. An etiological strategy, in contrast to the other two, would rely on a clinician's judgment as to whether the symptoms should be considered attributable to depression or to anemia and, therefore, whether the diagnosis of major depressive disorder should be given.

Assessment and Management of Psychiatric Problems and Nursing Home Reform

The widespread misuse of both psychotropic drugs and of physical restraints was instrumental in galvanizing attention to the need for nursing home reform on a national level. This misuse demonstrates how failure to recognize the high prevalence of mental disorders in nursing homes and to provide appropriate treatment can lead to poor, even inhumane, care.

Use of Psychotropic Drugs in the Nursing Home

One of the primary motivations for nursing home reform has been widespread concern regarding the overuse of psychotropic drugs in nursing home residents. Historically, studies have reported that about 50% of residents have orders for these agents, with 20%–40% taking neuroleptics, 10%–40% taking anxiolytics or hypnotics, and 5%–10% taking antidepressants (Avorn et al. 1989; Beers et al. 1988; Buck 1988; Burns et al. 1988; Cohen-Mansfield 1986; Custer et al. 1984; DeLeo et al. 1989; Ray et al. 1980; Teeter et al. 1976; Zimmer et al. 1984). This high prevalence means that a substantial proportion of nursing home residents are at risk for adverse drug effects.

Psychotropic drugs have frequently been prescribed without adequate consideration of the psychiatric or medical status of the residents. One study reported that only 15% of residents receiving psychotropic drugs had received a psychiatric consultation (Zimmer et al. 1984). Others report that mental health services were available to less than 5% of those with a known psychiatric illness and that 21% of patients with no psychiatric diagnosis received psychotropic medication (Burns et al. 1988), that physician characteristics (rather than those of patients) predicted drug dosage (Ray et al. 1980), and that psychotropic drugs are often prescribed in the absence of any charted reference to patients' mental status (Avorn et al. 1989).

The use of neuroleptic drugs for the control of behavioral symptoms may present the greatest potential for inappropriate overuse. Although evidence exists for the efficacy of neuroleptics in managing agitation and related symptoms in nursing home residents with dementia, the effects are often not dramatic and placebo responses may be common (Barnes et al. 1982; Schneider et al. 1990). Other medications as well as behavioral or environmental treatments may be equally effective. Moreover, note that all of the evidence for the efficacy of antipsychotic medications comes from short-term studies, but the medications are frequently prescribed for long-term treatment. One classic, double-blind, neuroleptic-withdrawal study showed that only 16% of patients who had been receiving medications on a chronic basis exhibited significant deterioration when they were withdrawn (Barton and Hurst 1966). A more recent withdrawal study in patients who had been receiving neuroleptics for several months ($n = 9$) found that 22%

experienced increased agitation on withdrawal, 22% were unchanged, and 55% actually showed improvement (Risse et al. 1987). Thus, it is important to reevaluate the need for neuroleptic treatment with trials of drug withdrawal on a regular basis.

Although overprescribing antipsychotic medications in patients with dementia has been a major issue, the misuse of psychotropic drugs in the nursing home is not limited to excesses. The Institute of Medicine (1986) report that did much to stimulate nursing home reform highlighted both problems of the overuse of antipsychotic drugs and the underuse of antidepressants for treatment of affective disorders. Similarly, in reviewing epidemiological studies on the use of psychotropic drugs in nursing homes, Murphy (1989) noted that antidepressants were the one class of drugs that appeared to be underused and that, as a result, much of the major depression present in the nursing home went untreated.

Use of Physical Restraints

The use of mechanical restraints for the control of behavior makes the most dramatic case for increased mental health services in the nursing home. The 1977 survey of American nursing home residents found that 25% of 1.3 million people were restrained by geriatric chairs, cuffs, belts, or similar devices (National Center for Health Statistics 1979). Other surveys have reported prevalence rates as high as 85%. Patient factors predicting the use of restraints in nursing homes and other settings include age, cognitive impairment, risk of injuries to self or others (e.g., from falls or combative behavior), physical frailty, presence of monitoring or treatment devices, and the need to promote body alignment. Institutional and system factors include pressure to avoid litigation, staff attitudes, insufficient staffing, and the availability of restraint devices. Mechanical restraints are frequently used to control disruptive behavior. However, little research has been devoted to evaluating the benefits versus the risks of the use of restraints or for systematic investigations of alternatives. Potential adverse effects include an increased risk of falls and other injuries, functional decline, skin breakdown, physiological effects of immobilization stress, disorganized behavior, and emotional desolation. Cross-national studies suggest that it is possible to manage nursing home residents without them (Cape 1983; Evans and Strumpf 1989; Innes and Turman 1983). Most significantly, Werner et al. (1989) demonstrated that, although agitation is a frequent cause for the use of restraints, they do not decrease behavioral disturbances. Because mechanical restraints are used to control behavior, mental health professionals should be involved in decisions about their use, both in evaluating individual patients and in formulating institutional policy. To be able to do so, mental health professionals must be knowledgeable about both the behavioral disorders of elderly individuals and about the nature of the physical and social environment in the long-term care facility (Evans and Strumpf 1989).

Federal Regulations and Psychiatric Care in the Nursing Home

Several factors provided the impetus for the federal government to enact legislation that provides for nursing home reform. Concerns about the misuse of physical and chemical restraints as discussed above were emphasized by consumer advocacy groups such as the National Citizens Coalition for Nursing Home Reform, and the Alzheimer's Association, as well as by the 1986 Institute of Medicine Report. In addition, the General Accounting Office cited concerns that the states had a strong incentive for placing patients with psychiatric problems in Medicaid-certified nursing facilities where the federal government bears a substantial portion of the cost of their care. The Congressional House Committee on the Budget noted in 1987 that substantial numbers of mentally retarded and mentally ill residents were inappropriately placed at Medicaid expense in nursing homes where they often did not receive the active psychiatric treatment or services that they needed. Apparently in response to both sets of concerns, Congress enacted Nursing Home Reform Amendments as part of the Omnibus Budget Reconciliation Act of 1987 (OBRA 87). This legislation provides for government regulation of many aspects of the operation of nursing facilities and of the care that they provide (Elon and Pawlson 1992). The laws enacted by Congress mandated that the Health Care Financing Administration (HCFA) issue regulations (HCFA 1991) designed to operationalize the laws that in turn required that HCFA develop guidelines to assist federal and state surveyors in interpreting the regulations (HCFA 1992a); states are charged with responsibility for enforcing the laws by conducting surveys using operational criteria presented in the guidelines to ensure that the regulations are being followed.

The Nursing Home Reform Amendments hold nursing facilities rather than physicians responsible for compliance; however, the regulations affect numerous aspects of medical and mental health practice. Mental health screening, assessment, care planning, and treatment are addressed under sections of the regulations that pertain to resident assessment, resident rights and facility practices, and quality of care.

The regulations include provisions for Preadmission Screening and Annual Resident Review (PASARR) that require assessment of each resident before admission to any nursing facility that receives federal funds (HCFA 1992b). When an initial first stage screening reveals that a serious mental disorder (other than dementia) is present, a second stage evaluation requiring a psychiatric evaluation is mandated to ascertain whether the patient has a mental disorder, to make a specific psychiatric diagnosis, and to determine whether there is a need for acute psychiatric care that precludes adequate or appropriate treatment in a nursing home. Thus, preadmission screening is intended to prevent inappropriate admission of patients with severe psychiatric disorders to nursing homes and to help ensure that patients with disability attributable in large part to treatable psychiatric disorders (such as depression) are not placed in long-term care facilities before receiving the benefits of adequate psychiatric treatment. For patients deemed eligible who are admitted to a nursing home, annual reassessment is required to determine whether nursing home care remains appropriate.

Regulations requiring comprehensive assessment for all residents (HCFA 1991) have led to guidelines for the administration of the Minimum Data Set (MDS) (Morris et al. 1990) or an equivalent instrument on a regular basis by members of an interdisciplinary health care team, usually with a nurse, and ultimately the nursing home administrator, responsible for its completion (HCFA 1992c). Areas of assessment relevant to mental illness and behavior include mood, cognition, communication, functional status, medications, and other treatments. Responses on the MDS suggesting that there may be a need to reevaluate a patient's clinical status and treatment plan serve as triggers for Resident Assessment Protocols (RAPs) that define medical conditions, psychiatric disorders, adverse treatment effects, functional impairments, and disabilities that are common among nursing home residents; list differential diagnoses, and potential causal and aggravating factors; outline procedures for evaluation; and list key elements of management or treatment (HCFA 1992c). The MDS and RAPs together are designed as a two-stage assessment system, with a screening survey followed by a focused clinical evaluation. RAP problem areas related to mental disorders and behavior include delirium, cognitive loss/dementia, psychosocial well-being, mood state, behavior problems, psychotropic drug use, and physical restraints. The individual RAPs are designed to help nursing home staff recognize common signs and symptom clusters that are indicators of clinically significant problems, conduct in-depth evaluations according to standardized algorithms, and then determine whether it is necessary to alter the treatment plan. The regulations hold facilities responsible for ensuring that RAPs are followed appropriately. Although physicians have no mandated role in this process, physician involvement is necessary for proper diagnosis and treatment of conditions covered by the RAPs (Elon and Pawlson 1992). Psychiatrists may be involved in this process either if they are delegated by the facility to coordinate RAPs relevant to mental disorders and behavior problems or if they are consulted regarding patients for whom the RAPs indicate a need for reevaluation.

Regulations related to resident rights and facility practices restrict the use of physical restraints and antipsychotic drugs when they are "administered for purposes of discipline or convenience and not required to treat the resident's medical symptoms." Regulations related to quality of care also require that residents do not receive "unnecessary drugs" and specify that antipsychotic drugs may not be given "unless these are necessary to treat a specific condition as diagnosed and documented in the clinical record." An unnecessary drug is defined as any drug when used 1) in excessive dose (including duplicate therapy); 2) for excessive duration; 3) without adequate monitoring; 4) without adequate indications for its use; 5) in the presence of adverse consequences that indicate that it should be reduced or discontinued; or 6) any combination of the reasons above (HCFA 1991). The guidelines based on these regulations also limit the use of antipsychotic drugs, antianxiety agents, sedative hypnotics, and related drugs (HCFA 1992a). For each of these classes, the guidelines specify a list of acceptable indications, maximum limits for daily doses, requirements for monitoring treatment and adverse effects, and time frames for attempting dose reductions and discontinuation. To minimize concerns about federal interference with medical practice, the current guidelines include qualifying statements that recognize cases in which strict adherence to prescribing limits is "clinically contraindicated." Although the emphasis remains clearly on limiting the use of psychotropic drugs, the guidelines acknowledge that appropriate medical treatment can entail psychotropic drug regimens that depart from these limits. The guidelines instruct surveyors to allow nursing facilities the opportunity to present a rationale for the use of drugs prescribed contrary to the guidelines and to explain why such use is in the best interest of the resident before finding that the facility is not in compliance with the regulations on "unnecessary drugs." Thus, the physician's options for treating nursing home residents need not be restricted by the regulations as long as the clinical reasoning process demonstrates that the benefits to the patient (in terms of symptom relief, improved health status, or improved functioning) outweigh the risks, and the justification is clearly documented in the clinical record. Although the facility, not the physician, is accountable for compliance with the regulations, the physician's clinical reasoning and judgment still play a critical role in the process of ensuring quality care.

In addition to addressing the use of psychotropic drugs, the interpretive guidelines also outline conditions for the use of physical restraints. According to the guidelines, restraints may not be used unless there is documentation that 1) efforts were made to identify and correct preventable or treatable factors that cause or contribute to the problem; 2) that prior attempts to use less restrictive measures failed; and 3) that use of restraints enables the resident to achieve or maintain the highest practicable level of function. Physical or occupational therapists must be consulted if restraints are deemed necessary to enhance body positioning or improve mobility.

The unique and complex problems of geriatric patients together with the federal mandate to ensure quality of care in long-term care settings also define a need for geriatric mental health services in the nursing home (Smith et al. 1990). Under the provision designed to foster quality of care, the regulations require that "the facility must ensure that a resident who displays mental or psychosocial adjustment difficulties receives appropriate services to correct the assessed problem" (HCFA 1991). Despite the attempt to promote case-finding through screening and assessment and provisions for mental health services under quality of care requirements, OBRA legislation and regulations thus far have not addressed deficiencies in access to mental health services for nursing home residents (Conn et al. 1992) or problems related to inadequate funding for such services (Borson et al. 1987; Kane et al. 1991).

Impact of Nursing Home Reform

Positive effects of nursing home reform are becoming apparent. Evidence is beginning to accumulate that significant reductions in antipsychotic drug use can be accomplished without adverse effects. Complementing the process initiated by federal regulations, a number of investigators have developed and evaluated educational programs designed to reduce excessive use of medications in nursing homes. Ray et al. (1987) conducted a statewide controlled trial of the efficacy of an educational visit in reducing antipsychotic drug prescribing for nursing home patients. They found that the use of educational visits to frequent antipsychotic prescribers did not reduce antipsychotic drug prescribing and, consequently, advised that future interventions should address factors within the nursing home that predisposed to antipsychotic drug use. More recently, Ray et al. (1993) evaluated an educational intervention aimed at physicians and nursing staff based on a model of care that included evaluations of patients for reversible medical or psychosocial causes of behavior disorders, nonpharmacological techniques for prevention and management, use of low-dose antipsychotics for serious behavior disorders, and gradual withdrawal of antipsychotics when possible. In nursing homes receiving the intervention, a 72% reduction in antipsychotic use was observed compared with only 13% in control nursing homes. Avorn et al. (1992) also evaluated the efficacy of an educational program in geriatric psychopharmacology aimed at physicians, nurses, and aides. Scores on an index of psychoactive drug use, measuring both the magnitude and the probable inappropriateness of medication use, declined to a significantly greater extent in the experimental compared with control nursing homes. Rovner et al. (1992) evaluated changes in psychotropic prescribing practices and quality assurance data in 17 corporately owned nursing homes in which a pharmacy service provided educational materials about medication use and OBRA regulations to medical directors, primary care physicians, and directors of nursing. Over 6 months, a 36% reduction in neuroleptic use occurred with no increase in sedative-hypnotics or other psychotropic medications. Taken together, these studies provide evidence that reductions in antipsychotic drug use are attainable without significant increases in symptomatology; they support the hypothesis that a significant component of the use of neuroleptics in nursing home residents is unnecessary. Similarly, Schnelle et al. (1992) evaluated management procedures designed to improve staff adherence to federal regulations regarding physical restraints and found that a simple strategy for providing cues to staff was effective in increasing compliance.

Although this recent research demonstrates that methods are available to correct historical patterns of overuse of psychotropic drugs and physical restraints in nursing home residents, they do not address complementary concerns related to ensuring that mental health treatment is made available to those residents who would benefit from it. This becomes especially important when one recognizes that behavioral symptoms in patients with dementia can be more than management problems; they can be symptoms indicating that a patient is experiencing a psychiatric syndrome that is contributing to distress and excess disability.

For all their actual and theoretical limitations, the OBRA 87 regulations constitute a major broad public policy initiative intended to improve the lives of nursing home patients by explicitly recognizing the importance of psychological and social domains of their lives, restricting the use of psychotropic medications and physical restraints, and advocating for specialized rehabilitative services to attain or maintain patients' highest practicable physical, mental, and psychosocial well-being. These regulations both reflect and define a concern about basic contradictions in the conceptualization of nursing home care in this country with regard to the problems that are to be expected when institutions designed and staffed for the residential care of cognitively intact patients with disabling medical and surgical disorders serve a patient population with high levels of dementia. From this perspective, problems such as the misuse of physical restraints and psychotropic medications probably resulted from attempts to care for psychiatric patients in an unsuitable environment. These problems have prompted the comparison of current nursing homes to the primitive mental institutions of the past and have suggested the need for a basic restructuring of care, a paradigm shift, analogous to that through which Philippe Pinel in the late 18th century replaced physical restraints with clinical programs emphasizing the dignity of patients at the mental institutions of Paris. Following this analogy, we are beginning to unchain our patients, but we are only beginning to learn how to treat them effectively and to develop the appropriate resources to accomplish this goal.

Special Care Units: A Paradigm Shift?

Special care units for nursing home care of patients with dementia have evolved to address the specific needs of residents with dementia. Rabins (1986) presciently discussed the pros and cons of establishing special care units in nursing homes. He noted that, at their best, such units can provide informed, compassionate care by recognizing the deficits and strengths of the patients but that their disadvantages can include increased costs, greater stigma by segregation, and uncertain admission and discharge criteria, especially in relation to the changing needs of the population as the disease progresses. Ohta and Ohta (1988) discovered and discussed the heterogeneity of these units and emphasized the need for more research. Holmes et al. (1990) provided the first comprehensive longitudinal assessment of the characteristics of patients in special care units by comparing them with their counterparts with dementia in the same facilities. Although differences in patient characteristics were demonstrated with special care unit patients having more severe cognitive, behavioral, and functional deficits, no deleterious nor beneficial effects associated with special care unit residence were noted during a 6-month period. Gold et al. (1991) developed a typology of care settings that included eight distinct types of special care units and found that they were associated with higher quality care than were traditional units, although the quality of the special care unit was not uniformly outstanding. Sloane et al. (1991) conducted a case-control study of 31 specialized dementia units and 32 traditional units in five states to evaluate the use of physical and pharmacological restraints among 625 patients with dementia and found that residence in a special care unit was associated with reduced use of physical restraints but not with reduced "pharmacological restraint use." Other research (Coleman et al. 1990) has suggested that residence in special care units may be associated with a trend toward increased hospitalization, usually for hip fractures, and that after these hospitalizations, a trend occurred toward greater cognitive decline. Although none of the hospitalizations was judged to be "preventable," it appeared that one cost of personal freedom and encouragement to walk might be a higher risk of falls and fractures. In contrast, other studies have demonstrated that admission to a special care unit appears to provide greater psychological benefit to caregivers (Wells and Jorm 1987) and increased family involvement (Hansen et al. 1988). Some preliminary studies evaluating the benefit of special care units have indicated their value in promoting stability of functional abilities and providing a greater sense of security and well-being (Benson et al. 1987; Rovner et al. 1990a). Encouraged by the research and propelled by both human concerns and profits, 10% of all United States nursing homes had established a special care unit by 1991 (Office of Technology Assessment [OTA] Report: Special Care Units for Persons With Dementia. Personal communication, K. Maslow, 1991). The OTA report found that "existing special care units vary in virtually every respect, including their patient-care philosophies and goals, physical design features, staff-to-resident ratios, activity programs, use of psychotropic medications and physical restraints, admission and discharge practices, and charges." Taking their variability and the limitations of existing studies into consideration, the OTA concluded that little evidence existed to demonstrate the effectiveness of special care units and suggested that we do not know what constitutes effective nursing home care for individuals with dementia. Research designed to define the elements of treatment in special care units and to determine their effectiveness is underway to improve the quality of care for nursing home residents and to inform public policy.

Although the development of special care units has focused on the specific needs of patients with Alzheimer's disease and related disorders, other residents also have "special" needs. Little is known about how to establish an environment in which elderly, cognitively intact patients with disabling medical disorders can most easily find sources of meaning and pleasure in life or about how to deliver basic nursing care for dependent patients in a manner that encourages autonomy and self-respect. Research in these areas is also necessary.

Roles of the Psychiatrist in the Nursing Home

Realizing the goals of nursing home reform and improving the care of nursing home residents with psychiatric disorders must involve bringing the expertise of mental health professionals into the residential care settings. Although a need exists to complement research on the clinical course and treatment of psychiatric disorders in the nursing home with health services research designed to optimize methods for the delivery of mental health care, it is now possible to present a model for the role of the psychiatrist.

Psychiatrists may serve patients and facilities in a number of ways. In the nursing home, as in most practice settings, case-oriented care in which the psychiatrist provides consultations or assessment and treatment for individual residents is a key element of mental health service (Cohn and Smyer 1988). However, the nursing home is a unique setting in which psychiatrists also may establish an ongoing relationship with the facility that includes consultation-liaison activities, staff education, and administrative consultation (Bienenfeld and Wheeler 1989; Borson et al. 1987; Grossberg et al. 1990; Liptzin 1983; Sakauye and Camp 1992). Often a combination of these functions is required to meet the needs of patients, families, nursing home staff, and administrators. Regardless of the extent to which the role for the psychiatrist focuses on the relationship with the patient and family or the facility staff and administration, involvement of a psychiatrist is necessary to address both the psychiatric disorders of the patient and the needs, opportunities, and limitations for treatment that result from the high prevalence of psychiatric disorders within the nursing home setting.

Psychiatric training emphasizes case-oriented models in which the focus is on assessment and management of problems with patients. With case-oriented approaches, care may be provided by the psychiatrist directly through services provided to the patient or indirectly where the psychiatrist serves as a consultant to the patient's primary care physician or the nursing home staff who then, with support from the consultant, carry out recommendations for interventions (Cohn and Smyer 1988). Whether care is provided to patients directly or indirectly, case consultation includes assessment and accurate diagnosis (American Psychiatric Association 1989) in which the emphasis is often on making sense of somatic, affective, cognitive, or behavioral symptoms that may be attributed to underlying psychiatric disorders, medical conditions, medication effects, interpersonal and social variables, and environmental factors (Birkett 1991; Herst and Moulton 1985). These evaluations serve as a foundation for clinical decision making and treatment planning (Goldman and Klugman 1990) in which the relative risks and benefits of appropriate treatment options are considered and recommendations are made. This includes evaluation of whether needed treatment can be provided on-site in the nursing home, or whether services in other mental health care settings such as acute care hospitals or partial hospitalization programs are needed. Admission to the acute care hospital may be necessary as a result of the severity of the psychiatric disorder, the complexity of coexisting medical problems, or the need for specialized diagnostic procedures, close monitoring of pharmacological treatment, or the administration of electroconvulsive therapy.

The task force on nursing homes and mentally ill elderly individuals (American Psychiatric Association 1989) emphasized that "all currently accepted modalities of psychiatric treatment have a place in the treatment of nursing home residents." Treatment options include pharmacological, behavioral, and psychotherapeutic approaches. The process of treatment includes delivery of the intervention, monitoring outcome, anticipating risks, managing adverse effects, and when appropriate, making adjustments to the treatment regimen. Treatment monitoring involves ascertaining when interventions have been of benefit (Vernberg and Repucci 1986) and recommending alternative approaches as indicated when they have not. Another critical element of case consultation involves determining when continuation or maintenance treatment is necessary to maintain gains or prevent the recurrence of symptoms or deterioration in functioning.

Requests for case consultation in the nursing home frequently arise as a result of medicolegal issues. Federal and state regulations that protect the rights of nursing home residents as well as ethical concerns about preserving autonomy require that, as much as possible, residents be empowered to make their own decisions about medical treatments and other matters that affect their lives. However, the high prevalence of dementia and other psychiatric disorders in nursing homes frequently imposes a need for psychiatric consultation to evaluate residents' decision-making capacity. Psychiatric disorders such as dementia and depression can affect comprehension, insight, judgment, and communication; however, the presence of these disorders does not inevitably render patients unable to make decisions on their own (Appelbaum and Roth 1981; Roth et al. 1977). Psychiatric evaluation is therefore often required to evaluate cognitive abilities, language function, communication, and the extent to which the resident understands specific issues related to his or her care. In selected cases, the evaluation of decision-making capacity may include assessments conducted by others including neuropsychologists, speech pathologists, and occupational therapists. Although standardized approaches have been proposed, the clinical examination remains the gold standard and psychiatric consultation is often required to determine whether residents can appropriately make decisions on their own or whether there is a need for activating arrangements for surrogate decision makers, invoking advance directives or substituted judgments, or for advising that the nursing facility or the family petition the courts to arrange for legal guardianship (Janofsky 1990).

In working within nursing homes, psychiatrists function as part of an interdisciplinary care team that may include the primary care physician or the facility medical director, nurses, aides, social worker, rehabilitation and activities staff, dietitian, pharmacist, and administrators who are involved in the process of care (Bienenfeld and Wheeler 1989; Cohn and Smyer 1988; Liptzin 1983; Sakauye and Camp 1992). The relationship of the psychiatrist to each member of the team and to the facility at large may vary from facility to facility. In contrast to the acute inpatient setting in which the psychiatrist generally serves as director or coordinator of the interdisciplinary team, the role in the nursing home may not be well defined initially, as many nursing homes do not have established mechanisms for integrating the functions of the psychiatrist with the rest of the team or for coordinating psychiatric, medical, nursing, and rehabilitation care (Borson et al. 1987). This often constitutes a barrier to the delivery of psychiatric care in the nursing home. In this setting, a wide variety of arrangements may be negotiated or may evolve between the psychiatrist and the nursing home staff or administration to facilitate communication between practitioners of different disciplines and to coordinate care. In response to the administrative and cultural differences between facilities, the psychiatrist may, for example, adopt the role of team member, consultant to the team or to individual team members, or either coordinator or supervisor of mental health services provided more directly by other clinicians.

Regardless of the resultant role of the psychiatrist, a collaboration between the psychiatrist and other members of the treatment team is necessary. Staff consultation is an important component of psychiatric care in the nursing home. Many programs have been described in which nurses and aides rely on consulting psychiatrists to provide guidance in assessing, understanding, and managing patients with psychiatric symptoms and behavioral disturbances (Colthart 1974; Liptzin 1983; Loebel et al. 1991; Sakauye and Camp 1992; Tourigny-Rivard and Drury 1987). However, in collaborative practice, the psychiatrist also relies on the staff for help. The nursing home staff who provide daily direct care for the patients, including supervision or assistance with activities of daily living, have numerous opportunities to participate in the psychiatric assessment process by making observations of clinical signs and symptoms, the context in which behavior problems occur, and the patient's involvement in social, recreational, and therapeutic activities. The psychiatrist needs to incorporate clinical information from staff in conducting evaluations, in formulating psychiatric diagnoses, and in interpreting the outcome of treatment intervention. Through this reciprocal process, staff help the psychiatrist by providing data from patient observations, and the psychiatrist helps the staff to become more skilled in their clinical assessments and teaches them to recognize and understand the characteristic features of the cognitive, affective, and behavior problems of nursing home residents.

Staff consultation also can be used to develop the role of nursing home staff in mental health treatment. Daily direct care provides numerous opportunities for negative as well as positive interactions between staff and patients, and the frequency and intensity of staff-patient contact can either be an important factor in the pathogenesis of psychopathology and behavior problems or a key component in their treatment. Through staff consultation, the psychiatrist can help promote therapeutic staff-patient interactions, and can guide the staff in reducing maladaptive responses and in supporting adaptive behaviors and independent functioning in nursing home residents (American Psychiatric Association 1989; Moses 1982). Similarly, the psychiatric consultant can assist staff in making observations regarding treatment outcome. Thus, staff consultation is a vehicle by which the consulting psychiatrist can help to improve psychiatric assessment and management by facilitating clinical observations and therapeutic interventions during the many hours of direct contact between staff and residents.

Another role for the psychiatrist in the nursing home is to provide staff education (Herst and Moulton 1985). Although case-oriented staff consultation is an effective approach for education (Bienenfeld and Wheeler 1989), case conferences, workshops, and seminars also are potentially useful formats for in-service training (Liptzin 1983; Sakauye and Camp 1992; Smith et al. 1990; Westlake and Rubano 1983). The goals of these educational efforts are usually to increase knowledge about the cognitive, affective, and behavioral disorders that are common in the nursing home (Chartock et al. 1988) and to enhance the staff's ability to recognize psychiatric symptoms, to know when to request consultation, to participate in the management of behavioral disturbances, to help track the effects of treatment, and to monitor patients for adverse drug effects. Dangerous or disruptive behaviors are usually apparent to staff and are likely to prompt requests for psychiatric consultation (Birkett 1991; Loebel et al. 1991). However, education is often necessary to help staff recognize the importance of less drastic presentations of psychiatric disorders with subtle behavioral symptoms such as withdrawal, decreased initiative, diminished activity, or loss of functional abilities (American Psychiatric Association 1989).

The psychiatrist also can serve a role as mental health consultant for administrative matters such as policy formulation, program development, and environmental design. Because the high prevalence of psychiatric disorders can be a source of significant distress for nursing home staff, most of whom do not have specific training in mental health, other goals of administrative consultation may be to improve staff effectiveness and job satisfaction, reduce absenteeism and staff turnover (Cohn and Smyer 1988), and recognize and prevent abuse of nursing home residents. Finally, the psychiatrist's expertise is essential in helping nursing homes comply with federal and state regulations regarding resident rights, assessment of mental health, evaluation of decision-making capacity, and quality of care (including issues related to the use of physical restraints and psychotropic drugs). Beyond the roles of the psychiatrist as a case consultant and provider of clinical care, the psychiatrist can provide administrative consultation regarding systems that ensure appropriate clinical observation by nursing home staff, assessment of psychiatric and behavioral symptoms, monitoring of treatment responses, and documentation in the clinical record.

The development of special care units for patients with Alzheimer's disease and related disorders suggests additional roles for psychiatrists. In these units, where patients are usually admitted because they experience disability resulting primarily from a psychiatric disorder, the physicians with the training and experience to best perform the administrative role of medical director may well be geriatric psychiatrists. Furthermore, for these patients, geriatric psychiatrists could serve a primary care role providing basic medical care as well as specialized psychiatric services.

Conclusions

The prevalence of psychiatric disorders in nursing homes has been estimated to be 80%–90%; the disorders that are most common include the dementias, primarily Alzheimer's disease, and depressions accompanying medical illness. In a real sense, nursing homes are psychiatric institutions, not because they house deinstitutionalized chronic psychiatric patients, but because the frail, elderly patients who require nursing home care have profound needs for psychiatric services. Recent federal regulations and educational initiatives show promise in reducing the misuse of psychotropic drugs and physical restraints that resulted from the mismatch between the design and staffing of nursing homes as sites for the care of patients whose disability is ascribed simply to injury or medical illness and the reality of the nursing home population, in which most patients have mental health needs. The development of special care units for patients with Alzheimer's disease and related disorders represents one approach for revising the basic concepts that underlie nursing home care, but a need exists to define these programs and to determine what elements contribute to effectiveness. Although all nursing homes should have the availability of psychiatric consultation, traditional consultative services alone are not sufficient to meet their needs for mental health expertise. Mental health services should include direct treatment (pharmacological, behavioral, and psychotherapeutic), development of screening programs for case identification, staff education, input into the design of activities and the therapeutic milieu, medicolegal advice, and administrative consultation.

References

American Psychiatric Association: Diagnostic and Statistical Manual of Mental Disorders, 3rd Edition. Washington, DC, American Psychiatric Association, 1980

American Psychiatric Association: Diagnostic and Statistical Manual of Mental Disorders, 3rd Edition, Revised. Washington, DC, American Psychiatric Association, 1987

American Psychiatric Association: Nursing Homes and the Mentally Ill Elderly (Task Force Report No 28). Washington, DC, American Psychiatric Association, 1989

American Psychiatric Association: Diagnostic and Statistical Manual of Mental Disorders, 4th Edition. Washington, DC, American Psychiatric Association, 1994

Ames D: Depression among elderly residents of local-authority residential homes: its nature and the efficacy of intervention. Br J Psychiatry 156:667–675, 1990

Ames D: Epidemiological studies of depression among the elderly in residential and nursing homes. Int J Geriatr Psychiatry 6:347–354, 1991

Ames D, Ashby D, Mann AH, et al: Psychiatric illness in elderly residents of part III homes in one London borough: prognosis and review. Age Aging 17:249–256, 1988

Appelbaum PS, Roth LH: Clinical issues in the assessment of competency. Am J Psychiatry 138:1462–1467, 1981

Ashby D, Ames D, West CR, et al: Psychiatric morbidity as prediction of mortality for residents of local authority homes for the elderly. Int J Geriatr Psychiatry 6:567–575, 1991

Avorn J, Dreyer P, Connelly K, et al: Use of psychoactive medication and the quality of care in rest homes. N Engl J Med 320:227–232, 1989

Avorn J, Soumerai SD, Everitt DE, et al: A randomized trial of a program to reduce the use of psychoactive drugs in nursing homes. N Engl J Med 327:168–173, 1992

Baker FM, Miller CL: Screening a skilled nursing home population for depression. J Geriatr Psychiatry Neurol 4:218–221, 1991

Barnes R, Veith R, Okimoto J, et al: Efficacy of antipsychotic medications in behaviorally disturbed dementia patients. Am J Psychiatry 139:1170–1174, 1982

Barnes RD, Raskind MA: DSM-III criteria and the clinical diagnosis of dementia: a nursing home study. J Gerontol 36:20–27, 1980

Barton R, Hurst L: Unnecessary use of tranquilizers in elderly patients. Br J Psych 112:989–990, 1966

Beardsley RS, Larsen DB, Lyons JS, et al: Health services research in nursing homes: a systematic review of three clinical geriatric journals. J Gerontol Med Sci 41:30–35, 1988

Beers M, Avon J, Soumerai SB, et al: Psychoactive medication use in intermediate-care facility residents. JAMA 260:3016–3020, 1988

Benson DM, Gambert SR: The impact of misdiagnosis on nursing home placement. Psychiatr Med 1:309–316, 1984

Benson DM, Cameron D, Humbach E, et al: Establishment and impact of a dementia unit within the nursing home. J Am Geriatr Soc 35:319–323, 1987

Berrios GE, Brook P: Delusions and psychopathology of the elderly with dementia. Acta Psychiatr Scand 75:296–301, 1985

Bienenfeld D, Wheeler BG: Psychiatric services to nursing homes: a liaison model. Hosp Community Psychiatry 40:793–794, 1989

Birkett PD: Psychiatry in the Nursing Home. Binghamton, NY, Haworth, 1991

Blazer D, Williams CD: Epidemiology of dysphoria and depression in an elderly population. Am J Psychiatry 137:439–444, 1980

Blessed G, Tomlinson BE, Roth M: The association between quantitative measures of dementia and of senile change in the cerebral grey matter of elderly subjects. Br J Psychiatry 114:797–811, 1968

Borson S, Liptzin B, Nininger J, et al: Psychiatry and the nursing home. Am J Psychiatry 144:1412–1418, 1987

Braun JV, Wykle MH, Cowling WR: Failure to thrive in older persons: a concept derived. Gerontology 28:809–812, 1988

Brink TL, Yesavage JA, Lum O, et al: Screening tests for geriatric depression. Clin Gerontol 1:37–43, 1982

Buck JA: Psychotropic drug practice in nursing homes. J Am Geriatr Soc 36:409–418, 1988

Burke WJ, Houston MJ, Boust SJ, et al: Use of the geriatric depression scale in dementia of the Alzheimer type. J Am Geriatr Soc 37:856–860, 1989

Burke WJ, Nitcher RL, Roccaforte WH, et al: A prospective evaluation of the geriatric depression scale in an outpatient geriatric assessment center. J Am Geriatr Soc 40:1227–1230, 1992

Burns BJ, Larson DB, Goldstrom ID, et al: Mental disorder among nursing home patients: preliminary findings from the national nursing home survey pretest. International Journal of Geriatric Psychiatry 3:27–35, 1988

Campion EW, Ban A, May M: Why acute-care hospitals must undertake long-term care. N Engl J Med 308:71–75, 1983

Cape RD: Freedom from restraint. Gerontologist 23 (special issue):217, 1983

Chandler JD, Chandler JE: The prevalence of neuro-psychiatric disorders in a nursing home population. J Geriatr Psychiatry Neurol 1:71–76, 1988

Chartock P, Nevins A, Rzetelny H, et al: A mental heath training program in nursing homes. Gerontologist 28:503–507, 1988

Cohen-Cole SA, Stoudemire A: Major depression and physical illness:

special considerations in diagnosis and biologic treatment. Psychiatr Clin North Am 10:1–17, 1987

Cohen-Mansfield J: Agitated behaviors in the elderly: preliminary results in the cognitively deteriorated. J Am Geriatr Soc 34:722–727, 1986

Cohen-Mansfield J, Billig N: Agitated behaviors in the elderly: a conceptual review. J Am Geriatr Soc 34:711–721, 1986

Cohen-Mansfield J, Marx MS, Rosenthal AS: A description of agitation in a nursing home. J Gerontol 44:M77–M84, 1989

Cohn MD, Smyer MA: Mental health consultation: process, professions, and models, in Mental Health Consultation in Nursing Homes. Edited by Smyer MA, Cohn MD, Brannon D. New York, New York University Press, 1988

Coleman EA, Barbaccia JC, Croughan-Minihane MS: Hospitalization rates in nursing home residents with dementia: a pilot study of the impact of a special care unit. J Am Geriatr Soc 38:108–112, 1990

Colthart SM: A mental health unit in a skilled nursing facility. J Am Geriatr Soc 22:453–456, 1974

Conn DK, Lee V, Steingart A, et al: Psychiatric services: a survey of nursing homes and homes for the aged in Ontario. Can J Psychiatry 37:525–530, 1992

Custer RL, Davis JE, Gee SC: Psychiatric drug usage in VA nursing home care units. Psychiatric Annals 14:285–292, 1984

DeLeo D, Stella AG, Spagnoli A: Prescription of psychotropic drugs in geriatric institutions. International Journal of Geriatric Psychiatry 4:11–16, 1989

Elon R, Pawlson LG: The impact of OBRA on medical practice within nursing facilities. J Am Geriatr Soc 40:958–963, 1992

Evans LK, Strumpf NE: Tying down the elderly: a review of the literature on physical restraint. J Am Geriatr Soc 37:65–74, 1989

Folstein MF, Folstein SE, McHugh PR: "Mini-Mental State" a practical method for grading the cognitive state of patients for the clinician. J Psychiatr Res 12:189–198, 1975

Foster JR, Cataldo JK, Boksay IJE: Incidence of depression in a medical long-term care facility: findings from a restricted sample of new admissions. International Journal of Geriatric Psychiatry 6:13–20, 1991

German PS, Shapiro S, Kramer M: Mental Illness in Nursing Homes: Agenda for Research. Edited by Harper MS, Lebowitz, BD. Rockville, MD, National Institute of Mental Health, 1986, pp 21–40

Gold DT, Sloane PD, Matthew LJ, et al: Special care units: a typology of care settings for memory impaired older adults. Gerontologist 31:

467–475, 1991

Goldman LS, Klugman A: Psychiatric consultation in a teaching nursing home. Psychosomatics 31:277–281, 1990

Grossberg GT, Rakhshanda H, Szwabo PA, et al: Psychiatric problems in the nursing home. J Am Geriatr Soc 38:907–917, 1990

Hansen SS, Patterson MA, Wilson RW: Family involvement on a dementia unit: the resident enrichment and activity program. Gerontology 28:508–514, 1988

Harrison R, Savla N, Kafetz K: Dementia, depression, and physical disability in a London borough: a survey of elderly people in and out of residential care and implications for future developments. Age Aging 19:97–103, 1990

Health Care Financing Administration: Medicare and Medicaid: Requirements for Long-Term Care Facilities, Final Regulations. Federal Register 56:48865–48921, September 26, 1991

Health Care Financing Administration: State Operations Manual: Provider Certification (Transmittal No 250). Washington, DC, U.S. Government Printing Office, April 1992a

Health Care Financing Administration: Medicare and Medicaid Programs: Preadmission Screening and Annual Resident Review. Federal Register 57:56450–56504, November 30, 1992b

Health Care Financing Administration: Medicare and Medicaid: Resident Assessment in Long-Term Care Facilities. Federal Register 57:61614–61733, December 28, 1992c

Herst L, Moulton P: Psychiatry in the nursing home. Psychiatr Clin North Am 8:551–561, 1985

Holmes D, Teresi J, Weiner A, et al: Impact associated with special care units in long-term care facilities. Gerontology 30:178–181, 1990

Horiguchi J, Inami Y: A survey of the living conditions and psychological states of elderly people admitted to nursing homes in Japan. Acta Psychiatr Scand 83:338–341, 1991

Hyer L, Blazer D: Depressive symptoms: impact and problems in long term care facilities. International Journal of Behavioral Gerontology 1:33–44, 1982

Innes EM, Turman WG: Evolution of patient falls. QRB Qual Rev Bull 9:30–35, 1983

Institute of Medicine, Committee on Nursing Home Regulation: Improving the Quality of Care in Nursing Homes. Washington, DC, National Academy Press, 1986

Janofsky JS: Assessing competency in the elderly. Geriatrics 45:45–48, 1990

Kane RL, Garrard J, Buchanan JL, et al: Improving primary care in nursing homes. J Am Geriatr Soc 39:359–367, 1991

Kaplitz SE: Withdrawn, apathetic geriatric patients responsive to methylphenidate. J Am Geriatr Soc 23:271–276, 1975

Katz IR, Parmelee PA: Depression in elderly patients in residential care settings, in Diagnosis and Treatment of Depression in Late Life: Results of the NIH Consensus Development Conference. Edited by Schneider LS, Reynolds CF III, Lebowitz BD, et al. Washington, DC, American Psychiatric Press, 1993, pp 437–461

Katz IR, Lesher E, Kleban M, et al: Clinical features of depression in the nursing home. Int Psychogeriatr 1:5–15, 1989a

Katz IR, Simpson GM, Jethanandani V, et al: Steady state pharmacokinetics of nortriptyline. Neuropsychopharmacology 2:229–236, 1989b

Katz IR, Simpson GM, Curlik SM, et al: Pharmacological treatment of major depression for elderly patients in residential care settings. J Clin Psychiatry 51:41–48, 1990

Katz IR, Parmelee PA, Brubaker K: Toxic and metabolic encephalopathies in long term care patients. Int Psychogeriatr 3:337–347, 1991

Katz IR, Beaston-Wimmer P, Parmelee PA, et al: Failure to thrive in the elderly: exploration of the concept and delineation of psychiatric components. J Geriatr Psychiatry Neurol 6:161–169, 1993

Kramer M, German PS, Anthony JC, et al: Patterns of mental disorders among the elderly residents of eastern Baltimore. J Am Geriatr Soc 33:236–245, 1985

Larsen DB, Lyons JS, Hohmann AA, et al: A systematic review of nursing home research in three psychiatric journals, 1966–1985. International Journal of Geriatric Psychiatry 4:129–134, 1989

Lesher E: Validation of the Geriatric Depression Scale among nursing home residents. Clin Gerontol 4:21–28, 1986

Liptzin B: The geriatric psychiatrist's role as consultant. J Geriatr Psychiatry 16:103–112, 1983

Loebel JP, Borson S, Hyde T, et al: Relationships between requests for psychiatric consultations and psychiatric diagnoses in long-term care facilities. Am J Psychiatry 148:898–903, 1991

Mann AH, Graham N, Ashby D: Psychiatric illness in residential homes for the elderly: a survey in one London borough. Age Aging 13:257–265, 1984

Marin RS: Differential diagnosis and classification of apathy. Am J Psychiatry 147:22–30, 1990

Marin RS: Apathy: a neuropsychiatric syndrome. J Neuropsychiatry Clin Neurosci 3:243–254, 1991

McCarthy P: Why one nursing home and not another? Senior Patient, May/June, 1989, pp 97–102

Morris JN, Hawes C, Fries BE, et al: Designing the national resident assessment instrument for nursing homes. Gerontology 30:293–307, 1990

Moses J: New role for hands-on caregivers: part-time mental health technicians. J Am Health Care Assoc 8:19–22, 1982

Murphy E: The use of psychotropic drugs in long term care (editorial). International Journal of Geriatric Psychiatry 4:1–2, 1989

National Center for Health Statistics: The National Nursing Home Survey. (DHEW Publ No PHS 79-1794). Washington, DC, U.S. Government Printing Office, 1979

National Center for Health Statistics: Use of Nursing Homes by the Elderly: Preliminary Data from the 1985 National Nursing Home Survey (DHHS Publ No PHS 87-1250). Hyattsville, MD, National Center for Health Statistics, 1987

Ohta RJ, Ohta BM: Special units for Alzheimer's disease patients: a critical look. Gerontologist 28:803–808, 1988

Omnibus Reconciliation Act of 1987: P.L. 100-203

Parmelee PA, Katz IR, Lawton MP: Depression among institutionalized aged: assessment and prevalence estimation. J Gerontol 44:M22–M29, 1989

Parmelee PA, Katz IR, Lawton MP: The relation of pain to depression among institutionalized aged. Journal of Gerontology: Psychology Sciences 46:15–21, 1991

Parmelee PA, Katz IR, Lawton MP: Incidence of depression in long term care settings. Journal of Gerontology: Medical Sciences 47:M189–M196, 1992a

Parmelee PA, Katz IR, Lawton MP: Depression and mortality among institutionalized aged. Journal of Gerontology: Psychology Sciences 47:P3–P10, 1992b

Rabins PV: Establishing Alzheimer's disease units in nursing homes: pros and cons. Hosp Community Psychiatry 37:120–121, 1986

Rabins PV, Rovner BW, Larsen DB, et al: The use of mental health measures in nursing home research. J Am Geriatr Soc 35:431–434, 1987

Ray WA, Federspiel CF, Schaffner W: A study of antipsychotic drug use in nursing homes: epidemiologic evidence suggesting misuse. Am J Public Health 70:485–491, 1980

Ray WA, Blazer DG, Schaffner W, et al: Reducing antipsychotic drug prescribing for nursing home patients: a controlled of the effect of an educational visit. Am J Public Health 77:1448–1450, 1987

Ray WA, Taylor JA, Meador KG, et al: Reducing antipsychotic drug use in nursing homes: a controlled trial of provider education. Arch Intern Med 153:713–721, 1993

Risse SC, Cubberley L, Lampe TH, et al: Acute effects of neuroleptic withdrawal in elderly dementia patients. Journal of Geriatric Drug Therapy 2:65–67, 1987

Roth LH, Meisel A, Lidz CW: Tests of competency to consent to treatment. Am J Psychiatry 134:279–284, 1977

Rovner BW, Katz IR: Psychiatric disorders in the nursing home: a selective review of studies related to clinical care. International Journal of Geriatric Psychiatry 8:75–87, 1993

Rovner BW, Kafonek S, Filipp L, et al: Prevalence of mental illness in a community nursing home. Am J Psychiatry 143:1446–1449, 1986

Rovner BW, German PS, Broadhead J, et al: The prevalence and management of dementia and other psychiatric disorders in nursing homes. Int Psychogeriatr 2:13–24, 1990a

Rovner BW, Lucas-Blaustein J, Folstein MF, et al: Stability over one year in patients admitted to a nursing home dementia unit. International Journal of Geriatric Psychiatry 5:77–82, 1990b

Rovner BW, German PS, Brant LJ, et al: Depression and mortality in nursing homes. JAMA 265:993–996, 1991

Rovner BW, Edelman BA, Cox MP, et al: The impact of antipsychotic drug regulations (OBRA 1987) on psychotropic prescribing practices in nursing homes. Am J Psychiatry 149:1390–1392, 1992

Sabin TD, Vitug AJ, Mark VH: Are nursing home diagnosis and treatment inadequate? JAMA 248:321–322, 1982

Sakauye KM, Camp CJ: Introducing psychiatric care in to nursing homes. Gerontologist 32:849–852, 1992

Schneider L, Pollock VE, Liness SA: A meta-analysis of controlled trials of neuroleptic treatment in dementia. JAGS 38:553–563, 1990

Schnelle SF, Simmons SF, Ory MG: Risk factors that predict staff failure to release nursing home residents from restraints. Gerontology 32: 767–770, 1992

Sloane PD, Mathew LS, Scarborough M: Physical and pharmacologic restraint of nursing home patients with dementia: impact of specialized units. JAMA 265:1278–1282, 1991

Smith M, Buckwalter KC, Albanese M: Geropsychiatric education programs: providing skills and understanding. J Psychosoc Nurs Ment Health Serv 28:8–12, 1990

Snowdon J: Dementia, depression, and life satisfaction in nursing homes. International Journal of Geriatric Psychiatry 1:85–91, 1986

Snowdon J, Donnelly N: A study of depression in nursing homes. J Psychiatr Res 20:327–333, 1986

Spagnoli A, Forester G, MacDonald A, et al: Dementia and depression in Italian geriatric institutions. International Journal of Geriatric Psychiatry 1:15–23, 1986

Steele C, Rovner BW, Chase GA, et al: Psychiatric symptoms and nursing home placement in Alzheimer's disease. Am J Psychiatry 147:1049–1051, 1990

Tariot PN, Podgorske CA, Blazina L, et al: Mental disorders in the nursing home: another perspective. Am J Psychiatry 150:1063–1069, 1993

Teeter RB, Garetz FK, Miller WR, et al: Psychiatric disturbances of aged patients in skilled nursing homes. Am J Psychiatry 133:1430–1434, 1976

Tourigny-Rivard MF, Drury M: The effects of monthly psychiatric consultation in a nursing home. Gerontologist 27:363–366, 1987

Trichard L, Zabow A, Gillis LS: Elderly persons in old age homes: a medical, psychiatric and social investigation. S Afr Med J 61:624–627, 1982

Vernberg EM, Repucci ND: Behavioral Consultation, in Handbook of Mental Health Consultation (DHHS Publ No [ADM] 86-1446). Edited by Mannino FV, Trickett EJ, Shore MF, et al. Washington, DC, U.S. Government Printing Office, 1986

Wells Y, Jorm FA: Evaluation of a special nursing home unit for dementia suffers: a randomized controlled comparison with community care. Aust N Z J Psychiatry 21:524–531, 1987

Werner P, Cohen-Masfield J, Braun J, et al: Physical restraint and agitation in nursing home residents. J Am Geriatr Soc 37:1122–1126, 1989

Westlake RJ, Rubano GL: Psychogeriatric seminars for nursing home nurses. Hosp Community Psychiatry 34:1056–1058, 1983

Zimmer JG, Watson N, Treat A: Behavioral problems among patients in skilled nursing facilities. Am J Public Health 74:1118–1121, 1984

Jürgen Unützer, M.D., M.A.
Gary W. Small, M.D.

Geriatric Consultation-Liaison Psychiatry

Consultation psychiatry in general hospitals has always involved a large number of geriatric patients, and some experts have asked for the fields of geriatric psychiatry and consultation-liaison psychiatry to be integrated (Lipowski 1983). Considering the small number of physicians trained in geriatric psychiatry (Small 1993) and the growing number of elderly patients, consultation skills will become increasingly important for geriatric psychiatrists who will often function as consultants rather than primary care physicians.

This chapter concentrates on the challenges presented to the psychiatrist consulting for medically ill elderly patients, the settings in which such work takes place, and models of consultation with some preliminary evidence of their efficacy. This chapter also discusses some commonly encountered problems and suggests practical solutions.

Nature of the Problem

Studies of the hospitalized elderly (Lipowsky 1983; Rabins et al. 1983; Rapp et al. 1988) have found the prevalence of psychiatric problems to range from 27% to 55%, which are rates significantly higher than those found in community-dwelling elderly individuals (George et al. 1988; Weissman et al.

1985). In a prospective study of 102 men older than age 65 years (mean age, 69.3) admitted to the medical wards of a Department of Veterans Affairs hospital, Rapp et al. (1991) found a 27% prevalence of mental disorders. Patients with comorbid psychiatric disorders had greater physical impairment than other medical patients, and only 35% of patients diagnosed with mental disorders at intake received any mental health treatment during a 1-year follow-up.

Elderly patients often have multiple medical conditions that can cause psychiatric symptoms, exacerbate a preexisting psychiatric illness, or complicate necessary treatment. Common psychiatric conditions such as depression and mania can present in an atypical fashion (Goldberg 1989).

The hospital environment presents psychological challenges to medically ill elderly individuals, including the unfamiliar environment, the need to share a room with other patients, frequent interruptions by staff that may change often, little distinction between day and night, and multiple tests and procedures that the patient may not understand. Such situations can be frightening and overwhelming even for those with considerable coping skills and social support. Elderly individuals may have additional stressors such as the loss of autonomy and independent functioning or the recent loss of a loved one. Such stressful situations can lead to regression, maladaptive behaviors, adjustment disorders with various emotional and behavioral features, and, in severe cases, posttraumatic stress disorder. Clinicians often fail to recognize such complex problems or request psychiatric consultation late in the course of the hospitalization.

Demand for Consultation Services

Although only 12% of the population or about 30 million Americans are more than age 65, this group occupies about 30% of all acute hospital beds and consumes about 30% of all expenditures for health care (Allen et al. 1986; Guilford 1988; U.S. Bureau of the Census 1987; U.S. Senate Special Committee on Aging 1984). Over the next 30 years, the demand for hospital care by elderly people is going to rise as this group will likely double or even triple in size.

Most elderly individuals receive treatment for their psychiatric problems from primary care physicians and not from mental health specialists (Regier et al. 1978; Schurman et al. 1985). Some studies suggest that medically ill elderly patients are referred for psychiatric consultation less often than their younger counterparts (Popkin et al. 1984; Rabins et al. 1983).

In a study of 651 consecutive psychiatric consultations, Rabins et al. (1983) found that although 28.5% of hospital beds were occupied by patients 60 years and older, only 21% of the consultations were done on this age group. An explanation for this proportionately lower referral rate may be that primary care physicians consider cognitive dysfunction and behavioral abnormalities a normal part of aging. Clinicians also may overlook psychiatric problems because acute medical problems demand a higher priority, because they are uncomfortable with treating such problems, or believe that treatment is ineffective. Other factors include financial concerns, patient refusal, and a belief that other mental health professionals are more available, can do as well at lower cost, or carry less stigma than psychiatrists (Thompson et al. 1989, 1990). In many instances, older patients are seen as "hopeless drains on the medical system" (Ruskin 1990). Such ageist biases exist among both referring physicians and psychiatrists (Butler 1990; Ford and Sbordone 1980; Sullivan 1989; Traines 1991). The recent finding that age alone is not an adequate predictor of long-term survival and quality of life in critically ill elderly patients challenges such biases (Chelluri et al. 1993).

Settings and Models for Geriatric Psychiatric Consultations

Setting

Most of the literature on geriatric consultation psychiatry focuses on the acute medical/surgical services of general hospitals. Small and Natterson (1988) have described the special challenges presented to patients and consultants in the intensive care unit. Thienhaus et al. (1988) have pointed out that elderly individuals make less use of psychiatric emergency services than younger persons but that they are frequently seen in general hospital emergency rooms and often have significant psychiatric comorbidity. Other settings for consultations include the whole range of psychiatric service settings from outreach to a patient's home (Brown and Lieff 1982; Gurian 1982) to work in a primary care setting, outpatient clinic, day treatment program, retirement community (Rabins et al. 1992), or nursing home. The role of psychiatrists in medical settings is similar to and different from that in long-term care facilities. In a comparative study, Lippert et al. (1990) showed that nursing home patients who are referred for psychiatric consultation are older, more likely to be female, and have dementia more often than patients in general hospitals who receive consultations.

Models of Consultation and Their Effectiveness

In the classic consultation model, the primary physician refers the patient for a psychiatric consultation. Allen et al. (1986) found that a geriatric psychiatry consultation team achieved a much higher rate of compliance with their recommendations than a general psychiatric consultation service (77% versus 21.7%), and the authors speculated that specific expertise in geriatric psychiatry partly explained these differences. Some programs have attempted to generate such expertise by training consultation-liaison psychiatrists in geriatric psychiatry (Lipowsky 1983; Schneider and Plopper 1984; Shulman et al. 1986).

Most studies demonstrating the effectiveness of psychiatric consultations include only limited economic analysis (Ackerman et al. 1988; Boone et al. 1981; Levitan and Kornfeld 1981; Lyons et al. 1986, 1988; Mumford et al. 1984). In a randomized controlled trial, Levitan and Kornfeld (1981) found that elderly patients with a hip fracture who received psychiatric consultation spent 12 fewer days in the hospital and were discharged home rather than placed in a nursing home twice as frequently when compared with the patients who did not receive a consultation. Cole et al. (1991) showed that the differences between a treatment group who received consultations and a control group who received usual medical care were not statistically significant. The most effective consultation services seem to be targeted at high-risk patients likely to benefit from psychiatric intervention such as elderly patients with hip fractures (Shamash et al. 1992). Strain et al. (1991) showed that routine psychiatric screening of elderly patients with hip fractures at admission resulted in an earlier discharge and significant cost savings to the hospital when compared with traditional referrals for consultations.

In the liaison model, the consulting psychiatrist is assigned to a specific clinical setting and performs consultations but also is involved in other ward activities such as staff education and regular meetings with the medical team. Although the liaison model can improve patient access to psychiatric services, provide "meaningful involvement with other medical disciplines" (Folks and Kinney 1991), and is intuitively attractive, current reimbursement mechanisms generally do not compensate for such services and data on their cost-effectiveness are limited.

Small and Fawzy (1988) have described a collaborative model of care practiced at a large university teaching hospital in which primary care physicians, specialists in geriatric medicine, consultation-liaison psychiatrists, and geriatric psychiatrists interact. This interaction is based on shared training experiences with a focus on the elderly patient. Although initial data look promising, this model has not been studied in a clinical trial with adequate controls. Arie and Jolley (1982) also have described the value of such cooperation among multiple professional disciplines in the care of elderly patients.

Another approach has been to establish geriatric assessment units in general hospitals. Although all of these units do not include geriatric psychiatrists, most use general psychiatric consultation services. Preliminary studies indicate that such units may improve health outcomes and level of functioning and contain costs (Arie and Dunn 1973; Rubenstein 1984; Rubenstein et al. 1982; Swenson and Perez 1986).

In recent years, many hospitals have developed inpatient units that care for medically ill psychiatric patients. In such units, geriatric psychiatrists may work together with specialists in geriatric medicine (Fogel 1985; Koran and Barnes 1982). So far, information on the cost-effectiveness of such units is limited but early findings appear promising (Fogel 1989; Fogel et al. 1985; Lewis et al. 1993; Stoudemire et al. 1987).

One of us (GWS) has developed a telephone consultation service to rural Department of Veterans Affairs medical centers. Given the lack of geriatric psychiatrists, such arrangements can be used for consultation and as a means of disseminating the current state of knowledge in the field. Unfortunately, such services are generally not reimbursed under current funding mechanisms.

Data on the cost-effectiveness of the above-mentioned models are limited but vital in advocating for the inclusion of geriatric psychiatry consultation services in any health plan. We need to determine referral criteria, find ways of identifying at-risk patients, improve the efficacy and quality of consultations, and devise strategies to maximize the compliance with recommendations, while always remaining conscious of the costs of these services.

Reimbursement for Geriatric Psychiatry Consultations

In the past, Medicare has reimbursed psychiatric consultations on a one-time basis with limited reimbursement for follow-up visits, which were usually billed as medical psychotherapy (American Psychiatric Association

1993). Such financial constraints have made it difficult to provide comprehensive consultation services on an inpatient basis (Hales et al. 1984) and adequate postdischarge follow-up, one of the strongest predictors of favorable outcome (Cole 1991). Reimbursement is even lower for psychiatrists working in nursing homes, but several proposed policy changes provide reasonable Medicare payments for such services (American Psychiatric Association 1993).

Working With the Medical Team

Establishing a Working Relationship

An effective working relationship with the referring clinician is essential for the success of a consultation. Criticisms of psychiatric consultations often mention a perception that psychiatrists isolate themselves from the rest of the medical community and do not keep up with developments in general medicine. Other criticisms include confusion about what a psychiatrist does and a feeling that psychiatrists often cannot agree on diagnostic or treatment issues (Baker 1987; Thompson et al. 1990; West and Walsh 1975). Psychiatrists working with medically ill elderly individuals should keep up with developments in general medicine and be able to "speak the consultee's language." Use of standard terminology as described in DSM-IV (American Psychiatric Association 1994) often reduces concerns about the unreliability of psychiatric diagnoses. Consultants also should try to use clear and practical language that patients, family members, and nonpsychiatric physicians can understand. The consultation can be an opportunity to teach other clinicians about geriatric psychiatry. Pasnau's (1985) "ten commandments of medical etiquette for psychiatrists" urge the consultant to communicate in person with the clinicians that requested advice, to respect them as fellow physicians and colleagues, to be available and prompt, to give concrete suggestions, to follow-up, and "not to preach." Such etiquette builds and maintains harmonious relationships with medical colleagues and ultimately improves psychiatry's image.

Defining the Question

Compared with younger patients, medically ill elderly individuals are referred more often for agitation and competency assessment (Levitte and

Thornby 1989; Popkin et al. 1984; Rabins et al. 1983; Ruskin 1985; Small and Fawzy 1988). Other common requests involve the assessment of depression, anxiety, psychosis, and organic mental disorders, or help with medication management, treatment compliance (Thompson et al. 1989), and psychiatric follow-up (Small and Fawzy 1988). The request may be limited, asking for transfer of a patient to a psychiatric unit or for help with arranging psychiatric follow-up. At other times, the request points to a comprehensive assessment with detailed recommendations for treatment and follow-up.

Consultation requests usually contain "stated and unstated questions" (Baker 1987) with considerable discrepancy between the consultee's initial question and the underlying problem. In such cases, the consultant can often help redefine and reframe the question, while respecting and addressing the referring physician's initial request. The consultant may assist the referring physician, the ward staff, or the family in understanding and coping with psychological aspects of a patient's illness (Karasu et al. 1977). The consultant should also attempt to address the concerns and agendas of such "informal consultees" as family members, caregivers, case managers, and ward staff (Baker 1987).

Recommendations

The written report should not contain all of the information gathered but instead focus on data pertinent to the case. The report should be concise and easily understood by nonpsychiatric colleagues. Table 32–1 gives a format for organizing the information.

The summary can be arranged in a problem list format that includes the questions asked, major psychiatric syndromes detected with a differential diagnosis, recommendations for further diagnostic evaluation, and suggestions for management, disposition, and follow-up. Recommendations should be specific (e.g., list specific drug doses and side effects) and clear about who will be responsible for the proposed interventions. Whenever possible, the consultant should provide answers to the questions asked, but other important issues and "unstated" questions should be addressed as well.

Direct communication with the referring physician, other team members, the patient, and family members is usually as important as the written consultation. This communication can clarify any questions about the purpose of the consultation or the treatment recommendations and improve compliance.

Table 32–1. Elements of a geriatric psychiatry consultation

Identification of patient and referral source; reason for consultation
History of the presenting problem(s) with prior treatments
Psychiatric review of systems and functional assessment
Past psychiatric history
Family history
Past medical history; medications; allergies
Developmental and social history; assessment of social support
Mental status examination: Mini-Mental State Exam score and depression
    rating scale
Physical examination
Laboratory data
Assessment with differential diagnosis
Recommendations: include forensic issues, diagnostic workup, medications,
    psychotherapy, behavior and environmental management, disposition, and
    follow-up, as needed

Evaluation

Approach to Medically Ill Elderly Individuals

Sensory and cognitive deficits, pain, noise, frequent interruptions, and limited privacy can make the evaluation of elderly people in the general hospital a difficult task. Elderly patients often view the consulting psychiatrist with guardedness, as this generation grew up during a time when the stigma attached to mental illness was even greater than it is today. The patient may fear that a psychiatric consultation means that someone thinks that they are "crazy" or wants to "put them away." To overcome such barriers, the psychiatrist needs to speak clearly, convey the purpose of the evaluation, and address the patient's fears and concerns in a sensitive manner.

Ruskin (1990) has noted that visual and hearing impairments occur in 40% and 30% of hospitalized elderly individuals, respectively. To cope with these impairments, Goldberg (1989) recommends that the psychiatrist always stay in full view of the patient and speak in low deep tones because high-frequency hearing is often diminished in elderly individuals. Consultants should remember, however, that not all elderly people either experience or have hearing impairment.

Age-related bias, ageism, and countertransference can cloud clinical judgment, and consultants should show respect for elderly patients by addressing them by their surnames (Goldberg 1989). Yager (1989) suggests beginning the consultation by providing "tangible" help such as adjusting the patient's pillow or position in bed or asking about pain.

Diagnostic Workup

Because of frequent cognitive impairment in medically ill elderly individuals, the consultant often depends on collateral sources such as relatives, caregivers, other clinicians, or old medical records. In addition to the usual thorough psychiatric assessment, the following elements are particularly relevant in evaluating the medically ill elderly.

In the history, the patient's presenting problems, symptoms, and functional limitations are detailed with their development over time and treatment history. This includes neurovegetative signs and symptoms of depression. Any recent psychosocial stressors or medication changes that may correlate with the onset or exacerbation of psychiatric symptoms should be pursued. Queries about alcohol or substance use and an assessment of suicidal risk should be routine.

A functional assessment should concentrate on changes from baseline functioning and activities of daily living (ADLs). Ruskin (1990) pointed out that as many as 60% of hospitalized elderly individuals are impaired in at least one ADL, and 10% depend on others for all of their ADLs. Cohen et al. (1992) found that ADL measures were stronger predictors of mortality after hospitalization than medical diagnoses. Pinholt et al. (1987) showed that physicians and nurses often miss moderately significant impairments in mental status, nutrition, vision, and continence. Standard tools for functional assessment can assist clinicians in identifying impairments that may be improved through early intervention.

The past medical history includes all medications taken (prescription and over-the-counter). This history may require a review of the hospital medication records, the help of a family member who can bring in medications from home, or a call to the patient's outside physician or pharmacist. The problem of polypharmacy in elderly individuals is significant, with one study finding 83% of elderly patients in the community taking 2 to 6 drugs while 14% were taking between 7 and 15 drugs daily (Chien 1979). The consultant also should consider possible medical causes of psychiatric symptoms (Table 32–2) and pay attention to gait, continence, nutritional history, hearing, vision, and other sensory losses.

The developmental/social history covers important life events such as recent losses. It also addresses educational level, work history and retirement, financial and legal problems, current living situation, relationships, social contacts, and supports.

The mental status examination should include a thorough assessment of cognitive functioning and may use standard cognitive screening instruments (Nelson et al. 1986). Such instruments as the Mini-Mental State

Table 32–2.   Some causes of organic mental disorders in medically ill
                  elderly individuals

Drugs	Multiple sclerosis
Alcohol (abuse, withdrawal, and	Normal pressure hydrocephalus
dependence)	Parkinson's disease
Antiarrhythmics (lidocaine,	Postanoxia
procainamide)	Stroke and transient ischemic attack
Anticonvulsants	Subdural hematoma
Antihypertensives (reserpine,	Tumor and paraneoplastic
clonidine, methyldopa,	syndromes
β-blockers)	**Collagen vascular disorders**
Antineoplastic agents	Systemic lupus erythematosus
Antiparkinsonian agents	Temporal arteritis
(amantadine, bromocriptine,	**Deficiency states**
levodopa)	Folate
Atropine and other anticholinergic	Thiamine
medications	Vitamin B_{12}
Barbiturates	**Infection**
Benzodiazepines	Hepatitis
Caffeine	Influenza
Cimetidine	Pneumonia
Digoxin	Tuberculosis
Illicit drugs (abuse, withdrawal, and	Meningitis (fungal, syphilis,
dependence)	carcinomatous)
Isoniazid	Encephalitis (HIV, herpes, Epstein-
Narcotic analgesics	Barr, other viruses)
Nonsteroidal anti-inflammatories	**Metabolic and endocrine disorders**
Psychotropic medications (also	Addison's disease
consider withdrawal)	Cushing's disease
Steroids (e.g., prednisone,	Fluid and electrolyte disturbances
estrogen)	Hypomagnesemia
Sympathomimetics	Parathyroid disorders
Theophylline	Pheochromocytoma
Thyroid hormones	Thyroid disorders
Central nervous system	**Organ failure**
Alzheimer's disease	Anemia
Amyotrophic lateral sclerosis	Renal failure
Epilepsy	Liver failure
Head injury	Congestive heart failure
Huntington's disease	Myocardial infarction

Exam (MMSE) (Folstein et al. 1975) have norms for age and educational level (Crum et al. 1993) and can be useful in screening for cognitive impairment in delirium or dementia and in following such functioning over time. The numerical ratings also provide a way of standardizing and communicating one's assessment to others. Such brief scales can miss mild cognitive deficits, especially in patients with focal lesions in the right hemisphere, and false-positive findings can occur in patients with little formal education. Screening instruments for depression include the Geriatric Depression Scale, a 30-item self-rating scale (Yesavage et al. 1983), the Cornell Scale for Depression in Dementia (Alexopoulos et al. 1988a, 1988b), and an 8-item clinician-rated Extracted Hamilton Depression Rating Scale (XHDRS) (Rapp et al. 1990). These scales provide quantitative measures of the degree of depression and are useful in assessing antidepressant drug response.

At times, the consultant performs a limited physical examination concentrating on vital signs, a neurological examination to evaluate abnormal movements (e.g., extrapyramidal symptoms from parkinsonism or neuroleptics), focal weakness, abnormal deep tendon reflexes, or on other areas as clinically indicated. Especially when patients are agitated and uncooperative, the referring physician may miss an important finding.

The utility of routine laboratory studies in psychiatric inpatients is limited (Anfinson and Kathol 1992; Sheline and Kehr 1990), but in medically ill elderly people, such tests may be useful in ruling out potentially reversible medical causes of psychiatric symptoms. They include a chemistry panel with liver and renal function tests; calcium, magnesium, and phosphorous evaluation; a complete blood count; thyroid function tests; and a urinalysis. Other useful tests include vitamin B_{12} and folate levels, blood or urine toxicology screens, a test for syphilis, an electrocardiogram, arterial blood gases, and screens for heavy metals. Structural imaging such as computed tomography or magnetic resonance imaging are helpful in evaluating the possibility of an intracranial mass or lesion when there are focal neurological signs or symptoms. A lumbar puncture is indicated for patients with suspected central nervous system infection. In certain instances, neuropsychological testing and functional imaging such as positron-emission tomography or single-photon emission computed tomography are useful in the evaluation of dementia. An electroencephalogram can be useful in evaluating a possible seizure disorder or organic mental disorder and in diagnosing and following patients with delirium.

Clinical Applications

Frequently Encountered Clinical Syndromes and Problems

The psychiatric disorders diagnosed most frequently among elderly patients in general hospitals include organic mental disorders, mood disorders, and adjustment disorders (Grossberg et al. 1990; Levitte and Thornby 1989; Mainprize and Rodin 1987; Popkin et al. 1984; Ruskin 1985; Small and Fawzy 1988) (Table 32–3). Compared with younger patients, medically ill elderly individuals are less often diagnosed with somatoform, anxiety, and personality disorders (Popkin et al. 1984; Small and Fawzy 1988). At times, the diagnosis is clear, but at other times the consulting psychiatrist is called to assess and treat a clinical syndrome such as agitated or disruptive behavior that may have a broad differential diagnosis.

Agitation and Disordered Behavior

Consultants are often called to see patients who are exhibiting agitated, disruptive, and sometimes dangerous behaviors on the medical/surgical wards. Such behaviors can include screaming, wandering, refusing treatment, assaulting staff, or self-destructive action, and they are often frightening to the patient, the family, and the hospital staff. The causes for the disordered behavior range widely from longstanding personality disorders to delirium and organic mental disorders, early or late-onset schizophrenia, delusional disorders or mood disorders, all of which are discussed in more detail below. The consultant should first ensure the safety of the patient and staff and then try to discern the underlying cause of the problem behavior.

Table 32–3. Primary psychiatric diagnoses for elderly patients receiving psychiatric consultations in general hospitals

Study	N	Disorder frequency (%)			
		Organic mental	Affective	Adjustment	Psychotic
Grossberg et al. 1990	147	37	28	26	2
Levitte and Thornby 1989	384	37	25	—	5
Small and Fawzy 1988	88	47	55	22	16
Mainprize and Rodin 1987	238	51	17	15	7
Ruskin 1985	67	37	24	—	16
Popkin et al. 1984	266	46	23	9	—

In some cases, the disturbance results from miscommunication between patient and staff that can be resolved by a meeting of all parties (Ruskin 1990). Such efforts at simplifying and improving communication patterns also can help patients with underlying personality disorders by maximizing their sense of control and information. These situations also may call for ongoing psychotherapy and a behavior management program that provides structure, clarifies the basic rules and conditions of treatment, allows more effective limit setting, and minimizes splitting. Sometimes psychiatrists must help the staff tolerate a patient's feelings of anger and entitlement.

Severely disturbed or psychotic behavior often requires pharmacological treatment. In such cases, a high-potency neuroleptic such as haloperidol or droperidol is safe and effective even with severely medically ill patients (Santos et al. 1992; Tesar and Stern 1988; Ziehm 1991). Although haloperidol does not have U.S. Food and Drug Administration approval for intravenous administration, this route is generally safe and has almost no effect on pulmonary or cardiovascular parameters (Sos and Cassem 1980). Metzger and Friedman (1993), however, reported three cases of prolongation of the corrected Q-T interval or torsades de pointes arrhythmia during treatment with intravenous haloperidol. Small doses (e.g., 0.5–1 mg intravenously or intramuscularly) can be doubled every 20 minutes until the patient is sedated. Once sedation is adequate, the amount needed to sedate the patient is used in calculating a schedule for a standing daily dose (e.g., 1 mg intravenously every 6 hours) with extra doses as needed to control further agitation. One should minimize the cumulative dose and observe for the development of extrapyramidal symptoms and akathisia that can worsen the agitation. These side effects may be less severe when haloperidol is administered intravenously (Menza et al. 1988; Sanders et al. 1989). Benzodiazepines such as 0.5 to 1 mg of lorazepam also can be useful in the treatment of acute agitation and anxiety and can reduce the total dose of neuroleptic required. Treatment of underlying medical problems such as hypoxia, hypoglycemia or hypertension, withdrawal states, and pain often reduces agitation (Tesar 1993). Anticholinergic medications or β-blockers are sometimes effective for agitation secondary to akathisia but may be contraindicated in medically ill elderly individuals because of their cognitive and cardiovascular side effects. In such cases, low doses of benzodiazepines may be preferable. The treatment of chronic aggression and agitation is discussed elsewhere (Colenda 1988; Gleason and Schneider 1990; Risse and Barnes 1986; Sakauye et al. 1993; Yudofsky et al. 1990).

When agitated behavior is refractory to behavioral and psychopharmacological management and is threatening the safety of the patient or staff, physical restraint may become necessary. In many cases, consultants are called after a patient is already restrained. Physical restraint is an infringement of patients' rights and may expose the physician to charges of battery if used inappropriately. Physical restraint also may worsen the patient's frustration, anxiety, and agitation. Consequently, it should be used only when necessary and when other less-restrictive alternatives have failed. Personnel must be trained in the proper technique for the use of the equipment and monitoring of the patient's safety.

Organic Mental Disorders

Organic mental disorders are the most commonly diagnosed psychiatric conditions in the general hospital (Table 32–1). They include delirium, dementia, organic affective and anxiety disorders, psychoses, and other psychiatric presentations of underlying medical problems (see Table 32–2). The resulting cognitive impairments are often associated with an increase in the length of hospital stay (Binder and Robins 1990).

Delirium

Delirium is one of the most commonly encountered problems in a medical setting and is also referred to as "confusion," "sundowning," and "ICU psychosis." It can be described as an acutely developing global cerebral dysfunction that manifests clinically by fluctuating consciousness, sleep-wake disturbances, disorientation, decreased attention span, perceptual disturbances, and agitation or lethargy. For elderly patients on medical and surgical wards, the frequency of delirium ranges from 10% to 50% (Williams-Russo et al. 1992). It is common in the intensive care unit and after open heart surgery, hip surgery, and other major orthopedic procedures (Gustafson et al. 1988; Smith and Dimsdale 1989; Williams-Russo et al. 1992). Delirium is frequently caused by a number of organic factors, although the exact pathogenesis often cannot be established. Erkinjutti et al. (1986) showed that delirium occurs more frequently in patients with compromised cerebral functioning such as patients with a preexisting dementia. In the treatment of delirium, the consulting psychiatrist may recommend additional diagnostic evaluation of underlying medical conditions and psychopharmacological management with high-potency neuroleptics such as haloperidol or droperidol and environmental modifications as described earlier.

Psychosis

Psychotic symptoms in hospitalized elderly individuals are common and can be the result of a preexisting psychiatric disorder, dementia, or delirium. Other causes include loss of vision (Holroyd et al. 1992), hearing (Post 1980), other medical conditions, and medications (see Table 32–2). Psychotic symptoms, for example, frequently occur in the treatment of Parkinson's disease. If no prior history of psychosis exists, an organic cause must be strongly suspected and pursued.

At times, elderly patients who may be mistrustful, suspicious and fearful when entering the hospital can become paranoid, especially after a few nights of sleep deprivation. In such cases, reassurance, improving the communication with the medical team, and rest may be sufficient, but if the psychotic symptoms become severe and disabling and interfere with proper medical care, a high-potency neuroleptic such as haloperidol or fluphenazine in small doses should be considered. Compared with lower potency neuroleptics, these agents have a lower incidence of anticholinergic side effects and orthostatic hypotension, a major risk factor for falls and fractures in medically ill elderly individuals.

Alcohol, Substance, and Prescription Drug Abuse

Elderly patients often underreport alcohol use (Atkinson 1990), and physicians in the emergency department or in an inpatient setting frequently fail to detect alcohol abuse (Adams et al. 1992), which may range from 15% to 50% in elderly inpatients (Adams et al. 1992; Bristow and Clare 1992; Curtis et al. 1989). In a nationwide analysis of claims data, Adams et al. (1993) found high rates of alcohol-related hospitalizations in elderly people (54.7 per 10,000 population for men and 14.8 per 10,000 population for women) despite the problem with underrecognition and underreporting of alcohol use. These rates were similar to those for myocardial infarction.

Alcohol, illicit drugs, and prescription and over-the-counter drugs may contribute to psychiatric symptoms such as depression, anxiety, and psychosis or cause serious withdrawal symptoms in medically ill elderly patients (Beresford et al. 1988). Alcohol withdrawal is treated with short- to intermediate-acting benzodiazepines, and attention to associated medical problems such as thiamine deficiency, dehydration, and electrolyte abnormalities is essential. Detoxification should not be attempted until concomitant medical conditions have been treated and are stable.

Spectrum of Depressive Disorders

Koenig et al. (1988) found that the prevalence of depressive disorders among medically ill geriatric inpatients ranged from 25% to 50%. Major depression in this population ranges from 6% to 45% and is strongly associated with impaired physical health and function (Koenig et al. 1993). Depression is often not noted or treated by primary physicians and persists after discharge in a majority of cases (Koenig et al. 1992). Comorbid depression has been associated with greater mortality (Katz et al. 1988; Rovner et al. 1991), lower rates of functional recovery (Gurland et al. 1986; Harris et al. 1988), worse functional outcomes after hip fractures (Mossey et al. 1990), and longer hospital stays (Ackerman et al. 1988; Verbosky et al. 1993). Reding et al. (1986) showed that stroke patients treated with nortriptyline had better functional outcomes. In their sample of depressed inpatients, Verbosky and associates (1993) found that depressed patients treated with antidepressants and supportive therapy stayed 31.8 days less than patients with untreated major depression.

The diagnosis of depression in medically ill elderly individuals can be complicated because depression often presents with cognitive and somatic complaints, sleep disturbance, appetite disturbance, decreased libido, poor energy, psychomotor retardation, and poor concentration and without the classic changes in mood and affect (Folks and Kinney 1991). Stoudemire (1985) refers to such patients who deny affective or emotional symptoms and focus predominantly on somatic complaints as having a "masked depression." Such vegetative and somatic symptoms, however, are common in all medically ill patients and the relationship between physical illness, somatic symptoms, and depression is far from clear (Cavanaugh 1984; Kathol and Petty 1981; Pelchat 1992). Endicott (1984) has emphasized the difficulty of applying standard sets of diagnostic criteria for depression in cancer patients and suggested modified research diagnostic criteria. Kathol et al. (1990) found that these modified criteria diagnosed depression less frequently than DSM-III-R criteria for major depression. Another concern is that patients and physicians alike may incorrectly attribute depressive symptoms to the normal aging process or feel that it is a "natural response" to the illness and therefore not treatable (Endicott 1984).

Kennedy et al. (1991) found, in a sample of randomly selected Medicare recipients, that untoward changes in physical health and disability contributed substantially to the onset of depressive symptoms and to the chronicity of depression. In studies of nursing home residents, Parmelee et al. (1991) showed a significant association between pain and depression in a sample of randomly selected Medicare recipients and suggested that depressed elderly patients may be more sensitive to somatic pain. Although additional studies are needed, many clinicians emphasize cognitive symptoms of depression (e.g., excessive pessimism and guilt) when diagnosing depression in the context of physical illness and treat symptoms empirically if the diagnosis remains unclear. By contrast, Small et al. (1986) found guilt expression to be less frequent and less severe in a sample of physically healthy elderly patients with major depression when compared with young adults with depression.

Medical conditions that cause organic affective disorders with depressive symptoms include stroke (Robinson et al. 1986; Starkstein et al. 1988; Stern and Bachman 1991), Parkinson's disease (40% of patients show depressive symptoms) (Cummings 1992), dementia, and other neurological illnesses. Lipsey et al. (1986) has shown that the phenomenology of poststroke depression does not differ from that of primary major depression. Early studies have pointed out an association between left anterior stroke and depression (Eastwood et al. 1989; Robinson and Starkstein 1990; Robinson et al. 1984; Sinyor et al. 1986). Poststroke depression also has been associated with a higher 10-year poststroke mortality (Morris et al. 1993) and higher rates of impairment of both physical activities and language functioning at 2-year follow-up (Parikh et al. 1990). Hypothyroidism, a condition found in 9.4% of hospitalized elderly individuals (Livingston et al. 1987), is another common cause. Table 32–2 lists others such as malnutrition, cancer, and metabolic disturbances.

The dementia syndrome of depression, a condition sometimes encountered in medically ill elderly individuals, can have signs and symptoms similar to a primary dementia but is secondary to depression and may be reversible with antidepressant treatment (Caine 1981; Cummings and Benson 1992; Wells 1979). In practice, this differential diagnosis is sometimes difficult. In many cases, the consultant recommends a therapeutic trial of antidepressant drugs and follow-up of the cognitive deficits over time.

The differential diagnosis of depression in hospitalized elderly individuals also includes adjustment disorders and grief reactions. Folks and Kinney (1991) point out that grief may occur as a reaction to the loss of a significant other or the loss of one's health and independence. The treatment of acute or prolonged grief usually involves psychotherapy, but in cases when there are suicidal thoughts, anhedonia, or weight loss, the patient may have a major depressive disorder that requires treatment with antidepressants (Brown and Stoudemire 1983; Folks and Ford 1985; Folks and Kinney 1991; Zisook and Shuchter 1993).

The pharmacological treatment of depression in medically ill elderly individuals has been reviewed by the recent National Institutes of Health consensus development conference on the diagnosis and treatment of depression in late life (Katz 1993; Reynolds et al. 1993). The panel concluded that "the evidence is contradictory whether concurrent medical illness has an adverse effect on response to pharmacotherapy" but goes on to suggest that "although medical comorbidity probably results in increased vulnerability to side effects, vigorous but careful treatment is still indicated." Such treatment includes secondary amine tricyclic antidepressants (e.g., nortriptyline, desipramine) (Small 1989b, 1991) and the newer antidepressants such as bupropion (Kane et al. 1983; Roose et al. 1991) and the selective serotonin reuptake inhibitors (Altamura et al. 1989; Cohn et al. 1990; Dunner et al. 1992; Feighner et al. 1988; Holliday and Plosker 1993; Hutchinson et al. 1992; Preskorn 1993), although the experience with the newer antidepressants in medically ill elderly individuals is still limited. In patients with insomnia, the sedating side effects of trazodone can be useful, but this drug can cause significant orthostatic hypotension. When antidepressants are contraindicated for medical reasons and a rapid effect is desired, psychostimulants such as methylphenidate can be useful, particularly in withdrawn, apathetic, and anergic patients (Ayd 1985; Kaufmann et al. 1982; Pickett et al. 1990). Anecdotal reports indicate efficacy using doses of 5–10 mg of methylphenidate orally twice or three times per day (Gurian and Rosowsky 1990; Roccaforte and Burke 1990), although little evidence exists for a long-term antidepressant effect. Electroconvulsive therapy is another highly effective and safe treatment for medically ill depressed patients (Welch 1993). Electroconvulsive therapy may be particularly useful if antidepressants are medically contraindicated, if the patient is psychotic or suicidal, or if the patient's physical health is severely compromised (e.g., inability to eat because of depression).

Anxiety

Using a random sample of the general population, Wells et al. (1988) have shown that people with chronic medical conditions had a 15.3% prevalence of anxiety disorders during a 6-month period compared with 6.6% for control subjects without such medical conditions. Estimates for anxiety disorders in medical inpatients range from 5% to 20% (Strain et al. 1981; Wise and Rieck 1993).

Anxiety in hospitalized elderly individuals often can be severe and disabling. Anxiety can result from the stress of hospitalization, the pain and suffering from a serious medical illness, or the impending loss of autonomy, health, or life. Other patients may have preexisting anxiety disorders or anxiety secondary to medical conditions such as cardiovascular and pulmonary disease, hyperthyroidism, medications, or drug intoxication and withdrawal. Patients with chronic obstructive pulmonary disease, for example, have a higher incidence of panic attacks that decreases as respiratory function is improved (Wise and Rieck 1993). Anxiety also may be a manifestation of depression and delirium.

The consultant should approach the anxious patient with an empathic and supportive attitude and attempt to understand the patient's concerns and fears. Sometimes this calls for efforts to improve the communication between a patient and the treatment team. Underlying medical conditions should be eliminated or treated. Pharmacological treatments for anxiety in the medically ill include short-acting benzodiazepines or buspirone (Stoudemire and Moran 1993; Wise and Rieck 1993). Benzodiazepines in low doses are generally safe but can cause paradoxical disinhibition and excitement, cognitive impairment, ataxia and falls, and dependence. They also can impair respiratory functioning at high doses, or worsen sleep apnea, particularly in patients with preexisting lung disease. Other useful treatments for anxiety include relaxation techniques, hypnosis, guided imagery, and biofeedback.

Somatization Disorders

When considering the possibility of a somatization disorder, the consultant should take a thorough history of any prior somatization disorders and explore the nature of the signs and symptoms as well as possible stressors, symbolic meanings of the symptoms, and secondary gains. The consultant also should consider the relationship of the patient to the referring physician (Ruskin 1990). Somatization can be seen as an effort to relieve anxiety in response to emotional discomfort and distress (Sakauye 1986) and as an effort to legitimize one's need for attention. In medically ill elderly individuals, the consultant must ensure that the referring physician has not overlooked an underlying medical problem or a major depression manifesting with somatic complaints. For additional discussion of somatopsychic symptoms and hypochondriacal behavior see Folks and Kinney (1991), Folks and Ford (1985), and Folks et al. (1990).

Suicidal Behavior

Severe and terminal medical illness, loss, chronic pain, and substance abuse are among the risk factors for elderly individuals that attempt suicide. In a retrospective study of 246 individuals who completed suicide at age 50 or older and who were divided into four age groups, Conwell et al. (1990) found that with increasing age physical illness and loss were the most common stressors associated with completed suicide, whereas other stressors such as job and financial pressures, family and relationship problems, and alcohol abuse became less frequent. Lyness et al. (1992) studied 168 consecutive patients age 60 years and older admitted to an adult psychiatric inpatient unit at Yale–New Haven hospital. Of these patients, 25 had made a suicide attempt, and 80% of those had a major depressive syndrome. Patients who had made more severe suicide attempts were more likely to have a psychotic depression, although this trend was not statistically significant. No significant differences were noted in symptomatic and functional outcomes between attempters and the entire cohort of elderly individuals in this study. Although depression is common in medically ill elderly individuals, its signs and symptoms can be atypical, and it is frequently not recognized or treated. Elderly individuals that attempt suicide are more likely to be successful (Richardson et al. 1989) and less likely to communicate their suicidal intentions than younger individuals (Bock 1972). At times, suicides can be masked as accidental overdoses or age-related deaths.

In the case of "passive suicide," a patient may attempt to starve to death or stop life-sustaining medication or treatments. When confronted with such a situation, clinicians must be careful not to engage in therapeutic nihilism because of ageism or other biases.

Competency and Capacity

The question of competency is frequently encountered by the consultation-liaison psychiatrist and usually arises when a patient's wishes conflict with the plans of the treatment team. A psychiatric consultant may be called to determine the patient's competency to consent to or refuse treatment. In such cases, psychiatrists find the patient incompetent in 75% of cases (Ruskin

1990) but must be careful not to deprive elderly patients of their right to choose or refuse a particular treatment (Small and Natterson 1988).

The consultant should clarify the specific area of competency in question (Folks and Kinney 1991) and remind the consultee about the difference between competency and capacity. The question of competency is a legal one that cannot be answered by a psychiatrist but is determined by judicial review. If a court rules that a patient is incompetent, it may appoint a substitute decision maker. The consulting psychiatrist can, however, give an expert opinion about the patient's capacity to give informed consent to a specific procedure or treatment, to refuse treatment, and to make advance directives (including do not resuscitate orders) or a will. Such advance directives may become activated when a patient loses the capacity to make such decisions.

In patients with fluctuating mental status, an effort should be made to assess them while they are lucid and able to express their wishes (Ruskin 1990). In true medical emergencies when there is a question of the patient's ability to give informed consent, most jurisdictions allow for care to be delivered against a patient's will.

Additional Treatment Considerations

Medications

Although primary care physicians are still by far the largest prescribers of psychotropic medications to elderly individuals (Larson et al. 1991), a geriatric psychiatrist can be helpful with the complex task of using these medications in medically ill elderly people (Small 1989; Small and Natterson 1988; Stoudemire and Moran 1993; Stoudemire et al. 1987, 1990, 1991). Several studies have shown that psychiatrists consulting for elderly patients in the general hospital commonly recommend psychotropic medications (Popkin et al. 1984; Rosse et al. 1986; Ruskin 1985; Small and Fawzy 1988). Medical illness can further exaggerate altered pharmacokinetics in elderly individuals, and, in general, clinicians should "start low and go slow," follow target symptoms, carefully monitor for the emergence of side effects, and allow sufficient time for the drug to reach effective plasma and receptor site concentration (Abernethy 1992). Medically ill elderly individuals often take several medications that can cause or worsen psychiatric problems or have undesirable interactions with psychotropic medications (Salzman 1992). Tune et al. (1992) found that 10 of the 25 drugs most commonly prescribed for elderly individuals have anticholinergic side effects that could be associated with impairments in memory and attention even in normal elderly individuals. Patients with organic mental syndromes may be particularly susceptible to the cognitive impairment from benzodiazepines and anticholinergic medications or the extrapyramidal symptoms from neuroleptics. In some cases, consultants have to recommend a simplification of the patient's current medication regimen rather than adding another drug.

In many cases, patients have medical conditions that complicate the pharmacological management of a psychiatric condition. Patients with underlying pulmonary disease and respiratory insufficiency, for example, may be particularly sensitive to benzodiazepines, which can depress respiration and may worsen sleep apnea (Garner et al. 1989; Thompson and Thompson 1993). Buspirone, which has been found to be an effective anxiolytic in elderly patients (Bohm et al. 1990; Feighner 1987; Napoliello 1986; Robinson et al. 1988; Salzman 1992), does not cause cognitive impairment, sedation, respiratory depression, or withdrawal symptoms and thus may be a safer anxiolytic in patients with respiratory disease and sleep apnea (Mendelson et al. 1991). Preliminary evidence suggests that buspirone may have stimulatory effects on respiratory drive (Garner et al. 1989; Mendelson et al. 1990) and may be useful in patients being weaned from a respirator (Gammans et al. 1989; Hart et al. 1991; Stoudemire et al. 1990). Kiev and Domantay (1988) have shown that buspirone is effective and well tolerated in combination with pulmonary medications such as terbutaline and theophylline.

Antidepressants have little or no effect on respiratory status. Borson et al. (1992) have successfully used nortriptyline in 32 depressed patients with chronic obstructive pulmonary disease. The drug was well tolerated without worsening of pulmonary disease and with significant improvement in anxiety and certain respiratory symptoms. Thompson and Thompson (1985) have reported the safe use of other tricyclic antidepressants in patients with respiratory diseases. Reviews of fluoxetine in the treatment of elderly patients with depression do not report any adverse effects of this drug in conjunction with pulmonary medications (Cooper 1988; Feighner et al. 1988).

In addition to their use in medically ill patients with depression, psychostimulants may be useful in the treatment of elderly patients with apathy and anergy associated with physical illness and dementia. Maletta and Winnegarden (1993) reviewed the literature and reported the successful use of methylphenidate to reverse anorexia in three elderly, severely demented patients with apathy who had stopped eating. Methylphenidate is generally well tolerated even in people over age 80 (Gurian and Rosowsky 1993) and can be given sublingually in patients who cannot eat. Side effects include insomnia, which can be avoided by giving doses early in the day, anorexia, headaches, tachycardia and palpitations, and a feeling of jitteriness that can be treated with low doses of benzodiazepines (Spar and LaRue 1990). Stimulants also can worsen psychotic symptoms and suicidal thinking.

Psychotherapy

The literature on the effectiveness of psychotherapy in elderly individuals is limited (Weiss and Lazarus 1993), but most clinicians agree that psychotherapy can be beneficial for the hospitalized elderly patient. Supportive individual psychotherapy aimed at minimizing the patient's distress and maximizing a sense of autonomy, control, and self-esteem by building on remaining strengths and adaptive skills is often used. Common patient concerns include fear of pain, disability, abandonment, loneliness, and dependency. The consultant should try to address such issues, help the patient grieve and adjust to losses, and try to understand the psychological meaning of the illness and the hospitalization. Other techniques such as cognitive or interpersonal therapy (Snyderman and Thompson 1993), guided imagery, or hypnosis also can be useful. Consultants can provide education about the illness and help patients cope with intellectual deficits. Other times, psychotherapy may involve work with the family or staff, helping them deal with emotions such as anger, guilt, frustration, and helplessness. Other characteristics of psychotherapy with hospitalized elderly individuals include brief sessions and frequent interruptions and invasions of the usual privacy of the doctor-patient relationship.

Behavior Management and Environmental Modification

Although psychotherapy is not always indicated in the treatment of a hospitalized patient, the consulting psychiatrist can sometimes help to coordinate efforts for behavior management and environmental modification. Such measures may include frequent reorientation and reassurance, the presence of family members and familiar faces or objects. They also may involve reducing noise, light, interruptions, and other disturbances in an intensive care setting. The consultant may work with the ward staff to generate a behavioral management program for particularly difficult patients.

Disposition and Follow-Up

To help with disposition, the consulting psychiatrist should be knowledgeable about different services and placements available to elderly individuals such as retirement communities, nursing homes, meals on wheels organizations, homemaker services, visiting nurses, outpatient and day treatment programs, and supportive services for caregivers. Psychiatrists unfamiliar with this area should work with discharge planners or social workers with appropriate expertise. Geriatric psychiatrists also can help patients and families negotiate the difficult task of placing a patient in a care setting outside the home.

A psychiatric follow-up during the patient's hospitalization ensures the maximum effect of the consultation. Allen et al. (1986) found that the ability to provide follow-up and to help with discharge planning improves compliance with the recommendations of consultants. Postdischarge follow-up also can be an important predictor of a consultation's long-term effectiveness (Cole 1991). In their study of depressed elderly medical/surgical patients, Sadavoy and Reiman-Sheldon (1983) attributed high relapse rates to ineffective follow-up. In an ideal setting, the consulting psychiatrist could arrange for psychiatric follow-up on an outpatient basis or make a home visit (Folks and Kinney 1991). If the psychiatric or behavioral symptoms are severe, a transfer to an inpatient psychiatric unit for further evaluation and treatment may be indicated.

References

Abernethy DR: Psychotropic drugs and the aging process: pharmacokinetics and pharmacodynamics, in Clinical Geriatric Psychopharmacology, 2nd edition. Edited by Salzman C. Baltimore, MD, Williams & Wilkins, 1992, pp 61–76

Ackerman AD, Lyons JS, Hammer JS, et al: The impact of coexisting depression and timing of psychiatric consultation on medical patients' length of stay. Hosp Community Psychiatry 39:173–176, 1988

Adams WL, Magruder-Habib K, Trued S, et al: Alcohol abuse in elderly emergency department patients. J Am Geriatr Soc 40:1236–1240, 1992

Adams WL, Zhong Y, Barboriak JJ, et al: Alcohol-related hospitalizations of elderly people. JAMA 270:1222–1225, 1993

Alexopoulos GS, Abrams RC, Young RC, et al: Cornell Scale for depression in dementia. Biol Psychiatry 23:271–284, 1988a

Alexopoulos GS, Abrams RC, Young RC, et al: Use of the Cornell Scale in nondemented patients. J Am Geriatr Soc 36:230–236, 1988b

Allen CM, Becker PM, McVey LJ, et al: A randomized, controlled clinical trial of a geriatric consultation team: compliance with recommendations. JAMA 255:2617–2621, 1986

Altamura AC, DeNovelis F, Guercetti G, et al: Fluoxetine compared with amitriptyline in elderly depression: a controlled clinical trial. Int J Pharmacol Res 9:391–396, 1989

American Psychiatric Association: Selected Models of Practice in Geriatric Psychiatry: A Task Force Report of the American Psychiatric Association. Washington, DC, American Psychiatric Association, 1993

American Psychiatric Association: Diagnostic and Statistical Manual of Mental Disorders, 4th Edition. Washington, DC, American Psychiatric Association, 1994

Anfinson TJ, Kathol RG: Screening laboratory evaluation in psychiatric patients: a review. Gen Hosp Psychiatry 14:248–257, 1992

Arie T, Dunn T: A "do it yourself" psychiatric geriatric joint patient unit. Lancet 2:1313–1316, 1973

Arie T, Jolley D: Making services work: organization and style of psychogeriatric services, in The Psychiatry of Late Life. Edited by Levy R, Post F. London, Blackwell Scientific, 1982, pp 222–251

Atkinson RM: Aging and alcohol use disorders: diagnostic issues in the elderly. Int Psychogeriatr 2:55–70, 1990

Ayd F: Psychostimulant therapy for depressed medically ill patients. Psychiatric Annals 15:462–465, 1985

Baker FM: Consultation-liaison activities with geriatric patients. J Natl Med Assoc 79:1259–1262, 1987

Beresford T, Blow F, Brower K, et al: Alcoholism and aging in the general hospital. Psychosomatics 29:61–72, 1988

Binder EF, Robins LN: Cognitive impairment and length of hospital stay in older persons. J Am Geriatr Soc 38:759–766, 1990

Bock EW: Aging and suicide: the significance of marital, kinship, and alternative relations. Fam Coord 21:71–79, 1972

Bohm C, Robinson DS, Gammans RE, et al: Buspirone therapy in anxious elderly patients: a controlled clinical trial. J Clin Psychopharmacol 10 (suppl 3):47S–51S, 1990

Boone C, Coulton C, Keller S: The impact of coexisting depression and timing of psychiatric consultation of medical patients' length of stay. Soc Work Health Care 7:1–9, 1981

Borson S, McDonald GJ, Gayle T, et al: Improvement in mood, physical symptoms, and function with nortriptyline for depression in patients with chronic obstructive pulmonary disease. Psychosomatics 33:190–201, 1992

Bristow MF, Clare AW: Prevalence and characteristics of at-risk drinkers among elderly acute medical inpatients. Br J Addict 87:291–294, 1992

Brown R, Lieff JD: A program for treating isolated elderly patients living in a housing project. Hosp Community Psychiatry 33:147–150, 1982

Brown JT, Stoudemire A: Normal and pathologic grief. JAMA 250:378–381, 1983

Butler RN: A disease called ageism (editorial). J Am Geriatr Soc 38:178–180, 1990

Caine E: Pseudodementia: current concepts and future directions. Arch Gen Psychiatry 38:1359–1364, 1981

Cavanaugh SV: Diagnosing depression in the hospitalized patient with chronic medical illness. Clin Psychiatry 45:13–16, 1984

Chelluri L, Pinsky MR, Donahoe MP, et al: Long-term outcome of critically ill elderly patients requiring intensive care. JAMA 269:3119–3123, 1993

Chien CP: Substance use and abuse among the community elderly: the medical aspect, in Drug Abuse Among the Aged. Edited by Peterson DM. New York, Spectrum, 1979

Cohen HJ, Saltz CC, Samsa G, et al: Predictors of two-year post-hospitalization mortality among elderly veterans in a study evaluating a geriatric consultation team. J Am Geriatr Soc 40:1231–1235, 1992

Cohn CK, Shrivastava R, Mendels J, et al: Double-blind, multicenter comparison of sertraline and amitriptyline in elderly depressed patients. J Clin Psychiatry 51 (suppl 12B):28–33, 1990

Cole MG: Effectiveness of three types of geriatric medical services: lessons for geriatric psychiatric services. Can Med Assoc J 144:1229–1240, 1991

Cole MG, Fenton FR, Engelsmann F, et al: Effectiveness of geriatric psychiatry consultation in a acute care hospital: a randomized clinical trial. J Am Geriatr Soc 39:1183–1188, 1991

Colenda CC: Buspirone in treatment of agitated demented patients. Lancet 1:1169, 1988

Conwell Y, Rotenberg M, Caine ED: Completed suicide at age 50 and over. J Am Geriatr Soc 38:640–644, 1990

Cooper GL: The safety of fluoxetine—an update. Br J Psychiatry 3:77–86, 1988

Crum RM, Anthony JC, Bassett SS, et al: Population-based norms for the Mini-Mental State Examination by age and educational level. JAMA 269:2386–2391, 1993

Cummings JL: Depression and Parkinson's disease: a review. Am J Psychiatry 149:443–454, 1992

Cummings JL, Benson F: Dementia: A Clinical Approach, 2nd Edition. Stoneham, MA, Butterworth-Heineman, 1992

Curtis JR, Geller G, Stokes EJ et al: Characteristics, diagnosis, and treatment of alcoholism in elderly patients. J Am Geriatr Soc 37:310–316, 1989

Dunner DL, Cohn JB, Walshe T III, et al: Two combined, multicenter double-blind studies of paroxetine and doxepin in geriatric patients with major depression. J Clin Psychiatry 53:57–60, 1992

Eastwood MR, Rifat SL, Nobbs H, et al: Mood disorder following cerebrovascular accident. Br J Psychiatry 154:195–200, 1989

Endicott J: Measurement of depression in patients with cancer. Cancer 53 (suppl 10):2243–2249, 1984

Erkinjutti T, Wikstrom J, Palo J, et al: Dementia among medical inpatients: evaluation of 2000 consecutive admissions. Arch Intern Med 146:1923–1926, 1986

Feighner JP: Buspirone in the long-term treatment of generalized anxiety disorder. J Clin Psychiatry 48 (suppl 12):3–6, 1987

Feighner JP, Boyer WF, Meredith CH, et al: An overview of fluoxetine in geriatric depression. Br J Psychiatry 3:150–158, 1988

Fogel BS: A psychiatric unit becomes a psychiatric-medical unit: administrative and clinical implications. Gen Hosp Psychiatry 7:26–35, 1985

Fogel BS: Med-psych units: financial viability and quality assurance. Gen Hosp Psychiatry 11:17–22, 1989

Fogel BS, Stoudemire A, Houpts JL: Contrasting models for combined medical-psychiatric inpatient treatment. Am J Psychiatry 142:1085–1089, 1985

Folks DG, Ford CV: Psychiatric disorders in geriatric medical/surgical patients, I: report of 195 consecutive consultations. South Med J 78:239–241, 1985

Folks DG, Kinney FC: Consultation-liaison in the general hospital, in Comprehensive Review of Geriatric Psychiatry. Edited by Sadavoy J, Lazarus LW, Jarvik LF. Washington, DC, American Psychiatric Press, 1991

Folks DG, Ford CV, Houck CA: Somatoform disorders, factious disorders, and malingering, in Clinical Psychiatry for Medical Students. Philadelphia, PA, JB Lippincott, 1990

Folstein MF, Folstein SE, McHugh PH: Mini-Mental State: a practical method for grading the cognitive state of patients for the clinician. J Psychiatr Res 12:189–198, 1975

Ford CV, Sbordone RJ: Attitudes of psychiatrists toward elderly patients. Am J Psychiatry 137:571–575, 1980

Gammans RE, Westrick ML, Shea JP, et al: Pharmacokinetics of buspirone in elderly subjects. J Clin Pharmacol 29:72–78, 1989

Garner SJ, Eldridge FL, Wagner PG, et al: Buspirone, an anxiolytic drug that stimulates respiration. Am Rev Respir Dis 139:946–950, 1989

George LK, Blazer DG, Winfield-Laird I, et al: Psychiatric disorders and mental health service use in later life: evidence from the Epidemiological Catchment Area Program, in Epidemiology and Aging. Edited by Brody J, Maddox GL. New York, Springer, 1988

Gleason RP, Schneider LS: Carbamazepine treatment of agitation in Alzheimer's outpatients refractory to neuroleptics. J Clin Psychiatry 51:115–118, 1990

Goldberg RL: Geriatric consultation/liaison psychiatry, in Issues in Geriatric Psychiatry, Vol 19. Edited by Billig N, Rabins PV. Basel, Karger, 1989, pp 138–150

Grossberg GT, Zinny GH, Nakra BRS: Geriatric psychiatry consultations in a university hospital. Int Psychogeriatr 2:161–168, 1990

Guilford DM (ed): The Aging Population in the Twenty-first Century. Washington, DC, National Academy Press, 1988

Gurian B: Mental health outreach and consultation services for the elderly. Hosp Community Psychiatry 33:142–147, 1982

Gurian B, Rosowsky E: Low-dose methylphenidate in the very old. J Geriatr Psychiatry Neurol 3:152–154, 1990

Gurian B, Rosowsky E: Methylphenidate treatment of minor depression in very old patients. American Journal of Geriatric Psychiatry 1:171–174, 1993

Gurland BJ, Golden R, Lantigua R, et al: The overlap between physical conditions and depression in the elderly: a key to improvement in service delivery. in The Patient and Those Who Care: The Mental Health Aspect of Long-Term Physical Illness. Edited by Nayer D. Nantucket, MA, Watson Publishers International, 1986

Gustafson Y, Berggreen D, Brännström B, et al: Acute confusional states in elderly patients treated for a femoral neck fracture. J Am Geriatr Soc 36:525–530, 1988

Hales RE, Holtz JL, Cassem EH: Issues in reimbursement for consultation-liaison psychiatry. Hosp Community Psychiatry 35:1195–1198, 1984

Harris RE, Mion LC, Patterson MB, et al: Severe illness in older patients: the association between depressive disorders and functional dependency during the recovery phase. J Am Geriatr Soc 36:890–896, 1988

Hart RP, Colenda CC, Hamer RM: Effects of buspirone and alprazolam on the cognitive performance of normal elderly subjects. Am J Psychiatry 148:73–77, 1991

Holliday SM, Plosker GL: Paroxetine: a review of its pharmacology, therapeutic use in depression and therapeutic potential in diabetic neuropathy. Drugs and Aging 3:278–299, 1993

Holroyd S, Rabins PV, Finkelstein D, et al: Visual hallucinations in patients with macular degeneration. Am J Psychiatry 149:1701–1706, 1992

Hutchinson DR, Tong S, Moon CA, et al: Paroxetine in the treatment of elderly depressed patients in general practice: a double-blind comparison with amitriptyline. Int Clin Psychopharmacol 6 (suppl 4):43–51, 1992

Kane JM, Cole K, Sarantakos S, et al: Safety and efficacy of bupropion in elderly patients: preliminary observations. J Clin Psychiatry 44:134–136, 1983

Karasu TB, Plutchnik R, Conte H, et al: What do physicians want from a psychiatric consultation service? Compr Psychiatry 18:73–81, 1977

Kathol RG, Petty F: Relationship of depression to medical illness: a critical review. J Affect Disord 3:111–121, 1981

Kathol RG, Mutgi A, William J, et al: Diagnosis of major depression in cancer patients according to four sets of criteria. Am J Psychiatry 147:1021–1024, 1990

Katz IR: Drug treatment of depression in the frail elderly: discussion of the NIH consensus development conference on the diagnosis and treatment of depression in late life. Psychopharmacol Bull 29:101–108, 1993

Katz IR, Curlik S, Nemetz P: Functional psychiatric disorders in the elderly, in Essentials of Geriatric Psychiatry. Edited by Lazarus LW. New York, Springer, 1988

Kaufmann M, Murray G, Cassem N: Use of psychostimulants in medically ill depressed patients. Psychosomatics 23:817–819, 1982

Kennedy GJ, Kelman HR, Thomas C: Persistence and remission of depressive symptoms in late life. Am J Psychiatry 148:174–178, 1991

Kiev A, Domantay AG: A study of buspirone coprescribed with bronchodilators in 82 anxious ambulatory patients. J Asthma 25:281–284, 1988

Koenig HG, Meador KG, Cohen HJ, et al: Depression in elderly hospitalized patients with medical illness. Arch Intern Med 148:1929–1936, 1988

Koenig HG, Veeraindar G, Shelp F, et al: Major depression in hospitalized medically ill elder men: documentation, management, and outcome. International Journal of Geriatric Psychiatry 7:25–34, 1992

Koenig HG, O'Connor CM, Guarisco SA, et al: Depressive disorder in older medical inpatients on general medicine and cardiology services at a university teaching hospital. Am J Geriatr Psychiatry 1:197–210, 1993

Koran LM, Barnes L: The Stanford comprehensive medicine unit: integrating psychiatric and medical care, in New Directions for Mental Health Services: Treatment for Psychosomatic Problems No 15. Edited by Kuldan J. San Francisco, CA, Jossey-Bass, 1982

Larson DB, Lyons JS, Hohmann AA, et al: Psychotropics prescribed to the US elderly in the early and mid 1980s: prescribing patterns of primary care practitioners, psychiatrists, and other physicians. International Journal of Geriatric Psychiatry 6:63–70, 1991

Levitan S, Kornfeld D: Clinical and cost benefits of liaison psychiatry. Am J Psychiatry 138:790–793, 1981

Levitte SS, Thornby JI: Geriatric and nongeriatric psychiatry consultation: a comparison study. Gen Hosp Psychiatry 11:339–344, 1989

Lewis LD, Wohlreich GM, Mintzer J: Admission to a geropsychiatric behavioral intensive care unit. Am J Geriatr Psychiatry 1:263–264, 1993

Lipowsky Z: The need to integrate liaison psychiatry and geropsychiatry. Am J Psychiatry 140:1003–1005, 1983

Lippert GP, Conn D, Schogt B, et al: Psychogeriatric consultation: general hospital versus home for the aged. Gen Hosp Psychiatry 12:313–318, 1990

Lipsey JR, Spencer WC, Rabins PV, et al: Phenomological comparison of poststroke depression and functional depression. Am J Psychiatry 143(4):527–529, 1986

Livingston EH, Hershman JM, Sawin CT, et al: Prevalence of thyroid disease and abnormal thyroid tests in older hospitalized and ambulatory persons. J Am Geriatr Soc 35:109–114, 1987

Lyness JM, Conwell Y, Nelson JC: Suicide attempts in elderly psychiatric inpatients. J Am Geriatr Soc 40: 320–324, 1992

Lyons JS, Hammer JS, Strain JJ, et al: The timing of psychiatric consultation in the general hospital stay. Gen Hosp Psychiatry 8:159–168, 1986

Lyons JS, Larson DB, Burns BJ, et al: Psychiatric co-morbidities and patients with head and spinal cord trauma: effects on acute hospital care. Gen Hosp Psychiatry 10:292–297, 1988

Mainprize E, Rodin G: Geriatric referrals to a psychiatric consultation-liaison service. Can J Psychiatry 32:5–9, 1987

Maletta GJ, Winnegarden T: Reversal of anorexia by methylphenidate in apathetic, severely demented nursing home patients. American Journal of Geriatric Psychiatry 1:234–243, 1993

Mendelson WB, Martin JV, Rapoport DM: Effects of buspirone on sleep and respiration. Am Rev Respir Dis 141:1527–1530, 1990

Mendelson WB, Maczaj M, Holt J: Buspirone administration to sleep apnea patients. J Clin Psychopharmacol 11:71–72, 1991

Menza MA, Murray GB, Holmes VF, et al: Controlled study of extrapyramidal reactions in the management of delirious, medically ill patients. Heart Lung 17:238–241, 1988

Metzger E, Friedman R: Prolongation of the corrected QT and torsades de pointes cardiac arrythmia associated with intravenous haloperidol in the medically ill. J Clin Psychopharm 13:128–132, 1993

Morris PL, Robinson RG, Andrzejewski P, et al: Association of depression with 10-year poststroke mortality. Am J Psychiatry 150(1):124–129, 1993

Mossey JM, Knott K, Craik R: The effects of persistent depressive symptoms on hip fracture recovery. J Gerontol 45:163–168, 1990

Mumford E, Schlesinger HJ, Glass GV, et al: A new look at evidence about reduced cost of medical utilization following mental health treatment. Am J Psychiatry 141:1145–1148, 1984

Napoliello MJ: An interim multicentre report on 677 anxious geriatric out-patients treated with buspirone. Br J Clin Pract 40:71–73, 1986

Nelson A, Fogel BS, Faust D: Bedside cognitive screening instruments: a critical assessment. J Nerv Ment Dis 174:73–83, 1986

Parikh RM, Robinson RG, Lipsey JR, et al: The impact of poststroke depression on recovery in activities of daily living over a 2-year follow-up. Arch Neurol 47:785–789, 1990

Parmelee PA, Katz IR, Lawton MP: The relation of pain to depression among institutionalized aged. J Gerontol 46:15–21, 1991

Pasnau RO: Ten commandments of medical etiquette for psychiatrists. Psychosomatics 26:128–132, 1985

Pelchat RJ: Presentations and management of depression in medical-surgical patients. New Dir Ment Health Serv 57:19–27, 1992

Pickett P, Masand P, Murray G: Psychostimulant treatment of geriatric depressive disorders secondary to medical illness. J Geriatr Psychiatry Neurol 3:146–151, 1990

Pinholt EM, Kroenke K, Hanley JF, et al: Functional assessment of the elderly: a comparison study of standard instruments with clinical judgment. Arch Intern Med 147:484–488, 1987

Popkin MK, Mackenzie TB, Callies AL: Psychiatric consultation to geriatric medically ill inpatients in a university hospital. Arch Gen Psychiatry 41:703–707, 1984

Post F: Paranoid, schizophrenia-like and schizophrenia states in the aged, in Handbook of Mental Health and Aging. Edited by Birren JE, Sloane RB. Englewood Cliffs, NJ, Prentice-Hall, 1980

Preskorn SH: Recent pharmacologic advances in antidepressant therapy for the elderly. Am J Med 94 (suppl 5A):2–12, 1993

Rabins P, Lucas MJ, Teitelbaum M, et al: Utilization of psychiatric consultation for elderly patients. J Am Geriatr Soc 31:581–585, 1983

Rabins PV, Storer DJ, Lawrence MP: Psychiatric consultation to a continuing care retirement community. Gerontologist 32:126–128, 1992

Rapp SR, Parisi SA, Walsh DA: Psychological dysfunction and physical health among elderly medical inpatients. J Consult Clin Psychol 56:851–855, 1988

Rapp SR, Smith SS, Britt M: Identifying comorbid depression in elderly medical patients: use of the Extracted Hamilton Depression Rating Scale. J Consult Clin Psychol 2:243–247, 1990

Rapp SR, Parisi SA, Wallace CE: Comorbid psychiatric disorders in elderly medical patients: a 1-year prospective study. J Am Geriatr Soc 39:124–131, 1991

Reding MJ, Orto LA, Winter SW, et al: Antidepressant therapy after stroke: a double-blind trial. Arich Neurol 43:763–765, 1986

Regier DA, Goldberg ID, Taube CA: The de facto US mental health services system: a public health perspective. Arch Gen Psychiatry 35:685–693, 1978

Reynolds CF III, Lebowitz BD, Schneider LS: Diagnosis and treatment of depression in late life: The NIH consensus development conference on the diagnosis and treatment of depression in late life: an overview. Psychopharmacol Bull 29:83–100, 1993

Richardson R, Lowenstein S, Weissberg M: Coping with the suicidal elderly: a physician's guide. Geriatrics 9:43–51, 1989

Risse SC, Barnes R: Pharmacological treatments of agitation associated with dementia. J Am Geriatr Soc 34:368–376, 1986

Robinson RG, Starkstein SE: Current research in affective disorders following stroke. Journal of Neuropsychiatry and Clinical Neurosciences 2:1–14, 1990

Robinson RG, Kubos KL, Starr LB, et al: Mood disorders in stroke patients: importance of lesion location. Brain 107:81–93, 1984

Robinson RG, Lipsey JR, Rao K, et al: A 2-year longitudinal study of poststroke mood disorder: a comparison of acute-onset with delayed onset depression. Am J Psychiatry 143:1238–1244, 1986

Robinson D, Napoliello MJ, Schenk J: The safety and usefulness of buspirone as an anxiolytic drug in elderly versus young patients. Clin Ther 10:740–746, 1988

Roccaforte WH, Burke WJ: Use of psychostimulants for the elderly. Hosp

Community Psychiatry 41:1330–1333, 1990

Roose SP, Dalack GW, Glassman AH, et al: Cardiovascular effects of bupropion in depressed patients with heart disease. Am J Psychiatry 148:512–516, 1991

Rosse RB, Ciolino CP, Gurel L: Utilization of psychiatric consultation with an elderly medically ill inpatient population in a VA hospital. Milit Med 151:583–586, 1986

Rovner BW, German PS, Brant LJ, et al: Depression and mortality in nursing homes. JAMA 265:993–996, 1991

Rubenstein L: Effectiveness of a geriatric evaluation unit: a randomized clinical trial. N Engl J Med 309:1664–1670, 1984

Rubenstein L, Rhee L, Kane RL: The role of geriatric assessment units in caring for the elderly: an analytic review. J Gerontol 37:513–521, 1982

Ruskin P: Geropsychiatric consultation in a university hospital: a report on 67 referrals. Am J Psychiatry 142:333–336, 1985

Ruskin P: Principles of consultation-liaison, in Verwoerdt's Clinical Geropsychiatry, 3rd Edition. Edited by Bienenfeld D. Baltimore, MD, Williams & Wilkins, 1990

Sadavoy J, Reiman-Sheldon E: General hospital geriatric psychiatric treatment: a follow-up study. J Am Geriatr Soc 31:200–205, 1983

Sakauye KM: Interface of emotional and behavioral conditions with physical disorders in nursing homes, in Mental Illness in Nursing Homes: Agenda for Research. Rockville, MD, National Institute of Mental Health, 1986

Sakauye KM, Camp CJ, Ford PA: Effects of buspirone on agitation associated with dementia. American Journal of Geriatric Psychiatry 1:82–84, 1993

Salzman C: Clinical Geriatric Psychopharmacology, 2nd Edition. Baltimore, MD, Williams & Wilkins, 1992

Sanders K, Minnema AM, Murray GB: Low incidence of extrapyramidal symptoms in treatment of delirium with intravenous haloperidol and lorazepam in intensive care unit patients. J Intensive Care Med 4:201–204, 1989

Santos AB, Wohlreich MM, Pinosky ST: Managing agitation in the critical care setting. J S Carolina Med Assoc 88:386–391, 1992

Schneider L, Plopper M: Geropsychiatry and consultation-liaison services. Am J Psychiatry 141:721–722, 1984

Schurman RA, Kramer PD, Mitchell JB: The hidden mental health network. Arch Gen Psychiatry 42:89–94, 1985

Shamash K, O'Connell K, Lowy M, et al: Psychiatric morbidity and outcome in elderly patients undergoing emergency hip surgery: a one year follow-up study. International Journal of Geriatric Psychiatry 7:505–509, 1992

Sheline Y, Kehr C: Cost and utility of routine admission laboratory testing for psychiatry inpatients. Gen Hosp Psychiatry 12:329–334, 1990

Shulman KI, Silver IL, Hershberg RI, et al: Geriatric psychiatry in the general hospital: the integration of services and training. Gen Hosp Psychiatry 8:223–228, 1986

Sinyor D, Jacques P, Kaloupek P: Poststroke depression and lesion location: an attempted replication. Brain 109:537–546, 1986

Small GW: Tricyclic antidepressants for medically ill geriatric patients. J Clin Psychiatry 50 (suppl):27–31, 1989

Small GW: Recognition and treatment of depression in the elderly. J Clin Psychiatry 52 (suppl):11–22, 1991

Small GW: Geriatric psychiatry fellowship recruitment: crisis or opportunity? American Journal of Geriatric Psychiatry 1:67–73, 1993

Small GW, Fawzy FI: Psychiatric consultation for the medically ill elderly in the general hospital: need for a collaborative model of care. Psychosomatics 29:94–103, 1988

Small GW, Natterson B: The elderly critically ill patient. Problems in Critical Care 2:101–115, 1988

Small GW, Komanduri R, Gitlin M, et al: The influence of age on guilt expression in major depression. Int J Geriatric Psychiatry 1:121–126, 1986

Smith LW, Dimsdale JE: Post cardiotomy delirium: conclusions after 25 years. Am J Psychiatry 146:452–458, 1989

Snyderman DA, Thompson WL: Specific psychotherapy approaches to medical-surgical patients. New Dir Ment Health Serv 57:9–17, 1993

Sos J, Cassem NH: Managing postoperative agitation. Drug Ther 10:103–106, 1980

Spar JE, LaRue A: Concise Guide to Geriatric Psychiatry. Washington, DC, American Psychiatric Press, 1990

Starkstein SE, Robinson RG, Price TR: Comparison of patients with and without poststroke major depression matched for size and location of lesion. Arch Gen Psychiatry 45:247–252, 1988

Stern RA, Bachman DL: Depressive symptoms following stroke. Am J Psychiatry 148:351–356, 1991

Stoudemire A: Masked depression in a combined medical-psychiatric unit. Psychosomatics 26:221–228, 1985

Stoudemire A, Moran MB: Psychopharmacologic treatment of anxiety in the medically ill elderly patient: specific considerations. J Clin Psychiatry 54 (suppl):27–36, 1993

Stoudemire A, Hales RE, Thomas CF: Medical psychiatry units: an economical alternative for consultation-liaison psychiatry? Hosp Community Psychiatry 38:815–818, 1987

Stoudemire A, Moran MG, Fogel BS: Psychotropic drug use in the medically ill, I. Psychosomatics 31:377–391, 1990

Stoudemire A, Moran MG, Fogel BS: Psychotropic drug use in the medically ill elderly, II. Psychosomatics 32:34–46, 1991

Strain JJ, Liebowitz MR, Klein DF: Anxiety and panic attacks in the medically ill. Psychiatr Clin North Am 4:333–350, 1981

Strain JJ, Lyons JS, Hammer JS, et al: Cost offset from a psychiatric consultation liaison intervention with elderly hip fracture patients. Am J Psychiatry 148:1044–1049, 1991

Sullivan P: Doctors guilty of "ageism and indifference," MD tells General Council. Can Med Assoc J 141:720, 725, 727, 1989

Swenson JR, Perez EL: The impact of a geriatric assessment unit on a psychiatric consultation service in a general hospital. Psychiatric Hospital 17:121–125, 1986

Tesar GE: The agitated patient, II: pharmacologic treatment. Hosp Community Psychiatry 44:627–629, 1993

Tesar GE, Stern TA: Rapid tranquilization of the agitated intensive care unit patient. J Intensive Care Med 3:195–201, 1988

Thienhaus OJ, Rowe C, Woellert D, et al: Geropsychiatric emergency services: utilization and outcome predictors. Hosp Community Psychiatry 39:1301–1305, 1988

Thompson WL, Thompson TL: Psychiatric aspects of asthma in adults. Adv Psychosom Med 14:33–47, 1985

Thompson WL, Thompson TL: Pulmonary disease, in Psychiatric Care of the Medical Patient. Edited by Stoudemire A, Fogel BS. New York, Oxford University Press, 1993

Thompson TL, Mitchell WD, House RM: Geriatric psychiatry patients' care by primary care physicians. Psychosomatics 30:65–72, 1989

Thompson TL, Wise TN, Kelley AB, et al: Improving psychiatric consultation to nonpsychiatrist physicians. Psychosomatics 31:80–84, 1990

Traines M: Ageism among physicians: fundamental questions. Rhode Island Med J:74:87–88, 1991

Tune L, Carr S, Hoag E, et al: Anticholinergic effects of drugs commonly prescribed for the elderly: potential means for assessing risk of delirium. Am J Psychiatry 149:1393–1394, 1992

U.S. Bureau of the Census: An Aging World, International Population

Reports, Series P-95, no 78, Washington, DC, U.S. Government Printing Office, 1987

U.S. Senate Special Committee on Aging in Conjunction With the American Association of Retired Persons: Aging America: Trends and Projections. Washington, DC, 1984

Verbosky LA, Franco KN, Zrull JP: The relationship between depression and length of stay in the general hospital patient. J Clin Psychiatry 54:177–181, 1993

Weiss LJ, Lazarus LW: Psychosocial treatment of the geropsychiatric patient. International Journal of Geriatric Psychiatry 8:95–100, 1993

Weissman MM, Myers JK, Tischler GL, et al: Psychiatric disorders (DSM-III) and cognitive impairment among the elderly in a United States urban community. Acta Psychiatr Scand 71:366–379, 1985

Welch CA: ECT in medically ill patients, in The Clinical Science of Electroconvulsive Therapy. Edited by Coffey CE. Washington, DC, American Psychiatric Press, 1993

Wells C: Pseudodementia. Am J Psychiatry 136:895–900, 1979

Wells KB, Golding JM, Burnam MA: Psychiatric disorder in a sample of the general population with and without chronic medical conditions. Am J Psychiatry 145:976–981, 1988

West ND, Walsh M: Psychiatry's image today: results of an attitudinal survey. Am J Psychiatry 12:1318–1319, 1975

Williams-Russo P, Urquhart BL, Sharrock NE, et al: Post-operative delirium: predictors and prognosis in elderly orthopedic patients. J Am Geriatr Soc 40:759–767, 1992

Wise MG, Rieck SO: Diagnostic considerations and treatment approaches to underlying anxiety in the medically ill. J Clin Psychiatry 54 (5 suppl):22–26, 1993

Yager J: Specific components of bedside manner in the general hospital psychiatric consultation: 12 concrete suggestions. Psychosomatics 30:209–212, 1989

Yesavage JA, Brink T, Rose T, et al: Development of a geriatric depression rating scale: a preliminary report. J Psychiatr Res 17:37–49, 1983

Yudofsky SC, Silver JM, Hales RE: Pharmacologic management of aggression in the elderly. J Clin Psychiatry 51 (suppl):22–32, 1990

Ziehm SR: Intravenous haloperidol for tranquilization in critical care patients: a review and critique. Clinical Issues in Critical Care Nursing 2:765–777, 1991

Zisook S, Shuchter SR: Uncomplicated bereavement. J Clin Psychiatry 54:365–372, 1993

C H A P T E R   3 3

Marie-France Tourigny-Rivard, M.D.,
 F.R.C.P.C., D.A.B.N.P.
Walter M. Potoczny, M.D., F.R.C.P.C.

Acute Care Inpatient and Day Hospital Treatment

I n this chapter we review acute care inpatient and day hospital treatment for elderly patients with psychiatric problems.

Overview

In the principles for good psychogeriatric care outlined by the World Health Organization (Skeet 1983), acute care inpatient treatment is seen as an important component of the comprehensive services that should be available to elderly psychiatric patients. Apart from allowing safe and rapid treatment of elderly patients who have severe psychiatric illnesses, inpatient treatment can contribute to the prevention of chronic institutionalization by ensuring that patients receive adequate diagnosis, treatment, and care leading to clinical improvement, rehabilitation, and resocialization. The value of geriatric psychiatry acute care inpatient and day hospital programs has been reaffirmed in governmental guidelines for services (Health and Welfare Canada 1988; Royal College of Physicians of London 1989), where both are listed as essential resources for patient care. The United States does not have published guidelines that are specific for geriatric psychiatry inpatient care. The Council on Aging has not prepared such a document; furthermore, the Joint Commission on Accreditation of Healthcare Organizations, which accredits health facilities in this country, does not have specific standards or guidelines for geriatric psychiatry programs; instead, the standards for geriatric patients are scattered through their general guidelines (Joint Commission on Accreditation of Healthcare Organizations 1993).

Principles applicable to geriatric psychiatry inpatient and day hospital treatment programs include 1) multidisciplinary staffing, 2) preadmission screening, 3) maintaining the patient in the community, 4) beginning discharge planning at admission, and 5) collaborating with community agencies (Health and Welfare Canada 1988; Skeet 1983; Royal College of Physicians of London 1989). These principles emphasize the need to consider acute care inpatient and day hospital treatment as part of a continuum of care that should be available to elderly patients with psychiatric problems.

Multidisciplinary staffing. The efficient running of a psychogeriatric service starts with a psychogeriatric team that has a special interest in the psychiatry of old age, is able to provide a full range of psychiatric skills, and has good knowledge of general medicine and social interventions (Pitt 1982). Multidisciplinary staffing is required to address concurrently the physical, psychological, and social problems that can contribute to the psychiatric illnesses of elderly patients. The majority (75% or more) of psychogeriatric patients admitted to the hospital have at least one of the common medical illnesses seen in old age (Conwell et al. 1989; Harrison et al. 1988). In fact, most geriatric psychiatry inpatients have more than one concurrent medical problem (Meier et al. 1992), and Zubenko et al. (1992) reported an average of 4.4 medical problems in their inpatient dementia population. Furthermore, most elderly patients admitted to the hospital will have acquired multiple age- and disease-related deficits; utilization data show that elderly Americans admitted to the hospital have an average of three medical diagnoses, the most common being atherosclerosis (Garnick and Short 1985). Weingarten et al. (1982) also emphasized the role of physical illness in precipitating psychiatric admissions and complicating treatment. In more than half of their sample ($N = 49$), medical illness precipitated the psychiatric decompensation, and 25% had significant previously unrecognized medical problems (e.g., vitamin B_{12} and folate deficiency, hyperparathyroidism, congestive heart failure, "sick sinus" syndrome, postanoxic encephalopathy). Medical problems affected psychiatric care negatively in most instances, delaying or preventing psychiatric intervention. In 14 cases, the medical problems had a positive impact on psychiatric outcome when treated successfully, and in 9 cases they had a negative outcome, including 3 deaths. The multidisciplinary team therefore includes members of the core mental health disciplines and other health professionals, including nonpsychiatric physicians, to ensure that patients receive comprehensive needs assessment and care (Arie and Jolley 1982).

Preadmission screening. Whenever possible, screening evaluations should take place prior to hospitalization, including partial hospitalization. These are often most informative if done at the patient's residence to give a better idea of the physical and social assets or liabilities of the individual and to see how the person relates to his or her family and caregivers in the natural setting (Arie and Jolley 1982; Pitt 1982; Whanger and Busse 1975). This screening helps to establish proper prioritization, prevent unnecessary or inappropriate admissions, and prepare realistic plans for discharge.

Maintaining the patient in the community. This principle is dictated not only by the economic pressures associated with expensive treatment settings (e.g., inpatient units), but also by the fear that the longer the hospital admission, the less likely the patient will successfully return home owing to loss of supports and friends. Discharge from hospital care may occur sooner if

- The treatment team is committed to getting the patient well enough to return home as quickly as possible
- Relatives and friends are provided useful information about the psychiatric problems of the patient and are encouraged to participate, as appropriate, in the inpatient care
- A well-organized network of mental health services is available in the community
- Coordination and cooperation exist between the inpatient unit and community support services that will be required by the patient after discharge (Royal College of Physicians of London 1989; Skeet 1983)

Meier et al. (1992) listed similar factors (rehabilitation approach, community caregiver involvement, availability of community resources, and coordination of aftercare) as contributing to the early discharge of elderly patients treated by a psychogeriatric team. Knight and Carter (1990) also demonstrated that an intensive case management program (which included a clear commitment to getting the patient well as quickly as possible, combined with active coordination of aftercare) was successful in reducing the length of stay from 27 to 12 days for older adults admitted to their psychiatric inpatient unit.

Similarly, one of day hospital's most frequently cited goals is to allow patients to remain in their own home while receiving the specialized care they need.

Beginning discharge planning at admission.   Discharge planning starts at admission, with a good understanding of the patient's living situation prior to admission, maintaining the patient's community resources (e.g., living accommodation, support of family and friends) and dealing with potential obstacles to returning or staying at home. Advice to patients and families on the need for placement in supervised facilities or on the need for a change in residence is given only after an adequate evaluation is done and a clear prognosis established. This caution is particularly important for depressed patients, who may feel hopeless and unable to care for themselves at the time of admission but should have a good prognosis and be able to continue to live at home after treatment. In fact, the majority of geriatric patients with functional disorders treated in specialized inpatient services (Conwell et al. 1989; Harrison et al. 1988; Spar et al. 1980) or in day hospital programs (Greene and Timbury 1979) are able to return to their preadmission residences.

Collaborating with community agencies.   Pitt (1982) and Skeet (1983) both felt that collaboration with community agencies and coordination of aftercare are two important principles that may help reduce hospital length of stay and readmission rates and make reinsertion/maintenance into the community successful. Although collaboration and coordination are very difficult to measure and comparative studies of services with and without such support do not seem to exist, most authors describing psychogeriatric inpatient care seem to agree with these principles (Harrison et al. 1988; Meier et al. 1992; Spar et al. 1980).

Geriatric Psychiatry Inpatient Units

Types of Units

In general hospitals, a geriatric psychiatry unit can be either part of the general psychiatric unit, with specific staff and programming for the elderly population, or a separate, usually small, unit (Health and Welfare Canada

1988). Advantages of mixed (or age-integrated) acute care wards are that elderly patients can benefit from the interactions and physical assistance sometimes provided by the younger population (Billig and Leibenluft 1987). The disadvantages are the risk of injury from acutely ill younger patients and being frightened by their language and behavior. It may also be more difficult to create a therapeutic milieu that actively addresses the problems related to aging unless there are staff, programming, and rooms provided specifically for elderly individuals. We believe it is easier to create a milieu that encourages patients to deal with issues related to aging and attract staff with a special interest in and knowledge about the psychiatric disorders of later life in age-segregated wards. Sexually integrated wards are currently the norm, and problems of improper behavior toward members of the opposite sex are infrequent (Pitt 1982).

Geriatric psychiatry units are sometimes located close to geriatric medicine units, with part of the staff having joint appointments to both units to facilitate cross-consultation and joint teaching. Such "joint units," described by Arie and Jolley (1982), can come under one department (e.g., the Department of Health Care of the Elderly at Nottingham University, which combines geriatric medicine and psychiatry) or under separate geriatric medicine and psychiatry departments in which there is agreement on the basic principles of joint care.

Several psychiatric hospitals have "acute care" psychogeriatric units (often called *psychogeriatric admission* or *assessment wards*) where patients are admitted for a period of 1 to 3 months and then discharged to the community or transferred to a rehabilitation or long-term care ward.

Design of Units

Acute care inpatient and day hospital treatment units are most suitable for geriatric patients if the environment minimizes the impact of problems frequently associated with aging. Because wandering and agitated patients are often admitted to geriatric psychiatry units, optimally the design of the unit should allow for safe wandering and adequate exercise levels. Visual impairment dictates good lighting throughout the unit, large-print reading material, and easy-to-read signs. Because hearing impairment is common, sound proofing of interviewing rooms allows privacy, and sound amplifying electronic systems facilitate individual and group therapy. Minimizing extraneous noises that tend to get amplified by hearing aids is also important (Hyatt 1987). Psychotropic medications will increase the risk for falls as a result of orthostatic hypotension, parkinsonism, or cerebellar toxicity, as well as through the worsening of preexisting risk factors for falls (e.g., arthritis, weakness, and urinary incontinence or urgency) (Janken et al. 1986). To minimize falls, nonskid flooring, wide corridors with handrails, an adequate number of well-located washrooms, and uncluttered rooms that allow easy access for wheelchairs or walkers are ideal. Equipment that encourages patients to maintain their everyday skills and personal appearance enhances the therapeutic effort (e.g., full-length mirrors and laundry and kitchen facilities).

Safety Considerations

For safety, inpatient units may have to be locked periodically for patients who are acutely suicidal or psychotic and for wandering patients who present a high risk for elopement (Billig and Leibenluft 1987). Electronic and remote control locks can contribute to making the locks as unobtrusive as possible. If the unit cannot be locked, wandering patients may have to be confined to a small area where they can be easily observed or may need costly individual supervision until they no longer present an elopement risk.

Staffing

Staffing ratios are very difficult to establish. There are few guidelines available regarding inpatient psychiatric care of elderly individuals, except for those of the Royal College of Physicians of London (1989). Overall, staffing should ensure that adequate evaluations take place and that a variety of treatment programs are available to respond to the needs of the inpatient population.

Indications for Inpatient Treatment

While considering inpatient treatment, the physician should keep alternatives in mind, such as day hospital and intensive outpatient crisis intervention, which can be used to prevent psychiatric admissions. Whanger (1989) has provided a good review of indications for psychiatric inpatient treatment; these are summarized in Table 33–1.

Although it is widely recognized that manic patients require admission, we recommend that admission also be considered for elderly patients with hypomania to minimize the risk of cardiovascular complications and prevent the painful consequences of hypomanic behavior.

Table 33–1. Indications for geriatric acute care inpatient treatment

Imminent danger to self or others	Intensive evaluation or treatment is required	Failure of the caregiving system
Suicidal or potentially harmful behaviors	Difficult diagnostic issues requiring close observation	Principal caregiver dies, leaves, or needs temporary relief
Homicidal, violent, or aggressive behavior	Psychiatric illness complicated by drug or alcohol addiction	Depletion of care resources without alternatives
Threatening behavior while acutely psychotic	Acute psychosis with unpredictable behavior	Lack of community resources or respite care beds
Fire hazard	Need for intravenous or frequent intramuscular injections	
Inability to attend to basic or essential care needs	Need for electroconvulsive therapy	
Dangerous wandering behavior	Multiple medical problems or drug sensitivities requiring close monitoring	
	Good prognosis but intensive treatment required	

Inappropriate Admissions

The most common forms of inappropriate admission include the following:

- Patients who clearly require an urgent admission to a medical ward
- Patients who are comatose or moribund
- Patients who require only placement or other social support services
- Patients who could have been treated easily in less intensive, less expensive settings that do not take them away from home and do not impose the financial burden and stigma of a psychiatric hospitalization

Population Served

Psychiatric diagnoses responsible for admission.   Redick and Taube (1980) reported on the diagnosis of all patients admitted to psychiatric facilities in the United States who were older than 65. Statistics related to private psychiatric hospitals and psychiatric inpatient units located in general hospitals likely describe the population that will require admission on acute geriatric psychiatry inpatient units. Redick and Taube (1980) found that 51.1% of patients admitted to private psychiatric hospitals and 46.1% of those admitted to general hospital psychiatric units had a diagnosis of depression, indicating that depression accounts for the majority of admissions to acute care inpatient units. Organic brain syndromes, excluding those related to alcohol and substance abuse, were the next most common diagnosis (25% and 28%, respectively), followed by alcohol-related disorders (7.5% and 6%, respectively), schizophrenia (4.6% and 3.3%, respectively), psychoneuroses (2.7% and 5.1%, respectively), and other disorders (9% and 11.5%, respectively). More recently, Andrews et al. (1994) reported on the diagnoses responsible for admission of Medicare patients to short-term general inpatient programs in the United States. Psychiatric diagnoses ranked in the following order: depression and affective disorders (30th over 186), alcohol-related disorders (53rd), organic disorders and dementia (56th), and schizophrenic disorders (62nd). Spar et al. (1980) and Weingarten et al. (1982) found that the most frequent diagnoses responsible for admission of elderly patients to acute care geriatric psychiatry wards were depression (51.6% and 57%, respectively) and dementia (27.1% and 18%, respectively). Harrison et al. (1988) reported that 29% of their patients had dementia; 29% had major depressive episodes; 19% had delirium; 10% had schizophrenia; and 8% had other psychoses, including acute manic episodes. Conwell et al. (1989) reported that 76% of their 168 patients had a primary affective disorder (19 of these had a bipolar disorder); organic brain syndrome was the second most common diagnosis: 24.5% had dementia, and 10.1% had delirium.

Gender distribution.   In 1980, women accounted for roughly two-thirds of all geriatric admissions to psychiatric wards of general hospitals and private psychiatric facilities, but according to demographic surveys, they should have accounted for only 58% of admissions (Redick and Taube 1980). Studies continue to report a higher percentage of female admissions, ranging from 65% (Harrison et al. 1988) to 75% (Spar et al. 1980).

Inpatient Assessment, Diagnosis, and Treatment

Assessment and Diagnosis

It is axiomatic that a thorough medical, psychiatric, and functional assessment should be part of every admission. Inpatient admission is useful in allowing more accurate observation of a variety of psychiatric signs and symptoms, including sleep patterns, food intake, intensity of somatic complaints, and functional ability. These observations are particularly useful for patients who tend to exaggerate or minimize their difficulties and patients with mild to moderate dementia who demonstrate their deficits more clearly in unfamiliar surroundings.

Multidisciplinary, multiaxial evaluation according to the biopsychosocial model is necessary, and each team member contributes to the assessment according to his or her expertise. Typically the treating physician will focus initial assessment on the medical and psychiatric problems of the patient, taking a careful history and performing appropriate medical and laboratory investigations. Nurses, occupational therapists, and physiotherapists usually focus on functional assessment, identifying problem areas and encouraging patients to use their abilities or accessory tools to compensate for their deficits. Standard instruments, such as the Older American Resources and Services Research (OARS) (Duke University Center for the Study of Aging and Human Development 1978), are available to assess instrumental activities of daily living and can provide useful information about patients' baseline level of functioning and degree of improvement at discharge. Social workers provide much needed details on the patient's familial and social resources, identifying problem areas that will have to be addressed urgently during hospitalization. Psychologists help document the cognitive abilities and deficits of the patients and add perspective on the patient's potential to respond to specific forms of psychotherapy.

Treatment Modalities

Each patient should have an individualized treatment plan that takes into account his or her physical, psychiatric, and social problems and makes optimal use of his or her abilities. Clear goals are set according to the treatability of the patient's psychiatric and medical illnesses and the patient's best previous level of functioning. As much as possible, both the patient and the caregivers are included in the formulation of the treatment plan—formally, by inviting the patient and caregivers to participate in multidisciplinary patient conferences, or informally, by discussing the treatment plan with patient and family, with due and appropriate regard for confidentiality.

Many of the treatment modalities used on the inpatient unit are described in detail in other sections of this book and are briefly mentioned here only to highlight how they may have to be adjusted to the inpatient setting.

Milieu. An important component of treatment in an inpatient setting is the possibility of creating a milieu that will, in itself, have therapeutic value to the patient. In general, a mixture of therapy groups, ward meetings, and activity groups contribute to the daily schedule of the unit. Group and ward meetings serve to facilitate communication and give a sense of community. Activity groups provide opportunities for observation of specific skills and social interactions. On a geriatric psychiatry unit, the milieu should be conducive to dealing with problems common to its population, such as adjusting to losses (including loss of health or youthfulness), adjusting to retirement, difficulties in finding worthwhile activities and maintaining self-esteem, adapting to changes in family relationships or changes in residence, and dealing with increased dependency needs.

The milieu also must be conducive to an eventual return home or to good integration in one of the community facilities. Wearing their own clothes, getting dressed as they would at home, using kitchen facilities, planning and preparing meals (at least snacks), using instruments such as the clothes washer and dryer, and carrying on responsibilities for self-care are all important for patients who will be discharged home. Implementing a schedule of ward activities and regulations similar to those the patient will have to follow when discharged to a nursing home or extended care facility is also important.

Individual psychotherapy. Individual psychotherapy using such modalities as cognitive, insight-oriented, and supportive psychotherapy is an integral part of treatment on inpatient units. Although many inpatients are near discharge before they become suitable candidates for insight-oriented psychotherapy, the treatment team should have a sufficient understanding and familiarity with psychodynamic therapeutic interventions to provide empathic listening, gentle confrontation (e.g., pointing out obvious avoidance), and clarification to help patients recognize feeling states they may be unaware of, links between current events and personal history, and reasons for avoidance (i.e., fears). Interpretation of unconscious process is a rare intervention on most short-term treatment units, however, because some time is usually required before the patient is ready to tolerate the emotional impact of the revealed thought or feeling (Rogoff 1986). Cognitive psychotherapy is probably a useful component of the treatment of depressed nonpsychotic inpatients, but studies of its efficacy have been done in outpatient rather than inpatient geriatric populations (Steuer 1982).

Behavior therapy. Various techniques of behavior therapy and behavior modification can be useful for selected inpatients. These techniques have been studied mostly in long-term care or outpatient settings but can be applied to a limited extent to the inpatient, acute care population. The most commonly used forms of behavior therapy are relaxation training and desensitization for anxiety-related disorders; habit retraining for incontinence; and biofeedback, which may be helpful in the management of chronic pain. Behavior modification techniques, which can be applied by staff in the overall approach of the patient, include positive reinforcement of adaptive behavior, removal of reinforcements for maladaptive behavior, counterconditioning, and reciprocal inhibition (Yates 1975).

Group therapy. This modality of treatment is fully discussed in Chapter 29.

Family therapy. On inpatient units, family therapy includes involving and evaluating families to negotiate appropriate goals for family intervention. Common goals as described for families of inpatients (Glick and Clarkin 1986) include the following:

- Accepting the reality of the illness and understanding the current episode
- Identifying the stresses that precipitated the current episode
- Identifying likely future stressors, both within and outside the family
- Elucidating family interaction sequences that stress the identified patient and seem to trigger symptoms, providing the family with better ways to relate to the patient
- Planning strategies for managing and/or minimizing future stresses
- Accepting the need for continued treatment following discharge from the hospital

Fears and anxiety can be reduced by keeping the family properly apprised of progress and supporting them in their efforts to help. When family problems are present, it is important to determine whether they are mostly related to the current illness of the patient or a reflection of more serious ongoing problems that will have to be addressed with formal therapy. Although patients often report stressful family relationships as a contributing factor to their illness, the clinician must keep in mind that the illness of the patient has often contributed greatly to the strained relations. In their study of elderly psychiatric inpatients, Liptzen et al. found that relatives of depressed and demented patients reported similar levels of burden (as measured by the Burden Interview [Zarit and Zarit 1982] and the Memory and Behavior Problem Checklist of Zarit [Teri et al. 1992]) at admission and at follow-up 2 to 4 months after discharge. This reinforces the fact that severe depression and dementia produce great stress for relatives and caregivers and suggests that the treatment team can help reduce this stress through appropriate family interventions.

Physical therapies.   Because medical illnesses and physical disabilities are common among geriatric psychiatry inpatients, physiotherapy, exercise programs, and teaching on the appropriate use of physical aids are important aspects of care.

Electroconvulsive therapy is an important physical treatment modality on geriatric psychiatry inpatient units and is covered in detail in Chapter 26.

Occupational and recreational therapy.   The occupational therapist can provide individual and group therapeutic activities to 1) provide structure and good contact with reality for the confused patient, 2) improve self-esteem and remotivate depressed patients, 3) develop interactional and social skills, 4) encourage patients to maintain or resume their usual activities, 5) develop vocational interests, and 6) increase patients' awareness of community resources. This therapy is done through a variety of activities tailored to match the abilities of the patient and his or her previous interests.

Recreational activities provide an opportunity to assess the patient's strengths, weaknesses, and customary modes of adapting. Frequent themes addressed in recreation therapy include adjustment to retirement, finding worthwhile activities such as volunteer work or hobbies, setting personal goals in areas such as personal fitness, and learning about community activities or resources available to seniors. The recreation therapist provides information and encourages patients to experience some of the suggested leisure activities by organizing exercise groups, community outings, music groups, card games, craft classes, or parties that stimulate socialization and provide pleasure and satisfaction.

Outcome of Short-Term Inpatient Care

The majority of elderly patients admitted to acute care psychiatric inpatient units are able to return home (or to their preadmission residence) at the time of discharge. Conwell et al. (1989) reported that 82% of their patients ($N = 168$) were discharged home alone or with relatives; 3.9% were transferred to other hospitals, and 14.4% were discharged to structured settings such as group homes and nursing homes. Harrison et al. (1988) reported that 54 of their 100 inpatients were discharged to the same level of accommodation or to a more independent level. Spar et al. (1980) reported that 62% of their 122 inpatients were discharged home; 2.5%, to the care of relatives; and 35.5%, to institutional care (7.5% were in institutions prior to admission); therefore, approximately 70% of their patients were discharged to the same level of accommodation as on admission. Weingarten et al. (1982) reported that 71% of their 49 patients were discharged home, albeit with some additional support (i.e., day care or caretaker) in 18% of these cases. Wells et al. (1993) reviewed the records of 2,746 depressed elderly inpatients in acute care general hospitals and reported that 9% of patients who were admitted from their home or a retirement home were discharged to a hospital or nursing home after implementation of the Medicare prospective payment system.

Elderly patients admitted to short-term care general hospitals tend to stay longer than younger adults, regardless of diagnosis (Garnick and Short 1985). In the literature regarding geriatric psychiatry acute care units, variable lengths of stay are reported: 32 days (Harrison et al. 1988), 44.5 days (Spar et al. 1980), 53.3 days (Conwell et al. 1989), and 59 days (Weingarten et al. 1982). These geriatric units clearly provided assessment and enough treatment to allow the majority of their patients to be discharged home, with almost no transfers to other inpatient or long-term care facilities. Studies reporting shorter lengths of stay also report a lower percentage of patients being able to return home: 50% of Harrison et al.'s patients (1988) who were admitted from a house or flat (living alone or with others) were able to return home after an average length of stay of 32 days; only 27.7% of patients in Sheline's (1990) study were able to return home (to self-care or the care of family) after an average length of stay of 23 days. Most acute care units strive toward short lengths of stay. However, the costs of premature discharge—for example, costs associated with the inability to return to independent living owing to significant residual symptoms, cost of readmission for the same diagnosis within 1 year, and costs associated with the need for adjunct services or institutionalization—have not been systematically studied and compared with the costs of longer inpatient admissions. In the study by Wells et al. (1993), the relatively high 1-year readmission rate of 52.4% (with a mean additional 17 days in the hospital) for their elderly depressed inpatients and the fact that 37% of their patients were considered unimproved at discharge could be considered possible costs associated with short-term admissions. Avoiding long-term hospitalization or institutionalization is associated with substantial savings that can easily offset the cost of a short-term admission. A brief case example will illustrate this point:

> Mrs. X was a 77-year-old caregiver to her legally blind husband at the time of her admission for treatment of refractory depression. Both she and her husband had applied to go to a nursing home, as she was no longer able to care for herself or her husband. A 6-week inpatient admission allowed successful treatment of her depression and full recovery. Maintenance medication and minimal follow-up treatment allowed this woman and her husband to stay home for 4 years, enjoying good quality of life. The savings in government subsidies for the nursing home more than covered the cost of this first admission. Mrs. X then had a major stroke and was not recovering well because of severe poststroke depression; a transfer to a long-term care hospital was requested. Meanwhile, her husband had been temporarily placed in a nursing home. With a 16-week inpatient psychiatric admission, Mrs. X again made a full recovery from her depression and nearly full recovery from her stroke. She returned home with the aid of minimal housekeeping services. She and her husband enjoyed another 3 years of quality life together at home until she died suddenly of another stroke.

A study of the effect of the creation of a psychogeriatric team in a long-term care hospital showed a decrease in waiting lists, an increase in discharges to the community, a decrease in the number of deaths, and a decreased proportion of patients staying more than 1 year in the hospital. Readmission rates increased from 30% to 40%, but most patients did not need to return to the hospital (Pitt 1982). This seems to indicate that a specialized team with an active interest in the care of elderly individuals can contribute to lower health care costs and improved quality of life. Unfortunately, there are no published data on the evaluation of the cost-effectiveness of acute care geriatric psychiatry inpatient units, although Conwell et al. (1989) did attempt to evaluate the outcome of treatment with a three-point scale to measure response (i.e., good response, partial response, no response), length of stay, and characteristics of their patients.

To properly evaluate the cost-effectiveness of a geriatric psychiatry inpatient unit, the clinician must consider the average cost of admission (average per diem cost for the unit multiplied by the average length of stay), the number of patients treated (taking into account readmission rates), and the outcome with and without admission. Outcome measures should include measures of psychopathology, functional capacity, level of distress, and quality of life; suicide rates; and need for placement or admission to a long-term care facility (which could have possibly been avoided or postponed with a timely admission). In addition, units with comparable case mix should be compared in cost-effectiveness studies. It is clear that much research remains to be done to develop realistic methods of calculating cost-effectiveness of inpatient psychiatric treatment (English and McGarrick 1986), starting with reliable appraisal of case mix, objective measures of improvement, and likely morbidity without treatment.

Limited Accessibility of Geriatric Psychiatry Inpatient Treatment

Elderly Canadians and Americans face different accessibility problems because of the vastly different methods of funding in the United States and Canada. In the United Sates, accessibility is limited to a great extent by one's personal financial resources and limited coverage of Medicare and private insurance plans. Currently Medicare offers full coverage for the first 60 days, with a decrease to 75% for the next 30, and to 50% for the next 60 days; there is a ceiling of 150 days for a single spell of illness and of 190 days over a lifetime. A more detailed review of these financial issues is offered in Chapter 37. Elderly Canadians have Universal Health Coverage, paid through the income tax system and administered by each province. Accessibility to psychiatric inpatient treatment is limited by the number of beds funded by each province for psychiatric care and their uneven distribution in different regions. Where geriatric psychiatry inpatient services exist, the needs usually exceed the supply, forcing the teams who run these units to establish priorities for admission and utilize ambulatory services as much as feasible. However, because geriatric psychiatry inpatient units are relatively rare, most geriatric patients who need psychiatric inpatient care are admitted to general psychiatry or medical units. Tax payers and governments are currently reluctant to fund additional beds because of their high operational costs and rapidly rising health expenditures.

Day Hospital Treatment

Historical Review of Day Hospitals

The development of day hospital services clearly antedates the current trend toward community-based medical care. The first adult psychiatric day hospital was started in Moscow in 1933 as a result of a shortage of inpatient facilities and was utilized for the treatment of large numbers of severely impaired psychotic patients (Kramer 1962). The first documented adult day hospitals in the English-speaking world were established by Cameron in Montreal in 1946 and by Bierer in Hampstead, England, in 1947 (Bierer 1959; Edwards 1982). In the United Kingdom, adult psychiatric day hospital services were legislated in the 1962 Hospital Plan for England and Wales, and it was envisaged that day hospitals would contribute significantly to the running down of the large mental hospitals (Vaughan 1985). Geriatric psychiatry day hospitals are an accepted part of the health care delivery system in the United Kingdom, where established government guidelines recommend 2 to 3 geriatric psychiatry day hospital places per 1,000 elderly population (Peace 1982).

In the United States, partial hospitalization was mandated in the community mental health model as of 1963 in the Mental Retardation Facilities and Community Mental Health Centers Construction Act (Casarino et al. 1982). The increased interest in partial hospitalization treatment led to the establishment of the American Association of Partial Hospitalization in 1979 and the inaugural issue of the *International Journal of Partial Hospitalization* in 1982.

Outside of the United Kingdom, the development of specific day hospital treatment programs for elderly patients with psychiatric problems has been more sporadic. Goldstein and Carlson reported on the establishment in 1968 of a psychogeriatric day hospital at the Maimonides Hospital in Montreal, Canada. The authors stated, "this appears to be a new facility because a survey of psychiatric day hospitals showed none for the aged in North America at that time" (Goldstein et al. 1968, p. 955). A common mechanism for the establishment of geriatric psychiatry day hospital services frequently involved the conversion of run-down and dilapidated hospital facilities. Examples of this include the use of war-damaged houses (Bierer 1959), and Goldstein's own day hospital program, which was started in a small cafeteria adjacent to an inpatient unit in 1973 (Goldstein and Carlson 1976) and had its first permanent home in an old frame building initially designed for tuberculosis patients and deemed unsuitable for inpatient care by the fire marshall.

In the United States, partial hospitalization units for elderly psychiatric patients were developed to bridge the gap between state psychiatric hospitals and nonpsychiatric senior citizen centers (Berger and Berger 1971). A review by Parker and Knoll pointed out that despite proven therapeutic and economic advantages, partial hospitalization has relatively low utilization and poor third-party reimbursement in the United States. Another factor relating to suboptimal program development and utilization is the lack of training and exposure to partial hospitalization in postgraduate psychiatric training programs (Parker and Knoll 1990).

Definition of Services

There continues to be ambiguity about what constitutes a day hospital facility and what differentiates a day hospital from day treatment and day care centers. Day care centers are at one end of the spectrum in that they provide a less comprehensive and less intensive level of care. Standards set for adult day care by the National Council on the Aging in 1984 identified a target population consisting of two main groups. The first group consisted of adults with physical, emotional, or mental impairment who require assistance and supervision, and the second, of adults who need restorative or rehabilitative services to achieve the optimal level of functioning. The emphasis in day care centers is on assistance and supervision; these centers do not provide the diagnostic or treatment facilities necessary to deal with major psychiatric disorders.

A simple but easily applied definition was offered by Craft, who stated, "A day hospital may be defined as one where full hospital treatment is given under medical supervision to patients who return to their homes each night" (Craft 1959, p. 251). A lack of guidelines early in the history of partial hospitalization programs in the United States resulted in a "kitchen sink" approach, in which all types of treatment were offered to all types of patients of all ages, with no attempt to match treatment to the patient characteristics (Klar et al. 1982). The American Association for Partial Hospitalization (quoted in Casarino et al. 1982) set out the following definition in 1980: "Partial hospitalization is an ambulatory treatment program that includes the major diagnostic, medical, psychiatric, psychosocial and prevocational treatment modalities for serious mental disorders which require coordinated, intensive, comprehensive and multidisciplinary treatment not provided in an outpatient clinic setting. It allows for a more flexible and less restrictive treatment program by offering an alternative to inpatient treatment" (p. 9).

These principles are applicable, for the most part, to the geriatric population with psychiatric disorders, and indeed, elderly patients with psychiatric problems may be found in general adult day hospitals, geriatric medical day hospitals, and more specialized geriatric psychiatry day hospital treatment facilities. A review of the literature gives a general impression that in the United States, very few elderly patients are treated in adult psychiatric day programs (Salzman et al. 1969) when compared with the United Kingdom, where a larger number of elderly geriatric patients are in general adult day programs (Hassall et al. 1972). The question as to whether elderly patients with psychiatric problems can do well in a general adult day hospital or in a partial hospitalization program remains unresolved, and the admission of such patients to these facilities may be determined more by fiscal and economic realities.

Elderly individuals with concurrent medical and psychiatric illness may also be found in medical geriatric day hospitals. In 1980 Brocklehurst and Tucker reported on an extensive review of 302 medical geriatric day hospitals in Great Britain. They found that separate provision of psychiatric assessment and treatment was found in only 36% of programs surveyed. This study supported the view that "separate day hospital accommodation is required for geriatric and psychogeriatric patients" (Brocklehurst and Tucker 1980, p. 179). The authors further stated, "where separate accommodation is not available, a possible method of providing some relief to the relatives of demented old people might be for the day hospitals to devote its facilities 1 day a week for this purpose alone" (Brocklehurst and Tucker 1980, p. 179). This conclusion is highly influenced by the fact that studies from the United Kingdom tend to show higher rates of patients with dementia than of patients with functional psychiatric disorders in geriatric psychiatry day hospital programs (Ballinger 1984; Farndale 1961; Gilleard 1985; Hassall et al. 1972), unlike in physical rehabilitation programs, which remain the domain of the medical geriatric day hospital.

Applications of Day Hospital Treatment

Health care planners usually perceive day hospitals as a cost-effective alternative to inpatient facilities; however, day hospitals can also provide a number of other services. These include a role in transition from inpatient services, rehabilitation of long-term patients, an alternative to outpatient treatment, maintenance of long-term patients, and assistance in cases that pose diagnostic difficulties (Voineskos 1976). The day hospital milieu helps maintain the social skills of elderly patients, who frequently become isolated in the community, and the regular contact with staff and peers may improve compliance with treatment. Wagner (1991) alluded to seven guiding principles in specialized partial hospitalization for older adults: 1) services that meet a continuum of needs of older adults, 2) services that are cost effective and economically viable, 3) services that are accessible and acceptable, 4) programs that provide an interdisciplinary orientation, 5) individualized assessment and treatment planning, 6) enhancement of family and community supports, and 7) the restitution of capacity.

To fulfill these guidelines, the geriatric psychiatry day hospital ideally should consist of a multidisciplinary team consisting of geriatric psychiatrists, psychiatric nurses, psychologists, occupational therapists, recreation therapists, and psychiatric social workers. All members of the multidisciplinary team should have extensive experience in individual assessment and the ability to carry out treatment programs within a group setting. Members of the team must be flexible in their approach to the elderly patient with psychiatric problems and able to tolerate the many areas of overlap of function among various team members. The underlying bond that holds multidisciplinary teams together consists of a genuine concern for the elderly individual and treatment planning that is always in the best interest of the patient.

Population Served

The two most common psychiatric conditions undergoing assessment and treatment in a geriatric psychiatry day hospital are depression and dementia. The therapeutic nihilism usually associated with geriatric patients may be related to the focusing of attention on patients who have dementia. However, functional disorders such as depression cause significant morbidity in the geriatric population and can be treated if active measures are instituted sufficiently early (MacMillan 1967). There are large variations in the rates of depression and dementia found in geriatric day hospital populations, as indicated in Table 33–2. The descriptive studies identified in Table 33–2 show high rates of patients with dementia in geriatric psychiatry day hospital programs in the United Kingdom. In contrast, day hospital reports from the United States, Canada, and Germany (Bergener et al. 1987) reflect higher rates of depression and other functional psychiatric disorders in the geriatric psychiatry day hospital population under treatment. The staffing, structure, and therapeutic milieu of a day hospital program are greatly influenced by the nature of the patient population. This led Goldstein and Carlson in 1976 to refer to their facility as an "active psychogeriatric day hospital" in that it provided short-term treatment with an emphasis on reactivation and

Table 33–2. Percentages of diagnoses in geriatric psychiatry day hospital patients

	Dementia	Mood disorders	Schizophrenia	Paranoid state	Anxiety disorder	Adjustment disorders	Other
United Kingdom							
Robertson and Pitt 1965	18	56	1	13	1		11
Hassall et al. 1972	39.6	33.5	18.8		0.5		7.6
Greene and Timbury 1979	46						54[a]
Gilleard 1987	86						14[a]
Canada							
Goldstein and Carlson 1976	11	81		6			2
Germany							
Bergener et al. 1987	17.3	55.4	9.9	6.8			10.5
United States							
Wagner 1991		62		2	13	19	4
Plotkin and Wells 1993		77			5	11	7

[a]Includes all functional disorders.

resocialization and functioned as a "bridge to the community" (Goldstein and Carlson 1976, p. 115).

Admissions to geriatric psychiatry day hospital programs generally fall into the categories outlined in Table 33–3.

Patients with cognitive impairment can be managed in a day hospital program, provided that they can orient themselves to their surroundings and that caregivers provide an appropriate amount of supervision in the community (Bergener et al. 1987).

The demographic data in most descriptive studies identify a much higher percentage of female patients than male patients (approximately a 2:1 ratio), regardless of the diagnostic makeup of the treatment population. Because of the large variations in the diagnostic groups found in geriatric psychiatry day hospitals, universally applicable admission and discharge criteria are not readily formulated; this is an area that requires further study. Short durations of day hospital treatment for elderly patients may be associated with specific psychological sequelae. For example, elderly patients who are initially reluctant to seek psychiatric care quickly develop dependence on the program and may experience a sense of rejection when nearing discharge (Goldstein 1971). Discharge planning is an important component of day hospital treatment, as programs that strive for short-term treatment of functional psychiatric disorders often end up with a cadre of patients requiring long-term treatment (Arie 1975).

Another unique and potentially complicating factor in the treatment of elderly patients with psychiatric disorders is their requirement for transportation to and from the day hospital. The practical problem in collecting a dozen or more elderly patients from their homes with a single vehicle may result in elderly patients spending as much time on the road as in the day hospital; this has led to the description of "transport therapy" as a new type of community-based psychiatric treatment. "In transport therapy, in keeping with the fashionable emphasis on keeping people out of hospital, the hospital becomes irrelevant and to travel happily becomes more important than to arrive. Meals can be taken at a friendly transport cafe, always provided there is a greater-than-average provision of functioning lavatories" (Arie 1975, p. 37).

Outcome of Day Hospital Treatment

Variability in goals of treatment, staffing, patient population, and treatment modalities makes generalizations concerning the effectiveness of day hospital

Table 33–3.   Guidelines for patient selection for psychogeriatric day
                    hospitals

Patients with acute psychiatric disorders who can be safely treated in an
    ambulatory care setting. This does not include patients who are an active
    suicidal risk or whose physical disabilities preclude their active participation
    in the program.
Patients who present with atypical or multidimensional psychiatric problems
    and require a period of observation in a multidisciplinary setting in order to
    establish a clear diagnosis.
Patients with chronic or recurrent psychiatric disorders who require a more
    intensive period of active treatment to stabilize their illness and develop
    coping mechanisms.
Patients who can be discharged earlier from inpatient care with additional
    support and treatment during the vulnerable transition period from hospital
    to home.

treatment difficult (Guy and Gross 1967; Moscowitz 1980). Studies of adult
day hospitals dealing with younger patients suggest that day hospital treatment is comparable or superior to standard inpatient treatment (Davis et
al. 1978; Hamilton and Ramaiah 1986; Herz et al. 1971, 1975; Penk and Van
Hoose 1978). A number of methodological problems, including small numbers of patients, selection bias, partial or lack of randomization, and lack of
control over variables such as diagnosis, medication, and follow-up treatment continue to complicate the findings with regard to the efficacy of day
hospital treatment (Creed et al. 1989). One study attempted to deal with the
methodological problem of randomization of patients and found that day
hospital treatment was "completely unfeasible" for 40% of the cohort under
study (Kluiter et al. 1992). Negative factors related to feasibility of day hospital treatment were the requirement of a certain level of surveillance, the
presence of physical illness, and ongoing depressive symptoms.

Outcome studies of elderly patients with psychiatric disorders treated
in a day hospital program must be reviewed carefully with respect to the
patient population. Patients with the diagnosis of dementia inevitably show
long-term attendance, very high rates of admission to long-term care institutions, and high mortality rates as a result of concurrent disease
(Christie and Train 1984; Gilleard 1985; Gilleard et al. 1984; Jones 1980;
Robertson and Pitt 1965). Greene and Timbury demonstrated in 1979
that if priority is given to organic mental disorders, the cases of dementia
increased from 46% to 90% in a geriatric psychiatry day hospital population over a 5-year period. In their study, 83% of patients with dementia
were living in their home at the time of admission to the day hospital, and
only 12% could be discharged back to their homes at the end of treatment,

with the vast majority being admitted to long-term care institutions. During the same 5-year period the authors treated 80 elderly patients with a functional psychiatric disorder. Sixty-six percent of these patients were living in their home at the time of admission, and 57% remained in their homes at the time of discharge from the day hospital program. This study is evidence that within the same geriatric psychiatry day hospital program, elderly patients with functional psychiatric disorders can be maintained in the community, whereas patients with dementia frequently require long-term institutional care.

Two studies have focused on the outcome of day hospital treatment for elderly patients with functional psychiatric illness. In 1992, Steingart described a geriatric psychiatry day hospital treatment program for depressed older adults over age 55. Clinical improvement was demonstrated on standardized rating scales for depression and led to the conclusion that the psychiatric day hospital is a "potent treatment modality for elderly depressed patients" (Steingart 1992, p. 348). Plotkin and Wells reported on a review of 100 geriatric patients in a partial hospitalization program over a 5-year period. Seventy-seven percent of the patients studied had a mood disorder. Fifty-seven percent of patients were rated on an ordinal scale as showing minimal to moderate improvement after an intensive phase of treatment lasting 3 months. Variables associated with a positive outcome included the diagnosis of a mood disorder, higher functional status, ongoing social support, and regular attendance at the program (Plotkin and Wells 1993). Both of these reports are well-documented descriptive studies; however, the lack of a control group attests to the ongoing methodological difficulties in outcome studies dealing with effectiveness of day hospital programs.

Although geriatric psychiatry day hospitals may function as an alternative to inpatient facility for some patients, they are part of a continuum of treatment and cannot be considered as a substitute for inpatient treatment. Studies with psychiatrically ill elderly patients treated in a day hospital setting have consistently demonstrated the need for inpatient treatment of a significant minority (21% [Fottrell et al. 1980] to 25% [Plotkin and Wells 1993]) of patients initially admitted to a day hospital program.

Cost-Effectiveness

In the absence of any scientific scrutiny, the statement could be made that day hospital treatment is more expensive than outpatient treatment or no treatment at all. Studies with younger psychiatric patients have demonstrated that day hospital treatment can reduce hospitalization rates

(Bateman 1985) and result in less utilization of medical facilities in a follow-up interval when compared with the pretreatment interval (Comstock et al. 1985). Other authors have pointed out that cost-effectiveness studies that consistently demonstrate day hospital treatment to be less expensive than inpatient treatment do not include costs such as nursing and housekeeping care in the home, basic pensions, rent or maintenance costs of the home, and various government subsidies. In 1989, Smith and Marshall demonstrated that, after the introduction of a psychogeriatric day hospital and closure of 100 inpatient beds, 38 long-term care patients who had been institutionalized for many years could be discharged back into the community (Smith and Marshall 1989). This report did not include a financial analysis demonstrating the cost-effectiveness of the day hospital as an alternative to long-term inpatient care; however, the high cost of inpatient care would likely support such a hypothesis.

Caregiver Stress

Outcome studies in geriatric psychiatry patients are highly dependent on the patient population that is under study. Standard measures that are usually applied to a general adult population, such as turnover rates, reduction in psychopathology on standardized rating scales, and mortality rates may be less valid indicators in an elderly day hospital population with high rates of dementia. Even though our therapeutic armamentarium cannot reverse the core cognitive impairment in most cases of dementia, day hospital treatment can result in a significant reduction in emotional distress and caregiver burden for the majority of relatives and friends (Gilleard et al. 1984). Studies regarding the reduction of stress in caregivers of elderly patients treated for mood disorders in day hospitals are lacking; however, providing relief and hope to close relatives of severely depressed patients is one of the intangible yet real positive effects of day hospital treatment.

References

Andrews RM, Fox S, Elixhauser A, et al: The national bill for diseases treated in United States hospitals: 1987 (AHCPR Publ No 94-0002). Division of Provider Studies Research Note 19. Rockville, MD, Agency for Health Care Policy and Research, Public Health Service, 1994

Arie T: Day care in geriatric psychiatry. Gerontol Clin (Basel) 17:31–39, 1975

Arie T, Jolley D: Making services work: organisation and style of psychogeriatric services, in The Psychiatry of Late Life. Edited by Levy R, Post F. Oxford, England, Blackwell Scientific Publications, 1982, pp 222–251

Ballinger BR: The effects of opening a geriatric psychiatry day hospital. Acta Psychiatr Scand 70:400–403, 1984

Bateman JK: Efficacy and cost effectiveness of partial hospitalization. Int J Partial Hosp 3:59–64, 1985

Bergener ME, Kranzhoff EU, Husser J, et al: The psychogeriatric day hospital: definition, historical development, working methods and initial efforts in research, in Psychogeriatrics: An International Handbook. Edited by Berenger ME. New York, Springer, 1987, pp 432–438

Berger MM, Berger LF: An innovative program for a private psychogeriatric day center. J Am Geriatr Soc 19:332–336, 1971

Bierer J: Theory and practice of psychiatric day hospitals. Lancet 21:901–902, 1959

Billig N, Leibenluft E: Special considerations in integrating elderly patients into a general hospital psychiatric unit. Hosp Community Psychiatry 38:277–281, 1987

Brocklehurst JC, Tucker JS: Progress in Geriatric Day Care. London, England, King's Fund Publishing Office, 1980

Casarino JP, Wilner M, Maxey JT: American Association for Partial Hospitalization (AAPH) standards and guidelines for partial hospitalization. Int J Partial Hosp 1:5–21, 1982

Christie AB, Train JD: Change in the pattern of care for the demented. Br J Psychiatry 144:9–15, 1984

Comstock BS, Kamilar SM, Thornby JI, et al: Crisis treatment in a day hospital impact on medical care-seeking. Psychiatr Clin North Am 8:483–499, 1985

Conwell Y, Nelson JC, Kim K, et al: Elderly patients admitted to the psychiatric unit of a general hospital. J Am Geriatr Soc 37:35–41, 1989

Craft M: Psychiatric day hospitals. Am J Psychiatry 116:251–254, 1959

Creed F, Black D, Anthony P: Day hospital and community treatment for acute psychiatric illness, a critical appraisal. Br J Psychiatry 154:300–310, 1989

Davis JE, Lorei TW, Caffey EM: An evaluation of the Veterans Administration day hospital program. Hosp Community Psychiatry 29:297–302, 1978

Duke University Center for the Study of Aging and Human Development: Multidementional Functional Assessment: the OARS Methodology.

Durham, NC, Duke University, 1978

Edwards MS: Psychiatric day programs, a descriptive analysis. J Psychosoc Nurs Ment Health Serv 20:17–21, 1982

English JT, McGarrick RG: The economics of inpatient psychiatry, in Inpatient Psychiatry: Diagnosis and Treatment, 2nd Edition. Edited by Sederer LI. Baltimore, MD, Williams & Wilkins, 1986, pp 367–382

Farndale J: The Day Hospital Movement in Great Britain. Elmsford, NY, Pergamon, 1961

Fottrell E, Spy T, Mearns G, et al: "Asset stripping" the declining mental hospital. Br Med J 280(6207):89–90, 1980

Garnick DW, Short T: Utilization of hospital inpatient services by elderly Americans. Research note 6 (DHHS Publ No [PHS] 85-3351). Washington, DC, 1985

Gilleard CJ: Predicting the outcome of psychogeriatric day care. Gerontologist 25:280–285, 1985

Gilleard CJ: Influence of emotional distress among supporters on the outcome of psychogeriatric day care. Br J Psychiatry 150:219–223, 1987

Gilleard CJ, Gilleard E, Whittick JE: Impact of psychogeriatric day hospital care on the patient's family. Br J Psychiatry 145:487–492, 1984

Glick ID, Clarkin JF: The family, in Inpatient Psychiatry, Diagnosis and Treatment, 2nd Edition. Edited by Sederer LI. Baltimore, MD, Williams & Wilkins, 1986, pp 296–307

Goldstein S: A critical appraisal of milieu therapy in a geriatric day hospital. J Am Geriatr Soc 19:693–699, 1971

Goldstein S, Sevruk J, Graver H: The establishment of a psychogeriatric day hospital. Can Med Assoc J 98:955–959, 1968

Goldstein SE, Carlson S: Evolution of an active psychogeriatric day hospital. Can Med Assoc J 115:874–876, 1976

Greene JG, Timbury GC: A geriatric psychiatry day hospital service: a five year review. Age Ageing 8:49–53, 1979

Guy W, Gross GM: Problems in the evaluation of day hospitals. Community Ment Health J 3:111–118, 1967

Hamilton P, Ramaiah RS: An evaluation of objectives of a psychiatric day hospital as a planning process. Hosp Health Serv Rev May:114–117, 1986

Harrison AW, Kernutt GJ, Piperoglou MV: A survey of patients in a regional geriatric psychiatry inpatient unit. Aust N Z J Psychiatry 22:412–417, 1988

Hassall C, Gath D, Cross KW: Psychiatric day-care in Birmingham. Br J Prev Soc Med 26:112–120, 1972

Health and Welfare Canada: Guidelines for Comprehensive Services to Elderly Persons With Psychiatric Disorders, Cat No H39-120. Ministry of Supply and Services, Ottawa, Ontario, Canada, Health and Welfare Canada, 1988

Herz MI, Endicott J, Spitzer RL, et al: Day versus inpatients hospitalization: a controlled study. Am J Psychiatry 127:1371–1381, 1971

Herz MI, Endicott J, Spitzer RL: Brief hospitalization of patients with families: initial results. Am J Psychiatry 132:413–418, 1975

Hyatt LG: Supportive design for people with memory impairments, in Confronting Alzheimer's Disease. Edited by Kalicki A. Owings Mills, MD, National Health Publishing, 1987, pp 138–163

Janken JK, Reynolds BA, Swiech K: Patient falls in the acute care setting: identifying risk factors. Nurs Res 35:215–219, 1986

Joint Commission on Accreditation of Health Care Organizations: Accreditation Manual for Mental Health, Chemical Dependency and Mental Retardation/Developmental Disorders Services. Oakbrook Terrace, IL, Joint Commission of Accreditation of Health Care Organization, 1993

Jones IG: An evaluation of a day hospital for the demented elderly. Health Bull 40:11–15, 1980

Klar H, Frances A, Clarkin J: Selection criteria for partial hospitalization. Hosp Community Psychiatry 33:929–933, 1982

Kluiter H, Giel R, Nienhuis FJ, et al: Predicting feasibility of day treatment for unselected patients referred for inpatient psychiatric treatment: results of a randomized trial. Am J Psychiatry 149:1199–1205, 1992

Knight BG, Carter PM: Reduction of psychiatric inpatient stay for older adults by intensive case management. Gerontologist 30:510–515, 1990

Kramer BM: Day hospital, a study of partial hospitalization in psychiatry. New York, Grune & Stratton, 1962

Liptzin B, Grob MC, Eisen SV: Family burden of demented and depressed elderly psychiatric inpatients. Gerontologist 28:397–401, 1988

MacMillan D: Problems of a geriatric mental health service. Br J Psychiatry 113:175–181, 1967

Meier HMR, Besir M, Sylph JA: Psychogeriatric hospitalization: terminable or interminable. Can J Psychiatry 37:157–162, 1992

Ministry of Health: A Hospital Plan for England and Wales. London, Her Majesty's Stationery Office, 1962

Moscowitz IS: The effectiveness of day hospital treatment: a review. J Community Psychol 8:155–164, 1980

National Council on Aging Inc: Standards for Adult Day Care. Washington, DC, April 1984

Parker S, Knoll JL: Partial hospitalization: an update. Am J Psychiatry 147:156–159, 1990

Peace SM: Review of day hospital provision in psychogeriatrics. Health Trends 14:92–95, 1982

Penk WE, Van Hoose TA: Comparative effectiveness of day hospital and inpatient psychiatric treatment. J Consult Clin Psychol 46:94–101, 1978

Pitt B: Psycho-Geriatrics: An Introduction to the Psychiatry of Old Age. Edinburgh, Scotland, Churchill Livingstone, 1982, p 224

Plotkin DA, Wells KB: Partial hospitalization (day treatment) for psychiatrically ill elderly patients. Am J Psychiatry 50:266–271, 1993

Redick RW, Taube CA: Demography and mental health care of the aged, in Handbook of Mental Health and Aging. Edited by Birren JE, Sloane RB. Englewood Cliffs, NJ, Prentice Hall, 1980, pp 57–71

Robertson WMF, Pitt B: The role of day hospital in geriatric psychiatry. Br J Psychiatry 111:635–640, 1965

Rogoff J: Individual psychotherapy, in Inpatient Psychiatry: Diagnosis and Treatment, 2nd Edition. Edited by Sederer LI. Baltimore, MD, Williams & Wilkins, 1986, pp 240–262

Royal College of Physicians of London: Care of elderly people with mental illness: specialist services and medical training. A joint report of the Royal College of Physicians and the Royal College of Psychiatrists. London, Royal College of Physicians of London, 1989, p 29

Salzman C, Strauss ME, Engle RP, et al: Overnight guesting of day hospital patients. Compr Psychiatry 10:369–375, 1969

Sheline, YI: High prevelence of physical illness in a geriatric psychiatric inpatient population. Gen Hosp Psychiatry 12(6):396–400, 1990

Skeet M: Protecting the Health of the Elderly. Copenhagen, Denmark, World Health Organization Regional Office for Europe, 1983, p 125

Smith SA, Marshall WL: Alternative programs in a psychogeriatric hospital. Dimensions in Health Service 66920:17–19, 33, 1989

Spar JE, Ford CV, Liston EH: Hospital treatment of elderly neuropsychiatric patients, II: statistical profile of the first 122 patients in a new teaching ward. J Am Geriatr Soc 28:539–543, 1980

Steingart AB: Geriatric psychiatry day hospital: a treatment program for depressed older adults, in Aging and Mental Disorders. Edited by Bergener ME. New York, Springer, 1992, pp 338–355

Steuer J: Psychotherapy with the elderly. Psychiatr Clin North Am 5:195–210, 1982

Teri L, Truax P, Logsdon R, et al: Assessment of behavioral problems in dementia: the revised Memory and Behavior Problems Checklist. Psychol Aging 7(4):622–631, 1992

Vaughan PJ: Developments in psychiatric daycare. Br J Psychiatry 147:1–4, 1985

Voineskos G: Part time hospitalization programs: the neglected field of community psychiatry. Can Med Assoc J 114:320–324, 1976

Wagner BD: Specialized partial hospitalization for older adults: a clinical description of an intermediate-term program. Psychiatr Hosp 22:69–76, 1991

Weingarten CH, Rosoff LG, Eisen SV, et al: Medical care in a geriatric psychiatry unit: impact on psychiatric outcome. J Am Geriatr Soc 30:738–743, 1982

Wells KB, Rogers WH, Davis LM, et al: Quality of care for hospitalized depressed elderly patients before and after implementation of the Medicare prospective payment system. Am J Psychiatry 150:1799–1805, 1993

Whanger AD: Inpatient treatment of the older psychiatric patient, in Geriatric Psychiatry. Edited by Busse EW, Blazer DG. Washington, DC, American Psychiatric Press, 1989, pp 593–633

Whanger AD, Busse EW: Care in hospital, in Modern Perspectives in the Psychiatry of Old Age. Edited by Howells JG. New York, Brunner/Mazel, 1975, pp 450–485

Yates AJ: Theory and Practice in Behavior Therapy. New York, Wiley, 1975, p 243

Zarit JM, Zarit SH: Measurement of burden and social support. Paper presented at the Annual Scientific Meeting of the Gerontological Society of America, San Diego, CA, November 1982

Zubenko GS, Rosen J, Sweet RA, et al: Impact of psychiatric hospitalization on behavioral complications of Alzheimer's disease. Am J Psychiatry 149:1484–1491, 1992

Carl I. Cohen, M.D.

Integrated Community Services

P sychiatric treatment of the geriatric patient generally cannot be conducted in isolation. Consequently, the psychiatrist may be called on to orchestrate the various components of the treatment plan. Even if the psychiatrist does not assume a coordinating role, it is nevertheless incumbent on the clinician to assist the patient, family, and other health care professionals in identifying those services that will help optimize the patient's level of functioning. The description of services provided in this chapter is designed to provide the geriatric psychiatrist with the basic information that is critical to educating patients, families, and other health professionals about the types of support services available in the community.

In addition to helping patients negotiate the formal support system, clinicians often work with the patient's and family's informal support networks, which comprise relatives, friends, clergy, storekeepers, letter carriers, and so forth. These members of the informal network may be important informants and may provide or help to secure crucial support to the patient, such as food, household chores, and shopping. In recent years, community outreach efforts have spawned the development of network techniques—that is, teaching persons to better utilize their existing networks or encouraging them to broaden their support system to obtain additional emotional and material support (Biegel et al. 1984; Collins and Pancoast 1976; Gottlieb 1983).

In examining which factors inhibit or facilitate access to community services, a variety of structural and individual barriers have been identified. Structural barriers thought to be important are 1) inconvenient locations for services; 2) a relative lack of services in a community; 3) the financial cost of obtaining services; 4) negative professional attitudes and behaviors; 5) bureaucratic orientation of programs; and 6) the lack of any real coordination, integration, or organization within and among agencies servicing elderly individuals (Krout 1985; Reed 1980). Impediments to obtaining help at the individual patient level include 1) fear for personal safety, 2) poor health, 3) lack of knowledge about the availability of services, 4) negative attitudes toward services, and 5) fear of becoming too dependent on such services (Krout 1985). Finally, sources of information may play a significant role. Silverstein (1984) found that information that elderly individuals obtained through formal sources (e.g., senior centers, medical facilities) was the best predictor of service utilization. However, elderly individuals cited such formal sources much less frequently than television, newspapers, friends/relatives, and brochures as preferred channels of information (Goodman 1992).

Gerontological practitioners, planners, and researchers are frequently required to impose some order on the myriad of services and facilities available to community-dwelling elderly individuals (Golant and McCaslen 1979). Although there is no consensus or well-accepted rationale for any existing classification schema, Table 34–1 represents a synthesis of a classification schema proposed by Golant and McCaslen (1979) and Cantor and Little (1985). (The items listed in Table 34–1 will be described later in the chapter.) On the vertical axis of the table is a measure of independence and self-functioning divided into three categories: well, moderately impaired, and frail or severely impaired. On the horizontal axis are three broad categories of needs: a basic level consisting of health needs; an intermediate level comprising self-maintenance needs such as dressing, grooming, cooking, transportation, cleaning, and handling money; and a complex level involving social needs such as work roles, friendship, intimacy, and education. Thus, for example, a comparatively well older person who has recently lost several close friends might be helped by referrals to social and vocational services listed in the upper right corner of Table 34–1. Similarly, a moderately impaired person with Alzheimer's disease might benefit from the self-maintenance and social services contained in the center and right cells of the middle row of Table 34–1.

Organizationally, in this chapter the hierarchical model of Table 34–1 will be followed, with descriptions of items moving from those at the lowest levels of functioning to those at the highest levels. The items have been placed under two broad headings—"Community Services" and "Community Housing"—that will serve as the main subdivisions of the chapter.

Community Services

In this section an overview of the principal geriatric community services is provided. More detailed descriptions are available elsewhere (Gelfand 1993; Huttman 1985). The reader should note that the intensity and level of services will vary between services that are primarily aimed at clinical populations (e.g., day care, nursing homes) and those that are psychosocially supportive (e.g., mutual aid groups, volunteer groups). The latter may serve a preventive function by ensuring that elderly individuals do not become socially isolated and, if disease develops, that they are already part of a network that makes clinical care accessible. Table 34–2 summarizes the principal governmental programs and their related services and benefits. Clinicians should also be aware that a variety of private health insurance policies have emerged that may cover the costs of home care and nursing homes. Moreover, some health maintenance organizations (HMOs) may provide home and institutional care in their prepaid plans. Increasingly, social health maintenance organizations (SHMOs) are being introduced. These offer older persons prepaid long-term care and social services (e.g., homemaker, case management, day care) along with traditional acute health services (Skolnick and Warrick 1985). Finally, elderly veterans may be eligible for a variety of residential long-term care services (e.g., nursing home, domiciliary care) provided by the Veteran's Administration.

Assistance and Protection

Information and referral (assistance) services. The Older Americans Act (OAA) was enacted in 1965 to assist aging individuals by providing funds to states for services, training, and resources. These activities are coordinated through the Administration on Aging (AOA), which is an independent agency in the Department of Health and Human Services. Title III of the OAA provides for each state to designate an agency for aging services. In about half the states, an independent office on aging has been established; in the remaining states, aging programs are part of a human services department. In most states, aging agencies designate smaller geographic service centers, termed *area*

Table 34–1.   Types of services available to elderly individuals

Function level	Physical and mental health needs
Well elderly (60% of population)	Mutual help groups Consumer health education Health insurance Health screening
Moderately impaired (30% of population)	Outreach services Visiting nurse Crisis intervention teams
Frail or severely impaired (10% of population)	Mutual help groups for family Outreach services Visiting nurses Crisis intervention teams Inpatient psychiatric and medical care

Note.   ECHO = Elder Cottage Housing Opportunity.
Source.   Modified from Golant and McCaslen (1979) and Cantor and Little (1985).

agencies on aging (AAA), to provide local communities with information and referral services. The AAAs are forbidden to provide direct services, unless absolutely necessary. In 1990, there were 680 AAAs throughout the country (Gelfand 1993).

Whereas the AAAs are public agencies, there are a variety of voluntary and private resources that provide information and assistance; these include

Table 34–1. Types of services available to elderly individuals (*continued*)

Self-maintenance needs	Social needs
Shared housing	Senior center
Converted boarding homes	Voluntary associations
ECHO units and "granny flats"	Retired seniors
Section 8 and Section 202 housing	Volunteer program
Elderly apartment complexes	Foster parents and grandparents
Retirement community	Senior companions
Congregate meals program	Service Corps of Retired Executives
Nutrition education	Green Thumb
"Brown bag" programs	Senior aides
	Adult education
Case management	Friendly visiting
Home care services	Telephone reassurance
Domiciliary care	Strengthen informal social support
Foster care	network
Vocational rehabilitation	
Assisted living	
Board and care homes	
Congregate housing	
Meals-on-Wheels	
Transportation services	
Escort services	
Chore services	
Day care	Friendly visiting
Respite care	Telephone reassurance
Home care services	Strengthen informal social support
Hospice	network
Nursing home	
Meals-on-Wheels	
Protective services	
Case management	

family services facilities, senior centers, and mental health associations. About 85% of information and assistance programs are part of public agencies, approximately half of which are AAAs and the remainder are usually part of local social services departments (Huttman 1985). Problems most often requiring referrals are financial, social security, and transportation problems; health problems and care; housing, food and nutrition, and homemaker

Table 34–2.   Summary of principal governmental programs relevant to community services

Program	Services and benefits	Eligibility
Old Age Survivors and Disabled Insurance (OASDI) (1935)	Social Security benefits	All persons ages 65 and older, disabled workers, and dependent survivors when worker dies. Reduced amounts for retirees age 62
Supplemental Security Income (SSI) Program (1972)	Supplemental payments to bring persons up to poverty threshold; states have option to pay for domiciliary care homes and personal home care	Indigent persons 65 and older, disabled, and blind
Title XVIII of the Social Security Act (1965)	Medicare, which includes hospital costs, physicians' fees, skilled nursing facility (limited), home health care, and hospice care	Persons ages 65 and older and those under 65 who receive Social Security disability payments
Title XIX of the Social Security Act (1965)	Medicaid, which includes medical services, skilled nursing care (unlimited), and home health care Optional by state: Adult day care, drugs, intermediate care facility	Indigent elderly, disabled, and blind persons
Social Services Block Grant (1981) (formerly Title XX of the Social Security Act [1975])	Varying levels by state: Chore services, congregate meals, home-delivered meals, homemaker, senior centers, protective services	Indigent persons (all ages) up to 115% of state median income

Program	Services	Target Population
Older Americans Act (OAA) (1965), Title III	Services vary by state: Congregate meals, home-delivered meals, home health care, chore services, senior centers, friendly visiting	All persons ages 60 and older; low-income persons are special targets
Frail Elderly Act (1991)	Varies by state: An optional Medicaid program to provide homemaker/home health aide services, chore services, respite care, day care, nursing care	Indigent persons
Older Americans Act (OAA) (1965), Title V	Community employment (e.g., senior aides, Green Thumb)	Indigent persons ages 55 and older
ACTION (1971)	Federal agency established to coordinate volunteer programs, programs for elderly persons include Foster Grandparents, RSVP, Senior Companions	Some programs open only to indigent persons
Section 202 of Housing Act (1959)	Low-interest loans for construction of low-rent housing	Nonprofit sponsors
Section 8 of Housing and Community Development Act (1974)	Rent subsidies to cover difference between fair market rent and 30% of participants' income	Low-income persons
Food Stamp Program (1964)	Department of Agriculture program to purchase foods at lower prices	Low-income persons

Note. RSVP = Retired Seniors Volunteer Program.
Sources. Huttman (1985), Maddox (1987), and Skolnick and Warrick (1985).

services; employment; consumer needs; legal problems; companionship; and nursing home care (Huttman 1985).

Funding for information and referral programs generally comes from governmental sources, with state governments providing the largest shares. Nonprofit organizations, religious groups, and foundations are also important sources of revenues. Gelfand (1993) observed that because of their lack of expense and wide availability, information and referral programs are used by a disproportionate number of persons who are already connected to the system in some way. Unfortunately, direct outreach to underserved individuals is usually too expensive for most programs.

How to Access Services

With the dramatic expansion of geriatric services and varying eligibility requirements needed to obtain such services, the most expeditious way for clinicians and consumers to learn about a particular type of service in their community is by contacting their state or local agency on aging. Community agencies such as United Way, Family Service America, Catholic Charities, or Jewish Family Services can also assist with information and referrals. On the national level, the National Health Information Clearinghouse is designed to bring together consumer and health information resources. One of the best ways to secure services is through the local Yellow Pages, looking under appropriate headings such as "Social Services Organizations," "Home Health Services," "Senior Services," and "Nursing Services."

Case or care management.   The primary aim of case management is to help clients and family deal with a fragmented and complex system by locating and coordinating existing resources through a process that includes screening, assessment, case planning, linkage to services, advocacy, monitoring, and, in some instances, therapeutic counseling (Huttman 1985). Much of the growth in case management services has been spurred by the expanding need for in-home services for persons with mental or physical impairments and the variety of funding sources and eligibility requirements. Thus, various health and welfare agencies such as public agencies, social services agencies, HMOs, health care facilities, or insurance carriers that provide services to elderly individuals currently use case management (Westhoff 1992). Moreover, consumers may enlist the assistance of a private case management to obtain the appropriate mix of in-home services. Fees generally vary from $50 to $100 for an initial consultation (American Association of Retired Persons 1986b).

There are three case management approaches that are commonly used to secure and coordinate services (Westhoff 1992):

1. The *brokering model*, in which case managers identify the appropriate service package from resources in the community; case managers do not have dollars to allocate, but negotiate and advocate with providers for various services
2. The *service management model*, in which the case manager authorizes both the services provided and the clients' service budget, with the funding source influencing what services can be recommended
3. The *managed care model*, in which the carrier of a high-risk group of clients or a group of enrollees in a health care program prospectively pays the organization providing managed care

White (1987) observed that the popularity and success of case management is evidenced by its proliferation in all types of health and social services settings, especially in programs serving long-term care populations. However, a major evaluation of two models of case management— variants of the brokering and the service management models—using 10 demonstration sites was largely disappointing (Carcagno and Kemper 1988). The overall impact on rates of institutionalization and cost savings was small (Thornton et al. 1988). Although caregivers had somewhat higher levels of satisfaction and well-being than controls, there were no differences in perceived emotional, physical, or financial strain, nor did programs affect client mortality or functioning. One important finding was that, although the service system may be fragmented and confusing, families are generally able to find services on their own. Zarit and Teri (1991) speculated that case management may be more effective for older persons without involved caregivers.

Protective services. These services serve persons who are 1) incapable of performing functions necessary to meet basic physical and health requirements, 2) incapable of managing finances, 3) dangerous to self or others, or 4) exhibiting behavior that brings them into conflict with the community. Such agencies may facilitate hospitalization or assist with various legal actions. In general, these services have been provided by public departments of social services and legal service centers (Beattie 1976). The effectiveness of the protective casework model in use since the 1960s has been questioned (Zborowsky 1985), and several demonstration projects were found to be no more effective than the usual community control services (Blenkner et al.

1974). Studies of elder abuse programs have also raised questions about the ability of professionals to successfully resolve the abuse problem (Zborowsky 1985). Despite the controversy that exists over these findings (Berger and Piliavin 1976), Zborowsky (1985) argues that a continued search for more effective protective social services is needed.

Community Care

Noelker and Bass (1989) developed a useful typology to examine how community-based services are supposed to benefit caregivers. They delineated four patterns:

1. *Complementary*, in which formal and informal helpers (e.g., kin, neighbors) provide different but complementary services
2. *Supplementary*, in which formal services augment the efforts of the informal caregivers
3. *Substitution*, in which formal agencies take the place of informal helpers
4. *Kin independence*, in which the informal helpers provide all the assistance

The impact of formal services will vary depending on the pattern. For example, if introduction of services results in a complementary pattern, informal caregivers may feel relief that new services are being provided; however, these caregivers will be still giving the same level of assistance.

Respite care.   Respite care is care provided on a short-term basis (usually several hours to several weeks) to a dependent person in the community to relieve the caregiver of responsibility for the constant care of that person (Abrahams et al. 1991). Hegeman (1989) identifies five major categories: 1) in-home (e.g., home companions, homemakers), 2) in-the-community (e.g., adult day care), 3) institutions caring for elderly individuals (e.g., adult homes, overnight stays), 4) hospitals, and 5) combination models. Services may be organized by religious organizations, nursing homes, home health care agencies, and voluntary agencies.

Evaluation of specific respite approaches is discussed in later sections. An examination of respite services as a general approach has shown mixed effects. A study from Duke University (Gwyther 1989) of both in-home and overnight respite care found a positive effect on caregivers' mood. Nevertheless, many persons eligible for respite services did not use them because of their financial costs and because of complaints about the lack of dependability of in-home respite care providers. Lawton et al. (1989)

found that respite services only slightly decreased rates of institutionalization and afforded no benefits in caregivers' subjective burden or well-being. A drawback of these studies is that experimental subjects received only very small amounts of respite (e.g., often as little as 1 hour per week of in-home respite and 10 days of respite over a year) (Zarit and Teri 1991). Zarit and Teri (1991) concluded that the first-generation studies of interventions and services for caregivers have demonstrated "an expectably modest amount of improvement, given the complexity of caregivers' lives and the relatively limited magnitude of the interventions" (p. 304).

In-home health care services.   This covers a wide array of services offered in the home that can be grouped under three categories (Gelfand 1993):

1. *Intensive or skilled services* (e.g., assistance with open wounds, catheters, or tube feedings) that are ordered by a physician and are under the supervision of a nurse
2. *Personal care* or *intermediate services,* which are for medically stable individuals who require assistance with activities of daily living such as bathing, prescribed exercises, and ambulation
3. *Homemaker, chore,* or *basic services* (e.g., light housekeeping, meal preparation, or other maintenance activities), which are offered to persons who have difficulties caring for their personal environment, but who are able to do more basic activities of daily living such as toileting or bathing

Whereas intensive services usually require visits by a physician, nurse, or physical therapist, services in the other two categories are generally provided by a homemaker/home health aide. Home health care services must be provided by a home health agency that is certified by the state health department. Five types of home health agencies exist: government-sponsored agencies (e.g., Department of Social Services), nonprofit agencies (e.g., Visiting Nurse Service), for-profit agencies, hospital-based programs, and community health centers (Gelfand 1993). There are six ways to pay for in-home services:

1. Medicaid, which will pay for almost all costs of home health care for indigent persons
2. Medicare, which is available to those ages 65 and over who are confined to home and who require skilled nursing care, physical therapy, or speech therapy under a plan established by a physician

3. Supplemental private insurance, such as "Medigap" insurance, which covers certain home health care services, and may provide supplement benefits that exceed Medicare limits
4. Social Services Block Grants (formerly Title XX of Social Security Act), which have provided limited funds to state departments of social services to reimburse public and private home care agencies for home-based services to the indigent
5. Title III of the OAA funnels funds to public and private agencies through local AAAs for services to persons ages 60 and over who are generally indigent
6. Out-of-pocket fees, which range from $10 to $17 per hour for a home-maker/home health aide to $12 to $50 per visit for a registered nurse or $50 per visit for a physical therapist (Abrahams et al. 1991; American Association of Retired Persons 1986a)

Although home care services are gaining ardent supporters, the cost-effectiveness of such services is unclear because cost-effectiveness depends on which factors are included in the equation (Ellis 1984). There is general consensus that home care is more humane and improves the older person's quality of life. Gurland et al. (1983) propose that home care services could be made even more efficacious by making the family, rather than the disabled person, the primary focus of intervention and by including in the repertoire of home care skills the capacity to provide emotional support for the family and dependent elderly persons, in addition to more material services.

Related in-home services.   There are a variety of services for homebound elderly individuals that can complement or substitute for the in-home services described in the preceding section. In most instances these services are offered by senior centers or agencies that provide other services to elderly individuals. Such services include the following:

- *Friendly visiting.* A volunteer visits the home usually 1–2 times per week for general conversation, to inquire about needs, to help with errands, and so forth. There is no charge for this service, which is usually offered by a volunteer group or religious organization. The usual aims of friendly visiting are to reduce social isolation, increase morale and well-being, and delay the onset of institutionalization (Korte and Gupta 1991). The few studies that have been done are generally supportive of the effectiveness of friendly visiting (Korte and Gupta 1991). Seniors receiving friendly visiting showed higher morale and better health, mental status, grooming, and apartment upkeep than their nonvisited counterparts (Korte and Gupta 1991; Mulligan and Bennett 1977).

- *Telephone reassurance.* Clients are given a number to call if they feel lonely or have a request for help. Volunteers also call to check on the client.
- *Emergency response systems.* This program provides a reliable contact by telephone or electronic device to police or rescue squads in the event of an emergency.
- *Chore services.* These services offer minor household repairs, household cleaning, and yard work. Costs average $7.50 an hour, plus materials; some agencies may offer assistance at reduced costs (American Association of Retired Persons 1986a).

Adult day care.   These programs are designed for at-risk persons who are mentally, physically, or socially impaired and who need day services to maintain or improve their level of functioning so that they can remain in or return to their own home. Such programs also provide some respite for families. Patients attend for 3–7 hours for as many as 5 days per week. Two decades ago, day care centers could be categorized into two broad types: health-oriented and social services–oriented (Weissert 1976). Although these divisions remain to some extent, some of these distinctions have become blurred. Weissert et al. (1989) suggested that it is more profitable to examine programs based on their affiliations. Thus, Auspice Model 1 includes outpatient day centers affiliated with nursing homes and rehabilitation centers that cater to physically dependent, older populations. Services are generally health-oriented and include nursing; health assessments; social services; and physical, occupational, and speech therapies. Auspice Model 2 is situated in an outpatient unit of a general hospital or a social services or housing agency. Most patients are younger than those in Model 1 and can perform activities of daily living; however, more than 40% have mental disorders. Services are proportionately more social and supportive and include case management, professional counseling, transportation to and from centers, nutrition, education, and health assessment. Auspice Model 3 involves special purpose centers that serve a single type of clientele, such as blind or mentally ill persons, those with dementia, or veterans.

All programs rely on a combination of federal, local, and private funds. Most governmental funds are provided through patients' Medicaid reimbursement, although programs may obtain additional funds through Title III and Social Services Block Grants. Medicare provides only a very small fraction of funding, usually for specific rehabilitative therapies. When not reimbursed by Medicaid, out-of-pocket daily costs range from $10 to $105, with a median of $30 for 6 hours of service (Zelman et al. 1991).

Research on adult day care has been generally positive although its cost-effectiveness has been more equivocal (Weiler 1987). Compared with a community control group, day care participants showed higher levels of physical and emotional functioning (Weiler et al. 1976). The median daily cost for day care—$30—is lower than costs for nursing homes (Capitman and Gregory 1984; Rathbone-McCuan and Elliot 1976–1977) and compares favorably with the cost of a home visit from a home health nurse ($40) or a 4-hour visit from a homemaker ($25+). Nevertheless, for persons less at risk for nursing home placement, the cost benefits of day care are thought to be modest (Skellie et al. 1982).

Community Mental Health Services

Of the more than 600 community mental health centers in the United States, only half have services for elderly individuals (Lebowitz 1987). The Community Mental Health Centers Act of 1963 was revised in 1975 to include specialized services for elderly individuals as one of 12 required service components; however, the block grant program of 1981 eliminated elderly services as a required component (Morrissey and Goldman 1984). Moreover, switching federal mental health funding from separate categorical funding to block grants to states allowed the states to determine at what level mental health services to elderly individuals should be funded. Data indicated a decline in specialized services to elderly individuals in the years immediately following the institution of block grants (Gelfand 1993). Currently, mental health services for older persons are reimbursed through Medicare and supplemented by Medicaid if the person is indigent. Mental health centers may also receive additional funding from state and local sources.

Lebowitz and colleagues (Lebowitz 1988; Lebowitz et al. 1987) identified several factors that may enhance mental health service utilization by elderly individuals, the most critical being the existence of a unit for elderly individuals within an outpatient clinic staffed by professionals with specialized training in geriatric mental health and that has cooperative affiliations with local area agencies on aging. Lebowitz (1987) further recommended that programs be made more accessible and that, rather than relying on referrals and self-identification, programs engage in aggressive outreach. In later sections, several specialized community programs for elderly individuals are described.

Mental health crisis intervention services. The aim of these services is to provide rapid restabilization of a person's psychiatric symptoms and social adjustment (Phipps and Liberman 1988). Crisis services are often hospital based or tied to community mental health centers. Services may be delivered in the patient's home or at a designated place outside the home. Mobile units or home treatment teams may visit the home or maintain daily telephone contact (Reifler et al. 1982; Sherr et al. 1976). Alternatively, patients may receive crisis care in the hospital or emergency department or leave their homes to live in a respite home or in crisis lodging.

Community outreach. Community outreach programs have proven to be especially successful in meeting the mental health needs of traditionally underserved and disadvantaged populations, such as rural elderly individuals (Buckwalter et al. 1993; Raschko 1991), homeless elderly individuals (Cohen et al. 1993), elderly persons in public housing (Roca et al. 1990), or mentally ill older adults in suburban communities (DeRenzo et al. 1991). One comprehensive outreach program in a suburb of Baltimore addressed the mental health needs of an elderly population by dividing its program into thirds: one-third of staff time is devoted to efforts in senior centers, one-third to assessment and on-going treatment in the homes of elderly individuals, and one-third to services provided in community mental health centers (DeRenzo et al. 1991). A rural outreach team in Iowa estimated annual costs to be half those of mental health services provided by professionals in private practice (Buckwalter et al. 1993), and Parish and Landsberg (1984) found that their outreach efforts (e.g., home visits and work with family and community support networks) in a rural community reduced psychiatric hospitalization by 60%. Funding for these programs commonly comes from mixes of federal, state, and local funds.

Psychiatric vocational rehabilitation. Although older patients are underserved by these programs, such programs should be considered as a treatment option for aging psychiatric patients. Two basic types of programs exist:

1. *Sheltered employment,* also known as *sheltered workshops* or *compensated work therapy programs,* provides work opportunities for individuals who are not ready for competitive employment. Work days may be decreased, tasks simplified and structured, and on-job pressures reduced. Some programs are based in psychiatric treatment centers, but most are managed by nonprofit agencies such as Goodwill Industries or Jewish Vocational Services. Patients receive either piecework pay or hourly pay according to their abilities and the specific contract (Jacobs 1988).

2. *Transitional employment* provides real-work jobs with commercial establishments that are supervised by psychiatric or rehabilitation professionals. The vocational rehabilitation program contracts with local businesses for jobs and assumes responsibility for their completion. Patients earn the same pay as regular workers. These programs are operated by various nonprofit agencies (e.g., Fountain House in New York City, and Thresholds in Chicago, Illinois).

Funding for rehabilitation programs are most often provided through special state Medicaid reimbursement rates or through funds from state offices of vocational rehabilitation; information about referrals can be obtained from the latter.

Senior Centers

In 1990, 5–8 million older persons were participating in 10,000–12,000 centers nationwide (Krout et al. 1990). Participation in senior centers is 4–12 times greater than reported for any other community-based service for elderly individuals (Krout et al. 1990). Senior centers have been conceptualized as being organized around two models (Litwin 1987). One model views the center as an informal social club or voluntary organization. The other model depicts the center as a multipurpose service provider or social services agency designed to meet a range of needs of frail elderly individuals, particularly poor and disengaged persons. A survey of senior center staff and participants (Gelfand et al. 1991) indicated six core programs—crafts, exercise, information and assistance, meals, opportunities for socializing, and transportation—that were thought to be essential for all centers. Five supplemental programs—arts (music, drama, painting), community college courses, health services, support groups, and trips—were considered highly desirable.

Although centers for older people can be traced back to a program in New York City begun in 1943, until the 1970s most relied on nonprofit agency or local government support. An amendment to the OAA in 1973 identified "multipurpose senior centers" as a unique and separate program (Gelfand 1993). Title III of the OAA provides for the acquisition, renovation, or construction of senior centers, as well as for their operation. Additional federal legislative support has been provided by Title XX of the Social Security Act. On average, senior centers currently receive 30% of their funding from federal sources (Krout et al. 1990).

Although considerable controversy exists about those variables that correlate with senior center participation, survey data of nearly 14,000 elderly persons from the 1984 National Health Interview Survey have provided the most reliable information to date (Krout et al. 1990). This survey indicated that higher participation was correlated with being female, increasing age until age 84, increasing education until college, lower family income, living alone, fewer difficulties with activities of daily living, and living in suburbs and rural nonfarm areas. Contrary to some earlier findings, race was not correlated with participation. Krout et al. (1990) concluded that senior centers are generally used by "less advantaged" but not the "least advantaged" elderly individuals (e.g., those unable to perform activities of daily living or the very old).

Social Network Interventions and Mutual Aid (Self-Help) Groups

A growing number of community mental health programs have begun to recognize the important roles that the informal social network plays in providing individuals with material and emotional assistance. The social network techniques most commonly used include 1) helping clients expand their networks, 2) assisting individuals to increase the support and exchange within existing networks, 3) identifying natural helpers and gatekeepers (e.g., clergy, letter carriers, physicians) who can assist clients, and 4) teaching service personnel to work with existing networks (Pancoast et al. 1983). Two distinct network approaches have emerged in work with older persons. One approach involves the actual convening of members of the individual network into a "network session" in which a treatment plan is developed and sponsored by network members themselves (Garrison and Howe 1976). A second approach (Cohen 1991) involves the clinician utilizing the network on the client's behalf, usually by working with network members to elicit their involvement in the client's treatment. Although most reports have been descriptive and anecdotal, the more systematic studies have tended to be favorable, with several important stipulations (Cohen and Adler 1984). Cohen and Adler (1984) concluded that network interventions are not suitable for every problem or for every person. Transactions that have long been part of a population's cultural world are most likely to yield successful network outcomes. In other words, service workers should not expect to undertake network tasks that clients are not already familiar with. They also cautioned that natural supports should not be used to justify public policies that might result in the withholding of professional services.

Self-help or mutual help groups are one of the most popular network modalities. These groups provide mutual assistance by creating a personal, intimate, face-to-face environment where elderly individuals with similar experiences can exchange ideas and coping techniques. Examples include informational and emotional support groups, such as Alzheimer's caregivers groups, and political action groups, such as the Gray Panthers. Self-help groups have been organized with the financial assistance of churches, community organizations, and community mental health centers. Indirect funding may come from foundations and governmental support. The fluidity of membership and the difficulty of controlling the number of complex variables has limited the scope of evaluative research (Lieberman and Borman 1979). Evaluation of self-help groups has been sparse, especially with respect to "hard" data (Gartner and Riessman 1977; Maddox 1987). According to Spiegel (1982), the widespread acceptance and apparent effectiveness of self-help groups stem from commonality of experience, mutual support, receiving of help through giving it, collective willpower, information sharing, and goal-directed problem solving. Self-help groups provide assistance to individuals who may have never availed themselves of professional help.

In recent years, support groups, especially for caregivers, have evolved from a self-help modality into a more formal method of intervention, generally conducted by trained group leaders. Toseland and Rossiter (1989) have identified seven common themes found among caregiver support groups: 1) information, 2) development of the group as a support system, 3) emotional impact of caregiving, 4) self-care, 5) improving interpersonal relations and communications, 6) development of outside support systems, and 7) the improvement of home care skills. Summarizing the evaluative literature on group intervention, Zarit and Teri (1991) made the following three conclusions:

1. Improvement has been more consistently reported for heterogeneous samples of caregivers than for caregivers of dementia patients.
2. Although positive gains have been reported on measures of mood, mental health, and subjective burden, the magnitude of treatment effect is modest.
3. There were often discrepancies among the goals of interventions, the goals of participants, and measure of outcome.

Zarit and Teri (1991) proposed that intervention studies must identify carefully targeted groups and problems that require sophisticated interventions (e.g., management of specific behavior problems, depression among caregivers).

Nutritional Services

In 1973, the original thrust of the National Program on Nutrition was not only to provide older persons with meals, but also to offer outreach and services such as education, counseling, and recreation. Austin (1987) argues that because of insufficient funding, the focus over time has been primarily on serving meals, and the other goals have largely evaporated. Moreover, even the former goal has been elusive in that the average program participant receives 7 meals per 10-week period—a level of participation that can barely contribute to the client's nutritional status (Austin 1987). Beginning in 1983, budgetary cutbacks at the federal level have further weakened these programs.

Home delivery program ("Meals on Wheels"). Nonprofit agencies or congregate meals programs prepare, package, and deliver midday meals and occasionally cold suppers or snacks to homebound (according to accepted medical criteria) persons of any age. Funding is primarily provided by Title III of the OAA; however, United Way, churches, community groups, and fees from clients are other sources of revenue. For-profit home-delivered meal services also exist.

Congregate meals program. All persons ages 60 and older are eligible to receive inexpensive meals at nearby centers such as churches, senior centers, and schools. Funding comes primarily from Title III of the OAA, although clients are encouraged to contribute something for the meal. The nutrition program is currently the largest single component in OAA funding and served 2.7 million people in 1990 (Gelfand 1993). The original legislation also provided for nutrition education, information and referral, social services counseling, and recreational activities.

Nutrition education program.   Also funded under OAA, it is designed to provide nutrition education as part of a meal program or separately.

"Brown bag" program.   Various community groups provide volunteers who fill shopping bags for low-income elderly individuals.

Food stamp program.   Started in 1964 by the Department of Agriculture, this program allows low-income Americans of all ages to purchase, at less than face value (or, if they are very indigent, obtain for free), food stamps that substitute for cash in buying specified kinds of food at grocery stores. Applications can be obtained by mail or at local Social Security offices. A large proportion of elderly individuals who are eligible do not utilize the program.

Transportation and Escort

Transportation services.   These services are generally funded by the Urban Mass Transportation Act and the OAA. Communities provide three modes of transport to assist elderly persons with physician visits and errands: subsidized taxis, minibuses, and private cars.

Escort services.   Community agencies and police provide escorts to assist frail elderly individuals with errands and other activities.

Shopping assistance.   Senior centers and other senior organizations provide transport service to help elderly persons get to shopping centers.

Volunteer and Employment Programs

Cnaan and Cwikel (1992) noted that since the early 1960s, there has been roughly a two- to threefold increase in volunteer activity among persons ages 65 and older, with approximately one-fourth of elderly individuals engaged in volunteering. This proportion of elderly individuals is lower than— or at best equal to—that in other age groups, and the percentage who volunteer with formal organizations has plateaued over the past 15 years.

Most of the publicly funded volunteer programs in the country are administered under ACTION, the federal volunteer agency that also includes the Peace Corps, or under Title V of the OAA. These programs include the following:

- *Retired Seniors Volunteer Program (RSVP)*. Originated under OAA, RSVP is currently funded through ACTION. Volunteers ages 60 and older work in hospitals, nursing homes, and senior centers. Local senior centers sponsor a variety of RSVP programs, such as friendly visiting. RSVP volunteers also work with children and juvenile delinquents.
- *Foster Grandparents.* Subsidized through ACTION, this program provides a small stipend to low-income elderly individuals to work with youths in need of supportive and affectionate adults; the program is conducted in schools, care centers, and hospitals.
- *Senior Companions.* This is another ACTION-supported program that provides a stipend for low-income older persons to visit other elderly individuals in nursing homes, hospitals, and private homes.
- *Service Corps of Retired Executives (SCORE)*. This program, funded by ACTION, gives retired professionals an opportunity to assist small business owners who lack funds to pay for such services.
- *Green Thumb.* Funded under the Senior Community Service Employment Program (SCSEP) of OAA (Title V), this program employs retired farmers and other low-income rural elderly individuals to work part-time in parks and other beautification programs.
- *Senior Aides.* Another program of SCSEP, this offers small stipends for part-time work in community service jobs as homemakers, home health aides, food program assistants.

In general, studies have demonstrated that older volunteers derive substantial benefit in life satisfaction, self-esteem, and mood (Carp 1968; Cutler 1976; Hunter and Linn 1980–1981). Stevens (1991) found four factors that predicted satisfaction and likelihood that volunteers stay on the job longer: 1) a pattern of providing community service throughout adulthood, 2) a congruence between the volunteer's role expectations and actual experiences on the job, 3) social contact on the job, and 4) perceived recognition and appreciation for their volunteer work.

Adult Education

There has been considerable growth in the number of specialized educational programs for older adults offered by public schools, colleges, government, industry, libraries, museums, and voluntary and religious organizations (Pearce 1991). Increasing numbers of elderly individuals are enrolling in tuition-waiver programs in colleges, adult education courses, and elder hostel programs. The last program sponsors 1-week courses on college campuses; the costs of transportation, tuition, and room and board are paid by the participant.

Studies in educational gerontology have indicated that several factors—being female, being in the 60- to 64-year-old age group, higher educational attainment, higher socioeconomic status, and good health—correlate with increased participation (Heisel et al. 1981; Pearce 1991). The principal motivations for attending courses are intellectual, social, and recreational interests (Heisel et al. 1981). The few rigorous investigations of the effects of educational programs have indicated that such programs enhance personal growth and quality of life (Brady 1983; Russ-Eft and Steel 1980). Scanlan and Darkenwald (1984) identified six factors that deter participation in educational courses: 1) lack of confidence, 2) lack of course relevance, 3) time constraints, 4) low personal priority, 5) cost, and 6) personal problems. Pearce (1991) concluded that the literature suggests two main thrusts for the future: 1) improved matching of course content to the interests and daily needs of elderly individuals and 2) elimination of barriers to participation such as poor health or financial costs.

Community Housing

Long-Term Care Facilities

Long-term care facilities provide medical and psychosocial care to individuals who have relatively severe, chronic impairments.

Nursing homes.   These institutions can be divided into two broad categories: 1) skilled nursing facilities, which provide 24-hour nursing care and medical coverage for persons who require extensive care (reimbursement is provided by Medicaid and time-limited coverage by Medicare), and 2) intermediate care facilities, which provide health-related care for persons who are more stabilized but require some medical and nursing supervision (not full time); costs are covered by Medicaid but not Medicare. It is possible to buy long-term care insurance policies that will reimburse at part or full cost any subsequent nursing home placement.

Domiciliary care residences. These facilities are also known as personal care residences, custodial care, homes for the aged, rest homes, sheltered care facilities, and adult homes. These homes are primarily nonprofit and are often church sponsored; their capacity ranges from 50 to 300 (Gelfand 1993). They are nonmedical institutions for persons who do not have major health problems or injuries but need supervision. Services include food, some personal care, and usually recreational and social work. These residences are often used for chronic mentally ill individuals to provide them with a protective environment. Because these facilities are considered nonmedical, they are licensed by state departments of social services, and health care benefits such as Medicare or Medicaid benefits are not available to pay for stays in such facilities. However, qualified residents may receive additional reimbursement from Supplemental Security Income (SSI). With respect to efficacy, one study found that elderly participants in a Pennsylvania domiciliary program were more optimistic, engaged in more social activities, expressed greater satisfaction with living conditions, and had lower costs than a matched community control group (Vandivort et al. 1984).

Hospice. Hospices provide a setting of comfort, friendship, familiar possessions and relief from pain in a person's last weeks of a terminal illness. Hospices may be found as 1) a hospital unit, 2) a free-standing facility, 3) an outpatient unit for counseling and medical visits, or 4) a home care program. Care averages about 1 month. Medicare provides benefits to those who are diagnosed as having 6 months or less to live. Benefits under Medicaid vary by state. Some private insurance policies also provide reimbursement.

Specially Designed Housing for Elderly Individuals in Need of Varying Levels of Support Services

The aim of this type of housing is to include a variety of supportive services to help older persons compensate for physical decline and more effectively deal with the special health problems of advanced age (Huttman 1985; Lawton 1981).

Assisted living. This is a new form of community-based residential care facility that has been defined as a "transition level of care between independent living and the lowest level of nursing care" (Sherman 1988, p. 2). These facilities are generally operated by for-profit developers who cater to middle- and upper-class elderly individuals (Kalymun 1992) and consist of 50–100 self-contained apartments, with meals and social activities provided centrally. Care is provided by trained resident assistants, with available nursing personnel. These facilities generally offer a more extensive package of services than congregate care facilities (see later discussion), and unlike board and care facilities that typically provide care for persons who had lived previously in institutions such as mental hospitals or nursing homes, assisted living facilities aim to delay the onset of institutionalization. Under the Frail Elderly Act of 1991, these facilities may become eligible for Medicaid funds to be used for homemaker/home health aide services (Pristic 1991). Currently, licensing requirements vary among states. The average monthly costs are between $860 and $1460.

Congregate housing.   Congregate housing consists of apartment houses or group accommodations that provide limited health services and other support services (e.g., meals in a central dining room, heavy housekeeping, social services, recreational activities) to functionally impaired older persons who do not need routine nursing care. Such support services enable persons to continue an independent lifestyle. These facilities are somewhat less institutionalized than domiciliary care residences. They are usually operated by government agencies or nonprofit groups; many received funding for construction from the Section 202 federal housing program, which provides low-cost loans to develop residences that include support services (Gelfand 1993). Costs vary widely. Ruchelin and Morris (1987) reported that monthly service costs were $563 per tenant, which they considered cost-effective in comparison to nursing home placement.

Board and care homes.   These facilities are dominated by small "mom and pop" operations and by some larger homes operated by charitable nonprofit organizations (Kalymun 1992). The numbers of residents range from 1 to more than 100. Homes typically provide three meals a day, laundry service, and 24-hour supervision; many also provide transportation services, cleaning of living areas, personal assistance, and arrangement of medical appointments (Eckert and Lyon 1991). A high proportion of older residents in these facilities have physical limitations or a history of mental illness, often in combination, along with low income and lack of family support (Eckert and Lyon 1991). The National Board and Care Reform Act (1989) required that every facility with two or more recipients of social security or SSI meet minimum health and safety standards, with states being allowed to control the specifics thereof. In some states, homes may be able to operate without licenses. Average monthly fees are between $240 and $1150. SSI may provide supplementary case payments.

Foster care.   For older persons (particularly those with chronic mental illness) in need of care and protection in a substitute family, foster care can provide socialization, stimulation, support, and protection. The number of paying residents is usually limited to four. Evaluation of foster care programs have been favorable. One study (Newman and Sherman 1979) found that elderly participants interacted to a moderate degree with family and community, and several investigators (Braun and Rose 1986; Oktay and Volland 1987; Vandivort et al. 1984) have reported generally favorable levels of well-being and equal improvements in activities of daily living functions in elderly foster care participants compared with nursing home patients. Importantly, the annual cost of foster care is approximately $8400 (Abrahams et al. 1991), which is substantially less than nursing homes. Foster care programs are usually administered by local departments of social services using Title XX funds and therefore are primarily targeted to lower income elderly individuals (Gelfand 1993).

Elder cottage housing opportunity (ECHO).   Also known as granny flats, accessory housing, and second-unit ordinances, these are ancillary structures for elderly individuals (e.g., mobile minihouses or small attached units) that are permitted by special zoning variances to be placed on land belonging to the children of these individuals, thereby enabling the older person to receive informal care and support from his or her kin (Friedman and Harris 1991).

Continuing care and life-care facilities.   These facilities, operated by nonprofit and for-profit organizations, offer multiple levels of care ranging in setting from one's own home to a nursing home (Friedman and Harris 1991). These communities provide private living units with ancillary services such as meals, mail services, and health care. When there is a need for more intensive care, the resident may be transferred to a nursing home, often on the same site.

Currently three levels of continuing care are available (Friedman and Harris 1991):

1. *Unlimited care* (or *life-care*), which guarantees a full level of care for the resident's lifetime. Entrance fees range from $50,000 to $150,000, and monthly fees average $1,000.

2. *Limited care*, which provides a basic level of medical care with extra care available for additional fees. Entrance fees average $30,000 to $100,000, and monthly fees are about $700.

3. *"Pay-as-you-go" care* provides a living unit with meals and medical care available on a "menu" basis. There is no guarantee of future services. Entrance and monthly fees are relatively low ($20,000 to $50,000 and $500, respectively).

Retirement communities. These are nonlicensed, age-segregated communities of apartments or free-standing homes. Services are generally of a social nature (e.g., clubhouses, tennis courts) and do not routinely include health services. To remain age-segregated and satisfy requirements of the Fair Housing Law, these retirement communities must have at least 80% of units occupied by someone at least 55 years old, they should offer facilities and services especially designed for elderly individuals, and the age restriction must be a specific policy of the complex (Friedman and Harris 1991).

Elderly apartment complexes. These include public, nonprofit, and privately owned buildings for elderly individuals, many of which have been built with Section 202 federal funds. They do not routinely provide health care. Section 8 housing allowances (i.e., a federally subsidized program administered by a local housing authority for low-income elderly individuals) have frequently provided a rent supplement to Section 202 housing.

Shared housing ("senior matching"). A social services agency matches occupant (owner/renter) with renter, or the agency buys or rents units and then rents these units to others. Results have been favorable. One study of apartment- or house-sharing elderly individuals found that two-thirds of these arrangements were still functioning after 1 year (Lawton 1981).

Summary

Because treatment of the geriatric patient, particularly the moderately or severely impaired patient, requires a comprehensive array of services, it is essential that geropsychiatrists familiarize themselves with the principal community services described in this chapter. Moreover, as outlined in Table 34–1, the psychiatrist should be able to match services with the patient's level of functioning and then link the patient to the appropriate services. Assistance with the latter is usually available from local area agencies for the aging and/or from a social worker.

There has been a relative dearth of evaluative studies of community programs. Much of the evaluative research that has been done has been too generalized, and the next generation of research must be better able to define groups to be served and goals to be achieved. Most needed are studies that identify older populations that are inadequately served by existing programs, and that develop and test methods for outreach and overcoming barriers to services. Although cost-effectiveness has not always been demonstrated, community programs generally have been judged to be at least clinically equivalent to institutional programs and considerably more humane. However, to make the case for community care more compelling, future research will have to 1) broaden traditional economic measures to include hidden economic costs and burdens to families and society and 2) consider the economic equivalences of quality-of-life measures. Finally, community research must be conducted with the input of and in close collaboration with elderly individuals for whom services are developed.

References

Abrahams R, Bishop C, Hernandez W: Respite service delivery: learning from current programs. Pride Institute Journal of Long-Term Health Care 10:16–28, 1991

American Association of Retired Persons: Making Wise Decisions for Long Term Care. Washington, DC, AARP, 1986a

American Association of Retired Persons: Miles Away and Still Caring. Washington, DC, American Association of Retired Persons, 1986b

Austin C: Nutrition programs, in The Encyclopedia of Aging. Edited by Maddox GL. New York, Springer, 1987

Beattie WM: Aging and social services, in Handbook of Aging and the Social Sciences. Edited by Binstock RH, Shanas E. New York, Van Nostrand Reinhold, 1976

Berger RM, Piliavin I: The effect of casework: a research note. Social Work 21:205–208, 1976

Biegel DE, Shore BK, Gordon E: Building Support Networks for the Elderly. Beverly Hills, CA, Sage, 1984

Blenkner M, Bloom M, Nielsen M, et al: Final Report: Protective Services for Older Adults. Cleveland, OH, Benjamin Rose Institute, 1974

Brady EM: Personal growth and the elder hostel experience. Lifelong Learning 7(3):11–26, 1983

Braun KL, Rose CL: The Hawaii geriatric foster care experiment: impact, evaluation, and cost analysis. Gerontologist 26:516–524, 1986

Buckwalter KC, Abraham IL, Smith M, et al: Nursing update: nursing outreach to rural elderly people who are mentally ill. Hosp Community Psychiatry 44:821–823, 1993

Cantor M, Little V: Aging and social care, in Handbook of Aging and the Social Sciences, 2nd Edition. Edited by Binstock RH, Shanas E. New York, Van Nostrand Reinhold, 1985

Capitman JA, Gregory KL: Supplemental Report in the Adult Day Health Care Program in California: A Comparative Cost Analysis. Sacramento, CA, Department of Health Services, 1984

Carcagno GJ, Kemper P: The evaluation of the national long-term care demonstration: an overview of the channeling demonstration and its evaluation. Health Serv Res 23:1–22, 1988

Carp F: Differences among older workers, volunteers, and persons who are neither. J Gerontol 23:497–501, 1968

Cnaan RA, Cwikel JG: Elderly volunteers: assessing their potential as an untapped resource. Journal of Aging and Social Policy 48:125–147, 1992

Cohen C, Onserud H, Monaco C: Outcomes for the mentally ill in a program for older homeless persons. Hosp Community Psychiatry 44:650–656, 1993

Cohen CI: Social network therapy with inner-city elderly, in New Techniques in the Psychotherapy of Older Patients. Edited by Myers WA. Washington, DC, American Psychiatric Press, 1991, pp 79–93

Cohen CI, Adler A: Network interventions: do they work? Gerontologist 24:16–22, 1984

Collins AH, Pancoast DL: Natural Helping Networks. Washington, DC, National Association of Social Workers, 1976

Cutler SJ: Membership in different types of voluntary associations and psychological well-being. Gerontologist 16:335–339, 1976

DeRenzo EG, Byer VL, Grady HS, et al: Comprehensive community-based mental health outreach services for suburban seniors. Gerontologist 31:836–840, 1991

Eckert JK, Lyon SM: Regulation of board-and-care homes: research to guide policy. Journal of Aging and Social Policy 3:147–161, 1991

Ellis NB: Sustaining frail disabled elderly in the community: an innovative approach to in-home services. Journal of Gerontological Social Work 7:3–15, 1984

Friedman JP, Harris JC: Keys to Buying a Retirement Home. New York, Barrons, 1991

Garrison JE, Howe J: Community intervention with the elderly: a social network approach. J Am Geriatr Soc 24:329–333, 1976

Gartner A, Riessman F: Self-Help in Human Services. San Francisco, CA, Jossey-Bass, 1977

Gelfand DE: The Aging Network Programs and Services, 4th Edition. New York, Springer, 1993

Gelfand DE, Bechill W, Chester RL: Core programs and services at senior centers. Journal of Gerontological Social Work 17:145–161, 1991

Golant SM, McCaslen R: A functional classification of services for older people. Journal of Gerontological Social Work 1:187–209, 1979

Goodman RI: The selection of communication channels by the elderly to obtain information. Educational Gerontology 18:701–714, 1992

Gottlieb BH: Social Support Strategies. Beverly Hills, CA, Sage, 1983

Gurland B, Copeland J, Kuriansky J, et al: The Mind and Mood of Aging. New York, Haworth Press, 1983

Gwyther LP: Overcoming barriers: home care for dementia patients. Caring, August 1989, pp 12–16

Hegeman CR: Geriatric Respite Care: Expanding and Improving Practice. Albany, NY, Foundation for Long-Term Care, 1989

Heisel MA, Darkenwald GG, Anderson RE: Participation in organized educational activities among adults age 60 and over. Educational Gerontology 6:227–240, 1981

Hunter KI, Linn MW: Psychosocial differences between elderly volunteers and non-volunteers. Int J Aging Hum Dev 12:205–213, 1980–1981

Huttman ED: Social Services for the Elderly. New York, The Free Press, 1985

Jacobs HE: Vocational rehabilitation, in Psychiatric Rehabilitation of Chronic Mental Patients. Edited by Liberman RP. Washington, DC, American Psychiatric Press, 1988, pp 245–284

Kalymun M: Board and care versus assisted living: ascertaining the similarities and differences. Adult Residential Care Journal 6:35–44, 1992

Korte C, Gupta V: A program of friendly visitors as network builders. Gerontologist 31:404–407, 1991

Krout J, Cutler S, Coward R: Correlates of senior center participation: a national analysis. Gerontologist 30:72–79, 1990

Krout JA: Service awareness among the elderly. Journal of Gerontological Social Work 9:7–19, 1985

Lawton MP: Alternative housing. Journal of Gerontological Social Work 3:61–80, 1981

Lawton MP, Brody EM, Saperstein AR: A controlled study of respite services for Alzheimer's patients. Gerontologist 29:8–16, 1989

Lebowitz B: Mental health services, in the Encyclopedia of Aging. Edited by Maddox GL. New York, Springer, 1987

Lebowitz B: Correlates of success in community mental health programs for the elderly. Hosp Community Psychiatry 39:721–722, 1988

Lebowitz BD, Light E, Bailey F: Mental health center services for the elderly: the impact of coordination with area agencies on aging. Gerontologist 27:699–702, 1987

Lieberman M, Borman L: Self-Help Groups for Coping With Crisis. San Francisco, CA, Jossey-Bass, 1979

Litwin H: Administrative correlates of senior center programs. J Appl Gerontol 6:201–212, 1987

Maddox GL: Mutual support groups, in The Encyclopedia of Aging. Edited by Maddox GL. New York, Springer, 1987

Morrissey JP, Goldman HH: Cycles of reform in the care of the chronically mentally ill. Hosp Community Psychiatry 35(8):785–793, 1984

Mulligan M, Bennett R: Assessment of mental health and social problems during multiple friendly visits: the development and evaluation of a friendly visitor program for the isolated elderly. Int J Aging Hum Dev 8:43–65, 1977

Newman ES, Sherman SR: Community integration of the elderly in foster family care. Journal of Gerontological Social Work 1:175–186, 1979

Noelker LS, Bass DM: Home care for elderly persons: linkages between formal and informal caregivers. Journal of Gerontology Social Services 44:S63–S72, 1989

Oktay JS, Volland P: Foster homecare for the frail elderly as an alternative to nursing home care: an experimental evaluation. Am J Public Health 77:1505–1510, 1987

Pancoast DL, Parker P, Froland C: Rediscovering Self-Help. Beverly Hills, CA, Sage, 1983

Parish B, Landsberg G: Developing a geriatric mental health outreach unit in a rural community. Journal of Gerontological Social Work 7(3):75–82, 1984

Pearce SD: Toward understanding the participation of older adults in continuing education. Educational Gerontology 17:451–464, 1991

Phipps C, Liberman RP: Community support, in Psychiatric Rehabilitation of Chronic Mental Patients. Edited by Liberman RP. Washington, DC, American Psychiatric Press, 1988, pp 285–311

Pristic S: Assisted living in the spotlight. Contemporary Long-Term Care

February 1991, pp 40–42

Raschko R: Spokane community mental health center elderly services, in the Elderly With Chronic Mental Illness. Edited by Light E, Lebowitz BD. New York, Springer, 1991

Rathbone-McCuan E, Elliot W: Geriatric day care in theory and practice. Social Work in Health Care 2:153–170, 1976–1977

Reed WL: Access to services by the elderly: a community research model. Journal of Gerontological Social Work 3:41–52, 1980

Reifler BV, Kelhley A, O'Neill P, et al: Five-year experience of a community outreach program for the elderly. J Am Geriatr Soc 139:220–223, 1982

Roca RP, Storer DJ, Robbins BM, et al: Psychogeriatric assessment and treatment in urban public housing. Hosp Community Psychiatry 41:916–920, 1990

Ruchelin HS, Morris JN: The congregate housing services program: an analyses of service utilization. Gerontologist 27:87–91, 1987

Russ-Eft DF, Steel LM: Contributions of education to adult quality of life. Educational Gerontology 5:180–209, 1980

Scanlan CS, Darkenwald GG: Identifying deterrents to participation in continuing education. Adult Education Quarterly 34:155–166, 1984

Sherman FJ: Overview: Retirement Housing Industry. Philadelphia, PA, Laventhol and Horwath Publications Department, 1988

Sherr VT, Eskridge OC, Lewis L: A mobile, mental-hospital-based team for geropsychiatric service in the community. J Am Geriatr Soc 24:362–365, 1976

Silverstein NM: Informing the elderly about public services: the relationship between sources of knowledge and service utilization. Gerontologist 24:37–40, 1984

Skellie AF, Mobley GM, Coan RE: Cost-effectiveness of community-based long-term care: current findings of Georgia's alternative health services project. Am J Public Health 72:353–358, 1982

Skolnick B, Warrick P: The Right Place at the Right Time: A Guide to Long-Term Care Choices. Washington, DC, American Association of Retired Persons, 1985

Spiegel D: Self-help and mutual support groups: a synthesis of the recent literature, in Community Support and Mental Health. Edited by Biegel D, Naparstek A. New York, Springer, 1982

Stevens ES: Toward satisfaction and retention of senior volunteers. Journal of Gerontological Social Work 16:33–41, 1991

Thornton C, Dunstan SM, Kemper P: The evaluation of the national long-term care demonstration: the effect of channeling on health and long-term care costs. Health Serv Res 23:129–142, 1988

Toseland RW, Rossiter CM: Group interventions to support family caregivers: a review and analysis. Gerontologist 29:438–448, 1989

Vandivort R, Kurren G, Braun K: Foster family care for frail elderly: a cost-effective quality care alternative. Journal of Gerontological Social Work 7:101–114, 1984

Weiler PG: Adult day care, in the Encyclopedia of Aging. Edited by Maddox GL. New York, Springer, 1987

Weiler PG, Kim P, Pickard LS: Health care for elderly Americans: evaluation for an adult day health care model. Med Care 14:700–708, 1976

Weissert WG: Two models of geriatric day care findings from a comparative study. Gerontologist 16:420–427, 1976

Weissert WG, Elston JM, Bolda EJ, et al: Models of adult day care: findings from a national survey. Gerontologist 29:640–649, 1989

Westhoff LJ: Care management: quelling the confusion. Health Prog 73:43–46, 1992

White M: Case management, in The Encyclopedia of Aging. Edited by Maddox GL. New York, Springer, 1987

Zarit SH, Teri L: Interventions and services for family caregivers. Annu Rev Gerontol Geriatr 11:287–310, 1991

Zborowsky E: Developments in protective services: a challenge for social workers. Journal of Gerontological Social Work 8:71–83, 1985

Zelman WM, Elston JM, Weissert WG: Financial aspects of adult day care: national survey results. Health Care Financ Rev 12:27–36, 1991

Medical-Legal, Ethical, and Financial Issues

George T. Grossberg, M.D.
George H. Zimny, Ph.D.

Medical-Legal Issues

P sychiatrists commonly may be asked by a court of law to attest to the competency of their geriatric patients. In this chapter we examine definitions and evaluative guidelines for competency in geriatric patients; the types of disorders that may commonly affect mental competence in elderly individuals; and, once an older adult is considered to be incapacitated, what types of surrogate management arrangements are available, with a particular focus on guardianship. Laws and regulations vary from country to country. The focus of this chapter is on accepted practice and regulations in the United States.

Competency Versus Decisional Capacity

Parry (1988), in his analysis of the selected recommendations from the National Guardianship Symposium held in July 1988, pointed out that there has been considerable "vagueness or lack of precision" relative to the definition of competency or incapacity. Kapp (1990, p. 25) highlighted the importance of distinguishing between decisional capacity and competency, with the former relating to "the opinion of a clinical evaluator concerning an individual's functional ability to make autonomous, authentic decisions about his own life" and the latter referring to "the judgement of a court of law about the same issue." This is usually the "prelude to the appointment of a proxy decisionmaker."

The Uniform Probate Code defines a mentally incapacitated person as: "[one] who is impaired by reason of mental illness, mental deficiency, physical illness or disability, advanced age, chronic use of drugs, chronic intoxication or other abuse to the extent that he lacks sufficient under-standing or capacity to make or communicate responsible decisions con-cerning his person" (Fisher 1994, p. 198). In his review of legal consensus, Parry (1988) stated that "five elements should be included in any accept-able notion of incapacity." These are listed in Table 35–1. In addition, the cognitive elements of impairment (i.e., the person's ability to make a deci-sion/decisions) are important.

Competency Evaluation

Psychiatrists may be involved in helping to determine mental competence in geriatric patients who refuse needed hospitalization or lifesaving pro-cedures or whose testamentary capacity (e.g., to write a will) is being ques-tioned, or in patients who are being considered for guardianship or conservatorship (Baker 1986). The court relies heavily on the physician's input in determining whether a patient is deemed incompetent and may require some form of surrogate management (Juretic et al. 1993). This places a significant amount of responsibility on the psychiatrist, especially if guardianship is to be recommended. The appointment of a guardian essentially strips the patient of any and all decision-making abilities and may be subject to potential abuse, such as misuse of financial resources or inappropriate institutionalization (Iris 1990; Kapp 1994).

Table 35–1.   Key components of incapacity

Incapacity may be partial or complete.

Incapacity is a legal, not a medical, term.

Incapacity should be supported by evidence of an increase in functional impairment over time.

Incapacity should include the notion of the respondent being likely to have substantial harm by reason of inability to manage his or her personal or financial affairs.

Incapacity should not be based solely on descriptive or diagnostic labels (e.g., advanced age, Alzheimer's disease).

Source.   Adapted from Parry (1988).

Unfortunately, physicians are rarely trained in competency evaluation. According to a study of 40 competency cases involving geriatric patients (>60 years old) in Harris County, Texas, Probate Court, 10 (25%) of the 40 physician letters did not even contain a medical or psychiatric diagnosis. In addition, 92.5% of the letters did not include results of a formal mental status evaluation, and nearly half (47.5%) of the letters consisted mainly of unsupported statements of incompetence (Juretic et al. 1993). The essentials of a thorough competency evaluation are outlined in Table 35–2.

The psychiatrist must establish a diagnosis and rule out potentially reversible causes of cognitive impairment in elderly individuals, whether medical or psychiatric (e.g., delirium or other remediable disorders) that may temporarily affect mental capacity. Once a reversible disorder is ruled out, the psychiatrist must determine the degree of impairment as measured by neuropsychological testing and/or a functional evaluation focusing on activities of daily living (Nolan 1984; Scogin and Perry 1986). The mere presence of a psychiatric diagnosis "is insufficient to warrant a finding of incompetency requiring the appointment of a guardian or a conservator" (Goldstein 1987, p. 273). The evaluating psychiatrist also must determine to what extent the patient has problems with financial, medical, and other day-to-day personal decisions.

A variety of psychiatric disorders can affect competence in elderly individuals. Those most commonly seen are listed in Table 35–3.

Alzheimer's disease is the most commonly seen cause of incompetency in elderly individuals (Mann 1992). However, even with probable Alzheimer's disease, it is important to evaluate the stage of the illness and

Table 35–2. Competency evaluation in elderly individuals

Thorough history up to present time (use family or other informants)
Review of pertinent medical and psychiatric records
Review of prescription and nonprescription medications, including alcohol history
Physical/neurological examination
Psychiatric assessment, including a formal mental status evaluation
Laboratory tests, including blood chemistry, a complete blood cell count, thyroid function tests, tests to determine vitamin B_{12} and folate levels, urinalysis, chest radiograph, and electrocardiogram, if indicated
Neuroimaging (computed tomography and magnetic resonance imaging scans, electroencephalogram), if warranted
Neuropsychological testing, if indicated
Functional evaluation

Table 35–3.   Psychiatric disorders that may lead to incompetence in elderly individuals

Progressive dementias (Alzheimer's disease, vascular dementia)
Delirium (temporary)
Mood disorders (e.g., major depression, bipolar affective disorder)
Psychotic disorders (e.g., schizophrenia)

determine which functional abilities the patient may retain. Indeed, the patient's degree of impairment will determine whether the psychiatrist can recommend a less restrictive form of surrogate management than guardianship.

Surrogate Management Arrangements

As the cognitive deficits that constitute incompetency become more pronounced, elderly persons may find it increasingly difficult to manage their lives in a way that maintains their health, safety, comfort, and enjoyment. The widespread concern in many jurisdictions over abuse of elderly individuals in its many forms underscores the issue of protection of elderly persons, particularly mentally incompetent individuals, both from themselves and from others (Gest 1985; Quinn and Tomita 1986; Subcommittee on Health and Long-Term Care 1990; Topolnicki 1989).

As the capacity for self-management decreases, the need for surrogate management increases. Surrogate management is "a formal relationship established for the purpose of allowing another person or entity to make decisions for an adult who has or expects to have significantly limited physical or mental capacity" (Gilchrist and Zimny 1993, p. 258). A variety of surrogate management arrangements can be established by and for elderly persons. The geriatric psychiatrist should know what these arrangements are and the advantages and disadvantages of each, to be able to answer basic questions about them and to provide appropriate advice to elderly patients and their families. It is also important to be aware that state laws affecting surrogate management arrangements vary from state to state.

Before turning to formal arrangements, it should be acknowledged that informal arrangements involving the families and close friends of elderly persons are usually the most desirable means of providing surrogate decision making for elderly persons. However, this is not always the case. One study found that "about 40 persons per 1,000 elderly population recently experienced some serious form of maltreatment in their own home, at the hands of a partner, relative, or significant others" (Podnieks 1992, p. 5). Formal surrogate management arrangements as defined previously thus have an important and sometimes lifesaving role to play in protecting elderly persons, particularly as they lose the capacity to care for themselves and become increasingly vulnerable.

Before Incompetency: Advance Directives

The two broad types of formal surrogate management arrangements are those established by the elderly person for himself or herself while still competent, and those established by someone else for the elderly person who is presumed to be incompetent.

Arrangements of the first type are advance directives, in that the person gives directions for what is to be done in the event of incompetency. The major advantage of advance directives is that the person is able to specify who is to make what kinds of decisions when the time comes that he or she is not able to make those decisions. A measure of control and autonomy is thus retained by the person even on becoming incompetent. Some advance directives have particular disadvantages or limitations, and these are noted in the discussion that follows.

Wills. A will is probably the best known advance directive. It is written in advance of death (or a state of complete incompetency) by a person who is competent. It is a formal legal document that is processed in a court of law, and it directs what is to be done with the person's possessions after his or her death. Certain legal requirements must be met to make a valid last will and testament. One requirement is that the person making the will have testamentary capacity (Baker 1986). Although varying somewhat from state to state, testamentary capacity commonly requires that the person, or testator, know who the natural heirs are, the amount of the assets, and that a will is being made.

A will can be made or changed by an adult of any age, but the question of testamentary capacity is more likely to be raised with elderly than with younger persons. Because of this likelihood, it may be advisable for the testator or the attorney drawing up the will to obtain information or documentation of the testator's capacity. This can be done by having an evaluation made by a psychiatrist and/or a videotape made of the testator at the time the will is being prepared or signed. The evaluation should include inquiries designed to elicit information relevant to the specific requirements for testamentary capacity designated by the law of the particular state (Sadoff 1991).

A *living will* expresses a person's desires and instructions concerning the use of life-prolonging medical procedures at a time when he or she is unable to make or convey decisions concerning the procedures. The forms and wording for living wills differ from state to state and are subject to change. A form prepared by the Missouri Bar, for example, contained the following wording. "I make this health care directive to exercise my right to determine the course of my health care and to provide clear and convincing proof of my wishes and instructions about my treatment. If I am persistently unconscious or there is no reasonable expectation of my recovery from a seriously incapacitating or terminal illness or condition, I direct that all of the life-prolonging procedures I have initialled below be withheld or withdrawn" (Missouri Bar Association 1991, p. 11). The procedures listed included artificially supplied nutrition and hydration, heart-lung resuscitation, mechanical ventilator, and "all other 'life prolonging' medical or surgical procedures that are merely intended to keep me alive without reasonable hope of improving my condition or curing my illness or injury" (Missouri Bar Association 1991, p. 11).

The force of living wills is not totally clear. Controversy still exists about provisions in living wills, state laws differ and change, and state and federal supreme court decisions continue to appear. However, the existence of a living will makes it more likely that the wishes and preferences of an elderly person concerning his or her health care will be implemented when he or she is incompetent. More people are becoming familiar with living wills and their rights regarding health care as a result of the Patient Self-Determination Act (PSDA), which became effective December 1, 1991. According to the provisions of the PSDA, persons entering a health care facility such as a hospital or nursing home must be asked if they have an advance directive. If they do, that directive should be included in their record. If they do not, the fact that they do not must be entered in their record. The facility must explain to the person its policy concerning which directives it will and will not implement. The PSDA is likely to affect large numbers of elderly persons, because they are the most frequent users of health care facilities and are facing end-of-life issues.

Power of attorney. The power of attorney is a document in which the principal—the elderly person in this case—gives the agent—a person or institution—the power or authority to act on his or her behalf. The actions are identified in the document and may be very specific (e.g., "sell all my stock and bonds and put the proceeds in a specified money market fund") or very broad (e.g., "handle all my financial affairs").

Three types of power of attorney exist, and each must be prepared while the elderly person is competent. *General power of attorney* takes effect on its completion but ceases when the principal becomes incompetent. *Springing power of attorney* becomes effective only when the principal becomes incompetent. *Durable power of attorney* encompasses both of these types; it becomes effective on its completion and remains in effect when the principal becomes incompetent.

Each type is rather easily established, can effectively transfer authority, and can be revoked by the principal at any time as long as he or she is competent. However, there are two major problems. One is the determination of competency or incompetency. Who determines, and by what criteria, that the principal was competent at the time the document was written, is no longer competent to invoke or to revoke any powers in the document, or is incompetent, with the result that the general power of attorney ceases to be effective and the springing power becomes effective? This is an extremely difficult question to answer in the context of a particular state law, the wording of a particular document, and a particular principal and agent. Hopefully, the principal selected an agent whom he or she knows and trusts so that, as the principal begins to lose capacity, the transfer of power from the principal to the agent can begin and then accelerate as the loss of capacity increases. If the principal denies loss of capacity while the agent or family claims it, then a psychiatrist can provide an assessment of the principal's capacity and serve as a mediator in the dispute.

The second problem is the lack of monitoring of the agent and the consequent opportunity for abuse by the agent of the powers given in the document. "Because there is no ongoing court supervision, there is greater potential for abuse than with guardianship. Powers of attorney are therefore most appropriate when trust is fully warranted" (Chavkin 1990, p. 276).

Joint ownership. Joint ownership is another surrogate management arrangement that is very easy to establish and can be very helpful to an elderly person. However, like power of attorney, it is subject to abuse because of lack of monitoring. Joint ownership involves two or more people as co-owners of any investment that has a title. For example, an elderly man may put his daughter's name on a joint bank account or make her co-owner of his car or house. Each of the two has full control over the investment and full rights of ownership. The daughter can write a check withdrawing all of the funds from the account even though she did not put any funds into it.

Trusts.   In a trust arrangement, assets are transferred to a trustee according to the terms set forth in what is often an extensive trust document. Trusts are technical arrangements and are prepared by experienced professionals. Because of the terms set forth in the document, a trust is generally a safe and reliable, although often expensive, form of surrogate management of assets; it continues to function even if the grantor becomes incompetent.

After Incompetency

Representative payeeship and guardianship are two surrogate management arrangements that can be established by someone for an elderly person who is behaving in ways indicating incompetence.

A *representative payee* is a person or institution to whom certain government agencies, including the Social Security System, Veterans Administration, and Railroad Retirement Board, will send an elderly person's benefit checks when it has been established to the agency's satisfaction that the recipient is not capable of managing his or her public benefit money. This arrangement is rather easily established and can be a useful, although limited, form of money management. The danger, of course, is that the payee may not use the money to the benefit of the elderly person. This is a real concern, because the annual questionnaire that the payee must complete provides little effective monitoring of the payee's performance.

Guardianship is the most complicated, expensive, and drastic surrogate management arrangement. In guardianship, a judge in court adjudicates an elderly person to be fully or partially incompetent to care for his or her personal needs and/or financial affairs. Personal needs include health, nutrition, housing, clothing, and hygiene. Financial affairs include investments, real estate, business transactions, personal property, income, and expenses.

Power and authority to provide the personal and/or financial care for the incompetent person, called the *ward,* are taken from the ward and given by the court to a guardian. The effect on the ward is drastic. "Depending on the law of the state and extent of authority given to the guardian, the ward may lose many of her or his legal and civil rights as an adult citizen and be reduced to the legal status of a child—being deprived of the rights to control almost every aspect of life, including the right to manage finances, to write cheques, to contract, to sue and be sued, to travel, and to choose what medical treatment to receive, where to live, and with whom to associate" (Subcommittee on Housing and Consumer Interests 1989, p. 11).

Guardianship is a matter of state law. Each state as well as the District of Columbia has a different guardianship statute with its particular terms and procedures defined and described. In California, guardianship is only for minors, and conservatorship is only for adults. In Minnesota, guardianship provides full power for a guardian, whereas conservatorship provides only limited powers for the conservator. In Missouri, guardianship provides power over the person of the ward, whereas conservatorship provides power over the finances of the ward. In addition, the state guardianship law can change each time the state legislature meets.

Steps in Guardianship

Even though the scope of guardianship is state specific, the sequence of steps in guardianship cases is generally similar from state to state.

Petition. The first step is to file a petition with the court, usually the probate court, requesting that an allegedly incompetent person, the respondent, be adjudicated incompetent and guardian be appointed.

The geriatric psychiatrist may be involved in a guardianship petition for an elderly respondent in two ways. First, because petitions are usually filed by relatives of the respondent who are concerned about the seemingly irresponsible and even dangerous behavior of the respondent, they wisely may request an evaluation by a geriatric psychiatrist to help them determine the condition of the elderly person and what should be done. Based on the evaluation of the elderly person and discussions with the family members, the geriatric psychiatrist may recommend guardianship as the best way to proceed for the welfare of the elderly person. In some cases the court may appoint a psychiatrist or other health professional to conduct an evaluation of a respondent.

Second, the petitioner may request that the geriatric psychiatrist submit a deposition or interrogatory to the court to be used as evidence at the court hearing on the petition. The deposition contains questions to elicit the results of the evaluation of the elderly person and an opinion about the necessity for the court to appoint someone to care for the person's personal and/or financial needs.

Notice served.   After the petition is accepted by the court, a notice of the petition for guardianship is sent to the respondent and other interested parties. An attorney, either the respondent's attorney or an attorney appointed by the court, is responsible for meeting with the respondent to explain the petition and its implications.

Hearing.   A hearing on the petition is held in the courtroom and the case decided by either a judge or a jury. The petitioner and the respondent are each represented by an attorney. The respondent can attend the hearing, but few do so unless they are contesting the petition. Evidence in the form of exhibits, such as letters or depositions, and testimony of witnesses called by either attorney are presented at the hearing. The respondent may also be called to provide testimony.

Adjudication and appointment.   The adjudication or decision by the court concerning the competency/incompetency of the respondent is based on the evidence presented and can take one or a combination of forms, such as competent, fully or partially incompetent with respect to personal care, or fully or partially incompetent with respect to financial affairs. For example, if the respondent is adjudicated to be partially incompetent personally and fully incompetent financially, then the court will appoint a limited guardian of the person and a full conservator of the estate (or whatever terms are used in the particular state). Most guardians and conservators appointed by the court are relatives of the petitioner, but, depending on the state, they may also be unrelated individuals; agencies, such as social service agencies; institutions, such as banks; or professional guardian/conservator companies.

Monitoring.   An important safety feature of guardianship is that courts are required by the state statute to monitor the performance of guardians and conservators with respect to the care they provide for their wards. The monitoring process varies from state to state (Hurme 1991; Zimny et al. 1991b), but a common requirement is that each year the guardian must submit a report to the court describing the care provided to the ward, such as a change in residence or medical treatment, and the conservator must submit a report describing the ward's finances, such as income and expenses and the sale of real estate (Zimny et al. 1991a).

Termination.   Virtually all guardianships are terminated by the death of the elderly ward. A very few, however, are terminated as a result of the ward being restored to competency by the court. A petition for restoration must be filed with the court, and the subsequent proceeding is similar to that for guardianship. Restoration to competency may occur because the physical or mental condition underlying incompetency has been reversed. In one such case, a 67-year-old man had become quite cognitively impaired as a result of alcohol abuse. He was adjudicated to be fully incompetent, and a guardian and conservator were appointed by the court. The guardian had the ward admitted to a nursing home, and after several months of proper care, his alcohol-induced impairment reversed. He was subsequently evaluated by a geriatric psychiatrist, who recommended that he be declared fully competent with respect to his personal care and partially competent with respect to his financial affairs.

Summary

Psychiatrists have a major role to play in appropriate diagnostic evaluation of competency in elderly individuals. Familiarity with reversible syndromes as well as the most common causes of progressive impairment is essential, as is familiarity with the various forms of surrogate management, including, but not limited to, guardianship.

References

Baker FM: Legal issues affecting the older patient. Hosp Community Psychiatry 37:1091–1093, 1986

Chavkin DF: Planning for the future: legal and financial considerations, in Dementia Care: Patient, Family and Community. Edited by Mace N. Baltimore, MD, Johns Hopkins University Press, 1990, pp 270–293

Fisher JW: Legal aspects of the psychosocial management of the demented patient. Psychiatric Annals 24:197–201, 1994

Gest T: Ripping off estates—an epidemic of abuse. U.S. News and World Report, February 25, 1985, pp 53–56

Gilchrist BJ, Zimny GH: Surrogate management, in Problem Behaviors in Long-Term Care: Recognition, Diagnosis, and Treatment. Edited by Szwabo PA, Grossberg GT. New York, Springer, 1993

Goldstein RL: Non compos mentis: the psychiatrist's role in guardianship and conservatorship proceedings involving the elderly, in Geriatric Psychiatry and the Law. Edited by Rosner R, Schwartz H. New York,

Plenum, 1987, pp 269–278

Hurme SB: Steps to Enhance Guardianship Monitoring. Chicago, IL, American Bar Association, 1991

Iris MA: Threats to autonomy in guardianship decision making. Generations 14:39–41, 1990

Juretic MC, Martin DL, Taffet GE, et al: Physician input into guardianship cases involving the elderly. International Journal of Geriatric Psychiatry 8:1009–1013, 1993

Kapp MB: Evaluating decision making capacity in the elderly: a review of recent literature. Journal of Elder Abuse and Neglect 2:15–29, 1990

Kapp MB: Ethical aspects of guardianship. Clin Geriatr Med 10(3):501–512, 1994

Mann CK: Alzheimer's and multi-infarct dementia—incapacity to execute will, in American Jurisprudence Proof of Facts,Vol 17, 3rd Series. New York, Lawyers Cooperative Publishing, 1992, pp 219–310

Missouri Bar Association: Durable Power of Attorney for Health Care and Health Care Directive. Jefferson City, MO, Missouri Bar Association, 1991

Nolan BS: Functional evaluation of the elderly in guardianship proceedings. Law Med Health Care 12:210–218, 1984

Parry J: Selected recommendations from the national guardianship symposium at Wingspread. Mental and Physical Disability Law Reporter 12:398–406, 1988

Podnieks E: National survey on abuse of the elderly in Canada. Journal of Elder Abuse and Neglect 5–58, 1992

Quinn M, Tomita S: Elder Abuse and Neglect: Causes, Diagnosis and Intervention Strategies. New York, Springer, 1986

Sadoff RL: Medical-legal issues, in Comprehensive Review of Geriatric Psychiatry. Edited by Sadavoy J, Lazarus LW, Jarvik LF. Washington, DC, American Psychiatric Press, 1991, pp 637–651

Scogin F, Perry J: Guardianship proceedings with older adults: the role of functional assessment and gerontologists. Law and Psychology Review 10:123–128, 1986

Subcommittee on Health and Long-Term Care, Select Committee on Aging: Elder abuse: a decade of shame and inaction (Committee Publ No 101-768). 101st Congress, 2nd Session. Washington, DC, U.S. Government Printing Office, 1990

Subcommittee on Housing and Consumer Interests, House Select Committee on Aging: Model standards to ensure quality guardianship and representative payeeship services, a report by the chairman (Committee

Publ No 101-729). 100th Congress, 1st Session. Washington, DC, U.S. Government Printing Office, 1989

Topolnicki DM: The gulag of guardianship. Money, March 1989, pp 114–152

Zimny GH, Gilchrist BJ, Grossberg GT, et al: Annual reports by guardians and conservators to probate courts. Journal of Elder Abuse and Neglect 3(2):61–74, 1991a

Zimny GH, Gilchrist BJ, Diamond JA: A National Model for Judicial Review of Guardians' Performance. St. Louis, MO, St. Louis University, 1991b

CHAPTER 36

Steven H. Miles, M.D.
Gabe Maletta, M.D.

Clinical Ethics

C linical ethics is about the role of values in clinical decision making. At its most basic level, ethics examines the question, "What ought to be done?" Should the respirator be disconnected? Should the man be placed in a nursing home despite his objection? At a broader level, ethics asks, "Who decides?" "What should be decided?" "How are these competing goods weighed?" and "Why is this a good or bad decision?" At a more fundamental level, ethics asks," "What are the implications of respecting the patient, of trying to do good, or of trying to be fair?" Ethics is not about law. Laws are relevant to clinical setting, but they usually suggest due process procedures and standards and do not specify precise clinical decisions.

Geropsychiatric ethics may be distinguished from the clinical ethics of psychiatric medicine by special features of the geropsychiatry practice environment, age-related clinical problems, and the important presence of personal caregivers to aging persons. The practice environment includes institutions (e.g., nursing homes, liaison geropsychiatry) that are particularly likely to intersect the lives of older persons. The proper conduct of these institutions requires ethical reflection. Some ethics problems, such as end-of-life care or the care of persons with acquired cognitive and decision-making dysfunction, are particularly frequent in the care of aging persons. Finally, caregivers play such an important role in the lives of older persons that they merit special attention.

This chapter is topical and clinically focused. A comprehensive theory of clinical ethics or a complete review of all of the ethics issues that arise in geropsychiatry is not presented.

The Practice Environment of Geropsychiatry

Geropsychiatrists typically function in two major kinds of consulting roles. Traditionally, they respond to cases referred from other clinicians. Alternatively, they may be retained as an ongoing consultant to all the residents of a long-term care setting.

The hospital geropsychiatric liaison-consultant is usually consulted by an internist and is most often asked to address affective and adjustment disorders, dementia, and psychotropic medication (Grossberg et al. 1990). Consultants are also asked to perform the role of clinical ethicists (Hayes 1986; Webb 1987). The range of ethical issues arising in the care of geriatric patients includes those that are seen in adult psychiatry, such as problems related to respect for confidentiality, evaluation of informed consent, and ensuring proper oversight of decisions to administer psychotropic medications to persons without decision-making capacity.

The geropsychiatrist who is a house consultant in a long-term care setting, where 80%–90% of persons can have a secondary psychiatric diagnosis (Rovner et al. 1990; Tariot et al. 1993), has complex ethical duties related to the general nature of the nursing home environment. First, the consultant faces the dehumanization implicit in the diagnostic or labeling use of terms such as *wanderer, uncooperative,* or *assaultive.* Such behavioral descriptors can sometimes divert attention away from underlying etiologies or, worse, lead to stigmatization as exemplified by the punitive or abusive use of restraints (Berland et al. 1990; Schnelle et al. 1992). Second, there are ethics issues that are sometimes taken for granted by nursing home staff but are of great importance to nursing home residents. These include regulations about bedtimes, rising times, bath times, and meal times; roommate choice; marriage and sexual life; private telephone access; passes to leave the facility; and liquor rules (Ambrogi 1989; Hofland 1988; Kane and Caplan 1990). The scale of personal control in a total care institution such as a nursing home is needlessly dehumanizing. This is an appropriate theme for a geropsychiatric house consultant to engage. To engage these questions, the geropsychiatrist will have to participate in education at all levels of the facility's staff and administration.

Clinical Problems in Geropsychiatry

Competence and Decision-Making Ability

Geropsychiatrists are frequently asked to assess a person's decision-making capacity, to assess the authenticity of a patient's particular decision, or to recommend a decision-making process for a person who is unable to make decisions. This may occur when a person is refusing a recommended medical treatment (e.g., antidepressants or life-sustaining medical care), when a caregiver cannot manage a patient (e.g., a frail person who is unable to live in the community and refuses nursing home placement or home care), or when a family caregiver disagrees with a patient's decision (e.g., a dementia patient's decision to drive). When a request for psychiatric consultation regarding a treatment refusal raises a question of the patient's decision-making capacity, the patient often has organic mental disease or alcoholism, which can adversely affect the person's ability to live independently (Golinger and Federoff 1989; Mahler et al. 1990; Mebane and Rauch 1990). By contrast, when decision-making ability is not challenged in a treatment refusal psychiatric consultation, the dispute about the treatment can be successfully resolved by brief counseling focusing on the situational reasons for the refusal (Howanitz and Freedman 1992).

Competence, decision-making ability, and informed consent are different concepts. Competence or incompetence is a legal status. Incompetence is a *court finding* that places a person under the legal control of a court-appointed guardian. By contrast, decision-making ability is a *clinical finding*. Although these terms are often used interchangeably, the difference emphasizes the limited authority of a clinician over patients who have not yet been declared incompetent and the definitive authority of a designated guardian for a person who has been found incompetent. Both of these terms differ from a forensic finding of responsibility for a crime.

For decision-making ability to be present, patients must be able to 1) receive and communicate information after attempts to reverse or overcome sensory or speech disorders have failed, 2) appreciate the personal implications of risks and benefits, and 3) provide a cogent explanation of how he or she weighs them or relates them to personal goals. The clinical conclusion that a patient lacks decision-making ability may lead to the decision to seek a legal finding that a patient is incompetent and in need of a legal guardian, to use emergency medical holds or treatment powers, to use a proxy decision maker named in an advance directive, or perhaps to use certain human services (e.g., nursing home placement or a home health aide to dispense medications).

Decision making should be assessed as a process, rather than simply in relation to the strangeness of the person's decision. Thus, a person's decision making should not be deemed impaired simply because it is unusual or supported by unconventional premises. However, individuals should be able to give an account of their decision making, describing the major grounds for a decision and relating the decision to those grounds. Major decisions should not change arbitrarily, although they may evolve with further discussion, experience, or in relation to how the issue or information is framed.

Decision-making incapacity may be limited in time and scope. It may be transient and reversible when caused by medical conditions (e.g., delirium), by social situations (e.g., learned dependence), or by risk averse life-orientations or when a person is temporarily overwhelmed by an unfamiliar situation. Decision-making incapacity may be limited to a small set of decisions. For example, a person may be unable to evaluate a particular treatment while being fully capable of deciding that a daughter, rather than a husband, should be the proxy decision maker. Similarly, a person may need a financial conservator even though otherwise capable of making his or her own medical decisions and living independently.

The doctrine of informed consent holds that a patient or proxy with decision-making capacity must be given sufficient information and freedom to make an authentic treatment decision. Patients should be given information that will be "material" to how they make decisions. This includes information on why a therapy is proposed, the likelihood of benefit, the range and incidence of undesirable side effects, and alternatives to the recommended course. Material information is defined in relation to the patient's values. For example, the rare possibility of a blood transfusion should certainly be disclosed when obtaining consent to remove a colonic polyp from a Jehovah's Witness with a strong religiously grounded objection to receiving blood.

Forgoing Life-Sustaining Treatment

Geropsychiatrists become involved in decisions to withdraw or withhold life-sustaining treatment by 1) evaluating a patient's decision-making capacity, 2) assessing whether depressive symptoms are influencing decision making, and 3) counseling patients and families about decisions to forgo treatment. The withdrawal or withholding of life-sustaining treatment precedes 1.5 million deaths in the United States each year (about 75% of hospital inpatient deaths and a higher percentage of nursing home deaths). Half of these persons do not make the decision to withdraw or withhold treatment, often because clinicians have deferred discussing this issue, thus passing decisions on to family members and the physician.

There is a legal and clinical standard of care for these decisions (Council on Ethics and Judicial Affairs 1992; Meisel 1991). This standard includes the following:

- All life-sustaining treatments are elective.
- Medically provided food and fluid are life-sustaining treatment.
- There must be consent to any life-sustaining treatment by the patient or a person who can speak for the patient's interest.
- The right to consent to or refuse treatment is not conditional to having a terminal or irreversible illness.

States vary as to the degree of proof that is required for evidence of an incompetent person's preference to forgo treatment. States also vary in procedures pertaining to selecting and empowering proxy decision makers and with regard to decisions for persons under state guardianship or in state-owned health care facilities. Court involvement is rare (i.e., about 100 appeals court decisions since 1976). Patients usually perceive discussions with physicians about the limited use of life-sustaining treatments as positive experiences that give patients a sense of being cared for, address fears, and decrease depressive symptoms (Finucane et al. 1988; Kellogg et al. 1992; Lo et al. 1986; Stolman et al. 1990). A small minority of persons find this counseling to be upsetting or saddening or to lead to a sense of resignation or health-related fear. Successful counseling focuses on enhancing the patient's sense of control as well as on the goal of continuing the treatment relationship. It must avoid the implicit suggestion that a patient is being abandoned, which can arise if the discussion is focused on the limitation of treatment.

Psychiatrists participating in these decisions should address both the affective and cognitive components of decision making. They should consider the possibility of depression, undertreated pain, or adjustment disorders to catastrophic illness that might affect a patient's request to forgo life-sustaining treatment. Depressive symptoms alone, as opposed to clinical depression, do not disqualify or appear to affect these decisions (Cohen-Mansfield et al. 1991; Shmerling et al. 1991). Older persons' preferences for cardiopulmonary resuscitation (CPR) are influenced by their overly optimistic estimate of the efficacy of resuscitation. About one of seven persons who receives hospital CPR survives to discharge, but this decreases substantially when cardiac arrest occurs in persons who are chronically ill or who have multiorgan system disease. Survival after nursing home resuscitation is very rare. These outcomes should be discussed with patients in the course of counseling about treatment plans.

Physicians should encourage patients to make advance directives to clarify future decisions about life-sustaining treatment in the event the patient loses decision-making capacity.

A *living will* specifies an individual's values and preferences for medical care. One form creates a "values history," in which personal questions in everyday language define the person's values; these should guide medical care (Lambert et al. 1990). Other living wills require persons to choose treatments for hypothetical terminal illness, coma, or dementia (Emanuel and Emanuel 1989). This format offers clinicians more specific guidance about the patient's wishes but uses more technical medical language.

A *durable power of attorney* for health care enables a person to appoint someone to make treatment choices in the event of loss of decision-making ability. In effect, this enables a person to appoint his or her own guardian. A durable power of attorney is particularly useful when a person wants an unrelated friend or a distant relative to supersede the immediate family. Durable power of attorney has an advantage over a living will in that it empowers a person who can interpret the patient's past statements and values (Annas 1991). Most patients want living wills interpreted flexibly (Sehgal et al. 1992). Studies show that surrogate decision makers, including physicians, have a very limited ability to exactly estimate a person's treatment preferences (Seckler et al. 1991).

Proxy decision makers should be chosen on the basis of their intimate familiarity with the patient's values rather than simply on the basis of the closeness of their kinship, as is done when identifying persons to consent for autopsies or donate organs. They should be encouraged to discuss the patient's preferences for care rather than their own.

Comfort Care for Persons With End-Stage Dementia

The comfort care of persons with profound dementia is like other forms of hospice care. It rests on the foundation of a thorough medical evaluation and conscientious decision making about the goals of treatment (Miles and Moss 1988). It may be based on an advance directive or on the conclusion that the patient is not experiencing the benefit of the life-sustaining therapy that is being provided. It may follow a recognition that a patient is anorectic and that life-sustaining food or fluids could be provided only by the unacceptable use of permanent enteral nutrition. It is usually possible to conduct family meetings to arrive at a reasonable consensus between health care providers and family members (Volicer et al. 1986). Like discussions with patients, such counseling should be grounded on how the patient will be cared for and what the patient's interests are; such positive foundations give an essential context to family members, who may feel that they are being asked to abandon a loved one.

A comfort-care-only treatment plan entails a comprehensive review of medications and therapies. Routine laboratory tests or medications that prolong life but do not comfort (e.g., antiarrhythmics, lipid-lowering agents) are not indicated. Life-sustaining medications may be appropriate if they minimize suffering (e.g., some diuretics for congestive heart failure). Calorie counts are misleading in patients who are expected to die and who have refused a feeding tube; the chart should note that patients have been offered food or fluids to satisfy their hunger or thirst. Other measures, such as physical therapies, skin care, and new hearing aid batteries, should be provided as needed to optimize quality of life and prevent suffering. Hospitalization is ordinarily not indicated except for palliative treatment that is beyond the capability of a personal caregiver or long-term care facility. If a patient is transferred to a hospital, especially via an ambulance, the physician should ensure transmission of the comfort-care-only treatment plan to the ambulance, emergency department, and inpatient providers (Sachs et al. 1991).

The Unsafe Driver

Although most older drivers are safe drivers, older drivers as a group are more likely than younger drivers to have accidents and have driving-related injuries (Retchin and Anapolle 1993). These accidents are attributed to age-related sensory, neuroleptic, and musculoskeletal disorders and to the effects of medications. Geropsychiatrists are especially likely to be asked to evaluate persons whose driving is impaired by dementia or psychoactive drugs. Alzheimer's disease is not of itself sufficient cause for the summary withdrawal of driving privileges. For such persons, periodic and individualized evaluations of the functions and skills needed for safe driving should be undertaken (Donnelly and Karlinsky 1990; Odenheimer 1993). The progression of dementia is correlated with a deterioration in driving performance (Hunt et al. 1993).

The responsibilities of geropsychiatrists with regard to impaired drivers are imprecisely defined. First, the patient must be informed so that he or she is empowered to protect him- or herself and others. Second, the geropsychiatrist with others should identify and address reversible causes of impaired driving. With the patient's permission, the clinician can also work with caregivers to identify alternatives to driving. Third, the duty to report an impaired driver to the state falls within the "duty to warn" ethic, which is widely known by psychiatrists. A physician may be obligated to report reasonably foreseeable dangers but need not personally prevent the person from driving (Retchin and Anapolle 1993). Six states mandate physician reporting of this information to their motor vehicle department, whereas others require more frequent reporting based on age (Metzner et al. 1993). This individualized and stepwise set of intervention—informing, rehabilitating, providing voluntary restrictions, and imposing external restraints—exemplifies a widely used ethical framework known as the *least restrictive alternative.*

Finally, older persons may perceive the loss of driving privileges to be objectionable, insulting, inconvenient, and even disabling if it prevents them from performing some household management activities of daily living (e.g., shopping), especially for persons who live in a rural area. The geropsychiatrist has a role in supportive counseling and assistance with these issues.

Nursing Home Placement

Nursing home placement entails a radical change in a patient's definition of self and in others' perceptions of the patient. Fear of nursing home placement is a common precipitant of suicide (Loebel et al. 1991). It can disrupt the conduct of marital and social relationships and impoverish the patient, a noninstitutionalized spouse, or other family member. These consequences of nursing home placement justify a high standard of patient advocacy on the part of geropsychiatrists involved in these decisions. First, there must be diligent efforts to keep the person at home by optimizing biopsychosocial functioning through health and social services. Second, there should be supportive counseling of persons who are at risk of nursing home placement. Finally, placement should be based on a demonstrated, rather than predicted, failure to care for one's self. There should be proper legal authority to institutionalize a person who is opposed to nursing home placement.

Research Ethics

Institutionalization and cognitive dysfunction, not age, define the vulnerability of elderly research subjects and their corresponding need for greater protection (Sachs and Cassel 1990; Sachs et al. 1993). Older or vulnerable persons should not lose the opportunity to participate in research. Older research subjects may differ historically from younger persons in education, familiarity with technical or scientific terms, willingness to participate in research, or willingness to assume risk. Older subjects have a greater prevalence of sensory disorders that require time-consuming ways of presenting information about the research.

The vulnerability of persons with impaired decision-making ability poses special issues in research design that have not been definitively addressed by law or professional standards. There is consensus that proxy decision makers should be used to authorize consent to research, as is done with consent to treatment. Subjects who do not assent to the research, as evidenced by signs of being frightened by or resisting research procedures, should usually be dropped from the study, even if permission for participation from a properly empowered proxy has been obtained.

Research in long-term care is problematic. Adequate independent oversight of research design and subject recruitment is difficult in facilities that do not fall within the purview of an institutional research review board. Privacy is difficult to maintain. Research participation should not be the only means by which a subject may secure needed or adequate health care. The possibility of coercion by trusted caregivers or by financial inducements to indigent persons for research participation merits careful oversight.

Even so, there are many issues relevant to the well-being of older persons that can be studied only in nursing homes and with persons with impaired decision-making ability. There is no consensus on whether individuals with impaired decision-making ability or those who are institutionalized should be used for studies that do not pertain to their cognitive disorder or the medical conditions that are nearly unique to persons in nursing homes. Caution and broad consultation are urged in such matters. Geropsychiatrists may play a leading role in consultation regarding the capacity for insight of potential research subjects.

Physician-Assisted Suicide

The potential legalization of physician-assisted suicide is widely debated. This practice must distinguished from two approved practices: 1) honoring a patient's (or proxy's) refusal of life-sustaining treatment and 2) providing palliative treatments that may, when provided in a manner or dose sufficient to relieve suffering, have the unintended consequence of shortening a patient's life. For example, it is legal and proper to honor an end-stage emphysema patient's request for medications to treat the anxiety of dyspnea, even though the drugs may have the side effect of depressing respiration. This person may also direct that a ventilator not be used if respiratory failure ensues.

Theorists presently distinguish physician-assisted suicide, in which a physician dispenses a drug to a patient that the patient then self-administers to effect death (Quill 1991), from voluntary active euthanasia, in which a physician administers the lethal drug with the patient's immediate preceding consent and cooperation (Orentlicher 1989). At this time, these acts violate standards of practice and may be illegal, although they are rarely successfully prosecuted. Geropsychiatrists will likely be asked to evaluate persons requesting physician-assisted suicide, if the practice is legalized. The distinction between "rational" suicidal intention and mental illness is unclear (Conwell and Caine 1991). The preference to be killed is very uncommon in terminally ill patients and often indicates clinical depression, which is common in chronically ill persons (Brown 1986).

Truth Telling and the Diagnosis of Alzheimer's Disease

The diagnosis of Alzheimer's disease has profound implications for both patients and their caregivers. Aside from being a grave condition in itself, the diagnosis can affect how a patient is seen by others. It can affect the price or ability to purchase health and long-term care insurance, admission to some retirement facilities, authority over personal affairs, and the standing of wills and contracts. Emerging genetic tests may enable a clinician to predict a high likelihood of acquiring Alzheimer's disease if death from other causes does not occur in the years or decades between the test and old age.

It is currently obligatory to tell patients of diagnoses. One study has shown that more than 90% of adults would want to be told of the diagnosis of Alzheimer's disease in order to be able to make plans for their own care, to settle family matters, and to obtain a second opinion (Erde et al.

1988). People with early Alzheimer's disease can be harmed by not being told; they may be deprived of the opportunity to make a will, appoint a proxy decision maker, or leave instructions for their family. The uncertain nature of most early Alzheimer's disease diagnoses is a part of this important information. To respect patients and enhance their choices, patients should be told of this diagnosis as they would be told of any other.

The Role of Caregivers

Geropsychiatrists will meet caregivers for many frail, disabled, or cognitively impaired older persons. These caregivers play complex roles in the lives of older persons. First, they provide essential services, making the older person uniquely dependent on and vulnerable to the caregiver. Some older persons tolerate physical, emotional, or financial abuse by a caregiver out of fear of being moved to an institutional setting. In such instances, geropsychiatrists must consider whether an intervention is required over the abused persons objection. Second, caregivers have a unique intimate relationship with older persons, attending and sometimes speaking for the person during encounters with physical therapists, social workers, or visiting family. Needing a caregiver entails a loss of privacy and, depending on the caregiver, the acquisition of a more articulate voice or a silencing interloper.

The most powerful role of caregivers is as proxies for older persons, making decisions when a person has impaired decision-making ability and often being asked to ratify (and thus being empowered to veto) decisions for competent persons. Numerous studies show that proxy decision makers' decisions imperfectly correlate with the patient's own views and in fact may overestimate the degree of aggressive treatment an elderly dementia patient or one who is unconscious would want (Danis et al. 1991; Tomlinson et al. 1990; Zweibel and Cassel 1989). There is no consensus on how to clinically manage such situations, although the ethical consensus is that the decision should center on the patient's preferences and values. A geropsychiatrist may help a caregiver 1) become more aware of how the caregiver's emotions are affecting the decisions and 2) sort out the patient's interests from the caregiver's own fears and needs.

The caregiver's life is often profoundly affected by the experience of caregiving. Conflict between the caregiver's needs and the caregiver's sense of obligation to the older person receiving care are stated as ethical problems: the extent of family mutuality, as conflicts between obligations to one's career and family versus obligations to the older person, or a family resource sharing (Pratt et al. 1987). However, these ethical problems are often experienced as stress. The geropsychiatrist should recognize and address this stress but also provide supportive counseling to help these families address the important ethical debates that underlie it.

References

Ambrogi DM: Legal issues in nursing home admissions. Law Med Health Care 18:254–262, 1989

Annas GJ: The health care proxy and the living will. N Engl J Med 324:1210–1213, 1991

Berland B, Wachtel TJ, Kiel DP, et al: Patient characteristics associated with the use of mechanical restraints. J Gen Intern Med 5:480–485, 1990

Brown J: Is it normal for terminally ill patients to desire death? Am J Psychiatry 143:208–211, 1986

Cohen-Mansfield J, Rabinovich BA, Lipson S, et al: The decision to execute a durable power of attorney for health care and preferences regarding the use of life-sustaining treatments in nursing home residents. Arch Intern Med 151:289–294, 1991

Conwell Y, Caine ED: Rational suicide and the right to die: reality and myth. N Engl J Med 325:1101–1102, 1991

Council on Ethics and Judicial Affairs: Decisions near the end of life. JAMA 267:2229–2233, 1992

Danis M, Southerland LI, Garrett JM, et al: A prospective study of advance directives for life-sustaining care. N Engl J Med 234:882–888, 1991

Donnelly R, Karlinsky H: The impact of Alzheimer's disease on driving ability: a review. J Geriatr Psychiatry Neurol 3:67–72, 1990

Emanuel LL, Emanuel EJ: The medical directive: a new comprehensive advance care document. JAMA 261:3288–3293, 1989

Erde E, Nodal E, Scholl T: On truth-telling and the diagnosis of Alzheimer's disease. J Fam Pract 26:401–403, 1988

Finucane TE, Shumway JM, Powers RL, et al: Planning with elderly outpatients for contingencies of severe illness: a survey and clinical trial. J Gen Intern Med 3:322–325, 1988

Golinger RC, Federoff JP: Characteristics of patients referred to psychiatrists for competency evaluations. Psychosomatics 30:296–299, 1989

Grossberg F, Zimny G, Zakra B: Geriatric psychiatry consultations in a university hospital. Int Psychogeriatr 2:161–168, 1990

Hayes J: Consult-liaison psychiatry and clinical ethics: a model for consultation and teaching. Gen Hosp Psychiatry 8:415–418, 1986

Hofland BF (ed): Autonomy and long term care. Gerontologist 28 (suppl): 2–96, 1988

Howanitz EM, Freedman JB: Reasons for refusal of medical treatment by patients seen by a consultation-liaison service. Hosp Community Psychiatry 43:278–279, 1992

Hunt L, Morris J, Edwards D, et al: Driving performance in persons with mild senile dementia of the Alzheimer type. J Am Geriatr Soc 41:747–753, 1993

Kane RA, Caplan AL (eds): Everyday Ethics: Revolving Dilemmas in Nursing Home Life. New York, Springer, 1990

Kellogg FR, Crain M, Corwin J, et al: Life-sustaining interventions in frail elderly persons: talking about choices. Arch Intern Med 152:2317–2320, 1992

Lambert P, Gibson JM, Nathanson P: Values history: an innovation in surrogate medical decision making. Law Med Health Care 18:202–212, 1990

Lo B, McLeod GA, Saika G: Patient attitudes to discussing life-sustaining treatments. Arch Intern Med 146:1613–1615, 1986

Loebel JP, Loebel J, Dager SR, et al: Anticipation of nursing home placement may be a precipitant of suicide among the elderly. J Am Geriatr Soc 39:407–408, 1991

Mahler JC, Perry S, Miller F: Psychiatric evaluation of competency in physically ill patients who refuse treatment. Hosp Community Psychiatry 41:1140–1141, 1990

Mebane AH, Rauch HB: When do physicians request competency evaluations? Psychosomatics 31:40–46, 1990

Meisel A: Legal myths about terminating life support. Arch Intern Med 151:1497–1502, 1991

Metzner J, Dentino A, Godard S, et al: Impairment in driving and psychiatric illness. J Neuropsychiatry Clin Neurosci 5:211–220, 1993

Miles SH, Moss R: Evaluating life-sustaining treatments for demented persons. Clin Geriatr Med 4(4):917–924, 1988

Odenheimer GL: Dementia and the older driver. Clin Geriatr Med 9:349–364, 1993

Orentlicher D: From the office of the General Counsel: physician participation in assisted suicide. JAMA 262:1844–1845, 1989

Pratt C, Schmall V, Wright S: Ethical concerns of family caregivers to dementia patients. Gerontologist 27:632–638, 1987

Quill TE: Death and dignity: a case of individualized decision making. N Engl J Med 324:691–694, 1991

Retchin SM, Anapolle J: An overview of the older driver. Clin Geriatr Med 9:279– 296, 1993

Rovner B, German P, Broadhead J, et al: Prevalence and management of dementia and other psychiatric disorders in nursing homes. Int Psychogeriatr 2:13, 1990

Sachs GA, Cassel CK: Biomedical research involving older human subjects. Law Med Health Care 18:234–243, 1990

Sachs GA, Miles SH, Levin R: Limiting resuscitation: emerging policy in the emergency medical system. Ann Intern Med 114:151–154, 1991

Sachs GA, Rhymes J, Cassel CK: Biomedical and behavioral research in nursing homes: guideline for ethical investigations. J Am Geriatr Soc 41:771–777, 1993

Schnelle JF, Simmons SF, Ory MG: Risk factors that predict staff failure to release nursing home residents from restraints. Gerontologist 32:767–770, 1992

Seckler AB, Meier DE, Mulvihill M, et al: Substituted judgement: how accurate are proxy predictions? Ann Intern Med 115:92–98, 1991

Sehgal A, Galbraith A, Chesney M, et al: How strictly do dialysis patients want their advance directives followed? JAMA 267:59–63, 1992

Shmerling RH, Bedell S, Lilienfeld A, et al: Discussing cardiopulminary resuscitation: a study of elderly outpatients. J Gen Intern Med 3:317–321, 1988

Stolman CJ, Gregory JJ, Dunn D, et al: Evaluation of patient, physician, nurse and family attitudes toward do-not-resuscitate orders. Arch Intern Med 150:653–658, 1990

Tariot PN, Podgorski CA, Blazina L, et al: Mental disorders in the nursing home: another perspective. Am J Psychiatry 150:1063–1069, 1993

Tomlinson T, Howe K, Notman M, et al: An empirical study of proxy consent for elderly persons. Gerontologist 1:54–64, 1990

Volicer L, Rheaume Y, Brown J, et al: Hospice approach to the treatment of patients with advanced dementia of the Alzheimer type. JAMA 256:2210–2213, 1986

Webb W: The ethics of the consultation process. Psychosomatics 28:278–279, 1987

Zweibel NR, Cassel CK: Treatment choices at the end of life: a comparison of decisions by older patients and their physicians, selected proxies. Gerontologist 615–621, 1989

CHAPTER 37

Gary L. Gottlieb, M.D., M.B.A.

Financial Issues

Financing strategies have shaped the development of psychiatric services for older adults (Goldman and Frank 1990; Goldman et al. 1987). Payment mechanisms and associated policy influence the identification of patient populations, the organization of services, the site of service delivery, the type and behavior of providers, and the process of evaluation and treatment.

For the most part, government has driven the economic prerogatives and incentives of geriatric mental health care: As financial responsibility shifted from local to state government, older adults who were cared for in the almshouses and asylums of the 19th century helped to fuel the growth of the state hospital systems of the early and middle 20th century (Grob 1983). In 1965, the implementation of Medicare and Medicaid shifted a substantial proportion of the financial responsibility for the psychiatric care of elderly individuals from the states to the federal government. The fee-for-service framework of these programs and the growth of private indemnity insurance stimulated the rapid growth of private and general hospital psychiatric settings (Goldman et al. 1987). Simultaneously, deinstitutionalization and the combined federal and state support provided by Medicaid fostered the expanded use of nursing homes for the care of the chronically mentally ill (Goldman et al. 1986). Similarly, limited reimbursement of outpatient specialty mental health services by Medicare and other third parties has helped to fortify the general health care sector as the dominant source of psychiatric services, particularly for elderly individuals (Regier et al. 1978; Schurman et al. 1985). Prospective payment and nursing home reforms, implemented in the 1980s, are currently affecting the process and content of psychiatric care for older adults (English et al. 1986; Freiman et al. 1989; Goldman et al. 1987; Wells et al. 1993).

Providers and policymakers who seek to optimize the psychiatric well-being of elderly individuals require an understanding of the economic context of aging in late 20th century America. In addition, a working knowledge of the organization of the geriatric mental health delivery system and mechanisms for payment for health and mental health services for elderly individuals is fundamental to this effort. In this chapter, I highlight key financial issues that affect the psychiatric care of older adults. Essential details specific to reimbursement of geropsychiatric services are provided, and relatively recent changes in third-party payment schemes are described. An understanding of the terminology and subtleties of this system should help providers to cope with some of the systematic barriers to the care of this exceptionally needy population. In addition, fundamentals of reforms in the mechanisms for payment for services provide a framework for appreciation of the landscape that is driving the development of health care reform.

Economic and Health Policy Issues

The size, need, and diversity of the aging population shape the economic environment of geriatric mental health care. In the mid-1950s, only 1 of every 11 Americans was older than 65. By the end of the 1980s, slightly less than 1 in 8 Americans was older than 65. The elderly population grew by 23% to nearly 31 million during the 1980s (U.S. Bureau of the Census 1987). This increase is somewhat smaller than the 28% growth experienced during the 1970s. As a result of relatively small Depression Era birth rates, the older population should grow by only about 10% in the 1990s and by 12% in the first decade of the next century. This rate of projected expansion will yield about 39 million older Americans by 2010. Shortly thereafter, the aging of the post–World War II baby boom cohort will cause dramatic growth in the over-65 population segment: By the year 2030, about one-fourth of the population (approximately 66 million people) will be in this age group.

Differences in life expectancy between the sexes and the distribution of minorities among elderly individuals have important economic consequences. There are approximately 1.5 women for every man older than 65 and about 2.5 women for every man older than 85 (U.S. Bureau of the Census 1987). Traditional work roles and Social Security and pension provisions affect surviving women adversely. In general, continued earning potential from work and from pension income in late life is less for women than it is for men. Generally, older women have more limited financial assets. Inasmuch as they usually live longer than their spouses, they are more likely to become dependent on adult children and on the health care establishment to meet social and medical needs (Soldo and Agree 1988).

Ethnic minorities make up a growing segment of the older population. In 1990, about 11% of persons older than 65 were nonwhite. However, by the year 2025, about 15% of elderly individuals are expected to be from minority groups (National Center for Health Statistics 1992). Although life expectancy at birth for whites exceeds that for blacks by about 8%, at age 75, mortality rates for blacks are lower than those for whites (National Center for Health Statistics 1992). However, very old blacks have considerably higher rates of poverty and illness than whites in the same age group (Soldo and Agree 1988). Economic and social discrimination and underprivilege associated with minority status in the United States are exacerbated by the socioeconomic realities of older age: Accrued social and financial resources are limited, barriers to preventive and acute health care are more substantial, and the need for non–health care governmental services, including housing, transportation, meals, and income maintenance, is greater (Furino and Fogel 1990; Markides and Mindel 1987). Cultural differences may also affect the expression of illness and the ways in which American health care, designed for a predominantly white population, is accessed (Hazzard 1989).

The distribution of wealth and income among older adults is highly variable. The degree of this variability has impeded the development of rational policy, thereby affecting reimbursement and delivery of health and mental health services to older adults.

Retirement is generally associated with a one-third to one-half reduction in personal income (Soldo and Agree 1988). Many individuals retire in their late 50s or early 60s. In 1986, close to 90% of men in their early 50s participated in the labor force, while only about 45% of men between the ages of 62 and 64 were still working (Schulz 1988). This rate declines remarkably with age; after age 70, only about 10% of men and 4% of women are in the labor force. Elimination of a mandatory retirement age and the shift of the American economy from heavy industry to less physically demanding service and technology production may extend the working longevity of the population in the near future. In addition to the emotional consequences of retirement, leaving the work force may affect health insurance premium costs, the type of insurance available, and the possibility of participating in some health delivery systems (e.g., some health maintenance organizations [HMOs] and other managed care systems).

The reduction of income associated with retirement may affect standard of living adversely. Most older adults derive postretirement income from a combination of Social Security benefits, public and/or private pensions, and income from savings or investments (Soldo and Agree 1988). The magnitude of these earnings depends almost entirely on preretirement income. For many, these relatively fixed sources may be inadequate, and older adults may suffer the consequences of poverty for the first time in their lives (Furino and Fogel 1990). In 1986, one in eight Americans older than 65, or about 3.5 million people, had income below the established poverty level. About 10% of the younger population were in that income category. Indigence appears to increase with age: about one-fifth of those who live past the age of 85 had incomes at or below the poverty level. These rates are even more dramatic for women and for minorities. For example, a remarkable 60% of black women older than 65 not living with their families had incomes below the poverty level in 1986 (Soldo and Agree 1988).

Poverty and aging are not synonymous, however. Almost 13% of households headed by individuals older than 65 have net assets in the top 5% of American families.

This disparity in distribution of wealth has an important effect on health and welfare policy. Lawmakers frequently do not recognize the socioeconomic heterogeneity of the older population. Therefore, programs such as Social Security and Medicare do not address completely the financial and health care needs of all older adults. Resulting gaps are filled unevenly by programs for indigent individuals. These inequities are particularly important in mental health and long-term care, where out-of-pocket payments make up a substantial component of costs to consumers (Letsch 1993).

Since 1970, the older population has grown twice as rapidly as the rest of the population. In addition, the older population is aging at an extraordinary rate: By the year 2000, 45% of the older population will be at least 75 years old, with the number of those older than 85 growing at a faster rate than any other segment of the population (Soldo and Agree 1988). Growth in the absolute number of older people continues to augment demand for the products that elderly individuals are likely to consume.

Because many of the programs that benefit older adults depend on contributions from the younger population, the growing ratio of older Americans to younger persons may affect society's ability to supply the goods, services, and payments necessary to meet this expanding demand. There are currently about 19 Americans older than 65 per 100 people ages 18–64. This so-called "dependency ratio" is expected to double by 2050 (U.S. Bureau of the Census 1992). Therefore, emerging policy is likely to require the older generation to support its own needs.

The first government program requiring older adults to support financially the increased medical needs of their own generation was the Catastrophic Coverage Act (CCA) of 1988. This legislation provided compulsory insurance for Medicare beneficiaries to defray catastrophic health care costs. The CCA required beneficiaries (predominantly individuals older than 65) to pay an additional premium to cover the cost of increased coverage. Among other factors, the shifting of financial responsibility to potential recipients made the CCA unacceptable politically, and it was repealed in 1989. Despite the current political environment, growth in the dependency ratio will influence policy strategy long into the future and will affect the labor market and national productivity. Therefore, medical and psychiatric interventions that promote the health and productivity of older workers may have social benefits that mirror individual improvements in function and quality of life (Furino and Fogel 1990; Hazzard 1989).

The Medicare System

Enacted in 1965 and initiated on July 1, 1966, under Title XVIII of the Social Security Act, Medicare is a social insurance program first designed to provide medical care benefits for Americans older than age 65 (Cutler and Fine 1985; Iglehart 1992; U.S. Senate Committee on Finance 1978). The program was developed in response to years of debate regarding national health insurance policy and to data derived from comprehensive evaluation of the needs of elderly individuals provided by the Senate Select Committee on Aging. In 1972, the program was expanded to include younger disabled individuals and older adults who are not eligible for social security but who are willing to pay a monthly premium for coverage. In 1973, Medicare coverage was extended to provide medical coverage for individuals experiencing end-stage renal disease. About 36 million people are currently covered by Medicare; 90% of these individuals are elderly (Iglehart 1992).

Despite aggressive efforts to contain costs, expenditures for health care have grown remarkably, and Medicare outlays have made an important contribution to this expansion. In 1991, total health care expenditures accounted for about 13% of the U.S. Gross Domestic Product (Letsch 1993). The more than $130 billion of federal spending for Medicare in 1992 accounted for approximately 17% of total health care expenditures (Iglehart 1992). Adjusted for inflation and age, the average annual growth rate for Medicare expenditures per beneficiary was 5% during the 1970s and more than 5.5% for most of the 1980s (Long and Welch 1988). During these same time periods, health care costs for the general population grew at rates of 3.6% and 4.3%, respectively.

Specialty mental health services for older adults account for only a tiny fragment of Medicare expenditures. Outlays for treatment of psychiatric disorders are about 2.5% of total Medicare spending. These data are more striking when one considers that more than half of all Medicare-covered psychiatric hospitalizations are for nonelderly disabled individuals (Goldman et al. 1987). The relative underutilization of specialty mental health services by older Medicare beneficiaries results from the reinforcement of long-standing provider- and patient-induced barriers to care by economic disincentives and systematic stigmatization.

Medicare benefits are designed to cover acute care services primarily. Preventive services, long-term care, and dental services are excluded. Some services, including mental health care, are subject to limitations in coverage and substantial copayments. Under current conditions, Medicare covers only about 75% of elderly hospital care, 2%–3% of nursing home care, and about 58% of physician services, totaling slightly less than half of geriatric health care costs (Iglehart 1992; Physician Payment Review Commission 1989; Waldo and Lazenby 1984).

Medicare has two components: Part A, the Hospital Insurance program, covers inpatient hospitalization, limited home care, skilled nursing facility services, and hospice care. The Supplemental Medical Insurance program, Part B, covers physician services and provides additional benefits for clinical laboratory tests, durable medical equipment, and some outpatient hospital care.

Hospital Insurance (Part A)

By virtue of participation in the Social Security system, most Americans older than 65 are entitled to Part A coverage. The Part A Hospital Insurance trust fund is underwritten through Social Security payroll taxes paid by employers and employees.

Part A hospital coverage is intentionally limited to coverage of relatively brief inpatient stays, presumably for stabilization of acute conditions. Regulations provide coverage for "spells" of illness. A spell is defined as an inpatient episode that begins with inpatient admission and ends with the close of the first period of 60 consecutive days after discharge. It is possible for a patient to be discharged and readmitted on several occasions during a given episode of illness and still be considered to be in the same spell, as long as 60 days have not elapsed between discharge and admission. For admission to general hospitals, there is no limit on the number of spells or "total lifetime" days covered. However, the maximum number of covered days during a single spell is 150.

The first 60 days of coverage for each episode are fully paid after a deductible equal to the average cost of 1 day of hospitalization ($736 in 1996) has been met. The next 30 inpatient days are subject to a daily coinsurance payment equal to 25% of the hospital deductible, and the last 60 days of covered hospitalization require a copayment equal to half of the deductible amount. These last 60 days of a spell of illness (days 91–150) are designated as *lifetime reserve days.* Coverage for these days may be used electively during any episode but can be used only once during a patient's lifetime. For example, if a patient requires three hospitalizations totaling 110 days with no period of discharge as great as 60 days, he or she would have 40 reserve days of remaining coverage in his or her lifetime for subsequent spells lasting more than 90 days. Patients may elect to save these days for future prolonged hospitalizations and use other financial resources for payment of any part of the costs of days 91–150. Medicare regulations require that a hospital or skilled nursing facility notify a beneficiary of this right at least 5 days prior to the end of coverage. If a facility is not informed that an individual has exhausted all coverage, including lifetime reserve days, Medicare regulations guarantee payment for up to 6 days of hospitalization. Since the repeal of CCA, there is no annual limitation on the out-of-pocket liability of Medicare recipients (American Psychiatric Association [APA], Office of Economic Affairs 1986; Gottlieb 1988; Iglehart 1992).

Although there is no limit on the total number of hospitalizations or inpatient days covered for medical or surgical diagnoses or for psychiatric care in general hospitals, coverage for inpatient psychiatric care in facilities recognized by the Health Care Financing Administration (HCFA) as free-standing psychiatric hospitals is limited to a total of 190 days during an individual's lifetime. In addition, if an individual becomes eligible for Medicare during the course of a first episode of psychiatric hospitalization, Medicare's local intermediary may elect to cover less than the full 150 benefit days of that spell of illness. This provision is designed to restrict

Part A psychiatric benefits to the active component of treatment and to prevent full reimbursement for a person who may have been institutionalized for long periods of time.

Part A also provides limited coverage for care in skilled nursing facilities. Services provided by domiciliary, personal care, and intermediate care facilities are not reimbursable by Medicare. To obtain skilled nursing facility benefits, an individual must have been hospitalized for at least 3 consecutive days, and admission must occur within 30 days of hospital discharge. Hospital Insurance covers up to 100 days of skilled nursing facility care. The need for continued skilled care must be reassessed and documented regularly. Similarly, home health care services are limited and must be related to acute and remediable conditions (APA, Office of Economic Affairs 1986; Gottlieb 1988; Waldo and Lazenby 1984).

From 1966 until late 1983, Part A of Medicare paid for all inpatient care through a retrospective cost-based reimbursement system. In an effort to prevent depletion of the Hospital Insurance trust fund, Congress and the Reagan administration enacted the Tax Equity and Fiscal Responsibility Act (TEFRA) of 1982. TEFRA emphasized cost containment, providing for limits on all inpatient operating costs and establishing target rates for cost increases. Incentives were developed providing for reduced hospital reimbursement if targets were not met and extra payments if limits were not exceeded. Reimbursement limits were adjusted to reflect patient mix, geographic location, and training costs. TEFRA mandated legislation to replace cost-based reimbursement with a prospective payment system (English et al. 1986; Frazier et al. 1986; Scherl et al. 1988; Wells et al. 1993).

Public Law 98-21 of the Social Security Amendments of 1983 established a prospective payment system for Medicare. The prospective payment system is based on a patient-discharge classification system using diagnosis-related groups (DRGs) to cluster patients who presumably require similar care. The DRG system categorizes patients into 23 relatively general major diagnostic categories and then assigns the discharge to one of 468 DRGs derived from principal and secondary diagnoses, procedures rendered, and, to a lesser degree, age, sex, comorbidity, complications, and discharge status. Hospitals are paid a predetermined amount for each case according to the DRG assigned. This sum is independent of actual costs incurred. Therefore, payment is considered to be an incentive for efficient utilization of resources. If patients consume extraordinary resources or require prolonged inpatient care, they are classified as "outliers," and Medicare provides additional payments to the hospital, but at a rate considerably less than actual cost.

Fourteen of the DRGs apply to discharges related to treatment of psychiatric disorders. Concerns regarding the ability of DRGs to accurately predict resource consumption for psychiatric disorders led to a temporary exemption from this payment method for free-standing psychiatric hospitals and for distinct psychiatric units in general hospitals. However, treatment of primary psychiatric patients in "scatter" beds on general medical and surgical units is reimbursed through the DRG system.

Research regarding the application of DRGs to treatment of patients with principal psychiatric diagnoses has substantiated their inaccuracy in prediction of resource consumption. DRGs have been shown to account for only a limited proportion (16%–40%) of the variation in individual lengths of stay for all diagnoses. Moreover, they are considerably less accurate in predicting psychiatric utilization, generally accounting for less than 8% of the variance (English et al. 1986; Frank and Lave 1985; Goldman 1988). The American Psychiatric Association's comprehensive assessment of DRG data (English et al. 1986) suggests that the similarity among patients within a given psychiatric DRG is extremely limited. Patients who require very brief hospitalizations are frequently clustered with individuals in need of much longer hospital stays. Analysis of study data indicates that DRGs favor less severely ill patients and settings that provide short-term evaluation and limited treatment.

Free-standing psychiatric hospitals and exempted psychiatric units in general hospitals continue to be paid retrospectively by Medicare. However, TEFRA modified and substantially limited these reimbursements. Medicare reimbursement for treatment in these sites is capped at a target rate established for each facility based on resource utilization during a "base" year (the first full fiscal year of operation after October 1, 1983). If the actual cost per case exceeds the target rate, the hospital must absorb the loss. If the cost is less than the TEFRA capped rate, the hospital may retain 50% of the difference up to 5% of the target rate. For hospitals that care for a substantial number of geriatric patients with complex problems, this payment scheme is even more arbitrary than DRGs: As geriatric psychiatry expands as a field, recognition and aggressive treatment of acute mental disorders in Medicare recipients are also growing. This will likely translate into greater resource consumption in acute care settings. Therefore, the employment of relatively old utilization experience (i.e., 1984 or 1985 for established institutions) to set payment limits can easily become de facto per-case reimbursement at a rate that has nothing to do with the patient (or even with the patient's diagnosis!).

The nature of psychiatric disorders in elderly individuals makes these incentives worrisome. Incomplete evaluation of complicated patients in settings that are discouraged from employing expensive but often necessary diagnostic technologies may add unnecessary disability and ultimately generate substantially greater costs (Fogel et al. 1990). In addition, the high prevalence of medical disorders among older adults with psychiatric diagnoses makes both DRGs and TEFRA caps even less appropriate. Patients with active medical diagnoses treated by psychiatric personnel in scatter beds and/or in exempt units have not been considered in research assessing these payment mechanisms.

Wells et al. (1993) evaluated the effects of the prospective payment system on various aspects of quality of care and other outcomes for older adult depression patients who required hospitalization. They compared data for patients who were hospitalized for depression in acute care general medical hospitals just prior to TEFRA (1981–1982) with those collected shortly after its full implementation (1985–1986). This analysis determined that the quality of "psychological" components of care improved after implementation of the prospective payment system. However, even in light of the improvements noted, the authors determined that the overall quality of care received by geriatric depression patients was in the low to moderate range. The authors recognized that some of the improvement noted could have been attributable to the development of geriatric psychiatry as a field and improvements in treatment technology. In addition, the authors found no improvement in the quality of nonpsychological, medical care provided. An assessment of more recent data that can more effectively determine the importance of the maturity of geriatric psychiatry, the advent of new treatment approaches, and longer term functional and psychiatric outcomes is necessary.

A number of alternative mechanisms have been proposed to allow implementation of a prospective payment system for psychiatry. Although several methods substantially improve predictability of length of stay and other measures of resource consumption, no system has been tested with adequately large data sets in a way that reflects the extremely differentiated nature of the mental health care delivery system (Goldman 1988). Research in this area remains active, and potential improvements in policy in the near future are possible.

Supplemental Medical Insurance (Part B)

The Supplemental Medical Insurance benefit program of Medicare Part B is voluntary. Participation requires payment of a monthly premium ($46.10

in 1995). About 97% of Medicare Part A recipients elect to purchase Supplemental Medical Insurance benefits. The Part B trust fund is financed by general revenues from the federal treasury, trust fund interest, and participant premiums. The Part B premium is set by law at 25% of the average monthly benefit per enrollee, and premiums cover about one-fourth of program expenditures (Iglehart 1992; Physician Payment Review Commission 1989).

Part B benefits are subject to an annual deductible ($100 in 1994) and a copayment. For nonpsychiatric physician services and psychiatric inpatient services, a 20% copayment is required. Coverage of medical and surgical visits has never been limited by number of visits or costs of resources consumed. However, when Part B psychiatric benefits were designed, mental illness was depicted as "lacking precise diagnostics and established treatment protocols expected to lead to specified outcomes within a defined period of time" (Cutler and Fine 1985, p. 20). Therefore, coverage for outpatient psychiatric treatment was limited severely. From the initiation of Medicare in 1966 through early 1988, total annual reasonable charges were set at $500, and the law required that the maximum annual Medicare reimbursement for outpatient psychiatric services was $312.50 or 62.5% of reasonable charges, whichever was lower. The 80% federal share, which was the maximum amount paid by Medicare to the psychiatrist, was only $250 per year.

The Omnibus Budget Reconciliation Act of 1987 (OBRA 87) (Public Law 100-203) recognized, in part, the discrimination against services for mental disorders inherent in the Supplemental Medical Insurance benefit. Coverage for outpatient psychiatric services was increased to $2,200 annually by 1989. However, the 50% copayment remained. In addition, services for the medical management of psychiatric disorders were exempted from the $2,200 limit and are subject to the same 20% copayment required for nonpsychiatric outpatient services. The Omnibus Budget Reconciliation of 1989 (OBRA 89) (H.R.3299 Report 101-386) provided further improvement of the psychiatric benefit (Omnibus Budget Reconciliation Act of 1989 Reform). Effective July 1, 1990, the annual dollar limit for outpatient mental health services was eliminated. However, the discriminatory 50% copayment and 190-day lifetime psychiatric hospital utilization limit were unaffected by the new law.

OBRA 89 was also revolutionary in its expansion of coverage provided by nonphysician providers. Until the enactment of this legislation, necessary services delivered by psychologists, social workers, therapists, nurses, and aides were reimbursable only if performed under the "direct supervision" of a physician. Direct supervision was defined as immediate availability to provide assistance at the time of service. Exceptions to this rule included psychological testing and services provided by psychologists in some community mental health settings. The new law provided for direct reimbursement of psychologists in all settings. Direct reimbursement of clinical social worker services at a rate of 80% of the actual charge or 75% of the amount paid to a psychologist, whichever is less, is also provided, except when services are provided to an inpatient of a hospital or skilled nursing facility as required for the facility's participation in Medicare. OBRA 89 also described criteria regarding consultation with a physician for these nonphysician providers. These criteria are vague and somewhat superficial: The provider must document that the patient has been informed of the desirability of consultation with the patient's primary care physician to consider potential medical conditions that may contribute to the patient's condition. In addition, the provider must document written or verbal communication with the primary physician regarding the patient's treatment, unless the patient specifically refuses such contact. The law makes no provision for assessment or consultation with a psychiatrist. Reimbursement of services provided by psychiatric nurses and other therapists continues to require direct physician supervision (Omnibus Budget Reconciliation Act of 1989 Reform).

For the most part, direct patient treatment or evaluation is required to bill Medicare. Services rendered by telephone and patient contacts that do not involve evaluation of patient status (e.g., renewing a prescription) are not reimbursable. However, charges for obtaining treatment information from relatives or close associates of a patient who is unreliable or uncommunicative are allowable. Family counseling services are covered only when the purpose of counseling is to facilitate treatment of the identified patient.

There are currently two procedures available for Medicare beneficiaries to receive benefits for provider services under Part B:

1. A provider may agree to accept assignment from Supplemental Medical Insurance and thereby accept the Medicare-approved fee as payment in full. The Fiscal Intermediary (FI) pays the approved amount, less copayment and deductible, to the provider directly. The copayment and deductible must be collected from the patient.
2. A provider may elect not to accept assignment. Nonparticipating providers may charge only up to 115% of the Medicare-approved fee for the procedures they perform. Medicare reimburses nonparticipating providers 95% of the Medicare-approved fee, less copayments and deductibles. Providers must bill patients directly for the balance of

the limited charge. In addition, since April 1, 1990, all providers are required to accept assignment from Medicare beneficiaries who are also recipients of Medicaid and from all Medicare recipients who are at or below the federal poverty level (OBRA 89 Physician Payment Reform Summary Draft).

From the time of implementation of the prospective payment system for hospital services through 1991, the annual growth rate for costs of physicians' services was more than twice the rate of growth for inpatient hospital services (Letsch 1993). Rising prices for services and increases in the number of services consumed per beneficiary were the greatest contributors to this growth. Part B expenditures grew about 17% per year during the 1980s and currently account for about a one-third of Medicare expenditures (Letsch 1993). This growth concerned policymakers, and, in addition to the aforementioned expansion of coverage for mental health services, OBRA 89 stipulated the implementation of significant reform in methods of physician payment under Medicare.

OBRA 89 provided for the development of expenditure targets, or volume performance standards, to control growth in physician services. The Secretary of Health and Human Services is mandated to recommend to Congress an overall volume performance standards growth rate before the beginning of each fiscal year. The volume performance standards should be related to fee increases, growth in the size of the Medicare population, changes in service volume and intensity, and a volume performance factor. At the end of the year, the Secretary compares actual growth in outlays with the volume performance standards and uses those data to determine if and by how much fees should be increased or decreased (Iglehart 1992; Omnibus Budget Reconciliation Act of 1989 Reform). The law requires separate determinations of growth in surgical and nonsurgical expenditures and respective recommendations for fee schedule modifications.

In addition, OBRA 89 provided for the development of a uniform Medicare fee schedule to replace Medicare's traditional method of payment based on determination of customary, prevailing, and reasonable charges ascertained for individual physicians. The new fee schedule is based on a resource-based relative value scale (RBRVS), developed after extensive research led by Hsiao et al. (1988, 1992) and substantial input from the Physician Payment Review Commission (1989) and professional groups nationally. The RBRVS was used to determine the relative values of about 7,000 physician services. The relative value for each procedure has three measurable components: the work required to perform the procedure, associated practice and malpractice expenses, and the amortized value of the opportunity costs for training in a specialty. (This last component is not included in fee determination.) These proportions are based on a weighted average of specialty-specific practice expense and malpractice data. Approximately 60% of each fee is adjusted for geographic variations in cost (Hsiao et al. 1992). The product of each relative value and a monetary conversion factor determines the fee for each service.

The transition to the new fee schedule began in 1990 with reductions in payments for "overvalued procedures." Existing fee schedules for anesthesia and radiology were adjusted to conform to the RBRVS fee schedule. For most other specialties, the RBRVS fee schedule was implemented on January 1, 1992, with a gradual phase-in of adjustments scheduled to occur until 1996.

In an effort to correct for perceived overvaluation of noncognitive procedures, the RBRVS emphasizes cognitive assessment, patient management, and caring activities performed by providers (Hsiao et al. 1988, 1992). The work component of relative values is based largely on time, intensity, and stress associated with delivery of services. Case vignettes were assessed by panels of providers in each specialty so that appropriate values could be assigned. Procedure codes from the *Current Procedural Terminology* (CPT) (American Medical Association 1990) were then employed to describe the procedure performed.

Unfortunately, efforts to apply the RBRVS to psychiatry were seriously flawed. The vignettes employed were simplistic and unrepresentative of psychiatric practice. Measurements of clinical work performed and of practice costs were inconsistent, and efforts to develop work scenarios comparable to those encountered in other specialties considered the circumstances of psychiatric care poorly. In addition, the CPT codes for psychiatry are extremely broad and therefore difficult to map onto the activities associated with specific vignettes (Fogel et al. 1990; Sharfstein 1990). Despite several technical surveys, the Medicare fee schedule for psychiatric services did not result in an improved valuation for these predominantly cognitive services. Notably, just prior to implementation, a modification in the fee schedule did result in increased payment for psychotherapy codes without adjustment to other psychiatric codes that reflect similar work.

Medicaid

Medicaid is a social insurance program enacted in 1965 to pay for medical care for indigent Americans by providing matching funds to the states.

Although states must provide certain minimum basic benefits to receive these matching funds, the program allows states to impose some restrictions on the types of services funded and the level of reimbursement for specific services. Therefore, Medicaid services for mental health care and for specific services for indigent older adults vary substantially by state (Chulis et al. 1993; Letsch 1993).

Between 3 and 4 million individuals older than 65 receive Medicaid benefits annually. Older adults represent about 16% of all Medicaid beneficiaries and account for about 40% of program expenditures (Chulis et al. 1993; Waldo and Lazenby 1984). Most older Medicaid recipients also have Medicare. In addition, many state Medicaid programs have Part B buy-in provisions. This allows these states to reduce their risk for payment of physician services by paying for Medicare Supplemental Medical Insurance on behalf of their older Medicaid recipients. Therefore, Medicaid is principally a coinsurer for many older adults. The program covers Medicare deductibles, copayments, uncovered physician services, and other services after Medicare benefits have been exhausted (Chulis et al. 1993). Fees for all Medicaid services are set at the state level and are generally unrelated to other fee schedules.

State governments have some discretionary power in the development of local Medicaid programs. Local needs often influence the nature of services offered. Numerous programs that are not covered by Medicare may be available to indigent older adults. These include day treatment programs (which are often longer term and broader than partial hospitals that meet guidelines for cost-based reinbursement by Medicare), home mental health services, and prescription drugs.

The Medicaid program is most important in its role as payer for long-term care services. Medicaid pays for about 42% of skilled and intermediate level nursing home care, and Medicare pays for only 2% of all long-term care costs. The balance of these expenses is borne out of pocket by patients and their families. Most states require that individuals have limited income and that they spend down their assets below an established level before they become eligible for Medicaid benefits (Letsch 1993; Levit et al. 1985).

The nursing home is probably the most important site of care for older adult psychiatric patients, particularly those with severe and chronic disorders such as dementia, depression associated with medical illness and disability, and schizophrenia (Goldman et al. 1986). Deinstitutionalization has left the nursing home as the last resort for care of many chronically psychiatrically ill younger and older adults. From the federal government's perspective, this phenomenon has effectively shifted costs from the states (i.e., for state hospitals) to federally supported Medicaid nursing home beds. In the nursing home reform provisions of OBRA 87, the federal government required preadmission screening of nursing home applicants for psychiatric illness. Referral for active treatment is required if such treatment cannot be provided in the nursing home. These requirements may simultaneously improve psychiatric care for disabled indigent older adults in nursing homes while creating significant barriers to admission for others.

Private Insurance and Out-of-Pocket Expenditures

Out-of-pocket expenditures are those health care costs that older adults must pay from personal or family income or savings. Out-of-pocket expenses include premiums for Supplemental Medical Insurance and private "Medigap" policies; copayments and deductibles for Parts A and B; charges that exceed Medicare-approved limits imposed by providers who do not accept assignment; and charges for uncovered services, including much of long-term care. In 1988, out-of-pocket expenditures for health care accounted for 12.5% of after-tax household income for older adults (Iglehart 1992). Older adults with psychiatric disorders are affected even more adversely, as copayments are higher, total psychiatric hospital days are limited, and the ability to continue to work to provide income may be even more impaired.

To reduce risk related to out-of-pocket expenditures, 75% of older adults have some kind of private insurance to supplement Medicare. About 38% of older adults supplement Medicare with private insurance sponsored by employers. Employers continue to provide primary health insurance to older employees who work. When a person who is 65 or older retires, Medicare becomes his or her primary insurer and the former employer's policy becomes a secondary payer. This combination of insurances may be beneficial to the recipient, as the employer may continue to pay all or part of the supplemental insurance premium, and the benefit package is often more comprehensive than Medicare (Chulis et al. 1993).

The most common form of Medicare supplementary coverage is individually purchased "Medigap" insurance. Nearly 42% of older adults purchased these policies in 1991 (Chulis et al. 1993). As of July 30, 1992, the market for Medigap insurance was standardized. Federal regulations currently allow insurers to offer as many as 10 different supplemental policies. Each vendor must offer a basic policy that covers a core benefits package including coinsurance for Part A and coverage for 365 additional days after Medicare benefits are exhausted; Part B coinsurance, including payment for the full 50% copayment required for outpatient psychiatric services; and the first three pints of blood that may be required for transfusion each year. The other nine policies include these core benefits plus coverage for other services not covered by Medicare, including outpatient prescription drugs, preventive services, and some in-home and long-term care services at incrementally higher premiums. In 15 states thus far, insurers may also offer a Medigap plan that may require beneficiaries to receive their services through a preferred provider network in exchange for a lower premium and/or some reduction in copayments and deductibles (Grimaldi 1992).

TEFRA contains a provision that facilitates the use of health maintenance organizations (HMOs) by elderly Medicare recipients (Iglehart 1985). This policy allows qualified managed care programs to contract directly with Medicare. Each month Medicare pays the contractor a premium equal to 95% of the estimated per capita cost for Medicare services in the local market to provide the complete Medicare benefit to subscribers. The program allows HMOs to earn normal profit margins. However, cost savings above a predetermined rate must be used to provide extra services for elderly members. In regions with a high penetration of managed care, Medicare HMO products are marketed aggressively, often offering potential subscribers membership without incremental premium costs. Because marketing efforts generally focus on healthier segments of the geriatric population, costs of care are usually dramatically below premiums that are derived from utilization rates for the overall Medicare population, providing substantial operating margins for insurers. As a result, traditional indemnity Medicare in these regions continues to cover adversely selected, more chronically ill populations. The HCFA is currently reevaluating the entire Medicare HMO program to assess the effects of this phenomenon.

The market for long-term care insurance has exploded since the mid-1980s. This market has been poorly regulated, and prices and products vary remarkably. Policies frequently cover 2 to 3 years of institutionalization in a variety of facilities. Some also cover home care services. Many of these policies exclude patients with psychiatric disorders and patients with preexisting dementia. Premiums are often five times higher than those for Medigap policies, and deductibles and copayments can be substantial.

Conclusion

The economic and health care needs of older adults are extensive and diverse. Health and mental health policy for elderly individuals has been a patchwork that has left extraordinary gaps despite massive and growing expenditures. For nearly 30 years, Medicare policy has been the most important force in the organization and delivery of geriatric psychiatric services. Stigmatization and discrimination, reflected in exceptionally poor reimbursement of services and perverse incentives to employ expensive inpatient services, have reinforced existing barriers to care for this important and needy population.

Legislation has provided somewhat improved access to mental health services for older adults. Innovative cost containment methods may supply incentives to provide greater continuity of care. However, limited scrutiny of the quality of managed mental health care by policymakers may put some of the improvements in psychiatric care created by the growth of the field of geriatric psychiatry at substantial risk. The greatest challenges in this dynamic environment lie ahead. It is hoped that proactive policy development will facilitate the delivery of higher quality services to this population as it grows.

References

American Medical Association: Current Procedural Terminology, 4th Edition. Chicago, IL, American Medical Association, 1990

American Psychiatric Association, Office of Economic Affairs: The Coverage Catalog. Washington, DC, American Psychiatric Association, 1986, pp 403–420

Chulis GS, Eppig FP, Hogan MD, et al: Health insurance and the elderly. Health Affairs 12:111–118, 1993

Cutler J, Fine T: Federal health care financing of mental illness: a failure of public policy, in The New Economics of Psychiatric Care. Edited by Sharfstein SS, Beigel A. Washington, DC, American Psychiatric Press, 1985, pp 17–37

English JT, Sharfstein SS, Scherl DJ, et al: Diagnosis-related groups and general hospital psychiatry: the APA study. Am J Psychiatry 143:131–139, 1986

Fogel BS, Gottlieb GL, Furino A: Present and future solutions, in Mental Health Policy for Older Americans: Protecting Minds at Risk. Edited by Fogel BS, Furino A, Gottlieb GL. Washington, DC, American Psychiatric Press, 1990, pp 257–277

Frank RG, Lave JL: The psychiatric DRGs: are they different? Med Care 23:1148–1155, 1985

Frazier SH, Goldman H, Taube CA: Psychiatry, Medicare, and prospective payment (editorial). Am J Psychiatry 143:198–200, 1986

Freiman MP, Ellis RP, McGuire T: Provider response to Medicare's PPS: reductions in length of stay for psychiatric patients treated in scatter beds. Inquiry 26:192–201, 1989

Furino AF, Fogel BS: The economic perspective, in Mental Health Policy for Older Americans: Protecting Minds at Risk. Edited by Fogel BS, Furino A, Gottlieb GL. Washington, DC, American Psychiatric Press, 1990, pp 23–36

Goldman HH: Overview of studies on psychiatric hospital care under a prospective payment system, in Prospective Payment in Psychiatric Care. Edited by Scherl DJ, English JT, Sharfstein SS. Washington, DC, American Psychiatric Association, 1988, pp 81–89

Goldman HH, Frank RG: Division of responsibility among payors, in Mental Health Policy for Older Americans: Protecting Minds at Risk. Edited by Fogel BS, Furino A, Gottlieb GL. Washington, DC, American Psychiatric Press, 1990, pp 85–95

Goldman HH, Feder J, Scanlon W: Chronic mental patients in nursing homes: reexamining data from the National Nursing Home Study. Hosp Community Psychiatry 37:269–272, 1986

Goldman HH, Taube CA, Jencks SJ: The organization of the psychiatric inpatient services system. Med Care 25 (9 suppl):S6–S21, 1987

Gottlieb GL: Financial issues affecting geriatric psychiatric care, in Essentials of Geriatric Psychiatry. Edited by Lazarus L. New York, Springer, 1988, pp 230–248

Grimaldi P: Medigap insurance policies standardized. Nurs Manage 23:20–24, 1992

Grob GN: Mental Illness and American Society, 1875–1940. Princeton, NJ, Princeton University Press, 1983

Hazzard WR: Geriatric medicine: life in the crucible of the struggle to contain health care costs, in The Medical Cost Containment Crisis. Edited by McCue JD. Ann Arbor, MI, Health Administration Press, 1989, pp 263–264

Hsiao WC, Braun P, Dunn D, et al: Resource-based value scale. JAMA 260:2347–2353, 1988

Hsiao WC, Braun P, Dunn DL, et al: An overview of the development and refinement of the resource-based relative value scale: the foundation for reform of U.S. physician payment. Med Care 30:NS1–NS12, 1992

Iglehart JK: Health policy report: Medicare turns to HMOs. N Engl J Med 312:132–136, 1985

Iglehart JK: Health policy report: the American health care system. N Engl J Med 327:1467–1472, 1992

Letsch SW: National health care spending in 1991. Health Aff 12:94–110, 1993

Levit KR, Lazenby H, Waldo DR, et al: National health expenditures, 1984. Health Care Financ Rev 7:731–734, 1985

Long SH, Welch WP: Are we containing costs or pushing on a balloon? Health Aff 7:113–117, 1988

Markides KS, Mindel CH: Aging and Ethnicity. Newburg Park, CA, Sage, 1987, pp 31–35

National Center for Health Statistics: Health, United States, 1991 (DHHS Publ No [PHS] 92-1232). Washington, DC, U.S. Government Printing Office, 1992

Omnibus Budget Reconciliation Act of 1989 Reform: Annual Report to Congress. Washington, DC, U.S. Government Printing Office, 1989

Physician Payment Review Commission: Annual Report to Congress. Washington, DC, U.S. Government Printing Office, 1989, pp 7–28

Regier DA, Goldberg ID, Taube CA: The de facto U.S. mental health services system. Arch Gen Psychiatry 35:685–693, 1978

Scherl DJ, English JT, Sharfstein SS (eds): Preface, in Prospective Payment and Psychiatric Care. Washington, DC, American Psychiatric Association, 1988, pp xv–xxii

Schulz J: Economics of Aging, 4th Edition. Dover, MA, Auburn House Publications, 1988

Schurman RA, Kramer PD, Mitchell JB: The hidden mental health network. Arch Gen Psychiatry 42:89–94, 1985

Sharfstein SS: Payment for services: a provider's perspective, in Mental Health Policy for Older Americans: Protecting Minds at Risk. Edited by Fogel BS, Furino A, Gottlieb GL. Washington, DC, American Psychiatric Press, 1990, pp 97–107

Soldo BJ, Agree EM: America's elderly population. Population Bulletin 43(3):1–53, 1988

U.S. Bureau of the Census: An aging world. International Population Reports, Series P-95, No 78. Washington, DC, U.S. Government Printing Office, 1987

U.S. Senate Committee on Finance: Background material on health insurance. Washington, DC, U.S. Government Printing Office, 1978

Waldo DR, Lazenby HC: Demographic characteristics and health care use by the aged in the United States: 1977–1984. Health Care Financ Rev 6:1–29, 1984

Wells KB, Rogers WH, Davis CM, et al: Quality of care for hospitalized, depressed elderly patients before and after implementation of the Medicare prospective payment system. Am J Psychiatry 150:1799–1805, 1993

Self-Assessment:
Questions & Answers

Self-Assessment Questions

Chapter 1: Epidemiology of Psychiatric Disorders

Choose the one best response:

1. Among all noninstitutionalized persons in the United States ages 65 years or older, 1-month prevalence rates of depression, including major depression, dysthymia, cyclothymic disorder, atypical depression, *and* other depressive symptomatology of clinical interest, are

    a. <1%
    b. 1%–2%
    c. Somewhere between 3% and 10%
    d. Over 10%

2. Among all noninstitutionalized persons in the United States ages 65 years or older, 1-month prevalence rates of phobic disorders are

    a. <1%
    b. 1%–2%
    c. Somewhere between 3% and 10%
    d. Over 10%

3. Among all noninstitutionalized persons in the United States ages 65 years or older, 1-month prevalence rates of Alzheimer's disease are

    a. <1%
    b. 1%–2%
    c. Somewhere between 3% and 10%
    d. Over 10%

4. Among all noninstitutionalized persons in the United States ages 65 years or older, the relative 1-month prevalence rates of Alzheimer's disease and multi-infarct dementias are

    a. Higher for Alzheimer's disease
    b. Higher for multi-infarct disease
    c. More or less equal
    d. Variable

5. Among all residents of nursing homes in the United States ages 65 years or older, the relative 1-month prevalence rates of major depression are

    a. <1%
    b. 1%–2%
    c. Somewhere between 3% and 10%
    d. Over 10%

6. The Omnibus Budget Reconciliation Act of 1987 (OBRA 87) attempted sweeping changes in admission and retention criteria for residents in Medicare- or Medicaid-certified nursing homes. A likely result of OBRA 87 is that nursing homes will have

    a. More persons with schizophrenia
    b. More demand for intensive mental health care
    c. Little need for psychiatric treatment
    d. Fewer persons with solely physical disorders

7. In clinics delivering primary medical care, psychiatric problems of patients 65 years of age or older include >10% point prevalence rates of

    a. Major depression
    b. Other types of depressive disorders
    c. Excess alcohol consumption
    d. Schizophrenia

8. Lifetime risk of developing Alzheimer's disease or a related dementia for men who survive to 85 years of age is

    a. <15%
    b. Between 15% and 19%
    c. Between 20% and 30%
    d. >30%

9. Onset of schizophrenia occurs after age 45

   a. Very rarely (<5% of all cases)
   b. Quite often (6%–30% of all cases)
   c. As often as an earlier onset (~50% of all cases)
   d. Never, by definition

10. The later in life that a first episode of schizophrenia occurs, the more likely it is to

    a. Have an unfavorable untreated outcome
    b. Have distinctive brain abnormalities on neuroimaging
    c. Occur in a male
    d. Be resistant to treatment

11. Where cognitive impairment sufficient for a diagnosis of dementia occurs together with the symptoms of major depression, the outcome is likely to be

    a. Typical of major depression in >90% of cases
    b. Typical of a progressive dementia in >90% of cases
    c. Usually a mild form of dementia
    d. Often (20%–60%) resembling major depression initially and later typical of dementia

12. Rates of Alzheimer's disease type of dementia are reported as being relatively low in the following group:

    a. Chinese
    b. Italians
    c. Illiterate
    d. African Americans

13. Recently bereaved widows are more likely to have clinically significant depression lasting longer than a year in all the following situations *except* where they

    a. Had symptoms of depression in the months prior to bereavement
    b. Have a physical illness of their own
    c. Have minor feelings of guilt and worthlessness
    d. Have close relatives and friends

14. The strongest of the following predictors of major depression in persons 65 years or older is

    a. Deterioration in physical health
    b. Lack of a confidant or other close friend
    c. Being female
    d. Advanced age (80 years or older)

Chapter 2: Genetics of Geriatric Psychopathology

Choose the one best response:

1. All of the following characterize the polymerase chain reaction (PCR) *except*

    a. A technique in which a specific DNA sequence can be amplified several millionfold in a few hours
    b. A technique with wide applicability to the diagnosis of human diseases
    c. A technique that allows the separation of DNA on the basis of size
    d. A revolutionary technique used in DNA studies for which Kary Mullis won the 1993 Nobel Prize in Chemistry
    e. A technique that can be used on frozen or fixed postmortem specimens to study DNA

2. Which of the following factors has *not* been implicated in Alzheimer's disease?

    a. Autosomal dominant inheritance
    b. CAG trinucleotide repeats
    c. ApoE-e4 allele
    d. Tau protein
    e. β-amyloid protein

3. Patients with Down's syndrome who live beyond age 35 have been found at autopsy to exhibit the characteristic neuropathologic lesions of the following disorder:

    a. Huntington's disease
    b. Amyotrophic lateral sclerosis

   c. Alzheimer's disease
   d. Creutzfeldt-Jakob disease
   e. Schizophrenia

4. In 1993, researchers successfully cloned and sequenced the gene responsible for

   a. Alzheimer disease
   b. Schizophrenia
   c. Huntington's disease
   d. Pick's disease
   e. Parkinson's disease

5. The following have all been identified as possible risk factors for late-onset Alzheimer disease *except*

   a. Age
   b. ApoE-e4 allele
   c. Linkage to chromosome 19 markers
   d. Positive family history of dementia
   e. Amyloid precursor protein mutations

6. Autosomal recessive mode of inheritance underlies all of the following diseases *except*

   a. Wilson's disease
   b. Huntington's disease
   c. Phenylketonuria
   d. Von Gierke's disease
   e. Hurler's disease

7. Gene mutations responsible for the transmissible dementias of Creutzfeldt-Jakob and Gerstmann-Straussler-Scheinker diseases have been identified in the PRNP gene located on chromosome

   a. 20
   b. 11
   c. 21
   d. 4
   e. 14

8. Family and twin studies have indicated a role for genetic factors in

     a.   Schizophrenia
     b.   Bipolar disorder
     c.   Alcoholism
     d.   None of the above
     e.   All of the above

9. Family studies of schizophrenia indicate that the risk for family members is

     a.   Higher in late-onset than early-onset families
     b.   Higher in late-onset families than in the general population
     c.   Lower in late-onset families than in the general population
     d.   The same in late-onset families as in the general population
     e.   None of the above

Questions 10–14: Match the following genetic findings with their specific disease(s):
     a.   Valine to isoleucine amino acid substitution, codon 717
     b.   CAG trinucleotide repeats
     c.   Glutamic acid to lysine amino acid substitution, codon 200
     d.   ApoE-e4 allele
     e.   Trisomy 21

10. Creutzfeldt-Jakob disease
11. Early-onset familial Alzheimer's disease
12. Huntington's disease
13. Late-onset Alzheimer's disease
14. Down's syndrome

Chapter 3:   Biology of Aging

For questions 1–4

Answer   a.   if 1, 2, and 3 are correct
               b.   if 1 and 3 are correct
               c.   if 2 and 4 are correct
               d.   if only 4 is correct
               e.   if all are correct

1. In biological senescence, there is a quantitative loss of cells as well as changes in many of the enzymatic activities within cells. Which of the following statements are true?

    1. Most enzymatic syntheses continue, although some rates of production and clearance may decline.
    2. There may be diminution in receptor number or affinity for transmitters.
    3. The aging individual may be unable to respond to the demands for increased activity.
    4. Of the organ systems, the normal kidney, lung, and skin age much more rapidly than the heart and liver.

2. Changes in the heart and resiliency of blood vessel walls have been thought to be the major determinants of decreased exercise tolerance leading to loss of conditioning. Which of the following statements about age-related changes in exercise capacity are true?

    1. Loss of energy reserve depends on interactions between the musculoskeletal and the cardiovascular systems.
    2. Changes in the vascular system are major factors contributing to feelings of agedness and overall decline in physical strength.
    3. Loss of energy depends on activity level and lifestyle.
    4. Loss of exercise tolerance is minimally dependent on pulmonary aging.

3. Regular physical activity is associated with higher levels of plasma epinephrine and norepinephrine. The following statements about adrenergic transmitters are true:

    1. Institutionalized elderly people show increased activity tolerance with vigorous conditioning programs.
    2. The highest levels of norepinephrine are seen in fit old women.
    3. Aged organisms are capable of making homeostatic adjustments even in the absence of physiological stressors such as exercise.
    4. Regular exercise acts to activate resting sympathetic nervous system tone.

4. Degenerative joint disease is the most common and debilitating disease of elderly people. It is responsible for limiting the enjoyment of recreation and interfering with activities of daily living as well as re-

stricting job-related functions. Which of the following clinical issues are frequent problems for the practitioner?

1. There is no difference in delay patterns between younger and older patients with similar complaints.
2. Joint and muscle aches and stiffness characteristic of the arthritides are frequently ascribed to getting old and the attribution of symptoms to "getting old" delay the seeking of health care.
3. These symptoms lead to use of both prescription and nonprescription analgesics, which are generally safe with few adverse side effects.
4. Analgesics can have psychotropic side-effects such as depression.

Choose the one best response:

5. Most ingested drugs as well as metabolites that are absorbed from the small intestine and stomach pass through the liver. They are either unchanged or undergo metabolic detoxification by microsomal enzymes.

    a. Aging causes no changes in the rate of Phase I type hepatic microsomal enzyme synthesis.
    b. There are losses in cellular microsomal enzyme activity, primarily CYP2D6 and CYP1A2 isoenzymes of cytochrome P450.
    c. There is a decrease in blood flow.
    d. Most psychotropic drugs undergo single-pass glucuronidation in the liver and are then excreted through the kidneys.

6. Changes in thyroid physiology occur with advancing age, but

    a. An euthyroid status is maintained.
    b. There are *no* age-related changes in circulating hormone levels.
    c. There is diminished availability of T_4 in peripheral tissues and decreased T_4 disposal rate.
    d. Basal thyroid-stimulating hormone (TSH) secretion increases in persons over 60 years of age while maintaining the euthyroid state except in very old men.

7. All of the following statements about age-related sensory changes is false *except*

    a. Visual acuity is significantly related to loss of the ability to accommodate.
    b. Loss of high tone perceptions and the ability to discriminate words are classic symptoms of presbycusis.

   c.   There are no gender differences in hearing loss patterns across the life span in current cohorts over the age of 65.

   d.   Retinal degeneration is a common sign of normal aging in the eye.

8. Impaired glucose tolerance

   a.   Is a common presentation of mild diabetes mellitus in elderly people

   b.   Is related to altered peripheral responsiveness to insulin

   c.   May be related to chlorpromazine use

   d.   Reflects impaired insulin synthesis in elderly people

9. Organs age at different rates; some remain minimally affected across the life span, whereas others show dramatic structural and functional declines. Which of the following statements about the kidney is true?

   a.   Glomerular filtration rate declines by 40%–50% across the life span.

   b.   The kidney does not lose the ability to compensate for abnormalities of acid, base, electrolyte, and free water clearance.

   c.   There is no reduction in the capacity to conserve sodium along with a decline in levels of vasopressin leading to water retention.

   d.   The decline in renal function has serious implications for the dosing of drugs such as lithium and buspirone.

10. Synaptic markers in the nucleus basalis of Meynert are interesting to study in individuals without dementia or chronic illness because

   a.   The nucleus has few radiations to cortical and subcortical targets

   b.   This area is linked to memory impairments in patients with dementia

   c.   Significant declines in dopamine, serotonin (5-HT) and metabolites, 5-hydroxyindoleacetic acid, 5-HT binding, choline acetyltransferase and acetylcholinesterase activities, and dopamine turnover are noted before the age of 40

   d.   There are long projections of the ventral tegmental and substantia nigra dopamine cell groups to neostriatal and limbic targets

11. Women enjoy greater longevity because of the gender specific advantages of

   a.   Reversal of osteoporotic bone loss by use of estrogens, progesterone, calcium supplementation of the diet, and fluoride ingestion

   b.   Premenopausal protection from coronary artery disease and stroke

    c. Better utilization of informal and formal health resources

    d. Decreased vulnerability to diabetes mellitus because of high pre-menopausal levels of estrogen and insulin

12. Aerobic exercise in elderly persons

    a. Is of questionable utility because they are prone to fracture and have a high incidence of degenerative joint disease

    b. Is effective in improving conditioning as measured by increased VO_2, and anaerobic threshold

    c. Can lead to lower levels of total and low-density lipoprotein cholesterol and elevations in high-density lipoprotein levels

    d. Is as effective as weight-bearing exercise on bone maintenance

Chapter 4:   Normal Aging: Changes in Sensory/ Perceptual and Cognitive Abilities

Choose the one best response:

1. Spar and La Rue (1990) have concluded that the following cognitive functions remain preserved in older adults:

    a. Intellectual ability, wisdom, and creativity

    b. Attention, concentration, overlearned skills, and crystallized learning

    c. Everyday communication skills; lexical, phonological, and syntaxic processing; discourse comprehension; attention; and simple visual perception

    d. There is no preservation of cognitive function

2. A cohort effect may be responsible for

    a. Difficulties interpreting studies in intelligence because of specific characteristics of the sample

    b. The finding that the five senses decrease in older adults as a function of decreased acuity of receptor cells

    c. Differences between woman and men in terms of their threshold perception

    d. A major confound in studies of aging

3. The literature on global intellectual function indicates that

   a. All cognitive abilities diminish after age 30
   b. Crystallized intelligence diminishes before age 50 and sometimes in the 30s and 40s
   c. Most people plateau in their 50s and 60s and begin a slow but increasingly rapid decline in their late 70s
   d. People are so variable that a global determination is not currently possible

4. Which of the following is true?

   a. "You can't teach an old dog new tricks."
   b. Fluid intelligence diminishes before crystallized intelligence.
   c. Dementia is a normal consequence of aging.
   d. Cognitive decline in older adults is not as extensive as once thought.

5. Reserve capacity has been used to explain why

   a. The variability in cognitive skills increases with age
   b. Studies of autonomic responsivity have found response inhibition among older men
   c. Younger people have more reserves than do older individuals
   d. None of the above

6. Which type of memory is the most sensitive to aging?

   a. Primary memory
   b. Secondary memory
   c. Remote memory
   d. Tertiary memory

7. What percentage of persons over age 65 will have at least one chronic disease?

   a. 50%
   b. 60%
   c. 65%
   d. 80%

8. Functional abilities in the normal elderly person are

    a.   Impaired for their instrumental activities of daily living by age 70, but their ability to perform their activities of daily living is not impaired

    b.   Are not particularly important to evaluate

    c.   Typically not impaired, although the speed of performance declines

    d.   Impaired as a result of age-related changes in cognitive abilities

9. With regard to cultural issues in assessment:

    a.   There are inadequate normative databases for the older adult.

    b.   A number of tests given to older adults are culturally biased.

    c.   Neither a and b are true.

    d.   Both a and b are true.

10. The relationship between normal aging and creativity

    a.   Suggests increasing creativity with age

    b.   Shows no relationship between creativity and age

    c.   Needs to be determined by further well-designed studies

    d.   Has not been studied

Chapter 5:   Sociodemographic Aspects

Choose the one best response:

1. When examining the older population in the United States, one can say that

    a.   It is growing older but doing so at a decelerating rate

    b.   The United States leads the industrialized world in life expectancy at birth in 1990

    c.   On the whole, women live longer than men

    d.   The median age increased in mid-century and is now decreasing

2. With regard to retirement and work it is true that

    a.   There is a decreasing acceptance of retirement as a desired social status

b. Labor force and retirement patterns have been similar for men and women
c. Among the professions, job satisfaction decreases after mid-career, encouraging early retirement
d. Most workers retire when they feel that they can afford to do so
e. There has been a trend away from early retirement toward later retirement since World War II

3. Concerning the economic status of elderly people, which statement is not true?

a. Persons ages 65 and older tend to have lower incomes than those under 65.
b. The median family income is about one-third more for elderly people than for younger adults as a whole.
c. A high proportion of older persons feel that their income is adequate even when objectively it is low.
d. Case income is less in old age but in-kind income is more.
e. The income disparity between whites, blacks, and Hispanics carries over into old age.

4. It is a fact that

a. Older men and women are similarly distributed among types of living arrangements
b. Most older women live in family settings
c. Nearly half of all men over 65 in 1990 were widowers
d. Over three-fourths of older men live alone
e. There is a long-term trend away from intergenerational living arrangements among elderly people

5. In terms of their geographical distribution and mobility, it is true that

a. Today's older adults tend to remain where they have spent most of their adult lives
b. About 10% of all persons over 60 will move in any 5-year period
c. The suburbs are not aging because retirees tend to move from suburbs to small towns
d. Of the older persons who moved across state lines, half of them go to only 10 states
e. Most long-distance moves among elderly people are motivated by health problems

6. Disease of the heart, cerebrovascular disease, and atherosclerosis together account for what proportion of all deaths in the United States
among those 85 years and older?

    a.   One-fourth
    b.   One-half
    c.   Two-thirds
    d.   Three-fourths
    e.   The total

7. Recent evidence suggests that the disability rate among the elderly in
the United States is _____, and the absolute number of
disabled elders is _____.

    a.   Increasing; increasing
    b.   Decreasing; decreasing
    c.   Increasing; decreasing
    d.   Decreasing, increasing
    e.   Holding steady; holding steady

8. Self-assessed health status is a _____ predictor of mortality among elderly people.

    a.   Strong
    b.   Weak
    c.   Ambiguous
    d.   Vacillating
    e.   Soft

9. Which of the following statements regarding the social environment
and the health of older adults is true?

    a.   Low levels of social contact are associated with higher mortality
         because of cardiovascular diseases but lower mortality because of
         cancer.
    b.   Low levels of social contact are not independently associated with
         mortality, regardless of cause.
    c.   Low levels of social contact are associated with higher mortality
         as a result of all causes.
    d.   Low levels of social contact are highly associated with disability
         but not with mortality.
    e.   Low levels of social contact are associated with lower mortality as
         a result of stress-related causes.

10. Most older Americans perceive their physical health to be

   a. Abominable
   b. Very poor
   c. Poor
   d. Fair
   e. Good to excellent

Chapter 6: Self and Experience Across the Second Half of Life

Choose the one best response:

1. Although aging is sometimes understood simply in terms of chronological age, it might be best to understand aging as

   a. Changing biological capacity
   b. Changing ability to maintain adaptation to the environment
   c. Changing place within the socially defined life course
   d. All of the above

2. When it occurs in late life rather than middle adulthood, role losses such as widowhood or retirement

   a. Have a more adverse impact on health and morale because they are likely to be accompanied by other losses
   b. Have a less adverse impact on health and morale because they are anticipated and shared
   c. Have a more negative impact on physical health and morale because age peers are facing losses of their own
   d. Have neither greater or less negative impact on physical health and morale

3. For men, changes in middle adulthood include

   a. Increased concern with personal mortality
   b. A more outward-focused psychological orientation
   c. Reduction in actual social ties
   d. Lessened concern with self

4. In later life, reminiscence provides

    a.   Comfort and solace
    b.   The means to come to terms with one's own life
    c.   A sense of personal coherence
    d.   All of the above

5. Role strain that results from family members' need for care and support may be greatest among

    a.   Young adult women
    b.   Middle-aged women
    c.   Middle-aged men
    d.   Late adult women

6. In later life, health problems

    a.   May be minimal, but subjective health decreases
    b.   Increase, and subjective health decreases
    c.   May increase, but subjective health remains positive
    d.   None of the above

7. Wisdom may be a matter of

    a.   Acquiring procedural knowledge about living
    b.   Acquiring factual knowledge about living
    c.   Preserving fluid intelligence
    d.   None of the above

8. In later life, artistic activities

    a.   May provide a medium for life review
    b.   Tend to produce less creative works because of cognitive losses
    c.   Are usually preferable to less visible forms of meaning creation
    d.   All of the above

9. The understanding of later life has been limited by its dependence on the study of a particular historical cohort because

    a.   The lives of the members of a cohort were affected by a unique set of macro-historical events
    b.   Levels of education have changed

   c. Health practices and levels of nutrition have changed
   d. All of the above

10. In relying on others for support, older family members especially prefer

   a. Own offspring
   b. Formal community services
   c. A few confidants
   d. All of the above

Chapter 7:   Ethnocultural Aspects

Choose the one best response:

1. What factors are linked to misdiagnosis in the culturally different?

   a. Language barriers
   b. Different idioms or concepts of illness
   c. Lower socioeconomic status and education
   d. Ethnocentric bias of diagnosticians
   e. None of the above
   f. All of the above

2. In judging the potential scope of problems, the 1990 census found what approximate percentage of the total United States elderly population (over age 65) was a racial minority (African American, Asian American, or Hispanic American)?

   a. 7%
   b. 14%
   c. 21%
   d. 28%

Matching set. Choose the correct lettered answer for each of questions 3–5 (each answer can only be used once).

A common stereotype is that racial groups have different dosing requirements for psychotropic medications. Pharmacokinetic differences seem to explain many differences.

    a.   Asian Americans
    b.   African Americans
    c.   Hispanic Americans
    d.   Whites

3. Lithium tends to be effective at lower blood levels.
4. The frequency of poor metabolizer variants of cytochrome P450 IID6 is higher than other racial groups.
5. Poor metabolizers of mephenytoin hydroxylase may exceed 20%.

Choose the one best response:

6. Suicide rates for African American and Hispanic American elderly are

    a.   Double that of whites
    b.   Only higher for men
    c.   Only higher for women
    d.   Lower than that of whites

7. In testing for dementia, areas that seem most vulnerable to language and cultural effects are

    a.   Digit span
    b.   Orientation
    c.   Verbal comprehension and verbal fluency
    d.   a and c
    e.   a, b, and c

Chapter 8:   Comprehensive Psychiatric Evaluation

Choose the one best response:

1. All of the following statements regarding cognitive assessment are true *except*

    a.   The pattern of cognitive dysfunction can reveal clues about the etiology of the illness.
    b.   A single "cross-sectional" examination of cognitive function can determine the course and prognosis of the illness.

    c. Assessment of the quantity and pattern of cognitive dysfunction is essential to determine how much care or supervision a patient requires.

    d. The cognitive assessment can help the clinician decide if a more detailed neuropsychological assessment is required.

2. All of the following statements regarding the cognitive assessment are true *except*

    a. The cognitive assessment should always be left until the end of the comprehensive psychiatric examination.

    b. The cognitive assessment should be carefully documented, including noting the quality of the errors.

    c. The cognitive assessment should be introduced appropriately in a nonthreatening manner.

    d. Specific tests should be chosen that take into account the characteristics of the particular age cohort.

3. All of the following are examples of communication problems *except*

    a. Anomia
    b. Aprosodia
    c. Paraphasias
    d. Dysarthria
    e. Apraxia

4. Frontal systems tasks

    a. Are rarely impaired in extrapyramidal disorders
    b. Do not involve higher-order functions such as abstraction and insight
    c. Can elicit signs of perseveration
    d. Include having the patient copy a series of multiple loops to elicit concrete thinking

5. All of the following statements about standardized assessment instruments are true *except*

    a. Certain rating scales can be used to solve specific clinical problems.

    b. Rating scales should be avoided when communicating with colleagues because of their poor reliability.

c. Standardized assessments are helpful for documenting treatment response.
d. Standardized assessments can be used for teaching purposes.

6. On the mental status exam, an elderly person looking vacantly into space, dressed in ill-fitting, stained clothes, with buttons missing and smelling of urine, suggests the presence of a(n)

a. Affective disorder
b. Anxiety disorder
c. Cognitive disorder
d. Paranoid disorder

7. Which of the following statements is true about the Geriatric Mental Status Examination?

a. The Mental Status Examination is best completed at the end of the psychiatric interview.
b. The examination begins as soon as the clinician meets the patient in the waiting room.
c. Depressed geriatric patients seldom require a careful review of suicide ideation and intent.
d. The best test of judgment is to ask the patient what he or she would do if he or she saw a fire in a theater.

8. Which of the following is true about an assessment for competence?

a. Competence is best viewed as a task-specific assessment.
b. Geriatric psychiatrists are seldom required to assess a patient's capacity to make decisions.
c. If a patient is competent to give consent for treatment, then he or she is competent to change a will.
d. Patients with delusions are always incompetent to give consent for treatment.

9. All of the following is true about an interview with the informant *except*

a. The quality of the informant's relationship with the patient some-times interferes with obtaining an accurate history.
b. Most geriatric psychiatry assessments require taking a history of the patient's problems from a significant other.

c. If the informant is the caregiver, it is important to inquire about caregiver burden.
d. The interview with the informant is usually unnecessary when the patient has a dementia.

10. The following are true about history taking in geriatric psychiatry patients *except*

a. The purpose of the history of presenting illness is to document the events and arrange them in the order in which they happened.
b. Knowledge of the patient's past almost always sheds light on the vulnerabilities and strengths of each patient.
c. A sexual history is seldom necessary in geriatric history taking.
d. An inquiry into a patient's activities, religious affiliation, and hobbies is useful in assessing each individual's social vulnerabilities and strengths.

Chapter 9: Medical Evaluation and Common Medical Problems

Choose the one best response:

1. A 70-year-old woman is being treated in your clinic for depression. During a routine visit she reports that her arthritis has been bothering her and she has doubled her prescribed dose of a nonsteroidal anti-inflammatory drug (NSAID) without consulting a physician. You express to her your concern over this action. In explaining features of NSAID therapy to her, all of the following are true *except*

a. There is risk of severe gastric mucosal injury with NSAIDs.
b. Older women are at increased risk of major gastrointestinal complications of NSAIDs.
c. Alternative analgesics such as acetaminophen have been demonstrated to be ineffective in the treatment of osteoarthritis.
d. There is risk of renal insufficiency with NSAIDs.
e. Patients who develop major gastric complications from NSAIDs may be asymptomatic on these drugs before the complication.

2. The following statements regarding vitamin B_{12} deficiency are true
except

a. The anemia of B_{12} deficiency is usually macrocytic.
b. Neurological changes of B_{12} deficiency can occur before hemato-
    logic changes.
c. Patients with B_{12} deficiency generally can be treated with a
    3-month course of intramuscular B_{12} injections.
d. The most frequent cause of B_{12} deficiency in elderly people is per-
    nicious anemia.

3. Match the following conditions to the statements below:

a. Apathic hyperthyroidism
b. Euthyroid sick syndrome
c. Hypothyroidism
d. Myxedema coma
e. Subclinical hypothyroidism

1. Elevated thyroid-stimulating hormone with normal T_4 and FTI
2. Characterized by anorexia, fatigue, weight loss, and general de-
    cline with laboratory evidence of hyperthyroidism
3. Definitive treatment in older patients is usually accomplished with
    radioactive iodine therapy
4. Medical emergency requiring intravenous L-thyroxine therapy

4. A 72-year-old man returns to your office after 1 week of treatment
with a tricyclic antidepressant. He reports bladder fullness and involuntary loss of urine. You do not have supplies to perform straight
catheterization. You should

a. Stop the tricyclic antidepressant
b. Add bethanechol
c. Order a urinalysis
d. Make no changes because this is a common and minor complica-
    tion of tricyclic antidepressants

5. During routine screening for potentially reversible causes of dementia in a 75-year-old woman, you find the patient has positive venereal
disease research laboratory (VDRL) testing. The following statements
are true *except*

a. VDRL is a nonspecific reagin antibody test with a high false-positive rate.

b. In one-third of patients with latent or tertiary syphilis, the VDRL titer can spontaneously decline over time.

c. VDRL will usually remain positive after successful treatment of syphilis.

d. General paresis is a form of neurosyphilis characterized by progressive dementia, alterations in speech, and generalized weakness with hyperreflexia.

e. Penicillin is the treatment of choice for all stages of syphilis.

6. You are considering electroconvulsive therapy (ECT) for a 75-year-old man with depression. You know ECT is an effective treatment in older patients. The patient is concerned about rumors he has heard regarding ECT. In explaining the risks of ECT to him, which of the following statements would be correct?

a. Contraindications to ECT therapy include brain tumor.

b. Pretreatment with atropine prevents post-ECT tachycardia.

c. Pacemaker patients cannot receive ECT therapy.

d. Cardiac events are the major cause of mortality reported from ECT.

7. You wish to choose an antidepressant medication for an 80-year-old woman with osteoporosis and a history of vertebral compression fractures. The best predictor of postural hypotension occurring with antidepressant therapy is

a. A history of hypertension

b. Preexisting orthostatic hypotension

c. A history of vertebral compression fractures

d. An abnormal electrocardiogram

8. Many psychoactive medications have anticholinergic effects. Typical anticholinergic effects include all of the following *except*

a. Urinary retention

b. Confusion

c. Increased salivation

d. Constipation

e. Tachycardia

9. In an elderly patient with a history of cardiac disease you obtain an electrocardiogram before instituting treatment for depression. Changes in the electrocardiogram that warrant caution before instituting tricyclic antidepressant therapy include all of the following *except*

   a. Bifascicular block
   b. Second-degree heart block
   c. First-degree AV block
   d. QT prolongation

Chapter 10:   The Neurological Evaluation

Choose the one best response:

1. The following statement best characterizes cerebrovascular disease in elderly people:

   a. Transient monocular blindness (amaurosis fugax) represents a vertebrobasilar circulation transient ischemic attack.
   b. Hypertensive hemorrhage is more common in the putamen than in the cerebral cortex.
   c. Nausea and vomiting are rare in subarrachnoid hemorrhage.
   d. Minor head trauma is an unlikely cause of subdural hematoma in elderly patients.

2. Features of Parkinson's disease include

   a. Bradykinesia, myoclonus, and ataxia
   b. Characteristic loss of noradrenergic neurons in the locus ceruleus
   c. Age-associated increase in prevalence, rising rapidly with each decade after age 40
   d. Behavioral disorders such as depression or dementia in less than half of cases

3. Neurological changes associated with normal aging include all of the following *except*

   a. Loss of ankle jerks
   b. Spontaneous buccolingual dyskinesias
   c. Dysmetria on finger-to-nose testing
   d. Impaired lateral gaze

4. The following clinical feature helps distinguish motor systems dysfunction of different etiologies:

   a. Neuroleptic-induced parkinsonism is associated with more resting tremor than idiopathic Parkinson's disease.
   b. Psychomotor retardation in depression usually produces less rigidity than idiopathic Parkinson's disease.
   c. Neuroleptic-induced akathisia usually produces less shifting from foot to foot than psychogenic hyperactivity.
   d. Progressive supranuclear palsy frequently exhibits both rigidity and ophthalmoplegia.

5. Which of the following statements is correct?

   a. Unilateral resting tremor is seen in idiopathic Parkinson's disease.
   b. Brain tumors usually produce papilledema in elderly subjects.
   c. Gait disorders effect <5% of elderly people.
   d. Unilateral temporal lobe pathology usually produces bilateral anosmia.
   e. Alcoholic cerebellar degeneration produces more appendicular than truncal ataxia.

6. Frontal release signs

   a. Reveal frontal lobe pathology
   b. Are common in healthy older people
   c. Include patellar hyperreflexia
   d. Do not occur with frontal lobe pathology
   e. Can distinguish basal ganglia from frontal lobe pathology

Chapter 11:   Neuropsychological Testing

Choose the one best response:

1. Patients' learning ability can be assessed in the course of interviewing by

   a. Asking them how they would find their way to a familiar location
   b. Observing whether they keep their mind on the conversation
   c. Asking them to interpret a common proverb

d. Asking them to describe their favorite recipe
e. Discussing current events

2. The most commonly used mental status screening tests all assess

a. Conceptualization
b. Figure copying
c. Naming
d. Verbal fluency
e. Memory

3. Persons with low educational achievement who are administered a mental status screening test

a. Can perform below cutoffs for impairment even when they have not declined in cognitive ability
b. Are rarely identified as being impaired when they are not
c. Are as frequently misidentified as showing impairment as well-educated persons
d. Are likely to refuse some of the items
e. Are less likely to fail than well-educated persons

4. A dementing disease that is known for its rapid rate of progression is

a. Alzheimer's disease
b. Pick's disease
c. Creutzfeldt-Jakob disease
d. Progressive supranuclear palsy
e. Binswanger's disease

5. A dementing disease that has been associated with early evidence of personality change is

a. Pick's disease
b. Alzheimer's disease
c. Wilson's disease
d. Etat lacunaire
e. Normal pressure hydrocephalus

6. In most cases, fewer cognitive tasks can be performed well if there is an impairment in

   a. Memory
   b. Spatial ability
   c. Conceptualization
   d. Attention
   e. Language

7. The language dimension that is most commonly assessed when dementia is suspected is

   a. Comprehension
   b. Repetition
   c. Reading
   d. Writing
   e. Naming

8. The most important thing to include in the assessment of memory for the differential diagnosis of dementia is

   a. Immediate recall
   b. The difference between immediate and delayed recall
   c. Remote memory
   d. Procedural memory
   e. None of the above

9. The examination of conceptualization includes tasks that evaluate

   a. Concept formation
   b. Set shifting
   c. Abstraction
   d. Set maintenance
   e. All of the above

10. If patients have difficulty learning new information, then

    a. They will, in most cases, have difficulty remembering things from the remote past
    b. They will, in most cases, have lost the ability to carry out well-learned skills

    c.   They can still have the ability to carry out well-learned skills

    d.   They will, in most cases, have attentional deficits

    e.   They will, in most cases, have language deficits

11. Neuropsychological testing can assist in

    a.   The initial diagnosis of a patient

    b.   The development of a treatment plan

    c.   Assessing change in function over time

    d.   Measuring response to treatment

    e.   All of the above

Chapter 12:   Neuroimaging

Choose the one best response:

1. Which of the following is a structural imaging technique?

    a.   Positron-emission tomography (PET)

    b.   Single-photon emission computer tomography

    c.   Magnetic resonance imaging (MRI)

    d.   Computerized electroencephalography (CEEG)

2. The imaging technique that has the best spatial resolution is

    a.   MRI

    b.   PET

    c.   SPECT

    d.   CEEG

3. The most widely accessible type of scan is

    a.   PET

    b.   CEEG

    c.   CT

    d.   MRI

4. The best MRI image type for detecting white-matter pathology is

    a. T1-weighted
    b. T2-weighted
    c. MR spectroscopy
    d. Inversion recovery

5. Advantages of PET over SPECT include all of the following *except*

    a. PET is quantitative
    b. PET is more widely accessible
    c. PET can image a wider variety of physiological processes
    d. PET has better spatial resolution

6. PET and SPECT findings in multi-infarct dementia include

    a. Isolated frontal lobe hypermetabolism/blood flow
    b. Bilateral parietal lobe hypermetabolism/blood flow
    c. Flow or metabolism reductions in the infarcted areas
    d. Interictal hypometabolism with ictal increase

7. Commonly reported types of white-matter lesions on MRI include all of the following *except*

    a. Periventricular hyperintensity
    b. Discrete deep white matter focal hyperintensity
    c. Focal decreases in intensity on T2-weighted images
    d. Confluent patches of increased signal in the deep white matter

8. Common dementing disorders diagnosable by neuroimaging include those caused by

    a. Folate deficiency
    b. Brain tumors
    c. Drug intoxication
    d. Subdural hematoma

For questions 9 and 10, match the best lettered item. Each lettered item can be used once, more than once, or not at all.

    a.   Bilateral parietal lobe decrease in metabolism (hypometabolism)
    b.   Caudate hypometabolism
    c.   Frontal lobe atrophy and localized frontal hypometabolism
    d.   Interictal hypometabolism

  9. Huntington's disease
10. Pick's disease

Answer   a.   if only 1 and 3 are correct
                 b.   if only 2 and 4 are correct
                 c.   if only 1, 2, and 3 are correct
                 d.   if only 4 is correct

11. Reasons why functional imaging might be better than structural imaging in psychiatric disorders include

    1.   Functional tissue disturbances occur earlier than structural disturbances.
    2.   Most psychiatric disorders do not have obvious associated structural abnormalities.
    3.   The pathophysiology of major psychiatric disorders includes physiological dysfunctions amenable to functional neuroimaging.
    4.   Functional neuroimaging is so much less expensive than structural imaging that it is a cost-effective screening tool.

Chapter 13:   Electroencephalography

Choose the one best response:

 1. The EEG in elderly people

    a.   Does not differ at all from that of young adults
    b.   May be used to diagnose dementia
    c.   May be used to rule out seizures
    d.   May normally show temporal slow waves
    e.   Should be routinely performed in depressed patients

2. Common "normal" findings in the EEG of elderly people include

    a. A posterior dominant rhythm of <10 Hz
    b. Isolated temporal slow waves
    c. Spike-and-wave foci
    d. All of the above
    e. a and b only

3. In the evaluation of confusion, an EEG should be performed

    a. Only when delirium is suspected
    b. Whenever there are focal neurological signs
    c. To document the presence of a secondary mental disorder
    d. Only to rule out possible seizures
    e. Even when the diagnosis of dementia is clear

4. A normal EEG in an elderly patient

    a. Is inconsistent with the presence of dementia
    b. Rules out the presence of an encephalopathy
    c. Is seen rarely after the age of 90
    d. Is frequently of lower voltage than that in a young adult
    e. Usually lacks an alpha rhythm

5. The EEG in delirious patients

    a. Is almost invariably abnormal
    b. Often shows slowing that is proportional to the level of confusion
    c. May appear similar to that of a patient with dementia
    d. All of the above
    e. b and c only

6. Normal EEGs may be seen in

    a. Dementia
    b. Delirium
    c. Aging
    d. Seizure disorders
    e. All of the above

For questions 7–10 choose the correct lettered response (answers may be used more than once or not at all).

    a. Repeated loss of consciousness with generalized tonic-clonic movements

    b. Spike-and-wave complexes in the EEG

    c. Frontally predominant intermittent rhythmic delta activity

    d. Occipital spikes

    e. Focal slowing

    f. Posterior dominant rhythm of <10 Hz

    g. Psychomotor variant

    h. Bancaud's phenomenon

7. Which is the most common EEG abnormality seen following stroke?

8. What is the single most reliable indicator of a seizure disorder?

9. What finding most reliably distinguishes between the EEGs of normal older and young adults?

10. Which is the most common EEG abnormality in multi-infarct dementia?

Chapter 14:   Alzheimer's Disease

Choose the one best response:

1. At which level of incapacity are patients with Alzheimer's disease most likely to achieve scores above zero on the Mini-Mental State Exam (MMSE)?

    a. Unable to sit up without assistance

    b. Unable to speak

    c. Unable to toilet without assistance

    d. Unable to dress without assistance

    e. Unable to smile

2. Which of the following reflexes are frequently observed in an immobile Alzheimer's disease patient?

    a. Babinski reflex

    b. Sucking reflex

    c. Grasp reflex

    d. All of the above

    e. None of the above

3. Agitation, including violence, is most likely to be observed in which of the following Alzheimer's disease patients?

   a. A patient with an MMSE score of 28
   b. A patient with an MMSE score of 23
   c. A patient with an MMSE score of 18
   d. A patient with an MMSE score of 8
   e. A patient with an MMSE score of 0

4. Agitation, including violence, is most likely to be observed in which of the following Alzheimer's disease patients?

   a. A patient who is having difficulty paying his or her rent on time
   b. A patient who is having difficulty preparing Thanksgiving dinner for her grandchildren
   c. A patient who must be supervised in proper dress and bathing procedures
   d. A patient who can no longer speak or walk and is falling over in the chair
   e. A patient who is having difficulty continuing to work as a primary school teacher

5. Which of the following delusions is most commonly seen in Alzheimer's disease patients?

   a. The delusion that the place in which one is residing is not one's home
   b. The delusion that the spouse is plotting to institutionalize the patient
   c. The delusion that the FBI, CIA, or similar agencies are after the patient
   d. The delusion that the spouse is having a sexual liaison with the caregiver
   e. The delusion that persons are stealing things from the patient

6. Sleep disturbance in Alzheimer's disease is most commonly marked by

   a. Initial insomnia
   b. Fragmented sleep
   c. Terminal insomnia
   d. Hypersomnia
   e. Narcolepsy

7. Depressive disorder and Alzheimer's disease have many similarities in clinical presentation. However, there are some symptoms that are much more common in one condition than the other. Which of the following symptoms is most characteristic of depressive disorder in contrast to early Alzheimer's disease?

   a.   Paucity of speech
   b.   Slowing of walking speed
   c.   Emotional withdrawal
   d.   Anxiety
   e.   Repeated suicidal attempts

8. Which of the following apolipoprotein allelic genotypes is associated with the greatest risk of developing Alzheimer's disease in whites?

   a.   Homozygous Apo E2
   b.   Homozygous Apo E3
   c.   Homozygous Apo E4
   d.   Heterozygous Apo E2 and Apo E3
   e.   Heterozygous Apo E3 and Apo E4

Chapter 15:   Vascular Dementias

Choose the one best response:

1. All of the following statements about the epidemiology of vascular dementia are true *except*

   a.   The incidence of vascular dementia increases with increasing age.
   b.   Vascular disease is the second most common cause of dementia.
   c.   The incidence of vascular dementia appears to be declining.
   d.   Alzheimer's disease is more prevalent than vascular dementia in all nations for which reports are available.
   e.   In North America vascular dementia is likely to coexist with dementia as a result of Alzheimer's disease.

2. The Ischemia Scale, developed by Hachinski et al., is the most commonly used instrument for assessing vascular dementia. Which of the following risk factors for vascular dementia is *not* included in the Ischemia Scale?

a. History of stroke
b. Sudden onset of dementia
c. Hypertension
d. Atrial fibrillation
e. Associated atherosclerosis

3. Which of the following antidepressants is the most thoroughly established in treatment of poststroke depression?

a. Trazodone
b. Nortriptyline
c. Bupropion
d. Amitriptyline
e. Desipramine

4. All of the following laboratory tests are recommended in the assessment of vascular dementia *except*

a. Complete blood count
b. Sedimentation rate
c. Liver function tests
d. Thyroid function tests
e. Fasting glucose level

5. Which of the following tests of cardiac function are currently recommended for all patients with vascular dementia?

a. Electrocardiogram (ECG)
b. 24-hour Holter monitor
c. Echocardiogram
d. Treadmill test
e. Arterial oxygen saturation

6. All of the following may be considered insignificant on magnetic resonance imaging (MRI) of brain in an elderly patient *except*

a. Ventricular enlargement
b. Basal ganglia hyperintensities
c. Multiple subcortical lacunes
d. White matter hyperintensities
e. Enlarged cortical sulci

7. All of the following can assess functional brain deficits in vascular dementia *except*

   a. X-ray computed tomography
   b. Single photon emission computed tomography (SPECT)
   c. Positron-emission tomography (PET)
   d. Neuropsychological testing
   e. Quantitative electroencephalography (QEEG)

8. All of the following are recognized subtypes of vascular dementia *except*

   a. Lacunar state
   b. Hypoperfusion dementia
   c. Cerebral atherosclerosis
   d. Binswanger's disease
   e. Multi-infarct dementia

9. All of the following subcategories have been added in DSM-IV as available modifiers for vascular dementia *except*

   a. With hallucinations
   b. With perceptual disturbance
   c. With behavioral disturbance
   d. With communication disturbance
   e. With delirium

10. The psychiatrist managing a patient with vascular dementia will usually be required to integrate all of the following in his or her treatment plan *except*

    a. Medications for concomitant medical illness
    b. Referral to community support services
    c. Psychoanalytic psychotherapy
    d. Psychotropic medication
    e. Supportive psychotherapy

Chapter 16: Delirium

Choose the one best response:

1. The hallmark of delirium is

    a. Memory
    b. Thought disorder
    c. Mood disturbance
    d. Impairment of consciousness with an attentional disturbance

2. All of the following symptoms are characteristic of delirium *except*

    a. Change in orientation
    b. Hallucinations
    c. Obsessions
    d. Illusions
    e. Fluctuation over the course of the day

3. All of the following symptoms are characteristic of a "hyperactive" delirium *except*

    a. Lethargy
    b. Hyperalertness
    c. Restlessness
    d. Excitability
    e. Loud, pressured speech

4. The prevalence of delirium in medical inpatients is

    a. 0%–10%
    b. 10%–20%
    c. 20%–30%
    d. 30%–40%
    e. 40%–50%

5. All of the following can cause delirium *except*

    a. Drug toxicity
    b. Drug withdrawal
    c. Metabolic disturbance
    d. Stroke
    e. Obesity

6. All of the following are independent risk factors for delirium *except*

    a. Prior cognitive impairment
    b. Age over 80 years
    c. Loss of spouse
    d. Fracture
    e. Symptomatic infection

7. Delirium is associated with all of the following *except*

    a. Higher rates of nursing home admissions
    b. Longer hospital stays
    c. Higher mortality rates
    d. Complete resolution of symptoms within 24 hours

8. In most patients with delirium the EEG will show

    a. Diffuse slowing
    b. Increased alpha activity
    c. No correlation with severity of symptoms
    d. No difference from depressed patients

9. All of the following are critical in the evaluation of a delirious patient *except*

    a. History of present illness
    b. Physical exam
    c. Mental status exam
    d. Information from family members
    e. MRI

10. The most important treatment for a delirious patient is

    a. Use of anticonvulsants
    b. Reversing the underlying medical cause
    c. Use of a neuroleptic
    d. Bright light therapy

Chapter 17: Other Dementias and Mental Disorders Due to General Medical Conditions

Choose the one best response:

1. Which of the following diagnostic terms does not appear in DSM-IV?

    a. Amnestic disorder
    b. Delirium
    c. Organic delusional syndrome
    d. Mental retardation
    e. Hallucinogen-related disorders

2. Pick's disease usually begins between the ages of

    a. 20 and 30
    b. 30 and 40
    c. 40 and 60
    d. 60 and 70
    e. 70 and 80

3. In Huntington's disease the CT scan often shows atrophy of the

    a. Hippocampus
    b. Caudate nuclei
    c. Nucleus basalis of Meynert
    d. Corpus callosum
    e. Parietal lobes

4. Progressive supranuclear palsy is characterized by all of the following clinical features *except*

    a. Pseudobulbar palsy
    b. Axial rigidity
    c. Supranuclear gaze paresis
    d. Dementia
    e. Hallucinations

5. The proportion of patients with normal pressure hydrocephalus (NPH) who have a history of subarachnoid bleeding is about

     a. One-half
     b. One-third
     c. One-fourth
     d. One-eighth
     e. One-tenth

6. The annual incidence of Creutzfeldt-Jakob disease is about 1 per

     a. 1,000
     b. 50,000
     c. 120,000
     d. 250,000
     e. 1,000,000

7. In Creutzfeldt-Jakob disease, 50% of patients die within

     a. 2 months
     b. 6–9 months
     c. 12–18 months
     d. 24 months
     e. 36 months

8. According to Robinson et al., depression is most likely to develop following a stroke involving

     a. Anterior-right hemisphere
     b. Anterior-left hemisphere
     c. Posterior-right hemisphere
     d. Posterior-left hemisphere
     e. Brain stem

9. In DSM-IV, subtypes of "personality change due to a general medical condition" include all of the following *except*

     a. Dependent
     b. Aggressive
     c. Disinhibited
     d. Apathetic
     e. Paranoid

10. Which of the following is most likely to help a patient with Wernicke's encaphalopathy?

    a. Niacin (vitamin B$_3$)
    b. Ascorbic acid (vitamin C)
    c. Thiamine (vitamin B$_1$)
    d. Cyanocobalamin (vitamin B$_{12}$)
    e. Pyridoxine (vitamin B$_6$)

Chapter 18:   Grief and Bereavement

Choose the one best response:

1. All of the following statements are true about the duration of grief *except*

    a . It is not uncommon for symptoms of depression to last as long as 2 years after the death of a loved one.
    b. According to C. M. Parkes, most widows, 13 months after the death of a spouse, describe themselves as happy and well adjusted, rarely think of their deceased husbands, and have completed their grief.
    c. Symptoms of anxiety may last 1–2 years, or more, after the death of a loved one.
    d. Some aspects of grief work never end for many otherwise normal widows and widowers.
    e. Grief is almost always briefer for widows than for widowers.

2. Emotional and cognitive experiences often noted after the death of a husband or wife include

    a. Shock and denial
    b. Symptoms of somatic distress
    c. Preoccupation with the deceased
    d. Relief
    e. All of the above

3. Frequently seen aspects of uncomplicated bereavement include all of the following *except*

    a. Anticipating the deceased will suddenly reappear
    b. Hearing the voice of the deceased or seeing his or her image

    c.   Carrying on conversations with the deceased
    d.   Social withdrawal
    e.   Preoccupation with suicide plans

4. Known complications of bereavement and grief in late life include all of the following *except*

    a.   Chronic grief
    b.   Cognitive decline
    c.   Major depression episodes
    d.   Complaints of somatic symptoms and increased medical health care utilization
    e.   Protracted symptoms of anxiety

5. Known risk factors for grief complications include all of the following *except*

    a.   A long and loving relationship with the deceased
    b.   Multiple sudden or unexpected deaths
    c.   Loss of a child
    d.   Poor health, depression, or substance abuse before the death
    e.   Multiple concurrent life stressors

6. All of the following are true about absent, delayed, or inhibited grief *except*

    a.   Most likely to occur in young children and elderly people
    b.   Almost always portends later depression, severe anxiety, or medical complications
    c.   Most likely to occur when the relationship with the deceased had been unduly dependent or ambivalent
    d.   Not uncommon when the bereaved has a severe narcissistic personality disorder
    e.   May be caused or perpetuated by a major psychiatric disorder

7. Regarding increased mortality rates during bereavement, all of the following are true *except*

    a.   Widows and widowers appear to have a higher mortality rate than their married counterparts.
    b.   Suicide, accidents, and heart disease likely are the predominant causes of the excess mortality.

    c. Moving into a chronic care facility, social isolation, and lack of social support are risk factors.

    d. Widowers who remarry shortly after their wife's death are at particularly high risk.

    e. Widowed or divorced mothers who lose a son in war have an increased mortality rate.

8. Regarding major depressive syndromes during widowhood, all of the following are true *except*

    a. The risk for having a major depressive syndrome remains elevated, compared with married individuals, for at least 2 years after the death.

    b. Depressions occurring within the first 2 months of the death are benign, not associated with psychosocial dysfunction, and have an excellent prognosis.

    c. During the first year of widowhood, the frequency of major depressive episodes and intensity of symptoms is lower in late life than in mid-life.

    d. Elderly widows with major depression display abnormal sleep architecture comparable to nonbereaved women with major depression.

    e. Poor prior medical and mental health are risk factors for developing a major depressive episode after the death of a spouse.

9. Regarding treatment for grief-related difficulties, all of the following are true *except*

    a. Mutual support programs have been shown to decrease morbidity in bereaved individuals, especially those at high risk for complications.

    b. Brief individual psychotherapy has been shown to benefit adults with postbereavement adjustment disorders.

    c. Dynamic psychotherapy has been shown to benefit adults with postbereavement adjustment disorders.

    d. Antidepressant medications given after the first 6 months of bereavement have been found to attenuate depressive symptoms in widows and widowers with major depression.

    e. Antidepressant and antianxiety medications should not be given in the first 6 months of bereavement because they will interfere with the process of grief.

10. A 78-year-old man in excellent health has been manifesting persistent crying, anhedonia, anorexia, early morning awakening, poor concentration, anxiety, hopelessness, self-deprecation, and a wish to be dead for the 3 months since his wife's death. Which of the following should his psychiatrist do?

   a.   Don't worry about him. He'll get over it.
   b.   Tell him that this is normal grief and that he should join a support group.
   c.   Evaluate and consider treatment just as you would with anyone presenting with this constellation of symptoms.
   d.   Seize the opportunity to confront him about his guilt and anger.
   e.   Provide support and encouragement and have him return in 1 month for a follow-up assessment.

Chapter 19:   Affective Disorders

Choose the one best response:

1. The overall prevalence of major depression in persons ages 65 or older is estimated to be

   a.   0.1%
   b.   1%
   c.   2%–5%
   d.   3%–5%
   e.   4%

2. Compared with the general elderly population, depression is more frequent in

   a.   Women
   b.   Medically hospitalized patients
   c.   Medical outpatients
   d.   Nursing home patients
   e.   All of the above

3. Which of the following statements is correct for depression of Alzheimer's disease patients?

a. Major depression occurs in about 17% of Alzheimer's disease patients.
b. Depression is elicited often when reports of relatives are used.
c. Family history for depression is associated with high rate of depression in Alzheimer's disease patients.
d. Subsyndromal depression may be found in almost 50% of patients.
e. All of the above.

4. Poststroke depression is associated with

a. Low socioeconomic level
b. Degree of paresis
c. Lesion in the left frontal pole and the head of the left caudate
d. Recent adverse life events
e. None of the above

5. Which of the following is true for patients with the dementia syndrome of depression or pseudodementia who cognitively improve after successful antidepressant treatment:

a. Frequent depressive relapses are anticipated.
b. A high percentage of patients will meet criteria for irreversible dementia 2–4 years later.
c. They are at low risk for development of irreversible dementia at follow-up.
d. None of the above.

6. Compared with elderly people with depression who experience onset of illness in early life, late-onset depression patients have

a. Less frequent family history of mood disorders
b. Greater enlargement of lateral brain ventricles
c. More white-matter hyperintensities
d. All of the above
e. None of the above

7. In geriatric psychiatric patients, the dexamethasone suppression test is

    a. Highly sensitive in geriatric depressives
    b. Nonspecific for geriatric depression
    c. Frequently abnormal in Alzheimer's disease patients
    d. All of the above
    e. None of the above

8. It has been reported that late-onset mania is associated with

    a. Medical disorders or drug treatment
    b. Coarse brain disease
    c. Low rate of mood disorders in the family
    d. All of the above
    e. None of the above

Chapter 20: Psychoses

Choose the one best response:

1. Which *one* of the following statements is correct? Auditory hallucinations

    a. Occur more often than delusions in patients with Alzheimer's dementia
    b. Are pathognomonic of "paranoia," as defined by Kraepelin
    c. May be inferred from the behavior of a patient with Alzheimer's disease
    d. Do not occur in late-onset schizophrenia
    e. Are none of the above

2. A 67-year-old male patient with dementia is given thioridazine to reduce his agitation. Which of the following statements is true concerning this medication?

    a. The medication may cause a delirium to worsen.
    b. The patient will likely require higher doses of the drug than would a 30-year-old woman.

   c. The drug produces extrapyramidal symptoms in the majority of patients.

   d. The drug is likely to improve cognitive functioning.

   e. None of the above.

3. All of the following are true statements about late-onset schizophrenia *except*

   a. Onset can be after age 55.

   b. Premorbid schizoid personality may be associated with this disorder.

   c. Patients may respond to low doses of neuroleptics.

   d. Men are more likely than women to develop this disorder.

   e. None of the above.

4. Prevalence of schizophrenia in first-degree relatives of probands with late-onset schizophrenia is

   a. The same as that in families of normal control subjects

   b. Greater than that in families of normal control subjects

   c. The same as that in families of earlier-onset schizophrenic patients

   d. Greater than that in families of earlier-onset schizophrenic patients

   e. None of the above

5. Alzheimer's dementia is most commonly associated with

   a. Bizarre delusions

   b. Alcoholism

   c. Olfactory hallucinations

   d. Isolated psychotic symptoms

   e. All of the above

For questions 6–10

Answer   a. if 1, 2, and 3 are correct
             b. if 1 and 3 are correct
             c. if 2 and 4 are correct
             d. if 4 is correct
             e. if all are correct

6. Delusional disorder

   1. Usually presents in middle to late adulthood
   2. Occurs in about 8%–15% of the psychiatric population
   3. Has a somewhat earlier age at onset in men than in women
   4. Is characterized by the presence of bizarre delusions

7. Regarding the elderly delusional patient and neuroleptic medications:

   1. The elderly patient usually requires lower doses than younger patients.
   2. A relatively high risk of tardive dyskinesia may be expected.
   3. Noncompliance is a common problem.
   4. The high-potency neuroleptics are superior to low-potency neuroleptics.

8. Schneiderian first-rank symptoms characterize

   1. Late-onset schizophrenia
   2. Alzheimer's disease with psychosis
   3. Early-onset schizophrenia
   4. Delusional disorder

9. Duration of active psychotic symptoms of longer than 2 months is *inconsistent* with a diagnosis of

   1. Delusional disorder
   2. Schizophreniform disorder
   3. Schizophrenia
   4. Brief reactive psychosis

10. Aging of the schizophrenic patient taking a neuroleptic is usually accompanied by

1. Increased severity of positive symptoms
2. Appearance of visual hallucinations
3. Development of new types of delusions
4. Remission of illness in one-third of patients

Chapter 21: Anxiety Disorders

Choose the one best response:

1. Studies of serotonin function in normal aging indicate

   a. An increased risk of developing panic disorder
   b. An increased risk of developing generalized anxiety disorder
   c. An increased risk of developing obsessive-compulsive disorder
   d. An increased risk of developing posttraumatic stress disorder
   e. None of the above

2. All of the following statements regarding the use of anxiety rating scales in elderly patients are true *except*

   a. These rating scales can be useful aids to clinical evaluation.
   b. They can serve as outcome measures for various treatments.
   c. Beck Anxiety Inventory is a self-rated scale.
   d. Hamilton Anxiety Rating Scale is preferable for use in elderly populations because of its ease of use.
   e. State-Trait Anxiety Inventory (STAI) is a self-rated scale.

3. All of the following may be effective in panic disorder *except*

   a. Buspirone
   b. Sertraline
   c. Imipramine
   d. Phenelzine
   e. Alprazolam

Chapter 22:   Somatoform and Personality Disorders

Choose the one best response:

1. The majority of data indicate that

   a. Increased age correlates positively with the presence of somatoform disorders.
   b. Diagnosis of depression correlates positively with the presence of somatoform disorders.
   c. Gender correlates positively with the presence of somatoform disorders.
   d. Physical illness correlates positively with the presence of somatoform disorders.
   e. All of the above.

2. In somatoform disorders,

   a. Personality and developmental factors are unlikely to be etiologic factors.
   b. A learned sick role in childhood is a precursor.
   c. Gender, ethnicity, education, and social class are poorly correlated factors.
   d. Patients express anger easily.
   e. None of the above is true.

3. A 78-year-old woman has new-onset, clear-cut symptoms of somatoform disorder. She has no prior history of this disorder. After full work-up and consideration of all diagnoses, which of the following medications is the therapist most likely to prescribe?

   a. Haloperidol
   b. Tacrine
   c. Nortriptyline
   d. Carbamazepine
   e. None of the above

4. Somatoform disorder in elderly people is commonly associated with all of the following comorbid features *except*

   a. Suicide
   b. Gastrointestinal disturbance

    c.   Paranoid delusions

    d.   Personality disorder

    e.   Alexithymia

5. Choice of treatment of somatoform disorder in elderly patients is commonly based on

    a.   Neuropsychological findings

    b.   Patients' willingness to accept the diagnosis

    c.   Presence of comorbid dementia

    d.   Long-standing history of substance abuse

    e.   None of the above

6. Antisocial personality symptoms

    a.   Inevitably burn out in old age

    b.   Tend to decline in middle age

    c.   Are associated with increased incidence of dementia

    d.   Are often associated with depression in elderly patients

    e.   Include none of the above

7. All of the following statements about personality changes in the elderly are true *except*

    a.   Cluster A disorders remain stable to midlife.

    b.   Neurological disorder often affects personality function.

    c.   There are almost no studies that have followed patients with personality disorders from mid-life to early old age.

    d.   The Epidemiologic Catchment Area (ECA) study provided a reliable estimate of all three personality disorder clusters in elderly subjects.

    e.   DSM-IV has no Axis II diagnostic provisions specific to elderly people.

8. Studies of the epidemiology of personality disorders show

    a.   The prevalence of antisocial personality is 0.8% in individuals over age 65.

    b.   Borderline and histrionic diagnoses are rarely applied to elderly subjects.

    c.   10%–20% of older psychiatric patients have a comorbid personality disorder diagnosis.

    d.   All of the above.

    e.   None of the above.

Chapter 23:　Substance Abuse

Choose the one best response:

1. Common symptoms of chronic salicylate toxicity in elderly people include all of the following *except*

    a.　Cognitive impairment
    b.　Pill-rolling tremor
    c.　Tinnitus
    d.　Irritability

2. The over-the-counter drugs least often used by elderly patients are

    a.　Vitamins
    b.　Laxatives
    c.　Over-the-counter sleep remedies
    d.　Over-the-counter analgesics
    e.　Antacids

3. Which one of the following is most characteristic of elderly long-term users of benzodiazepines (daily use for more than 1 year)?

    a.　Most ingest these drugs for euphoriant effects.
    b.　A majority gradually increase the drug dosage over time and develop high-dose dependence.
    c.　A majority are likely to have discontinuance symptoms (withdrawal and rebound) if the drug is stopped abruptly.
    d.　Most are polysubstance abusers.
    e.　Most do not return to see the physician who prescribed the benzodiazepine.

4. An 82-year-old woman comes to you saying that she has taken 3 mg of lorazepam daily for 8 years. She was prescribed this medication for sleep difficulties and anxiety that developed after her husband died. She recently read that this drug may be addictive and she would like to discontinue it. Which of the following best states the advice you should give to her?

    a.　Reassure her that she is not an addict, that the drug is safe in this dose, and that she should continue to take it.
    b.　Reassure her that she is not an addict and that she can discontinue the drug as she likes.

    c.   Tell her that it is likely that she is dependent and that her chances of successfully discontinuing the medication are so low that it is best not to try.

    d.   Tell her that it is likely that she is dependent on the drug but with a prescription of propranolol she will be able to discontinue the medication successfully and with a minimum of side effects.

    e.   Tell her that she may be dependent on the drug; however, with close observation it is worth trying to discontinue the drug with a slow taper over 1–2 months.

5. Compared with young benzodiazepine-dependent patients, which of the following statements most accurately characterizes elderly benzo-diazepine-dependent patients?

    a.   They are likely to have more severe withdrawal even if they are taking a similar dosage and have a similar duration of benzodiaz-epine use.

    b.   They are more likely to successfully complete benzodiazepine with-drawal protocols.

    c.   Following successful withdrawal, they have a lower rate of relapse to benzodiazepine dependence.

    d.   They are more likely to have the symptoms of benzodiazepine withdrawal overlooked by their physician and attributed to an-other medical illness.

Chapter 24: Sleep Disorders

Choose the one best response:

1. Age effects on sleep include all the following *except*

    a.   Decreasing stages 3 and 4 sleep with increasing age

    b.   Increasing stage 1 sleep with advancing age

    c.   Decreasing percentage of REM sleep with increasing age

    d.   Increasing numbers of arousals after sleep onset with increasing age

    e.   Relative age stability of sleep latency

2. Which *one* of the following is *not* characteristic of obstructive sleep apnea?

   a. Complications include first- and second-degree heart block
   b. Morning headache, confusion, depression, and impotence
   c. NREM apneas last longer than REM apneas
   d. Is more common in men than in women and in elderly people than in young
   e. May respond to protriptyline, progestational agents, or tracheotomy

3. All of the following characterize sleep changes in Alzheimer's dementia *except*

   a. Decreased phasic activity (spindles, K complexes) during NREM sleep
   b. Increased phasic rapid eye movements during dream sleep
   c. Increased prevalence of sleep apnea
   d. Loss of sleep-wake consolidation (i.e., polyphasic sleep-wake patterns)
   e. Relatively normal circadian temperature rhythmicity

4. All of the following statements about the pharmacotherapy of late-life insomnia are true *except*

   a. A sedating phenothiazine probably has less behavioral toxicity than a benzodiazepine in an agitated patient with dementia.
   b. Long-acting benzodiazepines probably have less behavioral toxicity than shorter-acting benzodiazepines.
   c. Benzodiazepines may exacerbate sleep apnea.
   d. Low-dose sedating antidepressant medication probably retains its sedating efficacy longer and has less behavioral toxicity than a benzodiazepine.
   e. Some nonpsychotropic drugs such as α-methyldopa or diphenhydramine can cause daytime sedation and disrupt sleep-wake rhythms.

5. Snoring has been shown to be a risk factor for which of the following:

   a. Sleep apnea
   b. Hypertension
   c. Ischemic heart disease
   d. Stroke
   e. All of the above

Answer   a. if only 1, 2, and 3 are correct
              b. if only 1 and 3 are correct
              c. if only 2 and 4 are correct
              d. if only 4 is correct
              e. if all are correct

6. Physiological differences between REM and NREM sleep include the following:

   1. During REM sleep, heart rate, respiratory rate, and blood pressure tend to decrease.
   2. The onset of REM sleep is mediated by the firing of cholinergic cells in the pontine tegmentum.
   3. Ventilatory response to increased concentrations of inhaled CO_2 is enhanced during REM sleep compared with NREM sleep.
   4. The occurrence of REM sleep is more likely near the nadir or throughout the circadian temperature rhythm.

Chapter 25:   Sexuality and Aging

Choose the one best response:

1. Secondary impotence

   a. May occur transiently at any age
   b. May be related to alcohol excess
   c. May be related to conflict, divorce, or grief
   d. Is commonly psychogenic, but organic causes must be ruled out because both may coexist
   e. Is all of the above

2. Orgasmic dysfunctions in women

   a. Rarely occur
   b. May present at any age
   c. Are almost always caused by urinary tract infections
   d. Are nonresponsive to brief sex therapy
   e. Are all of the above

3. The following ingested substances may cause reversible impotency and or ejaculatory difficulties:

    a. Ethanol
    b. Hypnotics
    c. Propranolol
    d. Antihypertensives
    e. All of the above

4. A 53-year-old man is being discharged after coronary bypass surgery. He asks about resuming sexual relations. The physician's best response is to tell him that

    a. He should forget sex because of danger to his heart.
    b. He may have sex as soon as he can walk up two flights of stairs comfortably.
    c. He should substitute light jogging to avoid sex.
    d. He should try to suppress sexual urges.
    e. All of the above.

5. Brief sex therapy

    a. Relies primarily on anxiolytic medications
    b. Is primarily didactic sex education
    c. Requires a period of abstinence from all sexual contact
    d. Reverses a high percentage of nonorganic sex symptoms
    e. Is none of the above

6. Premature ejaculation

    a. Is at times followed by secondary impotence
    b. Is refractory to brief sex therapy
    c. Is related to anxiety about career performance
    d. Usually improves after age 50
    e. Is all of the above

7. Dyspareunia in women over 50 years

    a. Is almost unknown in those with children
    b. May relate to menopausal atrophic vaginitis
    c. Is usually caused by unconscious rejection of men

    d. Rarely responds to local or systemic hormone replacement or lubrication for coitus

    e. Is all of the above

Chapter 26: Electroconvulsive Therapy

Choose the one best response:

1. All of the following diagnoses are appropriate indications for ECT in elderly patients *except*

    a. Severe organic affective disorder

    b. Delirium

    c. Major depression

    d. Depressive pseudodementia

    e. Mania

2. ECT can be considered a first choice treatment *most frequently* for

    a. Mania

    b. Major depression

    c. Schizoaffective disorder

    d. Delusional depression

    e. Depression with drug-induced parkinsonism

3. In elderly patients, the condition associated with the *greatest* ECT complication risk is

    a. 6 weeks post–myocardial infarction

    b. 6 weeks poststroke

    c. Atrial fibrillation

    d. Chronic obstructive pulmonary disease

    e. Increased intracranial pressure

4. The *least* amount of memory loss after ECT occurs with which type of stimulation?

    a. Sine wave, bilateral

    b. Brief-pulse, right unilateral

    c. Sine wave, right unilateral

    d.   Sine wave, left unilateral
    e.   Brief pulse bilateral

5. Informed consent for ECT with an elderly patient requires preferably

    a.   Durable power of attorney
    b.   Lack of refusal by the patient
    c.   Understanding and acceptance of the treatment by the patient
    d.   Understanding and agreement by the family of the patient

6. An absolutely essential pre-ECT assessment for all elderly patients is

    a.   EEG
    b.   Spinal X rays
    c.   Inspection of dentition
    d.   MRI
    e.   Neurology consultation

7. The following electrical stimulation parameters are acceptable:

    a.   Fixed dose—below threshold
    b.   Dosage titration
    c.   Fixed dose—at threshold
    d.   Fixed dose—above threshold
    e.   b and d

8. Which is the best statement regarding the laterality of ECT stimulation?

    a.   Bilateral ECT is clinically the most effective.
    b.   Unilateral treatments result in less memory loss or confusion.
    c.   Those patients who do not respond clinically to unilateral ECT should be treated with bilateral ECT.
    d.   Unilateral ECT at 75% or greater of the ECT machine capacity will come closest to equaling the efficacy of bilateral ECT.
    e.   All of the above are equally true.

9. Regarding stimulation dosage, all of the following are correct *except*

    a.   A traditional ECT series in the United States is three times per week; in Great Britain it is twice a week.
    b.   Seizure duration decreases with age.

c. Multiple monitored ECT allows for greater safety of the ECT procedure.

d. Seizure threshold increases with age.

e. Seizure duration decreases with the number of treatments in the series.

10. The following statements regarding premedication and anesthesia for ECT in elderly patients are all true *except*

a. The anesthetic of choice by most is methohexital, given its shorter sleep time, fewer incidences of arrhythmia, and less postictal confusion.

b. The most frequently recommended pretreatment antihypertensives, because of their relatively shorter duration of action, are labetalol and esmolol.

c. Pulse oximetry is not necessary for ECT because it is such a short procedure.

d. When safely possible, a pretreatment atropinic should be used if a β-blocker may be administered during ECT.

e. Pretreatment of premature venticular contractions with low dose lidocaine may raise the seizure threshold and prevent the induction of the seizure.

11. All of the following statements regarding management of concurrent medication during ECT are true *except*

a. Benzodiazepines should be tapered and discontinued when possible because they raise the seizure threshold and also reduce the clinical efficacy of the seizure.

b. Coadministration of tricyclic antidepressants or selective serotonin reuptake inhibitors during the treatment series has been shown to increase the efficacy of ECT.

c. Anticoagulants can continue during the ECT series as long as dosage is carefully calculated and prothrombin times are regularly assessed.

d. Theophylin should be avoided if possible because it may prolong the seizure and can lead to status epilepticus.

e. Coadministration of lithium may result in the need for prolonged ventilation of the patient and also increases the potential for a post-ECT confusional state.

12. All of the following statements regarding continuation and maintenance ECT are correct *except*

   a. Continuation ECT is defined as the ongoing application of ECT
after the completion of a series, with a decreasing frequency and
increasing interval, usually on an outpatient basis.

   b. Maintenance ECT is defined as the reinitiation of ECT treatments
after a patient has undergone a series, been placed on maintenance medications, and then relapsed.

   c. Continuation and maintenance ECT can be accompanied by antidepressant medication.

   d. For those individuals with a history of multiple prior relapses of
severe major depression, continuation ECT may be preferable to
waiting to see whether maintenance ECT is required.

   e. Continuation ECT is carried out for a minimum of 1 year.

Chapter 27: Psychopharmacology

Choose the one best response:

1. Which of the following results from the decreased renal function associated with increased age?

   a. Increased hepatic metabolism of neuroleptics

   b. Decreased volume of distribution of lipid-soluble drugs

   c. Decreased excretion of hydroxylated tricyclic antidepressant (TCA)
metabolites

   d. Increased gastrointestinal absorption of lithium

2. Which of the following characterizes secondary amine TCAs, as contrasted with tertiary amine TCAs?

   a. Greater orthostatic hypotensive effects

   b. Less anticholinergic effect

   c. Higher plasma concentrations per milligram dose

   d. Less efficacy in elderly patients

3. Which of the following is suggested by very low plasma concentration
of TCA in depressed nonresponders?

   a. Rapid hepatic metabolism

   b. Good compliance

    c.   Inflammatory state
    d.   Hypothyroidism

4. Pharmacodynamics can be altered by all of the following *except*

    a.   Drug interactions at the tissue level
    b.   Diseases
    c.   Aging
    d.   Decreased absorption

5. Which of the following is true of high-potency neuroleptics compared with low-potency neuroleptics?

    a.   Fewer extrapyramidal side effects
    b.   Greater sedation
    c.   Less orthostatic hypotension
    d.   Greater anticholinergic effect

6. Which of the following is a risk of benzodiazepine use in elderly patients?

    a.   Cognitive dysfunction
    b.   Hypothyroidism
    c.   Quinidine-like prolongation of intracardiac conduction effects
    d.   Hypertension

7. Assessment of blood pressure in association with antidepressant and neuroleptic treatment should include which of the following?

    a.   Exercise stress values
    b.   Sitting values only
    c.   Orthostatic measurement
    d.   Bedtime measurement

8. Adequate drug treatment of delusional depression most often requires which of the following?

    a.   Neuroleptic treatment alone
    b.   Antidepressant drug treatment alone
    c.   Combined lithium and antidepressant treatment
    d.   Combined neuroleptic and antidepressant treatment

9. Use of anticholinergic agents is most often associated with which of the following side effects?

   a. Urinary retention
   b. Bradycardia
   c. Altered thyroid function
   d. Diarrhea

10. Which of the following will enhance compliance with pharmaco-therapy in elderly patients?

   a. Divided dose regimens
   b. Cognitive impairment
   c. Using the fewest drugs
   d. Putting responsibility on the patient alone

11. The following statements are true of quinidine-like prolongation of intracardiac conduction *except*

   a. It is a toxic effect of TCAs.
   b. It is potentiated by type I antiarrhythmics used with TCAs.
   c. It is correlated with plasma TCA concentrations.
   d. It occurs more often with monoamine oxidase inhibitors than TCAs.

12. Neuroleptic side effects that occur frequently in elderly patients include all of the following *except*

   a. Dystonia
   b. Pseudoparkinsonism
   c. Tardive dyskinesia
   d. Akathisia

13. Which of the following statements is true of monoamine oxidase inhibitors?

   a. They produce orthostatic blood pressure effects within a few days if they are likely to occur at a given dose.
   b. They are clinically useful in combination with fluoxetine.
   c. They are effective in maintaining symptom remission in major depression.
   d. Their anticholinergic effects are 10-fold greater that those of TCAs.

14. Any drug interactions are an important concern in elderly patients. In using lithium salts, which of the following drug interactions can occur?

    a. Benzodiazepine increases volume of distribution.
    b. Antidepressants decrease absorption.
    c. Diuretics decrease clearance.
    d. Nonsteroidal anti-inflammatory drugs increase clearance.

Chapter 28:   Individual Psychotherapy

Choose the one best response:

1. During psychotherapy with elderly outpatients, the psychotherapist will sometimes do all of the following *except*

    a. Encourage reminiscence
    b. Support patient's attempts to maintain self-esteem
    c. Support the patient's healthier defense mechanisms
    d. Provide education about normative aspects of aging
    e. Quickly stop the first signs of an idealizing transference by interpretation

2. Each of the following approaches is useful in the initial psychotherapy sessions with elderly patients *except*

    a. Conveying an attitude of hope
    b. Maintaining a neutral, reflective therapeutic attitude
    c. Actively exploring and working through resistances to treatment
    d. Interviewing significant others, such as family
    e. Conveying in a real and symbolic way the therapist's acceptance and desire to help

3. Developmental tasks of later life include all of the following *except*

    a. Adapting to biopsychosocial losses
    b. Accepting shifts in traditional masculine or feminine strivings
    c. Turning to adolescent modes of coping
    d. Maintaining self-esteem and a sense of continuity with one's past
    e. Accepting the finitude of life

4. Which of the following statements about cognitive therapy with elderly patients is true?

   a. Depressed patients with endogenous signs respond better than those without endogenous signs.

   b. Cognitive therapy is less effective when modified for elderly patients.

   c. Cognitive therapy is especially efficacious for the depressed, cognitively impaired patient with a concomitant personality disorder.

   d. Positive features of cognitive therapy with elderly patients include its time-limited nature, the patient's active participation, and integration with other treatment modalities.

   e. A potential strength of cognitive therapy is its tendency to produce intellectualization.

5. All of the following psychotherapeutic techniques are appropriate to use during the early stage of brief psychotherapy with elderly patients *except*

   a. Confirmation of the patient's perception of his or her present problems

   b. Confrontation of character defenses

   c. Working through of resistances to psychotherapy

   d. Maintaining an engaged attitude toward the patient

   e. Forming an agreement regarding the goals of treatment

6. Indications for dynamic psychotherapy of elderly patients

   a. Are highly age specific

   b. Exclude mild cognitive impairment

   c. Generally include the frail elderly

   d. Exclude patients emerging from a crisis

   e. None of the above

7. Of the following choices the most significant barrier to dynamic psychotherapy with elderly patients is

   a. Overloading of outpatient services by elderly patients

   b. Resistance of elderly patients to family pressure to seek help

    c.   The child's desire to control the aging parent
    d.   The elderly patient's acceptance of depression and anxiety as normal
    e.   All of the above

8. The following are important principles of individual psychotherapy *except*

    a.   The therapist individualizes therapeutic interventions regardless of the form of therapy used.
    b.   Psychotherapy is frequently impeded by the need for medication.
    c.   The psychotherapist maintains a family perspective.
    d.   Exploration of reactions and resistance to therapy precedes active intervention.
    e.   The therapist is active and engaging of the patient during the assessment.

9. In the psychotherapy of crisis situations of elderly patients,

    a.   The first goal is intrapsychic adaptation to the effects of the crisis.
    b.   The therapist's goal is return of full function.
    c.   The therapist promotes the best attainable level of function.
    d.   Understanding of unconscious root causes of distress is the primary goal.
    e.   All of the above are true.

10. The transference that emerges during dynamic psychotherapy of elderly patients

    a.   Generally casts the therapist in the role of the patient's child
    b.   Contains elements of significant adult relationships
    c.   Differs in form and content from younger patients
    d.   Rarely contains eroticized components
    e.   Contains none of the above

Chapter 29:   Group Therapy

For questions 1–7

Answer   a. if only 1, 2, and 3 are correct
                  b. if only 1 and 3 are correct
                  c. if only 2 and 4 are correct
                  d. if only 4 is correct
                  e. if all are correct

1. Objectives of psychodynamic group therapy with elderly patients include

    1. Grieving and adaptation to loss
    2. Reducing social isolation
    3. Acquiring interpersonal skills
    4. Restoring a sense of self-esteem and self-worth

2. Possible adverse effects of a reminiscence focus in group therapy with elderly patients include

    1. Preoccupation with the past
    2. Increased morbid self-absorption
    3. Increased guilt over poor decisions made in life
    4. Increased focus of the group on the here-and-now

3. Behavioral group approaches with elderly patients employ

    1. Role playing
    2. Relaxation exercises
    3. Log books and homework assignments
    4. Interpretation of conflict

4. Groups for burdened caregivers provide opportunities for

    1. Education about dementing process
    2. Problem solving
    3. Validation of the caregiver's efforts
    4. Grieving

5. Effects of pregroup preparation for patients entering group therapy include

   1. Facilitation of the therapeutic alliance
   2. Increased patient anxiety
   3. Increased patient hopefulness
   4. Reduced patient adherence to the group task

6. Important components of effective group psychotherapy with cognitively impaired elderly patients include

   1. Therapist interpretation of group dynamics and group process
   2. Active reinforcement of interpersonal and cognitive skills
   3. Discouraging reminiscence
   4. Ongoing reality orientation on the ward

7. Positive outcome in group therapy with elderly patients rarely correlates with

   1. Interpersonal engagement and interaction
   2. Acquisition of interpersonal skills
   3. Interpersonal competence and effectiveness
   4. Unstructured group formats

Choose the one best response:

8. Therapy groups for elderly people should aim to achieve homogeneity of group composition regarding

   a. Age
   b. Level of physical functioning
   c. Marital status
   d. Level of cognitive functioning
   e. Gender

9. Group intervention with cognitively impaired elderly patients produces all of the following *except*

   a. Improved socially appropriate behavior
   b. Improved verbal orientation

    c.   Durable cognitive improvements
    d.   Improved staff morale
    e.   Improved patient socialization

10. Therapist "prizing" of patients in group therapy

    a.   Increases patient dependency
    b.   Enhances patient self-concept
    c.   Reflects therapist countertransference
    d.   Interferes with group cohesion
    e.   Is contraindicated

Chapter 30:   Families of Older Adults

Choose the one best response:

1. Family therapy for the treatment of frail elderly patients

    a.   Is generally only effective in home health care
    b.   Can improve quality of life in all medical settings where elderly patients are treated
    c.   Is not appropriate as a consultation-liaison service
    d.   Is reimbursed by Medicare in cases of adult maltreatment syndrome
    e.   Is none of the above

2. Family therapy can contribute to

    a.   Role definition and boundary setting between family members
    b.   Improved knowledge of level of dependence and autonomy of the elderly relative
    c.   Improved activities of daily living and driving ability of elderly patients
    d.   Prevention of abusive behaviors
    e.   All of the above

3. For persons ages 65 and older the following is correct:

    a.   There are 25–30 unmarried men per 100 unmarried women.
    b.   70% have grandchildren.

   c.   10% have living parents.

   d.   40% have great grandchildren.

   e.   All of the above.

4. Mutual support groups for families of impaired elderly patients usually

   a.   Take the place of family therapy

   b.   Resolve marital conflict

   c.   Reduce isolation

   d.   Address the mourning process

   e.   Do none of the above

5. Family therapy for the elderly patient with progressive dementia includes

   a.   Education about the course of dementia

   b.   Facilitation of acceptance of repetitive speech

   c.   Recognition of family contribution to improvement of patient's quality of life

   d.   Role definition of each family member in the care of the elderly patient with dementia

   e.   All of the above

6. Manifestations of caregiver strain include

   a.   Depression

   b.   Elevated sedimentation rate

   c.   Higher rate of retirement

   d.   Increased incidence of hypertension

   e.   All of the above

7. Theoreticians whose models of family structure and development can be applied in family therapy for individuals in late life include

   a.   Borszormenyi-Nagy

   b.   Nemiroff

   c.   Butler

   d.   Salzman

   e.   All of the above

Chapter 31:　Psychiatric Aspects
of Nursing Home Care

Choose the one best response:

1. The prevalence of psychiatric disorders in nursing homes is

    a.　Under 25%
    b.　Approximately 33%
    c.　40%–60%
    d.　80%–95%

2. The prevalence of delirium among nursing home residents has been demonstrated to be

    a.　0.1%–0.3%
    b.　1%–2%
    c.　6%–7%
    d.　Over 10%

3. The most common reason for a psychiatric consultation in a nursing home is

    a.　Evaluation of causes for cognitive impairment in patients with dementia
    b.　Evaluation of depressive symptoms in cognitively intact patients
    c.　Evaluation of behavioral symptoms in patients with dementia
    d.　Competency evaluations in patients with possible impairments in decision-making capacity

4. The prevalence of behavioral symptoms in nursing home residents with dementia is

    a.　5%–10%
    b.　One-third to one-half
    c.　Two-thirds to three-quarters
    d.　80%–95%

5. The prevalence of major depression in cognitively intact nursing home residents is

    a.　2%–4%
    b.　5%–10%

c. 20%–25%
d. Over 33%

6. In patients with significant physical illness, the approach to the diagnosis of major depression that maximizes sensitivity (over specificity) is

a. Etiologic
b. Inclusive
c. Exclusive
d. Substitutive

7. Depression in the nursing home has been shown to be associated with all of the following *except*

a. Increased mortality
b. Increased rates of depression in first-degree relatives
c. Increased pain complaints
d. Biochemical evidence for subnutrition

8. Issues that led the federal government to enact nursing home reform legislation in 1987 included all of the following *except*

a. Concerns about the overuse of physical restraints
b. Concerns about the overuse of psychoactive drugs as chemical restraints
c. Concerns about the overuse of mental health services by nursing home residents
d. Concerns about states shifting the costs for the care of chronic psychiatric patients to the federal government

9. Federal regulations and surveyor's guidelines regarding the use of psychoactive medications in nursing homes specify all of the following *except*

a. Psychoactive medications should not be given except for treatment of a specific condition diagnosed and documented in the clinical record.
b. Medications cannot be given for purposes of discipline or convenience.
c. Psychoactive medications can never be given at doses that exceed specified limits.
d. Psychoactive medications cannot be given in excessive doses, for excessive duration, or without adequate monitoring.

10. Physical restraints

    a. Were used in approximately 10% of nursing home residents before OBRA 87 reforms

    b. Decrease the risk of falls and injuries

    c. Are used to a similar degree in all countries

    d. Have been used primarily in patients with cognitive impairment

Chapter 32: Geriatric Consultation-Liaison Psychiatry

Choose the one best answer:

1. The prevalence of psychiatric disorders among elderly patients admitted to general medical-surgical hospitals is

    a. 0%–5%

    b. 5%–15%

    c. 15%–25%

    d. 25%–55%

    e. 55%–75%

2. The hospital environment frequently presents all of the following challenges to the medically ill elderly *except*

    a. An unfamiliar environment

    b. The need to share a room with strangers

    c. Unavailability of medical care in emergency situations

    d. Frequent staff turnover

    e. Frequent interruptions by medical staff

3. There is evidence that elderly medical-surgical patients receive psychiatric consultations less frequently than their younger counterparts. Explanations that have been suggested for this include all of the following *except*

    a. Referring physicians consider cognitive dysfunction and behavioral abnormalities a part of normal aging and refer these patients less often.

    b. Elderly patients have a lower prevalence of psychiatric disorders.

c. Elderly patients refuse psychiatric consultation more often.
d. Referring physicians feel that acute medical problems demand a higher priority.
e. Financial constraints make it difficult for psychiatrists to provide comprehensive consultation services to this population.

4. Regarding the use of services by elderly patients, all of the following statements are true *except*

a. Elderly patients receive treatment for their psychiatric problems more often from primary care physicians than from psychiatrists.
b. Elderly patients use psychiatric emergency services more frequently than younger persons.
c. Over the next 30 years, the demand for hospital care by elderly patients is likely to rise as this group will likely double or even triple in size.
d. The stigma of mental illness can make elderly patients resistant to a psychiatric consultation.
e. Only a minority of elderly medical-surgical patients diagnosed with mental disorders in the general hospital receive adequate treatment for these conditions.

5. Psychiatric consultations in the nursing home differ from those in the general hospital in all of these factors *except*

a. Patients in the nursing home are older.
b. Patients in the nursing home are more often diagnosed with delirium.
c. Patients in the nursing home are more likely to be female.
d. Patients in the nursing home are more often diagnosed with dementia.
e. Referrals in the nursing home are usually less urgent.

6. The cost-effectiveness of psychiatric consultations in a general hospital has been demonstrated most clearly in elderly patients with

a. Hip fractures
b. Diabetes mellitus
c. Chronic heart disease
d. Arthritis
e. Decubitus ulcers

7. Common psychiatric consultation requests for elderly medical-surgical patients include all of the following *except*

   a. Assessment and treatment of agitation
   b. Assessment of competency
   c. Assessment and treatment of depression
   d. Disposition, including transfer to a psychiatric unit
   e. Family therapy

8. Essential elements in the psychiatric evaluation of elderly medical-surgical patients include all of the following *except*

   a. Routine neuroimaging assessment
   b. A functional assessment
   c. An assessment of medications taken
   d. An assessment of medical problems and treatments
   e. A careful mental status examination

9. All of the following statements about depression among elderly patients in general hospitals are true *except*

   a. It is rare because most of the symptoms can be accounted for by comorbid medical illnesses.
   b. It is frequently not recognized or treated.
   c. It is associated with greater mortality and lower functional outcomes.
   d. It can be secondary to medical conditions such as stroke or Parkinson's disease.
   e. It sometimes produces cognitive difficulties.

10. The following statements about psychotherapy with elderly medical-surgical patients are correct *except*

   a. Dependency and loss of autonomy are prominent issues.
   b. Sessions are usually longer than with younger outpatients.
   c. Sessions are frequently interrupted.
   d. Psychotherapy may also involve work with the family or the medical staff.
   e. Supportive psychotherapy can help increase a sense of autonomy and self-esteem.

Chapter 33: Acute Care Inpatient and Day Hospital Treatment

Choose the one best response:

1. When elderly patients are admitted to acute care psychiatric inpatient units, discharge planning should start at admission and include all of the following *except*

   a. A good understanding of the patient's living situation before admission
   b. Identifying potential obstacles to discharge
   c. Maintaining community resources
   d. Encouraging families to look for a supervised facility or nursing home
   e. Establishing a clear prognosis

2. On "Joint Geriatric Medicine/Psychiatry units," as described by Arie and Jolley,

   a. Elderly patients with acute medical problems and patients with acute psychiatric illness are admitted side by side to the same ward.
   b. All staff members have to have dual qualifications in medicine and psychiatry because they will have to care for patients with acute medical and psychiatric illness.
   c. Every patient is seen by a geriatrician and a geropsychiatrist several times during admission.
   d. Students can learn about medical and psychiatric care of elderly patients through joint teaching.
   e. All patients are screened by the geropsychiatrist and the geriatrician in charge before admission.

3. Statistics on the diagnosis responsible for admission of elderly patients to private psychiatric hospitals and psychiatric units of general hospitals reveal that

   a. Depression is the most common reason for admission.
   b. Dementia is the most common reason for admission.
   c. Alcohol-related disorders account for <5% of admissions.
   d. Schizophrenia accounts for <15% of admissions.
   e. Psychoneuroses account for approximately 15% of admissions.

4. In addition to patients who present an imminent danger to themselves or others, elderly patients who will need inpatient psychiatric admission include all of the following *except*

    a. Acutely psychotic patients
    b. Patients with psychiatric disorders who have multiple nonacute medical problems requiring close monitoring
    c. Patients addicted to alcohol or pain killers who require treatment for significant psychiatric symptoms
    d. Patients with psychiatric disorders who need intravenous fluids or frequent intramuscular injections
    e. Patients with dementia who need a higher level of care than can be provided in their current residence

5. Problems that are more common in the geriatric population and call for particular attention on the part of architects when they design inpatient units include all of the following *except*

    a. Falls
    b. Hearing loss
    c. Wandering
    d. Aggressive behavior
    e. Visual impairment

6. All the following patients would be appropriately admitted to a geriatric psychiatry inpatient unit *except*

    a. An elderly patient who suffers from an episode of psychotic agitated depression
    b. An elderly schizophrenic patient living in a group home who suddenly becomes agitated and aggressive
    c. An elderly patient known to a psychiatric service for major recurrent depressive episodes who presents with a new complaint of shortness of breath
    d. A 75-year-old man with diabetes and hypertension who presents with a first episode of hypomania

7. In the United States, geriatric psychiatry day hospital treatment programs are frequently affiliated with

    a. The YMCA
    b. Elder hostels

   c. American Association of Partial Hospitalization
   d. American Association of Retired Persons
   e. American Association of Gerontology

8. The most intensive diagnostic and treatment facilities for elderly patients with psychiatric disorders may be found in

   a. Day care centers
   b. Day treatment programs
   c. Community centers for seniors
   d. Geriatric psychiatry day hospitals
   e. The Alzheimer's Society "Day Away" programs

9. One of the factors related to underutilization of partial hospitalization for elderly psychiatric patients includes

   a. Decreasing numbers of elderly psychiatric patients
   b. Decreased incidence of psychiatric disorders with age
   c. Lack of exposure of psychiatrists during postgraduate training programs
   d. An increase in long-term psychiatric beds
   e. A decrease in long-term psychiatric beds

10. The American Association of Partial Hospitalization's definition of partial hospitalization includes which of the following treatment modalities?

   a. Diagnostic
   b. Psychiatric
   c. Psychosocial
   d. All of the above

11. Day hospitals for elderly psychiatric patients can provide all of the following services *except*

   a. A transition from inpatient services
   b. 24-hour respite care
   c. Rehabilitation of long-term patients
   d. Assistance in cases that present diagnostic difficulties
   e. Treatment of patients with moderately severe acute psychiatric disorders

12. The two most common conditions found in patients treated in geriatric psychiatry day hospital programs are

   a. Depression and grief reactions
   b. Depression and schizophrenia
   c. Depression and dementia
   d. Depression and substance abuse
   e. Depression and anxiety disorders

Chapter 34:   Integrated Community Services

Choose the one best response:

1. All of the following are typically performed by protective services *except*

   a. Service for persons incapable of performing functions necessary to meet basic physical and health requirements
   b. Service for persons incapable of managing finances
   c. Service for persons who have no formal support system
   d. Service for persons dangerous to self or others
   e. Service for persons exhibiting behavior that brings them into conflict with the community

2. Case managers typically provide all the following services *except*

   a. Assessment
   b. Vocational training
   c. Advocacy
   d. Linkage
   e. Monitoring

3. All of the following are considered examples of long-term care residences *except*

   a. Domiciliary care residence
   b. Intermediate care facilities
   c. Section 8 housing
   d. Hospice
   e. Skilled nursing facilities

4. Comprehensive in-home health services are most likely to be reimbursed by

a. Medicare
b. Medicaid
c. Social Services Block Grant (Title XX) funds
d. Title V funds of the Older Americans Act

5. Which of the following is most suitable for persons with no mental or physical deficits?

a. Assisted living
b. Congregate housing
c. Foster care
d. Retirement community
e. Board-and-care home

6. Which of the following services would be most suitable for a moderately impaired person with Alzheimer's disease?

a. Green Thumb
b. Mutual help group
c. Home care services
d. Section 8 housing
e. Hospice

7. Which of the following is *not* one of the principal models of geriatric day care?

a. A health-oriented model for physically dependent persons
b. A model that involves special purpose centers for a single type of client
c. A psychosocial-oriented model that often targets persons with mental disorders
d. A vocational model for those persons requiring work-skills training

8. Which of the following is *not* a senior volunteer or vocational program?

a. Green Thumb
b. Service Corps of Retired Executives

    c.   Senior Work Program

    d.   Foster Grandparents

9. All of the following are true about home health care *except*

    a.   It provides nursing care.

    b.   It provides personal care services.

    c.   It must be provided by a state-certified agency.

    d.   It provides friendly visiting.

Chapter 35:   Medical-Legal Issues

Choose the one best response:

1. The most commonly encountered cause of incompetency in elderly patients is

    a.   Schizophrenia

    b.   Alzheimer's disease

    c.   Bipolar affective disorder

    d.   Alcoholism

2. Which of the following statements about incompetency is not correct?

    a.   It is an all or none condition.

    b.   It is a legal term.

    c.   It is a condition that can result in harm to the elderly person.

    d.   It involves functional impairment.

3. All are important, but the essential cognitive process in competency/ incompetency is

    a.   Reasoning

    b.   Judgment

    c.   Decision making

    d.   Ideation

4. The Patient Self Determination Act

    a.   Varies from state to state

    b.   Provides freedom of choice in the selection of a health care facility

    c.   Deals with advance directives

    d.   Is a form of living will

5. The springing power of attorney springs into operation

   a. Upon written order of the principal
   b. When the principal becomes incompetent
   c. At the death of the principal
   d. When the principal's assets reach a specified amount

6. A major problem with any form of power of attorney is

   a. Cost
   b. Shortage of effective agents
   c. Death of the agent
   d. Possible abuse

7. Which of the following does not belong in the group?

   a. Trust agreement
   b. Joint ownership
   c. Representative payee
   d. Power of attorney

8. In guardianship cases, the sequence is

   a. Respondent, adjudication, ward, guardian
   b. Adjudication, respondent, ward, guardian
   c. Ward, respondent, adjudication, guardian
   d. Ward, adjudication, guardian, respondent

9. In guardianship cases, adjudication is an action taken by

   a. An attorney
   b. A judge
   c. A psychiatrist or other physician
   d. An agency or professional guardian

10. In guardianship cases, courts monitor

   a. Wards
   b. Attorneys
   c. Guardians
   d. Petitioners

Chapter 36:   Clinical Ethics

Choose the one best response:

1. Which of these acts would most closely fit the definition of physician-assisted suicide?

   a. A patient with end-stage emphysema is hospitalized for pneumonia. The patient has required a respirator for pneumonia twice in the past year and now appears to be going into respiratory failure. The patient asks not to be placed on a respirator again and to be given morphine to relieve his air hunger. The physician and patient both know that the normal doses of morphine needed to treat air hunger may suppress respiratory drive. The physician administers the morphine and the patient dies.

   b. A patient with leukemia requests a lethal amount of medication to keep at home just in case she should want to die. Meanwhile she is continuing to receive therapy. The physician gives her the drug and tells her how to use it. A few months later, she decides to end her life and takes the overdose.

   c. A patient with ovarian cancer is delirious with pain in a hospital. An on-call physician sees her and she begs him, "Please, lets get this over with." He administers a lethal dose of medication.

   d. A diabetic patient is dialysis dependent and has a long history of progressively severe multisystem disease, including congestive heart failure, blindness, and bilateral leg amputations. The patient has been diagnosed as being depressed and is on an antidepressant medication that has been helpful although he has remained unhappy with his quality of life. The patient requests that dialysis be discontinued and, at the request of his physician, agrees to suspend acting on this request for 2 months. During that time he appears to be competent and cooperating with therapy. At the end of 2 months, the primary care physician admits the patient for terminal care without dialysis.

   e. A patient has a long history of depression with multiple suicide attempts. His physician prescribes 2-week supplies of antidepressants. During a time when the patient is particularly sad, the patient calls twice for an early refill, claiming he lost his medication. The physician refills the medication and the patient commits suicide.

2. What is the difference between "lacks decision-making ability" and "incompetence"?

   a. There is no difference.

   b. Competence is a conclusion about global intellectual function. Decision-making capacity refers to circumscribed areas of dysfunction.

   c. Although often used interchangeably, competence refers to a court finding; decision-making capacity is the conclusion of a clinical assessment.

   d. Decision-making ability is an informal or colloquial usage. Competence is the term that psychiatrists should use in their reports.

   e. Neither term is in DSM-IV and thus neither has any standard meaning in geropsychiatry.

3. A researcher proposes to study the use of a new medication for treating urinary incontinence in persons with Alzheimer's disease. What statement best summarizes the current ethical standard for such studies?

   a. This study should go through routine institutional review board approval so long as there is family consent.

   b. Subjects with dementia may only be studied for conditions related to dementia. Other research uses of these persons is an unnecessary abuse of vulnerable subjects.

   c. There is no consensus on how to proceed with such a study. Therefore, research should be postponed.

   d. The vulnerable nature of subjects with dementia means that extra precautions, such as an oversight committee or consent auditor, should be established to review the risks and burdens of this study to the subjects.

4. Motor vehicle accidents involving older drivers primarily are attributed to what age-related problem?

   a. Sensory changes
   b. Musculoskeletal problems
   c. Neurological decline
   d. Medication effects
   e. All of the above

5. According to one small survey study, what percentage of adults want to be told by their physician that they have a diagnosis of Alzheimer's disease?

   a. 10%
   b. 25%
   c. 50%
   d. 75%
   e. 90%

6. Deteriorating driving performance in elderly people is best correlated with the progression of

   a. Joint disease
   b. Dementia
   c. Hearing dysfunction
   d. Visual dysfunction
   e. Dysphoria

7. The obligation of a physician to report to the motor vehicle agency patients who have driving impairments secondary to psychiatric problems is mandated by how many states?

   a. All of them
   b. 75% or less
   c. 50% or less
   d. 25% or less
   e. None of them

Chapter 37:   Financial Issues

Choose the one best response:

1. Medicare currently accounts for approximately how much of total payments for nursing home care?

   a. 42%
   b. 27%
   c. 12%
   d. 3%
   e. 19%

2. Medicare currently pays for about what percentage of total health care costs for elderly patients?

   a. 15%
   b. 50%
   c. 87%
   d. 75%
   e. 30%

3. The percentage of older adults living below the poverty level in the United States is about

   a. 12%
   b. 23%
   c. 5%
   d. 34%
   e. 45%

4. All of the following regarding care in skilled nursing facilities is true *except*

   a. Coverage by Medicare requires 3 days of hospitalization within 30 days of admission.
   b. Medicaid and out-of-pocket expenditures contribute the lion's share of payments.
   c. Preadmission screening for active mental disorders is required.
   d. TEFRA caps control expenditures for per diem reimbursement.
   e. Some states require patients to spend down personal assets to qualify for Medicaid reimbursement.

5. The current annual limitation for reimbursement of outpatient psychiatric treatment by Medicare is

   a. $1,100 as 50% payment for an annual limit of $2,200 of charges
   b. $250 as 50% payment for an annual limit of $500 of charges
   c. No annual limit in payments
   d. $1,500 annual limit on a maximum of 20 visits annually
   e. $750 as 50% payment for an annual limit of $1,500 of charges

6. The legal requirement for "core" Medigap insurance benefits includes

   a.   Payment for in-home services beyond those covered by Medicare
   b.   Payment for intermediate care facility days up to an annual total
        of 190
   c.   Payment for the 50% copay for outpatient psychotherapy services
   d.   Payment for physician charges in excess of the Medicare fee sched-
        ule up to 115% of the approved charge
   e.   Payment for inpatient psychiatric days over and above the 190-
        day lifetime limit in freestanding hospitals

7. Physician payment reform under OBRA 89 included all of the following *except*

   a.   Adaptation of a uniform fee schedule based on the RBRVS
   b.   The establishment of volume performance standards for annual
        expenditures for physician payments nationally
   c.   Limitations on all fees that may be charged to Medicare recipients
   d.   Requirements that all physicians accept Medicare assignment
   e.   Immediate fee reductions for "overvalued procedures"

8. Medicaid

   a.   Has universally adapted the RBRVS fee schedule
   b.   Requires needs testing for eligibility
   c.   Requires a 50% copayment for ambulatory psychiatric benefits
   d.   Serves as the primary carrier for beneficiaries who are also en-
        rolled in Medicare
   e.   Provides uniform benefits nationally

9. The "dependency ratio"

   a.   Is derived from a formula integrating activities of daily living func-
        tion and medical illness
   b.   Refers to the number of older adults per individuals ages 18–64 in
        the general population
   c.   Will remain stable over the coming 50 years
   d.   Is influenced only by changes in the size of the geriatric popula-
        tion
   e.   Has not changed remarkably over the past half century

10. The Catastrophic Coverage Act of 1988

    a.   Continues to provide stop-loss limitation on out-of-pocket liability for Medicare recipients

    b.   Provides for limits in premiums required by Medigap insurers and commercial long-term care insurance

    c.   Was repealed 1 year after enactment

    d.   Was designed to provide elective coverage of catastrophic cost

    e.   Was designed to be supported through general revenue taxes

Self-Assessment Answers

Chapter 1: Epidemiology of Psychiatric Disorders

Answers:
1.   d.   Over 10%
2.   c.   Somewhere between 3% and 10%
3.   c.   Somewhere between 3% and 10%
4.   a.   Higher for Alzheimer's disease
5.   d.   Over 10%
6.   b.   More demand for intensive mental health care
7.   b.   Other types of depressive disorders
8.   d.   >30%
9.   b.   Quite often (6%–30% of all cases)
10. b.   Have distinctive brain abnormalities on neuroimaging
11. d.   Often (20%–60%) resembling major depression initially and later typical of dementia
12. a.   Chinese
13. d.   Have close relatives and friends
14. a.   Deterioration in physical health

Chapter 2: Genetics of Geriatric Psychopathology

Answers:
1.   c.   A technique that allows the separation of DNA on the basis of size
2.   b.   CAG trinucleotide repeats

3. c. Alzheimer's disease
4. c. Huntington's disease
5. e. Amyloid precursor protein mutations
6. b. Huntington's disease
7. a. 20
8. e. All of the above
9. b. Higher in late-onset families than in the general population
10. c. Glutamic acid to lysine amino acid substitution, codon 200
11. a. Valine to isoleucine amino acid substitution, codon 717
12. b. CAG trinucleotide repeats
13. d. ApoE-e4 allele
14. e. Trisomy 21

Chapter 3:   Biology of Aging

Answers:
1. e. All are correct
2. b. 1 and 3 are correct
3. d. Only 4 is correct
4. c. 2 and 4 are correct
5. b. There are losses in cellular microsomal enzyme activity, primarily CYP2D6 and CYP1A2 isoenzymes of cytochrome P450.
6. d. Basal thyroid-stimulating hormone (TSH) secretion increases in persons over 60 years of age while maintaining the euthyroid state except in very old men
7. a. Visual acuity is significantly related to loss of the ability to accommodate.
8. a. Is a common presentation of mild diabetes mellitus in elderly people
9. c. There is no reduction in the capacity to conserve sodium along with a decline in levels of vasopressin leading to water retention.
10. b. This area is linked to memory impairments in patients with dementia
11. b. Premenopausal protection from coronary artery disease and stroke
12. d. Is as effective as weight-bearing exercise on bone maintenance

Chapter 4: Normal Aging: Changes in Sensory/Perceptual and Cognitive Abilities

Answers:

1. c. Everyday communication skills; lexical, phonological, and syntaxic processing; discourse comprehension; attention; and simple visual perception
2. a. Difficulties interpreting studies in intelligence because of specific characteristics of the sample
3. c. Most people plateau in their 50s and 60s and begin a slow but increasingly rapid decline in their late 70s
4. d. Cognitive decline in older adults is not as extensive as once thought.
5. a. The variability in cognitive skills increases with age
6. b. Secondary memory
7. d. 80%
8. c. Typically not impaired, although the speed of performance declines
9. d. Both a and b are true.
10. c. Needs to be determined by further well-designed studies

Chapter 5: Sociodemographic Aspects

Answers:

1. c. On the whole, women live longer than men
2. d. Most workers retire when they feel that they can afford to do so
3. b. The median family income is about one-third more for elderly people than for younger adults as a whole.
4. e. There is a long-term trend away from intergenerational living arrangements among elderly people
5. a. Today's older adults tend to remain where they have spent most of their adult lives
6. b. One-half
7. d. Decreasing, increasing
8. a. Strong
9. c. Low levels of social contact are associated with higher mortality as a result of all causes.
10. e. Good to excellent

Chapter 6:   Self and Experience
Across the Second Half of Life

Answers:
1. d. All of the above
2. b. Have a less adverse impact on health and morale because they are anticipated and shared
3. a. Increased concern with personal mortality
4. d. All of the above
5. b. Middle-aged women
6. c. May increase, but subjective health remains positive
7. d. None of the above
8. a. May provide a medium for life review
9. d. All of the above
10. c. A few confidants

Chapter 7:   Ethnocultural Aspects

Answers:
1. f. All of the above
2. b. 14%
3. b. African Americans
4. d. Whites
5. a. Asian Americans
6. d. Lower than that of whites
7. d. a and c

Chapter 8:   Comprehensive Psychiatric Evaluation

Answers:
1. b. A single "cross-sectional" examination of cognitive function can determine the course and prognosis of the illness.
2. a. The cognitive assessment should always be left until the end of the comprehensive psychiatric examination.
3. e. Apraxia
4. c. Can elicit signs of perseveration
5. b. Rating scales should be avoided when communicating with colleagues because of their poor reliability.

6. c. Cognitive disorder
7. b. The examination begins as soon as the clinician meets the patient in the waiting room.
8. a. Competence is best viewed as a task-specific assessment.
9. d. The interview with the informant is usually unnecessary when the patient has a dementia.
10. c. A sexual history is seldom necessary in geriatric history taking.

Chapter 9: Medical Evaluation and Common Medical Problems

Answers:
1. c. Alternative analgesics such as acetaminophen have been demonstrated to be ineffective in the treatment of osteoarthritis.
2. c. Patients with B_{12} deficiency generally can be treated with a 3-month course of intramuscular B_{12} injections.
3. 1. e. Subclinical hypothyroidism
    2. a. Apathic hyperthyroidism
    3. a. Apathic hyperthyroidism
    4. d. Myxedema coma
4. a. Stop the tricyclic antidepressant
5. c. VDRL will usually remain positive after successful treatment of syphilis.
6. d. Cardiac events are the major cause of mortality reported from ECT.
7. b. Preexisting orthostatic hypotension.
8. c. Increased salivation
9. c. First-degree AV block

Chapter 10: The Neurological Evaluation

Answers:
1. b. Hypertensive hemorrhage is more common in the putamen than in the cerebral cortex.
2. c. Age-associated increase in prevalence, rising rapidly with each decade after age 40
3. d. Impaired lateral gaze

4.   d.   Progressive supranuclear palsy frequently exhibits both rigidity and ophthalmoplegia.

5.   a.   Unilateral resting tremor is seen in idiopathic Parkinson's disease.

6.   b.   Are common in healthy older people

Chapter 11:   Neuropsychological Testing

Answers:

1.   e.   Discussing current events
2.   e.   Memory
3.   a.   Can perform below cutoffs for impairment even when they have not declined in cognitive ability
4.   c.   Creutzfeldt-Jakob disease
5.   a.   Pick's disease
6.   d.   Attention
7.   e.   Naming
8.   b.   The difference between immediate and delayed recall
9.   e.   All of the above
10.   c.   They can still have the ability to carry out well-learned skills
11.   e.   All of the above

Chapter 12:   Neuroimaging

Answers:

1.   c.   Magnetic resonance imaging (MRI)
2.   a.   MRI
3.   c.   CT
4.   b.   T2-weighted
5.   b.   PET is more widely accessible
6.   c.   Flow or metabolism reductions in the infarcted areas
7.   c.   Focal decreases in intensity on T2-weighted images
8.   b.   Brain tumors
9.   b.   Caudate hypometabolism
10.   c.   Frontal lobe atrophy and localized frontal hypometabolism
11.   c.   1, 2, and 3 are correct

Chapter 13: Electroencephalography

Answers:
1. d. May normally show temporal slow waves
2. e. a and b only
3. c. To document the presence of a secondary mental disorder
4. d. Is frequently of lower voltage than that in a young adult
5. d. All of the above
6. e. All of the above
7. e. Focal slowing
8. a. Repeated loss of consciousness with generalized tonic-clonic movements
9. f. Posterior dominant rhythm of <10 Hz
10. e. Focal slowing

Chapter 14: Alzheimer's Disease

Answers:
1. d. Unable to dress without assistance
2. d. All of the above
3. d. A patient with an MMSE score of 8
4. c. A patient who must be supervised in proper dress and bathing procedures
5. e. The delusion that persons are stealing things from the patient
6. b. Fragmented sleep
7. e. Repeated suicidal attempts
8. c. Homozygous Apo E4

Chapter 15: Vascular Dementias

Answers:
1. d. Alzheimer's disease is more prevalent than vascular dementia in all nations for which reports are available.
2. d. Atrial fibrillation
3. b. Nortriptyline
4. c. Liver function tests

5.   a.   Electrocardiogram (ECG)
6.   c.   Multiple subcortical lacunes
7.   a.   X-ray computed tomography
8.   c.   Cerebral atherosclerosis
9.   e.   With delirium
10. c.   Psychoanalytic psychotherapy

Chapter 16:   Delirium

Answers:
1.   d.   Impairment of consciousness with an attentional disturbance
2.   c.   Obsessions
3.   a.   Lethargy
4.   b.   10%–20%
5.   e.   Obesity
6.   c.   Loss of spouse
7.   d.   Complete resolution of symptoms within 24 hours
8.   a.   Diffuse slowing
9.   e.   MRI
10. b.   Reversing the underlying medical cause

Chapter 17:   Other Dementias and Mental Disorders Due to General Medical Conditions

Answers:
1.   c.   Organic delusional syndrome
2.   c.   40 and 60
3.   b.   Caudate nuclei
4.   e.   Hallucinations
5.   b.   One-third
6.   e.   1,000,000
7.   b.   6–9 months
8.   b.   Anterior-left hemisphere
9.   a.   Dependent
10. c.   Thiamine (vitamin B_1)

Chapter 18: Grief and Bereavement

Answers:
1. b. According to C. M. Parkes, most widows, 13 months after the death of a spouse, describe themselves as happy and well adjusted, rarely think of their deceased husbands, and have completed their grief.
2. e. All of the above
3. e. Preoccupation with suicide plans
4. b. Cognitive decline
5. a. A long and loving relationship with the deceased
6. b. Almost always portends later depression, severe anxiety, or medical complications
7. d. Widowers who remarry shortly after their wife's death are at particularly high risk.
8. b. Depressions occurring within the first 2 months of the death are benign, not associated with psychosocial dysfunction, and have an excellent prognosis.
9. e. Antidepressant and antianxiety medications should not be given in the first 6 months of bereavement because they will interfere with the process of grief.
10. c. Evaluate and consider treatment just as you would with anyone presenting with this constellation of symptoms.

Chapter 19: Affective Disorders

Answers:
1. b. 1%
2. e. All of the above
3. e. All of the above.
4. c. Lesion in the left frontal pole and the head of the left caudate
5. b. A high percentage of patients will meet criteria for irreversible dementia 2–4 years later.
6. d. All of the above
7. d. All of the above
8. d. All of the above

Chapter 20: Psychoses

Answers:

1. c. May be inferred from the behavior of a patient with Alzheimer's disease
2. a. The medication may cause a delirium to worsen.
3. d. Men are more likely than women to develop this disorder.
4. b. Greater than that in families of normal control subjects
5. d. Isolated psychotic symptoms
6. b. 1 and 3 are correct
7. a. 1, 2, and 3 are correct
8. b. 1 and 3 are correct
9. d. 4 is correct
10. d. 4 is correct

Chapter 21: Anxiety Disorders

Answers:

1. e. None of the above
2. d. Hamilton Anxiety Rating Scale is preferable for use in elderly populations because of its ease of use.
3. a. Buspirone

Chapter 22: Somatoform and Personality Disorders

Answers:

1. b. Diagnosis of depression correlates positively with the presence of somatoform disorders.
2. b. A learned sick role in childhood is a precursor.
3. c. Nortriptyline
4. c. Paranoid delusions
5. b. Patients' willingness to accept the diagnosis
6. b. Tend to decline in middle age
7. d. The Epidemiologic Catchment Area (ECA) study provided a reliable estimate of all three personality disorder clusters in elderly subjects.
8. d. All of the above.

Chapter 23:   Substance Abuse

Answers:
1. b. Pill-rolling tremor
2. c. Over-the-counter sleep remedies
3. c. A majority are likely to have discontinuance symptoms (withdrawal and rebound) if the drug is stopped abruptly.
4. e. Tell her that she may be dependent on the drug; however, with close observation it is worth trying to discontinue the drug with a slow taper over 1–2 months.
5. d. They are more likely to have the symptoms of benzodiazepine withdrawal overlooked by their physician and attributed to another medical illness.

Chapter 24:   Sleep Disorders

Answers:
1. c. Decreasing percentage of REM sleep with increasing age
2. c. NREM apneas last longer than REM apneas
3. b. Increased phasic rapid eye movements during dream sleep
4. b. Long-acting benzodiazepines probably have less behavioral toxicity than shorter-acting benzodiazepines.
5. e. All of the above
6. c. 2 and 4 are correct

Chapter 25:   Sexuality and Aging

Answers:
1. e. Is all of the above
2. b. May present at any age
3. e. All of the above
4. b. He may have sex as soon as he can walk up two flights of stairs comfortably
5. e. Is none of the above
6. e. Is all of the above
7. b. May relate to menopausal atrophic vaginitis

Chapter 26:   Electroconvulsive Therapy

Answers:
1.   b.   Delirium
2.   d.   Delusional depression
3.   e.   Increased intracranial pressure
4.   b.   Brief-pulse, right unilateral
5.   c.   Understanding and acceptance of the treatment by the patient
6.   c.   Inspection of dentition
7.   e.   b and d
8.   e.   All of the above are equally true.
9.   c.   Multiple monitored ECT allows for greater safety of the ECT procedure.
10.   c.   Pulse oximetry is not necessary for ECT because it is such a short procedure.
11.   b.   Coadministration of tricyclic antidepressants or selective serotonin reuptake inhibitors during the treatment series has been shown to increase the efficacy of ECT.
12.   e.   Continuation ECT is carried out for a minimum of 1 year.

Chapter 27:   Psychopharmacology

Answers:
1.   c.   Decreased excretion of hydroxylated tricyclic antidepressant (TCA) metabolites
2.   b.   Less anticholinergic effect
3.   a.   Rapid hepatic metabolism
4.   d.   Decreased absorption
5.   c.   Less orthostatic hypotension
6.   a.   Cognitive dysfunction
7.   c.   Orthostatic measurement
8.   d.   Combined neuroleptic and antidepressant treatment
9.   a.   Urinary retention
10.   c.   Using the fewest drugs
11.   d.   It occurs more often with monoamine oxidase inhibitors than TCAs.
12.   a.   Dystonia

13. c. They are effective in maintaining symptom remission in major depression.
14. c. Diuretics decrease clearance

Chapter 28: Individual Psychotherapy

Answers:
1. e. Quickly stop the first signs of an idealizing transference by interpretation
2. b. Maintaining a neutral, reflective therapeutic attitude
3. c. Turning to adolescent modes of coping
4. d. Positive features of cognitive therapy with elderly patients include its time-limited nature, the patient's active participation, and integration with other treatment modalities.
5. b. Confrontation of character defenses
6. e. None of the above
7. d. The elderly patient's acceptance of depression and anxiety as normal
8. b. Psychotherapy is frequently impeded by the need for medication.
9. c. The therapist promotes the best attainable level of function.
10. b. Contains elements of significant adult relationships

Chapter 29: Group Therapy

Answers:
1. e. All are correct
2. a. 1, 2, and 3 are correct
3. a. 1, 2, and 3 are correct
4. e. All are correct
5. b. 1 and 3 are correct
6. c. 2 and 4 are correct
7. d. 4 is correct
8. d. Level of cognitive functioning
9. c. Durable cognitive improvements
10. b. Enhances patient self-concept

Chapter 30:   Families of Older Adults

Answers:
1. b. Can improve quality of life in all medical settings where elderly patients are treated
2. e. All of the above
3. e. All of the above
4. c. Reduce isolation
5. e. All of the above
6. a. Depression
7. a. Borszormenyi-Nagy

Chapter 31:   Psychiatric Aspects of Nursing Home Care

Answers:
1.   d. 80%–95%
2.   c. 6%–7%
3.   c. Evaluation of behavioral symptoms in patients with dementia
4.   c. Two-thirds to three-quarters
5.   c. 20%–25%
6.   b. Inclusive
7.   b. Increased rates of depression in first-degree relatives
8.   c. Concerns about the overuse of mental health services by nursing home residents
9.   c. Psychoactive medications can never be given at doses that exceed specified limits.
10. d. Have been used primarily in patients with cognitive impairment

Chapter 32:   Geriatric Consultation-Liaison Psychiatry

Answers:
1. d. 25%–55%
2. c. Unavailability of medical care in emergency situations
3. b. Elderly patients have a lower prevalence of psychiatric disorders.

4. b. Elderly patients use psychiatric emergency services more frequently than younger persons.
5. b. Patients in the nursing home are more often diagnosed with delirium.
6. a. Hip fractures
7. e. Family therapy
8. a. Routine neuroimaging assessment
9. a. It is rare because most of the symptoms can be accounted for by comorbid medical illnesses.
10. b. Sessions are usually longer than with younger outpatients.

Chapter 33:   Acute Care Inpatient and Day Hospital Treatment

Answers:
1. d. Encouraging families to look for a supervised facility or nursing home
2. d. Students can learn about medical and psychiatric care of elderly patients through joint teaching.
3. a. Depression is the most common reason for admission.
4. e. Patients with dementia who need a higher level of care than can be provided in their current residence
5. d. Aggressive behavior
6. c. An elderly patient known to a psychiatric service for major recurrent depressive episodes who presents with a new complaint of shortness of breath
7. c. American Association of Partial Hospitalization
8. d. Geriatric psychiatry day hospitals
9. c. Lack of exposure of psychiatrists during postgraduate training programs
10. d. All of the above
11. b. 24-hour respite care
12. c. Depression and dementia

Chapter 34:   Integrated Community Services

Answers:
1. c. Service for persons who have no formal support system
2. b. Vocational training

3.   c. Section 8 housing
4.   b. Medicaid
5.   d. Retirement community
6.   c. Home care services
7.   d. A vocational model for those persons requiring work-skills training
8.   c. Senior Work Program
9.   d. It provides friendly visiting.

Chapter 35:   Medical-Legal Issues

Answers:
1.   b. Alzheimer's disease
2.   a. It is an all or none condition.
3.   c. Decision making
4.   c. Deals with advance directives
5.   b. When the principal becomes incompetent
6.   d. Possible abuse
7.   c. Representative payee
8.   a. Respondent, adjudication, ward, guardian
9.   b. A judge
10.   c. Guardians

Chapter 36:   Clinical Ethics

Answers:
1.   b. A patient with leukemia requests a lethal amount of medication to keep at home just in case she should want to die. Meanwhile she is continuing to receive therapy. The physician gives her the drug and tells her how to use it. A few months later, she decides to end her life and takes the overdose.
2.   c. Although often used interchangeably, competence refers to a court finding; decision-making capacity is the conclusion of a clinical assessment.
3.   d. The vulnerable nature of subjects with dementia means that extra precautions, such as an oversight committee or consent auditor, should be established to review the risks and burdens of this study to the subjects.
4.   e. All of the above

5.   e.   90%
6.   b.   Dementia
7.   d.   25% or less

Chapter 37:   Financial Issues

Answers:
1.   d.   3%
2.   b.   50%
3.   a.   12%
4.   d.   TEFRA caps control expenditures for per diem reimbursement.
5.   c.   No annual limit in payments
6.   c.   payment for the 50% copay for outpatient psychotherapy services.
7.   d.   Requirements that all physicians accept Medicare assignment
8.   b.   Requires needs testing for eligibility
9.   b.   Refers to the number of older adults per individuals ages 18–64 in the general population
10.   c.   Was repealed 1 year after enactment

Index

Page numbers printed in **boldface** *type refer to tables or figures.*